COMPREHENSIVE COMMUNITY HEALTH NURSING

Family, Aggregate,
& Community Practice

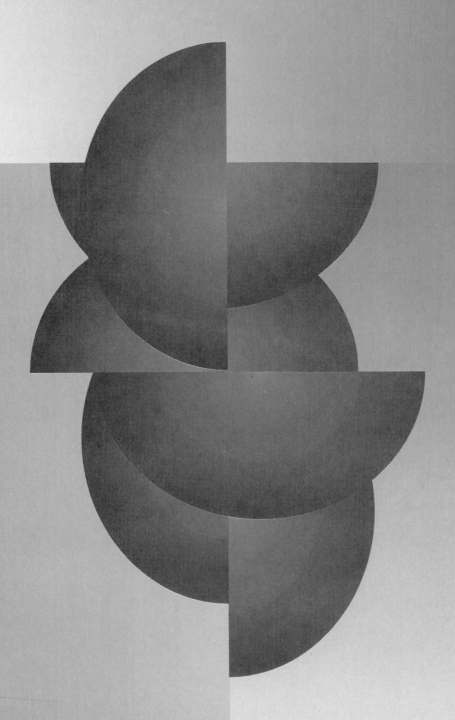

The logo for the book, interconnecting systems and subsystems on a continuum, emphasizes a major focus in community health nursing practice—helping clients to effectively fit together community systems and subsystems in their environment to maximize growth. Clients (individuals, families, aggregates at risk, and communities) frequently have not reached their maximum potential because the environment in which they are functioning does not enhance the growth process. Community health nurses can alter this occurrence; they have unique skills that assist them in bringing together in a meaningful way all of the systems encountered by their clients.

COMPREHENSIVE COMMUNITY HEALTH NURSING

Family, Aggregate, & Community Practice

Susan Clemen-Stone, RN, MPH
Associate Professor, Community Health Nursing,
Division of Health Promotion and Risk Reduction Programs,
School of Nursing, University of Michigan,
Ann Arbor, Michigan

Diane Gerber Eigsti, RN, MS
Assistant Professor, Department of Nursing,
Miami University, Oxford, Ohio

Sandra L. McGuire, RN, EdD
Associate Professor,
College of Nursing, University of Tennessee-Knoxville,
Knoxville, Tennessee

FOURTH EDITION

with 162 illustrations

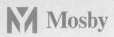 Mosby

St. Louis Baltimore Berlin Boston Carlsbad Chicago London Madrid
Naples New York Philadelphia Sydney Tokyo Toronto

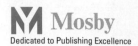

Mosby
Dedicated to Publishing Excellence

Publisher: Nancy Coon
Managing Editor: Loren Stevenson Wilson
Associate Developmental Editor: Brian Dennison
Project Manager: Karen Edwards
Production Editor: Cindy Deichmann
Designer: Liz Fett
Manufacturing Supervisor: John Babrick, Kathy Grone
Cover art: The Composing Room

FOURTH EDITION

Printed in the United States of America
Composition by Graphic World, Inc.
Printing/binding by R.R. Donnelley & Sons Company

Mosby–Year Book, Inc.
11830 Westline Industrial Drive
St. Louis, Missouri 63146

International Standard Book Number 0-8016-7940-0

95 96 97 98 99 / 9 8 7 6 5 4 3 2 1

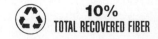

10%
TOTAL RECOVERED FIBER

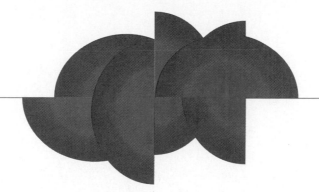

To Our Significant Others

Verna and Al J. Clemen, for their special love that promoted growth and family cohesiveness, and for encouraging and supporting independent thinking even when this was not the norm.

John and Sharon Clemen and **Sara and Henry Parks,** for their caring, friendship, and encouragement.

Denver Stone, for his love, unfailing support, and knowing just the right time to assist.

Teresa and Rick Stone, for their patience and understanding.

Holly Marie Huling, for bringing the joys of childhood into our life and for her loving ways.

To the memory of **Ike.**

Heiki-Lara Eigsti Nyce and Inge-Marie Eigsti, for their patience and loving.

To **John E. Gerber and his daughters,** for the new joy they brought when two families joined.

Joseph, Kelly and Kerry McGuire, and **Matthew Currin,** for their love, support, and encouragement.

Donald and Mary Lue Johnson, for their pride in this publication, their continued encouragement, and their love and interest.

Arthur and Sally Johnson, for the belief they instilled in the value of education, the role modeling they provided, and their constant love.

Judy Simpson, for her continued faith in and support of the nursing profession.

Alma Weale, for recognizing the importance of this publication and her unfailing encouragement.

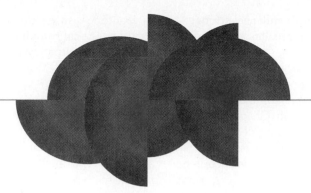

Preface

When the first edition of this book was published almost fifteen years ago, it was obvious that health care trends would make a significant impact on community health nursing practice. For community health nursing, the 1980s and early 1990s were indeed characterized by major changes such as the emphasis on cost containment, the shifting of health care delivery to the home and other community-based settings, more active consumer involvement in health care decision-making, the development of different models for providing community health nursing services, and the emergence of health problems that are posing a threat to the health of our society.

As we approach the year 2000, **health care reform** is in the forefront of public consciousness, providing many opportunities and challenges for community health nurses. It is apparent that society is no longer willing to pay for escalating health care costs, while the health needs of so many people in this country are neglected. Changes are occurring in all components of the health care delivery system in order to deal with the emerging health care crisis. Community health nursing is ready to make the needed changes; the struggles experienced during the past decade and a half were maturing ones. Much rethinking about the goals and values of community health nursing has taken place. Nurse-managed care in such settings as nursing centers, parish communities, homeless shelters, neighborhood centers, and home care is emerging rapidly.

THE FOURTH EDITION

Although *Comprehensive Community Health Nursing: Family, Aggregate, and Community Practice* adheres to the original purposes of previous editions, a substantial attempt has been made in the fourth edition to reflect the changes and innovations that have occurred within the field since it was first published in 1981. As originally designed, this text was presented to help students and practitioners gain an understanding of the unique role of the community health nurse and the exciting, challenging nature of a specialty field that integrates the knowledge and skills of professional nursing and the philosophy, content, and methods of public health. The fourth edition, however, places increased emphasis on examining how unprecedented changes in the health care delivery system have expanded the nature and scope of community health nursing practice. The role of the community health nurse in providing health promotion and disease prevention services in addition to home health care is stressed. The importance of achieving our nation's public health goals, as described in major policy documents such as *Healthy People 2000,* is examined carefully. Both the health promotion needs of groups across the life span and strategies to meet those needs are addressed. Neglected public health mandates and growing challenges in community health nursing practice have been expanded to increase the comprehensiveness of the text. A more thoroughly developed discussion on the role of the community health nurse in addressing these mandates and challenges strengthens students' abilities to develop relevant community health nursing interventions.

Numerous revisions in the book enrich its usefulness for students and practitioners. A separate chapter on environmental health (Chapter 6) and expanded content on community organization (Chapter 13) help to strengthen students' understanding of the importance of developing community partnerships to resolve contemporary health issues. Additional content on at-risk aggregates such as the homeless, rural populations, women, minority groups, those incarcerated, and persons with AIDS, tuberculosis, and other communicable diseases, provides the reader with a more complete base from which to develop multiple health promotion strategies for these aggregates. Providing "culturally competent" health care, a concept endorsed by the American Academy of Nursing, is stressed throughout the text. Moreover, significantly expanded discussion of cultural concepts in two chapters of the text—Chapter 7, "Family Assessment and Cultural Diversity: Tools and Concepts," and Chapter 9, "Use of Family-Centered Nursing Process with Culturally Diverse Clients"—provides the foundation for developing culturally relevant nursing skills.

In recent years significant philosophical, economic, social, political, and technological trends have dramatically influenced community health nursing practice. Revisions have been made throughout the text to reflect these trends by including the most current data related to major health care legislation, demographic characteristics of the population, health problems of at-risk aggregates, and advancements in nursing. Trends are well documented by recent literature. Extensive information about where community health nurses can obtain up-to-date statistical data related to the health needs of at-risk aggregates, with resources that assist them in meeting community health needs, has also been added. The appendices provide valuable assessment tools, legislative information, and data that facilitate the use of the nursing process with various client groups. Illustrations and design have been enhanced by the addition of color. In keeping with community health nursing's increased concern about our environment, this edition is printed on recycled paper. Significant additions to the *Instructor's Manual* will assist educators in planning relevant didactic and clinical learning activities and in preparing evaluation measures. The *Instructor's Manual* includes key concepts covered in each chapter, learning objectives, lec-

ture outlines, suggestions for learning activities that promote critical thinking, instructor resource materials, and approximately 1000 test questions.

Critical Thinking

An addition to each chapter in the fourth edition of this text is a section titled *An Exercise in Critical Thinking*. Critical thinking is what education is all about; it is learning to think about the content fundamental to community health nursing in order to make it an integral part of one's professional practice. The information essential to this specialty area of nursing becomes, for the nurse, a way of thinking and communicating about the world. Educated nurses know more than a collection of facts; they learn that community health nursing is a unique way of thinking about the processes in the field. Intentional problem solving and the clarification of ideas is essential to obtaining specialty knowledge.

At the core of critical thinking are two basic human abilities: analysis and communication (Loacker G, Cromwell L, Fey J, and Rutherford D: *Analysis and communication at Alverno: an approach to critical thinking,* Milwaukee, 1984, Alverno Productions). Analysis is something that we do; it is taking apart the elements of the content and examining them, be they concepts or scientific frameworks. Analysis is probing, questioning, and dissecting these concepts and frameworks. Communication involves synthesizing and connecting this content and sending and receiving messages via written materials, speaking, and listening. Communication challenges nurses to clarify their thinking and to work out solutions, all in the process of conveying conclusions. Thus communication is another process, not a product. It is a result of the nurse's thoughts, style, purpose, and audience.

Analysis and communication are interdependently basic to learning community health nursing. The purpose of this new edition is to aid readers in learning to analyze and communicate community health nursing practice. While the content of this book is crucial, it is critical that readers develop the ability to take apart the material and then communicate the unique processes of our specialty area; only then will they have truly "learned." The exercises are designed to help readers dissect the material in the chapter and then to "put it together" in a meaningful manner. Our goal as authors is to help you truly think critically about the material you have read.

Organization

The organization of this text stems from the philosophy of community and public health nursing practice delineated in the definitions of the American Nurses Association and the American Public Health Association. From these definitions the authors explore the unique aspects of community health nursing practice throughout the text. The reader is encouraged to examine the multiple factors that affect the health status of individuals, families, aggregates at risk, and communities and to seek improved ways for providing preventive health care services in an effective and efficient manner. Emphasis continues to be placed on how the community health nurse can provide **quality** nursing care for multiple client groups within the community setting. Major revisions in Chapter 23 were made to reflect current trends in total quality management.

The unique perspective that community health nurses bring to any health care team is a holistic philosophy derived from a synthesis of nursing and public health knowledge. Preventive activities at all three levels—primary, secondary, and tertiary—are implemented by community health nurses to enhance the state of wellness in a community. Community health nurses respect cultural differences and varying lifestyles and analyze sociocultural, political, economic, and environmental forces that influence consumer interests, needs, beliefs, and values. This text addresses the unique role of the community health nurse by:

- Analyzing the scope of community health nursing practice
- Integrating nursing and public health knowledge throughout the text
- Presenting the family-centered approach to nursing care with emphasis on examining significant structural and process parameters of family functioning
- Describing the health care planning and community organization processes as problem-solving approaches for communities
- Using a developmental approach to address the health needs of aggregates across the life span and to plan appropriate preventive health services for aggregates at risk
- Discussing in-depth health and welfare service systems and how the community health nurse can facilitate client usage of these resources

- Presenting the importance of examining environmental influences on the health of families, aggregates, and communities
- Integrating understanding about cultural diversity
- Presenting specific federal legislation that provides funding for health care services and affects the delivery of nursing services
- Discussing the emerging importance of home health and long-term care and the impact of this trend for community health nurses
- Including the principles of management and continuous quality improvement used by community health nurses to manage and evaluate the multiple responsibilities assigned to them
- Integrating theoretical concepts and clinical data in case situations to illustrate the application of nursing and public health theory in the practice setting
- Presenting tools currently being used by practitioners that assist them in delivering quality nursing services to clients
- Including selected bibliographies that expand on the theoretical concepts presented in the text that describe the multiple situations encountered by the community health nurse

The overall acceptance of the past three editions of this book has prompted us to retain the basic organization of the original text. The two major parts of this textbook explore how community health nurses use concepts from nursing and public health to provide comprehensive, continuous preventive health services for aggregates (families, populations at risk, and communities).

Part One presents a philosophical foundation for nursing practice in the community. It analyzes the origin, scope, and changing nature of current community health nursing practice and examines community dynamics and social, cultural, political, and economic factors that influence the delivery of health and welfare services. The focus is also on the direct service functions of the staff community health nurse. This part discusses why the family is viewed as the unit of service in community health and outlines relevant theoretical concepts essential for understanding family dynamics. Special emphasis is placed on analyzing how the community health nurse uses the nursing process to implement and evaluate intervention strategies with families.

Part Two stresses the value of working with aggregates at risk in the community. Population groups, delineated by age, are examined in terms of developmental characteristics, health needs, health and welfare services, barriers to the use of health and welfare services, and the role of the community health nurse in meeting the needs of high-risk aggregates. Long-term care, which has particular relevance for this specialty area, is discussed. The epidemiological process and the principles of health planning are presented as tools for studying the determinants of health and disease frequencies in populations and for planning health promotion and disease control programs. The need for health care providers to address the ethical dimension of practice and to become politically active during the health planning process is stressed. Management concepts and information systems are also included because they help community health nurses to integrate and handle their multiple professional commitments in a meaningful way.

ACKNOWLEDGMENTS

The authors are greatly indebted to family, friends, colleagues, students, and former faculty and associates for their support, guidance, and assistance as we revised this book. Special appreciation is extended to the following individuals:

- Beverly Smith, our administrative secretary and a special friend, whose painstaking efforts, patience, and dedication to our project made it a reality. This book could never have been published without her help.

- Bill Smith, whose "it only takes a little more to do it right" encouragement, as we began this process almost fifteen years ago, provided the impetus to move forward. His willingness to share his wife's time will never be forgotten.
- Shu-Chen Chang and Marilyn Franecki for their invaluable assistance with research of the literature.
- Leslie Davis and Henry Parks for helping us with our artwork and photography.
- Denver Stone, who willingly devoted considerable time to the tedious aspects of the manuscript preparation process. His commitment to quality was an inspiration to all of us.
- Colleagues from the service setting who have shared with us materials their staffs developed to facilitate the delivery of quality client services.
- Publishers and authors who graciously granted us permission to use information from their writings.
- The Mosby–Year Book staff, especially Darlene Como, Loren Stevenson Wilson, Brian Dennison, Rae Robertson, Cindy Deichmann and Liz Fett, for their support, understanding, and concrete assistance.
- All our friends and family members who "understood" and allowed us to postpone events and activities.

Susan Clemen-Stone
Diane Gerber Eigsti
Sandra L McGuire

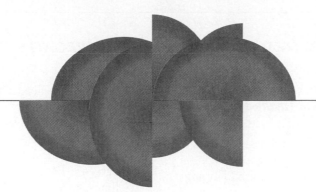

Contents

PART ONE

A FOUNDATION FOR COMMUNITY HEALTH NURSING PRACTICE

PART TWO

PLANNING HEALTH SERVICES FOR AGGREGATES AT RISK

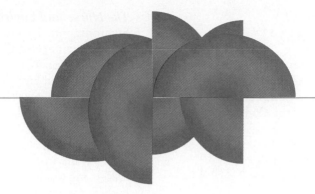

Detailed Contents

PART ONE

A FOUNDATION FOR COMMUNITY HEALTH NURSING PRACTICE

PART TWO

PLANNING HEALTH SERVICES FOR AGGREGATES AT RISK

COMPREHENSIVE COMMUNITY HEALTH NURSING

Family, Aggregate,
& Community Practice

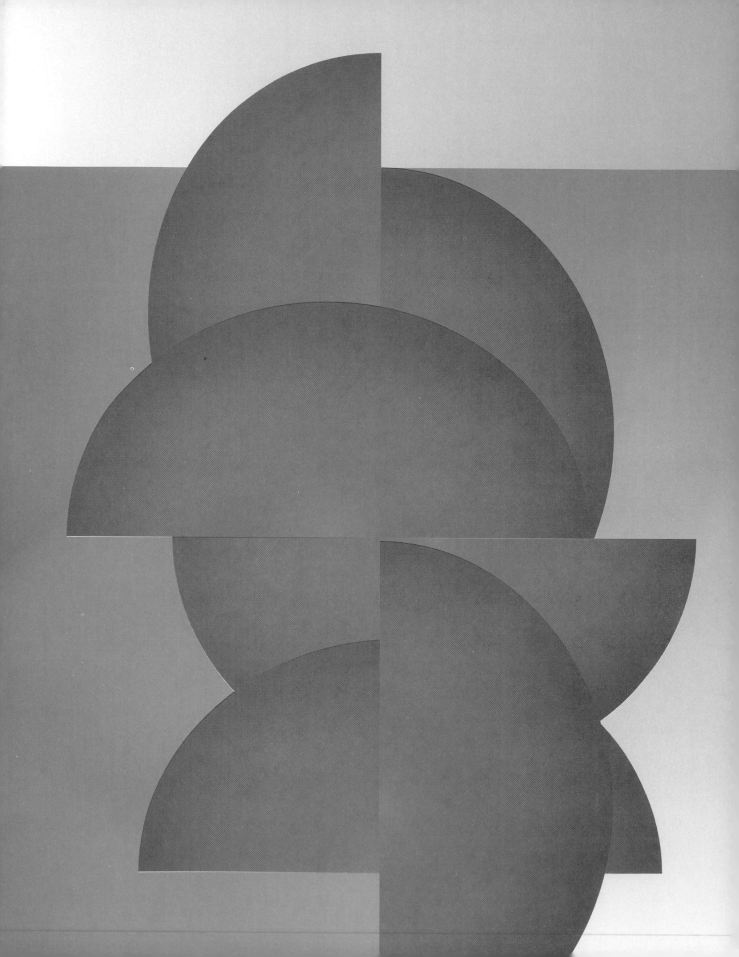

Part One

A FOUNDATION FOR COMMUNITY HEALTH NURSING PRACTICE

Public health nurses have been leaders in improving the quality of health care for people since the late 1800s. They have been the vanguard of change for both the nursing profession and society as a whole, stressing the importance of establishing standards for nursing practice and education and of social reform to improve the quality of life for all individuals. They quickly recognized the need to expand the concept of client beyond the individual and to examine the multiple forces that influence client health. Culturally sensitive, community-focused practice with an emphasis on addressing the needs of aggregates at risk and family-centered nursing care emerged as key principles in the specialty field of community health.

Our early leaders were role models for effective change. They dealt with community dynamics and worked to influence legislative processes that shape the direction of health, welfare, and environmental systems at local, state, and national levels. Using multiple intervention strategies, they empowered community residents for the purpose of promoting self-care.

Our heritage involves over a century of caring— caring for communities, aggregates, and families. In order to continue the progress made by their early leaders, community health nurses must understand where and how their specialty began, the nature of current community health nursing practice, and how community forces contribute to or distract from the health of families and aggregates at risk. Part One presents the theoretical concepts essential for understanding these aspects of community health nursing practice. It also helps the reader to identify current health issues in our society and needed health care reform by examining the *Healthy People 2000* mandates and the organization of our current health, welfare, and environmental systems. The challenges are great. The opportunities to promote the health of communities are endless.

1

Unit One

Historical and Current Perspectives on Community Health Nursing

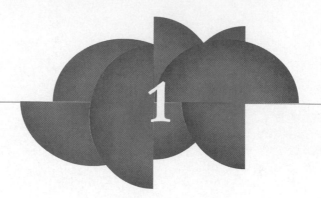

Historical Perspectives on Community Health Nursing

OBJECTIVES

Upon completion of this chapter, the reader should be able to:

1. Identify how early feminists shaped the development of public health nursing.
2. Relate how societal beliefs about women influenced the development and image of nursing.
3. Discuss how historical events have shaped the development of public health, nursing, public health nursing, and community health nursing.
4. Analyze the contributions of Lillian Wald and Florence Nightingale to nursing and public health.
5. Summarize historical events that influenced beliefs about educational preparation for community health nursing practice.
6. Analyze the development of a consciousness for the public's health.

Histories make women wise.

FRANCIS BACON

A century of caring—caring for communities, aggregates, and families! That was the history of tradition formally celebrated in 1993 by public health nurses across the United States. That year nursing practitioners, educators, and researchers came together to honor the accomplishments of their founders: nursing leaders like Lillian Wald, who established the Henry Street Settlement, the first organized public health nursing agency or settlement house. Henry Street was founded in New York City in 1893 to "assure that public health nurses would be available to those in need" (Division of Nursing, 1992). Serving those in need now and in the past involved family-centered nursing care as well as health planning to meet the needs of aggregates (populations at risk) and communities. As will be demonstrated in this chapter, nurses at all levels of practice throughout the past century have been challenged by the opportunity to change societal conditions detrimental to the health of people.

Today's nurse should be proud of the founders of public health nursing! They are heroines who are role models for persons committed to nursing and to working for the improvement of health care services. Lavinia Lloyd Dock, one early public health nurse pioneer, was picketing, parading, and protesting 75 years ago. Dock, a feminist, scholar, and accomplished musician, devoted 20 years of her life to helping women gain the right to vote (Christy, 1969).

To understand the role our legendary leaders played in establishing quality public health nursing and public health practice, it is important to examine significant historical events. Examining history helps us to understand how nursing as an occupation was a response to the needs of people. Public health nursing, now called community health nursing, was the reaction of women who understood that nursing care should be extended beyond the physical concerns of patients. The "whole person" needed to be nursed and illness could be prevented with health teaching and social services (Allen, 1991, p. 75). It was further believed that a patient's family, friends, neighbors, and the environment contributed to that person's illness and recovery. These early nurses built upon the advances made in scientific inquiry and the development of the public health sciences to reduce both morbidity and mortality rates. Community health nursing as we practice it today is a culmination of the work that extraordinary women and men accomplished over a great many years. Contemporary community health nurses owe them a great debt.

IN THE BEGINNING

Nursing began when humanity began.

The word *nurse* is a reduced form of the Middle English *nurice,* which was derived, through the old French norrice, from the Latin *nutricius* (nourishing). In Roman mythology, the Goddess Fortuna, in addition to her usual function as Goddess of Fate, was also worshipped as Jupiter's nurse (Fortuna Praeneste) and prayed to for hygiene in the public baths (Fortuna Balnearis). From the dawn of civilization, mankind has sought to acquire a knowledge of pain-relieving remedies and to discover additional means of preventing disease. To alleviate human suffering, man has also developed nursing roles. (Kalisch and Kalisch, 1986, p. 1)

In 1916 Mary Sewall Gardner, another public health nurse pioneer, published the "first really comprehensive and authoritative presentation on the subject of public health nursing" (Nelson, 1954, p. 38). Gardner wrote that "the true ancestors of the modern nurse are the noble abbesses and early Christian women who were trying to do for their day what the nurse of today is trying to do for her's" (Gardner, 1919, p. 3).

Visiting nursing, or the care of ill people at home by a specialized group, has probably existed through the ages. The New Testament is replete with stories of how the sick were visited. The Apostle Paul wrote of Phoebe in Rom. 16:1-2, "I commend to you our sister Phoebe, a deaconess of the church at Cenchreae, . . . help her in whatever she may require from you, for she has been a helper of many and of myself as well." In the same way, the visiting nurse helps clients with whatever is needed. Phoebe is probably the first visiting nurse we know by name.

The Middle Ages (500-1500 AD), with the subsequent rise of monasteries and convents, contributed a specialized effort to care for the ill. Specific convents and religious orders existed to provide nursing care to sick people. To perform acts of mercy for the well-being of one's eternal soul was a common and accepted reason for entering nursing convents. These early nurses included men who were drawn into military nursing orders as a result of the Crusades (1091-1291). The Crusades were religious wars between the Turks and the Christians that encouraged both the spread of disease and the exchange of ideas between East and West. It has been well documented that nurses of high intellectual capacity responded to the needs of society in times of war and persecution (Dolan, 1978).

The Renaissance (about 1500-1700) brought about great political, social, and economic expansion. Two names of this period that are important to public health nursing are St. Vincent de Paul and Mademoiselle Le Gras. Gardner says of de Paul that "there is no more prominent figure in the history of nursing and social welfare" (Gardner, 1919, p. 9).

In 1617 de Paul organized the Sisterhood of the Dames de Charité. The ladies went from home to home, visiting the sick. As the movement spread and its numbers increased, difficulties arose because of a lack of supervision of their work. St. Vincent reorganized this group by appointing Mademoiselle Le Gras as a supervisor. Together, their greatest contribution to the development of public health nursing was the idea of providing education for those persons helping the poor and the sick, as well as recognizing the need for professional supervision of caregivers. Taking care of ill people at home could not be accomplished simply with intuition; nursing practice must be based on principles somewhat akin to social work as we know it today. They felt that people could best be helped by "helping them to help themselves." De Paul and Le Gras also believed that one must find out the needs of the poor, investigate the causes, and then help supply possible solutions. Taken for granted by people today, these were entirely new concepts of charity for this time (Maynard, 1939).

THE PUBLIC HEALTH MOVEMENT

During the Middle Ages epidemics of communicable, infectious diseases such as bubonic plague, syphilis, scarlet fever, smallpox, influenza, and leprosy periodically swept civilization. For example, after an initial epidemic in 1348, plague raged in Europe for three centuries. "In 1359 and 1360, one third of the population in certain regions are said to have died; in 1360 and 1361, many Polish towns lost half their inhabitants; in 1361 there were 500 deaths a day in Montpellier . . . ." (Winslow, 1943, p. 115). Much earlier, the writings of Hippocrates offered five explanations for the terrible epidemics and included "(1) the wrath of the gods, (2) the epidemic constitution of the

atmosphere, (3) local miasmatic conditions due to climate, season, and organic decomposition, (4) contagion, and (5) variations in individual resistance" (Winslow, p. 181). The years between 1867 and 1882 were the years the germ theory of disease was finally understood; Louis Pasteur of France and Robert Koch of Germany are associated with this breakthrough.

"The first half of the nineteenth century was marked by the inception of the modern public health movement. Under the stimulus of a group of enthusiastic humanitarians, a campaign for sanitary reform was launched in England and spread throughout the world to lay the foundation for our modern war against disease" (Winslow, 1943, p. 236). By this time health problems were changing; plague and typhus fever had almost disappeared from Western Europe. Intestinal diseases, including cholera and typhoid, had become the menaces.

The title given to this period in public health history is "The Great Awakening," and the person whose name is associated with it is Edwin Chadwick. Chadwick related the lack of sewage and water systems to the prevalent diseases: "I found the whole area of the cellars of both houses were full of night-soil, to the depth of three feet, which had been permitted for years to accumulate from the overflow of the cesspools" (Winslow, 1943, p. 244). Connecting diseases with "atmospheric impurities produced by decomposing animal and vegetable substances, by damp and filth, and close and overcrowded dwellings" (p. 248) was a gigantic leap forward in the development of preventable problems and a positive change in the public's health as changes in the environment occurred.

By the end of the nineteenth century the germ theory could "account for all conditions under which disease was actually shown to arise" (Winslow, 1943, p. 363). It was an American, Charles Value Chapin, who in 1910 synthesized the scientific learning that had preceded him, and laid a "firm foundation for the modern public health campaign" (Winslow, p. 363). His work in Providence, Rhode Island, as the Superintendent of Health produced three direct public health contributions: he made the vital statistics reports in the city accurate and complete; he developed a hospital that applied the new (for that time) idea that germ diseases were spread by contact; and he conceptualized health administration as based on scientific planning and visualized health education as his primary concern (Winslow, p. 364). Advances in nursing theory and practice paralleled these advances in public health.

The Era of Sairy Gamp

It is difficult to imagine how nursing could have sunk to the low levels it did between the end of the seventeenth century to the middle of the nineteenth century. The change from nursing care given by devoted deaconesses to nursing care given by drunks and prostitutes is baffling. In *Martin Chuzzlewit,* originally published in 1844, Charles Dickens (1910) immortalized the prototype of the nurse of this era by describing a drunken, untrained servant, Sairy Gamp, as a nurse. In order to understand what persons such as Florence Nightingale and her peers accomplished, the reader must know the nursing conditions that were in existence when they began their efforts to professionalize nursing.

As previously noted, early nurses were often in convents. The basis for the nursing care given by Phoebe and her contemporaries was charity. Thus the care was only as good as the church organization that supported it. During the time of the Reformation (the 1500s), nursing care degenerated to the greatest extent in countries where Catholic organizations were overthrown. In England, for instance, 100 hospitals were closed, and for a period there was no provision for the institutional care of ill people who were poor (Deloughery, 1977, p. 23). When nursing lost the importance once lent it by the church, it also lost its social standing. Being a nurse was less socially desirable and thus it was necessary to recruit nurses from distinctly lower classes, because "respectable" people would no longer do the work.

The status of women also greatly affected the change in the status of nursing. The church had given women an opportunity for a career in nursing. Love for others was the basis of the Gospel, and women were considered to be persons of worth. The general social position of women reached a low level in the eighteenth century, paralleling the status of nursing.

The accompanying conditions in society during this time were also dismal. The slums of European cities were huge and bred disease. Life expectancy was short and mortality rates were high. Before the Industrial Revolution (about 1750-1850) the social and economic structure of the Western world was quite simple: there were only a few large cities and work

was largely agrarian. Social classes were rigidly stratified. During this time medicine was at a low level, largely because the scientific basis for it was unknown. Thus health care was based on folklore and superstition. To summarize the status of nursing:

Nursing existed in a low and dismal state indeed. It existed without organization and without social standing. No one who could possibly earn a living in some other way performed this service. Those who did so lost caste thereby, for as one is judged partly by the company one keeps, a woman who began to practice nursing was almost certain to become corrupted if she were not so already. (Deloughery, 1977, p. 24)

With this background, the contributions of Florence Nightingale to nursing, to public health, and to women are inestimable.

Florence Nightingale's Legacy

The family of this pioneer nurse leader was a wealthy one, and the environment into which she was born in 1820 became instrumental in her life's work. Nightingale was well educated by her father and, to her family's chagrin, longed to be a nurse. After a delay of many years, in deference to her family's wishes, she entered nurses' training with Pastor Fliedner at Kaiserswerth on the Rhine, Germany. Her subsequent work in the Crimean War at Scutari has been chronicled by many, among them Longfellow, in his "Santa Filomena." It was there that she demonstrated that thousands of lives could be saved by intelligent nursing care and that capable nurses were needed in military hospitals. She accomplished this in the face of overwhelming obstacles. The hospital at Scutari was built for 1700 patients. When Nightingale arrived, there were 3000 to 4000 wounded men in it, lying naked with no beds, no blankets, and no eating or laundry facilities. Within days of her appearance at Scutari, she had a food kitchen operating, as well as a laundry.

When Florence Nightingale began her career, it was a very dreadful thing to be a nurse. By helping establish the first modernly planned training school for nurses at St. Thomas Hospital in 1850, Nightingale set the example for Bellevue Hospital in New York City to follow in 1873. She also began the movement which led to the University Schools of Nursing at Western Reserve and Yale (Winslow, 1946, p. 331). Nightingale was the originator of the concept of the nursing process. She insisted that educated nurses were essential to perform the nurse's role. In this role she included assessment and intervention, followed by evaluation. In her famous *Notes on Nursing* she defined nursing as that care that puts a person in the best possible condition for nature to either restore or preserve health, to prevent or cure disease or injury (Nightingale, 1859). From the very beginning of her career, she visualized the nurse as not merely an attendant for the sick but also a teacher of hygiene. She described the nurse as a "health missioner," a guide and teacher of health to the individual in the home. She recognized that "from the very nature of the case, compulsion can under no conditions work the changes we want to see wrought by the obedience of consent" (Winslow, p. 331). This was a very early affirmation of the principle that individuals are responsible for their own health.

Florence Nightingale is considered by many to be the first nurse researcher. She emphasized the importance of systematic observation, data collection, and statistical analysis in relation to nursing care. Her statistical research in British military hospitals in the Crimea showed that nursing interventions could make a difference in the morbidity and mortality rates of the soldiers. Her research report, *Notes on Matters Affecting the Health, Efficiency and Hospital Administration of the British Army,* led to both attitudinal and organizational changes in health care practices. After Nightingale's work, nursing research lay dormant for almost a century. Any nursing research that was done usually focused on nursing education in terms of what should be taught, faculty and organization of nursing programs, and curricular comparisons.

THE ESTABLISHMENT OF VISITING NURSING

Visiting nursing, or district nursing, was the forerunner of public health nursing. The modern concept of a nurse who provides care to families in the home was visualized and established in 1859 by William Rathbone of Liverpool, England. "It is to Mr. Rathbone that we owe the first definitely formulated district nursing association and in that sense he may be called the father of the present movement" (Gardner, 1919, p. 14). Rathbone was a wealthy businessman and philanthropist. His wife died after a long illness, and he had been impressed and comforted by the skilled nursing care given to her in the months before she died. Rathbone had long been interested in helping the many poor people of Liverpool. If nursing care could

help his wife, who had everything that money could buy, how much more might it do for poor people, whose physical illnesses were made increasingly burdensome by their poverty. To test his idea, he employed Mrs. Mary Robinson, the nurse who had cared for his wife, to visit the "sick poor" in their homes. She was to give care, instruct both the patient and the family in the care of the sick, and teach hygienic practices to prevent illnesses. The experiment was so successful that Rathbone decided to establish a permanent system of district or visiting nursing in Liverpool (McNeil, 1967, p. 1).

Rathbone's first problem was that there were no nurses in Liverpool to do this difficult work. So, with the help and advice of Florence Nightingale, he founded a school in 1859 for the training of visiting nurses on the grounds of the Liverpool Infirmary. Within 4 years, 18 nurses were working in this same city, demonstrating dramatically the organization and success of the venture. Even at this early date, these visiting nurses were visualized not only as people who cared for the sick but also as social reformers.

THE PUBLIC'S HEALTH IN THE UNITED STATES

Organized public health efforts in the United States in the early nineteenth century were local ones, and took place in the port cities of the eastern United States, including Philadelphia and New York. The goal of these efforts was to protect the population from the epidemic catastrophes of yellow fever and cholera while simultaneously not disrupting international trade (Fee, 1991, p. 3). Threats to the public's health and welfare were increasing due to diseases such as smallpox, yellow fever, cholera, typhoid, tuberculosis, and malaria (refer to Figure 1-1). "In Massachusetts in 1850, for example, the tuberculosis death rate was 300 per 100,000 population. The infant mortality rate was 200 per 1000 live births, and smallpox, scarlet fever, and typhoid were the leading causes of death" (Pickett and Hanlon, 1990, p. 30).

The Civil War, fought from 1861 to 1865, was a tragedy demonstrating to the nation that epidemic disease was a greater killer than war: two thirds of the 360,000 Union soldiers who died were killed by infectious diseases, not bullets. Concerned citizens realized that the public's health went beyond local cities, and conventions discussing these problems were held in New York and Philadelphia.

In response to these problems, some larger cities,

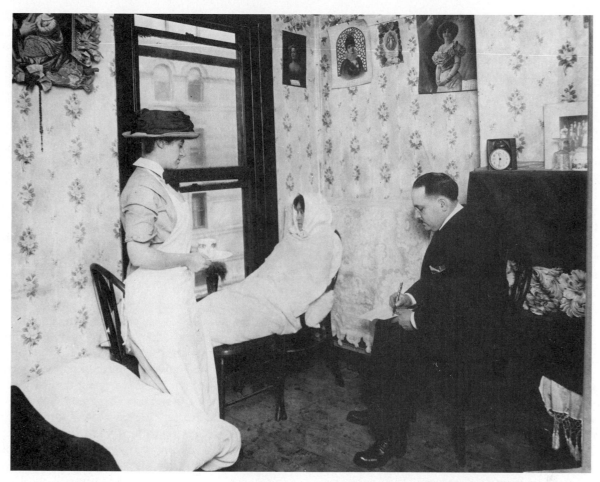

Figure 1-1   Convalescing from typhoid fever, New York City, 1912. (The Metropolitan Life Insurance Company of New York. Used with their permission.)

including Philadelphia and New York, established city health departments. In 1855 Louisiana set up what some historians call the first state health department. Its function was to deal with repeated outbreaks of yellow fever and other epidemic diseases. In terms of the more usual concept of the general functions of a state health department, Massachusetts is usually credited with founding the first such department in 1869 (Pickett and Hanlon, 1990, p. 33).

An early public health pioneer of this period was Lemuel Shattuck. In 1842 he helped to achieve passage of a Massachusetts law that resulted in the statewide registration of health-related statistics. In the next few years, Shattuck compiled shocking statistics about unbelievably high infant and maternal mortality rates. The Shattuck Report, one of the first public health

documents in the United States, was published in 1850. It recommended the establishment of state and local health departments and pointed out the need for sanitary surveys. It unfortunately lay unnoticed for 25 years, although much of it is relevant for today (Pickett and Hanlon, 1990, pp. 31-32).

Large numbers of affluent people became concerned with the poverty and misery experienced by so many people. Physicians, engineers, and public-minded people joined these efforts. Middle- and upper-class women who, to this point, had few opportunities to work in the public sector were influenced by feminists such as Dock, Wald, and Margaret Sanger to work for the abolition of child labor, decent housing, the organization of trade unions, and maternal and child health. At this point in our nation's history many voluntary organizations were founded, including the American Red Cross, the National Tuberculosis Association, and the American Society for the Control of Cancer. The formal organization of public health professionals, the American Public Health Association, was founded in 1872 (Fee, 1991, p. 5). It still exists today as a potent force in the health of our country.

Thus the concept of the public's health developed near the turn of the century. Personal health services played an increasingly important role in community health programs. A new era was reached when, in Los Angeles in 1889, a nurse was employed by the city's health department to provide home nursing care to the sick poor (Rosen, 1958, p. 380). At this point, public health nursing began to be officially recognized and tax supported. However, it was not until 1913 that the Los Angeles Health Department established a bureau of nursing.

Visiting Nurses in the United States

As is already evident from this historical overview, trends within nursing are directly influenced by trends in society. The development of visiting nursing in the United States was no exception.

By the later 1800s, organized nursing care in hospitals had been demonstrated to be effective. Germ theory was used as the basis for communicable disease control. Poverty was beginning to be seen as the result and cause of multiple social problems.

Florence Nightingale's work and the establishment of her school of nursing in England were well known. Her concept that better nursing care could be given if nurses were educated for the position became more clearly understood.

The growth of our nation's cities, as well as the waves of immigrants to America, the "land of opportunity," were two underlying reasons for the development of visiting nursing. Although every city had its rich people, the poor greatly outnumbered them (Kalisch and Kalisch, 1986, p. 262).

New York had the largest settlement of immigrants and thus faced the most problems concerning them (refer to Figure 1-2). Dismal tenement houses were built for this huge influx of people, and living conditions were horrible. Very young children were expected to work 12 to 14 hours a day in dark, airless factories.

Visiting nursing in the United States, just as in England, was begun by groups of people who were greatly distressed by the conditions in which many poor people lived. Then, as now, the most serious public health problems were in slum areas, and visiting nurse agencies were often located in buildings in low-income areas. Nurses from these organizations provided care to the sick in their homes and gave instruction to families as well. Buffalo, Boston, and Philadelphia developed such services during 1885 and 1886, about 25 years after Rathbone's experiment. The Philadelphia Visiting Nurse Society cared for the sick as well as for the poor and, at a very early date, established a fee for services given.

Visiting nursing in this country did not follow the English system established by Rathbone (Gardner, 1919, p. 29). In England, Queen Victoria's Jubilee Institute for Nurses was founded in 1889, and it set standards for the preparation of visiting nurses as well as for the care given by them. In 1890 in the United States, there were 21 separate organizations engaged in visiting nursing. These organizations had no connection with one another and also had no common standards of educational preparation for the caregivers. Each city and town established its own visiting nurse service so that there was great diversity in the quality of organization and care given.

In 1896 the Nurses' Associated Alumni (now the American Nurses Association) was formed and helped to organize the nurses of the country into a professional group. This was the beginning of "group consciousness" among the visiting nurses of the United States.

Enter Lillian Wald

The person who coined the expression *public health nursing* was Lillian Wald. Nightingale had originated the idea of "health nursing"; it was Wald who placed the word *public* in front of it so that all people would know that this type of service was available to them (Haupt, 1953, p. 81). Wald was the "predecessor of the modern public health nurse in the United States" (Christy, 1970, p. 50). *The House on Henry Street* is her story of the work she did as director of the Henry Street Settlement House. Lillian Wald's accomplishments are legendary and involve numerous "firsts" in nursing. She originated the idea of family-focused nursing and stressed the importance of health teaching in preventing disease and promoting health. She saw the value of, and helped to establish, school nursing as well as rural nursing in the Red Cross Town and Country Nursing Service. Wald truly promoted the

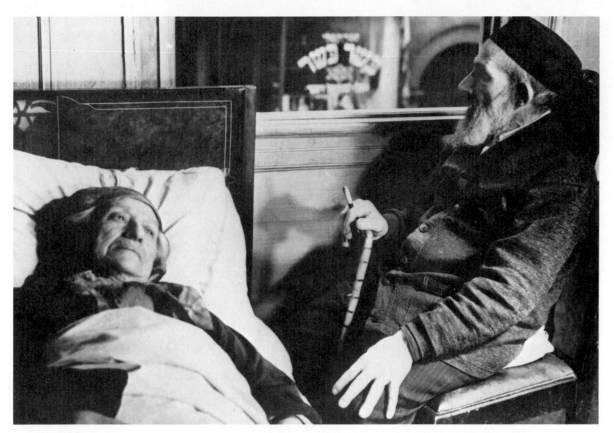

Figure 1-2 It was the year of the great blizzard, 1888, when this Russian blacksmith and his bride emigrated to the New World to build a life. Fifty years later, in sickness and in health, they were still together—thanks to a visiting nurse. (Courtesy Visiting Nurse Service of New York City.)

philosophy of professional nursing. She encouraged the teaching of courses for public health nursing at Teachers College of Columbia University and was founder and first president of the National Organization for Public Health Nursing (Kaufman, Hawkins, Higgins, and Friedman, 1988).

Lillian Wald has been honored for her social reform activities as well as her nursing achievements. She originated the idea of and then helped to establish the U.S. Children's Bureau. She was also instrumental in securing changes in child labor laws, better housing conditions in tenement districts, city recreation centers, more and better parks, pure food laws, graded classes for mentally handicapped children, and humanistic provisions for immigrants to the United States. What a role model for public health nurses today! And how appropriate the title, "predecessor of modern public health nursing" (refer to Figure 1-3).

Lillian Wald was born in 1867 and grew up in Rochester, New York. Though her family was not wealthy, her father, an optical goods dealer, provided a comfortable living for them. She studied at a private school and was an excellent student. Wald chanced to meet a graduate of the Bellevue Hospital Training School for Nurses who had assisted her sister during pregnancy. In this manner, Wald became interested in nursing and entered training at New York Hospital in 1891, where she spent two years.

After graduating she supplemented her nursing instruction with a period of study at a medical college. During this time of study, she was asked to give classes in home nursing and bedside care to a group of women in the Lower East Side tenement district. This was a turning point of Wald's career:

From the schoolroom where I had been giving a lesson in bed-making, a little girl led me one drizzling March morning.

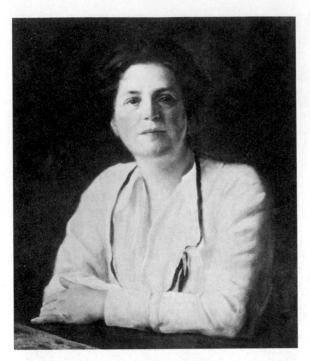

Figure 1-3 Lillian D. Wald, the nurse leader who was the "predecessor of modern public health nursing," was far ahead of her time. She promoted social reform at a time when it was not the norm for women to engage in such activity. Her accomplishments truly reflect the mark of a professional nurse. (Courtesy Visiting Nurse Service of New York City.)

She had told me of her sick mother, and gathering from her incoherent account that a child had been born, I caught up the paraphernalia of the bed-making lesson and carried it with me.

The child led me over broken roadways,—there was no asphalt, although its use was well established in other parts of the city,—over dirty mattresses and heaps of refuse,—it was before Colonel Waring had shown the possibility of clean streets even in that quarter,—between tall, reeking houses whose laden fire escapes, useless for their appointed purpose, bulged with household goods of every description. The rain added to the dismal appearance of the streets and to the discomfort of the crowds which thronged them, intensifying the odors which assailed me from every side. Through Hester and Division Streets we went to the end of Ludlow; past odorous fish-stands, for the streets were a marketplace, unregulated, unsupervised, unclean; past evil-smelling, uncovered garbage-cans; and—perhaps worst of all, where so many little children played—past the trucks brought down from more fastidious quarters and stalled on these already over-crowded streets, lending themselves inevitably to many forms of indecency.

The child led me on through a tenement hallway, across a court where open and unscreened closets were promiscuously used by men and women, up into a rear tenement, by slimy steps whose accumulated dirt was augmented that day by the mud of the streets, and finally into the sickroom.

All of the maladjustments of our social and economic relations seemed epitomized in this brief journey and what was found at the end of it. The family to which the child led me was neither criminal nor vicious. Although the husband was a cripple, one of those who stand on street corners exhibiting deformities to enlist compassion, and masking the begging of alms by a pretense at selling; although the family of seven shared their two rooms with boarders,—who were literally boarders, since a piece of timber was placed over the floor for them to sleep on,—and although the sick woman lay on a wretched, unclean bed, soiled with a hemorrhage two days old, they were not degraded human beings, judged by any measure of moral values.

In fact, it was very plain that they were sensitive to their condition, and when, at the end of my ministrations, they kissed my hands (those who have undergone similar experiences will, I am sure, understand), it would have been some solace if by any conviction of the moral unworthiness of the family I could have defended myself as a part of a society which permitted such conditions to exist. Indeed, my subsequent acquaintance with them revealed the fact that, miserable as their state was, they were not without ideals for the family life, and for society, of which they were so unloved and unlovely a part.

That morning's experience was a baptism of fire. Deserted were the laboratory and the academic work of the college—I never returned to them. On my way from the sickroom to my comfortable student quarters my mind was intent on my own responsibility. To my inexperience, it seemed certain that conditions such as these were allowed because people did not know, and for me there was a challenge to know and to tell. When early morning found me still awake, my naive conviction remained that, if people knew things,—and "things" meant everything implied in the condition of this family,—such horrors would cease to exist, and I rejoiced that I had had a training in the care of the sick that in itself would give me an organic relationship to the neighborhood in which this awakening had come (Wald, 1915, pp. 4-8).

This experience was the cause for the creation of the Henry Street Settlement House in 1893. Along with Mary Brewster, another New York Hospital graduate, Wald elicited funds from wealthy people and founded a place where care was offered to needy people.

Wald's settlement house changed the focus of nursing service: the only other visiting nurses during this period were those associated with sectarian organizations or free dispensaries. Wald felt that a nurse could be most effective if she were independent of any religious agency and not associated exclusively with one doctor. She insisted that nurses should be available to anyone who needed them, without the intervention of a doctor, establishing early in the history of nursing that the profession should be an independent one. She also believed that nurses should live in the neighborhood where they practiced so that they could identify with the needs of the families served, as Wald herself did.

School Nursing Develops

The nursing care of children in public schools began with an idea by Lillian Wald. In 1902 health conditions of school children in New York City were appalling. Thousands of students were sent home from school with diseases such as trachoma (an infectious eye disease), pediculosis, ringworm, scabies, and impetigo. They then played outside with the children from whom they had previously been excluded in the classroom (Wald, 1915, p. 51). Wald offered to show school officials in New York that with the assistance of a well-prepared nurse, fewer children would lose valuable school time and that it was possible to bring under treatment those who needed it.

Wald loaned a nurse to the New York City Health Department to accomplish these goals. The experiment was to be paid for with public funds. One month's trial with Lina Rogers, a nurse from Henry Street, proved to be immensely successful. The Board of Estimate and Apportionment approved $30,000 for the employment of trained nurses, the first municipalized school nurses in the world (Wald, 1915, p. 53). This was the first use of trained nurses in any large number in health departments. In 1903, this same health department appointed three nurses (annual salary $900) to visit tuberculosis patients at home. The nurses were to teach the patients about sputum disposal and other aspects of care. In 1905 the number of nurses serving tuberculosis patients was increased to 14. Alabama, in 1907, was the first state to legally approve the employment of public health nurses by local boards of health (Rosen, 1958, p. 380).

By 1912 public health nurses were supported by both private and public funds. The need for the skills and knowledge of this kind of professional was generally well recognized. They could be found in many kinds of agencies as well as in both rural and urban settings. Table 1-1, compiled by public health nurse

TABLE 1-1 Distribution of Public Health Nurses in 1912

Visiting nurse associations	205
City and state boards of health and education	156
Private clubs and societies	108
Tuberculosis leagues	107
Hospitals and dispensaries	87
Business concerns	38
Settlements and day nurses	35
Churches	28
Charity organizations	27
Other organizations	19

NOTE: This list, used by the author in 1912, as secretary of a joint committee of the American Nurses Association and the Society of Superintendents of Training Schools, to circulate names of the agencies then known to be engaged in public health nursing, probably gives a reasonably true picture of the general distribution of nursing work among the different types of agencies. There were 78 letters sent to nurses working in that number of counties in Pennsylvania and 204 to nurses independently employed by the Metropolitan Life Insurance Company.
From Gardner MS: *Public health nursing*, ed 3, New York, 1936, Macmillan, p. 40.

pioneer Mary Gardner, illustrates this distribution well.

Maternal-Infant Care Becomes a Concern

An appreciation of the needs of children, demonstrated in part by the rise of settlement houses like Henry Street, was a part of the social consciousness of the early 1900s. There were spasmodic efforts to help children to better health, and in 1909 these were united into action at a Conference on Infant Mortality called by the American Academy of Medicine. Finally in 1912, the Children's Bureau was created by Congress to draw the attention of the highest levels of government to the needs of children. Though many nurses and lay associations contributed to its formation, Lillian Wald's activities, initiative, and remarkable skill in securing support for new ideas was fundamental to the establishment of the Children's Bureau (Stewart and Austin, 1938, p. 197).

The passage of the Shepherd-Towner Act of 1921 was a historic milestone in the evolution of public

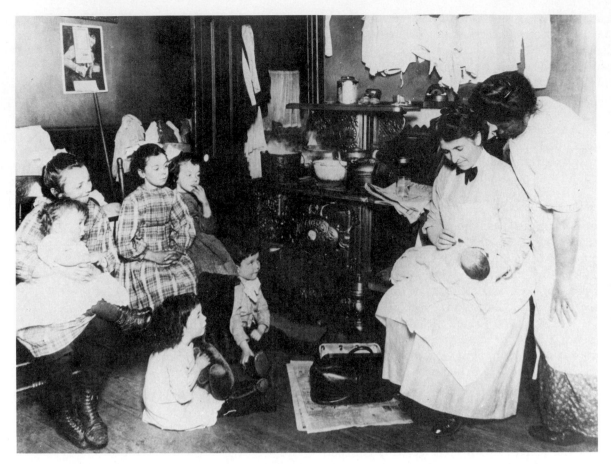

Figure 1-4 Involving the family in baby care, Boston, 1912. (The Metropolitan Life Insurance Company of New York. Used with their permission.)

health and public health nursing. Studies by the Children's Bureau at the federal level showed that the United States had a higher maternal death rate than most other developed countries. This act, administered by the Children's Bureau, gave grants to states to develop programs that provided care to that at-risk aggregate.

Marie Phelan was appointed in 1923 as the first nurse consultant to the federal government in peacetime. At the request of state health departments she helped to develop programs that promoted the health of mothers and children. Her work had the effect of creating a demand for nurses to work with established county or official agencies to begin demonstration programs with mothers and infants (refer to Figure 1-4). The results of these nurses' work are difficult to measure, but the maternal death rate was reduced

from 7.1 per 1000 live births in 1915 to 6.7 for the years between 1925 and 1929. In a final report on the program, the chief of the Children's Bureau noted that "a nurse working alone had frequently afforded a starting point for the development of full-time health departments" (Roberts, 1954, p. 196). As a result of strong political conservatism, the Shepherd-Towner Act was permitted to lapse in 1929 and was not renewed.

The original Shepherd-Towner Act was subsequently amended and broadened to include under its auspices a network of maternity and infant care programs, as well as child and youth programs, throughout the United States. Nurse-midwives, pediatric nurse practitioners, and family planning nurse practitioners were responsible for providing primary health care in many of these programs.

Metropolitan Employs PHN

In 1909 the first public health nursing program for policyholders of an insurance company was initiated (Haupt, 1953, p. 81). Lillian Wald and Lee Frankel, founder of the Metropolitan Life Insurance Company Welfare Division, convinced the board of directors at Metropolitan that healthier workers live longer and thus profit the company by purchasing insurance longer. Wald felt that nurses supplied by agencies such as Henry Street could provide skilled service needed to produce healthy workers. Increased efficiency on the workers' part could favorably influence the output of industry, which, in turn, would pay for the health services in cash and improve morale.

The two principles underlying this concept were that the company should utilize existing public health nursing services rather than employing their own nurses and that services should be available to anyone, with fees based on the ability to pay. Both of these ideas are used today in health agencies.

The Metropolitan project was terminated in 1953 after 44 successful years. The shifting of the voluntary responsibility for health care to professional community organizations was the basis for the change.

There were numerous contributions to public health nursing as a result of this project (Haupt, 1953). Among them are the following:

1. The extension of bedside nursing care on a fee-for-service basis.
2. The establishment of a cost-accounting system for visiting nurses, which is used to this day.
3. The recruitment of nurses, aides, and home nursing programs under the Red Cross by the use of advertisements in paper and radio. This was a new concept of recruitment.
4. The reduction of mortality rates from infectious diseases. Mortality rates were reduced by half in the 44 years of the program among the Metropolitan Life Insurance policyholders.
5. The demonstration of how nursing and a business organization can work together, despite each having an interest in the promotion of its own goals.

Public Health Nursing in Rural Areas

While public health nursing in cities and towns was developing at a rapid rate, work in rural areas was progressing slowly. In 1912, the same year the Children's Bureau was formed, Lillian Wald asked her wealthy friend, Jacob Shiff, to donate money to the Red Cross so that a system of rural nursing could be developed (Gardner, 1919, p. 37).

Wald had been a Red Cross member in 1904 and 1905. She expressed strong dissatisfaction at seeing an organization as potent as the Red Cross limited to the uncertainty and irregularity of service in war or calamity; she felt it simply wasteful to have a national organization inactive. Wald believed that the Red Cross was a logical facility to employ in promoting public health nursing in rural areas and scattered towns on a regular national scale (Dock, Pickett, Noyes, Clement, Fox, and Van Meter, 1922, p. 1212).

And so it happened that the Red Cross began a new department, the Town and Country Nursing Service, later named the Bureau of Public Health Nursing. The purpose of the department was to supply rural areas and small towns with trained public health nurses and to supervise their work. The Red Cross, however, did not assume the local financial responsibility for this work. Voluntary and charitable organizations, as well as fees for service, financed the nursing care given.

It is important to note that the early writings about the work of public health nurses with families and aggregates (i.e. mothers and infants, school-age children, and rural residents) referred to the poor:

> Perhaps the public health nurse pioneers were more innovative and community minded than the private duty nurses as a group. An alternative explanation may lie in the greater openness and vulnerability of the poor to official intervention as compared with the middle and upper classes. Because the homes of the poor were considered "ill regulated" nursing saw a need to expand its services and broaden its educational base, that is, to adopt a holistic perspective in addressing the problematic aspects of rendering care to the poor. The interconnectedness of their health problems and the lack of sanitation, and so on spurred the interest in social knowledge and the emphasis on philanthropic methods of investigation (Allen, 1991, p. 76).

The accomplishments of the early public health nurses led naturally to a desire on their parts to formally organize and develop standards for those entering the field.

ORGANIZING PUBLIC HEALTH NURSES

Leaders among public health nurses, including Lillian Wald, Mary Beard, Ellen Phillips Crandall, Jane Delano, and Mary Gardner, soon realized the need to develop professional standards for this expanding professional group. Although most agencies employing nurses were attempting to do conscientious work, there were no overall professional and ethical guidelines. These same leaders clearly felt that only a new organization "whose sole object should be public health nursing would adequately meet the need" (Gardner, 1919, p. 41).

June 7, 1912, was a momentous day in the history of American public health nursing: at the annual meeting of the American Nurses Association and the Society of Superintendents of Training Schools, the National Organization for Public Health Nursing (now the National League for Nursing) was voted into existence with Lillian Wald as president. The two purposes of the National Organization for Public Health Nursing (NOPHN) were the stimulation and standardization of public health nursing and the furthering of relationships among all people interested in the public's health. It was the first national nursing organization to have a headquarters and paid staff. For a long period in the development of nursing, it grew in power, set standards for practice, and influenced education by requiring certain curriculum content as a basis for employment (Fagin, 1978, p. 752). One of the unique features of the NOPHN was that membership was open to public health nursing agencies and other interested people as well as to nurses. Collaborative relationships among health and social agencies has always been a strength among those who work in public health nursing.

The area of public health nursing grew to meet the needs of society in addition to the needs of its practitioners. Allen (1991) describes how the development of district nursing and, later, public health nursing, spawned the concepts of holistic nursing. This meant nursing the whole person and including family, friends, neighbors, and the environment in the influence on illness and health. "The ideas of wholeness implicit in the public health nursing movement were important in providing its direction, significant in the notion that it was a type of nursing somehow set apart and above other specialties, and crucial to the movement of nursing education into the university and nursing's recognition as a profession" (Allen, p. 75).

Education for Public Health Nurses

The education of public health nurses presented special problems because, traditionally, all nurses were prepared in apprentice-type programs in hospitals. Their curriculum was determined by the needs of the hospital and was controlled by the physicians whose primary responsibility was service to patients rather than the education of nurses. The education was illness- and individual-oriented and did not adequately prepare (or even claim to prepare) a person to work in the community setting, where the care delivered differed from hospital care. In the community setting nurses had a greater degree of independence; they did health teaching, carried out case finding, and made referrals, and their responsibility was to population groups or aggregates.

The first course in public health nursing was offered by the Boston Instructive Nursing Association in 1906 (McNeil, 1967, p. 4). However, considering the broad scope of a public health nurse's work, it soon became apparent that education for this group was a function of the university. Because of the nurse's concern with social and educational problems, most of the early university public health nursing programs were in teacher's colleges or university departments of sociology or social work. By 1921, courses in public health nursing, which met standards developed by the NOPHN, were offered by 15 colleges and universities. These courses taught "preventive medicine," covering topics such as how to examine a class of children, how to find those who were developing measles, and how to visit in a home and evaluate tuberculosis contacts (Jensen, 1959, p. 236).

Public Health Nursing Magazine

On the very day that the NOPHN was formed, the Cleveland Visiting Nurses' Association presented its magazine, *The Quarterly,* to the group as a gift. *The Quarterly* later became *Public Health Nursing* and, still later, *Nursing Outlook.* It was an essential element to the development and dissemination of the public health nursing movement in the United States.

The Goldmark Report

In 1919, under the auspices of the Rockefeller Foundation and at the urging of concerned nursing leaders, the Committee for the Study of Public Health Nursing Education, with C-E.A. Winslow as chairman, began a 2-year investigation. Josephine Goldmark was secretary of the committee and the study was later to bear her name.

The purpose of the committee was to look at typical examples of public health nursing education and service, and to study the education afforded by hospital training schools, graduate courses for public health nurses, and special schools of a non-nursing type (Committee for the Study of Nursing Education, 1923, p. 2). The study was expanded the following year to look at the entire field of nursing education. Ten conclusions were reached that have profoundly affected the course of public health nursing, as well as of all nursing (Committee for the Study of Nursing Education). These conclusions are in the box on p. 18.

The significance of this very early study is, even today, not fully understood and implemented. However, some positive changes were slowly made: poor schools were closed, qualified faculty members were hired, and the money allotted to education programs was increased.

Changes in Nursing Education

Until World War II it was believed that nurses could be prepared for public health only after they graduated from a hospital (diploma) school of nursing. It became evident, however, that graduates of collegiate schools of nursing did not need the same additional content in public health nursing as did graduates of diploma schools, because the broader background of a liberal arts education helped prepare one for this area of nursing. Content in public health became increasingly evident in collegiate schools of nursing. Finally, in 1944, the first basic collegiate program in nursing was accredited as including adequate preparation for public health nursing, so that graduates did not need additional study to practice public health nursing after graduation from the basic nursing program (National Organization for Public Health Nursing, 1944, p. 371).

During the next 30 years there were drastic changes in nursing education. Like most major changes, they were met with resistance from many sources and caused severe distress for some individuals. These changes included the following:

1. One-year practical nursing programs were established and the numbers of schools and graduates increased rapidly. More than half of these programs were offered under vocational education.
2. Two-year programs in nursing were established (1952), most of them in junior colleges. These graduates were qualified to take the examination to become registered nurses.
3. After 1963 no baccalaureate nursing program was accredited unless it prepared its graduates for public health nursing.

4. Universities assumed more responsibility for clinical field instruction, which enriched both field and classroom teaching.
5. In 1965 members of the American Nurses Association approved a position paper on the educational preparation for nurse practitioners, which stated that education for all those licensed to practice nursing should take place in institutions of higher education.
6. In 1978 the American Nurses Association, after years of debate, resolved again that the baccalaureate degree should be the minimum preparation for entry into professional nursing practice.

The Effects of World War I on Public Health Nursing

By 1915 the role of the public health nurse was well established and the pioneer stage of this specialized area was drawing to a close. However, with the advent of World War I in 1917 and the involvement of thousands of nurses in military service, public health nursing services were threatened. The American Red Cross (which had been founded in 1882 by Clara Barton to supply nurses for war service), along with a committee chaired by Adelaide Nutting, the "farseeing dean of American nurses," investigated methods to deal with the situation (Roberts, 1954, p. 131).

The efficient use of the limited supply of public health nurses was ensured by the Red Cross, which set up a roster of nurses who could be called upon to coordinate and supplement health resources. Emphasis was placed upon educational programs for the community as well as the control of communicable diseases.

During World War I, a nurse was loaned to the U.S. Public Health Service from the National Organization of Public Health Nursing to develop a public health nursing program for the military outposts. This was the first public health nursing service to be established within the federal government (Gardner, 1919, p. 44).

The committee was convinced that the standards for preparing nurses must be maintained and that quick "short courses" to prepare nurses could have a disastrous effect on war and postwar health programs. To alleviate the nursing shortage, and to ensure standards of care, they encouraged the development of a quality shortened program.

◀ *Conclusions of the Committee for the Study of Nursing Education, 1923* ▶

Conclusion 1. That, since constructive health work and health teaching in families is best done by persons:

(a) capable of giving general health instruction, as distinguished from instruction in any one specialty; and

(b) capable of rendering bedside care at need; the agent responsible for such constructive health work and health teaching in families should have completed the nurses' training. There will, of course, be need for the employment, in addition to the public health nurse, of other types of experts such as nutrition workers, social workers, occupational therapists, and the like.

That as soon as may be practicable all agencies, public or private, employing public health nurses, should require as a prerequisite for employment the basic hospital training, followed by a postgraduate course, including both class work and field work, in public health nursing.

Conclusion 2. That the career open to young women of high capacity, in public health nursing or in hospital supervision and nursing education, is one of the most attractive fields now open, in its promise of professional success and of rewarding public service; and that every effort should be made to attract such women into this field.

Conclusion 3. That for the care of persons suffering from serious and acute disease, the safety of the patient, and the responsibility of the medical and nursing professions, demand the maintenance of the standards of educational attainment now generally accepted by the best sentiment of both professions and embodied in the legislation of the more progressive states; and that any attempt to lower these standards would be fraught with real danger to the public.

Conclusion 4. That steps should be taken through state legislation for the definition and licensure of a subsidiary grade of nursing service, the subsidiary type of worker to serve under practicing physicians in the care of mild and chronic illness, and convalescence, and possibly to assist under the direction of the trained nurse in certain phases of hospital and visiting nursing.

Conclusion 5. That, while training schools for nurses have made remarkable progress, and while the best schools of today in many respects reach a high level of educational attainment, the average hospital training school is not organized on such a basis as to conform to the standards accepted in other educational fields; that the instruction in such schools is frequently casual and uncorrelated; that the educational needs and the health and strength of students are frequently sacrificed to practical hospital exigencies; that such shortcomings are primarily due to the lack of independent endowments for nursing education; that existing educational facilities are on the whole, in the majority of schools, inadequate for the preparation of the high-grade of nurses required for the care of serious illness, and for service in the fields of public health nursing and nursing education; and that one of the chief reasons for the lack of sufficient recruits, of a high type, to meet such needs lies precisely in the fact that the average hospital training school does not offer a sufficiently attractive avenue of entrance to this field.

Conclusion 6. That, with the necessary financial support and under a separate board or training school committee, organized primarily for educational purposes, it is possible, with completion of a high school course or its equivalent as a prerequisite, to reduce the fundamental period of hospital training to 28 months, and at the same time, by eliminating unessential, non-educational routine, and adopting the principles laid down in Miss Goldmark's report, to organize the course along intensive and coordinated lines with such modifications as may be necessary for practical application; and that courses of this standard would be reasonably certain to attract students of high quality in increasing numbers.

Conclusion 7. Superintendents, supervisors, instructors, and public health nurses should in all cases receive special additional training beyond the basic nursing course.

Conclusion 8. That the development and strengthening of University Schools of Nursing of a high grade for the training of leaders is of fundamental importance in the furtherance of nursing education.

Conclusion 9. That when the licensure of a subsidiary grade of nursing service is provided for, the establishment of training courses in preparation for such service is highly desirable; that such courses should be conducted in special hospitals, in small unaffiliated general hospitals, or in separate sections of hospitals where nurses are also trained; and that the course should be of 8 or 9 months' duration; provided the standards of such schools be approved by the same educational board which governs nursing training schools.

Conclusion 10. That the development of nursing service adequate for the care of the sick and for the conduct of the modern public health campaign demands as an absolute prerequisite the securing of funds for the endowment of nursing education of all types; and that it is of primary importance, in this connection, to provide reasonably generous endowment for university schools of nursing.

From Committee for the Study of Nursing Education: *Nursing and nursing education in the United States,* New York, 1923, Macmillan.

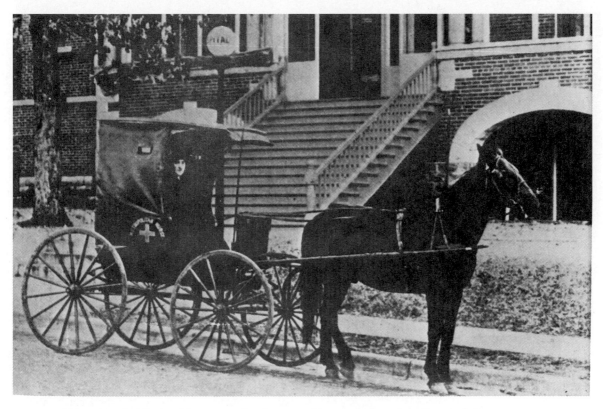

Figure 1-5 Public health nurse using horse and buggy before the advent of the automobile. (The Metropolitan Life Insurance Company of New York. Used with their permission.)

The Vassar Training Camp for Nurses

A unique experience in the annals of nursing education was the Vassar Camp School of Nursing. Begun in 1918 and supported by the American Red Cross and the Council of National Defense, the program was based on the principle that the 3-year nursing course could be shortened to 2 years for students who had graduated from college majoring in other subjects. It was modeled on the Plattsburg Military Camp at Plattsburg, New York, where college men were given intensive training to become army reserve officers. The purpose was to more rapidly fill the desperate need for nurses in wartime. Applicants to the program chose a college and were admitted into selected nursing schools across the country. Graduates of this program numbered 435; the program ended with the Armistice.

This patriotic opportunity attracted high-level faculty and students. The program produced distinguished nursing leaders of the next several decades, including people like Katherine Densford Dreves, who became dean of the University of Minnesota School of Nursing, president of the American Nurses Association, and second vice-president of the International Council of Nurses.

After World War I

Rapid changes came with peace. Economic prosperity, reaction to Prohibition, and the increasing use of the automobile created radical changes in the way people lived. These changes brought subsequent changes in public health nursing. The use of the automobile, for instance, permitted nurses to have easy access to rural areas and made once-closed areas accessible (refer to Figures 1-5, 1-6, and 1-7).

The poor physical condition of the nation's men, made evident in wartime, shocked the nation. About 29% of those called for service were unfit for military duty because of problems that in many cases were preventable (Roberts, 1954, p. 164). Health programs of both official and nonofficial private agencies grew as a result.

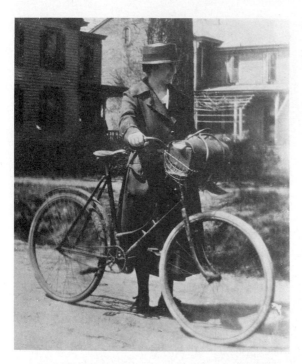

Figure 1-6   Public health nurse using a bicycle before the advent of the automobile. (The Metropolitan Life Insurance Company of New York. Used with their permission.)

Smillie says that

beginning in 1925 and extending through the present time (1952) is the extraordinary phenomenon of the nationalization of the public health. The public health was, for generations, a community affair administered under local self-government with some slight degree of state government supervision. Public health has now become a subject of nationwide interest and importance (Smillie, 1952, p. 10).

By 1920 there were 28 states with a statewide public health nursing program. However, only five had divisions of public health nursing within state health departments (Roberts, 1954, p. 168).

Two voluntary (non–tax-supported) agencies were very active during this time: the National Tuberculosis Association and the American Red Cross. The Red Cross supplemented but did not supplant the work of health agencies. Its goal was for public health nursing to be conducted as a public service by municipalities, counties, or states. In some states the public health nursing supervisors in state health departments also functioned as Red Cross supervisors. In 1921 state tuberculosis associations had supervising nurses in 28 states, the Red Cross in 31. In 29 states the state board of health had a director of public health nursing or a division of child hygiene (Fox, 1920, p. 180) (refer to Figure 1-8).

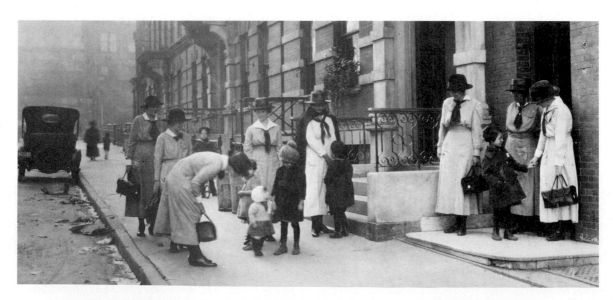

Figure 1-7   To these nurses of the 1930s, the city's streets were hospital corridors, and family bedrooms their wards. Each carried cakes of soap to protect themselves from germs and a whistle to guard themselves from danger. (Courtesy Visiting Nurse Service of New York City.)

The Effects of World War II on Public Health Nursing

The Depression of 1929, which preceded World War II, forced many hospitals and schools of nursing to close. The supply of nurses far exceeded the demand. In the health field as a whole, the financial crisis resulted in the wider use of national, state, and local tax funds for health and welfare services. An important aspect of this program on the national level was the passage of the Social Security Act in 1935, which introduced governmental involvement in health and welfare care on a larger scale. This meant that the federal government was taking on a new role in assuming responsibility for the health of people. The individualism that was important to the founding of this country was no longer sufficient to solve all problems. The Depression also led to the rapid growth of voluntary insurance plans for financing hospital and medical care (Stewart and Austin, 1938, p. 219).

In 1933 Pearl McIver, a well-qualified public health nurse in the U.S. Public Health Service, was assigned as a consultant for the placement of nurses on federal relief projects. Many of these nurses were formerly hospital nurses now assigned to public health agencies and clinics, and they became interested in this new field. Thus, when the Social Security Act of 1935 made money available for the education and employment of public health nurses, many of those working on relief projects seized the opportunity to study. Other educational funds followed that made it possible for nurses to complete their education in a shorter time. These included Training for Nurses for National Defense, the GI bill, the Nurse Training Act of 1943, and Public Health and Professional Nurse traineeships. Funds were also available to help prepare nurses at the graduate level for specialties such as tuberculosis, cancer, mental health, maternal and child health, and research (McNeil, 1967, p. 6).

After the war began in 1941, the nurse shortage became acute. The problem was more serious than in World War I because of the duration and scope of the war effort. The National Nursing Council, composed of six national nursing organizations, along with the aid of the U.S. Department of Education, requested $1 million to enlarge facilities for nursing education. The administration of this money was assigned to the U.S. Public Health Service.

In 1943 the Cadet Nurse Corps was authorized by the Bolton Act. Sixty million dollars was appropriated

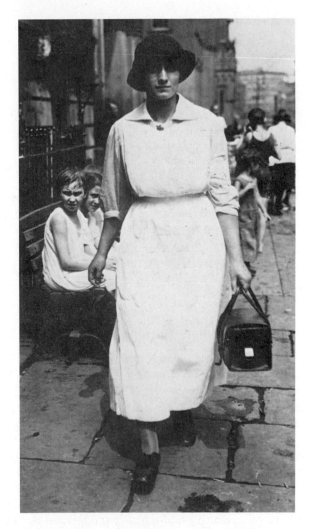

Figure 1-8 From the turn of the century on, the visiting nurse served as the first line of defense in the fight against diphtheria and other "killer" contagions of the era. (Courtesy Visiting Nurse Service of New York City.)

to recruit and educate 70,000 cadets in 1125 schools between 1944 and 1946. These nurses made up 90% of the total enrollment of basic nursing programs for this time. Lucille Petry, chief nurse officer, directed this remarkable program at a difficult time in our nation's history.

World War II, like World War I and the Depression, had a major impact on public health nursing. Specifically, the war influenced the following trends:

1. The importance of public health nursing service was recognized when public health nurses

were declared essential for civilian work, although many of them entered military service.

2. Maximum utilization of personnel was essential; official tax-supported public health nursing agencies combined with voluntary non–tax-supported agencies to avoid duplication.

3. Practical nurses were accepted as an important resource for nursing service.

4. The establishment of priorities for health care became more than a topic for discussion.

5. Additional funds for nursing education became available and the fear of governmental control of education decreased. After the war, the enrollment of nurses who were veterans or widows of veterans strained the resources of universities and agencies providing field experience.

The Birth of Modern Nursing Research

Sigma Theta Tau, the international honor society in nursing, awarded the first known grant for nursing research in the United States in 1936 (Hudgings, Hogan, and Stevenson, 1990, p. i). However, there was very little nursing research being done at this time.

The decade of the 1950s is considered by many to be the birth of modern nursing research. In this decade the American Nurses Association (ANA) and the National League for Nursing (NLN) became actively involved in promoting nursing research. In 1954 ANA formed a Committee on Research and Studies, and in 1959 NLN established a Research and Studies Service. In 1952 the first nursing research journal, aptly named *Nursing Research,* was published.

By the 1960s ANA and NLN were at the forefront of nursing research activities. In 1962 ANA established nursing research priorities and published "Blueprint for Research in Nursing" in the *American Journal of Nursing.* In the 1960s new journals with a nursing research focus emerged, such as *International Journal of Nursing Studies* and *IMAGE.* In 1965 ANA held the first nursing research conference. These conferences were held yearly from 1965 to 1973 and were funded by grants from the Division of Nursing in the United States Public Health Service. In 1969 the first Center for Nursing Research in a college of nursing was established at Wayne State University College of Nursing in Detroit, Michigan (Werley and Shea, 1973, p. 217). H. Harriet Werley was the director of this program.

FROM WORLD WAR II TO THE DECADE OF THE 1970s

The depressions before and after World War II, as well as the war itself, provided the milieu for the development of numerous programs designed to help the country renew itself. Chronic disease and accidents replaced infectious disease as the leading causes of death, a result of the effectiveness of new drugs and vaccines. Consequently, life expectancy increased.

The years between 1935 and 1965 produced much legislation that was aimed at improving the health, education, and housing of people, ending discrimination against minorities, and providing proper working conditions for wage earners. This legislation began with the Social Security Act of 1935; it provided monies for old-age benefits, state grants for aid to the blind and disabled, aid for dependent and crippled children, vocational rehabilitation programs, and unemployment compensation programs.

Title VI of the act focused on public health programs, and its overall purpose was to elicit a public health program that would protect and promote the nation's health. One part of Title VI provided money to states and counties to establish and maintain health services. Allocations in this part of the act provided money for nurses to study public health nursing. Prior to 1935, only one third of the states had a public health nursing section within the state health department, and only 7% of the public health nurses employed had taken an accredited course in public health nursing. During 1936, the first year that money became available through the Social Security Act, over 1000 nurses received money to study in a program accredited by the National Organization for Public Health Nursing.

Another part of Title VI provided money for research and the investigation of diseases and problems with environmental health. Title VI was directly responsible for expanding public health nursing programs and developing new ones. As a result of this legislation, the public health nurse became an integral part of local health departments: the maternal and child health programs of the Social Security Act made the nurse's work with families essential. By 1940, 3000 nurses had received public health training in accredited schools, 970 counties had developed full-time public health services, and 1150 clinics had been added to those already working on the problems of venereal diseases (Williams, 1951, p. 156).

Later, President Kennedy's New Frontier and President Johnson's Great Society epitomized the era in our nation's history when the government even more aggressively took on the role of guardian of the nation's health. The rugged individualism of the early 1900s had disappeared. John Kennedy's inaugural address in 1961 is remembered for the words, "Ask not what your country can do for you—ask what you can do for your country." A new social consciousness swept the country, and the differences between black and white, poor and rich became topics for scrutiny, worth dying for.

Citizens began to see health as a right rather than a privilege. This was a significant change from the beginning of the century, when families with large numbers of children were the norm so that at least some of them could be expected to live to adulthood. Parents realized that health should be the birthright of every child, not the privilege of a few.

The Constitution of the World Health Organization defined health as "complete physical, mental and social well-being and not just the absence of disease." This definition reflected inclusion of the mental and social aspects of health as well as its physical aspects.

The demand for health care services on the part of an increasingly sophisticated and informed public came about in part as the result of ideas generated through television, magazines, newspapers, and radio. The ability to pay for these services led to the quest for a national compulsory health insurance.

When the war was over in 1945, President Harry Truman presented to Congress a health message with the following proposals for a health care system (Kalisch and Kalisch, 1982, p. 21):

1. Prepayment of medical costs with compulsory insurance and general revenues.
2. Protection from loss of wages as a result of sickness.
3. Expansion of services related to the public's health and including maternal and child health services.
4. Governmental aid to medical schools for research.
5. Increased construction of hospitals, clinics, and medical institutions.

Charges of socialism from the American Medical Association ended the quest for national health insurance in 1949 and 1950 (Kalisch and Kalisch, 1986, pp.

568-573). Much later, in 1965, a health insurance program for people 65 and older, Medicare, financed under the Social Security Act, was enacted by President Johnson.

Hospital Survey and Construction Act, 1946

Only the last of Truman's proposals was enacted. The Hospital Survey and Construction Act, also called the Hill-Burton bill, provided a 5-year program to states for the purpose of assessing needs, and then planning and constructing needed hospitals and public health centers.

The federal government provided one third of the funds needed for the program, and each state provided the remaining two thirds of the money. This act gave some nurses an opportunity to help plan the areas where they worked.

Organizing Public Health Nursing Services

The concept of organized home care began with philanthropic people like Lillian Wald and Florence Nightingale, who cared about the poverty and pain of the working class. At the beginning of the 1900s, however, there was a growth in programs sponsored by federal, state, and local taxes. Public health nurses were "sent into homes of the poor to teach the ways of healthful living. Concepts of disease prevention, personal responsibility for health, and the methods of treatment derived from recent advances in both medical science and public health were the message of the 'public health nurse' in these new programs" (Buhler-Wilkerson, 1991, p. 9). Thus there were several different organizations in one city or county carrying out home care: visiting nurses from philanthropic charity organizations caring for the ill and teaching families, and public health nurses from official tax-supported health departments teaching disease prevention. Both kinds of nurses might visit the same home for differing reasons, with a resulting duplication of services and confusion on the part of families. To address these issues, a committee of representatives from numerous agencies interested in public health nursing published guidelines in 1946 on which this area of nursing should be organized (Desirable Organization, 1946, p. 387).

The guidelines adopted by the committee addressed this history and resulting problems. It was agreed that a population of 50,000 was needed to support an adequate health program and that there should be one public health nurse for every 2000 people. Other principles included:

- That each public health nurse should combine the functions of health teaching, control of disease, and care of the sick.
- That the community should adopt one of three patterns of organization that would best serve that community:
  1. All public health nursing service, including care of the sick at home, administered by the local health department
  2. Preventive services carried on by the health department with one voluntary agency, in close coordination with the health department, carrying responsibility for bedside nursing care
  3. A combination service jointly administered and financed by official and voluntary agencies, with all service given by a single group of public health nurses

The Nurse Shortage

Right after World War II a serious undersupply of nurses created critical situations in hospitals and health centers. This was a result of factors including the increase in the population, the increase in insurance plans such as Blue Cross, an increase in the sophistication of surgery and medicine, which kept people alive longer, and the different situations in which nurses were increasingly employed, such as industry and schools.

Also, during the 1940s and the 1950s societal norms placed women in the home with husband and children. Married nurses were affected by this philosophy, and careers came second. It was not until the late 1960s that nurses began to develop a consciousness about their possible role in shaping the health care policies of the country, as well as their role in the political arena. Nurses were finally beginning to see themselves as the very obvious answer to the health care problems in the United States (Grissum and Spengler, 1976). This rise in activism among nurses paralleled the feminist movement among women in general.

In 1972, Nurses for Political Action was organized with headquarters in Washington, D.C. It became affiliated with the American Nurses Association and later changed its name to N-CAP, Nurses' Coalition for Action in Politics. Its purpose as a nonpartisan, nonprofit association was to obtain support for nursing

from legislators, governmental officials, and the general public. At a time when a new national health care system was being developed and the present health care system was fragmented and dominated by the medical profession, nurses sought a place where they could make known their thoughts and ideas and help plan a system that comprehensively met people's health care needs. N-CAP is active today.

The Federal Government Prepares Nurses

The government became involved in preparing new nurses with the passage of the Health Amendments Act of 1956. Title II authorized monies to aid registered nurses in the full-time study of either administration, supervision, or teaching.

However, in 1963 the Surgeon General's Consultant Group on Nursing reported that there were still too few nursing schools and not enough capable people being recruited into nursing. Additional problems were the poor utilization of nursing personnel and the limited research being done in nursing (U.S. Public Health Service, 1963).

Based upon these conclusions, the Nurse Training Act of 1964 was passed. This act provided money for loans and scholarships and nursing school construction. With this act the federal government helped to improve greatly the quality of nursing in America.

The Expanding Role of the Nurse

By the 1960s the nursing profession began to look at new methods of meeting the health care needs of people, utilizing advanced nursing practice and extending the nursing role to take over some medical functions. The term *nurse practitioner* was first used at the University of Colorado in 1965 in a program that prepared nurses to provide comprehensive well-child care in ambulatory settings.

The concept of primary care nursing also became an important one. Primary care involves three important elements: first contact with the patient, continuity of care, and coordination of care. It is ambulatory care that views a person in relation to family and environment and emphasizes cure as well as prevention. Primary care can prevent both gaps and overlapping in health care services.

Public health nursing evolved from concern for the individual, the family, and the community. In fact, the early public health movement was the historical forerunner of today's primary care movement (Fagin, 1978, p. 752). Though presently other nursing specialties besides public health nursing work outside the hospital setting, and work with a person in terms of the family and the environment, public health nurses first used the concept that nursing could best meet the total health needs of people. The major difference between public health nursing and other areas of primary nursing is that public health nursing deals with the personal and environmental health of aggregates rather than only individuals and families. Public health practice must deal in concepts such as caseloads, clinics, counties, or census tracts to locate subgroups who have problems and are at risk. As the scope of public health nursing changed from the care of the sick poor to the care of the population as a whole, the community, it became time for a change in the title of this specialty area: the term *community health nurse* came into use to denote care for all people, not just those using public tax monies.

In 1971 a bronze bust of Lillian Wald was placed in the Hall of Fame for Great Americans. An editorial about this event stated:

The kind of health care Lillian Wald began preaching and practicing in 1893 is the kind the people of this country are still crying for. She demonstrated with no need to rest on formal research that nursing could serve as the entry point—not only for health care, but for dealing with many other social ills of which sickness is only a part. She felt that nurses should go to the sick, instead of expecting the sick to come to them (and waiting for physicians to refer them); that care of persons in the home, especially of children, was far more effective and much less expensive except perhaps for those needing, to use her own word, "intensive" care. (A Prophet Honored, 1971, p. 53)

There is still not total agreement in nursing on the definition of and preparation for the expanded role of the nurse. However, increasing numbers of people are viewing primary care as the major focus of nursing (Fagin, 1978, p. 753). Attractive federal funding has encouraged the growth of practitioner programs.

COMMUNITY HEALTH NURSING IN THE 1970s AND 1980s

With change and growth in health care, community health nursing, as well as all of professional nursing, was in a state of transition. The contribution of this specialty area to the health needs of people was less clear than it was in Lillian Wald's time. She and her

peers had no doubt about their mission and the goals of public health nursing. Through the 1920s and 1930s the public health nursing movement grew in power, set standards for practice, and influenced education by requiring certain content as a condition for employment.

In the 1970s all areas of nursing, including parent and child nursing, psychiatric nursing, and medical and surgical nursing, began discovering the community. These areas also began to emphasize the importance of the family to the patient, and the clear lines of distinction for what constituted public health nursing started to blur. At that time public health nurses had a difficult time agreeing on the nature, standards, and scope of public health nursing practice (Ruth and Partridge, 1978, p. 625). However, it must be re-emphasized that public health nursing was seen as a generalized area within nursing. Each of the other areas, medical-surgical nursing, psychiatric nursing, and parent and child nursing, had a specialized focus. Public health nursing had always been broad and comprehensive. Efforts were made to define the nature, standards, and scope of public health nursing practice.

Further, more non-health and allied health professionals began to work in the community. Social workers, physical therapists, occupational therapists, and physicians' assistants and home health aides, were seen in public health settings. To complicate the situation, there were numerous ways to become a "nurse"; associate degree programs, diploma programs, and baccalaureate programs all claimed to prepare a different level of nurse. How these levels functioned and were employed in the community setting varied from agency to agency.

Private agencies and health facilities multiplied, and many of them were not coordinated or designed with comprehensive health care plans in mind. Strong, effective official planning often was not evident on the state and local level. Health maintenance organizations, neighborhood health centers, free clinics, and numerous home health care programs based in hospitals and "for-profit agencies" represented the conglomeration of facilities that could spring up in any one community.

The rapid development of health services and specialties created even more confusion for people who found the existing health care system difficult to negotiate. People desperately needed someone to help them, and community health nurses offered hope.

The 1980s brought opportunities and threats to the health care setting. Unprecedented health care costs, health care delivery issues, an increasingly sophisticated consumer, and a recognition that more health care spending was not reducing health care needs spurred an emphasis on cost containment and quality assessment. Renewed interest in home care services emerged, as did a greater focus on health promotion and disease prevention. Consumers also became more involved in pressing for health care reform and in examining methods to reduce their own risks for disease and disability (Roberts and Heinrich, 1985).

Our nation's health status data reflected a dismal state of affairs during the 1980s. "Every key measure of maternal and child health in the United States worsened, failed to improve, or improved at a slower rate than in previous years. As a result the United States has fallen behind other countries with fewer resources on important health indicators such as infant mortality and low birthweight" (Children's Defense Fund, 1992, p. 1). Additionally, health care professionals and consumers were having to deal with immediate, enduring, and growing health care challenges such as AIDS, health and welfare access issues for the poor and near-poor, and increasing poverty and homelessness (Institute of Medicine, 1988). At this same time, funds for public health services were decreasing in many communities.

The 1980s were a time for reflection for consumer groups, health care professionals, and political leaders. Recognizing the serious state of affairs, all of these groups pushed for health care reform. Their efforts influenced the passage of significant federal legislation resulting in funds targeted for select high-risk populations. New models of care emerged and there was increasing integration of organizational efforts devoted to health care. Further, there was growing recognition that nurses are valuable resources in the health care system and can provide cost-effective preventive services. The Center for Nursing Research, established in 1985, placed a priority on research related to health promotion across the life span.

The Cyclical Nature of Issues in Community Health Nursing

The issues that faced CHNs relating to common practices and education in the 1980s were amazingly like those faced by Lillian Wald and her contemporaries. Babies were born to destitute parents; growing numbers of the elderly suffered from neglect, isolation, and lack of adequate care; and clients wished to die at home surrounded by family and familiar circumstances rather than in a hospital. Human needs do not change or diminish—only perhaps our methods of dealing with them do.

The economic crisis, with resulting cuts in the budgets of almost every agency, meant decreases in services provided, as well as reorganization of some of those services and agencies. Community health nursing agencies had to examine critically each program that they offered. Often programs lacked adequate documentation of the effectiveness of community health nursing intervention. Preventive efforts and those that are long-term in nature are difficult to evaluate; thus, CHNs must make such research a priority.

National Institute of Nursing Research Established

The National Center for Nursing Research [NCNR] was authorized under the Health Research Extension Act of 1985 (Public Law 99-158) and was established on April 18, 1986, as part of the National Institutes of Health [NIH] in the USPHS. Its major purpose was to conduct a program of grants and funding to support nursing research and research training, and expand the knowledge base in nursing. Through the efforts of ANA and NLN and the support of nurses across the nation, the Center is the first and only National Center for Nursing Research in the world. The nursing research priorities established by the NCNR are identified in the box on p. 27. The target dates for accomplishing these priorities are also delineated in this box after each priority.

With the establishment of NCNR, nursing research studies increased by leaps and bounds. NCNR became a major funding mechanism for nursing research. Other funding for nursing research includes the NIH's Institute of the Alcohol, Drug Abuse and Mental Health Administration, as well as many private funding resources (ANA, 1989).

On June 10, 1993, the NCNR became the *National Institute of Nursing Research* [NINR], the first and only one of its kind in the world. Nursing research studies in the United States are helping to shape international as well as national nursing practice; American nurses can be very proud of their research heritage.

◀ *Priorities Resulting from Second Conference on* ▶
Research Priorities in Nursing Practice

National Center for Nursing Research

1—Community-Based Nursing Models (1995)

Develop and test community-based nursing models designed to promote access to, utilization of, and quality of health services by rural and other underserved populations.

2—Health-Promoting Behavior and HIV/AIDS (1996)

Assess the effectiveness of bio-behavioral nursing interventions to foster health-promoting behaviors of individuals of different cultural backgrounds—especially women—who are at high risk for HIV/AIDS, incorporating bio-behavioral markers.

3—Cognitive Impairment (1997)

Develop and test bio-behavioral and environmental approaches to remediating cognitive impairment.

4—Living with Chronic Illness (1998)

Test interventions to strengthen individuals' personal resources in dealing with their chronic illness.

5—Bio-Behavioral Factors related to Immunocompetence (1999)

Identify bio-behavioral factors and test interventions to promote immunocompetence.

From National Center for Nursing Research: *Priorities resulting from second conference on research priorities in nursing practice, National Center for Nursing Research,* Bethesda, Md., February 1993, NCNR.

THE DECADE OF THE 1990s

As the decade of the 1980s came to an end, a number of trends in nursing's development became apparent (Lynaugh and Fagin, 1988): the acute-care model of care delivery and disease-focused insurance systems do not meet the needs of children, the old, the chemically dependent, and the dying. The profession of nursing must address the fact that the age of "delayed degenerative disease" means that aging citizens survive pneumonia to face a life in which they need help with the activities of daily living. Other vulnerable groups such as handicapped children and adults and minorities face this challenge at the same time that they strive to obtain access to health care. "Health Care for All"—a goal being promoted worldwide and discussed throughout this text—is not a reality for many people in our society.

Further, the United States is seeing a "Third Revolution in Medical Care," that of assessment and accountability (Relman, 1988, p. 1220). Rapid expansion of the entire health care system took place in the decades of the 1940s through the 1960s, followed by the era of cost containment of health care spending. Presently health care planners agree that we need to know more about the costs, effectiveness, quality, and safety of the methods we use for the prevention, diagnosis, and treatment of disease. Outcome management or methods to link health care management decisions to systematic information about outcomes of practice will improve the effectiveness of care and provide a firm basis for economic decision-making.

Challenges for the Future

The key issue that faced CHNs in the 1980s and that will continue to challenge the profession throughout the next decade is the spiraling cost of health care. For the federal government, medical costs are the fastest growing item in the budget, increasing at more than 8% annually at a time when inflation is only 5%. At the current rate of growth, spending for health care in the next 10 years will be in the trillions of dollars. If current rates of health care spending are maintained, problems with growing poverty, drug and alcohol abuse, teenage pregnancy, family violence, and the AIDS epidemic will have limited attention.

"Helping families to help themselves" was a creed of the earliest nurses who visited families in their homes. That creed is even more important for the contemporary community health nurse who cannot individually deal with the critical problems in our society. "In a free society public activities ultimately rest on public understanding and support, not on the technical judgment of experts. Expertise is made effective only when it is combined with sufficient public support, a connection acted upon effectively by the early leaders of public health" (Institute of Medicine, 1988). To be able to use the wealth of knowledge known about diseases and their prevention, we need to know more about how to communicate this to the public to mobilize their support. This is one of the major challenges for public health researchers and practitioners.

The challenges that need to be addressed in the 1990s are not insurmountable. Early public health nurse pioneers set the standards for the development of the nursing profession and reform in health care delivery. They were on the cutting edge of the suffragette movement, the birth control movement, and the social reform movement that brought health care and civil rights to women, children, immigrants, prisoners, and the mentally ill. They were not infrequently jailed for their beliefs. Their names are seen in the books that tell the story of our nation's history. Further, they worked independently in their profession and set standards for both nursing education and practice. Appendix 1-2 presents an overview of early nurse leaders whose lives we can celebrate today. We can use them as models for our own professional and personal growth.

In the first years of the 1990s there continue to be nurses at the cutting edge of nursing research, education, and practice and in local, state, and national politics. The following chapters tell some of their stories.

Summary

The beginnings of nursing can be traced to the beginnings of humankind, for there has always been a need for reducing pain with comfort measures. The early Christian church's contributions to nursing were significant, as were the organizational contributions of St. Vincent de Paul and Mademoiselle Le Gras to public health nursing. The influence of the status of women on nursing can be demonstrated by Sairy Gamp, a prostitute-nurse who cared for people in the 1700s when no "respectable" woman could take this position. Florence Nightingale's legacy to professional nursing and to public health, along with the contributions of William Rathbone, the founder of public health nursing in England, provided the basis for public health nursing in the United States. Events in society at large have shaped nursing as a whole and the development of public health nursing. The life and work of Lillian Wald, predecessor of the modern community health nurse, was powerfully influenced by the waves of immigrants to New York City and the desperate conditions in which they lived.

Public health nurses used advances in the public health sciences to deal with the problems they encountered. The title of community health nurse came into being to emphasize that this field was for the community, not just people who were poor enough to use public assistance programs. How community health nurses organized themselves along with methods of education for this area of nursing shaped not only the development of this specialty area but the entire field of nursing. Gradually the nation developed a consciousness about its collective health status; this was demonstrated by the formation of health services on the national, state, and local level. Both world wars and the Depression forced negative and positive changes in public health nursing. Emphases in community health nursing, as well as nursing in general, are changing; the health scene is chaotic because there is no overall health plan. Community health nursing, with its focus on the health of aggregates, can involve nurses in health planning and in the necessary task of bringing order out of chaos.

Appendix 1-1 presents some beginnings and significant developments to public health nursing in a chronological chart form. It is important to note other contemporary social events when reviewing the historical transition of community health nursing. Societal changes tremendously influence changes that occur in a profession.

◀ *An Exercise in Critical Thinking* ▶

"Nursing has reached a point at which it is ready to use its history. Nursing can better evaluate its values and goals and chart its course to fulfill them if nurses have a fuller understanding of who they are and what they do, wish to be, and need to know. If nursing is to continue to grow as a profession, knowledge of what has been done in the past and what factors influenced its growth are vitally important. It is in looking at nursing's history that safeguards can be established to ensure that the profession profits by its errors and recognizes its successes. If nursing does not study its history, its educational advances, its research, and its publications, it is doomed to repeat the same mistakes" (Hezel and Linebach, 1991, p. 272).

Examining nursing history and using it to analyze current trends and issues will help to ensure that community health nurses profit by errors and recognize successes. After reading this chapter, and considering the state of our current health care system, complete one of the following exercises:

1. Select a current societal issue such as environmental pollution and examine the progress or lack of progress made in addressing the problem since early recorded history. Note the writings on the environment of Edwin Chadwick, Florence Nightingale, and Lillian Wald in this chapter.

2. Examine the characteristics of the current immigrants to the United States and consider how they are similar to and different from the immigrants in the early part of the century. How can community health nurses assist recent immigrants with their health needs?

3. List the achievements of a nursing leader discussed in the chapter and identify factors that facilitated and hindered his or her ability to accomplish goals. How would you personally deal with these inhibiting factors today?

APPENDIX 1-1

Some Beginnings in and Developments of Significance to Public Health Nursing*

Nursing and public health nursing		Other significant events	
		1765	First school of medicine (Philadelphia)
		1798	Marine Hospital Service (became USPHS 1912)
			U.S. Treasury Department establishes an Act for the Relief of Sick and Disabled Seaman, imposing a 20 cent tax on seaman's wages to provide funds for their health care
1813	Ladies Benevolent Society, Charleston, South Carolina	1813	Act to Encourage Vaccination
		1839	First dental school (Baltimore)
		1848	Imports Drug Act becomes the first federal statute to ensure the quality of drugs
1851	Florence Nightingale (1820-1910) goes to Kaiserswerth		
1859	First District Nursing Association, Liverpool (William Rathbone and Mrs. Mary Robinson)		
1860	Nightingale Training School established, London		

*Some dates may be disputed.

Continued

Some Beginnings in and Developments of Significance to Public Health Nursing—cont'd

---

Nursing and public health nursing	Other significant events
	1861-1865 Civil War
	1864 International Red Cross (Henri Durant)
	1869 Massachusetts State Department of Health
1872 First schools of nursing in United States (New England Hospital for Women and Children, Boston, and Women's Hospital, Philadelphia)	1872 American Public Health Association founded by Stephen Smith
1873 Linda Richards, first nurse graduated in United States	
1877 New York City Mission sends trained nurses into homes of sick poor	
	1878 Act to Enforce Quarantine on Vessels and Vehicles
	1879 Act to Establish a National Board of Health for a 4-year period to cooperate with states on matters of public health
	1880 National Death Registration established by U.S. Bureau of the Census
	1882 American Red Cross (Clara Barton)
	1882-1884 Discovery of bacteria causing tuberculosis, diphtheria, and typhoid
1885 Buffalo District Nursing Association	
1886 Boston Instructive District Nursing Association and Philadelphia Visiting Nurse Association (VNA)	
1889 Chicago Visiting Nurse Association	
	1890-1910 "Golden Age of Bacteriology"
	1890 Pasteurization of milk developed
	Act to Prevent Interstate Spread of Disease passed
1892 School nursing, London (Amy Hughes)	
1893 Henry Street Visiting Nurse Service, New York (Lillian D. Wald and Mary Brewster); first milk station, New York City; American Society of Superintendents of Training Schools for Nurses (becomes National League for Nursing Education, 1912)	
	1894 School medical inspection, Boston
1895 Industrial Nursing, Vermont Marble Works (Ada Mayo Stewart)	
1897 Nurses' Associated Alumnae of United States and Canada (becomes American Nurses Association in 1911)	1897 University of Michigan grants Master of Science degree in Hygiene and Public Health
1898 Los Angeles Health Department pays public health nurses; Detroit Visiting Nurse Association established	1898 Course in social work, New York Charity Organization Society

APPENDIX 1-1

Some Beginnings in and Developments of Significance to Public Health Nursing—cont'd

Nursing and public health nursing		Other significant events	
1899	International Council of Nurses; University education for nurses, Teachers College, Columbia University (course in hospital economics)	1899	Association of Hospital Superintendents (becomes American Hospital Association in 1907)
1900	*American Journal of Nursing*	1900-1925	Expansion of voluntary agencies
1901	58 public health nursing associations; 130 public health nurses in United States		
1902	School nursing, New York City (Lina Rogers)	1902	Biologics Control Act
1903	Tuberculosis nursing, Baltimore; First Nurse Practice Acts		
1904	Visiting nurses have program at Conference of Charities and Correction	1904	National Organization for the Study and Prevention of Tuberculosis (becomes National Tuberculosis Association)
1905	200 public health agencies; 440 public health nurses in United States	1905	Medical social work, Massachusetts General Hospital
1906	Course in district nursing offered by Boston Instructive District Nursing Association	1906	Food and Drug Act
1907	Alabama law permitting employment of public health nurses	1907	Visiting teacher, Boston
1908	English health visitor; Detroit Health Department employs public health nurses		
1909	University of Minnesota School of Nursing Metropolitan Life Insurance Company contracts for visiting nurse service; The *Visiting Nurse Quarterly* published by Cleveland Visiting Nurse Association (later presented to NOPHN and becomes *Public Health Nursing* monthly until 1953)	1909	National Committee for Mental Hygiene; First White House Conference; American Association for the Study and Prevention of Infant Mortality
1910	Public health nursing program, Teachers College, Columbia University	1910	*Medical Education in the United States and Canada*, Abraham Flexner
		1911	Boston Instructive Visiting Nurse Association adds nutritional service; Joint Committee on Health Problems in Education, American Medical Association and National Education Association; county health departments in Guilford County, North Carolina, and Yakima County, Washington
1912	American Red Cross Rural Nursing Service (1200 services in 1922); National Organization for Public Health Nursing (NOPHN); U.S. Children's Bureau, Department of Labor	1912	Act to Establish a Children's Bureau (PL 62-116) establishes maternal and child health services on the federal level

Continued

APPENDIX 1-1

Some Beginnings in and Developments of Significance to Public Health Nursing—cont'd

---

Nursing and public health nursing		Other significant events	
1913	Division of Public Health Nursing, New York State Department of Health	1913	Harvard School of Public Health
1914	NOPHN suggests 4-month course in a visiting nurse association as essential preparation for public health nursing	1914	Harrison Narcotics Act (PL 62-223) establishes federal controls over narcotics
		1915	National Birth Registration Area established
		1915-1925	Wave of legislation of physical education and hygiene
1916	1922 public health nursing agencies; 5152 public health nurses: University of Cincinnati School of Nursing 5-year program leading to bachelor's degree		
		1917-1918	World War I
		1917	American Dietetic Association; Massachusetts and New York employ public health nutritionists Community chests and councils emerge
1918	USPHS organizes a division of public health nursing to work in extracantonment zones; Maternity Center Association, New York	1918	Compulsory education in all states; American Association of Medical Social Workers
1918-1923	Increased interest in combining local public health nursing agencies		
1919	*Public Health Nursing,* Mary S. Gardner; increase in public health nurses and public health nursing education; public health nursing program, University of Michigan	1919-1929	Demonstrations of child health and public health services
1920	NOPHN-approved university programs in public health nursing		
1921	Industrial and school nursing sections of NOPHN; NOPHN set 1 academic year as minimum for public health nursing certificate	1921	First university program in public health education, Massachusetts Institute of Technology, Harvard; National Health Council; American Association of Social Workers
		1921-1929	Shepherd-Towner Act—federal aid for maternal and child health
1922	4040 public health agencies; 11,548 nurses	1922-1935	American Child Health Association
1923	Public health nursing section, APHA; Nursing and Nursing Education in the United States ("The Winslow-Goldmark Report"); Yale and Western Reserve Universities establish collegiate schools of nursing		

Some Beginnings in and Developments of Significance to Public Health Nursing—cont'd

---

Nursing and public health nursing		Other significant events	
1924	U.S. Indian Bureau Nursing Service (Eleanor Gregg)	1924	Oil Pollution Act (PL 68-238) prohibits the dumping of oil in navigable waters
1925	Frontier Nursing Service—nurse-midwives (Mary Breckenridge); first NOPHN statement of qualifications for public health nurses; John Hancock Mutual Life Insurance Company Visiting Nurse Service		
1925-1926	Chicago Infant Welfare Society and Boston and East Harlem public health nursing agencies employ psychiatric social workers		
1926	Committee on Grading of Nursing Schools begins studies		
		1927-1931	Research by Committee on the Cost of Medical Care
		1929	Beginning of the Depression
1930	Unemployment of nurses	1930	Study of maternal mortality in New York City; Act to Establish a National Institute of Health (PL 71-251)
1931	4355 public health agencies; 15,865 nurses		
1932	Final report of Commission on Medical Education; Association of Collegiate Schools of Nursing; Lobenstine Midwifery Clinic and School (Maternity Center responsible for school 1934); 7% of nurses employed in public health nursing have completed a 1-year program		
1933	Pearl McIver appointed to USPHS as a public health nursing analyst	1933	U.S. Birth and Death Registration Areas complete
1934	*Survey of Public Health Nursing*, NOPHN, published		
1935	*Facts about Nursing*, American Nurses Association (ANA)	1935	Social Security Act (PL 74-721), designed to provide for the general welfare by establishing a system of federal old-age benefits, and by enabling the states to make provision for aged persons, blind individuals, dependent and crippled children, maternal and child welfare and the unemployed
		1935-1936	National Health Survey
		1937-1947	Beginning of federal appropriations for cancer, venereal diseases, tuberculosis, mental health, heart disease, etc.
		1938	Federal Food, Drug and Cosmetic Act (PL 75-717)

Continued

APPENDIX 1-1
Some Beginnings in and Developments of Significance to Public Health Nursing—cont'd

Nursing and public health nursing		Other significant events	
		1939	Reorganization of federal agencies; USPHS transferred from Treasury Department to Federal Security Agency
		1939-1945	World War II
1940	20,434 nurses employed in public health nursing; 22% have completed 1 or more years in an approved public health nursing program		
1941	Nurse Training Act (PL 77-146)		
1942	American Association of Industrial Nurses		
1943	Bolton-Bailey Act (PL 77-146) for nursing education and Cadet Nurse Program; Division of Nursing Education forms in USPHS [Lucile Petry (Leone)—Director]	1943-1947	Emergency Maternity and Infant Care Program
1944	Division of Nursing, USPHS [Lucile Petry (Leone)]; commissioned rank for nurses; NOPHN accredits only public health nursing programs with professional content of at least 1 year, which is part of program leading to a degree; Skidmore College basic nursing program approved for preparation of public health nurses	1944	Public Health Service Act (PL 78-410) consolidates all existing public health legislation into a single statute
		1945	End World War II; educational privileges provided for nurse veterans by GI Bill of Rights; publication of *Local Health Units for the Nation*; APHA accreditation of schools of public health
1946	Nurses classified as professional by U.S. Civil Service Commission	1946	Hospital Survey and Construction Act [Hill Burton](PL 79-725)
1947	Women's Medical Specialist corps (PL 80-36) establish permanent nursing corps in the army and navy		
1948	Publication of *Nurses for the Future* (Esther Lucile Brown)	1948	World Health Organization permanently established; meeting of World Health Assembly National Heart Act (PL 80-655) authorizes aid for research and training, and establishes the National Heart Institute at NIH; National Dental Research Act (PL 80-755) establishes the National Institute of Dental Research in NIH; and Water Pollution Control Act (PL 80-845) to help ensure clean water in the United States
1949	National Federation of Licensed Practical Nurses; national nursing organizations support legislation for federal financial aid for practical nursing education		

APPENDIX 1-1
Some Beginnings in and Developments of Significance to Public Health Nursing—cont'd

Nursing and public health nursing		Other significant events	
1950	25,081 nurses employed for public health work in the United States and territories; 34% have completed 1 or more years in an approved public health nursing program	1950	National Research Institutes Act (PL 81-692) expands NIH to include research and training related to arthritis, rheumatism, multiple sclerosis, cerebral palsy, blindness, and leprosy
1951	National League for Nursing recommendation that collegiate basic nursing education programs include preparation for public health nursing; National Association of Colored Graduate Nurses integrated with ANA		
1952	Reorganization of national nursing organizations, major functions transferred to American Nurses Association and National League for Nursing; Boston University program with a major in general nursing approved for preparation of public health nurses		
1952-1953	American Red Cross, Metropolitan Life Insurance Company, and John Hancock Mutual Life Insurance Company discontinue public health nursing services; *Public Health Nursing*, December 1952, last issue		
1953	*Nursing Outlook* published in January	1953	Department of Health, Education, and Welfare established with cabinet status
1955	27,112 nurses employed in public health work in the United States and territories; 37% have completed at least 1 year of approved public health nursing program; nursing programs preparing for public health nursing: Major in public health nursing 33 Baccalaureate basic 25 Major in general nursing 9	1955	National Association of Social Workers (seven associations combined); Air Pollution Control Act (PL 84-159); Mental Health Study Act (PL 84-182); and Polio Vaccination Assistance Act (PL 84-377)
		1956	National Health Survey Act (PL 84-652) provides for a continuing survey and special studies of sickness and disability in the U.S.
1959	NLN votes that no new specialized baccalaureate program be accredited and that after 1963 only baccalaureate programs that include public health nursing be accredited		
1960	*NLN Criteria for the Evaluation of Educational Programs in Nursing that Lead to Baccalaureate and Master's Degrees*	1960	International Health Research Act (PL 86-610) and Federal Hazardous Substance Labeling Act (PL 86-813)
		1961	First White House Conference on Aging

Continued

APPENDIX 1-1
APPENDIX 1-1
Some Beginnings in and Developments of Significance to Public Health Nursing—cont'd

Nursing and public health nursing		Other significant events	
		1962	11 accredited schools of public health in United States, 2 in Canada; National Institute of Child Health and Human Development (PL 87-838) and Vaccination Assistance Act (PL 87-868) aids programs to combat polio, diphtheria, whooping cough, and tetanus
1963	Report of Surgeon General's Consultant Group on Nursing	1963	Health Professional Educational Assistance Act (PL 88-129) and Clean Air Act (PL 88-206)
1964	*NLN Statement of Beliefs and Recommendations Regarding Baccalaureate Programs Admitting Registered Nurse Student*	1964	Economic Opportunity Act of 1964 (PL 88-452) enacted to mobilize the human and financial resources of the nation to combat poverty; it establishes the Office of Economic Opportunity, authorizes Volunteers in Service to America (VISTA), the Job Corps, Upward Bound, Neighborhood Youth Corps, Head Start, neighborhood health centers, and community action programs, assists small businesses, and is an impetus to antipoverty programs; Civil Rights Act of 1964 (PL 88-352) forbids discrimination based on race or sex in public accommodations, facilities, and educational settings; and Food Stamp Act (PL 88-525)
1964	Agencies and nurses employed for public health nursing:		

	Agencies	Nurses
Local	9,094	35,209
Board of Education	5,412	13,257
Official	2,712	14,738
VNA	682	3,826
Combination	51	1,478

Population per public health nurse in United States, 5586; 43.4% of full-time nurses had completed 30 or more hours in an approved public health nursing program; 39.7% had college degrees

Nurse Training Act of 1964 (PL 88-581)

| | | 1965 | Social Security Amendment of 1965 (PL 89-97) establishes Medicare and Medicaid; Federal Cigarette Labeling and Advertising Act (PL 89-92) designed to inform the public of the hazards of cigarette smoking |

Some Beginnings in and Developments of Significance to Public Health Nursing—cont'd

Nursing and public health nursing		Other significant events	
		1965	Heart Disease, Cancer and Stroke Amendments (PL 89-239); and Solid Waste Disposal Act (PL 89-272)
1966	NLN programs accredited for public health nursing—June 1966:	1966	Child Nutrition Act (PL 89-642) establishes a federal program of research and support for child nutrition, and Comprehensive Health Planning and Public Health Service Amendments (PL 89-749)
	Masters 42		
	Baccalaureate basic (students with no previous nursing preparation and registered nurses) 151		
	Baccalaureate basic (students with no previous nursing preparation) 91		
	Baccalaureate basic (registered nurses only) 6		
		1967	Air Quality Act (PL 90-148)
1968	Health Manpower Act (PL 90-490) extends Nurse Training Act of 1964		
		1969	Federal Coal Mine Health and Safety Act (PL 91-173) and National Environmental Policy Act (PL 91-190)
1970	National Commission on Nursing and Nursing Education—Abstract for Action published	1970	Family Planning Services and Population Research Act (PL 91-572); Occupational Safety and Health Act (PL 91-596); Comprehensive Alcohol Abuse and Alcoholism Prevention Treatment and Rehabilitation (PL 91-616); the Environmental Education Act (PL 91-516); Comprehensive Drug Abuse Prevention and Control Act (PL 91-513); Resource Recovery Act (PL 91-512); Health Training Improvement Act (PL 91-519); Emergency Health Personnel Act (PL 91-623); and Public Health Cigarette Smoking Act (PL 91-222)
1971	"Extending the Scope of Nursing Practice" report published Nurse Training Act of 1971 (PL 92-158) expands and continues nurse training provisions of the 1964 and 1968 acts	1971	Comprehensive Health Manpower Training Act (PL 92-218); National Cancer Act (PL 92-218); and Lead Based Poisoning Prevention Act (PL 91-695)
		1972	National Sickle Cell Anemia Control Act (PL 92-294); National Cooley's Anemia Control Act (PL 92-414); Federal Environmental Pesticide Control Act (PL 92-516); National Heart, Blood Vessel, Lung, and Blood Act (PL 92-423); National School Lunch and Child Nutrition Amendments (PL 92-433); Federal Environmental Pesticide Control Act (PL 92-516); Consumer Product Safety Act (PL 92-573)

Continued

Some Beginnings in and Developments of Significance to Public Health Nursing—cont'd

---

Nursing and public health nursing		Other significant events	
		1972	Noise Control Act (PL 92-574); Marine Mammal Protection Act (PL 92-522)
		1973	The Health Maintenance Organization (HMO) Act (PL 93-222) and Endangered Species Act (PL 93-205)
1974	Formation of Nurses Coalition for Action in Politics, N-CAP; first certification examinations by the ANA for excellence in practice	1974	Child Abuse Prevention and Treatment Act (PL 93-247); Sudden Infant Death Syndrome Act (PL 93-270); Narcotic Addict Treatment Act (PL 93-281); Research on Aging Act (PL 93-286); National Research Act (PL 93-348); National Diabetes Mellitus Research and Education Act (PL 93-354); Safe Drinking Water Act (PL 93-523); National Arthritis Act (PL 93-640)
		1975	National Health Planning and Resources Development Act (PL 93-641); Disabled Assistance and Bill of Rights Act (PL 94-103); and Health Services, Health Revenue, and Nurse Training Act [NTA] (PL 94-63)
		1976	Costs for health care in the United States rise 14% over 1975 Toxic Substances Control Act (PL 94-469)
1977-1978	Designated the "Year of the Nurse" by ANA to help the public better understand nursing	1977	Passage of the Rural Health Clinic Services bill (PL 95-210)
1978	Massachusetts becomes the seventh state to mandate continuing education as a requirement for relicensure of both registered and practical nurses; Robert Wood Johnson Foundation finances $5 million program to train nurses as school nurse practitioners and place them in areas where children now receive inadequate care	1978	President Carter vetoes the Nursing Training Act
1979	ANA board determines that future ANA conventions and conferences will be held only in states that have ratified the Equal Rights Amendment; Maryland passes law that requires insurance companies to provide reimbursement "for any service which is within the lawful scope of a duly licensed health care provider"; ANA sponsors a Study of Credentialing in Nursing, which spurs nationwide discussion and debate; N-CAP survey shows that nurses act on their political convictions and back candidates on the	1979	Due to antirecession lobbying by nurses and others, NTA funds were cut $15.75 million rather than Carter's $84 million; President Carter's fiscal 1980 budget cuts nursing education funds to $15 million in contrast to current levels of $122 million (only nurse practitioner programs fared well); President Carter sends Congress a national health insurance bill that would require minimum benefits for employed people and upgrade coverage for the poor, aged, and disabled; he becomes the first president to formally back a plan with the

APPENDIX 1-1
Some Beginnings in and Developments of Significance to Public Health Nursing—cont'd

Nursing and public health nursing		Other significant events	
	basis of issues, not party philosophy (they also vote and let officials know what they think)		underlying concept that health care is a basic human right President Carter's cost containment bill, designed to limit annual revenue for the nation's hospitals, runs into many snags and has a slim chance of passing
1980	"A Classification Scheme for Client Problems in Community Health Nursing," written by D. Simmons, provides the potential for systematically describing client needs in the community setting; Jo Eleanor Elliott named Director of the Division of Nursing, USPHS, replacing Jessie Scott; Colorado passes a new Nurse Practice Act that made it possible for nurses to practice independently in private settings; The Supreme Court declines to review the discrimination suit brought by NURSE (Nurses Underrepresented in Social Equality), which charged that the city of Denver paid women less than it did men who performed work of equal value; Maryland becomes the first state to pass the law that mandates reimbursement in all health insurance for services of nurses and other licensed providers	1980	Enrollments in higher education programs, including nursing, decline. The decline is expected to continue through the end of the century Civil Rights of Institutionalized Persons Act (PL 96-247)
1981	In a $5 million project to upgrade long-term care, the Robert Wood Johnson Foundation joined with the ANA to develop "teaching nursing homes"; Carolyn Davis becomes the first nurse to head the Health Care Financing Administration (HCFA) "The more an occupation is dominated by women, the less it pays" states a new report of the Equal Opportunity Employment Commission	1981	Ronald Reagan elected president and begins a period of retrenchment in numerous health and social programs California legislature passes a vote mandating that women in female-dominated jobs be paid in accordance with their ability to produce the same level or quality of work as men Omnibus Budget Reconciliation Act (PL 97-935); and Migrant and Seasonal Agricultural Worker Protection Act (PL 97-410)
1982	The nation's first directly elected board of nursing meets in Raleigh, N.C., for a swearing-in ceremony. North Carolina is the only state where RNs and LPNs nominate and vote for members of their own board of nursing To be licensed as RNs, students of nursing begin taking a new comprehensive test developed by the National Council of State Boards of Nursing over the past several years	1982	*Playboy* magazine abandons a plan to publish a pictorial feature on women in nursing when it meets with widespread protest by nurses across the country; The USPHS releases a report stating that exposure to other people's smoking may increase cancer risks to nonsmokers; With the nation's cities hard hit by the recession, major cities project the most declines in expenditures in the areas of health care

Continued

Some Beginnings in and Developments of Significance to Public Health Nursing—cont'd

---

Nursing and public health nursing		Other significant events	
1982	The ANA convention adopts a radically new organizational plan for the organization designed to make decisions more representative of the total membership Federal support for nursing education takes a massive blow from "Reaganomics"; hundreds of nurses and nursing students travel to Capitol Hill to protest the cutbacks; Faye Abdellah becomes the first nurse and the first woman to be promoted to rank of deputy surgeon general of the USPHS; May 6 voted National Recognition Day for Nurses by Congress The longest nurses' strike in the nation's history (2 years) ends February 8 when nurses at Ashtabula General Hospital vote to accept a 2-year contract; *Classification of Nursing Diagnoses*, the proceedings of the third and fourth national conferences for classification of nursing diagnoses, published; Nurses across the country work to ensure that the Equal Rights Amendment would be ratified by the necessary 38 states by June 30. The goal is not reached, and on July 14 the ERA amendment is reintroduced into the House and the Senate	1982	A 2-year drive by conservatives to ban voluntary abortions is blocked when the Senate votes to table a bill introduced by Senator Jesse Helms During a 1-year period, over 600 cases of Kaposi's sarcoma are reported to the Centers for Disease Control. The mortality rate is 40%; the disease is considered to be a manifestation of acquired immunodeficiency syndrome (AIDS) The first annual meeting of the National Association of Home Care is held in Atlanta, Ga. Its goal is to unite the rapidly growing ranks of home care providers in a single, national organization. Elsie Griffith, a nurse, is the founder of the association; The Third White House Conference on the Aging (held every 10 years) stresses the importance of nursing in the care of this population group Members attending the American Public Health Association convention vigorously oppose the Reagan administration's sizeable increases in military defense, which led to reduced spending in social and health programs November elections reveal that 83% of the political candidates endorsed by N-CAP were winners Tax Equity and Fiscal Responsibility Act of 1982 (PL 97-248) and Nuclear Waste Policy Act (PL 97-425)
1983	Ruth Freeman, a leader in the field of public health nursing, dies at the age of 76. For several decades, her writings helped to prepare nurses for CHN practice The state of Maine legislates a prospective reimbursement system that calls for regular reporting of nursing service data and the nursing costs of treating patients in similar classifications. For the first time anywhere, hospitals are compelled to break down nursing costs as a separate item in their accounting systems	1983	Dr. Barney Clark becomes the first recipient of an artificial heart The Reagan administration issues a regulation that would force 5000 family planning centers to inform parents when a teenager under 17 seeks birth control prescriptions or devices Health and Human Services (HHS), Division of Maternal and Child Health, develops projects to study the prevalence of ventilator-dependent children and to establish guidelines for a regional system for their care

APPENDIX 1-1

Some Beginnings in and Developments of Significance to Public Health Nursing—cont'd

Nursing and public health nursing		Other significant events	
1983	The final report of the National Commission on Nursing, sponsored by the American Hospital Association, states that future progress in the profession would mandate better-educated and more highly qualified nurses The Department of Public Health Nursing at the University of North Carolina's School of Public Health, a longtime leader in the field, is threatened with closure by the university. Nursing and public health leaders around the country move to block the plan Salaries for nurses in home and community health agencies increase 13.8% in the past year, to a median of $19,148 for official agencies and $17,480 for nonofficial agencies Institute of Medicine completes *Nursing and Nursing Education: Public and Private Action*, which concludes that the shortage of nurses has been eliminated and that funding for nursing education should be targeted for specialty groups	1983	AIDS is declared the number one priority of the USPHS Seven years into the study, over 100,000 nurses continue to participate in a Harvard project that examines health risks posing special threats to women President Reagan supports reductions in nursing education funding totaling $1.2 billion. His FY 84 budget represents an overall funding reduction of 75% for nursing programs *Deciding to For-go Life-Sustaining Treatment* was the report submitted by the President's Commission for the Study of Ethical Problems in Medicine and Biomedical Research Health Care Financing Administration (HCFA) set very low Medicare reimbursement rates for hospice care; critics argue that few agencies would be willing to sponsor hospices as a result; April 20, President Reagan signs Public Law 98-28, which changes payment for Medicare hospital stays. Hospital stays are now reimbursed by Medicare, based on prospectively established rates for 467 diagnosis related groups (DRGs); International Environmental Protection Act (PL 98-164)
1984	The Diamond Jubilee of the first school of nursing in the world to be located on a university campus where faculty held university appointments is celebrated. The University of Minnesota School of Nursing was founded in 1909	1984	That the risk of congestive heart disease (CHD) can be reduced by lowering serum cholesterol levels is conclusively demonstrated in a study by the National Heart, Lung, and Blood Institute; The Senate debates a bill that would create a National Institute of Nursing within the National Institutes of Health. The Institute would assume research responsibilities now assumed by the Division of Nursing, PHS "People Match" in Bristol, N.H., keeps people out of nursing homes by matching them with appropriate roommates President Reagan signs a bill authorizing the third Monday in January as Martin Luther King Day

Continued

APPENDIX 1-1

Some Beginnings in and Developments of Significance to Public Health Nursing—cont'd

---

Nursing and public health nursing		Other significant events	
		1984	The Missouri Supreme Court vindicates two obstetric/gynecologic nurse practitioners charged with unauthorized practice of medicine. They gave routine care under physician backup with written protocols to 5000 patients a year in a Title X neighborhood agency; Deficit Reduction Act of 1984 (PL 98-369); National Organ Transplant Act (PL 98-460)
1985	*Consensus Conference on the Essentials of Public Health Nursing Practice and Education: Report of the Conference, September 5-7, 1984* examines the critical issues confronting PHN; educational preparation needed to practice as a generalist and as a specialist; and collective goals for PHN in the future Patients are discharged "quicker and sicker" from hospitals under Medicare's DRG system NLN wages a fight to keep RN licensure for ADN graduates while the ANA strives to make the BSN the legal requirement for practice LPNs disappear from acute care settings with the shift to all-RN staffs across the country	1985	Food Security Act of 1985 (PL 99-198); "Live Aid," a 17-hour rock concert broadcast on radio and TV from Philadelphia to London to 152 countries, raises $70 million for starving people in Africa
1986	American Nurses Association revises the *Standards for Community Health Nursing Practice* and develops standards for *Home Health Nursing Practice* The National Center for Nursing Research is established at NIH North Dakota becomes the first state to require the BSN for RN licensure and the ADN for LPN licensure The NLN switches positions and backs two levels of nursing practice—professional and associate Certified nurse midwives form an independent mutual insurance firm to solve the malpractice insurance dilemma that threatened to shut down the profession; Major study in Institute of Medicine says that nursing homes need more RNs to upgrade care	1986	Comprehensive Smokeless Tobacco Health Education Act of 1986 (PL 99-252); Consolidated Omnibus Budget Reconciliation Act of 1986 (PL 99-272); Protection and Advocacy for Mentally Ill Individuals Act of 1986 (PL 99-319); Education of the Deaf Act (PL 99-371); Handicapped Children's Protection Act (PL 99-372); Comprehensive Anti-Apartheid Act of 1986 (PL 99-440); Radon Gas and Indoor Air Quality Research Act of 1986 (PL 99-499); Asbestos Hazard Emergency Response Act of 1986 (PL 99-519); Anti-Drug Abuse Act of 1986 (PL 99-570); Child Sexual Abuse and Pornography Act of 1986 (PL 99-628); Employment Opportunities for Disabled American Act (PL 99-643); Health Programs (PL 99-660)

Some Beginnings in and Developments of Significance to Public Health Nursing—cont'd

Nursing and public health nursing	Other significant events
	1986 In Chernobyl, Ukraine, a major accident at a nuclear power plant kills 23; 40,000 were evacuated The Gramm-Rudman Landmark Law cuts over $1 billion in the fiscal 1986 budget; AZT (azidothymidine), an antiviral drug now known as ZDV (zidovudine), was found to improve the health of some AIDS patients but was not a cure. Government officials predicted a tenfold increase in AIDS-related deaths in the next 5 years; Mounting use of illegal drugs (cocaine as "crack") causes passage of stiff antidrug laws
1987 *Public Health Nursing Education and Practice* document published by the USDHHS and addresses the congruence of public health baccalaureate education for practice in public health agencies National Center for Nursing Research created within NIH OSHA changes its rules, allowing OH nurses to have access to trade secrets in nonemergency situations UCLA's study of entering students finds sharp drop in number planning nursing careers The largest pay equity award in the history of nursing is won by the Pennsylvania Nurses' Association against that state	**1987** Stewart B. McKinney Homeless Assistance Act (PL 100-77); Wilbur J. Cohen Federal Building (PL 100-99); Developmental Disabilities Assistance and Bill of Rights Act Amendments of 1987 (PL 100-146); and Civil Rights Restoration Act of 1987 (PL 100-259) Condom ads become prominent in U.S. media, reflecting a concern for "safe sex" to prevent AIDS Biological father William Stern wins custody of Baby M, with parental rights terminated for Mary Beth Whitehead, who had contracted to bear Stern's child for $10,000
1988 Secretary's Commission on Nursing report confirms that the reported shortage of RNs is real, widespread, and of significant magnitude Candidates for nursing licensure take the first pass/fail test that replaced numerical scores BSN programs see a 7.8% decline in undergraduate enrollments Sigma Theta Tau begins building a $4 million center for Nursing Scholarship in Indianapolis	**1988** The Institute of Medicine's report *The Future of Public Health* examines America's public health system in detail—its mission, its current state, and the barriers to improvement—and makes recommendations for dealing with future public health challenges Medicare Catastrophic Coverage Act of 1988 (PL 100-360); School Asbestos Management (PL 100-368); Hearing Aid Compatibility Act of 1988 (PL 100-394); Technology-Related Assistance for Individuals with Disabilities Act of 1988 (PL 100-407); Hunger Prevention Act of 1988 (PL 100-435); Family Support Act of 1988 (PL 100-485)

Continued

Some Beginnings in and Developments of Significance to Public Health Nursing—cont'd

Nursing and public health nursing		Other significant events	
		1988	Health Maintenance Organization Amendments of 1988 (PL 100-517); Forest Ecosystems and Atmospheric Pollution Research Act of 1988 (PL 100-551); Lead Contamination Control Act of 1988 (PL 100-572); Native Hawaiian Health Care Act of 1988 (PL 100-579); Medical Waste Tracking Act of 1988 (PL 100-582); Health Omnibus Programs Extension of 1988 (PL 100-607); Water Resources Development Act of 1988 (PL 100-676); Ocean Dumping Ban Act of 1988 (PL 100-688); Anti-Drug Abuse Act of 1988 (PL 100-690); Federal Cave Resources Protection Act of 1988 (PL 100-691)
			A 3-year drive to boost a "thoroughly experienced" staff nurse salary to $50,000 started by The Pennsylvania Nurses' Association
			Nursing: Sixth Report to the President and Congress on the Status of Health Personnel in the United States addresses current developments in various health care practice settings, the increased movement of patients to the community, and future requirements for nursing personnel; Reagan Administration temporarily halts efforts to enforce new HHS regulations that would prohibit federally funded family-planning clinics from providing abortions; The AMA approves a proposal to train "registered care technologists" to assume a new role at the bedside, designed to carry out medical protocols, with special emphasis on technical skills
			The term "ecophobia" is coined to illustrate the nation's concern about polluted beaches and water, persistent drought, immense forest fires, and the worst air quality in decades
1989	*Strategies for a Collaborative Future: The Consensus Report from the National Consensus Conference on the Educational Preparation of Home Care Administrators* addresses the educational needs of practitioners preparing for leadership positions in home health care	1989	Whistleblower Protection Act of 1989 (PL 101-12) A draft of *Promoting Health/Preventing Disease: Year 2000 Objectives for the Nation* is distributed for public review and comment

APPENDIX 1-1
Some Beginnings in and Developments of Significance to Public Health Nursing—cont'd

Nursing and public health nursing		Other significant events	
1989	Nineteen hundred nurses are named in liability and malpractice suits yearly, 50% of those claims are upheld. The average claim against a nurse that results in payment is $145,397	1989	The revolutionary abortion pill, RU 486, is increasingly popular in France. Given anti-abortion pressures, it could take years before it becomes popular in other countries
	The majority of nurses had economic gains of 7% to 10% in 1988. The average pay for nurses rose 10.6% to $32,160, the largest maximum increase on record		George Bush is inaugurated President; he urges the nation to "use power to help people"
1990	The nursing shortage cripples emergency rooms; patient overloads cause waits of 12 hours for many people seeking emergency care	1990	Minimum wage is raised from $3.35 to $3.80; to become $4.25 in 1991; this impacts nursing homes, where 55% of aides and orderlies earn less than the minimum
	Nursing enrollments rebound and the quality of nursing students improves; The Public Health Service declares that no nursing student should graduate without a thorough education in AIDS care		Under new OSHA standards, hospitals must make hepatitis B vaccination and follow-up available to all people who are exposed
			Growing numbers of Medicaid and uninsured patients drain major urban hospitals financially
			Determining DNR (do not resuscitate) status in the home setting emerges as an important issue. New standards issued by JCAHO contain a statement about this issue
			The Florence Nightingale Museum, located underneath the same school of nursing at St. Thomas Hospital in London, opens; A measles epidemic spreads over the country; there is a 39.5% increase over 1989 in the first 6 months of the year; The Supreme Court rules 5-4 that Nancy Cruzan's parents cannot insist on removing the feeding tube that had kept her in a comatose state for 7 years; The Americans with Disabilities Act passes, making it illegal to discriminate against the physically and mentally disabled in employment, public accommodations, transportation, and telecommunications
1991	Six hospice nurses in Montana are placed on probation by their Board of Nursing for keeping narcotics in an unlocked place as an emergency supply for patients in sudden need	1991	Blue Cross-Blue Shield announces changes in the lifetime schedule of screening tests that a healthy adult should undergo

Continued

Some Beginnings in and Developments of Significance to Public Health Nursing—cont'd

---

Nursing and public health nursing		Other significant events	
1991	Active-duty and reserve RNs are sent to the Middle East when Iraq invades Kuwait. During the seven months of Operation Desert Shield, the Air Force deploys 1800 nurses to Saudi Arabia and Europe; the Navy sends 900 to run several 100-bed hospital ships; and 2300 RNs are sent to MASH stations, combat support hospitals, and evacuation hospitals Starting pay for a hospital RN in New York City is $40,000 "Nursing's Agenda for Health Care Reform" calls for a public/private system with a federally defined package of benefits and a central role for nurses; Margaret Daugherty Lewis is inducted into the Health Care Hall of Fame, sponsored by Modern Healthcare. She is credited as the driving force in linking public health agencies and VNAs by founding in 1970 the National Association of Home Health Agencies, which in 1982 becomes the National Association of Home Care; RNs volunteer to help heal Rumania's children and its devastated health care system created by the deposed dictator Ceausescu	1991	An initiative on the fall ballot in Washington State gives physicians the legal right to help a terminally ill person die Federally funded community health centers struggle with a shortage of immunization vaccines even as the country undergoes a measles epidemic Barbara Fassbinder, one of the first health care workers in the United States documented as becoming infected with the HIV virus by a patient, testifies in Congress against mandatory testing of health care workers for AIDS CDC encourages hospitals to test all patients for AIDS A Vietnam women's memorial receives a long-delayed stamp of approval from the Fine Arts Commission Some of the nation's VNAs produce their own brand name products, inspired by the rapid growth in hospital's use of prepackaged materials The ANA and the ANF join with the National Consumer's League to educate nurses and consumer advocates in health care public policy, economics, and management. The aim is to influence the debate about health care reform and to help nurses be part of that reform
1992	The American Nurses Association moves its offices to Washington D.C. to increase visibility with law makers and funding agencies	1992	The "gag" rule survives a campaign by healthcare groups to bar abortion counseling at federally funded family planning clinics Hurricane Andrew, one of the greatest natural disasters of the century, hits Florida; hospitals and health care workers struggle to restore health to the southern reaches of Miami and Dade County. The tragedy sparks renewed interest in disaster nursing as hundreds of nurses volunteer their services

Some Beginnings in and Developments of Significance to Public Health Nursing—cont'd

Nursing and public health nursing	Other significant events	
	1992	The National League for Nursing and the Joint Commission for Accreditation of Healthcare Organizations vie for deemed status, which means that agencies they accredit would not need to undergo annual Medicare surveys to be eligible for reimbursement. Both receive deemed status Legislators, healthcare professionals, and consumers are examining a national healthcare package to achieve "Health for All"
		The Centers for Disease Control in Atlanta, Georgia, are renamed the Centers for Disease Control and Prevention

Used by permission of Ella McNeil, Professor Emeritus of Public Health Nursing, School of Public Health, University of Michigan, Ann Arbor, Michigan. Original compilation of important beginnings has been updated to reflect significant changes in the 1970s, 1980s, and 1990s.

Selected Significant CHN/PHN Leaders

Leader	Contributions
Clarissa (Clara) Barton (1821-1912)	The first woman to take to the battlefield as a volunteer nurse and relief worker during the Civil War; founder of the American Red Cross
Mary Beard (1876-1946)	One of the founders of the National Organization for Public Health Nursing; an advocate of preventive health services and a worker for the Rockefeller Foundation
Mary Breckinridge (1877-1965)	Founder of the Frontier Nursing Service, public pioneer in nurse-midwifery and in bringing modern nursing to rural America
Ada M. Carr (*-1951)	Editor of the *Public Health Nurse* and the first nurse to conduct postgraduate studies in public health nursing
Charity Collins (1882-*)	The first black public health school nurse in the country
Ella Phillips Crandall (1871-1938)	One of the founders of the National Organization for Public Health Nursing and the Red Cross Rural Nursing Service
Annie Damer (1858-1915)	Instrumental in establishing tuberculosis nursing in New York City
Dorothy Deming (1893-1972)	Directed the National Organization for Public Health Nursing beginning in 1927 and a prolific author; among her books the *Penny Marsh* series for teenagers

*Dates unknown

Continued

APPENDIX 1-2
Selected Significant CHN/PHN Leaders—cont'd

Leader	Contributions
Dorothea Dix (1802-1887)	Crusader for the mentally ill and imprisoned, teacher and writer
Lavinia Lloyd Dock (1858-1956)	Helped develop the American Nurses Association; prolific author and educator; historian, advocate of social reform and women's rights
Margaret Dolan (1914-1974)	President of the ANA from 1962-1964 and the second nurse to be President of the American Public Health Association
Ruth Freeman (1906-1982)	Nurse, educator, and author, using an interdisciplinary outlook that related academic work to the real world, prolific author; worked to persuade personnel in public health to view nurses as team members
Mary Sewall Gardner (1871-1961)	Author of the first public health nursing text; founder of the National Organization for Public Health Nursing
Emma Goldman (1869-1940)	Used nursing as point from which to attack the problems in society; leader of the birth control movement; editor of *Mother Earth*, a radical journal; called the "mother of anarchy in America"; spent time in jail for birth control lectures in America; one of the most significant women in America in the years before WWI
Alma Haupt (1893-1956)	Graduate of the first class at the University of Minnesota in public health nursing; directed the Nursing Bureau of the Metropolitan Life Insurance company where she established a model home nursing program
Clara Maass (1876-1901)	A heroine in the war against yellow fever; volunteered to take part in the experiments in Cuba which proved that yellow fever was transmitted by mosquitoes; died from the disease
Pearl McIver (1893-1976)	The first nurse on the staff of the U.S. Public Health Service, which she expanded into a modern and extensive agency to serve the needs of the U.S. public
Mary Adelaide Nutting (1858-1948)	First professor of nursing in an American university, occupying the first endowed chair in nursing; a reformer of nursing education
Linda Richards (1841-1930)	America's first trained nurse; teacher
Margaret Sanger (1879-1966)	Pioneer in the birth control movement, launching the American Birth Control League, which became the Planned Parenthood Federation of America
Emilie Sargent (1894-1977)	Directed the Visiting Nurse Association of Detroit for 40 years, improving and diversifying its services; the first woman and public health professional to receive the University of Michigan Outstanding Achievement Award
Isabel Maitland Stewart (1878-1963)	Leader in the NLN and curriculum development; author of nursing history; avid supporter of the suffrage movement
Ada Mayo Stewart (1870-1945)	First occupational health nurse in the United States

APPENDIX 1-2
Selected Significant CHN/PHN Leaders—cont'd

Leader	Contributions
Lina Rogers Struthers (1870-1946)	First school nurse in the United States, chosen by Lillian Wald while a nurse at the Henry Street Settlement House
Stella Boothe Vail (1890-1926)	Implemented unique method for teaching health promotion and disease prevention; used entertainment techniques at county fairs to emphasize hygiene and public health
Lillian Wald (1867-1940)	Leader of the public health nursing movement in the United States; developed the Henry Street Settlement House in New York and improved the lot of immigrants on the Lower East Side; established playgrounds for children who had none; placed the first nurse in a public school setting; developed innovative financing for nursing services; helped to found the National Child Labor Committee; formed the New York State Bureau of Industries and Immigrations and the Joint Board of Sanitary Control to enforce basic sanitary rules; helped develop the forerunner of the ACLU; prolific writer and teacher

Modified from Kaufman M, Hawkins WJ, Higgins LP, and Friedman AH: *Dictionary of American nursing biography*, Westport, Conn, 1988, Greenwood Press; and Kalisch P and Kalisch BJ: *The advancement of American nursing*, ed 2, Boston, 1986, Little, Brown.

References

Allen CE: Holistic concepts and the professionalization of public health nursing, *Public Health Nurs* 8(2):74-80, 1991.

American Nurses Association: *Education for participation in nursing research*, Kansas City, 1989, The Association.

Buhler-Wilkerson K: Home care the American way: an historical analysis, *Home Health Care Services Quarterly* 12(3):5-17, 1991.

Christy TE: Portrait of a leader: Lavinia Lloyd Dock, *Nurs Outlook* 17:72-75, 1969.

Christy TE: Portrait of a leader: Lillian Wald, *Nurs Outlook* 18:50-54, 1970.

Children's Defense Fund: *The state of America's children 1992*, Washington DC, 1992, Author.

Committee for the Study of Nursing Education: *Nursing and nursing education in the United States*, New York, 1923, Macmillan.

Deloughery GL: *History and trends of professional nursing*, ed 8, St. Louis, 1977, Mosby.

Desirable organization of public health nursing for family service, *Public Health Nurs* 38:387-389, 1946.

Dickens C: *Martin Chuzzlewit*, New York, 1910, Macmillan.

Dock L, Pickett SE, Noyes CD, Clement FE, Fox EE, and VanMeter AR: *History of American Red Cross nursing*, New York, 1922, Macmillan.

Division of Nursing: *A century of caring: a celebration of public health nursing in the United States: 1893-1993*, Washington D.C., 1992, American Public Health Association.

Dolan JA: *Nursing in society: a historical perspective*, Philadelphia, 1978, Saunders.

Fagin CM: Primary care as an academic discipline, *Nurs Outlook* 26:750-753, 1978.

Fee E: The origins and development of public health in the United States. In Holland WW, Detels R, and Knox G, eds: *Oxford textbook of public health*, ed 2, Oxford, 1991, Oxford University Press, pp. 3-22.

Fox EG, ed: Red Cross public health nursing, *Public Health Nurs* 12:175-181, 1920.

Gardner MS: *Public health nursing*, ed 1, revised, New York, 1919, Macmillan.

Gardner MS: *Public health nursing*, ed 3, New York, 1936, Macmillan.

Grissum M and Spengler C: *Woman power and health care*, Boston, 1976, Little, Brown.

Haupt AC: Forty years of teamwork in public health nursing, *Am J Nurs* 53:81-84, 1953.

Hezel LF and Linebach LM: The development of a regional nursing history collection: Its relevance to practice, education, and research, *Nurs Outlook* 39(5):268-272, 1991.

Hudgings C, Hogan R, & Stevenson JS (eds.): *1990 directory of nurse researchers*, ed 3, Indianapolis, In., 1990, Sigma Theta Tau International.

Institute of Medicine: *Committee for the study of the future of public health: the future of public health*, Washington, D.C., 1988, National Academy Press.

Jensen DM: *History and trends of professional nursing*, ed 4, St. Louis, 1959, Mosby.

Kalisch P and Kalisch BJ: *Politics of nursing,* Philadelphia, 1982, Lippincott.

Kalisch P and Kalisch BJ: *The advancement of American nursing,* ed 2, Boston, 1986, Little, Brown.

Kaufman M, Hawkins JW, Higgins LP, and Friedman AH, eds: *Dictionary of American nursing biography,* Wesport, Conn., 1988, Greenwood Press.

Lynaugh JE and Fagin LM: Nursing comes of age, *Image: J Nurs Scholarship* 20:1184, 1988.

Maynard T: *The apostle of charity: the life of St. Vincent de Paul,* New York, 1939, Dial Press.

McNeil EE: *Transition in public health nursing,* John Sundwall Lecture, University of Michigan, 1967.

National Center for Nursing Research: *Priorities resulting from second conference on research priorities in nursing practice, National Center for Nursing Research,* Bethesda, Md, February 1993, NCNR.

National Organization for Public Health Nursing: Approval of Skidmore College of Nursing as preparing students for public health nursing, *Public Health Nurs* 36:371, 1944.

Nelson SC: Mary Sewall Gardner, *Nurs Outlook* 2:37-39, 1954.

Nightingale F: *Notes on nursing,* London, 1859, Harris and Sons; Philadelphia, 1859, Lippincott.

Pickett G and Hanlon JJ: *Public health administration and practice,* ed 9, St. Louis, 1990, Mosby.

A prophet honored, *Am J Nurs* 17:53, 1971 (editorial).

Relman A: Assessment and accountability. The third revolution in medical care, *N Engl J Med* 319:1220, 1988.

Roberts DE and Heinrich J: Public health nursing comes of age, *AJPH* 75:1162-1172, 1985.

Roberts MM: *American nursing, history and interpretation,* New York, 1954, Macmillan.

Rosen G: *A history of public health,* New York, 1958, MD Publications.

Ruth MV and Partridge KB: Differences in perception of education and practice, *Nurs Outlook* 26:622-628, 1978.

Shea FP and Werley HH: Research conducted at Wayne State University College of Nursing, *Nurs Res* 22:3, 268-270, 1973.

Smillie WG: *Preventive medicine and public health,* ed 2, New York, 1952, Macmillan.

Stewart IM and Austin AL: *A history of nursing,* ed 5, New York, 1938, Putnam.

U.S. Public Health Service: *Toward quality in nursing: needs and goals. Report of the Surgeon General's consultant group on nursing,* Washington D.C., 1963, U.S. Government Printing Office.

Wald L: *The house on Henry Street,* New York, 1915, Holt.

Werley HH and Shea FP: The first center for research in nursing: its development, accomplishments, and problems, *Nurs Res* 22(3):217-231, 1973.

Williams R: The United States public health service, Bethesda, Md, *Commissioned Officers Association of the US Public Health Service,* 1951.

Winslow, C-EA: *The conquest of epidemic disease: a chapter in the history of ideas,* Madison, 1943, University of Wisconsin Press.

Winslow C-EA: Florence Nightingale and public health nursing, *Public Health Nurs* 2:330-332, 1946.

Selected Bibliography

Bigbee JL and Crowder ELM: The Red Cross Rural Nursing Service: an innovative model of public health nursing delivery, *Public Health Nurs* 2:109-121, 1985.

Brainard AM: *The evolution of public health nursing,* Philadelphia, 1922, Saunders.

Carr AM: Development of public health nursing literature, *Public Health Nurs* 5:81-85, 1988.

Dock LL and Stewart IM: *A short history of nursing,* New York, 1931, Putnam.

Fiedler LA: *Images of the nurse in fiction and popular culture, literature and medicine,* Albany, N.Y., 1983, Albany State University of New York Press.

Frachel RR: A new profession: the evolution of public health nursing, *Public Health Nurs* 5:86-90, 1988.

Gardner MS: The National Organization for Public Health Nursing, *Visiting Nurse Quart* 4:13-18, 1912.

Gropper EI: Florence Nightingale: nursing's first environmental theorist, *Nursing Forum* 22:3, 30-33, 1990.

Hamilton D: Clinical excellence, but too high a cost: the Metropolitan Life Insurance Company Visiting Nurse Service (1909-1953), *Public Health Nurs* 5:235-240, 1988.

Hamilton D: Faith and finance, *Image: J Nurs Scholarship* 20:124, 1988.

Hermann EK: Clara Louise Maass: heroine or martyr of public health? *Public Health Nurs* 2:51-57, 1985.

Kalisch PA and Kalisch BJ: *The advance of American nursing,* Boston, 1986, Little, Brown.

Mereness DA: From there to here in fifty years, *Nurs Outlook* 39(5):222-225, 1991.

Pillitteri A: Documenting Lystra Gretteer's student experiences in nursing: a 100-year comparison with today, *Nurs Outlook* 39(5):273-279, 1991.

Pollitt P: Lydia Holman: community health pioneer, *Nurs Outlook* 39(5):230-232, 1991.

Rathbone W: *History and progress of district nursing,* New York, 1890, Macmillan.

Robinson KR: The role of nursing in the influenza epidemic of 1918-1919, *Nurs Forum* 25(2):19-26, 1990.

Watson J: The evolution of nursing education in the United States: one hundred years of a profession for women, *J Nurs Educ* 16:31-37, 1977.

Wuthnow S: Our mother's stories, *Nurs Outlook* 38(5):218-222, 1990.

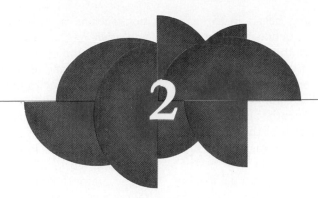

Defining Community Health Nursing

OBJECTIVES

Upon completion of this chapter, the reader should be able to:

1. Discuss how community health nursing differs from other specialty areas within nursing.
2. Formulate a personal definition of community health nursing practice, incorporating key concepts delineated by professional organizations.
3. Describe White's Conceptual Model for Public Health Nursing Practice and discuss terms specific to this model.
4. Discuss the mission of public health and how the concept of "Health for All" relates to this mission.
5. Identify the client groups in community health nursing practice and the roles nurses can assume when working with these groups.
6. Describe how community health nurses provide population-based nursing care.
7. Discuss various settings and modalities for providing community health nursing services.

When public health nursing began in the early 1900s, it was a simple matter to define it as a specialty area within nursing. Public health nursing took place outside the hospital setting; it was "nursing without walls," nursing that was community-focused and family- and group-oriented. Early public health nurses functioned relatively independently and worked to maintain and improve the health of the entire community. Thus, public health nursing was *"nursing for the public health"* (Brainard, 1921, p. 5).

Today, as the focus of health care continues to move outside the hospital setting and as more and more nurses assume expanded roles, defining community health nursing as a specialty area is less easily done. The definition becomes sharper and clearer, however, when one understands that the *nature of the practice,* not the *setting,* defines community health nursing as a specialty area. Nursing outside walls is not necessarily community health nursing; for example, pediatric nurses who do assessments of newborns in physicians' offices and nurses who counsel clients in mental health centers are probably functioning as specialty-focused nurse *practitioners* with advanced physical assessment skills and preparation to exercise independent and collaborative judgment in the health care management of clients. The holistic *community* focus characteristic of community health nursing practice is not a major emphasis of nurse practitioners in many ambulatory care and other community-based health care settings. These practitioners place emphasis on delivering care to individuals and are not necessarily oriented to the community (Goeppinger, 1984).

On the other hand, community health nursing is "nursing for the community's health." Its uniqueness lies in its emphasis on the health of the population as a whole. Community health nurses address both the personal and the environmental aspects of health and deal with community factors which either inhibit or facilitate healthy living. Personal health involves the biopsychosocial and spiritual aspects of individual, family, and group functioning, whereas environmental health deals with people's surroundings—settings such as homes, schools, workplaces, or recreational facilities. In community health nursing, nurses enter the environment in which people live and practice within that environment, in sharp contrast to the situation where the client enters the nurse's environment in a hospital or clinic. In addition to the one-to-one or single-family approach to health care, the community health nurse thinks in terms of popula-

tions such as caseloads, clinics, districts, census tracts, and cities. Aggregates at risk within these populations, including families at risk, are identified so that preventive measures and resources can be targeted for them. This kind of community focus involves educating individuals and groups and changing the social and physical environments that cue and reinforce the choices people make. Intervention strategies focus on providing services in health promotion settings such as school, work, or church. They also involve screening programs that are community based; environmental changes through persuasion, as illustrated by the public's use of seat belts; and regulation and the use of mass media (Shea, 1992, p. 787). The fact that smoking is now considered a health hazard and is no longer chic is a superb illustration of education at the community level through the mass media.

An example illustrates how the community health nurse expands the nurse practitioner role by focusing on aggregates at risk and the community:

▶ **Julie Cherry, a community health nurse working for an official health department, was assigned a census tract as her population to be served. This census tract was located in a decaying area of town with substandard housing and no transportation, playgrounds, or parks. A large industrial complex lay in the census tract, and consequently large numbers of young laborers and their families lived there. There was no hospital located in the area and only one physician. The community health nurse received numerous referrals from the physician and outlying hospitals to visit young mothers who needed support with parenting their newborn children. The nurse assessed the need for a parenting group by talking with the families whom she served as well as with her supervisors. She and the families she visited planned a weekly sharing and support group that met in a neighborhood church. The group was well attended and continued to function after the nurse left.**

The nurse in this illustration demonstrated several critical elements in community health nursing: providing care to the unit of service—the family—and concurrently planning preventive health measures for an aggregate at risk—young families needing parenting support. This is a step beyond providing primary health care to families who need that level of nursing intervention, and is different from the one-to-one focus of care to a sick person in the hospital or ambulatory care setting. Another illustration helps to clarify how community health nursing is "nursing for the community's health":

> Jack Webster is a community health nurse employed by a hospital-based home health agency. His caseload typically has a large percentage of people over 65 years of age with diagnoses such as congestive heart failure, diabetes, pneumonia, and hypertension. A common concern that Jack encounters with his clients is their inability to shop for food since they often cannot drive or walk to shop. It is difficult to rely on neighbors, and families frequently live long distances away from this inner-city neighborhood. Jack has worked with a local church to develop an organized cadre of volunteers who will grocery shop for those clients who need this service.

As was the situation with Julie Cherry, Jack Webster demonstrated how providing one-on-one care to ill clients was a window to the needs of an aggregate at risk within the community. Jack also utilized a community system to meet a crucial client need and to provide a long-term solution to the problem.

The World Health Organization has defined three necessary components of community health nursing practice that further delineate the uniqueness of this specialty area (WHO, 1974):

1. A sense of responsibility for coverage of needed health services in a community. It is not necessary for community health nursing to provide these services. The sense of responsibility for their provision, however, must be present.
2. The care of vulnerable groups in a community is a priority. The basis for involvement in the health care of aggregates is based upon their vulnerability. The long involvement of community health nursing in maternal-child health care is based upon this component.
3. The client (individual, family, group, community) must be a partner in planning and evaluating health care.

The unique aspects of community health nursing practice do not negate direct individual client care or practitioner-focused nursing. One-to-one clinical practice, illustrated by pediatric nurse practitioners and geriatric nurse specialists, certainly has a place in community health nursing when it is performed for the explicit purpose of improving the level of health in a community. Nurses in these roles can have the expertise needed to plan for aggregates at risk and are also very valuable consultants for other community health nurses. One official health department has, for example, a pediatric nurse practitioner who holds well-child conferences weekly in impoverished rural areas where there are almost no other health care resources available. This nurse is serving the high-risk aggregate of children, from birth through 5 years of age, in that county. Other staff nurses in the agency use her as a resource person when they have questions about the growth and development of the children they serve.

EVOLUTION OF TITLE OVER TIME

Historically, varying titles have been used to describe the type of nursing provided in the community setting, including district nursing, health nursing, visiting nursing, public health nursing, and community health nursing (McNeil, 1967). *District nursing,* which was the origin of our present concept of public health–community health nursing, was the title used by Rathbone when he hired nurses in England to care for the sick poor in their homes (refer to Chapter 1). When home nursing services were started in the United States, the term *visiting nursing* was used to identify the specialty area of practice that emphasized home-based nursing care. *Public health nursing* has its historical roots in Florence Nightingale's *health nurse* and Lillian Wald's *public health nurse.* Wald thought the word *public* denoted a service that was available to *all* people and, thus, coined the term *public health nursing* when she was director of the Henry Street Settlement in New York City. She hoped that by doing so the public would realize that the nursing services provided by the Henry Street Settlement were available to all individuals in the community. However, as federal, state, and local governments increased their involvement in the delivery of health services, the term *public health nursing* became associated with "public," or official, agencies and in turn with the care of poor people.

Home health nursing and *home care* were other titles that emerged with the development of the home health care industry. Governmental policy changes beginning in the 1970s, including Medicare's prospective payment system and the progressive use of third-party payments for noninstitutionalized care, fostered a rapid growth in home health care. The phrase *community health nursing* emerged out of an interest in reaffirming the original major thrust of public health nursing or community-based practice: nursing for the health of the entire public/community versus nursing only for the public who are poor. Some people use the terms *community health nursing* and *public health nursing* interchangeably. It must be remembered, however, that not every nurse who works in the community setting is a public health–community health nurse. Public, or community, health nurses have a definitive philosophy of practice that is described in the next section of this chapter.

In this text the authors have chosen to use the terms *community health nurse* and *community health nursing* because these terms help emphasize the major focus of the nurse's work—the community—as well as the services provided and the underlying philosophy. In addition to these terms, other titles (home health nursing, visiting nursing, and public health nursing) are still used in the practice setting.

DEFINING COMMUNITY HEALTH NURSING: PURPOSES AND GOALS

Throughout the history of community health nursing, leaders in the field have stressed the importance of defining beliefs about nursing practice and developing standards for practice that reflect these beliefs. The National Organization for Public Health Nursing (NOPHN) grew out of a concern for the rights and safety of clients. Community health nursing professionals were finding that as their specialty-based practice was rapidly expanding, "there were no generally accepted standards for anything" (Gardner, 1975). Gardner, a noted community health leader and an early president of the NOPHN, stated, when reminiscing about the development of the NOPHN, that "we realized that a body of poorly prepared and unsupervised nurses, some of whom might be without an ethical background for this work, were a dangerous element to let loose in the homes of the people and might easily jeopardize, in a short time, all the confidence we had been building throughout the country."

One of the major purposes of the NOPHN was to promote standardization of community health nursing practice. The first comprehensive statement of public health nursing objectives and functions was prepared by the NOPHN in 1931 (McIver, 1949, p. 65).

Since that time, community health nursing professionals have periodically reexamined their basic beliefs about community health nursing practice and have disseminated these beliefs to nurses across the country. Most recently, the ANA and APHA, the two professional organizations that represent community health nurses on the national level, have each published documents delineating their concept of community and public health nursing practice.

In its document *Standards of Community Health Nursing Practice,* the American Nurses Association (ANA) defines community health nursing practice as follows (ANA, 1986, pp. 1-2)*:

Community health nursing practice promotes and preserves the health of populations by integrating the skills and knowledge relevant to both nursing and public health. The practice is comprehensive and general, and is not limited to a particular age or diagnostic group; it is continual, and is not limited to episodic care. In the *Standards of Community Health Nursing Practice* document, the terms community health nursing and public health nursing are synonymous.

Community health nursing practice promotes the public's health. The programs, services, and institutions involved in public health emphasize promotion and maintenance of the population's health, and the prevention and limitation of disease. Public health activities change with changing technology and social values, but the goals remain the same: to reduce the amount of disease, premature death, discomfort, and disability (Milbank Memorial Fund Commission, 1976, p. 3).

While community health nursing practice includes nursing directed to individuals, families, and groups, the dominant responsibility is to the population as a whole. Nurses' efforts to promote and maintain the population's health entail the understanding and application of (a) concepts of public health and community; (b) skills of community organization and development; and (c) nursing care of selected individuals, families, and groups for health promotion, health maintenance, health education, and coordination of care.

The World Health Organization defines a community as a social group determined by geographical boundaries and/or common values and interests. Its members interact with each other. It functions within a particular social structure, exhibits and creates norms and values, and establishes social institutions (World Health Organization, 1978).

The nurse's actions reflect awareness of the need for comprehensive health planning in partnership with communities; the influence of social, economic, ecological,

*Reprinted with permission from *Standards of Community Health Nursing Practice,* © 1986, American Nurses Association, Kansas City, Mo.

and political issues; the needs of populations at risk; and the dynamic forces that stimulate change. Because the nurse's primary responsibility is to a population, some practice occurs through organization and coordination of the actions of others in response to health needs. When care is given to individuals, families, or groups, this responsibility dictates that the nurse's priorities concerning which clients to serve are determined by the needs of the population.

Professional community health nurses recognize that many local health issues are directly and profoundly affected by larger policy issues. Consequently, their practice reflects awareness of and responsiveness to legislative action and other means by which health and social policies are set at all levels within the health care system and the government.

The theoretical and factual context within which the community health nurse understands phenomena and their interrelationships derives from an interdisciplinary base including public health, the humanities, the social and behavioral sciences, epidemiology, and nursing science.

Community health nursing practice should be consistent with the World Health Organization's concept of primary health care as "essential health care made universally accessible to individuals and families in the community by means acceptable to them, through their full participation, and at a cost that the community and country can afford. Primary health care forms an integral part both of the country's health system (of which it is the nucleus) and of the overall social and economic development of the community" (World Health Organization, 1978). Embedded in this definition is the assumption that health care is a right and not a privilege.

The document lists nine standards; each standard is followed by rationale, as well as structure, process, and outcome criteria that validate the nurse's practice. Chapter 23 discusses these standards and criteria as a model for defining and measuring quality care.

The American Public Health Association's (APHA) position paper, *The Definition and Role of Public Health Nursing in the Delivery of Health Care,* was designed "to elucidate the essence of public health nursing practice and to clarify the role of public health nursing in the delivery of health care" (APHA, 1981, p. 3). This association's definition, emanating from the Public Health Nursing Section, is identified below (APHA, 1981, p. 4):

Public health nursing synthesizes the body of knowledge from the public health sciences and professional nursing theories for the purpose of improving the health of the entire community. This goal lies at the heart of primary prevention and health promotion and is the foundation for public health nursing practice. To accomplish this goal, public health nurses work with groups, families, and individuals as well as

in multidisciplinary teams and programs. Identifying subgroups (aggregates) within the population which are at high risk of illness, disability, or premature death and directing resources toward these groups, is the most effective approach for accomplishing the goal of PHN. Success in reducing the risks and in improving the health of the community depends on the involvement of consumers, especially groups experiencing health risks, and others in the community, in health planning, and in self-help activities.

The major concern of community health nurses, the health of the community, has not changed over time. In both the ANA and APHA definitions, emphasis is placed on "improving the health of the entire community" (APHA) or "the population as a whole" (ANA). In 1912, the NOPHN stated in its constitution that "the object of this organization shall be to stimulate responsibility for the health of the community" (NOPHN, 1975, p. 27).

A MODEL FOR COMMUNITY HEALTH NURSING PRACTICE

"While community health nursing practice includes nursing directed to individuals, families, and groups the dominant responsibility is to the population as a whole" (ANA, 1986, p. 2). Community health nurses, like all nurses, utilize the nursing process to ensure that the needs of clients are met. They use content and methods from nursing and public health in delivering *preventive* community health nursing services to populations and to establish priorities for care. The goal of community health nursing practice is health—that is, helping clients to obtain their maximum level of physical, mental, social, and spiritual functioning. The term *health* reflects the wellness orientation of the practice: a health orientation assumes that people always have the potential for higher levels of functioning and that people in all stages of living, including those who are dying, are growing and developing. The concept of health is further elaborated in Chapters 3, 9, and 10.

White's (1982) "Conceptual Model for Public Health Nursing Practice" pictorially presents the elements of this specialty area (refer to Figure 2-1). The community's health is determined by formal and informal public policy, and so to "practice nursing which seeks to enhance the public's health requires ethical and political involvement in defining the public, its health, and the policies that make the practice possible" (White, p. 527). On pp. 52 and 54

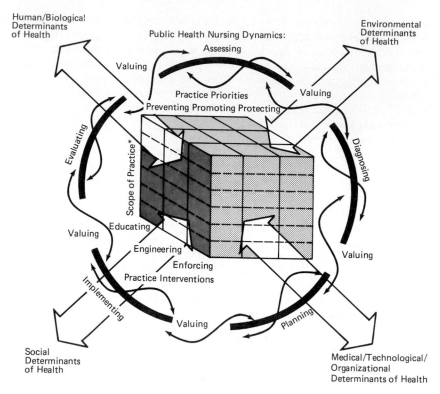

Figure 2-1 A Public Health Nursing Conceptual Model. The determinants of the health framework presented are modified from those in *Healthy People: The Surgeon General's Report on Health Promotion and Disease Prevention,* DHEW (PHS) Pub No 79-55071, 1979. (From White MS: Construct for public health nursing, *Nurs Outlook* 30:529, November/December 1982. Copyright 1982, American Journal of Nursing Company. All rights reserved.)

*The scope of practice is an open-ended continuum extending from individuals through such aggregates as groups, communities, entire populations to include the entire globe.

Julie Cherry, CHN, and Jack Webster, CHN, illustrated how they became involved in groups at a local level to define problems and create solutions to better the health of aggregates at risk for developing serious problems. Involvement in a professional nursing organization at either the student or staff level is a way of becoming politically involved in defining health and policies that make the "public's health" a sound one.

Multiple determinants in the environment influence how well clients function. *Environmental forces* encompass all of the internal and external factors that affect aggregate and individual functioning. Because people and their environments are dynamic and constantly changing, community health nurses must analyze interactions and mutual influences between humans and their environments. The concept of the environment is very broad and includes biological, sociocultural, ecological, and technological dimensions—all of which affect healthy functioning. These dimensions are discussed further in Chapters 6 and 11.

White's (1982) "Conceptual Model for Public Health Nursing Practice" depicts the relationships between the determinants of healthy functioning and the dynamics of public health nursing practice (see Figure 2-1). This model illustrates that the scope of public health nursing practice is very broad, extending from "one-to-one nursing intervention to a global perspective of world health. The overall focus of public health nursing is achieving and maintaining the public's health-at-all times" (White, 1982, pp. 527, 528). To accomplish this goal, preventive strategies ranging from health promotion to rehabilitation are used by the nurse in the community. Knowledge of what factors impact on health (health determinants), either positively or negatively, assists the community health nurse to plan appropriate prevention strategies. Intervention strategies are based on sound data and are planned in collaboration with the client. They include, but are not limited to, health education with individuals and aggregates, political action to promote effective public policy, and safety investigations to ensure a healthy environment.

The essential dynamics of this model consist of the nursing process and the valuing process (White, 1982, p. 529). The *nursing process* is a systematic approach to scientific problem solving, involving a series of circular dynamic actions—assessing, analyzing (diagnosing), planning, implementing, and evaluating (refer to Chapter 9). It is used to assess and diagnose client needs and to plan, implement, and evaluate effective nursing interventions.

According to White (1982), community health nursing interventions fall into three major categories: education, engineering, and enforcement. *Educative* nursing actions help clients to voluntarily acquire knowledge essential for understanding healthy functioning, to develop attitudes that foster preventive health behaviors, and to establish practices conducive to effective living. Educative strategies are commonly used in community health nursing practice. For example, community health nurses help families learn about normal growth and development and child care, conduct discussions related to sexuality issues in the school setting, and distribute health education materials in clinics, industrial plants, and other community health settings. Nurses visiting clients whose care is being reimbursed by Medicare teach the clients about their many medications, including why, when, and how to take them. They may also teach accurate wound care to clients and their families.

Because the community health nurse believes that clients and families are in charge of their own lives and will ultimately make the decisions that influence their own health, education is considered the most strategic intervention. Community health nurses work on the principle that when people are given a fish, their hunger is cured for several days. When people are taught how to fish their hunger is cured for many days. This concept is emphasized throughout the text, as are strategies to assist nurses in incorporating it into their practice.

Engineering strategies focus on environmental modification for the purpose of eliminating or managing environmental risk factors that affect healthy living. Campaigning against television advertisements that promote alcohol and cigarette use, conducting clinics for the treatment of sexually transmitted diseases, promoting actions to eliminate safety hazards in a schoolyard, and creating a system to help elderly clients safely take their many medications, are examples of engineering nursing actions.

Enforcement interventions are actions which impose regulatory controls and are designed to prevent disease, promote health, and protect society from harmful substances and conditions. Enforcement actions encourage the passage of regulations and legislation, such as seat belt, helmet, and drug abuse laws, which mandate health-promoting behaviors. These laws also mandate that high-risk clients with tuberculosis (the drug-addicted, those with failed TB treatment, the homeless, and those who have problems understanding the disease) take their pills under direct observation.

To intervene effectively in the community health setting, the nurse must engage in political activity. The political arena is where health care decisions are made for the public as a whole. Sound public policy is needed to eliminate or manage environmental risk factors, prevent disease, and promote public health. Political activism is emphasized in Chapters 13 and 24.

Valuing, the second dynamic process in White's model, guides nursing interventions and decision making and influences the development of goals and priorities for care. Valuing is "the process of assigning or determining the worth or merit of something" (White, 1982, p. 529). The influence that valuing has on decision-making becomes particularly evident during times of scarce resources. When resources are limited, professionals must critically examine their beliefs about practice and target resources so that they are used effectively and efficiently. Community health professionals place a high priority on targeting resources for at-risk aggregates in the community (APHA, 1981, p. 3). Their overall focus is "nursing for the health of the community." Identifying aggregates at risk and planning services to meet their needs benefits the community as a whole. *Aggregates at risk are those who engage in certain activities or who have certain characteristics that increase their potential for contracting an illness, injury, or health problem.* Individuals who smoke, for example, constitute an aggregate at high risk for developing cancer. The at-risk concept is basic public health practice; it guides epidemiological study and thus is discussed further in Chapter 11.

In order to "preserve and promote the health of populations" (or aggregates), White denotes three practice priorities: prevention, protection, and promotion. *Prevention* is a primary focus of community health nursing intervention. This focus entails a continuum of activities essential for preventing disease, prolonging life, and promoting health. These activities can be grouped under the three classic levels of prevention: primary, secondary, and tertiary (Leavell and Clark, 1965, p. 21). *Primary prevention* deals with health promotion and specific protection from health problems. *"Health promotion* begins with people who are basically healthy and seeks the development of community and individual measures which can help them to develop lifestyles that can maintain and enhance the state of well-being" (Surgeon General, 1979, p. 119).

Promotion strategies work in situations where one wants to decrease risks for disease by changing lifestyle patterns. Teaching caregivers of ill clients stress management techniques or providing respite services to prevent caregiver burnout are examples of health promotion strategies. Health promotion programs in the work setting designed to reduce the risk for cardiac disease, such as "Healthy Heart" meals in the employee cafeteria, are aggregate-focused promotion activities. *"Disease prevention* or specific protection begins with a threat to health—a disease or environmental hazard—and seeks to protect as many people as possible from the harmful consequences of that threat" (Surgeon General, 1979, p. 119). Following up the contact of a client who is diagnosed with a sexually transmitted disease such as syphilis is an illustration of the implementation of this strategy.

The significance of implementing health promotion activities is recognized worldwide. In 1986, the World Health Organization (WHO) institutionalized this concept through the development of *The Charter for Health Promotion.* WHO views health promotion as "a process of advocacy for health, encouraging a healthy lifestyle and mediating between different interests in society in the pursuit of health. Health promotion means building healthy public policy, creating supportive personal skills, and reorienting health services" (Turner, 1986).

Encouraging a healthy lifestyle is stressed because personal lifestyles play a critical role in the development of many serious diseases, injuries, and health conditions. It has long been recognized that if personal habits (e.g., regular exercise, adequate diet, no smoking, and appropriate use of alcohol and antihypertensive drugs) were changed, the mortality or death rate for seven of the ten leading causes of death could be substantially reduced (Surgeon General, 1979, p. 14). Immunizations, family planning services, antepartal care, classes for retirement preparation, smoking cessation, teaching, anticipatory guidance in family

health and child care, and counseling on accident prevention are all examples of activities which focus on primary prevention. Health promotion activities, such as regular exercise and adequate diet, and strategies for encouraging health promotion are discussed throughout the text.

Secondary prevention or health maintenance involves activities aimed at early diagnosis, prompt treatment, and disability limitation. Identification of health needs, health problems, and clients at risk is inherent in secondary prevention. The community health nurse who visits a client with congestive heart failure immediately after the client leaves the hospital and who teaches the client and family about dietary management of the disease is involved in secondary prevention. Conducting a health risk appraisal, observing for poor maternal-infant bonding, assessing for developmental delays in a young child, and reinforcing the need to carry out regular breast self-examination, are further examples of the concept of secondary prevention. The types of health needs a community health nurse should focus on when doing a health risk appraisal with individuals across the life span are discussed in Chapters 13 through 20.

Health risk appraisal is a process whereby a health history (refer to Chapter 9) is collected. Data obtained from this history are analyzed to identify characteristics that might make clients vulnerable to illness or premature death (e.g., personal and/or family history of hypertension and smoking), and educational nursing actions are instituted to help clients acquire knowledge about ways to reduce health risks. When conducting a health risk appraisal, community health nurses focus on collecting data about health problems that are likely to occur in a particular age group, such as inappropriate use of medication among the elderly, heart disease and cancer among well adults, and developmental delays among infants and children. Assessment tools and screening tests that facilitate risk appraisal are discussed in Chapters 14, 15, and 19. The ultimate goal of a health risk appraisal is to increase a client's self-care capabilities. *Self-care* is defined by Orem (1980) as "the practice of activities that individuals initiate and perform on their own behalf in maintaining life, health, and well-being."

Community health nurses focus on identifying at-risk populations as well as individuals at risk. Using the epidemiological process (Chapter 11), they collect and analyze community assessment data to identify which groups in the community are at risk for developing significant health problems. Pregnant women in a specific area of a community might, for example, be at risk for developing complications of pregnancy because of poor living conditions and inadequate health care resources. If this were found to be the case, the community health nurse would use the health planning process (refer to Chapter 13) to educate these women about their potential health risks and to develop health programs that better meet their needs.

Tertiary prevention has rehabilitation as its major focus. Rehabilitation activities assist clients to reach their maximum potential. The nurse who teaches an arthritic client how to rest at intervals throughout the day provides an example of tertiary prevention. Assisting a client who has had a cerebrovascular accident to continue with a physical and speech therapy regimen is also carrying out aspects of tertiary prevention. Chapter 18 discusses the role of the community health nurse in rehabilitation.

To achieve the goal of community health nursing— *optimal health*—all three levels of prevention— primary, secondary, and tertiary—must be implemented. Populations must develop behaviors that promote health as well as prevent disease to achieve an optimal level of functioning.

The dynamics and dimensions in White's model (Figure 2-1) stress the value of preventive activities. Preventing, promoting, and protecting are practice priorities. This model illustrates the community health nurse's use of the nursing process on the individual and aggregate level to provide preventive health services, and the multiple dimensions or determinants of health that must be addressed in order to successfully enhance individual and group health. It also illustrates the use of a range of intervention strategies, including political activism, to dilute or eliminate negative health determinants in the environment.

UNIQUENESS OF COMMUNITY HEALTH NURSING PRACTICE

Community health nursing's philosophy and scope of practice distinguish this practice field from other specialty areas in nursing. Community health nurses focus on providing *preventive* health services, as opposed to curative care, to enhance the health of individuals, families, and groups within the commu-

nity. Nursing service to individuals is viewed within the context of the family. It is recognized that the health of individuals can affect the health of all family members and that the family provides an environment that influences the health of its members. The family is seen as a natural unit of service (refer to Figure 2-2 on p. 60). It is also seen as a significant entry point from which to identify community strengths, needs, and resources related to the provision of health care services.

Community health nursing practice is general and comprehensive, not limited to a particular age group or diagnosis (ANA, 1980, p. 2). Community health nurses work with clients (individuals, families, and groups) across the life span. They are committed to improving *the health of the community* by identifying subgroups (refer to Figure 2-3 on p. 61) that are at high risk of illness, disability, or premature death and then directing resources toward these groups (APHA, 1981, p. 4). Determining specific populations at risk facilitates the identification of individuals and families at risk.

The words *client* or *consumer* rather than *patient* are used in community health nursing because they reflect a *wellness* orientation. In addition, they denote an active, independent relationship, in contrast to the passivity denoted by the word *patient*. The client asks questions and is a participant in assessing needs and in planning and implementing preventive health care. Care is not given to clients; rather, clients have a full part in their care. "Success in reducing the risks and in improving the health of the community depends on the involvement of consumers, especially groups experiencing health risks, and others in the community, in health planning and in self-help activities" (APHA, 1981, p. 4).

In order to assess needs and plan health services for individuals, groups, and the community as a whole, a public health knowledge base is mandatory. Community health nursing is a *synthesis of nursing and public health* practice. Community health nurses use the knowledge and skills of professional nursing and the philosophy, content, and methods of public health when delivering services in the community. The ANA, in its recent Social Policy Statement, defines nursing as "the diagnosis and treatment of human responses to actual or potential health problems" (ANA, 1980, p. 9). Nursing emphasizes assisting *individual* clients in dealing with responses to health problems. In contrast, public health focuses on the health of the *community*.

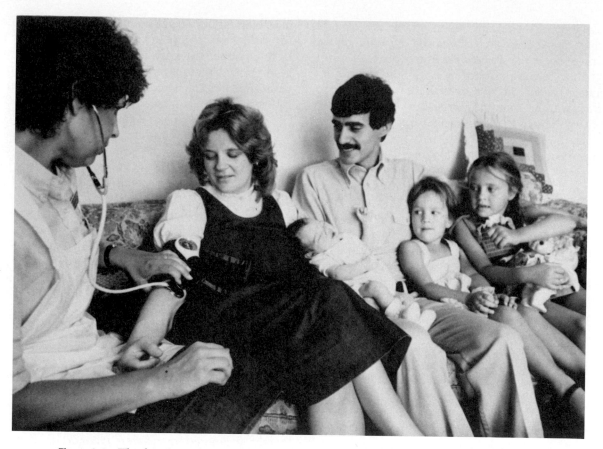

Figure 2-2 The family is the natural unit of service in community health nursing practice. During a home visit, the community health nurse determines the health status of all family members and assesses family dynamics as well. (Courtesy Genesee Region Home Care Association, Rochester, New York.)

Public health was described by Winslow (1952, p. 30) as follows:

[The] science and art of preventing disease, prolonging life, and promoting physical and mental health and efficiency through organized community efforts focused toward

1. maintaining a sanitary environment;
2. controlling communicable diseases;
3. providing education regarding principles of personal hygiene;
4. organizing medical and nursing services for early diagnosis and treatment of disease; and
5. developing social machinery to ensure everyone a standard of living adequate for health maintenance, so organizing these benefits as to enable every citizen to realize his birthright of health and longevity.*

*Reprinted by permission of Princeton University Press.

This includes the philosophy, content, and methods of epidemiology, biostatistics, social policy, health planning, public health organization and administration, and public health law. These topics are explored more fully in later sections of this text.

The values held by public health professionals when Winslow proposed this classic description of public health continue to guide the direction of practice in the field. A recent report prepared by the Institute of Medicine's Committee for the Study of Public Health reaffirms "the mission of public health as fulfilling society's interest in assuring conditions in which people can be healthy. Its aim is to generate organized community effort to address the public interest in health by applying scientific and technical knowledge to prevent disease and promote health" (Committee for the Study of the Future of Public

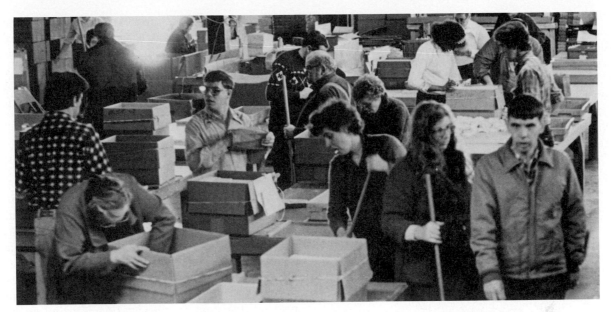

Figure 2-3 Aggregates as well as individuals are *clients* in community health nursing practice. An aggregate is a group of individuals having in common one or more personal or environmental characteristics (Williams, 1977). Community health nurses focus on identifying at-risk aggregates in the community in order to target resources more effectively. Individuals who are retarded, for example, make up a high-risk aggregate, because persons in this population group often need an array of community services in order to strengthen their self-care capabilities. (Courtesy Sunshine Workshop, a nonprofit voluntary agency sponsored by the Association of Retarded Citizens in Knox County, Tennessee. Photographer, Mary Louise Peacock.)

Health, 1988, p. 7). This report, entitled *The Future of Public Health* and known as the "IOM Report," addresses the need to deal with environmental health concerns, to control communicable disease, to provide personal health care services, and to encourage healthful behaviors through education and modification in the social environment.

HEALTHY PEOPLE 2000

Healthy People: The Surgeon General's Report on Health Promotion and Disease Prevention was published in 1979 and was based on the understanding that lifestyle and environmental factors are instrumental in health and disease. This landmark publication was the first national health promotion and disease prevention effort and set forth a course of action with five broad national goals for 1990, one for each of the five major stages of life. In 1990, *Healthy People 2000: National Health Promotion and Disease Prevention Objectives* was published,

building on the first effort (USDHHS, 1991). The report has 22 priority areas, with measurable goals for each area. Chapter 5 presents the areas and objectives; this text addresses the relevant areas and goals throughout the lifespan in Chapters 14 through 20.

HEALTH FOR ALL MANDATE

"What unites people around public (community) health is the focus on society as a whole, the community, and the aim of optimal health status" (Committee for the Study of the Future of Public Health, 1988, p. 39). This is the theme that guides community health action at all levels of national and international government. In 1978, 158 countries attending the International Conference on Primary Health Care, held in Alma-Ata, USSR, set for themselves a common goal, "Health for All by the Year 2000" (WHO, 1978). In committing themselves to this goal, countries did not mean that by the year 2000 disease and disability would no longer exist. The focus was placed on all people having access to health services that would assist them in leading socially and economically productive lives (Mahler, 1979). "The goal of Health for All by the Year 2000 is a vision founded on social equity; on the urgent need to reduce the gross inequality in the health status of people in the world, in developed and developing countries, and within countries" (Maglacas, 1988).

The Declaration of Alma-Ata specifies that primary health care is the key vehicle for attaining the "health for all" goal. Primary health care is a blend of essential health services, personal responsibility for one's own health, and health-promoting action taken by the community. It must include at least the following eight components (WHO, 1988, p. 23):

- Education concerning prevailing health problems and the methods of preventing and controlling them
- Promotion of food supply and proper nutrition
- An adequate supply of safe water and basic sanitation
- Maternal and child health care, including family planning
- Immunization against the major infectious diseases
- Prevention and control of locally endemic diseases
- Appropriate treatment of common diseases and injuries
- Provision of essential drugs

Primary health care facilitates client entry into the health care system, promotes integrated and coordinated services, requires client participation in the program planning and evaluation process and in policy making, and promotes self-reliance and self-determination (WHO, 1978). Community health nurses promote these types of services, activities, and values.

What is the status of "Health for All By the Year 2000"? "What is generally very clear is that every country, every member state of WHO has done something toward the attainment of 'health for all'. But unfortunately the level of achievement tends to be very unbalanced" (Little, 1992). Developing countries have basic concerns, such as food and water, and thus there has been a limited expansion of health budgets in many countries. Health care for all is a target; nurses as primary health care providers continue to play an instrumental role in making this happen.

No one discipline can address all of the health needs in the community. That is why community health nurses stress the importance of multidisciplinary planning. Multidisciplinary planning and cooperation can facilitate community diagnosis (Chapter 12) and health planning (Chapter 13). It also promotes effective and efficient use of resources.

SETTINGS, WORK FORCE, ROLES, AND SERVICES

Community health nurses implement a variety of roles in the practice setting and provide a broad range of services aimed at promoting individual and aggregate health. They work in diverse health and health-related organizations. Changing health care delivery trends have resulted in a need for increased numbers of nurses who can function in the community setting; deinstitutionalization is being stressed and community-based care is being advocated.

Settings in which Community Health Nurses Function

An exciting aspect of community health nursing is the existence of varied settings and modalities for practice. Community health nurses were first employed by visiting nurse associations, where they responded to the needs of people at greatest risk by nursing the sick in their homes and by providing instruction to both manage illness and remain well (refer to Figure 2-4). With the increase of home care this remains an important avenue. They have also been employed by health departments or other tax-supported agencies, visiting nurse associations or other non–tax-supported agencies, schools, and occupational health programs.

State and local health departments are mandated to protect the health of the community and, therefore, to provide a broad range of services that address the needs of groups across the life span. Visiting nurse associations primarily emphasize the delivery of home health care or bedside nursing services. Health programs in schools and occupational settings mainly serve a specific segment of the community. School-age children are the focus in school health programs, whereas the well adult is the target of service in the occupational health setting. Migrant health clinics, prisons, rural and urban nursing centers, homeless shelters, and senior citizen centers are other settings in

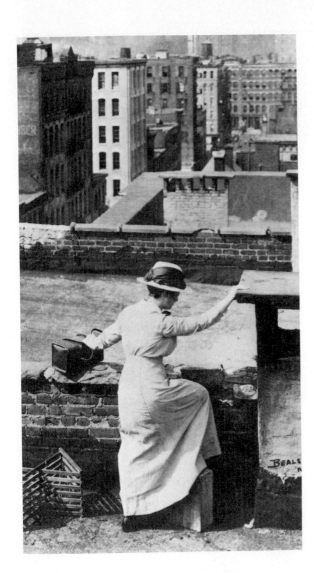

Figure 2-4 Community health nurses have traditionally gone into a variety of community settings to serve individuals, families, and groups. In this picture, a Henry Street nurse is climbing over a tenement roof on New York's Lower East Side to visit her clients in the home. Today, community health nurses usually do not need to climb over rooftops. They do, however, reach out to clients in all types of settings (e.g., homes, schools, rural clinics, neighborhood health centers, and sheltered workshops). (Courtesy Visiting Nurse Service of New York City.)

which the community health nurse works and where services are targeted for specific aggregates.

All of these settings have the following elements in common: an emphasis on independent practice by the practitioner; an understanding that the physical and social environment is critical to the state of health; and a focus on the concept that clients need to be taught how to fish rather than simply being given a fish to cure their hunger. Concepts of community assessment and intervention are less common in home health practice, where currently only illness care is reimbursed. However, there are encouraging signs that home health agencies are also realizing that it is at the community level that problems are both caused and solved and that community health nurses in all set-

tings need to support each other during the health care crisis that our nation faces (Green and Driggers, 1989; Zerwekh, 1992; Walcott-McQuigg and Ervin, 1992).

Size of the Work Force in Community Health Nursing

The earliest known count of public health nurses in the United States was reported by Harriett Fulmer at the International Congress of Nurses in Buffalo, N.Y., in 1901. At that time there were 58 public health nursing organizations, employing about 130 nurses. In 1912 Mary Gardner found that approximately 3000 nurses were engaged in community health nursing services. From 1916 to 1931, periodic enumerations of public health nursing agencies and the nurses they employed were recorded by the Statistical Department of the National Organization for Public Health Nursing. Since 1937 the state directors of public health nursing and the Division of Nursing, U.S. Public Health Service, have systematically collected and compiled data about numbers and educational preparation of nurses employed in public health work in the United States. State and local official and nonofficial (voluntary) public health agencies, boards of education, national agencies, universities, and, in some years, industries, have supplied the information (Source Book, 1975, p. 187).

In 1988 the Research Triangle Institute, under a contract with the Division of Nursing, Bureau of Health Professions, Health Resources and Services Administration, carried out a national survey of registered nurses. Previous surveys were completed in 1977, 1980, and 1984 (USDHHS, 1990, p. 10). Figure 2-5, on p. 66, depicts the fields of employment for RNs in 1984 and 1988. Though two thirds of the nation's 1,627

TABLE

2-1 Employment Setting of Primary Positions of Registered Nurses Employed in Nursing: March 1988

Employment setting	Number in sample	Estimated Number	Estimated Percent
Total	27,026	1,627,035	100.0
Hospital	18,284	1,104,978	67.9
Non-federal short-term hospital	16,399	996,143	61.2
Non-federal long-term hospital	741	46,430	2.9
Federal hospital	1,142	62,302	3.8
Other hospital	2	104	0.0
Nursing Home/Extended Care Facility	1,877	107,805	6.6
Nursing home unit in hospital	161	8,368	0.5
Other nursing home	1,598	92,246	5.7
Mentally retarded facility	83	4,680	0.3
Other extended care facility	35	2,510	0.2
Nursing Education	554	30,005	1.8
LPN/LVN program	70	3,878	0.2
Diploma program	50	2,872	0.2
Associate degree program	167	8,325	0.5
Baccalaureate or higher degree	266	14,914	0.9
Other nursing education	1	16	0.0
Community/Public Health	1,879	110,886	6.8
State health department	233	10,857	0.7
City or county health department	462	27,780	1.7
Combination nursing service	13	851	0.1
Visiting nurse service	314	20,076	1.2
Other home health agency (non–hospital-based)	453	26,993	1.7
Community mental health center	129	8,344	0.5
Neighborhood health center	84	5,283	0.3
Planned parenthood/family planning ctr	52	3,007	0.2
Rural health center	39	1,404	0.1
Day care center	27	1,510	0.1
Hospice	32	2,035	0.1
Retirement community center	32	2,534	0.2
Other community/public health	9	213	0.0
Student Health Service	772	47,792	2.9
Board of education (public school)	483	30,138	1.9
Private or parochial school	117	7,701	0.5
College or university	152	8,926	0.5
Other student health service	20	1,026	0.1
Occupational Health	366	21,857	1.3
Private industry	315	19,298	1.2
Government	51	2,559	0.2

TABLE 2-1 **Employment Setting of Primary Positions of Registered Nurses Employed in Nursing: March 1988—cont'd**

Employment setting	Number in sample	Estimated Number	Percent
Ambulatory Care Setting Employee	2,120	125,813	7.7
Solo practice (physician)	591	36,637	2.3
Partnership (one or more physicians)	386	20,625	1.3
Group practice (physicians)	477	27,376	1.7
Freestanding clinic (physicians)	351	20,489	1.3
Ambulatory surgical center (non–hospital-based)	121	6,716	0.4
Dental practice	20	1,137	0.1
Health maintenance organization	173	12,686	0.8
Other ambulatory care setting	1	146	0.0
Private Duty Nursing	263	19,988	1.2
Self Employed	217	13,203	0.8
Solo practice	137	8,441	0.5
Partnership with other nurses	31	1,895	0.1
Partnership with physicians	28	1,350	0.1
Partnership with other health professionals	21	1,516	0.1
Other	676	43,321	2.7
Central or regional federal agency	39	2,124	0.1
State board of nursing	12	630	0.0
Nursing or health association	22	1,332	0.1
Health planning agency	27	2,100	0.1
Prison or jail	90	6,570	0.4
Insurance company	162	11,099	0.7
Other	324	19,467	1.2
Not Known	18	1,386	0.1

NOTE: Estimated number and percent may not add to total because of rounding.
From U.S. Department of Health and Human Services, PHS, Health Resources and Services Administration: *1988: The registered nurse population. Findings from the national survey sample of registered nurses, March 1988*, Washington, D.C., June 1990, The Department, p. 44.

million RNs were working in hospitals, the number working in ambulatory care and community/public health settings grew at a faster rate than the number of those working in hospitals. The number working in nursing homes declined (USDHHS, p. 8).

Table 2-1 depicts the employment setting of primary positions of registered nurses employed in nursing for March 1988. The area of community/public health is broken down into 13 categories. The primary growth between 1984 and 1988 in these categories was among nurses working in non–hospital-based

home health agencies other than visiting nursing services (USDHHS, 1990, p. 20).

It is projected that in the years 2000 and 2020 the requirements for full-time-equivalent registered nurses will increase significantly in many health care settings, but that the highest percentage increase will occur in the community health setting. The RN community-health requirements represent increases of 75% and 205% in the years 2000 and 2020, respectively, over the 1985 requirements (Secretary of Health and Human Services, 1988).

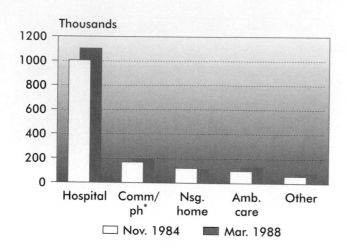

*Includes school and occupational health

Figure 2-5   Field of employment for registered nurses, 1984 and 1988. (From U.S. Department of Health and Human Services, PHS, Health Resources and Services Administration: *1988: The registered nurse population. Findings from the national survey sample of registered nurses, March 1988,* Washington, D.C., June 1990, The Department, p. 8.)

Roles of Community Health Nurses

A variety of roles can be assumed by nurses in providing community health nursing services (Green and Driggers, 1989; Gulino and La Monica, 1986; Riportella-Muller, Selby, Salmon, Quade, and Legault, 1991). Other chapters in this text discuss these roles in depth. Below is a partial listing of the types of roles community health nurses implement:

1. *Advocate.* Clients in the CHN setting frequently are unable to obtain needed health care services or to negotiate for change in the health care system. Community health nurses seek to promote an understanding of health problems, lobby for beneficial public policy, and stimulate supportive community action for health. This role is discussed in more detail throughout the text.

2. *Care manager.* Helping clients to make decisions about appropriate health care services and to achieve service delivery integration and coordination is a major role of the community health nurse. Chapter 10 focuses on this care manager role.

3. *Casefinder.* Community health nurses look for clients at risk among the population being served. Chapters 9, 10, and 13 through 21 discuss ways in which nurses serve as case finders.

4. *Counselor.* Clients in the community health setting frequently face difficult and complex health concerns and desire supportive and problem-solving assistance. Community health nurses are often in a unique position to help clients deal with stress related to health concerns. The counselor role of the CHN is highlighted in Chapter 8.

5. *Clinic nurse.* Chapter 21 expands on the role of the nurse in the ambulatory care setting. Clinic services are increasingly being expanded to meet the needs of aggregates at risk (e.g., noninsured groups of individuals).

6. *Epidemiologist.* The community health nurse uses the epidemiological method to study disease and health among population groups and to deal with community-wide health problems. Chapter 11 explains this role.

7. *Group leader.* Chapter 21 also discusses the role of the nurse who works with groups in practice.

8. *Health planner.* Providing health programs for aggregates at risk is described in Chapters 12 through 20.

9. *Home visitor.* Perhaps the most unusual aspect of this specialty is that the community health nurse enters the client's setting. The nurse not only assesses the environment but also works within it. Home visitors are able to gather environmental information, in addition to data about how a family system functions within its own setting. They also are able to provide direct care services in a situation familiar to the client.

10. *Occupational health nurse.* Chapter 17 presents this expanding and changing area of community health nursing.

11. *Researcher.* The goals for community health nursing practice are far from being realized. The critical need for research to assist health care professionals in reaching their goals is addressed throughout the text.

12. *School nurse.* Chapter 15 presents the role of the nurse with this vital aggregate.

13. *Teacher.* Application of teaching-learning principles to facilitate behavioral change among clients is a basic intervention strategy in community health. Chapter 8 presents the educative approach with families. Chapter 21 discusses the group educative approach.

Many of the roles listed above are carried out with all populations and within all community health nursing service delivery settings. For example, advocacy, case finding, and teaching are essential components of the community health nurse's activity whether in a clinic, home, school, workplace, or senior citizen center.

Many other roles are assumed by the community health nurse; those described above are by no means all-inclusive. The excitement of this specialty area lies in its diversity.

SERVICES PROVIDED BY COMMUNITY HEALTH NURSES

In order to accomplish their goals, community health nurses provide multiple and diverse direct and indirect client services. Direct client services usually involve a personal relationship between the nurse and client (which can be a person, a family, an aggregate, or the community). Teaching, hands-on bedside care, health risk appraisal, counseling, health planning with consumers, and the delivery of clinic services are examples of direct client services. Indirect client services include such things as record keeping, talking to a community agency about available resources to meet client needs, and supervising the care provided by a home health aide.

Following are stories that chronicle a day in the life of two community health nurses: Charlene is employed by a county health department, and John is employed by a large voluntary visiting nurses' association. The stories illustrate the range of services provided by nurses in various community settings (Haradine, 1978; George, 1991).

The community health nurses in these two stories illustrate several important concepts in community health nursing. The community health nurse is a generalist and serves all population groups. She or he works in the client's setting, utilizing principles of primary, secondary, and tertiary prevention. The community health nurse also serves population groups in clinics and schools; concepts from the public health sciences of biostatistics, epidemiology, and administration help the nurse to identify needs of these aggregates.

--- **A DAY IN THE LIFE OF A COMMUNITY HEALTH NURSE** ---

Her first stop by 8 AM each day is at her desk in the health department to pick up messages from the day before, make phone calls, and plan her day's schedule.

After morning coffee with the other nurses, which offers time for comparisons, she starts her calls.

"Sometimes you've had a dark day and you need input, you need to talk to someone," she explains. "I could get depressed if I allowed myself, but I realize whose problem it is. It's not my problem. It's only my place to help when I'm accepted."

Many calls start with a request from a school or another public health nurse, or Charlene's own case finding.

Her first stop on a gray, cheerless day recently was a happy one, to visit a new baby. Paul Daniel Conner had spent 2 months in a hospital nursery after being born prematurely, weighing only 3 pounds, 7 ounces. Now 2½ months old, he had adjusted easily to his mother's style in the 2 weeks he has been home.

"He's a perfect baby," says his mother, Julie. "He doesn't ever cry." But she does have a few questions, written on a scrap of paper.

"I was surprised how easy it has been. I've been just really relaxed with him," she tells Charlene.

The routine on a visit to a new baby includes leaving a sheaf of pamphlets for the mother's spare-time reading. Topics include first aid, exercises for the mother, feeding, birth control, and descriptions of the free services offered by the health department.

Charlene advises Mrs. Conner not to put Paul Daniel to bed with a bottle.

"A baby will get a pool of milk, juice or Kool-Aid in its mouth that causes tooth decay. I see children with nothing but little brown stubs left of their teeth," she explains.

"You can use your blender to make baby food from table food, then freeze it in an ice cube tray and put it in a bag. But be sure to freeze it."

The telephone number for the Western Michigan Poison Center and instructions on taking a baby's temperature are all part of the routine which ends with a full examination of the baby and measuring its height and weight.

Charlene tells Mrs. Conner she can take her baby to the health department's well-baby clinic, in the Belmont area, for children from birth to school age.

"It's one of your benefits as a taxpayer. You can take the baby in for his shots, but continue to see the doctor."

The idea appeals to Mrs. Conner. She takes the information, the telephone number she would use for an appointment.

"You can call me anytime," Charlene says as she leaves. "I'm usually in early in the morning."

Few newborns in Kent County are seen by a public health nurse. Many don't need it; more probably do. All it would take is a call—from the hospital, from the mother, or even from a relative.

"There are many out there I'm not getting, mothers who are having problems adjusting to a new baby, who didn't like children or babies before and now overcompensate," Charlene explains.

A stop at West Oakview School is squeezed in before the students' lunch break to check a girl with bites on her arms and legs (probably flea bites from a cat, Charlene thinks) and a progress report from a class for emotionally impaired youngsters.

At North Oakview School, after lunch, Charlene calls in to her office for messages. Then she visits a "readiness room" for 5- to 7-year-olds taught by Ann Westerhof.

"If Charlene didn't come in once a week, I don't know what I'd do," Mrs. Westerhof exclaims. "She's the go-between for me and the families. She helps me know what I can and can't do."

The "star" of this visit is Jim Fragale, 6, who is sporting a new brace, an unusual contraption with a tripod base and straps that keep his legs bent to aid healing of the hip joints.

The cause of Jim's hip problem is unknown, Charlene explains. "The ball joint of the hip softens, then starts coming back. But the regeneration is dependent on rest and nutrition."

Jim had a little trouble balancing when he was first fitted with the brace, and even fell backwards, Mrs. Westerhof explains. "And he was a little embarrassed by it at first. But now he can show the other students tricks they can't do."

Charlene's link was knowing what agency to contact to make the brace a reality. "So many times, parents can't afford the treatment needed, and Char knows how to get it," Mrs. Westerhof adds.

From the young to the old—that switch in thinking is typical for public health nurses.

Twice a month, Charlene is in charge of the well-baby clinic in Belmont. She sees humanity at its beginnings there, in the tots brought in for free care—routine physical examinations by a doctor, immunizations, and advice for parents.

Although the wait can be long, the time can be used to ask a public health nurse about the little doubts, those questions that seem too insignificant for the doctor.

"I thought he'd outgrow it by this time. I guess he won't," one mother was overheard commenting to one of the three nurses staffing the clinic.

These chats, informal and friendly, offer help on parenting to start the young out right.

When the young, at 14 or 15, stumble along the way, Charlene and the other public health nurses are there, just a telephone call away.

Sometimes it's the child's problem, and sometimes it's the parent's, spreading over to the child. "Rare is the teenager who will say, 'Hey, I've got a problem,' " Charlene notes. "Some social workers do refer kids to me.

"We see some child abuse cases and we see neglect, which is so hard to prove. It's insidious and camouflaged. Sometimes the parents are too wrapped up in themselves, or it might be a lack of resources, of money.

"We have to know what help is available from the different agencies."

The old pose a different problem, when loneliness and loss have taken their toll. Charlene pulls into a driveway along the Grand River, next to a small house with a tidy yard at 4566 Abrigador Trail NE. It's a call to the other end of life.

"They say I'll live to be 90, but I don't care to," says Josephine Robbins as Charlene takes her blood pressure.

"I know that," Charlene replies, acceptingly, as she removes the blood pressure cuff from the arm of the woman, who is 80.

The youngest of seven, Josephine says, "The others, they're all gone. My sister was 92."

Her husband, Lloyd, died in March. "What do I have to live for?" she asks.

In answer to Charlene's questions on her health, she reports only "a catch in my side" now and then. But she takes "just a little Lydia Pinkham's and it goes away."

An active woman now very lonely and anxious, Josephine looks forward to the weekly nurse visit. "You're not taking any of those pills, are you?" Charlene asks in a warning tone.

"No, I threw them out." A neighbor had given Josephine two drugs, Librium (a tranquilizer) and nitroglycerine (a heart drug), saying, "They always helped me. Maybe they'll help you."

Charlene had become aware of them on her last visit when she had asked what medications Josephine was taking.

Josephine worries about getting her things in order, her will, her records and being able to pledge her eyes and kidneys before she dies. "They said I had to come down and sign in front of two witnesses, but I can't get down there," she tells the nurse. Charlene explains, "Not necessary; just witnesses, here in your home."

Besides the decisions for her will, on the who and what of all she owns, Josephine must finish the mural she is painting on one wall, then paint a scene in a window and refinish some furniture. And then. . . .

"There's just an awful lot of red tape," the gray-haired woman comments sadly. "I'm never going to be through."

The public health nurse visits often when the need is great, then as the crisis eases, the visits taper off, to make time and room for someone else with other pressing needs.

Days are filled with joy and sadness. Charlene believes she gets as much as she gives in her 8-5 job. "I need people. I see myself as a helping person and they are fulfilling to me."

But in public health the rewards are seldom quick in coming. "You see something grow. You see a person who has never had any self-confidence make strides.

"I'm really in preventive medicine," Charlene says. "By educating others and by my intervention, I believe I'll make a difference."

From Haradine J: Public health nurse makes a difference, *Grand Rapids Press,* December 3, 1978, pp. 29-33.

A DAY IN THE LIFE OF A VISITING NURSE

Shortly before noon on yet another 90-plus-degree September day, John Roethke is praising automobile air-conditioning as he navigates the streets of West Philadelphia in search of a particular shopping center.

A few minutes later he finds it and, more importantly, the pay phone he uses to inform his next patient that he's just around the corner.

When Roethke pulls up to Derrick Smith's building at the Court Apartments in Yeadon, a family member already has a third-floor window open. Smith and his aunt have trouble climbing the three flights of stairs, so they have devised a ritual: Roethke calls when he gets close, honks his horn when he arrives, and they toss him the front-door key from the third floor.

Just another day for a home health care nurse.

Before joining the Visiting Nurse Association of Greater Philadelphia, Roethke worked in the trauma center at Albert Einstein Medical Center and as an emergency room nurse manager at Parkview Hospital.

"I thought I'd be bored silly working in home care after being in emergency rooms for so long." the 34-year-old Bethlehem native says. "But that hasn't happened. I'm working with a lot of high-tech equipment and teaching patients how to use it. It really astounds me that I'm teaching a 78-year-old woman how to work a CADD pump."

The computer-assisted delivery device, the size of a transistor radio, pumps medication into a patient's veins at a preset rate.

"It sounds kind of corny, but patients really do better at home where they are in familiar surroundings," Roethke says. "Hospitals in the 21st century won't be anything like they are today. They'll have an emergency room, a huge outpatient department and intensive-care units for surgery and that's it. Everything else will be home care."

Roethke's work day begins around 8 AM, when he contacts patients to let them know when he will be coming by.

His first stop on this oppressively hot day is in South Philadelphia, a few blocks from where Connie Mack Stadium once stood. The patient, 72-year-old Early Yearwood, suffers from cardiomyopathy—his heart is having a difficult time pumping fluid to his kidneys.

Roethke, who at 6-foot-6 is not the prototype nurse, attracts a few curious stares as he lifts his bag from the car's trunk.

Inside, Earl and his wife, Mary, are watching a television game show. The lights are off and two fans are oscillating in the heat.

"How do you feel today, Earl?" Roethke asks, as he checks Yearwood's blood pressure.

"Bad," he responds.

For a half-hour Roethke examines Yearwood and administers 50 milligrams of Lasix, a treatment for cardiomyopathy. At the same time he quizzes Yearwood's wife on how and when she should change

Yearwood's bandages. Home health aides are available to help patients get out of bed and dressed, but the idea, Roethke explains, is to have the family do as much as it can. If a nurse thinks the family can't handle the responsibility, a recommendation will be made to return the patient to the hospital.

Though Yearwood is stoic for most of the visit, Roethke gets him to smile occasionally.

"Now, no jogging around the block," Roethke says, as he packs up his equipment.

"I don't think I could do that," Yearwood answers with a grin.

On the way to his next patient, Derrick Smith, Roethke tells of two events that lead him to home health care.

He is going through a divorce and has joint custody of his children. Working as a home health care nurse allows him to set his own schedule so he can spend more time with his three daughters.

He also had the experience of becoming a patient after getting stuck with a needle and contracting Hepatitis B.

"When you become a patient they just don't strip away your clothes, they strip away your dignity," Roethke says. "I'm not trying to come down hard on the hospitals because they have a tremendous job to do."

But it made him an advocate for home care.

Roethke says he is unconcerned about visiting patients in high-crime areas, but he agrees maybe he should be.

"Some of the other nurses told me, in the drug-infested areas the drug dealers know you're there to care for the elderly in the neighborhood and they leave you alone," he says. "I don't bank on that, but I never had any problems."

Smith, the 44-year-old Yeadon patient, also suffers from cardiomyopathy.

"This is great," Smith says of being treated at home. "I've been in the hospital so much for so long. I don't want to go back."

"I've seen so much improvement." Roethke spent 40 minutes with Smith, checking his vital signs and administering about 200 milligrams of Lasix, seemingly oblivious to Smith's niece and nephew playing and yelling just a few feet away.

Before he leaves, the children hug Roethke, wrapping their arms around his knees.

"People are always giving you food or little gifts. It's amazing," Roethke says. "They're welcoming you into their home. When I worked in the emergency room it was often on patients who didn't want to be there. They'd fight you. If I didn't get called a MF at least once a shift I didn't feel loved."

Roethke's third visit on this day is a marked departure from the first two. His patient, Shirley Channick, lives in the Valley Forge Towers in King of Prussia.

The key isn't tossed out the window. The maid lets him in after a security guard buzzes him through the lobby.

Channick has rheumatoid arthritis and an infection stemming from a hip replacement. Her arthritis keeps Channick from administering medication to herself, so she is being treated with antibiotics delivered by a CADD pump.

Roethke's next stop is the office, where he will spend hours tackling the Medicare and Medicaid forms the job generates.

"I thought I'd find it difficult to work in long-term care where you don't always see improvement," he says. "I haven't found that to be the case. Maybe I should stop looking."

From George J: For John Roethke, the job of visiting nurse is anything but dull, *Philadelphia Business Journal,* October 7, 1991, pp. 1, 3-4.

Summary

Community health nursing is a synthesis of nursing and public health practice applied to promoting and preserving the health of populations (ANA, 1980). The community health nurse's philosophy and scope of practice distinguishes her or him from other nurses in the practice setting. Community health nurses serve individuals and aggregates (groups of people) across the lifespan on a continuing basis. Their major goal is to protect and promote the health of the community. Prevention is their primary focus in nursing practice. Identifying at-risk populations within the community assists community health nurses to effectively and efficiently provide preventive health care services.

Community health nurses work in a variety of settings and implement multiple roles such as case finder, teacher, group worker, and health planner. Changing health care delivery trends have increased the demand for community-based services and, in turn, the number of qualified community health nurses. The excitement of this specialty area lies in its diversity.

> ◀ *An Exercise in Critical Thinking* ▶
>
> The definition of community health nursing states that it is a synthesis of nursing and public health practice. Provide examples from the stories about a day in the life of a community health nurse and a day in the life of a visiting nurse (pp. 67-70) where elements of public health/community health nursing are practiced.

References

American Nurses Association: Community Health Nursing Division: *Standards of community health nursing practice,* Pub. No. CH-10, Kansas City, Mo., 1986, The Association.

American Nurses Association: *Nursing: a social policy statement,* Pub No. NP-63, Kansas City, Mo., 1980, The Association.

American Public Health Association. Public Health Nursing Section: *The definition and role of public health nursing in the delivery of health care,* Washington, D.C., 1981, The Association.

Brainard A: *Organization of public health nursing,* New York, 1921, Macmillan.

Committee for the Study of the Future of Public Health, Institute of Medicine· *The future of public health,* Washington, D.C., 1988, National Academy Press.

Gardner MS: Typewritten Reminiscences, Feb. 5, 1948, NOPHN Archive Microfilm H25. In Fitzpatrick ML, ed: *The national organization for public health nursing, 1912-1952: development of a practice field,* New York, 1975, National League for Nursing, p. 17.

George J: For John Roethke, the job of visiting nurse is anything but dull, *Philadelphia Business Journal,* October 7, 1991, pp. 1, 3-4.

Goeppinger J: Primary health care: an answer to the dilemmas of community nursing? *Public Health Nurs* 1:129-140, 1984.

Green JL and Driggers B: All visiting nurses are not alike: home health and community health nursing, *J Comm Health Nurs* 6:83-93, 1989.

Gulino C and La Monica G: Public health nursing: a study of role implementation, *Public Health Nurs* 3:80-91, 1986.

Haradine J: Public health nurse makes a difference, *Grand Rapids Press,* December 3, 1978, pp. 29-33.

Leavell HR and Clark EG: *Preventive medicine for the doctor in his community. An epidemiological approach,* ed 3, New York, 1965, McGraw-Hill.

Little C: Health for all by the year 2000. Where is it now? *Nurs Health Care* 13(4):198-204, 1992.

Maglacas AM: *Health for all.* Paper presented at a conference on international health, Ann Arbor, September 1988.

Mahler H: What is health for all? *World Health,* November 1979, p. 3-5.

McIver P: Public health nursing responsibilities, *Public Health Nurs* 41:65-66, 1949.

McNeil E: Transition in public health nursing, *U Michigan Medical Center J* 33:286-291, 1967.

Milbank Memorial Fund Commission: *Higher education for public health: a report,* Nantucket, Mass., 1976, Prodist.

National Organization for Public Health Nursing: Constitution of the National Organization for Public Health Nursing, Article 2, 1912, Wald: New York Public Library folder: NOPHN No. 1. In Fitzpatrick ML, ed: *The national organization for public health nursing, 1912-1952: development of a practice field,* New York, 1975, National League for Nursing, p. 27.

Orem D: *Nursing: concepts of practice,* ed 2, New York, 1980, McGraw Hill.

Riportella-Muller R, Selby ML, Salmon ME, Quade D, and Legault C: Specialty roles in community health nursing: a national survey of educational needs, *Public Health Nurs* 8:81-89, 1991.

Secretary of Health and Human Services: *Nursing sixth report to the President and the Congress on the status of health personnel in the United States, June, 1988,* NTIS Accession No. HRP-0907204, Springfield, Va., 1988, National Technical Information Service.

Shea S: Community health, community risks, community action, *Amer J Public Health,* 82(6):785-787, 1992.

Source Book, Nursing Personnel, December 1974, DHEW Publication No HRA 75-43, Bethesda, Md., 1975, U.S. Government Printing Office.

Surgeon General: *Healthy People: the Surgeon General's report on health promotion and disease prevention,* DHEW (PHS) Pub No 79-55071, Washington, D.C., 1979, U.S. Government Printing Office.

Turner J: Charter for health promotion, *Lancet* 2:1407, 1986.

U.S. Department of Health, Education, and Welfare: *Healthy people: the Surgeon General's report on health promotion and disease prevention,* Washington, D.C., 1979, Public Health Service.

U.S. Department of Health and Human Services: *Healthy People 2000: National health promotion and disease prevention objectives,* Washington, D.C., 1991, Public Health Service.

U.S. Department of Health and Human Services PHS, Health Resources and Service Administration: *1988: The registered nurse population. Findings from the national sample survey of registered nurses, March 1988,* Washington, D.C., The Department, June 1990.

Walcott-McQuigg J and Ervin NE: Stressors in the workplace: community health nurses, *Public Health Nurs* 9(1):65-71, 1992.

White MS: Construct for public health nursing, *Nurs Outlook* 30:527-530, 1982.

Williams CA: Community health nursing: what is it? *Nurs Outlook* 24:250-254,1977.

Winslow C-EA: *Man and epidemics,* Princeton, 1952, Princeton University Press.

World Health Organization: *Community health nursing,* 1974 WHO Expert Committee Report 558, Geneva, 1974, The Organization.

World Health Organization: *Alma-Ata 1978: primary health care: report of the International Conference on Primary Health Care,* Alma-Ata, USSR, Geneva, 1978, The Organization.

World Health Organization: *Four decades of achievement: highlights of the work of WHO,* Geneva, 1988, The Organization.

Zerwekh JV: Community health nurses: a population at risk, *Public Health Nurs* 9:1, 1992.

Selected Bibliography

Allen RJ and Allen J: A sense of community, a shared vision and a positive culture: care enabling factors in successful culture based health promotion, *Am J Health Prom* 1(3):40-47, 1987.

Archer SE: Synthesis of public health science and nursing science, *Nurs Outlook* 30:442-446, 1982.

Baldwin KA: The effectiveness of public health nursing services to prenatal clients: an integrated review, *Public Health Nurs* 6:80-87, 1989.

Barger SE: The nursing center. A model for rural nursing practice, *Nurs Health Care,* 12(6):290-294, 1991.

Becker M: The tyranny of health promotion, *Public Health Rev* 14:15-25, 1986.

Bernal B: Levels of practice in a community health agency, *Nurs Outlook* 26:364-369, 1978.

Consensus conference on the essentials of public health nursing practice and education, HRSA 84-564 (POLP), Rockville, Md., 1985, Health Resources and Services Administration.

Cross J, Northrop C, and Strasser J: How community health nurses spend their time, *Nurs Health Care* 4:314-317, 1983.

Culleton HF: Prisons. Logical innovative clinical nursing laboratories, *Nurs Health Care* 12(6):300-303, 1992.

Duffy M and Pender N, eds: *Conceptual issues in health promotion: report of proceedings of a Wingspread Conference,* Racine, Wi., 1987, Sigma Theta Tau.

Goodstadt M, Simpson R, and Loranger P: Health promotion: a conceptual integration, *Am J Health Prom* 1(3):58-63, 1987.

Hanchett E: *Nursing frameworks and community as client: bridging the gap,* Norwalk, Ct., 1988, Appleton and Lange.

Hollen P: A holistic model of individual and family based on a continuum of choice, *Adv Nurs Sci* 3(3):27-42, 1981.

Maglacas AM: Health for all: nursing's role, *Nurs Outlook* 36:66-71, 1988.

McKay R and Segall M: Methods and models for the aggregate, *Nurs Outlook* 31:328-334, 1983.

McLaughlin JS: Toward a theoretical model for community health programs, *Adv Nurs Sci* 4(2):7-28, 1982.

McNaughon Dunn A, and Decker SD: Community as client: appropriate baccalaureate and graduate-level preparation, *Journal of Community Health Nursing* 7:3, 131-139, 1990.

Salmon ME: Public health nursing . . . the neglected specialty, *Nursing Outlook* 37:5, 226, 1989.

Salmon ME, Riportella-Muller R, and Selby ML: Public health nursing education: a call for action, *Public Health Nurs* 8(2):68-73, 1991.

Shamansky SL and Clausen CL: Levels of prevention: examination of the concept, *Nurs Outlook* 28:104-108, 1980.

Shoultz JA, Harcher PA, and Hurrell M: Growing edges of a new paradigm: the future of nursing in the health of the nation, *Nurs Outlook* 40(2):57-61.

Sills G and Goeppinger J: The community as a field of inquiry in nursing. In Werley H and Fitzpatrick JJ, eds: *Annual Review of Nursing Research* ed 3, New York, 1985, Springer, pp. 4-23.

Smith JA: The idea of health: a philosophical inquiry, *Adv Nurs Sci* 3(3):43-51, 1981.

Smith JB: Levels of public health, *Public Health Nurs* 2:138-144, 1985.

Stevens PE and Hall JM: Applying critical theories to nursing in communities, *Public Health Nurs* 9(1):2-6, 1992.

Walker B: The future of public health: the Institute of Medicine's 1988 report, *J Public Health Policy* 10:19-31, 1989.

Whall AL: The family as the unit of care in nursing: a historical review, *Public Health Nurs* 3:240-249, 1986.

Witt BS: The homeless shelter, *Nurs Health Care* 12(6):304-307, 1991.

Unit Two

The Community and Its Health, Welfare, and Environmental Resources

73

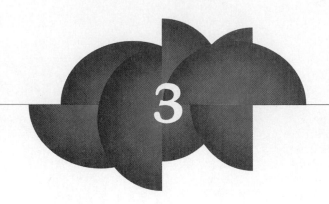

Community as Client

OBJECTIVES

Upon completion of this chapter, the reader should be able to:

1. Define the term *community.*
2. Discuss the meaning of community-as-client.
3. Describe the service areas of a community.
4. Discuss the functions of a community.
5. Discuss community dynamics.
6. Define the term *aggregate.*
7. Discuss the Healthy Cities Initiative.
8. Discuss some health problems of rural communities.
9. Differentiate between a community's normal line of defense and its flexible line of defense.
10. Discuss the relevance of community assessment to community health nursing practice.

There can be no health without community: that sense of mutual values and goals held by people regardless of geographic boundaries and their collective responsibility for nurturing their biophysical environment.

DR. NANCY MILIO (1990)

As previously discussed in Chapter 2, the uniqueness of community health nursing practice lies in the fact that nurses in this specialty area care for the "community." Community health nurses are committed to working with community residents to promote the health of all segments of the population. They view the community as client and work toward ensuring "health for all," a concept that promotes equal access to health services for everyone.

The importance of the community-as-client concept has long been recognized in community health nursing practice. Lillian Wald and other early community health nursing leaders realized that health problems, and their solutions, were deeply embedded in the structure of the community. These leaders promoted the idea that the dominant responsibility of the community health nurse was to the population as a whole (ANA, 1980; National Organization of Public Health Nurses, 1975). Today this responsibility to the population as a whole has been integrated into the American Nurses Association's definition of community health nursing practice and the American Public Health Association's definition for this specialty area (refer to Chapter 2). Nursing interventions in the community historically have focused on health promotion and disease prevention.

In its definition of community health nursing, the American Nurses Association has said that nursing efforts to promote and maintain the population's health entail the understanding and application of (1) concepts of public health and community; (2) skills of community organization and development; and (3) nursing care of selected individuals, families, and groups for health promotion, health maintenance, health education, and coordination of care (ANA, 1986, p. 1). This chapter addresses the concept of community, community dynamics, and nursing care of aggregates in the community.

Conceptualizing community-as-client can be difficult for the nurse. In acute care settings nurses often provide services to individuals and families, but not so often to aggregates or communities. The purpose of this chapter is to help the nurse develop an understanding of this concept. The concept of community is basic to public health practice and is a distinguishing feature of community health nursing (Turner and Chavigny, 1988, p. 118). Chapters 12 and 13 build on this understanding and discuss how community assessment, diagnosis, and health planning influence community health nursing practice.

DEFINING COMMUNITY

The word *community* has been in common use since its Latin origin as *communitas,* and there are no less than 100 definitions for the word *communis,* from which *community* was derived (Shamansky and Pesznecker, 1981, p. 182). Communities are frequently defined within one of two frameworks: (1) geographical area or (2) relational (McMillan and Chavis, 1986, p. 6).

Geographical definitions usually look at communities in terms of legal or geopolitical jurisdictions such as cities, towns, municipalities, or census tracts. In the United States, official public health services are offered through the geopolitical units of state and local governments.

Relational definitions are more abstract and examine how a group of people interacts to achieve common goals. Relational definitions are often more real for the populace, who frequently do not limit their personal definition of community to geographical boundaries. With relational definitions the boundaries of communities overlap and people often have membership in more than one community. An example of such overlapping boundaries is a person living in one community and working in another. This person has ties and relationships with both communities.

Health, social, urban, and political scientists have defined community from several different perspectives, and each perspective has merit and relevant applications (Lyons, 1988, p. 93). Nursing literature reveals diverse usages and definitions of the term community. It appears that no single definition of community can serve all its various contemporary applications (Bracht, 1990, p. 92). Characteristics that have emerged as being essential to a definition of community are (1) people, (2) social interaction, (3) area, and (4) common ties (Hillery, 1955, pp. 118-119; Wellman and Leighton, 1988, p. 58). People in a community share things in common such as land, history, culture, heritage, and even destiny (Moore, 1993).

A community is defined in a very broad sense as a

group of people living in an environment that has the ability to meet their major life goals and needs (e.g., food, shelter, and socialization). Sanders (1975, pp. 26-33; 1979; pp. 412-433) has described a community as a place to live, a collection of people, and a social system. Warren (1988, Observation on the State, p. 84) has described the community as a social system including people, spatial arrangements, shared institutions, interaction, and power structure.

The American Public Health Association (1991, p. 444) has said that the term community implies an entity from which the nature and scope of a public health problem, as well as the capacity to respond to that problem, can be defined; and that, depending on the problem area and response capacity, the definition of community may vary. According to the Association, for most instances of public health the community is defined as a geopolitical unit such as a town, city, or county.

The definition of community used in this text is the World Health Organization (WHO) definition that is incorporated into the American Nurses Association's (1986) *Standards of Community Health Nursing Practice.* This definition states that a "community is a social group determined by geographical boundaries and/or common values and interests; community members know and interact with one another; the community functions within a particular social structure; and the community creates norms, values, and social institutions" (WHO, 1974).

The American Community

The American community has been studied since the early 1900s. Early researchers on the American community were usually social scientists and included MacIver (1917), Hillery (1955), Sanders (1963), and Warren (1966). Many of these early studies have become classics in the field and are still cited in today's social science and nursing literature. Excerpts from these studies are included in this chapter. These early researchers recognized that there was a relationship between the community and the health of its members. One of them, Irwin T. Sanders, published in the community health nursing literature. His article "The Community: Structure and Function" appeared in *Nursing Outlook* (Sanders, 1963). For interested readers, *The Community: An Introduction to a Social System* (Sanders, 1958, 1966, 1975), *The Community in America* (Warren, 1963, 1972, 1978, 1987) and *Studying Your*

Community (Warren 1955, 1965) are considered classic works on the American community.

Early research on the American community focused on community as a *natural area.* This natural area is similar to the geographical definition of community mentioned earlier in this chapter. Contemporary research on community has been broadened to present a *natural network* approach (Hunter and Riger, 1986, p. 56). The natural network approach is more relational in nature and takes into account the widening scope of services and resources necessary to maintain the health and social well-being of a community in today's technological, complex, and diverse society. It creates an awareness of contemporary community health problems such as access to resources and resource distribution.

Communities as Social Units

Communities are social units that have characteristics similar to those of an individual person or family. In a community, people live together in such a way that they share not just a particular interest but the elements of a common life such as history, heritage, values, and culture (MacIver and Page, 1949, pp. 8-10).

A community is the basic unit of organization that transmits social and cultural values, beliefs, and attitudes to its members (Arensburg and Kimball, 1972, p. 15). It gives its members a sense of who they are and where they are going and perpetuates the culture and heritage of the community. These values, attitudes, and beliefs have an impact on the health care services in the community. For example, if a community does not value preventive health practices, and usually only seeks treatment for illness, it can be difficult to convince the families within it that immunizations and well-child health care services are necessary or important.

A community can be differentiated from other social units, such as groups, in that one's life can be lived within its bounds (MacIver and Page, 1949, pp. 8-10; Arensburg and Kimball, 1972; p. 17; Warren, 1978, p. 6). Being able to live one's life within its bounds is possible because of the various services and functions that the community carries out for its residents. Community service systems and functions are discussed later in this chapter under community dynamics.

The community has a life within which individuals define their own lives (Moore, 1993). It is where

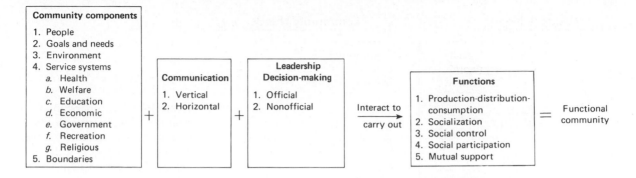

Figure 3-1 Community dynamics. (Service systems data from Sanders IT: *The community: an introduction to a social system,* ed 2, New York, 1966, Ronald Press. Communication and function data from Warren RL: *The community in America,* ed 2, Chicago, 1972, Rand-McNally, pp. 167, 237.)

people live, maintain their homes, earn their living, become educated, rear their children, and carry on day-to-day activities (Poplin, 1979, p. 8). A community is a setting for social action. As a setting for social action it can organize and mobilize its resources to promote health.

Communities as Part of a Larger Society

A community is part of, and has ties to, larger societies. These ties to the larger society are frequently on a county, state, regional, or national level. A community has patterns of communication and leadership that link it to the larger society and its resources. Patterns of communication and leadership are discussed later in this chapter.

In many communities health care resources are inadequate to meet the community's increasingly diverse health care needs, and people must go outside the community to the larger society to obtain the necessary health care. This is becoming increasingly evident in rural communities where health care resources are shrinking.

Community Autonomy

Some communities will have a greater sense of autonomy than others, and people will have varying degrees of loyalty to their communities. In some places a sense of community will exist, and in others it will not. The movement in the American community from natural area to natural network provides fertile ground for the loss of a sense of community within its

membership. Research has shown that a population base of 10,000 to 20,000 is preferred for maintaining a sense of community, that larger cities of up to 100,000 can still maintain this sense, and that cities or geographical areas larger than 100,000 often need to be broken down into target areas to maintain a sense of community and for effective health care delivery (Chamberlain, 1988, p. 302). This sense of community can be important in determining what health services are made available to community members.

COMMUNITY DYNAMICS

Community dynamics occur as a result of interactions within the community and between the community and the larger society. These interactions ultimately determine what public health services are offered in the community and the level of community health.

The dynamics of a community result in community action, change, and development and will determine the community's ability to promote health (Turner and Chavigny, 1988, p. 17). Critical to these dynamics are interactions between the community's people, goals and needs, environment, service systems, patterns of communication, leadership, and community functions.

Figure 3-1 is a flow chart illustrating how these elements work together to create a functional community. The figure summarizes the information on community dynamics presented in this chapter and assists the reader in visualizing and conceptualizing the discussion that follows.

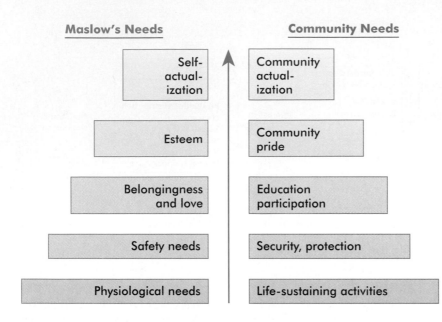

Maslow's Needs	Community Needs
Self-actualization	Community actualization
Esteem	Community pride
Belongingness and love	Education participation
Safety needs	Security, protection
Physiological needs	Life-sustaining activities

Figure 3-2   A comparison of Maslow's identification of basic needs of the individual with those of the community as a client. (From Higgs ZR and Gustafson DD: *Community as client: assessment and diagnosis,* Philadelphia, 1985, FA Davis, p. 12.)

Components of a Community

Communities have the common components of people in terms of shared goals, needs, and common life, and place in terms of environment, service systems, and boundaries. The community components of communication and leadership are discussed separately in relation to their unique impact on community dynamics. The nurse needs to be aware that the composition of these components will vary from community to community. Each community is unique.

People are a community's most important resource: they are its essence. People give the community its identity. They have responsibilities to the community and the community has responsibilities to them.

People have shared values that are an integrative force for cohesive, functional communities (McMillan and Chavis, 1986, p. 13). As these values change the community changes. Community health nurses need to be aware of, and respect, the values and attitudes that are part of the community in which they work. This is important to remember, especially when the nurse is working in culturally diverse communities.

In addition, knowledge of basic community population characteristics such as age, sex, ethnic origin, income level, and educational level is essential for the nurse to accomplish effective community health planning and action. Within communities, people will cluster or separate based on these characteristics, and they can influence the health status and needs of the community. For example, it has long been shown that people who live in poverty have poorer health status than those who do not. Also, by analyzing a community in relation to age distribution, the nurse would become aware that a community of predominantly school-age children and their families have different health care needs than a community of predominantly senior citizens. The *Community Assessment* in Chapter 12 gives specific assessment parameters to use in gathering data on the people of a community.

Goals and needs of a community are determined by its people. Each community will have community health goals and needs; however, it may not have the resources to meet them. In general, community health goals and needs follow Maslow's hierarchical order of basic needs (Meneshian, 1988, p. 116; Higgs and Gustafson, 1985, p. 12). Figure 3-2 shows a comparison of Maslow's hierarchical order of needs and the community's hierarchical order.

People often associate with others whose skills or competence can help them achieve their goals and needs (McMillan and Chavis, 1986, p. 13). Community health nurses' skills and competence make them a valuable resource in helping the community to assess, set, and achieve its health goals. The nurse can also serve as an advocate for the community in obtaining the health care resources and services necessary to achieve these goals.

Community environment has physical, biological, and sociocultural components. These components combine to make each community unique and have a major impact on the overall health of the community.

The *physical environment* of the community includes the geography, climate, terrain, natural resources, and structural entities (buildings such as schools, workplaces, and homes). The *biological environment* of the community includes various flora, fauna, bacteria, viruses, molds, fungi, toxic substances, and food and water supplies.

The *sociocultural environment* of the community reflects culture, values, attitudes, and demographic characteristics of the people of the community. As addressed in this chapter, it is an extremely important aspect of the community and significantly influences health care decision-making (Dean, 1986, p. 545).

The community's environment has a major impact on community health. For example, in many rural communities well water is the only source of fresh water. If children in these communities do not have regular, preventive dental fluoride treatments, they may develop serious dental problems. On a larger scale, environmental health concerns such as contaminated food and water supplies, air pollution, and toxic chemicals in landfills pose serious problems to public health. Environmental health concerns for the community health nurse are discussed in depth in Chapter 6.

Service systems of a community help its citizenry meet basic needs of daily living as well as special health and welfare needs. These service systems are represented by a multiplicity of agencies and organizations aimed at meeting some community need (Cottrell, 1977, p. 546). If there is a gap within a community service system, mechanisms should exist within the community to assist its members in finding the service elsewhere. In this way a "community of solution" is developed.

Sanders (1966, p. 170) viewed the major service systems of the community as (1) health, (2) social welfare, (3) educational, (4) economic, (5) governmental, (6) recreational, and (7) religious. Community service systems have the following identifiable characteristics (Sanders, 1966, pp. 175-180):

- A structure comprising a network of agencies, organizations, and establishments that frequently can be viewed as subsystems
- A set of functions, both manifest and latent
- Ideology or rationale, which provides the justification for the continuation of the system
- Norms and standardized procedures (standards of right and wrong)
- Functionaries, people charged with the responsibility of watching out for the interest of the system
- Paraphernalia, or the materials, resources, and artifacts required for system operation.

These community service systems form a network of resources that deliver services to community members. Each system is important and will in some way affect health. Not all systems have equal importance within the community, and they can become out of balance with one another. An example of this occurs when local government becomes so powerful that it uses a disproportionate amount of the tax dollars—tax dollars needed by other community systems such as education or health (Poplin, 1979, p. 167). Once this system equilibrium has been disturbed, it may never be restored, or it may take years to recover.

Community systems are extremely important to the community health nurse, because it is through them that services are provided to individuals, families, and aggregates. The nurse should assess all community systems, identify their resources and services, discover how each fits into the overall structure of the community, and then know how to utilize them effectively. All community systems are essential for maintaining and promoting community wellness.

Preserving and promoting the public's health is a major responsibility of the health care system. The health system is the central focus for the community health nurse. However, the economic system (economic sufficiency) has long been recognized as the usual focus for the citizenry and leadership of the community (National Commission on Community Health Services, 1966, p. 7). Until a community's basic economic needs are met, it is not likely that people will work diligently on other needs, such as health.

Boundaries of a community serve to regulate the exchange of energies between the community and its external environment. In general, boundaries may be *concrete* (definite, spatial) or *conceptual* (elusive, nonspatial). Concrete boundaries are more absolute and easier to see and to define. They include geographical boundaries (mountains, valleys, and deserts), political boundaries (cities, towns, counties, states, and nations), situational boundaries (home, school, and work), and combinations of these. For example, the service areas of many local health departments are

TABLE 3-1 Types of Community Leaders

Type	Basis for leadership	Area of authority	Examples
Institutional	Occupies a formal leadership position in the community and is elected or appointed to his or her post	Confined to routinized community actions	Mayor, city council, school principal, ministers, and labor union officials
Grassroots	Has personal influence and the ability to get other people interested in a "cause"	Confined to community actions of a spontaneous and/or initiated nature	Opponent of school desegregation, or leader of a campaign against water fluoridation
Power elite	Has wealth, economic power, and/or personal influence	Makes his or her influence felt in all areas of community action and decision-making	Wealthy business person, or top-echelon employee of a commercial, banking, or industrial firm

From Poplin DE: *Communities*, New York, 1979, Macmillan, p. 216.

determined by the geopolitical boundaries of cities, towns, or counties.

Conceptual boundaries are less definite and more relational in nature. They often do not fit into a neatly defined space. They include boundaries such as interest-area, problem-solving, or service-area boundaries, social ties, or social interactions. Service-area boundaries are of special interest to the community health nurse in relation to public health. For example, it is not uncommon for community health nurses to discover multiple service-area boundaries when working in rural settings. People in rural communities will often need to use health resources in the larger cities close to them. The nurse must remember that as the health goals and needs of a community change the service-area boundaries of the community change with them, and that these boundaries are flexible, dynamic, and ever-changing. Service-area boundaries for a community may cross several city and county boundaries.

Many public health services in the United States are provided through local health departments and appropriated strictly on the basis of a concrete boundary: residence in a geopolitical jurisdiction such as a city or county. Community health nurses working in these health departments must remember that even though their service area may be a specified geopolitical area, that area may not reflect "the community" for the populace.

Community Communication Patterns

Communities have both horizontal and vertical patterns of communication (Warren, 1978, pp. 163-164). *Vertical patterns* of communication link the community to the larger society (state, national, and international); *horizontal patterns* of communication link the community to its people, environment, and systems. The strength, cohesiveness, and ease with which these patterns operate will largely determine the extent to which the community is able to be self-sufficient and provide for the needs of its membership. The horizontal patterns of communication are especially important, because they influence the internal dynamics of the community. This communication within the community transmits community culture, tradition, values, and attitudes from generation to generation and helps to preserve the community.

Community Leadership

The leadership and decision-making processes within a community critically influence how well that community will function. Table 3-1 presents a summary of types of community leadership.

The community usually has elected and appointed leadership (official, institutional) such as a mayor or city council. This leadership is obvious to community members and other communities. However, much of a community's leadership is nonofficial.

Nonofficial community leadership is less obvious and may be more difficult to detect. However, this leadership often has more influence, power, and control over community action and decision-making than the elected, official leadership. In Table 3-1 nonofficial community leadership is represented as "grassroots" and "power elite."

The local community religious leader to whom people often go for advice and guidance and the wealthy philanthropist who heavily subsidizes community health activities are examples of nonofficial leaders. Nonofficial leaders are often the "heroes" of the community, those whom people in the community revere and respect. It is frequently laypeople in the community to whom others turn naturally for advice, emotional support, and assistance in daily living that can influence others to modify their health behaviors (Wiist and Flack, 1990, p. 381). The use of these natural helpers in health education activities can aid in the adoption of health promotion behaviors (Wiist and Flack, p. 381).

The community health nurse will find it useful to identify community leadership when doing an assessment of the community. This leadership needs to be assessed by the nurse because community leaders greatly influence what type of services will be available for community residents. The nurse should be aware of official leaders and their health and welfare responsibilities within a community, and the nonofficial leaders as well. Knowing these leaders and their patterns of functioning can facilitate the implementation of health care services in the community. An example of such facilitation is a research study by Wiist and Flack (1990) that showed how the support of religious leaders in a community made a large-scale cholesterol education program possible and successful. Nurses need to work with community leadership to foster community health care programs (Farley, 1993, p. 244).

Also, different community systems may have some form of leadership or authority over another. For example, the religious system may influence the health practices of its members. The religious practices of fasting, eating or not eating certain foods, and prohibiting the use of certain health care services, such as general medical care, blood transfusions, and family planning methods, are examples of how religious beliefs make an impact on the health care delivery system.

Many aspects of community life are in part controlled by leadership decisions made outside the community. These decisions are frequently in the form of state and federal laws and regulations. The community must adhere to such legal decisions even though they may be in conflict with its ideology.

Community Functions

In order to provide for the life goals and needs of its population, the community carries out a number of functions. Warren (1978, pp. 171-212) gives the following functions of a community:

1. *Production-distribution-consumption.* The community produces, distributes, and utilizes goods and services that are essential for meeting the health and welfare needs of its residents. This triad of activities provides opportunities that help community residents carry out activities of daily living, and it involves extensive resource coordination. Establishing and supporting local companies and businesses is an integral part of this function, because community residents need employment to meet their basic needs (food, clothing, and shelter) and the community needs funds from taxes to maintain its systems. Tax funds from industry and business significantly contribute to the economic stability of a community.

2. *Socialization.* This is the process by which prevailing knowledge, values, beliefs, customs, and behavior are transmitted to a community's members. It is a lifelong process that helps persons learn how to effectively relate in a social environment and to develop a philosophy of life. Educational services for the populace are included here.

3. *Social control.* The community influences the behavior of its members through norms and rules of social control. Social control has a legal component that is often enforced through law agencies, courts, and the government. It also has a social sanction component that is enforced by the family, neighborhood residents, friends, and the educational, religious, and recreational systems. Social control helps to safeguard and protect the community by providing mechanisms for safety and order.

4. *Social participation.* People have basic needs for self-expression and self-fulfillment. These

needs are largely met through interaction with others. Social participation is primarily carried out through the community's private sector. This function provides opportunity for members of the community to achieve psychosocial wellness, communication, social interaction, and support. Social networks evolve through social participation.

5. *Mutual support.* This involves people lending assistance to one another. It is frequently offered through family, friends, neighbors, and religious groups, as well as official health departments and departments of social service within the community.

These functions provide for the services and activities necessary for community life. The way in which a community carries out all of its functions makes an impact on how well the community health nurse will be able to meet the needs of the population. For example, if there is a gap in production-distribution-consumption, the community may not have the health resources to meet the health needs of its population. If people have not been socialized to value preventive health care, or if they have customs (such as religious fasting) that affect the delivery of health care services, the nurse's ability to implement preventive health care services can be hindered. If community health policy is inadequate, or if the health policy is not enforced, the health of the community may be in jeopardy. If the members of the community do not value social interaction and participation, the community's response to clinics, classes, and group activities may not be maximized. If a community does not offer much mutual support, there may be few health and welfare assistance programs for community members in need of them.

THE FUNCTIONAL COMMUNITY

Figure 3-1 illustrates that many forces interact to establish a functional, healthy community. According to Warren (1988, The good community, pp. 413-418) a functional community is one in which people interact (primary group relationships), participate, and have a degree of commitment to the community; the community has some autonomy from the larger society; people can confront their problems through concerted action (viability); decision making is relatively equally distributed throughout the population and not concentrated (power distribution); there is a balance of differences (degree of heterogeneity); and the degree of conflict is manageable.

Cottrell (1977, pp. 549, 554) has cited the variables of commitment and participation as necessities for a competent, functional community. Cottrell (pp. 551-556) further discussed the need of each segment of the community to be aware of its own interests and of how these relate to the interests of other elements (self-other awareness); the ability of each segment of the community to articulate its views, attitudes, needs, and intentions in relation to itself and the community at large (articulateness); the ability of the community to communicate with itself and the larger society (communication); the ability of the community to manage its relations with the larger society; and the ability of a community to utilize appropriate decision-making and leadership approaches so as to be representative of its membership. Communities with these characteristics can more successfully deal with stressors in their environment.

Community stressors are tension-producing stimuli that have the potential to cause disequilibrium and can result in disruption in the community (Anderson, McFarlane, and Helton, 1986, p. 221). Stressors often arise when service systems are unable to provide the necessary services for effective community functioning. An example of this is the inability of a community to maintain a tax base sufficient to adequately operate the local health department, or an absence of health care services to senior citizens. The reaction to these stressors may be reflected in community health statistics such as morbidity and mortality rates (Anderson, McFarlane, and Helton, 1986, p. 221).

A functional community can identify, prioritize, and address community needs and stressors. It provides health interventions at all three levels of prevention: primary, secondary, and tertiary. Such a community is capable of problem-solving and crisis resolution (Turner and Chavigny, 1988, p. 117). It maintains a high degree of system equilibrium while promoting growth and development.

AGGREGATES IN THE COMMUNITY

A community is made up of various aggregates. As discussed in Chapter 2, aggregates are groups of persons who have one or more shared personal or environmental characteristics (refer to Figure 3-3). The community health nurse's role in providing services to aggregates, based on age-related developmental tasks

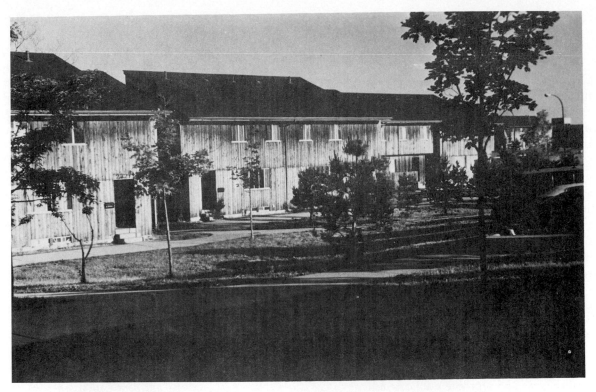

Figure 3-3 Residents of a university housing project for married students form an aggregate of persons who have shared personal and environmental characteristics. The environmental characteristics should not be overlooked, because people are identified according to the characteristics they share by living in a particular geographical area. Married students in university housing are frequently seen as an aggregate at risk, because they can experience multiple stresses such as crowded living conditions, financial difficulties, and educational pressures.

and at-risk characteristics, is discussed throughout this text.

By using the developmental approach, the community health nurse can assess the health needs of all individuals and groups within the community and can identify health promotion activities needed for people across the lifespan. Within this developmental framework, this text assists the reader in looking at services to aggregates such as preschool children, school-age children, adults, and the elderly. Examples of other aggregates in the community addressed in this text are workers, adults who are handicapped, people with long-term care needs, persons with AIDS, teenage parents, homeless individuals and families, victims of domestic violence, individuals and families living in poverty, disadvantaged groups, and ethnic and racial minority groups.

The developmental approach is based on the theory that individuals develop in their own way, yet conform to a common developmental pattern. It postulates that failure to accomplish developmental tasks at the appropriate time makes subsequent development more difficult. Erikson's (1978) eight stages of the life cycle (infancy, early childhood, play age, school age, adolescence, young adulthood, adulthood, and senescence) have been used widely in nursing and are integrated into the developmental framework for this text.

Community health nurses can use the developmental framework as a foundation for identifying existing or potential problems and determining health programs needed in a community for a particular developmental aggregate. For example, a major developmental task of aging is to adjust to changing sensory perceptions and self-care capabilities. These changes may increase the aging person's need for health care services and appliances such as glasses, hearing aids, and walkers, and decrease that person's ability to handle activities of daily living. The community health nurse would also want to be active in ensuring that resources in the community exist to address these needs and that the client has access to these services.

In these times of cost-containment it is much more cost-effective to serve a group of people than it is to visit people on an individual basis. Assessing and planning services for these aggregates at risk in the community are discussed in Chapters 12 and 13. Working with groups in the community is discussed in Chapter 21. A recent strategy, the Healthy Cities initiative, is one process to help ensure the health of aggregates in the community.

HEALTHY CITIES INITIATIVE

Two thirds of the world's populations live in cities (Flynn, 1993, p. 15). The Healthy Cities initiative is rather self-explanatory: its goal is to make cities healthier places and promote public health.

The Healthy Cities initiative had its origins in Canada in 1984 and was endorsed by the Canadian Public Health Association. In 1986, the World Health Organization actively endorsed the program as part of its overall move toward "Health Care for All," and designated the first 11 European cities that would participate in the program (Kickbusch, 1989, p. 77). From Europe the initiative spread to other cities in the United States, Canada, and Australia. We can be proud that in the United States the initiative has been led by community health nurses. The box on p. 85 lists the cities in the United States where a Healthy Cities initiative is in place.

A healthy city is defined as a city that is "continually creating and improving those physical and social environments and expanding those community resources which enable people to mutually support each other in performing all the functions of life and in developing to their maximum potential" (Hancock, 1987, p. 2; Hancock and Duhl, 1986). It creates supportive environments in which healthy living can occur (Flynn, Rider, and Ray, 1991, p. 332). Developing a city that promotes health requires the local creation of public policies that promote and enhance health, encourage health care for all, and work to reduce health inequities (Hancock, pp. 2-3). It also requires

coordination and communication between and within the governmental and private sectors.

Healthy Cities initiatives are designed to energize individuals to enact positive change and develop healthier communities through analysis, consensus, and social action (Flynn, 1993, p. 15). It enables and empowers local people to become more involved in the policy decisions that affect their future and create healthier cities (Flynn, Rider, and Bailey, 1992, p. 121). A major advantage to the Healthy Cities initiative is its ability to adapt to the unique needs of each community (Flynn, 1993, p. 18). The Healthy Cities initiative hopes to make major strides in promoting public health. Chapter 13 discusses the Healthy Cities initiative in relation to health planning.

Healthy Cities Indiana

The beginnings of Healthy Cities in the United States was the Healthy Cities Indiana project. This project is a collaborative effort between the Indiana University School of Nursing, Institute of Action Research for Community Health, Indiana Public Health Association, and six Indiana Cities (Flynn, Rider, and Bailey, 1992, p. 121). Dr. Beverly Flynn, a professor at Indiana University School of Nursing, is director of the Institute for Action Research for Community Health.

Flynn and Rider (1991, p. 510) state that the Indiana model of Healthy Cities emphasizes community leadership development in health promotion. The initiative supports local problem solving and action in health and the creation of supportive environments in which healthy living can occur. Flynn and Rider found that although community leaders exist in every city, they often do not know the potential they have for improving community health. The Healthy Cities initiative assists them in developing and acting on that potential.

In bringing community groups together to work toward community health, the project found that a major hurdle was for those involved to be concerned for the total community rather than their own special interests (Flynn, Rider, and Bailey, 1992, p. 123). The program fosters community awareness about health issues and helps place health as a priority on a city's or town's political agenda (Flynn, 1993, p. 15). The project has developed the Healthy Cities Indiana Resource Center to provide information about the program. The Healthy Cities Indiana initiative is

◄ *Healthy Cities on the Rise* ►

To date, there are more than 600 Healthy City initiatives taking place throughout the world, with the majority in Europe and Canada, and more recently in Africa, Australia and the United States. Interestingly, Healthy Cities currently is assisting in the democratization of Central and Eastern Europe.

The following cities and municipalities currently have initiated or adopted Healthy Cities programs within their communities:

Alaska	Anchorage	
California	Pittsburgh	Rohnert Park
	Santa Clarita	Pasadena
	Duarte	Monterey Park
	S. El Monte	Palm Desert
	W. Hollywood	Escondido
Colorado	Commerce City	Globeville
	Gunnison Basin	Las Animas County
	Mesa County	Montezuma County
	Northeast Colorado	Pueblo County
	Roaring Fork Forum	Delta and Montrose counties
	Telluride region	
	Gilpin County and the Nederland Mountain area	
	La Plata, San Juan and Archuleta counties	
Indiana	Clark County	Fort Wayne
	Gary	Indianapolis
	New Castle	Seymour
Iowa	Johnson County	
Massachusetts	Boston	
New Jersey	Atlantic City	
New Mexico	Mora County	Portalis
	Silver City	8 northern Indian pueblos
New York	Buffalo	
Pennsylvania	Philadelphia	

For further information on *Healthy Cities,* or how to bring the program to your community, write to: WHO Collaborating Center in Healthy Cities, Indiana University School of Nursing, 1111 Middle Drive, NU 236, Indianapolis, IN 46202, or phone (317)274-3319.

From Flynn BC: Healthy cities: the future of public health. Restructuring how we live, *Healthcare Trends and Transition* 4(3):16, 1993.

carried out in the following phases (Flynn and Rider, 1991, pp. 510-511):

Phase 1. City commitment

Phase 2. Formation of a Healthy Cities Committee

Phase 3. Community leadership involvement

Phase 4. City action

Phase 5. Provision of data base information to policymakers

Phase 6. Action research and evaluation

The box on p. 86 lists the different groups in each town that are represented in each Healthy Cities Indiana project. It is emphasized throughout these phases that community residents are active partici-

pants in the process, and strategies are used to empower the community to control decision making
(refer to Chapter 13).

The Healthy Cities initiative helps community
health professionals to address needs in diverse cultural communities. The Healthy Cities Committee
should have representatives from the predominant
cultural groups or aggregates residing in the community. With recent immigration patterns and demographic changes in the population, identifying the
cultural heritage of population groups in the community is imperative. Communities are becoming more
culturally diverse. The influence of cultural values,
attitudes, and beliefs on health practices in the community is discussed in Chapter 12.

Public health has long recognized the importance of
working with cities to resolve their problems (Hancock, 1987, p. 4). In the nineteenth century major
achievements in public health occurred in response to
the appalling health conditions in cities, and now the
new public health movement is focusing on improving
the health of cities (Hancock, p. 4). Public health helps
communities solve needs that are beyond any individual's ability to solve. For example, many health
problems are related to poverty and require community action to create new jobs, new housing, and
resources to assist families in dealing with their economic distress.

The Healthy Cities initiative demonstrates that

health is not just the responsibility of individuals or
health professionals, but is a mandate of the community as a whole (Flynn, 1993, p. 80). It will be interesting to watch the expansion of the Healthy Cities
initiative and its impact on public health across the
United States.

One important component of a city is neighborhoods. Since neighborhoods often form their own
culture, a Healthy Cities initiative must assess carefully which population groups or aggregates need to
be a part of the Healthy City Committee. To illustrate
the significant influence of neighborhoods on the
health of the community a discussion of neighborhoods follows.

Neighborhoods

Neighborhoods have a specific population and
boundaries and may provide resources to meet the
needs of residents, such as recreational facilities,
schools, and shops. A neighborhood is usually unable
to meet all the health and welfare needs of its population and must have ties with the larger community.
People may identify more closely with their neighborhood than with the community as a whole. Neighborhoods can be looked at in terms of interaction in the
neighborhood, identification with the neighborhood,
and connections outside the neighborhood (Warren
and Warren, 1975, pp. 72-76). Neighborhoods vary
greatly in leadership, cohesiveness, self-sufficiency,
and ties to the larger community. These neighborhood
variances play a significant role in relation to the health
services the community health nurse is able to provide
residents. Warren (1977, pp. 224-229) has elaborated
on the varying characteristics in neighborhoods by
using a classification schema to identify differences
between them; descriptions of these classifications are
given in the box on p. 87.

Identifying the type of neighborhood in which one
is working helps the community health nurse to assess
and plan for meeting health needs. For example, if a
community health nurse is working in a parochial
neighborhood, it would be imperative for her or him
to work closely with neighborhood leaders in the
delivery of health care services. The nurse may find
that the parochial neighborhood readily becomes
involved in providing services for its residents. However, there also may be more resistance in this neighborhood to health services proposed by the larger
community that do not coincide with neighborhood
values and beliefs. In an anomic neighborhood, on the

Classifications of Neighborhoods

Integral

The individuals in this setting have frequent face-to-face contacts. The norms, values, and attitudes of the neighborhood support those of the larger community. People are cohesive within the neighborhood but belong to other groups outside their area of residence. There is a form of power, authority, and leadership within this type of neighborhood which aids its members to reach out to the larger society for assistance when a problem arises that cannot be handled internally.

Parochial

People in this setting also have face-to-face contacts, but there is an absence of ties to the larger community. These neighborhoods tend to be protective of their status, to screen out values that do not conform to their own, and to enforce their own beliefs within the neighborhood. The power, authority, and leadership structure within this type of neighborhood encourages isolation from the larger community.

Diffuse

Neighbors within this type of environment interact infrequently with each other and have few ties with the larger community. There is often a lack of shared norms, values, and attitudes. A primary tie between these neighbors is geographic proximity to one another. There may be little or no leadership in these areas. When leadership exists, it is often not representative of the entire neighborhood, but is composed of an "elitist" leadership that ignores or subverts the values of most residents. Groups of residents, such as those living in a public housing unit, may be categorized and separated from the mainstream of the neighborhood.

Stepping-stone

This type of neighborhood is characterized by a rapid membership turnover and families who have a weak sense of identity with the neighborhood. Members are willing to give up the ties established in the neighborhood if other commitments arise; they strive to attain a higher social status. Residents of these areas do, however, have close ties to the larger community and do interact regularly with neighbors. Leadership is usually not effective because of the high rate of mobility; conflicts arise between the needs of the local neighborhood and the values of social mobility.

Transitory

Members of this kind of neighborhood fail to participate in or identify with the local community. There is an emphasis on people keeping to themselves, because links with others may interfere with the goals of the individual and the family. There may be a widespread feeling of mistrust in this type of neighborhood.

Anomic

Such a neighborhood is completely disorganized; its residents lack participation in and a common identification with the neighborhood or the larger community. This neighborhood reflects mass apathy and is not likely to influence or alter the values of its residents through any form of socialization. There is little interaction between people within the neighborhood or between the neighborhood and the larger community, and leadership activity is largely lacking.

Warren DI: Neighborhoods in urban areas. In Warren RL, ed: *New perspectives on the American community,* ed. 3, Chicago, 1977, Rand McNally, pp. 224-237.

other hand, the community health nurse may find little neighborhood leadership and may want to invest effort in developing this leadership to facilitate implementation of health care services. In addition, the nurse may find that the anomic neighborhood offers few services to its residents and that services need to be sought extensively from outside the neighborhood.

Whatever the type of neighborhood, its structure has implications for the activities of the community health nurse. Neighborhoods, as part of the commu-

nity, play an important role in providing for the needs of the population. Communities meet these population needs by carrying out specific functions.

RURAL VERSUS URBAN COMMUNITIES

Health care in rural America has been largely overlooked, and there is serious bias in resource allocation between rural and urban areas (Wakefield, 1990, pp. 83, 85). Until recently, little attention has been paid to the needs of at-risk groups in rural communities. An awareness of populations at risk and the general characteristics of rural communities will help the community health nurse differentiate them from their urban counterparts.

One in five rural Americans lives in poverty, and although the elderly account for 12% of the U.S. population as a whole they account for 25.4% of the rural population (Wakefield, 1990, p. 85). Rural communities are more sparsely populated than urban communities and often contain fewer health care resources, services, and practitioners. The number of rural hospitals declined 12% between 1980 and 1990 and is still declining (AHA study, 1990, p. 3). Over 9% of rural hospitals were closed in 1988 alone because of a shortage of registered nurses (Wakefield, p. 86). Rural areas have approximately one-half the physicians that urban areas do, and complicating this is the fact that many rural doctors are expected to retire or leave their practices by 1995 (Wakefield, p. 87). Additionally, rural shortages in public health professionals, psychologists, physical therapists, speech therapists, rehabilitation specialists, social workers, and other health care providers are drastically affecting the quality of health care available to rural communities.

Rural and urban areas also have differences in psychosocial characteristics and morbidity and mortality. A group of community health nurses became aware of this when they carried out a community assessment of adjacent rural and urban communities. The nurses assessed a rural county that included 760,000 people, or 578 people in each of its 1313 square miles. They also assessed an adjacent county that had 10,404 people in each of its 675 square miles and had a major industrial city.

The results of the community assessments surprised the community health nurses. The major health problem of the rural community was traffic deaths among males 16 to 24 years of age; the death rates for this age group were significantly higher than the death rates for the same age group in the urban community. After careful data analysis, reasons given for this were narrow, winding, two-lane roads with no shoulders; an image among the young rural males that fast cars were "macho"; no recreational facilities except bars; unlighted roads; and the necessity of driving very long distances to employment sites.

Rural communities are often more closely knit than urban communities, with many people on a first name basis with each other and having more frequent contact with community members. Conversely, urban communities are often known for the isolation that is evident when people living next to each other do not even know one another's names.

Rural communities are often classified on the basis of their dominant economic activity—farming, mining, or tourism (Poplin, 1979, p. 42). This activity often dominates community dynamics and action. Urban communities tend to have more diverse economic activity.

In some rural areas the tranquility of the environment (refer to Figure 3-4) can be deceiving; this tranquility makes health hazards less obvious. Statistics reveal that these environments are often not as healthy as they appear. Agricultural workers have some of the highest rates of occupational illness, injury, disability, and death in the nation. Also, coal mining communities often have high concentrations of workers with black lung disease and other respiratory diseases. These diseases may disable workers. Such conditions pose unique public health concerns for rural communities.

It is increasingly being recognized that many of our nation's rural areas have serious health problems that, because of the lack of needed health care resources and environmental surveillance, are not being resolved. The rural population groups most often in need of health services—farm workers, the poor, the elderly, persons with chronic illnesses, and migrant families—are often the ones with limited access to those services. The boxes on pp. 90 and 91 give some interesting facts and figures on health in rural communities and resources for information on rural health.

HEALTHY COMMUNITIES 2000

Healthy Communities 2000: Model Standards. Guidelines for Community Attainment of the Year 2000 National Health Objectives is a publication of the American Public Health Association (APHA, 1991). It assists U.S. communities in establishing achievable community health objectives in conjunction with the national health objectives in *Healthy People 2000*. Both documents are important to promoting community health and are discussed further in Chapter 5.

THE HEALTH SYSTEM AND THE COMMUNITY

The health system is a major community system. It consists of facilities, organizations, a work force, and

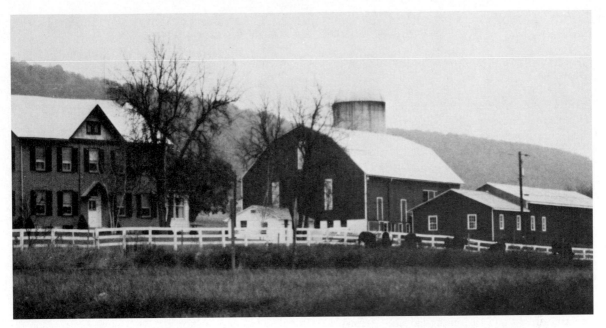

Figure 3-4   Some 60 million Americans, or 24% of the U.S. resident population, live in rural communities. Public health efforts need to be strengthened in these communities. Residents in rural settings are regularly exposed to environmental hazards such as pesticides, water pollution, soil pollution, and toxic chemicals. Many rural Americans lack access to regular and emergency health care services. The shortage of health care in rural communities presents serious problems for many rural Americans. (Photograph courtesy Henry Parks.)

funding to implement health care services. The health of a community depends on its ability to work toward common health goals and upon adequate distribution of health resources to all members (Hanchett, 1979, p. 46). Organized community effort to prevent disease and promote health is both valuable and effective (Committee for the Study of the Future of Public Health, 1988, p. 159).

The priority a community places on health varies and will affect health care resources and their distribution. Health care resources include individuals and groups or agencies, such as private health practitioners, volunteers, hospitals, clinics, pharmacies, nursing homes, health departments, and departments of social services.

Health resources are both governmental and private (refer to Chapter 4). Private-sector provision of health care services in the community is based on supply and demand and fee-for-service. The government (official) sector provides traditional public health services, such as communicable disease control, and preventive health services through official health de-partments at no or little cost to the consumer.

According to Anderson, McFarlane, and Helton (1986, p. 220), a community has a level of health reached over time that is called its *normal line of defense.* This line of defense can include characteristics such as high immunity and low infant mortality. They contrast this with the community's *flexible line of defense,* which represents a state of health that is more dynamic or in flux owing to temporary stressors such as environmental disasters and epidemics. It is important for the nurse to be aware of these normal and flexible lines of defense for community health, and to use the information for effective health planning, implementation, and evaluation.

The health service area for a community is the area within which a problem can be defined, dealt with, and solved (Ruybal, Bauwens, and Fasla, 1975, p. 365). A "community of solution" evolves. Within this health service area, the nurse must be familiar with the health needs of the people and available health resources and services. In order to meet client needs, the community health nurse often utilizes health resources outside the

◀ *Facts and Figures on Rural Communities* ▶

- Alcohol is by far the most widely abused drug in rural areas.
- Arrests for drug abuse violations in rural counties skyrocketed 54% from 1984 to 1988. In cities with a population of less than 100,000, arrests increased significantly, from close to 200,000 to 250,000.
- Prevalence rates for cocaine appear to be lower in rural than nonrural areas. Prevalence rates for other drugs, such as inhalants, may be higher in rural areas than elsewhere.
- Total alcohol and other drug abuse rates in rural States are about as high as those found in nonrural States.
- More than ever before, cocaine and heroin use is found in rural areas. Arrests for cocaine and heroin, two of the most highly addictive drugs, rose by almost 20% in rural areas between 1984 and 1988.
- Marijuana arrests are dropping but still outnumber cocaine arrests by 2 to 1 in rural areas.
- Most prison inmates in rural States have abused alcohol, other drugs, or both.
- Cocaine and opium have infiltrated the countryside. Cocaine and opium arrests have soared, increasing almost 20% in areas with populations under 100,000.
- Advertising has a strong influence on youth all over America. Consumer-oriented media messages glamorizing alcohol and tobacco reach rural youth as well as urban youth.
- Alcohol abuse treatment and arrests are higher in rural areas than in nonrural areas. In rural areas the rate is 1.4% and in nonrural areas it is 1.2%.
- Eighteen percent of rural youth are non-White, in contrast to 32% of urban youth. In rural areas, 82% of youth are White, 11% are African American, 5% are Hispanic, and 2% are Asian or other.
- Rural adolescents are less likely to be minorities, more likely to have both parents present, more likely to be poor in terms of absolute poverty levels, and more likely to live in the South.
- Rural children as young as 11 and 12 are drinking as many as 14 to 18 beers as part of their Friday and Saturday nights out. Excessive drinking by young people is extremely dangerous because alcoholism occurs far more quickly in children and adolescents and can take root in as little as 6 to 18 months.

- Snuff and chewing tobacco are being used more than ever before in rural areas by young men hoping to prove their "manhood." Many young men may begin using because of peer pressure and become addicted to the tobacco which causes mouth cancer, gum disease, and increased death rates.
- Rural areas may be ideal for manufacturing "crank," an extremely dangerous form of injectable methamphetamine which causes hallucinations, heart attack, and sometimes death. "Crank" is manufactured in rural, isolated labs where its strong odor cannot be detected.
- One third of rural children have had their first drink on their own by the age of 10 according to results of a survey conducted in one small middle-Atlantic town.
- It has been observed by several OSAP grantees that it is crucial that prevention occur in rural schools as opposed to other community settings because transportation is a hardship and youth are making their connections within school doors.
- Although males begin drinking earlier and drink more frequently than females, women are catching up quickly, according to a study of 650 students in one rural town. Close to one half of males have their first drink by age 10, while one fifth, still an extremely high number, of females do. By the age of 14, 82% of males and 80% of females have their first drink.
- For school-aged youth, the most powerful predictor of alcohol use is grade level. While 90% of 7th graders are light drinkers, by 12th grade, only 39% were light drinkers and 13% were heavy drinkers. Drinking in rural areas begins early and increases quickly.
- A survey of 600 junior and senior high school students in northwest Ohio revealed that 69% had used alcohol at least once and that 27% reported drinking four or more drinks at a sitting. Approximately 19% had driven under the influence of alcohol and 35% had ridden in a car with an intoxicated school-aged driver; 35% had refused a ride from a friend who was intoxicated, while 43% had tried to stop a drunk friend from driving.
- Rural youth in Michigan and Wisconsin were found to use alcohol at about three and a half times the rate of the national average for similar age groups.

Modified from USDHHS: *Prevention resource guide: rural communities,* Rockville, Md., 1991, USDHHS, pp. 1-3.

confines of a political jurisdiction. For instance, she or he may refer families to a medical center in another area, because the medical care needs of these persons cannot be met by local community resources.

Difficulties in the Community Health System

When the nurse analyzes the community's health system, there are several concerns that may become apparent. Communication between the health care system and the other community systems has historically been weak (refer to Chapter 5). In many communities, official local health departments have little contact with private health care resources and other official health and welfare resources. The health system of the community also may have little direct communication with the people of the community. The Healthy Cities initiative is trying to bridge these communication gaps.

No one agency has statutory (legal) responsibility for coordinating the health resources and services in the community, and thus the responsibility for management of these resources is often vague. Having one agency whose major role is to coordinate health services and to function as a health information center for the community could facilitate more effective delivery and utilization of community health resources. Local health departments are an excellent source of information on the health resources of a community.

Not only is the overall management of the health system weak, but the management skills of individual health practitioners may also be weak. Health practitioners frequently have not had educational experiences that prepare them to manage health care resources (refer to Chapter 22). Health care professionals must understand the principles of management if the health care system is to exist and carry out its functions effectively (National Commission on Community Health Services, 1966, p. 134).

Another problem community health nurses frequently experience is the community's adherence to traditional stands on health. American communities have historically reacted better to disaster and catastrophic health events than to providing ongoing, preventive community health services. There is usually general indifference to a health problem as long as no serious or long-term effects are apparent (Smolensky, 1982, p. 68). The feeling within the community

◀ *Rural Health* ▶
Information Resources

National Rural Health Association
301 E Armour Boulevard, Suite 420
Kansas City, MO 64111
(816) 756-3140
Robert Van Hook, Executive Director

Rural Information Center
U.S. Department of Agriculture
National Agricultural Library
10301 Baltimore Boulevard
Beltsville, MD 20705-2351
1-800-633-7701
(301) 344-5077

Office of Rural Health Policy
5600 Fishers Lane
Room 1422
Rockville, MD 20857
(301) 443-0835

ERIC Clearinghouse on Rural Education and Small Schools
Appalachia Educational Laboratory
1031 Quarrier
P.O. Box 1348
Charleston, WV 25325-1348
1-800-624-9120

that the responsibility for health concerns rests with official health departments, private health care practitioners, and health care facilities deters community involvement in health. This is unfortunate, because "health is a community affair" (National Commission on Community Health Services, 1966). Once again, the Healthy Cities initiative is trying to encourage communities to initiate health promotion activities instead of clinging to traditional treatment-oriented activities.

The community may not actively support health activities. This can occur for a variety of reasons, including other community priorities, a lack of information on health issues and resources, and a lack of understanding about the role the community can play in establishing and promoting positive health practices for its membership. The health system often does not include the community in health planning, implementation, and evaluation. Increased cooperation and collaboration between the community and the health care delivery system is needed; an appreciation of all aspects of health, as well as a plan to meet future health needs, could evolve from such efforts.

The National Commission on Community Health Services (1966) issued the following goals for community health systems that are still to be fulfilled:

All communities of this nation must take the action necessary to provide comprehensive personal health services of high quality to all people in the community. These services should embrace those directed toward promotion of positive good health, application of established preventive measures, early detection of disease, prompt and effective treatment, and physical, social, and vocational rehabilitation of those with residual disabilities. This broad range of personal health services must be patterned so as to assure full and intelligent use by all groups in the community.

Success in this endeavor will mean change. It will require removal of racial, economic, organizational, residential, and geographic barriers to the use of health services. It will require strengthened and expanded licensure and accreditation of services, manpower, and facilities. It will require maximum coverage through health insurance and other prepayment plans, and extension of such insurance to cover the broad range of services both in and out of hospitals. Finally, success will require citizenry that is sufficiently well informed and motivated to follow established principles conducive to good health services in all phases of prevention and treatment of illness and disability.

COMMUNITY ASSESSMENT FOR THE COMMUNITY HEALTH NURSE

The community health nurse is in the unique position of being able to see the community carry out its functions and activities on a day-to-day basis. Unlike many other health practitioners, the community health nurse is out in the community on a regular basis, working with its people and systems. She or he provides services in homes, schools, clinics, industry, and other settings and thus has multiple opportunities to collect data about community dynamics and to comprehensively assess the community. Chapter 12 addresses the community assessment process. Community assessment is briefly addressed here in relation to the concept of community-as-client.

Community Assessment

The Committee for the Study of the Future of Public Health (1988, p. 7) recommended that every public health agency regularly and systematically collect, assemble, analyze, and make available information on the health of the community. The community assessment process is often carried out by a multidisciplinary team of professionals, including nursing staff, in the local health department.

A community assessment provides a "window" through which to view the community. It provides the means for looking at community strengths, problems, and potential problems. It can identify aggregates at risk and gaps in community resources. It is the basis for community health planning and providing services to the community.

Various methods can be used to assess a community. It can be difficult for both neophytes and experienced professionals to collect all of the data that must be obtained when doing a community assessment. It is important to have assessment tools that help professionals to collect and organize community data. These tools will vary in their comprehensiveness.

A tool to assist the practitioner complete a brief assessment of the community is given in Appendix 3-1. This tool is based on a set of master categories that characterize community data (Stein and Eigsti, 1982). It provides observational information about a community's environment, mode of functioning, and social and health resources. Because community health nurses collect these data while driving through or walking around in a community, this form of community assessment has been termed a "windshield" survey of the community. A windshield assessment provides a beginning database about a community.

An in-depth, comprehensive assessment tool that assists health agencies to obtain a comprehensive profile of a community is presented in the appendix to Chapter 12. Other community assessment tools and frameworks from which nurses can assess the community are found in Allor (1983), Clark (1986), Edelman and Mandle (1990), Hanchett (1988), Martin (1988), Meneshian (1988), Rauckhorst, Stokes, and Mezey (1980), Rodgers (1984), and Ruffing-Rahal (1987). Through knowledge gained from a community assessment, the community health nurse has a data base for community diagnosis and health planning (refer to Chapters 12 and 13).

Summary

The community is not an easily or consistently defined entity. It is a nebulous, complex concept. However, it is within the confines of the community that nurses diagnose and solve health problems. Developing a conceptual understanding of the word *community* and how health problems are assessed and solved within the community is the first step in carrying out the unique responsibilities of the community health nurse.

Working with clients (individuals, families, aggregates at risk, and communities) becomes far more exciting when the community health nurse understands community concepts. This knowledge, coupled with flexibility in meeting the changing and diverse health needs of the community, facilitates the achievement of a high-level of community wellness. Understanding the concept of community-as-client helps the nurse to recognize the value of community-focused practice.

◀ *An Exercise in Critical Thinking* ▶

Look at the beginning of the chapter where the term *community* was defined and discussed. Conceptualize in your mind the community you lived in during high school or the community you live in now. Look at this community in terms of some of the major components of community dynamics, such as service systems, communication patterns, leadership, and community functions.

What were some of the major values held by this community? What were/are some of the major strengths of this community? What were some of the health needs of this community? How could a community health nurse build on these strengths and help meet these needs?

APPENDIX 3-1
University of Rochester School of Nursing: Categories for Recording Descriptive Community Data*

Find a place to eat in the community in which your caseload exists. After lunch, drive around or walk in the community in pairs, essentially observing on as many streets as possible for the following assessment categories, which are grouped according to community systems. Do not be concerned if all categories are not covered.

I. Physical environment
  A. Land use
    1. Open spaces (look for play areas, parks)
    2. Undeveloped space (vacant lots, fields)
    3. Residential space
      a. Single-family housing (note better or poorer housing)
      b. Multiple-family housing
    4. Commercial space
      a. Go into stores; note prices, atmosphere, selection

    b. Visit gas stations; find out where you could go for car repairs and gas, and what the costs are
    5. Industrial space
      a. Note location and condition
      b. Determine type of industry
    6. Water in area
      a. Note open ditches
      b. Stagnant water
      c. Bodies of water (lakes, rivers, or streams)
    7. Roads
      a. Note paved streets, condition
      b. Dirt roads, condition

*Areas currently found to be "essential" sources of data about communities. These areas are broad to allow you to add to or delete from categories, since some areas of community life may be of more concern than others in health assessment.
Modified from Christianson JZ: A community data base record (unpublished Master's of Public Health thesis), Houston, Tx, 1977, The University of Texas Health Science Center. In Stein KZ and Eigsti DG: Utilizing a community data base system with community health nursing students, *J Nurs Educ* 21:26-32, 1982.

Continued

University of Rochester School of Nursing: Categories for Recording Descriptive Community Data—cont'd

8. Boundaries
   a. Note any geographical boundaries which tend to separate communities, such as "the other side of the tracks"
9. Agriculture
   a. Note types of crops
   b. Note types of animals kept
B. Environmental status
   1. Sanitation
      a. Note debris, location
      b. Note garbage cans in area
      c. Waste disposal systems
   2. Air
      a. Note smell, color
      b. Note location of unusual odors
   3. Note utilities—note availability of water, gas, public telephones, telephone lines, and electricity
   4. Household pets—where kept, what type?
   5. Topography and geology
      a. Note general topography of land
      b. Obstacles to travel and hazards (such as rock slides)
II. Social and behavioral environment
   A. Education

1. Note church or synagogue schools: how many are there, what condition are they in? Types?
2. Alternative education systems: e.g., Montessori schools, encounter workshops, martial arts
B. Religion
   1. Locate churches, synagogues: How many are there, what condition are they in? Types?
C. Recreation and entertainment
   1. Movie house, auditoriums
   2. Bars—how many are there?
   3. Recreational centers
D. Health
   1. Services (clinics, hospitals, physicians)
   2. Status—do you get an overall impression of a "healthy" or "unhealthy" community? State rationale
E. Communications
   1. Public (radio, television)
   2. Informal: note "hangouts" and which groups congregate
F. Transportation and travel
   1. Availability and type of transportation
III. Government
   A. Note police protection: How are police transported?

References

AHA study reports changes, trends in 1980s, *Reflections* 16(2):3, 1990.

Allor MT: The "community profile," *J Nurs Educ* 22:12-17, 1983.

American Nurses Association, *Community Health Nursing Division: conceptual model of community health nursing,* Pub No CH-10, Kansas City, Mo., 1980, The Association.

American Nurses Association: *Standards of community health nursing practice,* St. Louis, 1986, The Association.

American Public Health Association: *Healthy communities 2000: model standards. Guidelines for implementing the year 2000 national health objectives,* Washington, D.C., 1991, The Association.

Anderson ET, McFarlane J, and Helton A: Community-as-client: a model for practice, *Nurs Outlook* 34:220-224, 1986.

Arensburg CM and Kimball ST: *Culture and community,* Gloucester, Ma., 1972, Peter Smith.

Bracht N: Health promotion at the community level, *Sage,* 1990, Newbury Park.

Chamberlain RW: *Beyond individual risk assessment: community wide approaches to promoting the health and development of families and children—conference proceedings,* Washington, D.C., 1988, National Center for Education in Maternal and Child Health.

Christianson JZ: A community data base record, Houston, Tx., 1977, unpublished Master of Public Health thesis, University of Texas Health Science Center.

Clark CC: *Wellness nursing: concepts, theory, research and practice,* New York, 1986, Springer, pp. 287-290.

Committee for the Study of the Future of Public Health-Institute of Medicine: *The future of public health,* Washington, D.C., 1988, National Academy Press.

Cottrell LS: The competent community. In Warren RL, ed: *New perspectives on the American community,* ed 3, Chicago, 1977, Rand McNally, pp. 546-560.

Dean PD: Expanding our sights to include social networks, *Nurs Health Care* 7:545-550, 1986.

Edelman CL and Mandle CL: *Health promotion throughout the lifespan,* ed 2, St. Louis, 1990, Mosby, pp. 139-143.

Erikson EH: *Childhood and society,* ed 2, New York, 1978, Norton.

Farley S: The community as partner in primary health care, *Nursing and Health Care* 14(5):224-249, 1993.

Flynn BC: Healthy cities: the future of public health. Restructuring how we live, *Healthcare Trends and Transition* 4(3):12-18, 80, 1993.

Flynn BC and Rider MS: Healthy cities Indiana: mainstreaming community health in the United States, *American Journal of Public Health,* 81(4):510-512, 1991.

Flynn BC, Rider MS, and Bailey WW: Developing community leadership in Healthy Cities: the Indiana model, *Nurs Outlook* 40(3):121-126, 1992.

Flynn BC, Rider MS, and Ray DW: Healthy cities: the Indiana model of community development in public health, *Health Education Quarterly,* 18(3):331-347, 1991.

Hanchett ES: *Nursing frameworks and community as client,* Norwalk, Conn., 1988, Appleton & Lange.

Hanchett ES: *Community health assessment,* New York, 1979, Wiley.

Hancock T: Healthy Cities: the Canadian project, *Health Promotion* 26(2):2-4, 27, 1987.

Hancock T and Duhl L: *Healthy Cities: promoting health in the urban context,* Copenhagen, 1986, WHO Europe.

Higgs ZR and Gustafson DD: *Community as client: assessment and diagnosis,* Philadelphia, 1985, FA Davis.

Hillery GA Jr.: Definitions of community: areas of agreement, *Rural Sociology* 20(2):118-120, 1955.

Hunter A and Riger S: The meaning of community in community mental health, *J Community Psychol* 14:55-71, 1986.

Kickbusch I: Healthy Cities: a working project and a growing movement, *Health Promotion* 4(2):77-82, 1989.

Lyons L: Choosing the best approach to the community. In Warren RL and Lyon L, eds: *New perspectives on the American community,* ed 5, Chicago, 1988, Dorsey Press, pp. 87-96.

MacIver RM: *Community,* London, 1917, MacMillan.

MacIver RM and Page CH: *Society: an introductory analysis,* New York, 1949, Rinehart.

Martin A: Community assessment: the cornerstone of effective marketing, *Pediatr Nurs* 14:50-53, 1988.

McMillan DW and Chavis DM: Sense of community: a definition and theory, *J Community Psychol* 14:6-23, 1986.

Meneshian S: Nursing assessment of a community. In Caliandro G and Judkins, eds: *Primary nursing practice,* Glenview, Ill., 1988, Scott, Foresman, pp. 111-118.

Milio N: Healthy cities: the new public health and supportive research, *Health Promotion International* 5(4):291-297, 1990.

Moore T: Conversation on the philosophy of community, Knoxville, Tennessee, June 29, 1993, University of Tennessee, College of Nursing.

National Commission on Community Health Services: *Health is a community affair,* Cambridge, Mass., 1966, Harvard University Press.

National Organization for Public Health Nursing (NOPHN): Constitution of the National Organization for Public Health Nursing, Article 2, 1912, Wald: New York Public Library folder: NOPHN No. 1. In Fitzpatrick ML, ed: *The National Organization for Public Health Nursing, 1912-1952: development of a practice field,* New York, 1975, National League for Nursing.

Poplin DC: *Communities: a survey of theories and methods of research,* ed 2, New York, 1979, Macmillan.

Rauckhorst LM, Stokes SA, and Mezey MD: Community and home assessment, *J Gerontol Nurs* 6:319-327, 1980.

Rodgers SS: Community as client—a multivariate model for analysis of community and aggregate health risk, *Public Health Nurs* 1:210-222, 1984.

Ruffing-Rahal MA: Resident/provider contrasts in community health priorities, *Public Health Nurs* 4:242-246, 1987.

Ruybal SE, Bauwens E, and Fasla MJ: Community assessment: an epidemiological approach, *Nursing Outlook* 23:365-368, 1975.

Sanders IT: *The community: an introduction to a social system,* New York, 1958, Ronald Press.

Sanders IT: *The community: an introduction to a social system,* ed 2, New York, 1966, Ronald Press.

Sanders IT: *The community: an introduction to a social system,* ed 3, New York, 1975, Ronald Press.

Sanders IT: The community: structure and function, *Nurs Outlook* 11:642-645, 1963.

Sanders IT: Health in the community. In Freeman HE, Levine S, and Reeder LG, eds, *Handbook of medical sociology,* ed 3, Englewood Cliffs, N.J., 1979, Prentice Hall, pp. 412-433.

Shamansky SL and Pesznecker B: A community is . . . , *Nurs Outlook* 29:182-185, 1981.

Smolensky J: *Principles of community health,* ed 6, Philadelphia, 1982, Saunders.

Stein KZ and Eigsti DG: Utilizing a community data base system with community health nursing students, *J Nurs Educ* 21:26-32, 1982.

Turner JG and Chavigny KH: *Community health nursing: an epidemiologic perspective throughout the nursing process,* Philadelphia, 1988, Lippincott.

United States Department of Health and Human Services: *Prevention resource guide: rural communities,* Rockville, Md., 1991, USDHHS.

Wakefield , MK: Health care in rural America: a view from the nation's capital, *Nursing Economics* 8(2):83-89, 1990.

Warren DI: Neighborhoods in urban areas. In Warren RL, ed: *New perspectives on the American community,* ed 3, Chicago, 1977, Rand McNally, pp. 224-237.

Warren RL: *Studying your community,* Chicago, 1955, Rand McNally.

Warren RL: *The community in America,* Chicago, 1963, Rand McNally.

Warren RL: *Studying your community,* Chicago, 1965, Rand McNally.

Warren RL: *Perspectives on the American community,* Chicago, 1966, Rand McNally.

Warren RL: *The community in America,* ed 2, Chicago, 1972, Rand McNally.

Warren RL: *The community in America,* ed 3, Chicago, 1978, Rand McNally.

Warren RL: *The community in America,* ed 4, Chicago, 1987, Rand McNally.

Warren RL: Observations on the state of community theory. In Warren RL and Lyon L, eds: *New perspectives on the American community,* ed 5, Chicago, 1988, Rand McNally, pp. 84-86.

Warren RL: The community in America. In Warren RL and Lyon L, eds: *New perspectives on the American community,* ed 5, Chicago, 1988, Rand McNally, pp. 152-157.

Warren RL: The good community—what would it be? In Warren RL and Lyon L, eds: *New perspectives on the American community,* ed 5, Chicago, 1988, Rand McNally, pp. 412-419.

Warren RL and Warren RB: Six kinds of neighborhoods, *Psychol Today* June 1975, pp. 72-76.

Wellman B and Leighton B: Networks, neighborhoods, and communities: approaches to the study of the community question. In Warren RL and Lyon L, eds: *New perspectives on the American community,* Chicago, 1988, Dorsey Press, pp. 57-72.

Wiist WH and Flack JM: A church-based cholesterol education program, *Public Health Reports* 105(4):381-388, 1990.

World Health Organization: *Community health nursing: report of a WHO expert committee,* Technical Report Series No. 558, Geneva, 1974, The Organization.

Selected Bibliography

American Nurses Association: *A guide for community-based nursing services,* Kansas City, Mo., 1985, The Association.

Anderson ET and McFarlane JM: *Community as client: application of the nursing process,* Philadelphia, 1988, Lippincott.

Archer SE and Fleshman RP: Community health nursing: a typology of practice, *Nurs Outlook* 23:358-364, 1975.

Braithwaite R and Lythcott W: Community empowerment as a strategy for health promotion for black and other minority populations, *JAMA* 261(2):282-283, 1989.

Brown RB: Community action for health promotion: a strategy to empower individuals and communities, *International Journal of Health Services* 21(3):441-456, 1991.

Buhler-Wilkerson K: Public health nursing: in sickness or in health? *Am J Public Health* 75:1155-1161, 1985.

Chalmers K and Kristajanson L: The theoretical basis for nursing at the community level: a comparison of three models, *J Adv Nurs* 14:69-574, 1989.

Colcord JC: *Your community,* New York, 1947, Russell Sage.

Drapo PJ, Patrick CR, and Kemp C: Addressing the needs of underserved populations in community health nursing education, *Public Health Nursing* 4(4):236-241, 1987.

Eigsti DG, Stein KZ, and Fortune M: The community as client for continuity of care, *Nurs Health Care* 3:251, 1982.

Eng W, Hatch J, and Callan A: Institutionalizing social support through the church and into the community, *Health Educ Q* 12:81-92, 1985.

Frost H: *Nursing in sickness and in health: the social aspects of nursing,* New York, 1939, Macmillan.

Goeppinger JE and Baglioni AJ: Community competence: a positive approach to needs assessment, *Am J Community Psychol* 13:507-523, 1986.

Hallman HW: *Neighborhoods. Their place in urban life,* Beverly Hills, 1984, Sage.

Heller K: The return to community, *Am J Community Psychol* 17:1-15, 1989.

Hanchett ES: *Nursing frameworks and community as client,* Norwalk, Conn., 1988, Appleton & Lange.

Jamieson MK: Block nursing: practicing autonomous professional nursing in the community, *Nurs Health Care* 11:250-253, 1990.

McKnight JZ: Regenerating community, *Social Policy* 54:54-58, 1987.

McLaughlin JS: Toward a theoretical model for community health programs, *Adv Nurs Sci* 5(1):7-28, 1982.

McMurray A: Advocacy for community self-empowerment, *International Nursing Review* 38(1):19-21, 1991.

Neufeld A and Harrison MJ: The development of nursing diagnoses for aggregates and groups, *Public Health Nursing* 7(4):251-255, 1990.

Nisbet RA: *The quest for community,* New York, 1953, Oxford.

Pender NJ, Barkauskas VH, Hayman L, Rice VH, and Anderson ET: Health promotion and disease prevention: toward excellence in nursing practice and education, *Nurs Outlook* 40(3):106-112, 1992.

Reiss AJ: The sociological study of communities, *Rural Soc* 24:118-127, 1959.

Schultz PR: When client means more than one: extending the foundational concept of person, *Adv Nurs Science* 10:71-86, 1987.

Selvy ML and Tuttle DM: Community health assessment and program planning in the nurse practitioner curriculum: evaluation of a guided design learning module, *Public Health Nurs* 4:160-165, 1987.

Sills GM and Goeppinger J: The community as a field of inquiry in nursing. In Werly HH and Fitzpatrick JJ, eds: *Annual review of nursing research,* vol 3, New York, 1985, Springer, pp. 4-23.

Steward M and White L: Nursing the community, *Canad Nurse* 77:32-33, 1981.

Stoner MH, Magilvy JK, and Schultz PR: Community analysis in community health nursing practice: the GENESIS model, *Public Health Nursing* 9(4):223-227, 1992.

Storfjell JL and Cruise PA: A model of community-focused nursing, *Public Health Nurs* 1:85-96, 1984.

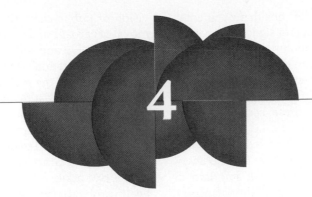

United States Health and Welfare Legislation and Services

OBJECTIVES

Upon completion of the chapter, the reader should be able to:

1. Summarize the development of health and welfare policy and legislation in the United States.
2. Discuss the purpose and mandates of significant health and welfare legislation in the United States.
3. Explain how the Social Security Act and the Public Health Service Act and their amendments have influenced health and welfare practices for half a century.

4. Discuss how health and welfare legislation affects community health nursing practice.
5. Discuss U.S. health care spending in relation to the Gross National Product (GNP).
6. Differentiate between private and governmental health and welfare services.
7. Explain methods of health care financing in the United States.
8. Give an overview of the welfare system in the United States.

Chapter 1 discussed the public health movement in the United States. This chapter is designed to create an awareness of the historical evolution of health and welfare *legislation* and *services* in the United States, as well as an understanding of current legislation and existing health and welfare programs. Chapter 5 will look at the organization of these services on the federal, state, and local levels.

The legislation and services discussed in this chapter help to ensure access to health care for all Americans, provide them with an adequate standard of living, and protect them from the possibility of income loss resulting from old age, unemployment, illness, or disability. Many clients with whom the community health nurse works use programs discussed in this chapter, such as Old Age, Survivors and Disability Insurance; Medicaid; Medicare; Aid to Families with Dependent Children; Supplemental Food Program for Women, Infants, and Children; Food Stamps; Unemployment Insurance; and Supplemental Security Income. Nurses need to be familiar with these programs, assist clients in using them, and understand that legislation influences the provision and availability of health and welfare services.

THE EVOLUTION OF HEALTH AND WELFARE PRACTICES

As was discussed in Chapter 1, health and welfare practices have evolved over time. Across civilizations, early public health habits focused on controlling communicable disease and prolonging life. Early societies used communicable disease control measures such as isolation (often in the form of quarantine or banishment), burial of the dead, and protection and conservation of food and water supplies.

Egyptians of 1000 BC were possibly the healthiest of all ancient civilized people (Pickett and Hanlon, 1990, p. 21). They had rigorous personal hygiene measures; isolation of lepers; elaborate sewage, drainage, and water supply systems; pharmaceutical preparations; and surgical treatments. The Romans practiced public health measures that included a periodic census; pro-

vision of public sanitation services including the removal of garbage and rubbish; protection of the public water supply; and supervision of public food and housing (Pickett and Hanlon, p. 22). It is known that as early as 1500 BC the Hebrews had a written hygienic code in *Leviticus* that dealt with personal and community hygiene (Pickett and Hanlon, p. 21).

Health and welfare practices and policies have continually changed to meet the demands and societal attitudes of the time. Throughout the history of public health, two major factors have determined how public health problems were solved: the level of scientific and technical knowledge, and the content of public values and popular opinions (Institute of Medicine, 1988, p. 1). Major improvements in the health of the American people have been accomplished through advances in scientific and technical knowledge, such as the development of antibiotics and immunizations and methods to ensure provision of safe food and water. Public values and popular opinions have greatly affected the passage of health and welfare legislation in this country and the provision of health and welfare services.

An examination of the historical evolution of health and welfare legislation and services in the United States demonstrates that their development has often been reactionary rather than preventive in nature. Historically, health and welfare programs are decentralized and operate at all levels of government and in the private sector. It was not until 1981 that U.S. national health objectives were developed. Today the President's Task Force on Health Care Reform is suggesting revisions that will shape health care in this country for decades to come.

Public health measures have prevented countless deaths and improved the quality of American life. Unfortunately, public health in the United States is often taken for granted, and areas in which we previously had made great strides, such as communicable disease control and infant mortality, are beginning to slip backward.

EUROPEAN INFLUENCE ON UNITED STATES HEALTH AND WELFARE POLICY

European influence has been singled out because of the significant impact it had on the development of United States health and welfare policy. Health and welfare policies in the United States reflect a background that is European, primarily English, in origin.

We are indebted to Professor Dorothy Donabedian, colleague and friend, whose efforts have stimulated both student and faculty awareness of the health and welfare systems as they apply to community health nursing practice. Her enthusiasm, encouragement, and suggestions in this work have been greatly appreciated.

Europe was not always a pacesetter in public health practices. Europeans of the Middle Ages (500-1500 AD) did not follow many of the health practices of previous times and cultures. They allowed refuse to accumulate in streets and dwellings, dumped human waste into public water supplies, improperly stored and prepared foods, often ignored personal hygiene, and practiced child labor. These practices did little to promote health; however, it is likely that they assisted in the development of European trade routes as the demand for perfumes and spices rose.

During this time epidemics of cholera, smallpox, typhoid, plague, and diphtheria raged. In the 1300s bubonic plague nearly exterminated the human race, reportedly killing up to one half of the world's population (Pickett and Hanlon, 1990, p.24). Epidemics of such magnitude have never been seen since, and public health practices evolved to control communicable diseases. At the time there was little governmental intervention in matters of public health.

During the Middle Ages the belief in *divine causation,* that conditions reflect the will and judgment of God, flourished and greatly influenced health and welfare policies and practices. Conditions such as poverty, illness, and disability were often viewed as having divine causation rather than societal causation. The sick, disabled, and poor were largely ignored as a public responsibility. *Self-help,* the responsibility of individuals or their responsible relatives to assume provision for care, was the prevailing policy. During this period poverty was often equated with crime, and beggars, vagrants, and the disabled could be physically punished or imprisoned. Welfare assistance was usually church-sponsored rather than government-sponsored. When assistance was given it was usually in the form of food and shelter rather than money. There was little governmental involvement in issues of public health and welfare. Governmental involvement was often more forced than voluntary. Economic depressions, wars, natural disasters, epidemics, the threat of government overthrow, and mass public indignation played an important role in shaping public policy. It was an economic depression that brought about the Elizabethan Poor Law of 1601.

The Elizabethan Poor Law of 1601

A severe economic depression spurred the enactment of the Elizabethan Poor Law of 1601. Large-scale involuntary unemployment and the fear of insurrec-

tion stimulated the government to provide welfare aid for select persons (Coll, 1969, p. 5). This law granted the right to assistance through taxation and established three major categories of dependent people: the vagrant, the involuntarily unemployed, and the helpless (Coll, p. 5). The helpless included widows, the disabled, and dependent children. The last two categories were deemed the "worthy" poor. Poor law concepts included:

1. *Local administration.* It was the responsibility of local government to aid and support those in need. The locality decided on the amount and type of aid to be given and who would receive it. Aid was often administered through the church.
2. *General aid.* Aid was usually available to the worthy poor, and others could be jailed or physically punished.
3. *Responsible relatives.* Relatives could be held responsible for the financial support of other family members.
4. *Restrictive residence.* The locality of the individual's origin was responsible for the financial support of the individual. An indigent who migrated from his or her locality of origin could be returned to it.
5. *Individual means test.* Aid was administered on an individual basis through determination of means and needs. Local jurisdictions exercised the right to use moral qualifications to determine who was worthy of assistance.
6. *Minimal subsistence.* A recipient was to receive no more assistance than necessary to exist.
7. *Compulsory work or service.* Work or service by the recipient was often compulsory to obtain assistance, and refusal to work could be a punishable crime. Workhouses for the indigent were commonplace.
8. *Funding through taxation.* Funds to administer the poor law were raised through local taxes.

The Elizabethan Poor Law was a forerunner of United States welfare policy, and all of the original 13 colonies adopted it in some form. Following poor law tradition, the United States left administration of assistance programs largely under local control, implemented responsible relative clauses, administered means tests, provided only minimal subsistence, encouraged or mandated work or service, imposed restrictive residency, and derived welfare revenues through taxation. Restrictive residency laws are now unconstitutional in the United States. However, many original poor law concepts are part of contemporary U.S. health and welfare policy. Another forerunner to U.S. health and welfare policy was a report written in England in the seventeenth century, the Chadwick Report.

The Chadwick Report

In 1832 the British Parliament appointed a royal commission to revise the poor law, and in 1834 the revisions were implemented. Edwin Chadwick was a member of this commission and later, in 1842, published the *Report of the Labouring Population and on the Means of Its Improvement,* often referred to as the Chadwick Report.

At the time of Chadwick's report one half of the children of working class parents died before their fifth birthday, and in large English cities the average age of death for laborers was 16, compared to 22 for tradesmen and 36 for the gentry (Richardson, 1887, cited in Pickett and Hanlon, 1990, p. 26). The report detailed the unsanitary conditions in which the laborers lived and the lack of proper refuse disposal, contaminated water supplies, high rates of morbidity and mortality, and generally poor living conditions of the laboring population. Chadwick's report helped to bring about the passage of the English Public Health Act of 1848, the establishment of a General Board of Health, and the writing of the Shattuck Report in the United States in 1850.

THE DEVELOPMENT OF UNITED STATES HEALTH AND WELFARE POLICY

The European traditions of belief in divine causation, self-help, minimal government intervention, and control of communicable disease prevailed in the United States. The word *health* was left out of the United States constitution, and each state was made responsible for providing for the health of its citizens and legislating its own health laws. Federal intervention in public health and welfare assistance programs was almost nonexistent in early America. At that time, when government health and welfare programs existed they were usually administered by the individual states. A major impetus to developing United States public health policy was the Shattuck Report.

The Shattuck Report

The *Shattuck Report* was written in 1850 by Lemuel Shattuck, a teacher, statistician, and legislator. This report recommended measures such as the creation of state and local boards of health; collection of vital statistics; supervision of housing, factories, sanitation, and foods; procurement of immunizations; community health control measures; and school health and health education (Pickett and Hanlon, 1990, p. 31). The majority of Shattuck's recommendations are accepted today as sound public health practice.

Before the Shattuck Report, local boards of health had begun to emerge in the United States. Some of the earliest of these were in Baltimore, Maryland (1798); Charleston, South Carolina (1815); Philadelphia, Pennsylvania (1818); and Providence, Rhode Island (1832). Following the Shattuck Report, the number of boards of health expanded. In 1869 Massachusetts established the first state board of health in line with Shattuck's recommendations (Pickett and Hanlon, 1990, p. 32). These state and local boards of health were the forerunners of today's state health authorities (SHAs) and local health departments (LHDs).

At the time of Shattuck's report institutions and almshouses (poorhouses) were the major form of welfare assistance in this country. These residential placements served to separate the poor, disabled, frail elderly, and ill from the population mainstream. Many people who were mentally ill or mentally retarded were placed in institutions; such institutions still exist in our country. The constitutionality of institutional placements for individuals, such as people who are mentally retarded, is being challenged in the U.S. court system.

The years following Shattuck's report saw significant strides worldwide in healthcare knowledge, technology, and practice: disease conditions were recognized and differentiated; the sciences of bacteriology, virology, immunology, and pharmacology emerged; antibiotics and sterile techniques were developed; the importance of vectors in disease transmission and control became known; and training for health professionals was expanded.

Development of Voluntary Agencies

When the term *voluntary* is used in relation to health and welfare services it can be somewhat confusing. Voluntary refers to private, nonprofit resources that

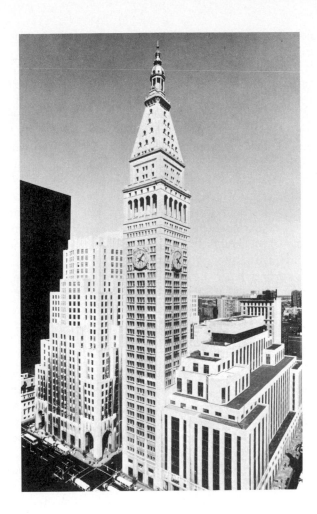

Figure 4-1   "For over 100 years, Metropolitan Life has been unique in performing a public health service in an insurance company setting. Its efforts have included the promotion of health and safety through publications, films, filmstrips, TV and radio, as well as demonstration projects, research and consultation and cooperation with local, state and national health organizations, both voluntary and governmental. Through the years, as various public health problems were brought under control and others arose, the Company's programs changed to meet the current health challenge." (From Metropolitan Life Insurance Company: *Brief History of Metropolitan Life's Health and Safety Activities 1871-1983,* New York, 1983, The Company. Photo courtesy Metropolitan Life Insurance.)

well-known *Control of Communicable Diseases in Man* (15th ed), *Healthy Communities 2000: Model Standards* (3rd ed), and the *American Journal of Public Health.* APHA is headquartered in Washington, D.C., and works diligently with federal and state governments to develop community health standards.

In 1882 one of our country's best-known voluntary organizations, the American Red Cross, was founded by Clara Barton. In 1892 the Anti-Tuberculosis Society of Philadelphia, a forerunner of today's American Lung Association, was established. Other voluntary organizations continued to develop, and by the early twentieth century groups such as the Rockefeller Foundation, the Commonwealth Foundation, and the Kellogg Foundation were established as private voluntary health and welfare organizations. At the same time private profit-making health organizations were emerging, some of which have made significant contributions to public health practice (refer to Figure 4-1). Today there are thousands of voluntary health and welfare organizations in the United States.

Voluntary organizations and individuals are an integral part of our health and welfare services. This voluntary tradition is to be applauded. Voluntary resources are discussed further in Chapter 5.

The Volunteer Tradition

The American volunteer tradition has early roots. The settlers who came to America were often trying to break from the traditional and sometimes oppressive influences of church and state from which they came. They were often mistrustful of governmental inter-

are not under the auspices of federal, state, or local government; are not tax supported; have no legal powers; and rely heavily on donations, endowments, grants, and fee-for-service as funding mechanisms. Voluntary resources traditionally represent people doing for people and a willingness to help others. These resources usually have a large volunteer staff. Nurses work extensively with voluntary agencies in the community.

Voluntary agencies have a long history. By the 1870s voluntary agencies were emerging to work with health and welfare issues in the United States. In 1872 the American Public Health Association was founded; its first president was Dr. Stephen Smith. Today it remains one of our foremost public health organizations, helping to protect and promote the nation's health. It has members in every state and produces numerous public health publications, including the vention into matters of personal health and welfare, and there were few material resources in the new and developing nation. People helped each other, charities developed, and voluntary organizations began to emerge.

The United States went through what is termed by some the *voluntaristic period,* the time between the Civil War and 1935. It was during this period that many voluntary resources were founded. The passage of the Social Security Act of 1935 signaled governmental involvement in the provision of health and welfare services and eliminated some of the need for voluntary programs (Tropman and Tropman, 1987, p. 827).

Volunteers are often the backbone of a voluntary agency. They provide direct services, promote change, act as advocates, serve on boards of directors, and assist administration. They are involved in many activities including telephone services, newsletters, transportation, public relations, fund-raising, and recruiting. Millions of Americans are involved in volunteer work each year.

Volunteers provide many important services that could not be offered otherwise or could only be provided at great time and expense. They work throughout the community in settings such as shelters for the homeless, safe houses for battered women and children, schools, and local health department clinics. They help to bring a human element to service provision. Volunteers should be treated with respect and given appropriate, meaningful roles. Negative experiences become barriers to people continuing volunteer work. In working with volunteers the nurse should promote an environment that fosters positive working relationships.

Establishing Government Involvement in the Delivery of Health and Welfare Services

Under the U.S. Constitution issues of health and welfare were left primarily to the states. Federal involvement in these issues emerged slowly and cautiously.

The federal Marine Hospital Service was established in 1798. In 1879 a National Board of Health was established; this Board was short-lived and disbanded in 1883. Today there is no National Board of Health in the United States. In 1912 the Marine Hospital Service became the United States Public Health Service (USPHS). At that time federal government involve-

ment in matters of public health and welfare was minimal, and health and welfare services were largely left to the states. The system of federal grant-in-aid to states originated in 1919 and supplied revenue to states for health and welfare programs.

By 1919 all states had a government branch dealing with health, often known as the state department of public health (Smolensky, 1977, p. 168). State public health programs focused on the control of communicable disease and maternal-child health problems. Also by this time many states had a government branch dealing with welfare, often a state department of social services. State welfare assistance programs focused on providing services to widows, dependent children, and the indigent elderly. State welfare insurance programs, in the form of workers' compensation, began to evolve in 1911. State and local taxes made up the major source of revenue for health and welfare assistance programs.

The Great Depression

The Great Depression started with the stock market crash of 1929 and peaked in 1933 when 13 million persons, 25% of the work force, were unemployed, and 19 million persons were on state relief rolls. Neither private nor government-funded health and welfare programs could handle the demands created by this event. Possibly no other single event has had such an impact on U.S. health and welfare policy. The Depression showed the general public that anyone could become poor. It dealt a mortal blow to the belief of divine causation, because many people whom the general public believed were not deserving of poverty became impoverished. There was considerable public pressure on the federal government to assist those in need.

A major concern that developed as a result of the Depression was the large, young, unemployed labor force. New jobs were hard to generate, and many jobs were held by older workers with seniority. There was no mandatory retirement age and few retirement pension plans. The idea of mandatory retirement of workers, with the retiree being eligible for a government pension, emerged. The federal government needed to assist the states with these concerns.

The Social Security Act of 1935

Out of the Depression, under the presidency of Franklin D. Roosevelt, came the federal Social Security Act of 1935. For the first time, federal welfare pro-

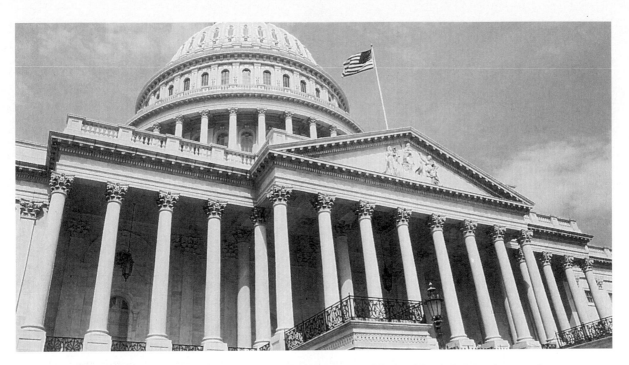

Figure 4-2 The Capitol Building, Washington, D.C. Public health professionals monitor the laws being proposed here to ensure that the needs of their clients are met.

grams were consolidated under one law. The passage of the Social Security Act gave the United States the dubious distinction of being the last of the major industrial nations to develop a federal welfare program (Institute of Gerontology, 1970, p. 2).

The Social Security Act established insurance programs (contributory) and assistance programs (noncontributory). Contributory programs are financed through both taxation and individual contributions, whereas assistance programs are financed only through taxation. It is a landmark piece of legislation, possibly the most important one of our time. Since 1935 the Social Security Act has been amended numerous times to incorporate other health and welfare programs.

UNITED STATES HEALTH AND WELFARE LEGISLATION

Each year numerous laws with health and welfare implications are enacted and many existing laws are amended (refer to Figure 4-2). Health and welfare legislation should be examined and understood in terms of its administration, funding, services offered, clients served, service delivery, and quality control. An in-depth perspective on laws can be obtained by reading materials specific to each piece of legislation in the *United States Code—Congressional and Administrative News* and the *United States Statutes at Large*. This type of information is needed in order for the community health nurse to effectively help clients obtain services available to them, as well as to identify gaps in the delivery of health and welfare services. When gaps or deficiencies are identified, the community health nurse uses the principles of health planning to correct these problems (refer to Chapter 13).

Administration of Health and Welfare Legislation

The organization of health and welfare resources is discussed in depth in Chapter 5. It is a complicated system, but one with which the community health nurse should be familiar in order to facilitate the utilization of health and welfare services by clients.

◀ *1965: The Turning Point in Health Law in the United States* ▶

1. Drug Abuse Control Amendments of 1965 (PL 89-74).
2. Federal Cigarette Labeling and Advertising Act (PL 89-92).
3. Mental Retardation Facilities and Community Mental Health Centers Construction Act Amendments of 1965 (PL 89-105).
4. Community Health Services Extension Amendments of 1965 (PL 89-109).
5. Health Research Facilities Amendments of 1965 (PL 89-115).
6. Water Quality Act of 1965 (PL 89-234).
7. Heart Disease, Cancer and Stroke Amendments of 1965 (PL 89-239).
8. The Clean Air Act Amendments and Solid Waste Disposal Act of 1965 (PL 89-272).
9. Health Professions Educational Assistance Amendments of 1965 (PL 89-290).
10. Medical Library Assistance Act of 1965 (PL 89-291).
11. The Appalachian Regional Development Act of 1965 (PL 89-4).
12. The Older Americans Act (PL 89-73).
13. The Social Security Amendments of 1965 (PL 89-97).
14. The Vocational Rehabilitation Act Amendments of 1965 (PL 89-333).
15. The Housing and Urban Development Act of 1965 (PL 89-117).

From Forgotson EH: 1965: the turning point in health law—1966 reflections, *Am J Publ Health* 57(6):934-935, 1967.

Health and welfare legislation is administered through many offices, staffs, agencies, and departments of government. The responsibility to carry out this legislation is often dispersed over several agencies at the federal, state, and local levels, with a resulting diffusion of responsibility and accountability (Institute of Medicine, 1988, p. 115). The complexity of this organization is presented in the next chapter.

Major United States Health and Welfare Legislation

Several acts of legislation had a major impact on the development of health and welfare policy and practices in the United States. The nurse needs to be aware of this legislation because it has significant impact on the availability of resources and services. When nurses examine new legislation, they will find that it is often an amendment to an existing law rather than an entirely new law, and that amendments to a law can significantly alter it. Federal laws are designated *public law* and are followed by the number of the congressional session and the sequential number of the law.

The Social Security Act of 1935 and the Public Health Service Act of 1944 are two of the most significant pieces of U.S. legislation ever enacted. Many newer laws are amendments to these two acts, and they provide numerous health and welfare services for clients.

The year 1965 has been called the turning point in U.S. public health law and federal involvement in matters of public health (Forgotson, 1967, p. 934). During 1965 more than a dozen important laws relating to health were passed (Forgotson, p. 934). The box above lists those laws. Discussion of some major U.S. health and welfare legislation follows.

Social Security Act of 1935 (Public Law 74-721) as Amended

The Social Security Act of 1935 provided for the general welfare by establishing a system of federal old-age benefits and by enabling the states to make adequate provision for aged persons, blind persons, dependent and crippled children, maternal and child welfare, public health, and the administration of state unemployment compensation laws. This act established a Social Security Board and mechanisms for raising revenue for retirement income and welfare purposes. The Social Security Act was a giant step toward safeguarding the health and welfare of Americans.

When the act was passed in 1935 it included both welfare insurance and welfare assistance programs. Originally its welfare insurance programs included the federal program of old age insurance (OAI) and the

TABLE 4-1 Some Major Social Security Act Programs and Their Source of Administration

| Type of benefits | Type of programs | | |
	Federal programs*	State-federal programs†	Federal-state programs‡
Welfare insurance (cash benefit)	Old Age, Survivors, and Disability Insurance (OASDI)	Unemployment Insurance [Department of Labor, Department of the Treasury]	None
Welfare assistance (cash benefit)	None	Aid to Families with Dependent Children (AFDC) [Social Security Administration]	Supplemental Security Income (SSI)
Health insurance	1. Medicare A—hospital insurance, prepaid through social security contributions 2. Medicare B—medical insurance, individual premium required	None	None
Health assistance	None	1. Medicaid [Health Care Financing Administration] 2. Miscellaneous maternal and child health programs (i.e., services to crippled children, PRESCAD)	None

*Administered federally through the Social Security Administration and/or the Health Care Financing Administration.
†Administered through the state government. Federal sharing agency may be indicated in brackets by program.
‡Administered federally through the Social Security Administration. State sharing agency or agencies will vary in each state.
Note: Programs such as workers' compensation, general assistance, and food stamps are not provided for under the Social Security Act of 1935 and are discussed later in this chapter.

state-federal program of unemployment insurance. Its categorical welfare assistance programs were originally the federal-state programs of Aid to the Blind (AB), Old Age Assistance (OAA), and Aid to Dependent Children (ADC). It also provided funds for services to crippled children and high-risk mothers and children. In 1939, the Act was amended to provide for Survivors Insurance (OASI); in 1950, to provide Aid to the Permanently and Totally Disabled (APTD); and in 1956, to include Disability Insurance (OASDI). Medicare and Medicaid were added to the act in 1965; in 1988 Medicare Catastrophic Health Insurance was added to Medicare coverage, but this coverage was repealed in 1989. Appendix 4-1 chronologically summarizes some of the major amendments to the Social

Security Act and the purpose of the amendments.

Today nearly every American family is involved with the Social Security Act in some form. Employers, employees, and the self-employed pay into the insurance programs of the act. Almost 95% of all U.S. workers contribute to these programs. The social security insurance protection (OASDI) earned by workers stays with them even in a new job or residence. The contributions made by a worker determine eligibility and the amount of benefits.

Table 4-1 summarizes major health and welfare insurance and assistance programs of the Social Security Act. Determination of eligibility for social security *assistance* programs is handled through a number of federal, state, and local agencies. Determining social security *insurance* eligibility is handled through local branches of the federal Social Security Administration. Social Security Administration offices are located throughout the country and representatives are sent to communities in which there are no offices. Applications for the insurance programs of Old Age, Survivors, and Disability Insurance (OASDI) and Medicare, as well as the assistance program of Supplemental Security Income (SSI) can be made at these offices. Persons should contact the office to determine what information is necessary to complete the application.

Public Health Service Act of 1944 (Public Law 78-410) as Amended

The Public Health Service Act of 1944 consolidated and revised the laws relating to the Public Health Service and has since served to consolidate national public health legislation. It is the major piece of public health legislation in the country but does not have administration over the health programs, Medicaid and Medicare, of the Social Security Act. Its provisions are comprehensive.

This act incorporates legislation on healthcare personnel, health facility construction and modernization, and services to specific population groups. Over the years this law has been frequently amended (refer to Appendix 4-2) to provide financing for traineeships for health care professionals (nurse training acts and traineeships for graduate students in public health); grants-in-aid to schools of public health; construction of community mental health centers and facilities; national comprehensive health planning and resource development; the development of health maintenance organizations (HMOs); health services for migratory workers; family planning services and communicable disease control; emergency medical services; and research and facilities for the prevention and control of conditions such as heart disease, cancer, stroke, kidney disease, sudden infant death syndrome, arthritis, Cooley's anemia, sickle-cell anemia, AIDS, and diabetes mellitus. Amendments such as the Heart Disease, Cancer, and Stroke Amendments gave research and service priority to some of the leading causes of death in this country.

Civil Rights Act of 1964 (Public Law 88-352)

Most states and many municipalities have enacted civil rights laws that forbid discrimination and ensure constitutional rights. Federal civil rights legislation was enacted in the United States in 1866, 1870, and 1871. Contemporary civil rights acts were enacted in 1957, 1960, 1964, and 1968. In 1980 the Civil Rights of Institutionalized Persons Act (Public Law 96-247) was enacted.

Of all the civil rights legislation, the Civil Rights Act of 1964 is frequently considered to be the most significant; it was designed to ensure fair and equal treatment for all. The act forbade discrimination on the basis of race or sex in public accommodations, public facilities, and public education. It also enforced the constitutional right to vote. In addition, it established a Commission on Equal Employment Opportunity and attempted to ensure fair employment practices. The original act covered private employers but not government employers; it was amended in 1972 to cover public employees. Since 1972, if a state or local government is found to be practicing discrimination, the federal Attorney General can sue to have that state's revenue-sharing funds cut off. The Civil Rights Restoration Act of 1987 (Public Law 100-259) clarified and enlarged the scope of coverage of the Civil Rights Act of 1964.

Economic Opportunity Act of 1964 (Public Law 88-452)

The Economic Opportunity Act of 1964 was designed to mobilize the human and financial resources of the nation to combat poverty. It included work training and study programs, established the Office of Economic Opportunity, authorized Volunteers in Service to America (VISTA), the Job Corps, Upward Bound, Neighborhood Youth Corps, Head Start, neighborhood health centers, and community action programs. An impetus to antipoverty programs, it also incorporated urban and rural community action programs and assistance to small businesses and work experience programs. The future of Public Law 88-452 is now questionable.

Older Americans Act of 1965 (Public Law 89-73)

This act was passed to provide assistance in the development of programs to help older Americans. It provided grants to states for community planning and services and for training and research in the field of gerontology and aging. It established the Administration on Aging, which is now located in the Department of Health and Human Services. This act gave national attention to the needs of the elderly and facilitated state and area planning on the needs of this aggregate, establishing state and local agencies on aging. It is extensively discussed in Chapter 19.

Occupational Safety and Health Act of 1970 (Public Law 91-956)

The Occupational Safety and Health Act is the most comprehensive piece of legislation on occupational health and safety in the United States. Championed by organized labor, its intent is to protect the health of the worker, and it made worker health a public concern. The United States was the last major industrial nation to enact such a law. This act is discussed in depth in Chapter 17.

Rehabilitation Act of 1973 (Public Law 93-112)

The Vocational Rehabilitation Act of 1920 (Public Law 66-236) was an outgrowth of the healthcare needs evidenced by veterans after World War I and was a forerunner of the 1973 act. The Rehabilitation Act of 1973 replaced the 1920 act but retained its major components. This new act extended and revised the authorization of grants to states for vocational rehabilitation services; emphasized services to those with severe handicaps; expanded federal responsibilities and training programs; defined services necessary for rehabilitation programs; established the National Architectural and Transportation Barriers Board to enforce legislation designed to remove architectural barriers for persons who are handicapped; and began affirmative action programs to facilitate employment of persons who are handicapped. Its ultimate goal was to help such persons become productive members of society. The Rehabilitation Act Amendments of 1974 (Public Law 93-516) transferred the Rehabilitation Services Administration to the Department of Health, Education and Welfare, strengthened services for the blind, and authorized a White House Conference on Handicapped Persons. This act is discussed further in Chapter 18.

Education for All Handicapped Children Act of 1975 (Public Law 94-142)

This act amended the Education of the Handicapped Act (Public Law 90-247). Through it the federal government took an active role in ensuring the educational rights of people who are handicapped. The law helps to provide free, public education for children who are handicapped (refer to Chapters 14 and 15). Before its passage, many children in the United States who were handicapped had been denied access to the public educational system. Recently the government has tried to deregulate the act and to become less involved in protecting the educational rights of persons who are handicapped. Active lobbying by parent groups and professionals has prevented this.

Omnibus Budget Reconciliation Act of 1981 (Public Law 97-35)

This was a major cost-containment law that had a great impact on services provided by health and welfare programs in the United States. It mandated cost containment in aspects of government including taxation, government operations, health and human services, veterans' affairs, consumer affairs, labor/employment, transportation, communications, energy, environment, agriculture, and foreign and military operations. The massive cutbacks in public spending will need to be monitored in the coming years to ascertain that needs of at-risk groups are not being neglected.

This act also provided for block grants and reduced the number of categorical aid programs. *Block grants* to states give the states increased flexibility in the manner in which money is spent but place individual programs and agencies in competition with one another for funding. This act places more responsibility on the states and localities for program provision.

Consolidated Omnibus Budget Reconciliation Act of 1985 [COBRA] (Public Law 99-272)

This act contained many Medicaid and Medicare amendments. A significant change in regard to public health is that it makes Medicaid coverage available to low-income pregnant women in two-parent families and thereby increases their opportunities for obtaining appropriate prenatal and postnatal care (refer to Appendix 4-1).

Omnibus Budget Reconciliation Act of 1986 [OBRA] (Public Law 99-509)

This act contained several Medicaid and Medicare amendments. Of significant interest to public health was the change in Medicaid to allow states the option of expanding Medicaid coverage to pregnant women, infants up to age 1, and children up to age 5 whose family incomes were below the federal poverty level. The act also required states to continue Medicaid coverage to disabled individuals who lost their eligibility for SSI as a result of work earnings, and clarified

Medicaid coverage for the homeless (refer to Appendix 4-1).

Stewart B. McKinney Homeless Assistance Act (Public Law 100-77)

This important and comprehensive act dealt with the increasing problem of homelessness in American society and provided urgently needed assistance to protect and improve the lives and safety of the homeless, with special emphasis on elderly persons, persons who are handicapped, and families with children. It established the Interagency Council on the Homeless, Emergency Food and Shelter Program National Board, Emergency Food and Shelter Grants, Supportive Housing Demonstration Program, Primary Health Services and Substance Abuse Services Grant Program, and Food Assistance for the Homeless Food Stamp Program. It authorized emergency food supplies for the homeless, HUD programs for emergency shelter, supportive housing, programs for primary health care, substance abuse services, community mental health care, adult education for the homeless, education for homeless children and youth, job training for the homeless, and studies of youth homeless and Native American homeless.

Medicare Catastrophic Coverage Act of 1988 (Public Law 100-360)

This act was a monumental piece of health legislation. In recognition of the rising costs of health care and the economically devastating impact catastrophic health care can bring, this act attempted to protect the elderly against catastrophic health care expenses under Medicare. It was financed through an increase in the part B premium and an income-related supplemental surtax. From the beginning the act met with much resistance, even though it had the backing of such major organizations as the American Association of Retired Persons (AARP). This act was repealed in 1989.

Americans with Disabilities Act (Public Law 101-336)

The Americans with Disabilities Act was signed into law on July 26, 1990. The act is one of the most significant pieces of legislation in this country to help guarantee the rights of the nation's 43 million disabled citizens. It includes a new definition of disability. The act's provisions help to ensure equal access and opportunity in employment, transportation, education, public accommodations, and telecommunications. This landmark act increased the opportunity for people who are disabled to be integrated into the mainstream of society. It is further discussed in Chapter 16.

Year 2000 Health Objectives Planning Act (Public Law 101-582)

This act amended the Public Health Service Act of 1944. It established a program of grants to states for the development of state plans for meeting the objectives established by *Healthy People 2000*.

Cancer Registries Amendments Act (Public Law 102-515)

This act also amended the Public Health Service Act of 1944. It assisted in cancer prevention, early detection, and statistics compilation. It established federal funding to states for state cancer registries. Each state is eligible for a grant and technical assistance from the federal government to operate a registry in which demographic data, industrial and occupational history information, pathological data, diagnosis, and date of diagnosis would be recorded. The act authorized a breast cancer study in a number of states with high incidence of breast cancer.

Preventive Health Amendments of 1992 (Public Law 102-531)

This act amended the Public Health Service Act of 1944. It emphasized and mandated major federal involvement in preventive health and primary prevention activities. It changed the name of the Centers for Disease Control to Centers for Disease Control and Prevention (CDC). The act authorized prevention programs including injury control; lead poisoning; preventable infertility from sexually transmitted diseases; vaccination services; screening and detection programs for breast, cervical, and prostate cancer; and international cooperation in preventive health measures. Further, the act provided for more comprehensive maternal and child health services and community education programs in Migrant Health Centers and established the National Foundation for the Centers for Disease Control and Prevention. The purpose of the foundation is to promote the public's health and support and implement activities for the prevention and control of diseases, disorders, injuries, and disabilities. Foundation activities include (1) programs of fellowships for state and local public health officials to work and study in association with the CDC, (2) international exchange programs for public health officials who are interested in working in a foreign country, (3) studies, projects, and research on prevention, (4) forums for government officials and private entities to exchange information, (5) meetings, conferences, courses, and training workshops, (6) programs to improve the collection and analysis of data on the health status of various populations, and (7) programs for writing, editing, printing, and publishing books and materials.

Family and Medical Leave Act (Public Law 103-5)

This law entitles an employee of a private employer with fifty or more employees to up to 12 weeks unpaid leave during a one-year period for the birth or adoption of a child; care of an ill child, spouse, or parent; or the employee's own illness. The employer must provide adequate protection of the employee's employment and health benefits during the leave.

State Workers' Compensation Acts

The state workers' compensations acts are the oldest form of government health and welfare insurance in this country. The first state act was legislated in 1911, and by 1948 all states had such acts. The federal government provides workers' compensation benefits for federal employees. Workers' compensation programs vary greatly from state to state in the amount of cash and health care benefits provided. State workers' compensation laws are usually administered by the state labor department or an independent workers' compensation agency. Court administration exists in a few states. Workers' compensation is discussed further under insurance programs in this chapter.

THE UNITED STATES HEALTH CARE SYSTEM

Silver (1974) provides what is possibly the best description of health care in America by using the following passage from the *Book of Common Prayer:*

We have left undone those things which we ought to have done and we have done those things which we ought not to have done, and there is no health in us.

In the United States, comprehensive health services exist, but they are unequally distributed, fragmented, and expensive. Almost any type of health care service is available in the United States, but often these services are neither accessible nor affordable. Health care resources and services are found in both government (official) and private sectors. There is often little coordination between health care resources, and there

is great complexity and diversity in the United States health care delivery system. This presents major problems for nurses when they attempt to coordinate available resources and services. Presently the federal government is looking at ways to improve coordination of health care resources and services, enhance access to health care services, make health care services more equitable, and provide more preventive health services. From these efforts a new system of national health care is expected to evolve.

For a variety of reasons (many of which are discussed in Chapter 10), many people are not using available health services. Ensuring accessibility to preventive health care services has become a national health goal in *Healthy People 2000.* Preventive services such as free or low-cost immunizations clinics are available throughout the country, yet many children and adults are not adequately immunized. Preventive health care and early diagnosis and screening services are available, but many people do not use them. Many preventable conditions such as heart disease, cancer, stroke, injuries, HIV infection, alcoholism, drug abuse, low-birth-weight infants, and communicable diseases continue to occur in the United States at great personal and economic expense (USDHHS, 1991, p. 5). Of the approximately half-million Americans who die of cancer each year, it is estimated that more than 100,000 could have been saved if they had had early diagnosis and treatment (American Cancer Society, 1993, p. 1).

Prevention and early diagnosis are too important to be ignored. Yet health care is sought and offered in this country largely on a treatment basis rather than a preventive one. In spite of this discrepancy, Americans continue to be among the healthiest people in the world. The average life expectancy of Americans continues to increase, the death rate is historically low, and childhood mortality continues to decline. Sometimes we appear to make advances in spite of ourselves.

Health Care Facilities and the Health Care Work Force

Health care resources in the United States are fragmented, unequally distributed, and increasingly expensive. Presently there is little coordination between health care resources, and not all Americans have equal access to health care.

The United States has an abundance of health care facilities. There are 5808 acute-care hospitals, 535 long-term hospitals, and 16,033 nursing homes in the United States (National Center for Health Statistics [NCHS], 1992, p. 141). Of these hospitals 311 are federally owned, 3233 are nonprofit, 769 are for-profit, and 1495 are run by state and local governments (NCHS, p. 255). There is a trend toward increased for-profit ownership of these facilities. The number of acute-care hospitals has been declining steadily since 1977, especially in rural areas (Health Insurance Association of America [HIAA], 1992, p. 80).

The U.S. government closed its Public Health Service hospitals at the end of fiscal year 1981. Government ownership of hospitals includes armed forces hospitals, prison hospitals, state long-term psychiatric care facilities, facilities for the mentally retarded, state university medical school hospitals, and city and county hospitals for the indigent. There are thousands of state and local health departments and departments of social services, as well as many private agencies and individuals who provide health care services.

Hospital care in the United States accounts for over 38% of the personal health care money spent each year (NCHS, 1992, p. 268). Hospitals are becoming increasingly competitive in the services and incentives they offer to clients; many are offering alternative health care services such as home care, occupational health services, rehabilitation services, decentralized services (minihospitals distributed throughout an area providing broad outpatient and emergency facilities), and alternative care programs similar to programs offered by health maintenance organizations.

Nursing homes are increasing in number in the United States, and their ownership is largely in the private profit-making sector. Approximately 5% of Americans aged 65 and over occupy a bed in a nursing or related home. Nursing homes are licensed by the state and are usually certified for Medicaid and Medicare funding. The average individual monthly cost for a nursing home is $1456 (NCHS, 1992, p. 280).

There are more than 9 million people employed in health care occupations in the United States (NCHS, 1992, p. 242). Health care is one of the nation's biggest businesses. There is federal funding available to train various health professionals including nurses, physicians, occupational health professionals, and public health professionals.

Education, certification, and licensing help to distinguish between various health care workers. For every 10,000 Americans there are approximately 23 physicians, 67 registered nurses, 6 dentists, 6 pharmacists, and 10 optometrists in practice today (NCHS, 1992, p. 247). However, there is a great disparity between the number of health care providers in urban, rural, and inner-city areas. Studies have consistently shown that rural and inner-city areas have a significantly smaller health work force than suburban areas and that more affluent areas often have more health care resources. The government offers financial incentives to universities and colleges that make a commitment to increase their output of health practitioners to areas with a shortage of health care personnel, and it offers financial incentives to students to practice in such areas.

Health Care Cost

In general, health care in the United States is uneconomical and disproportionately inflationary. Spending for health accounts for an increasing share of the nation's gross national product (GNP). Health care spending amounts to more than $666 billion each year in the United States. This represents 12.2% of the gross national product, and $2566 per person per year on health care (NCHS, 1992, p. 266). Despite 20 years of policy aimed at reducing health care costs, U.S. health care spending increases every year (Himmelstein and Woolhandler, 1992, p. 1). The United States spends more on health care than any other country in the world; most developed nations have been able to stabilize their health spending at about 8% to 9% of their GNP (Himmelstein and Woolhandler, p. 1).

The United States can no longer afford to pay such inflationary health care costs. Table 4-2 shows the rise in national health expenditures from 1940 to estimated year 2000 figures. The figures are astounding! It is obvious that national health care programs and legislation will need to be enacted to contain costs. Some cost controls implemented in recent years include health care deductibles and coinsurances, utilization reviews, rate-setting commissions, hospital reimbursement under Medicare diagnostic-related groups (DRGs), and managed care programs under Medicaid and health maintenance organizations. The federal government has influenced the financing of health care through tax subsidies and incentives, including provisions for deductions of medical expenses with personal income tax, allowing employer's contributions to health insurance plans to be tax-

TABLE 4-2 National Health Expenditures—United States: Selected Years			
Year	Cost (rounded to nearest billion)	Per capita cost	Percent of GNP
1940	$ 4	$ 29	4
1950	$ 13	$ 80	4.5
1960	$ 27	$ 143	5.3
1970	$ 74	$ 346	7.3
1980	$ 250	$1063	9.3
1990	$ 666	$2566	12.2
2000	$1616	$5712	16.4

From Health Insurance Association of America: *Source Book of Health Insurance Data*, Washington, D.C., 1992, The Association, p. 6; and National Center for Health Statistics: *Health, United States, and Prevention Profile 1991*, Washington, D.C., 1992, U.S. Government Printing Office, p. 266.

exempt, allowing income tax deductions for contributions to charitable organizations engaged in health care, and extending tax-exempt status to nonprofit health care resources.

Health care is financed through individual payment and governmental and private agencies. Methods of payment for health care in the United States are discussed in this chapter. The health services that an individual uses largely depend on the payment methods available to that person.

METHODS OF HEALTH CARE FINANCING IN THE UNITED STATES

The methods of health care financing in the United States are diverse, complicated, and confusing. Health care services often are not utilized because an individual is unable to afford them. Both governmental and private sector resources provide methods of health care financing. To help make this diverse system of financing clearer a discussion of financing methods follows; the box on this page summarizes methods of health care financing. Remember that the federal government is presently evaluating our health care system and in the near future the methods of

◀ *Methods of Health Care Financing in the United States* ▶

Individual Payment (direct, out-of-pocket)

Health Insurance
1. Governmental: Medicare, Workers' Compensation
2. Private: Blue Cross-Blue Shield, commercial insurance, self-insurance, health maintenance organizations (HMOs), and preferred provider organizations (PPOs)

Health Assistance
1. Governmental: Medicaid, Maternal-Child Health (MCH) Programs
2. Private: Numerous services offered by voluntary, community agencies and individuals, such as the American Heart Association, the American Lung Association, local churches, and individual donations

Health Service Programs
1. Governmental: Programs for veterans, military personnel, merchant marines, American Indians on reservations, native Hawaiians, and federal employees
2. Private: On-site employee health services and group health maintenance centers

financing health care in the United States may be significantly altered.

Individual Payment (Direct, Out-of-Pocket)

Individual payment for health care services is exactly what it says—the individual pays for the health care directly. For the 35 million Americans who are not covered under insurance and assistance programs, and for the underinsured, individual payment is a hard reality. The box on p. 112 gives some information on who the uninsured and underinsured are in the United States. These at-risk populations are growing rapidly.

Individuals and families with inadequate health insurance often seek only crisis health care, which presents serious consequences for personal and community health. This has significant implications for public health practice.

◀ ▶ *A Look at the Uninsured and Underinsured in the United States—*
Who Are They?

Almost 14% of the U.S. population, or 35 million people, are uninsured; more people than at any time since the passage of Medicare and Medicaid in 1965.

About ⅔ of the uninsured are employed workers and their families and about 13% of these workers are working full-time.

Men are more frequently uninsured than women.

Young adults are the age group most likely to be uninsured.

The poor are more likely than other socioeconomic groups to be uninsured: 22% of families with incomes of less than $25,000 are uninsured, while only 8% of families with incomes of greater than $50,000 are uninsured.

Professionals are not exempt from being uninsured: there are 29,900 uninsured physicians, 328,000 unin-

sured teachers and professors, 52,500 uninsured clergy, and 18,600 uninsured lawyers. However, no legislators or judges are uninsured.

33% of Hispanic Americans and 20% of African Americans are uninsured as compared to 10.7% of the white population.

Today there are 50 to 70 million Americans who, due to inadequate health insurance coverage, could likely become bankrupt or suffer severe financial distress in the event of a major illness.

5 million young women have insurance policies that exclude maternity care.

Many senior citizens are underinsured since Medicare only pays for about 50% of their medical expenses.

From Himmelstein DU and Woolhandler S: *The National Health Program Chartbook,* Cambridge, Mass., 1992, The Center for National Health Program Studies, Harvard Medical School/Cambridge Hospital, pp. 3-7, 13.

Even with health insurance, many people are involved in some form of individual payment because of insurance deductibles, insurance premiums, fixed payment amounts, and uncovered services. A *deductible* is a set expense that must be paid by the insured before the insurer will reimburse for services (e.g., a $500 deductible). With *coinsurance* the insured pays a percentage of the covered health care expenses, often in addition to a deductible (e.g., a 20% coinsurance rate). *Fixed payments* are arrangements whereby only a specified amount for a health service is paid by the insurer, regardless of the cost to the client (e.g., $300 for antepartal care). *Uncovered services* are services that the insurer does not pay for, and payment is left to the insuree (e.g., prescription medications). The rising costs of health insurance are prompting more employers to institute coinsurance plans or to limit covered services. This presents a real hardship for many individuals and families.

Direct payment accounts for approximately 22% of personal health care expenditures, more than $136 billion dollars each year (Health Insurance Association of America, 1992, p. 63). When direct payment for health care becomes excessive it can place the individual and family at great financial risk. A form of health care financing that helps to protect the indi-

vidual and family from the financial risk of health care is health insurance.

Health Insurance

Health insurance is a contractual agreement between an insurer and an insuree for the payment of health care costs. The insuree pays a prepaid premium for specified benefits; the benefits under the insurance program are variable. Health insurance is administered by both government and private agencies. Private health insurance programs serve the majority of the American people, whereas government programs are limited largely to serving the aged and disabled.

Most health insurance programs cover hospital and surgical costs for the insuree because these costs are the most predictable and insurable of health care costs. Many insurance plans do not include regular medical, major medical, disability, or dental insurance. Some insurance plans do not cover the cost of prescription medications or health care equipment. The box on p. 113 illustrates some forms of health insurance coverage.

Most people are vulnerable to the cost of long-term health care and catastrophic illness. Chapter 20 exam-

---

◀ *Forms of Health Insurance Coverage in the United States* ▶

Hospital

Insurance that covers the cost of inpatient hospital services

Surgical

Insurance that covers physicians' fees for surgical care

Regular Medical

Insurance that pays for physicians' fees for nonsurgical care; there are usually maximum benefit amounts for specified services

Major Medical

Insurance that helps protect against large, unpredictable medical costs; usually supplements an existing insurance

program, frequently has maximum benefit limits, and is subject to deductibles and coinsurance

Dental

Insurance that provides payment for the cost of specified dental care

Disability

Insurance that protects against wages lost from disability; may provide long-term or short-term benefits

Catastrophic

Insurance that protects against the high cost of acute or long-term illness that would otherwise not be covered by insurance

---

ines in depth the extent of this problem and actions needed to correct it.

Government Health Insurance

Federal government health insurance did not exist in any significant form until 1965 with the passage of Medicare under the Social Security Act. Government health insurance incorporates many of the same types of coverage as private health insurance. There are two major forms of government health insurance: Medicare and workers' compensation programs. Medicare is a federal program and workers' compensation is a state program.

Medicare is a federal health insurance program created by the 1965 amendments to the Social Security Act. It is a contributory program, paid into during the working years. Clients apply for Medicare at local branches of the federal Social Security Administration. Reimbursement for services is provided through private insurance companies, such as Blue Cross-Blue Shield organizations, under contract with the federal government.

Medicare insures almost 31 million Americans and provides health insurance for eligible persons age 65 and over and for qualifying people who are disabled (NCHS, 1992, p. 292). Medicare expenditures make up approximately 60% of federal fiscal spending for health care and almost $89 billion a year (NCHS, p. 276; SSA, 1993, Annual Statistical Supplement 1992,

p. 291). An excellent publication describing the Medicare program, *The Medicare Handbook,* is updated yearly by the Health Care Financing Administration. The Social Security Administration publishes *A Guide to the Medicare Program,* which can be obtained free of charge by calling the administration's toll-free number, 1-800-772-1213.

Medicare has two parts, Medicare A and Medicare B. *Medicare A* is a hospital insurance program, financed through individual social security contributions. In addition to inpatient hospital care, Medicare A covers selected posthospitalization home health care services, such as skilled nursing care, and physical or speech therapy on a qualifying basis. It sets limits on the number of hospital and extended care facility days that will be covered and is subject to yearly changes in services and deductibles.

Medicare B is a voluntary, supplemental medical insurance program. In 1994 the monthly premium is $41.10. It covers physicians' services; limited services by dentists, podiatrists, optometrists, and chiropractors; hospital outpatient services; some home health service visits; outpatient physical therapy and speech therapy; specified equipment; radiation therapy; hospice services; and other services on a qualifying basis. It excludes coverage for prescription drugs, glasses, dentures, hearing aids, yearly physical examinations, dental care, and routine foot care. Because of these exclusions, many persons 65 and older have obtained supplemental private health insurance policies to augment their Medicare benefits.

Workers' compensation benefits are provided to workers who have a work-related disability and to the dependents of workers whose death resulted from a job-related accident or occupational disease (Nelson, 1992, p. 51). Both income maintenance and health benefits are offered under the various state programs.

Approximately 95% of the U.S. work force is covered by workers' compensation legislation (SSA, 1993, Annual Statistical Supplement 1992, p. 9). Employees most likely to be excluded from coverage are domestic, agricultural, and part-time workers; and coverage is often incomplete for workers in small firms, nonprofit organizations, and state and local government (Nelson, 1992, p. 52).

Benefits are awarded regardless of who is at fault for the occurrence. This no-fault principle precludes legal suits against employers when the acquired injury, illness, disability, or death is covered under the workers' compensation program. The deadline for filing a claim is usually 1 or 2 years after the disability or death occurs (Nelson, 1991, p. 35).

All workers' compensation acts require that medical care be furnished to injured workers without delay and provide physical rehabilitation when needed. If the worker is injured on the job but suffers no loss of ability to work, such as with certain types of hearing loss, the injury may not be compensable. Loss of ability to work is generally a criterion for awarding a workers' compensation claim.

The employer is liable for the cost of the insurance program and the employee does not make contributions. Generally the methods available to employers to insure workers are private insurance, state-operated insurance funds, and self-insurance (Nelson, 1992, p. 54). In 1989 $19.9 billion was paid for workers' compensation through private insurance, $6.8 billion through state-operated insurance funds, and $6.4 billion through self-insurance (Nelson, p. 54).

The amount of the cash benefit awarded to the worker is related to the degree and permanence of the injury, the worker's earnings, and the number of the worker's dependents. In some states workers may receive benefits only for a specified period of time or for a specific monetary amount. Workers are often subject to waiting periods before the compensation can begin.

Each state sets a minimum and maximum payment range for workers' compensation benefits. Maximum weekly state workers' compensation payments range from $175 to $700, and minimum cash benefits can be as low as $20 weekly (Nelson, 1991, p. 31). Workers' maximum wage replacement averages about 67% of their take-home earnings before taxes. This reduction in pay can cause financial hardship for a family in addition to the other adjustments the family is making in relation to the disability.

Private Health Insurance

A forerunner of private health insurance in the United States was the Baylor University Plan of 1929. A group of teachers contracted with Baylor Hospital in Dallas, Texas, to provide specific health care services at a predetermined cost (Health Insurance Association of America, 1992, p. 1). The monthly premium was 50 cents, and the plan offered 21 days of semiprivate care at Baylor Hospital in Dallas, Texas (Wilner, Walkley and O'Neill, 1978, pp. 138-139). Out of this plan emerged the Blue Cross-Blue Shield concept of 1939. In 1940 less than 10% of the civilian population was covered by private health insurance (Health Insurance Association of America, 1983, p. 13). Today 73.2% of the U.S. population, 182 million Americans, are covered by private health insurance (Health Insurance Association of America, 1992, pp. 8, 24).

Health insurance plans are often provided as part of employee work benefits. The most common forms of health insurance in this country are Blue Cross–Blue Shield, commercial insurance, self-insurance, health maintenance organizations (HMOs), and preferred provider organizations (PPOs). Each of these forms is discussed here.

Blue Cross and Blue Shield organizations are nonprofit (voluntary) health insurance organizations serving both individuals and groups. They are tax-exempt organizations and exist through state legislation enabling them to provide health insurance. The state insurance commissioner usually has powers of regulation over these programs, with rate increases being approved by the commissioner and subject to public hearings. These organizations are allowed to contract with providers of service for agreed-upon fees, and payment is made directly to the service provider.

Blue Cross and Blue Shield organizations are legally independent of each other but usually work in close cooperation. Their boards of directors are composed of representatives from the public, providers of care, and their own organizations. These organizations pay almost $100 billion in insurance benefits and insure almost 71 million Americans annually (Health Insurance Association of America, 1992, pp. 25-26). Blue Cross provides protection against the cost of hospital care, and Blue Shield provides protection against the cost of medical and surgical care.

Commercial insurance companies are private profit-making organizations. They provide health insurance for almost 97 million Americans, and cover services similar to those offered under Blue Cross-Blue Shield plans. Commercial insurers compete with Blue Cross-Blue Shield and have pioneered several types of health insurance coverage now common to other carriers, including major medical care, prescription drugs, and posthospitalization home care services. Commercial insurers contract with clients for prepaid premiums and benefits. Clients are expected to pay the service provider and are then reimbursed by the insurer for the agreed-upon cost.

Self-insurance was stimulated by the passage of the Employee Retirement Income Security Act of 1974 (Health Insurance Association of America, 1978, p. 20). Under this act, corporations and organizations can establish self-funded, nonprofit health plans and escape the taxes and regulations of state insurance laws.

Health maintenance organizations (HMOs) provide a wide range of comprehensive health care services for a specified group at a fixed, prepaid cost to the insured. Health maintenance organizations combine the principles of health insurance and group health practice and stress the preventive aspects of health care. The Health Maintenance Organization Act of 1973 (Public Law 93-222), an amendment to the Public Health Service Act of 1944, provided financial and other assistance to aid in HMO development. There are hundreds of HMOs in the United States serving millions of Americans. These organizations are characterized by:

- Direct service provision to enrollees on a pre-payment basis, with each enrollee paying a fixed amount regardless of the volume or expense of the services used.
- Service provision through physicians, nurses, and other health care providers who are under contractual agreement with the HMO. Their practice is limited to the HMO, and subscribers to the HMO are limited to usage of the health workers employed by the plan.
- Comprehensive services that include both in-patient and outpatient care and emphasize preventive health practices.

- Internal, self-regulatory mechanisms to ensure quality of care and cost-control.

Today Medicare and Medicaid have authorized the use of HMOs as service providers. HMO growth has increased from less than 2 million subscribers in the early 1970s to 556 HMOs and more than 38 million subscribers today (Health Insurance Association of America, 1992, pp. 19, 21).

Preferred provider organizations (PPOs) are a form of prepaid health insurance similar to HMOs. PPOs began to develop in the 1980s and generally offer the subscriber more flexibility in choosing service providers. PPOs contract with providers who agree to provide health care services for a prenegotiated fee schedule. Listings of approved providers are given to subscribers, who are expected to use the PPO-approved service providers' health care services. If subscribers use a provider outside of the PPO, coverage is nonexistent or limited. Providers are usually selected for their emphasis on primary prevention, cost-effectiveness, and efficiency. There are 978 PPOs in the United States, serving 38 million people (Health Insurance Association of America, 1992, p. 22).

National Health Insurance

Teddy Roosevelt first attempted to have national health insurance enacted in 1912 (Harrington, 1989, p. 214). However, his efforts were unsuccessful, and there is still no form of national health insurance in this country. In the past proposed programs have varied as to whether they would be federally or privately administered, who would be covered, what would be covered, how they would be funded, and what quality control measures would be taken. One of the major barriers to passage of such a plan has been the proposed cost.

Today the Clinton administration is diligently working to develop a national health care reform package. "Two major proposals for health care reform have emerged as the leading contenders: a single-payer national health program and managed competition" (Clancy, Himmelstein and Woolhandler, 1993, p. 30). The managed care proposals have four key elements: (1) a standardized benefit package, which in many of the managed competition proposals will be established by a National Health Board; (2) tax reform that will allow a tax deduction for only the standard health care benefit package (health care benefits beyond the standard package would be considered taxable); (3) the establishment of health insurance purchasing cooperatives (HIPCs), which would be the source of health insurance for many or all purchasers of health coverage; and (4) health plans that will contract with HIPCs for enrollees, for whom the health plans will provide care on a capitation basis or a fixed rate for a package of services (Frisof, 1993; Kotelchuck, 1993, pp. 4-9). Kotelchuck and others (Frisof; McKenzie, 1993) believe that no reform proposal will ensure access to health care unless critical gaps in the infrastructure of health care delivery are addressed. As discussed previously in this chapter, many underserved communities lack basic primary and preventive care services. It is anticipated that some form of "managed competition" will be the immediate health care plan established under the Clinton Health Care Reform mandate. However, some health care analysts and professional groups, including the American Nurses Association, believe that this type of reform is inadequate to meet the needs of all Americans (Davis, 1993; Frisof; Kotelchuck; and McKenzie). Single-payer activists have spearheaded a grassroots coalition, the Universal Health Care Action Network (UHCAN), to keep in the forefront the need for a universal health plan (Frisof).

Health care professionals must monitor carefully all proposed national health programs to ensure that they actually provide the services needed by the population as a whole. The American Public Health Association (APHA) has championed the platform of "Health Care for All" in the United States by the year 2000. The American Nurses Association has developed a national health care agenda. *Nursing's Agenda for Health Care Reform* advocates universal coverage, stringent cost-containment initiatives, a restructured health care system, a federally defined standard package of essential health care services, insurance reform, case management for clients with continuing care needs, and provisions for long-term care, including public sector review. Forty-four nursing organizations support this agenda. Nursing is promoting new models of health care delivery that emphasize wellness and care versus illness and cure (ANA, 1991).

Health Assistance

Health assistance programs provide health services to qualifying individuals without the prepayment of premiums by the individual and generally without the individual participating in cost-sharing for the services rendered. These programs are largely noncontributory ones.

Government Health Assistance

The major government health assistance programs are the state-federal, state-administered program of Medicaid and a number of maternal-child health programs. The private sector health assistance programs are diverse and are found largely in the private non-profit (voluntary) sector.

Medicaid was created by the same 1965 Social Security Act amendments that created Medicare. It is a noncontributory health assistance program that provides health services for the medically indigent, people who are unable to meet their health care expenses and who fall within specified economic guidelines.

Each state administers its own Medicaid program through various offices of state government, often the state Department of Human or Social Services. Programs vary from state to state in relation to Medicaid eligibility and covered services. There are no age or residency requirements (legal aliens are eligible) for Medicaid.

Both federal and state funds pay for Medicaid services, with federal funding for the program varying from 50% to 83%, depending on the state's economic status (Waid, 1991, p. 51). On the average, states receive reimbursement for 57% of their Medicaid costs from the federal government (Waid, p. 51). In 1991 more than 28 million people participated in the program at a cost of more than $77 billion (SSA, 1993, Annual Statistical Supplement 1992, p. 310). Medicaid has provided millions of Americans with health services they would not otherwise have.

Federal law does not mandate that a state operate a Medicaid program. However, all states participate in the program. (Arizona provides medical assistance through a Medicaid demonstration project.) To receive federal funds the state Medicaid program must offer certain basic services, which are:

- Inpatient hospital services
- Outpatient hospital services
- Prenatal care
- Physician services
- Nursing facility services for individuals age 21 or older
- Home health care services
- Family planning services and supplies
- Pediatric and family nurse practitioner services
- Rural health clinic services

◄ *Who Is Eligible for Medicaid?* ►

Mandatory Coverage under Federal Medicaid Guidelines

- Recipients of Aid to Families with Dependent Children (AFDC) and Supplemental Security Income (SSI) recipients.
- Children under age 6 and pregnant women who meet the State's AFDC financial requirements or whose family income is at or below 133 percent of the Federal poverty level. (Effective July 1, 1991, States are required to extend Medicaid eligibility to all children born after September 30, 1983, and under age 19, in families with incomes at or below the Federal poverty level. This phases in coverage so that by the year 2002 all poor children under age 19 will be covered.)
- Infants born to a Medicaid-eligible woman must continue Medicaid eligibility throughout the first year of life so long as the infant remains in the woman's household and she remains eligible, or would be eligible if she were still pregnant.
- Recipients of adoption assistance and foster care under Title IV-E of the Social Security Act.
- Certain Medicare beneficiaries.
- Special protected groups such as people who lose AFDC or SSI payments due to earnings from work or increased Social Security Benefits.

Optional Coverage under Federal Medicaid Guidelines [States will receive matching federal funds for these groups]:

- Infants up to age 1 and pregnant women not covered under the mandatory rules whose family income is at or below 185 percent of the federal poverty level.
- Certain aged, blind, or disabled adults who have incomes above those requiring mandatory coverage, but below the federal poverty level.
- Children under age 21 who meet income and resources requirements for AFDC, but who otherwise are not eligible for AFDC.
- Institutionalized individuals with income and resources below specified limits.
- Persons receiving care under home and community-based waivers.
- Persons receiving only state supplementary SSI payments.
- "Medically needy" persons such as those with high medical costs who meet the eligibility requirements except that they have more income and/or countable resources than allowed under the mandatory or optional categorically needy levels. Such persons may "spend down" to Medicaid eligibility.

From Waid MO: Medicaid, *Social Security Bulletin* 54:49-50, 1991.

- Laboratory and x-ray services
- Nurse-midwife services
- Federally qualified ambulatory and health-center services
- Early and periodic screening, diagnosis, and treatment (EPSDT) for children under the age of 21

People who are on Aid to Families with Dependent Children (AFDC) and Supplemental Security Income (SSI) are automatically eligible for Medicaid but must apply for it. To receive federal funds states must make certain groups of people eligible for Medicaid. States have the option of providing Medicaid coverage for medically needy groups other than those mandated; they receive matching federal funds for these groups. The box above shows the mandatory Medicaid eligibility groups as well as the optional groups.

Persons who are eligible for both Medicaid and

Medicare are called "dual eligibles." Some aged, blind, and/or disabled people are eligible for both of these programs. The state's Medicaid program can pay the Medicare premiums for such individuals, and Medicaid supplements the Medicare coverage with services not available under Medicare, such as prescriptions, hearing aids, eyeglasses, and long-term care. Unfortunately, many people eligible for this dual status are not participating because they are not aware that they are eligible.

Maternal-child health programs (MCH) have traditionally been a major source of funding for activities that are carried out by local health departments to meet the needs of high-risk mothers and children. These activities include the nutrition and health programs for women, infants, and children (WIC), medical or dental care, and comprehensive preventive medical care services through centers such as

PRESCAD (Preschool, School-age, and Adolescent). These services are discussed more extensively in Chapter 14. The monies appropriated for these programs now are largely available through federal block grants.

Private Health Assistance

Health assistance in the private sector is primarily of a voluntary, nonprofit nature. This volunteerism is prevalent, with many people donating time, money, and effort to help procure health services for others. The candy stripers in the local hospital, volunteer respite workers, and the readers for the blind are examples of volunteers who are helping clients to obtain health care services.

Service groups such as the American Cancer Society, American Diabetes Association, American Heart Association, Associations for Retarded Citizens, Lions' Clubs, Rotarians, Goodfellows, Knights of Columbus, church groups, and Visiting Nurse Associations provide cash and service benefits in the health field. A majority of U.S. hospitals operate on a voluntary, nonprofit basis. The dedicated leadership, financial support, and personal service of volunteers and voluntary agencies (non–tax-supported) have greatly aided the health care delivery system in this country, and an extension of this voluntary tradition is essential to continuing health services. Refer to Appendix 18-2 for a listing of some privately funded voluntary organizations.

Health Service Programs

Some government and private health service programs are administered through an organization for the benefit of specific employees or service groups. These programs often encompass a combination of insurance and assistance benefits.

Government Programs

Government programs have been generally established to meet the health care needs of specific population groups. Health service programs have existed for veterans, military personnel, merchant marines, American Indians on reservations, native Hawaiians, and federal employees. These programs vary in relation to the type of services and benefits offered. Changes in these programs may occur with the Clinton administration's health care reform.

Private Programs

Private service programs are often part of a benefit package for employees in the work setting. In addition to payment of employee health insurance premiums, many industries provide on-grounds employee health services. These services are usually preventive and treatment-oriented for work-related disease and disability.

THE UNITED STATES WELFARE SYSTEM

The primary task of the welfare system is to alleviate the hardships of the most disadvantaged. Welfare programs reflect an effort to ensure a basic standard of living and to promote social well-being. Like the health care financing system, the welfare system is complex. In this text programs are arbitrarily divided into welfare insurance and assistance programs. The box at the top of p. 119 outlines these programs.

Welfare Insurance

Welfare insurance programs are contributory. The individual or someone on behalf of the individual, such as the employer or the government, pays a premium, and benefits are awarded by virtue of these past premium contributions. Welfare insurance programs are found in both the government and private sectors.

Government Welfare Insurance

The federal government became extensively involved in welfare insurance programs with the passage of the Social Security Act in 1935. This act and its amendments are the basis for many federal government welfare insurance programs today. The act has been discussed earlier in this chapter. State governments also provide welfare insurance. A discussion of the major government welfare insurance programs follows.

Old Age, Survivors, and Disability Insurance (OASDI) is commonly called "Social Security." A history of the term *Social Security* is given in the box on the bottom of p. 119.

OASDI is a Social Security Act program that provides cash benefits to a qualified worker and his or her family when the worker retires in old age, becomes severely disabled, or dies. Eligibility is based on the amount of time worked and the amount of contributions made to the program. The principles that have historically guided benefit provision with the program are given in a box on p. 120.

OASDI is the largest income maintenance program in the country. Presently almost 42 million Americans receive OASDI benefits (SSA, 1993, Annual Statistical Supplement, p. 13); $286 billion is paid in OASDI benefits each year (SSA, p. 13). Benefits must be applied for and are administered through 1300 local branches of the federal Social Security Administration. These local offices issue the familiar social security numbers, help workers and employers maintain contribution records, process applications and make benefit decisions, coordinate Social Security Act programs for beneficiaries, and give workers and their families the information necessary to understand their rights and obligations under the program (Schwartz and Grundmann, 1991, p. 19). Whenever a branch office makes an eligibility decision for Social Security benefits a letter is sent that explains the decision (SSA, Fast

---

◀ U.S. Welfare Insurance and Assistance Programs ▶

Welfare Insurance

Governmental
1. Old Age, Survivors, and Disability Insurance (OASDI)
2. Unemployment insurance
3. Worker's compensation
Private

Welfare Assistance

Governmental
1. Aid to Families with Dependent Children (AFDC)
2. Supplemental Security Income (SSI)
3. Food Stamps
4. Supplemental Food Program for Women, Infants, and Children (WIC)
5. General assistance
Private

◀ Origin of the Term "Social Security" ▶

Abraham Epstein is the person generally recognized as introducing the term "Social Security." He was a national leader in the social welfare movement in the first half of this century. Epstein authored three books. The most well known is *Insecurity, a Challenge to America* (1933).

From 1918 to 1927 Epstein served as the research director of the Pennsylvania Commission on Old Age Pensions and was instrumental in having the state adopt an old-age assistance law in 1923. When Epstein realized that the Pennsylvania Commission would not be continued, he decided to establish a national organization to boost public support for social legislation such as State old-age assistance and pension programs. In 1927 he founded the American Association for Old Age Security. In 1933 he changed the name of his organization to the American Association for Social Security.

When Epstein was asked by Wilbur Cohen, later

Secretary of the Department of Health, Education, and Welfare, why he chose the term "Social Security" he explained that at the time Germany was using the term "Social Insurance" and England was using the term "Economic Security," and he did not want to use either of these. Epstein responded that he wanted a term to convey a program that not only provided economic security for workers, but the type of security that would promote the welfare of society as a whole. In a letter to Cohen, Epstein stated, "I was convinced that no improvement in the conditions of labor can come except as the security of the people as a whole is advanced."

It was Epstein's term "Social Security" that became the title of one of our country's landmark pieces of legislation, the Social Security Act of 1935. It is a term that has become a household word and denotes economic security to millions of Americans.

From Origin of the term "Social Security," *Social Security Bulletin* 55(1):63-64, 1992.
Original article based on letters:
1. Cohen to Abraham Epstein, March 3, 1941, Abraham Epstein Papers, Columbia University Library, New York.
2. Epstein to Wilbur J. Cohen, March 4, 1941, Abraham Epstein Papers, Columbia University Library, New York.
3. Frankel to Wilbur J. Cohen, October 1949, Abraham Epstein Papers, Columbia University Library, New York.

◀   *Old Age, Survivors, and Disability Insurance (OASDI): Program Principles*   ▶

Work Related

Benefits grow out of the individual's own work history. The amount of cash benefits the worker and his/her family receive is related to work earnings and contributions and the amount of time worked.

No Means Test

Benefits are a qualifying insured worker's right and are paid regardless of other income.

Contributory

During work years, workers pay Social Security (FICA) taxes to finance benefits. These taxes are routinely deducted from employee earnings. In this way workers "contribute" to the program.

Universal Compulsory Coverage

95% of the U.S. workforce is covered under OASDI. Coverage is universal and compulsory.

Rights Defined by Law

A person's rights to OASDI benefits are clearly defined in federal law.

From Schwartz D and Grundmann H: Old-age, survivors and disability insurance, *Social Security Bulletin* 54(9):6, 9-10, 1991.

TABLE

4-3 Maximum Annual Worker Taxable OASDI Earnings and Annual Contributions

Year	Maximum annual worker taxable earnings	Maximum worker annual contributions
1937	$ 3,000	$ 30.00
1953	$ 3,600	$ 54.00
1963	$ 4,800	$ 162.00
1973	$10,800	$ 464.40
1983	$35,700	$1,704.68
1993	$57,600	$3,225.60

From: Social Security Administration: *Annual Statistical Supplement to the Social Security Bulletin, 1992,* Washington, D.C., 1993, The Administration, pp. 14-15.

Facts, 1993, p. 34). OASDI benefit decisions can be appealed.

Employers, employees, and the self-employed pay mandated contributions, or taxes, into OASDI. The maximum amount of taxable earnings and worker contribution is updated each year in proportion to national increases in the average wage. Table 4-3 illustrates the maximum annual worker taxable earnings and contributions to OASDI for selected years from 1937 to 1993. It is readily apparent that worker contributions have steadily increased over the years.

More than 25 million people receive OASDI retirement insurance benefits, and the average monthly benefit for a retired worker is $653 (SSA, 1993, Annual Statistical Supplement 1993, p. 13). Today workers usually begin to receive old age retirement benefits at age 65; if a worker starts to receive OASDI benefits before age 65, the amount of his or her check is permanently reduced. If a worker returns to work after beginning retirement benefits there is a limit on the amount that the worker can earn if he or she still wants to collect Social Security retirement benefits. If a worker delays retirement past age 65, certain financial rewards and incentives accrue through age 70. The retirement age under the program is gradually being raised to age 67. The Social Security Administration publishes a booklet, *A Guide to Social Security Retirement Benefits,* which can be obtained free of charge by calling the administration's toll free number, 1-800-772-1213. To see the age at which persons can retire and receive full OASDI benefits, refer to Table 4-4.

The *survivors' insurance* component of the act has been in place since 1939. It provides benefits to the family of a deceased or disabled qualifying worker. Ninety-five percent of American children and their surviving parent are eligible for benefits should the family breadwinner die. The Social Security Administration publishes a booklet, *A Guide to Social Security*

TABLE **4-4**	**Projected Year of Retirement with Full OASDI Benefits: Based on Year Person Becomes 62**

If you are an OSADI eligible worker who becomes 62 in:	you can retire with full benefits at
2000	65 and 2 months
2001	65 and 4 months
2002	65 and 6 months
2003	65 and 8 months
2004	65 and 10 months
2005-2016	66
2017	66 and 2 months
2018	66 and 4 months
2019	66 and 6 months
2020	66 and 8 months
2021	66 and 10 months
2022 and over	67

From Social Security Administration: *Annual Statistical Supplement to the Social Security Bulletin, 1992,* Washington, D.C., 1993, The Administration, p. 35.

Survivors Benefits, which can be obtained free of charge by calling the administration.

The *disability insurance* component of the act has been in place since 1956. It provides benefits to qualifying persons under 65 years of age on the basis of medical evaluations and the person's continued inability to work. After age 65 the disabled worker can apply for the old age component of the insurance program. More than 3 million disabled workers receive benefits under OASDI, with average monthly benefits of $626 (SSA, 1993, Annual Statistical Supplement 1993, p. 13). The Social Security Administration publishes a booklet, *A Guide to Social Security Disability Benefits,* which can be obtained free of charge by calling the administration.

The U.S. Social Security system is coordinated with the social security systems of various countries to help ensure benefits to people who have lived and worked in other nations. The United States presently has Social Security agreements with 16 nations: Austria, Belgium, Canada, Germany, Finland, France, Ireland, Italy, Luxembourg, the Netherlands, Norway, Portugal, Spain, Sweden, Switzerland, and the United Kingdom (SSA, 1993, Annual Statistical Supplement 1992, p. 10).

Unemployment insurance was one of the original components of the act in 1935. It is a state-federal program that provides benefits to regularly employed members of the labor force who are involuntarily unemployed and who are able and willing to seek employment (Schmulowitz and Bretz, 1991, p. 20). It is a Social Security Act program that is administered by the state, often by the state Department of Labor. The state decides the amount and duration of the benefits, eligibility requirements, and disqualification criteria (Schmulowitz and Bretz, p. 20).

Unemployment benefits are available to qualified unemployed workers in employment covered under the act (Schmulowitz and Bretz, 1991, p. 20). The worker must remain registered to work and must actively seek employment while collecting benefits. Most states provide a maximum of 26 weeks of benefits each year, with benefits being applied for each week and paid weekly. For workers who have exhausted state benefits, there is a federal program of extended benefits available during times of high unemployment. However, regular and extended benefits cannot exceed a maximum period of 39 weeks during a year. If employment has not been found when unemployment benefits are exhausted, the family is often left without means of financial support and will begin to look at available state or local assistance programs or job training programs.

Employers pay into the program on behalf of the employee while the employee is working for them. All contributions collected under the state laws must be deposited in the Unemployment Trust Fund in the U.S. Treasury, in which each state has an interest-drawing account. A state must pay into this trust fund; there is no commercial or self-insurance available. A state can withdraw funds only to pay benefits. The federal government pays the costs of administration of the program, and makes loans to states when their unemployment insurance accounts run low.

There is great variation in program benefits from state to state. Approximately 109 million workers are insured under state unemployment insurance programs (Schmulowitz and Bretz, 1991, p. 22). More than 2.6 million workers collect unemployment benefits each year, and the average weekly benefit amount is $164 (Schmulowitz and Bretz, pp. 22, 25). The maximum weekly benefit each state ranges from $116 to $293 and the minimum weekly benefit ranges from $5 to $64 (Schmulowitz and Bretz, p. 25).

Workers' compensation has already been discussed under the legislative section on state workers' compensation and the health insurance section in this chapter. Refer to those sections for information on this program. Workers' compensation provides cash benefits and health care benefits for insured workers.

Private Welfare Insurance

Private welfare insurance, often in the form of income replacement insurance, is available through a number of agencies. Major forms of private welfare insurance include retirement and disability insurance. Many of these programs are obtained through the workplace, whereas others are purchased individually by the consumer. Millions of American workers are covered by private retirement insurance through their place of employment. The Retirement Income Security Act of 1974 helped to safeguard the financial integrity of these private retirement programs.

Welfare Assistance Programs

Welfare assistance programs are noncontributory or minimally contributory programs for qualifying indigent individuals, and they provide cash and ser-

vice benefits (e.g., food, shelter, and clothing). They exist largely as a result of state and federal legislation and are locally administered. Once a person's eligibility for a categorical government welfare assistance program has been determined, he or she usually receives cash benefits, social service benefits, and medical benefits through Medicare or Medicaid. Welfare assistance programs include both governmental and private programs.

Government Welfare Assistance

Government welfare assistance programs provide subsistence benefits for those without other resources. Applicants often apply for these programs through local departments of social service or through the Social Security Office, depending on the program. An applicant is generally asked to provide the following information when applying for government assistance programs:

- Proof of residence
- Proof of gross income from all sources for all household members
- Record of all property, including savings accounts, checking accounts, bonds, and land owned
- Record of house payments or rent and also insurance and taxes
- Record of utility bills
- Record of current medical and dental expenses
- Birth dates and social security numbers of household members
- Records of child support and alimony
- Proof of tuition and other required educational expenses
- Records of child care payment for employment or training purposes

Some major categorical government welfare assistance programs include the AFDC and SSI. Other government assistance programs include general assistance, food stamps, and WIC. These programs are discussed below.

Aid to Families with Dependent Children (AFDC) is the state-federal program provided for under the Social Security Act of 1935 that helps needy families with children by authorizing federal matching grants to states. Families usually apply for AFDC at local branches of the state Department of Human or Social Services. In 1992 over four million families, almost 13 million people, received almost $21 billion in AFDC payments (SSA, 1993, Annual Statistical Supplement

1993, p. 15). An AFDC family with two children received approximately $4700 a year or $390 a month (SSA, 1993, Annual Statistical Supplement 1993, p. 15). This amount of financial assistance puts AFDC families below the poverty level of income. All AFDC families are eligible for food stamps and most receive them. Payments are usually made directly to AFDC recipients, but individuals who are physically or mentally incapable of managing their own funds can have their payments go to a representative on their behalf.

AFDC furnishes financial and other assistance to encourage the care of dependent children in their own homes, to help parents become capable of self-support, and to maintain family life. In order for a family to qualify for AFDC there must be children who are deprived of the financial support of one parent because of death, disability, absence from the home, or, in some states, unemployment. The family's income must fall below a "needs standard" set by each state, which is the dollar amount necessary to meet a minimum standard of living in that state. AFDC funds are available to pregnant women, and in most states a woman can apply for AFDC or for an increase in her present allotment once a physician has verified in writing that she is pregnant. The actual amount of the AFDC payment will depend on the number of persons in the family and the amount of other income.

Any United States citizen or any alien lawfully admitted for permanent residence can apply for AFDC; there is no age requirement. However, aliens sponsored by private individuals or public or private agencies are usually not eligible until 3 years after they enter the United States, because they are considered to have the resources of their sponsors.

The Family Support Act of 1988 (Public Law 199-485) made major revisions in the AFDC program to assist AFDC families in obtaining education, training, and employment to avoid long-term welfare dependence. It established the first federal requirement that AFDC recipients seek employment, and it required that each state have in place a job opportunity and basic skills (JOBS) training program and enforce child support efforts (refer to Appendix 4-1 for additional information on this act).

Supplemental Security Income (SSI) is federal-state assistance provided for under the Social Security Act, federally administered through the Social Security Administration. It provides aid to qualifying aged, blind, and disabled people who have limited financial resources. The objective for establishing this program was to develop a uniform national minimum cash income for the indigent aged, blind, and disabled. It builds on the Social Security disability insurance programs of the act. In 1993 the SSI payment standard was $434 per month for an individual and $652 per month for a couple (Social Security Administration, Fast Facts, 1993, p. 1). More than 5.5 million people receive SSI each year (Social Security Administration, Fast Facts, p. 24).

Federal monetary benefits under the program remain constant throughout the nation and are adjusted to reflect Social Security cost-of-living increases. Forty-eight states supplement the program with additional cash benefits. State supplementary benefits vary and may be made directly to the beneficiary or paid through the federal Social Security Administration. Adults are usually the beneficiaries of SSI, but a child may be eligible if he or she suffers from an impairment that is expected to last a year or longer, such as mental retardation, terminal illness, or blindness. Applications for SSI are made at local branches of the federal Social Security Administration offices. Qualifying United States citizens and legally admitted aliens are eligible. The Social Security Administration publishes a booklet, *A Guide to the Supplemental Security Income Program,* that can be obtained free of charge by calling the administration's toll-free number, 1-800-772-1213.

Food stamps were begun on a pilot basis in 1961 to improve the nutritional adequacy of low-income individuals and families. It was formally established by the Food Stamp Act of 1964. It is a federal-state program under state administration; the federal sharing agency is the Department of Agriculture. Application is made at the local office of the state department of human or social services.

An eligible family of four persons with no personal income receives approximately $370 per month in food stamps (Social Security Administration, 1993, Annual Statistical Supplement 1993, p. 15). The average food stamp recipient has approximately 65 cents worth of food stamps to use for each meal ($59 per person per month). More than 25 million Americans take part in this program at a cost to the government of almost $21 billion each year (SSA, p. 15). Persons qualify on the basis of financial need. A food stamp office must determine eligibility of an applicant within 30 days of submission of a signed application.

Food stamps are available across the nation. Coupons are given to those who are eligible and are used like money at participating stores. Food stamps can be used only to purchase edible items; no imported foodstuffs, alcoholic beverages, or tobacco products can be bought with them. They are not transferable to another person and must be used by the person to whom they were issued. Most grocery stores are authorized to accept food stamps.

Supplemental Food Program for Women, Infants, and Children (WIC) is a federal nutrition and health assistance program authorized under the Child Nutrition Act of 1966. It is administered by the Food and Nutrition Service of the U.S. Department of Agriculture. WIC is designed to help pregnant and postpartum women, infants, and children up to 5 years of age who have been identified by health professionals as being at nutritional risk and who meet certain age and income requirements. More than 30% of infants born in the United States participate (Loeff, 1991, p. 74). The program includes food distribution, health assessment, and mandatory nutrition education. Participants receive vouchers that are redeemable at participating grocery stores for items such as infant formula, cereal, and juices; milk; cereals; and cheese.

WIC programs are frequently administered through local health departments. However, any public or nonprofit health or welfare agency can apply for program funds. There are approximately 7600 approved WIC service agencies in the United States (Loeff, 1991, p. 74). The WIC program has been very successful in promoting adequate nutrition and nutrition education. It serves 4.5 million people each year at a cost of $2.1 billion (approximately $30.30 per person each month) (Loeff, p. 74). If a family is receiving food stamps, participation in WIC does not affect their food stamp eligibility. Other food programs in which the federal government is involved are school lunch programs, school breakfast programs, school milk programs, needy family commodity foods, and food programs for the elderly.

General assistance is a state and locally funded and administered program that is offered in 36 states. There are no federal monies involved. In approximately one fourth of the states it is financed by local funds (Kerns, 1991, p. 76). The program is often administered through the state Department of Human or Social Services. It is usually made available to indigent persons who do not meet the criteria for other forms of welfare insurance or assistance but who are unable to meet their basic survival needs of food,

shelter, and clothing. This may be the only form of government assistance available for individuals who are poor but who do not qualify for AFDC, unemployment insurance, OASDI, or SSI.

In many states general assistance is limited to emergency relief (e.g., a catastrophic event such as a flood), short-term relief, and burial benefits. Any citizen or legally admitted alien can apply. In some states people receiving general assistance do not receive cash benefits, but instead receive vouchers for food, rent, or clothing. In some states the program is called *direct assistance.* Approximately 1.2 million people received general assistance in the United States each year (Kerns, 1991, p. 76).

In addition to the cash benefit programs discussed, many state and local governments offer a number of other welfare services. The following is a list of some of these services:

- Adoption services: accepting and placing children for adoption, recruiting adoptive families, and supporting and evaluating the adoption placement
- Foster care: funding, licensing, and monitoring
- Day care: licensing, monitoring and maintaining a listing of such placements
- Counseling: counseling individuals and families with problems to strengthen family functioning and to help prevent family breakdown
- Chore services: paying part or all of the cost for unskilled help with household tasks, personal care, home maintenance, or other activities for qualifying aged and disabled
- Education or training: providing funds and counseling services so that persons can improve their job skills through education and training programs
- Employment: helping people find jobs
- Family planning: providing information and referral to appropriate agencies
- Homemaking: teaching people about home management
- Housing: subsidizing low-income housing and keeping lists of appropriate low-income housing
- Information and referral: helping people learn about community services
- Mental health treatment and rehabilitation: providing services to persons with mental health problems through community mental health agencies

- Money management: helping people learn to budget
- Placement: helping place youth and adults in appropriate living facilities with follow-up (often in the form of foster care)
- Problem services: investigating reports of abuse and neglect and providing counseling services to prevent recurrence of such problems, counseling services for runaway youth, housing in emergency situations, and protection of aging clients and children from abuse and neglect (protective services)

Private Welfare Assistance

The United States is one of the few countries in the world to offer so many private welfare assistance programs and so comprehensive an array of them. Most offer short-term (acute) relief but do not provide long-term assistance for chronic problems.

Historically the provision of social services and educational programs has been an important aspect of the private sector (Kerns and Glanz, 1991, p. 4). The private sector has played a significant and valuable role in the provision of social welfare programs to local communities in the United States. Provision of such services costs private social welfare agencies more than $730 billion a year and represents about 40% of the nation's social welfare expenditures (Kerns, 1992, p. 61).

A recent census survey involving a sample representing 106,000 social service agencies and establishments found numerous services are frequently provided by private welfare agencies in the areas of individual and family services, residential care, recreation and group work, civic and social activities, and job training and rehabilitation. Examples of these services are given in the box above.

Summary

Over the ages health and welfare practices and services have evolved. We have come a long way in our knowledge and practice of good public health measures.

Early public health and welfare services were usually voluntary and were sponsored by churches and local organizations. In this country the Shattuck Report was the impetus behind the development of public health practice, and many of its components are part of contemporary public health policy and practice.

In the United States the federal government was slow to get involved in health and welfare service provision. Two pieces of legislation that set the stage for this governmental involvement were the Social Security Act of 1935 and the Public Health Service Act of 1944. The health and welfare programs of the Social Security Act have been enlarged over the years and provide many of the services that are used by the clients of community health nurses today. Legislation in the 1980s and 1990s has significantly affected the provisions of these acts and the availability of funding for health and welfare services. More significant legislation is in the making under the Clinton administration Health Care Reform mandate.

Today health and welfare services are found at all

three levels of government—federal, state, and local—and in the private sector. These services are complicated, diverse, and often poorly coordinated. Keeping up with governmental services is facilitated by knowledge of legislation and ordinances. Keeping up with private-sector health and welfare services requires diligent effort on the part of the nurse because these services vary greatly from locality to locality.

In relation to health care, millions of Americans are uninsured or underinsured, and millions do not have access to necessary health services. For many community health nursing clients, basic welfare needs such as food and shelter are a higher priority than health needs; health needs may not be viewed as a priority until the nurse can assist the client in meeting existing welfare needs.

Knowledge of health and welfare legislation and services is essential when nursing a community. The time and effort spent learning them will equip the community health nurse to more effectively deal with client situations encountered daily in the practice setting. Through this knowledge nurses can help clients become aware of the services available to them and enhance their quality of life. The nurse needs to network with other care professionals, local leadership, service groups, and organizations to remain informed.

◀ *An Exercise in Critical Thinking* ▶

This chapter gives community health nurses an overview of the depth and scope of health and welfare services available to people in the United States. What were your thoughts as you read the chapter? Were you overwhelmed? Excited about what will occur with health care reform? Saddened by the present system of delivery? All of these? Many services were presented in this chapter. Think about a client you have served and ascertain the practical use of the service information presented. What services could the client be eligible for? As a knowledgable professional, you need to know about the service yourself before you can help others.

APPENDIX 4-1

The Social Security Act of 1935: Major Amendments and Changes

1935   *Social Security Act of 1935 (Public Law 74-721)*—An act arising out of the Great Depression and designed to provide for the general welfare by establishing a system of federal old age benefits, and by enabling the states to make more adequate provision for aged persons, blind persons, dependent and crippled children, maternal and child welfare, public health, and the administration of their unemployment compensation laws. It consolidated existing welfare legislation under one law and established both insurance (contributory) and assistance (noncontributory) programs. Its original welfare insurance programs were Old Age Insurance (OAI) and the state-federal program of unemployment insurance. Its original categorical welfare assistance programs included the federal-state programs of Aid to the Blind (AB), Old Age Assistance (OAA), and Aid to Dependent Children (ADC).

1939   *Social Security Amendments (Public Law 74-271)*—Provided for the payment of insurance benefits to qualifying survivors of workers. The insurance program under the act was Old Age and Survivors Insurance (OASI).

1950   *Social Security Amendments of 1950 (Public Law 81-734)*—Provided for federal aid to states for financial assistance to people who were disabled under Aid to the Permanently and Totally Disabled. Under a new title, Title XIV, Aid to Dependent Children was broadened to include the relative with whom the child was living and became known as Aid to Families with Dependent Children. The federal-state public assistance programs under the act were Old Age Assistance (OAA), Aid to Families with Dependent Children (AFDC), Aid to the Blind (AB), and Aid to the Permanently and Totally Disabled (APTD). Federal matching of state payments to providers of medical services to persons on public assistance (vendor payments) was added.

1956   *Social Security Amendments of 1956 (Public Law 85-880)*—Provided disability insurance benefits for qualifying disabled individuals, reduced to 62 the age at which benefits could be paid to women (the Social

Security Amendments of 1961, Public Law 87-64, would make this the age for men also). The insurance portion of the act was Old Age, Survivors and Disability Insurance (OASDI).

1960   *Social Security Amendments of 1960 (Public Law 86-778)*—Established grants to states for medical care for the indigent aged, improved unemployment compensation and disability insurance benefits, eliminated the waiting period for disability insurance, and increased the insurance benefits for children of deceased workers.

1963   *Maternal and Child Health and Mental Retardation Planning Amendments (Public Law 88-156)*—Amended the act to assist states and communities in preventing mental retardation through expansion and improvement of maternal child health and crippled children's programs. This amendment provided for prenatal, maternity, and infant care for individuals with conditions associated with child bearing that may lead to mental retardation; it also provided funds for planning efforts that would promote comprehensive action to combat mental retardation.

1965   *Social Security Amendments of 1965 (Public Law 89-97)*—Provided for Medicare *(Title XVIII)* and Medicaid *(Title XIX)*. The insurance program (Medicare) under the act became Old Age, Survivors, Disability and Health Insurance (OASDHI). Medicaid was added to the assistance programs under the act. This was a landmark piece of legislation and marked the advent of major federal government involvement in health care delivery. Medicare greatly influenced the expansion of home health care services (refer to Chapter 19).

1967   *Social Security Amendments of 1967 (Public Law 90-248)*—Consolidated all maternal and child health and crippled children programs under one authorization and provided for funding of family planning services. Initiated the Work Incentive Now (WIN) program. Provided for the coverage of outpatient physical therapy and the purchase of durable medical equipment (DME) under Medicare. Established the Early, Periodic, Screening and Development Testing (EPSDT) under Medicaid and allowed Medicaid recipients free choice in the selection of qualified medical facilities and practitioners.

1972   *Social Security Amendments of 1972 (Public Law 92-603)*—Mandated the establishment of Professional Standard Review Organizations (PSROs) in health care. Established the assistance program of Supplemental Security Income to replace the categorical assistance programs of Old Age Assistance, Aid to the Blind, and Aid to the Permanently and Totally Disabled. This change provided for more nationally uniform payment levels to people qualifying for these programs and set a minimum level of payment.

States were encouraged to supplement the federal Supplemental Security Income (SSI) payments. The assistance programs under the act were now Supplemental Security Income (SSI) and Aid for Families with Dependent Children (AFDC), along with the medical assistance program of Medicaid. Health insurance coverage for the disabled was made available under Medicare.

1974   *Social Services Amendments of 1974 (Public Law 93-647)*—Consolidated previous federal-state social service programs into a block grant that would incorporate a ceiling on federal matching funds while providing reasonable flexibility to the states in determining the services to be provided. Reduced the federal regulatory role in social service programs. Included child support enforcement provisions and established the Parent Locator System to aid in collecting child support.

1977   *Social Security Amendments (Public Law 95-216)*—Strengthened the financing of the Social Security system through increased rates of contribution; provided benefits to young fathers who have in their care qualifying surviving children of deceased mothers; reduced the duration of marriage requirements for benefits to divorced spouses from 20 years to 10 years, and set a limit on retroactive benefits for a period of up to 12 months before the month of filing. A significant attempt of these amendments was to eliminate sex bias from the act. The establishment of fathers' benefits was significant to maintaining the financial stability of a young family. The National Commission on Social Security was also established.

Medicare-Medicaid Antifraud and Abuse Amendments (Public Law 95-142)—Established regulations and procedures to help protect these health care programs from fraud and abuse.

Social Security Act-Rural Health Clinic Amendments (Public Law 95-210)—Provided payment for rural health clinic services and allowed for direct reimbursement for nursing services in these settings. Also allowed the National Institute for Occupational Safety and Health (NIOSH), upon written request, to obtain the mailing address of taxpayers for the purpose of locating individuals who are, or may have been, exposed to occupational hazards, in order to determine the status of their health or to inform them of the possible need for medical treatment.

1978   *Medicare Endstage Renal Disease Amendments (Public Law 95-292)*—Made improvements in the end-stage program for clients with renal disease and kidney donors. Authorized experiments and pilot projects for the purchase of new or used durable medical equipment for end-stage renal dialysis clients. Encouraged public participation in the donor programs and authorized studies and measures to look at the costs of the program.

1980   *Medicare and Medicaid Amendments of 1980 (Public Law 96-499)*—The 100-visit-a-year limit was removed from both Part A & B home health care service provisions. Alcohol detoxification facility services were added to Part A benefits. These amendments also provided for payment of nurse-midwife services.

1981   *Omnibus Budget Reconciliation Act (Public Law 97-35)*—An act separate from the Social Security Act but amending it. Made an impact on many matters of health and welfare in the United States. In relation to the Social Security Act, it changed the following:
Medicare and Medicaid Amendments of 1981—Title XXI of the Omnibus Budget Reconciliation Act eliminated payment for alcohol detoxification services and occupational therapy as a basis for home health services. The part B deductible under Medicare was increased to $75, and federal Medicaid payment was decreased by 3 percent in 1982, 4 percent in 1983, and 4.5 percent in 1984, setting the trend for future disengagement from the program on the part of the federal government.
Maternal and Child Health Block Grant Act—Title XXI of the act provided for the consolidation, into one block grant, of seven grant programs from Title V of the Social Security Act and programs from the Public Health Service Act. The consolidated programs include the maternal-child health and crippled children's programs, genetic disease research, adolescent pregnancy services, sudden infant death syndrome research, hemophilia research, SSI payments to crippled children, and lead poisoning research.
Social Service Block Grant—Retained foster care, adoption assistance, and child welfare services as categorical programs while incorporating most of the programs administered by the Community Services Administration into a single social services block grant. Categorical funding was continued for immunizations, tuberculosis, venereal disease, family planning, and migrant health programs.
Other—The Omnibus Budget Reconciliation Act phased out benefits for students under the Social Security Act after the age of 18 years (students who were survivors of a deceased, qualifying parent) and eliminated the minimum benefit available under the Social Security Act, except for those eligible before January 1982. In addition, it authorized states to establish community work experience programs for AFDC recipients that could require work on useful public projects in return for benefits.

1982   *Tax Equity and Fiscal Responsibility Act of 1982 (Public Law 97-248)*—An act separate from the Social Security Act but amending it. The mandates of this act

were designed to reduce Medicare and Medicaid payments by the federal government by more than $14 billion between 1983 and 1985. The act set forth a system of prospective payment for Medicare services called Diagnostic Related Groups (DRGs). The overall intent of the act was to save the federal government money. However, professionals need to look carefully at the benefits and losses that result in relation to client care and then address these issues.

1983   *Social Security Amendments of 1983 (Public Law 98-21)*—Strengthened the financial basis of the program by increasing contributions by employers, employees, and self-employed individuals. Beginning in 1984, a portion of the Social Security retirement benefits paid to higher-income recipients will be considered taxable income. Effective January 1, 1984, the Social Security system covers all employees of nonprofit organizations and all federal employees hired on or after that date. Prior to this time, these employees had their own retirement program. Under this amendment, state and local governments that have withdrawn from the Social Security system will be permitted to rejoin. This amendment increases the bonus for individuals who delay their retirement. Regular retirement age, at which time individuals can receive Social Security benefits, will be increased in steps from 65 to 67. This amendment also authorized extended interfund borrowing between the funds making up the Social Security system and established a prospective payment plan for hospital reimbursement under the Medicare program.
Medicare Hospice Reimbursement (Public Law 98-90)—Amended title XVIII of the Social Security Act to increase the cap amount allowable for the reimbursement of hospice services under the Medicare program to $6500 for accounting years that end after October 1984.

1984   *Deficit Reduction Act of 1984 (Public Law 98-369)*—An act separate from the Social Security Act but amending it. Directed the Secretary of Health and Human Services to establish a national fee schedule for *all* Medicare laboratory services, except those provided in hospital facilities; for 15 months (beginning July 1, 1984), Medicare-participating physicians *must* accept Medicare payments as payment in full; conducted a study to determine how more physicians can be induced to accept Medicare assignment; limited for a 2-year period (beginning October 1, 1984) the increase in hospital costs eligible for reimbursement under the Medicare program; provided for the operation of *mobile* intensive care units by Medicare-reimbursed hospitals; made for-profit hospitals eligible for research and demonstration grants; permitted Medicare benefit payment to a third party, a health benefits plan, if the physician or supplier accepts the plan's payment as payment in full; terminated the Health Insurance Benefits advisory council; required states to provide Medicaid benefits to first-time pregnant women meeting Aid to Families with Dependent Children (AFDC) requirements; increased the assets ceiling for SSI beneficiaries, the ceiling increasing in steps to $2000 for an individual and $3000 for a married couple in 1989; provided that, in cases of SSI overpayment of benefits not involving fraud, willful misrepresentation, or concealment, recoupment will not exceed 10 percent of the recipient's monthly salary; increased the gross income limitations for AFDC; made aliens basically *ineligible* for AFDC benefits for 3 years if entry into the United States had been sponsored by an agency or organization.

Child Support Enforcement Amendments of 1984 (Public Law 98-378)—Amended Title IV of the Act to ensure, through *mandatory* income withholding, incentive payments to states, and other improvements in the child support enforcement program, that all children in the United States who are in need of assistance in securing financial support from their parents will receive such assistance. This amendment included provisions for increasing the availability of federal parent locator services to state agencies and provides for collection of past-due support from federal tax refunds. It also provided for the inclusion of medical support in child support orders. In addition, it required that availability of child support enforcement services be publicized, encouraged state guidelines for child support awards, and directed state and local governments to focus on the problems of child custody, support, and related domestic issues.

Social Security Disability Benefits Reform Act of 1984 (Public Law 98-460)—Provided for reform in the Social Security disability determination process

1985   *Consolidated Omnibus Budget Reconciliation Act of 1985 [COBRA] (Public Law 99-272)*—Amended the Social Security Act under Medicaid to extend Medicaid coverage for prenatal and postnatal care to low-income women in two-parent families where the primary breadwinner is unemployed; expanded the Medicaid services available under home and community-based services waivers; permitted state to offer hospice services to the terminally ill as an optional Medicaid benefit; required states to formulate policies for Medicaid coverage of organ transplants; and enhanced third-party liability connections. Under Medicare it postponed full implementation of the prospective payment system until October 1, 1987; delayed for 1 year the transition from regional DRG rates to uniform national rates; established extra payment of up to 15 percent of the regular DRG rates for hospitals serving a dispropor-

tionate number of low-income persons in an effort to compensate for the higher costs of caring for low-income clients—"disproportionate share allowance"; made permanent a temporary provision in the law allowing Medicare reimbursement for hospice care of the terminally ill and increased by $10 per day the rate of hospice payment; restructured the way Medicare pays teaching hospitals for the direct costs of graduate medical education; established an 11-member committee to study ways to improve the system for physician reimbursement under Medicare; extended the fee freeze for nonparticipating physicians; authorized demonstration projects in at least five states to determine cost effectiveness of providing Medicare coverage for preventive services such as immunizations and drug-abuse prevention; and required Medicare patients to receive a second medical opinion before certain elective surgery, denying Medicare reimbursement to those who failed to do so. The "anti-dumping" provisions required hospitals that participated in Medicare to provide emergency services for people with an urgent need for care, including women in labor, regardless of their ability to pay, and prohibited transfers of such patients unless their condition had been stabilized or a doctor certified that the move would be beneficial. Hospitals that violated the "anti-dumping" provisions could be barred from participating in Medicare and both the hospital and the responsible physician could face civil penalties of up to $25,000 per violation. Also, provided for a study of physician payments; established a Council on Graduate Medical Education to assess long-term physician training issues; and required the Department of Health and Human Services to establish a task force to develop recommendations for insurance policies to offer long-term health care.

1986   *Omnibus Budget Reconciliation Act of 1986 [OBRA] (Public Law 99-509)*—Amended the Social Security Act under Medicaid to allow states the option of expanding coverage for pregnant women, infants up to age 1, and children up to age 5 who had incomes below the Federal poverty level; required states to continue Medicaid coverage to disabled individuals who lost their eligibility for SSI assistance as a result of work earnings; clarified Medicaid coverage policies with regard to aliens and homeless individuals; and gave states the option of expanding Medicaid coverage for respiratory care services in the home. Under Medicare it established the rate of increase in prospective payment for fiscal years 1987 and 1988; provided for reductions in expenditures for inpatient hospital services; required prompt payment for provider claims; limited the Part A deductible to $520 in 1987; made a number of requirements to protect the quality of patient services; modified payment for physician services; authorized payment for services of physician assistants; authorized direct reimbursement for the services of certified nurse anesthetists; established a new payment system for hospital outpatient services; limited payment for cataract surgery involving a lens implant; and expanded beneficiary appeal rights under the Part B program.

1987 *Medicare and Medicaid Patient and Program Protection Act of 1987 (Public Law 100-93)*—Amended Titles XI, XVII, and XIX of the Social Security Act to protect beneficiaries under the act's health care programs from unfit health care practitioners, and otherwise to improve the antifraud provisions relating to those programs.

Omnibus Budget Reconciliation Act of 1987 (Public Law 100-203)—Under Medicare specified allowable increases in payments for all physician services and provided for reductions in payments for certain overpriced surgical procedures; increased the "disproportionate share allowance" for hospitals caring for a large number of medically indigent and specified the increases in hospital payment rates for fiscal years 1988 and 1989; established a home health toll-free hotline and investigative unit; permitted disabled individuals to renew entitlement to Medicare after gainful employment without a 2-year waiting period; provided incentive payments for physician's services in underserved areas; and allowed for collection of past-due amounts owed by physicians who breached contracts under the National Health Service Corps Scholarship program. It also established the Boarder Babies Demonstration Project for the development of model projects to develop alternative care for infants who do not require hospitalization, but who would otherwise remain in hospital settings owing to parental inability to care for them for reasons such as drug or alcohol addiction. Infants under this program could remain with a parent who resides in community residential setting (e.g., alcohol or drug treatment) or be placed in foster care, the goal being to rehabilitate the parent and eliminate the need for such infant care. In addition, this act authorized the Study of Infants and Children with AIDS in Foster Care to determine the total number of infants and children in the United States diagnosed as having acquired immunodeficiency syndrome and placed in foster care, to determine the problems encountered in placing such children, and the potential increase over the next 5 years in the number of such children. Provided a vaccine compensation program to compensate victims of vaccine side effects.

1988 *Family Support Act of 1988 (Public Law 100-485)*—Reformed the federal welfare system. Revised the AFDC program to emphasize work, child support, and family benefits. Amended Title IV of the Social Security Act to encourage and assist needy children and their parents to obtain the education, training, and employment needed to avoid long-term welfare dependence. Established child support and withholding programs, job opportunities and basic skills and training programs, and supportive services for families. Established the first federal requirement that welfare recipients seek employment and restored the permanent work incentive. Ended the WIN (Work Incentive Now) Program as of fiscal year 1990. Required that each state establish an education, training, and work (NETWork) program for parents seeking assistance under the family support program, and required parental participation for children age 3 and over (provided child care is guaranteed for children under 6 years of age and that participation is part-time for parents with a child under age 6). Required states to offer a family support supplement to needy two-parent families in which the principal wage earner is unemployed. Required state Medicaid programs to provide 6 months of transitional coverage for families leaving AFDC roles and beginning employment that may not provide health insurance, and to offer an additional 6-month extension (for a 12-month total) at the family's option (with the state being allowed to impose a modest premium for the second 6 months and/or allowing the state to fund the family's enrollment in an employer health plan). Required that states provide Medicaid to two-parent families with an unemployed head that meet AFDC income standards—health insurance for the unemployed. Established rules regarding recipient rights.

Medicare Catastrophic Coverage Act of 1988 (Public Law 100-360)*—A controversial and comprehensive act that amended the Social Security Act to protect Medicare beneficiaries from catastrophic health care expenses related to acute illness. Coverage was financed through increased Medicare Part B monthly premiums and a supplemental premium or "surtax" based on yearly income. In addition to covering catastrophic health care expenses, it provided under Medicare the first broad coverage of outpatient prescription drugs, removed the limit on hospice coverage, limited the inpatient hospital deductible to one per year, eliminated the durational limits and coinsurance charges for inpatient hospital services, limited coinsurance charges for posthospital skilled nursing facility (SNF) service to the first 8 days, and

---

*As of 1-1-90 the Medicare provisions of this act were repealed by the Medicare Catastrophic Repeal Act of 1989 (Public Law 101-234). Many of the Medicaid provisions were retained.

provided for 150 days of posthospital SNF benefits each year. It prohibited the misuse of symbols, emblems, or names in reference to Social Security or Medicare. Under Medicaid it required states, on a phased-in basis, to pay Medicare premiums, deductibles, and coinsurance for elderly and disabled individuals with incomes below the federal poverty level, and resources at or below twice the SSI standard; by 1990 to provide Medicaid coverage to all pregnant women and infants up to 1 year old with family incomes below poverty level; increased the amount of income and assets that may be retained by one member of a couple when the spouse enters a nursing home; and established uniform standards relating to disposal of resources for less than their fair market value in order to gain Medicaid eligibility.

1989　*Medicare Catastrophic Coverage Repeal Act of 1989 (Public Law 101-234)*—This act repealed the Medicare provisions of the Medicare Catastrophic Coverage Act of 1988 (Public Law 100-360) effective as of January 1, 1990. The Medicaid provisions of the 1988 Catastrophic Act that were left intact were the spousal impoverishment adjustment, enabling a spouse of an institutionalized older person to protect up to $60,000 in jointly held liquid assets while receiving Medicaid assistance for nursing home bills; the Medicaid "buy-in" requirement that states buy into Medicare, and pay the Medicare premiums, copayments, and deductibles for impoverished individuals; and Medicaid benefits for low-income pregnant women and infants. The act included transitional assistance for those persons already receiving nursing home and hospital benefits under the 1988

Catastrophic Act. The act also provided for reinstatement of MediGap policies held by persons covered previous to the 1988 Act.
Omnibus Budget Reconciliation Act of 1989 (Public Law 101-239)—Increased individual Social Security contributions; established an outreach program to make families of children who are potentially eligible for SSI benefits aware of their eligibility; provided a Medicare buy-in for selected disabled individuals under age 65; and required that state Medicaid programs pay, on a sliding scale, the Medicare Part A premiums for disabled individuals who are eligible to purchase Medicare under Section 6012 of the Act, whose income under the SSI program does not exceed 200 percent of the official poverty line, and whose resources do not exceed twice the SSI limits.

1990　*Omnibus Budget Reconciliation Act of 1990 (Public Law 101-508)*—Provided for changes in Medicare to allow Medicare B premiums to be paid for Medicare beneficiaries with income below 125% of federal poverty level and assets of $4000 or less, and provided for a toll-free number for Medicare and Medigap information for the public. Increased Medicaid coverage for children 12 years old or younger in families with incomes at or below the federal poverty level (this increased coverage is expected to add 700,000 children to the Medicaid program by 1995) and mandated use of outreach locations other than welfare offices. Required extended hospice benefits. Expanded coverage of nurse practitioners in rural areas, and changed the fee schedule for reimbursement for certified nurse anesthetists.

APPENDIX 4-2

The Public Health Service Act of 1944: Some Major Amendments and Changes

1944　*Public Health Service Act (Public Law 78-410)*—Consolidated and revised the laws relating to the Public Health Service.

1946　*Hospital Survey and Construction Act (Public Law 79-725)*—Authorized grants to states for surveying their hospitals and public health centers and for planning and construction grants for facilities. This legislation is commonly referred to as the Hill-Burton Act; it was frequently amended over the years and was incorporated into the 1974 PHSA amendments of the National Health Planning and Resources Development Act—Title XVI.

1954　*Medical Facilities Survey and Construction Act (Public Law 83-482)*—Amended the Hill-Burton provisions of the act to provide for assistance to states in surveying the need for diagnostic or treatment cen-

ters, hospitals for the chronically ill and impaired, rehabilitation centers, and nursing homes. Provided construction assistance for such facilities through grants to public and nonprofit agencies.

1956　*Health Research Facilities Act (Public Law 84-835)*—Provided for grants-in-aid to nonfederal public and nonprofit agencies for constructing and equipping facilities for research in the health sciences.
National Health Survey Act (Public Law 84-652)—Provided for a continuing survey and special studies of sickness and disability in the United States and for periodic reports on the results.
Health Amendments Act (Public Law 84-911)—Improved the health of the people by assisting in increasing the number of adequately trained professional and practical nurses and professional public

health personnel and in developing improved methods of care and treatment in the field of mental health.

1958 *Grants-in-Aid to Schools of Public Health (Public Law 85-544)*—Authorized the Surgeon General to make certain grants-in-aid to public and nonprofit accredited schools of public health for training in the fields of public health and public health administration of state and local public health programs.

1960 *Graduate Training in Public Health (Public Law 86-720)*—Amended Title III of the act to authorize project grants for graduate education in public health.
Health Promoting Sciences-Grants-In-Aid (Public Law 86-798)—Authorized grants-in-aid to universities, hospitals, laboratories, and other public or nonprofit institutions to strengthen their programs of research and training in sciences related to health.

1961 *Community Health Services and Facilities Act (Public Law 87-395)*—Assisted in expanding and improving community facilities and services for the health care of the aged and other persons; provided grants for research, experiments, and demonstration projects. Amended the Hill-Burton portion of the act.

1962 *Migrant Health Act (Public Law 87-692)*—Amended Title III of PHSA to authorize grants for family clinics for domestic, agricultural migratory workers.

1963 *Health Professions Educational Assistance Act (Public Law 88-129)*—Amended Title VIII to increase the opportunities for training physicians, dentists, and professional public health personnel. Provided for grants for construction of medical, dental, pharmaceutical, optometric, podiatric, nursing, osteopathic, and public health teaching facilities. Established the National Advisory Council on Education for Health Professions.

1964 *Nurse Training Act (Public Law 88-581)*—Increased opportunities for training professional nursing personnel and for construction of nursing schools.
Hospital and Medical Facilities Amendments (Public Law 88-443)—Amended the Hill-Burton portion of the act to include long-term care facilities and rehabilitation facilities.

1965 *Health Profession Educational Assistance Amendments (Public Law 89-190)*—Improved the educational quality of schools of medicine, dentistry, and osteopathy by authorizing grants to such schools for the awarding of scholarships to needy students. It also extended expiring provisions of the act for student loans and for aid in the construction of teaching facilities for such schools.
Heart Disease, Cancer, and Stroke Amendments (Public Law 89-239)—Assisted in combating heart disease, cancer, stroke, and related diseases by providing for education, research, training, and demonstration projects.

1966 *Comprehensive Health Planning and Public Health Service Amendments (Public Law 89-749)*—An act to promote and assist in the extension and improvement of comprehensive health planning and public health services and to provide for a more effective use of available federal funds for such planning and services.
Allied Health Professions Personnel Training Act (Public Law 89-751)—An act to increase the opportunities for training of medical technologists and personnel in other allied health professions; to improve the educational quality of schools training such allied health professions' personnel; and to strengthen and improve the existing student loan programs for medical, dental, podiatry, pharmacy, optometric, and nursing students.

1968 *Public Health Service Amendments (Public Law 90-574)*—Extended and improved provisions of the PHSA relating to Title I regional medical programs. It also extended the authorization for Title II migratory agricultural workers and provided for construction of facilities for alcoholic and narcotic addict rehabilitation. Commonly referred to as the Alcoholic and Narcotic Addict Rehabilitation Amendments of 1968.
Health Manpower Act (Public Law 90-490)—A major amendment to the PHSA, it extended and improved programs relating to the training of nursing and other health professions and allied health professions personnel, and the programs relating to student aid for such personnel and research facilities authorization. It authorized the study of school aid and student programs to establish aid levels for the future, along with the adequacy of health care personnel to meet long-term needs. Increased the monies available for nursing training.

1970 *Medical Facilities Construction and Modernization Amendments (Public Law 91-296)*—Revised, extended, and improved the programs previously established by Title VI relating to medical facility construction and modernization, and increased appropriations. It amended the Hill-Burton portion of the act.
Communicable Disease Control Amendments of 1970 (Public Law 91-464)—Authorized grants for communicable disease control, vaccination assistance, and studies to determine community-based communicable disease needs and strategies. Supported communicable disease programs designed to contribute to national protection against tuberculosis, venereal disease, rubella, measles, RH disease, poliomyelitis, diphtheria, tetanus, pertussis, and other communicable diseases transmissible from state to state that are amenable to treatment.
Comprehensive Drug Abuse Prevention and Control (Public Law 91-513)—Provided for increased research

into, and prevention of, drug abuse and dependence; provided for treatment and rehabilitation of drug abusers and drug-dependent persons; and strengthened existing law enforcement authority in the field of drug abuse.

Heart Disease, Cancer, Stroke, and Kidney Disease Amendments of 1970 (Public Law 91-515)—Improved and expanded research, education and training, and demonstration programs in these areas.

Health Training Improvement Act (Public Law 91-519)—Established eligibility of new schools of medicine, dentistry, osteopathy, pharmacy, optometry, veterinary medicine, and podiatry for grants; extended the program related to training of personnel in allied health professions.

Family Planning Services and Population Research Act (Public Law 91-572)—Established Title X, Population Research and Voluntary Family Planning Programs, to promote public health and welfare by expanding, improving, and better coordinating the family planning services and population research activities of the federal government.

Emergency Health Personnel Act (Public Law 91-623)—Authorized assignment of commissioned officers of the Public Health Service to areas with critical medical manpower shortages, in order to encourage health personnel to practice in such areas.

1971 *Comprehensive Health Manpower Training Act (Public Law 91-157)*—Provided for increased funding for health personnel through loan guarantees to students, student subsidies, startup assistance to schools, assistance to schools in distress, and health personnel initiative awards. Established the National Advisory Council on Health Professions Education and the National Health Manpower Clearinghouse. Mandated studies to look at the cost of educating health personnel students.

Nurse Training Act (Public Health Law 92-158)—Provided for training increased numbers of nurses through construction grants and student loan guarantees, advanced training traineeships, scholarships, loan repayment and forgiveness, and capitaltion grants. Prohibited sex discrimination in student selection.

National Cancer Act (Public Law 92-218)—Strengthened the National Cancer Institute and National Institutes of Health in order to more effectively carry out national efforts against cancer.

1972 *National Sickle Cell Anemia Control Act (Public Law 92-294)*—Provided funding to aid in the control of sickle cell anemia.

National Cooley's Anemia Control Act (Public Law 92-414)—Provided funding to aid in the control of Cooley's anemia.

Communicable Disease Control Amendments Act of 1972 (Public Law 92-449)—Extended and revised the program of assistance to states for control and prevention of communicable disease, including grants for vaccinations, venereal disease prevention and control, and family planning services, grants and contracts.

1973 *Emergency Medical Services System Act (Public Law 93-154)*—Provided assistance and encouragement to states for the development of comprehensive area emergency medical services systems.

Health Maintenance Organization Act (Public Law 93-222)—Provided assistance and encouragement for the establishment and expansion of HMOs.

Safe Drinking Water Act (Public Law 93-253)—Significant environmental health legislation to assure safe drinking water in the United States.

1974 *Sudden Infant Death Syndrome Act (Public Law 93-270)*—Provided financial assistance for research, counseling, information, education, and statistical programs related to sudden infant death syndrome (SIDS).

National Cancer Program Improvement (Public Law 93-352)—Improved the national cancer program and reauthorized appropriations. Mandated an information dissemination program for professionals and the general public. Established the President's Biomedical Research Panel.

Health Services Research, Health Statistics and Medical Libraries Act (Public Law 93-353)—Revised programs of health services research and extended assistance for medical libraries. Established the National Center for Health Services Research.

National Diabetes Mellitus Research and Education Act (Public Law 93-354)—Provided for greater and more effective efforts in research and public education on diabetes mellitus. Established the National Commission on Diabetes within the National Institutes of Health and the Diabetes Mellitus Coordinating Committee to oversee federal activities on the subject. Authorized prevention and control programs and research and training centers.

National Arthritis Act (Public Law 93-640)—Expanded the authority of the National Institute of Arthritis, Metabolism, and Digestive Diseases in order to advance a national attack on arthritis.

National Health Planning and Resource Development Act (Public Law 93-641)—Authorized the development of national health policy and effective state and area health planning resources development programs. Established Titles XV and XVI. Title XV, National Health Planning and Development, dealt with national health policies and priorities, established health service areas and health systems agencies, and required state health planning and development agencies. Title XVI, Health Resources Development, dealt largely with construction and modernization of health care facilities. Existing Hill-Burton legislation was integrated into this act under Title XVI.

1975   *Public Health Service Act Amendments (Public Law 94-63)*—Revised and extended the revenue-sharing programs, family planning programs, community mental health programs, programs for migrant health centers, community health centers, hemophilia programs, the National Health Service Corps, and nurse training assistance. These amendments include: The Special Health Revenue Sharing Act, Family Planning and Population Research Act, and Community Mental Health Centers Amendments and Nurse Training Act of 1975. Established the National Center for the Prevention and Control of Rape.

1976   *National Consumer Health Information and Health Promotion Act (Public Law 94-317)*—Added Title XVII, Health Information and Promotion, to the act. Called for the development of consumer and community information programs related to health information, prevention, and promotion activities and health education.
Indian Health Care Improvement Act (Public Law 94-437)—Improved federal Indian health programs and dealt with provision of services, construction and renovation of facilities, insured safe water, promoted construction of sanitary waste disposal sites, promoted access to health care services and these services for urban Indians, and authorized an American Indian School of Medicine feasibility study.
Health Maintenance Organization Amendments of 1976 (Public Law 94-460)—Revised and extended the program for establishment and expansion of HMOs.
Health Professions Educational Assistance Act (Public Law 94-484)—Revised and extended the programs of assistance under Title VII for training in health and in allied health professions. New authorization for special projects for departments of family medicine and programs related to the recruitment and enrollment of disadvantaged students. Also authorized special project grants for schools of public health and graduate programs in health administration for enlarging programs in biostatistics, epidemiology, health administration, health planning, health policy, environmental and occupational health, and nutrition. Traineeships for students in schools of public health were initiated under Title VII.
Arthritis, Diabetes, and Digestive Diseases Amendments of 1976 (Public Law 94-562)—Established the National Arthritis Advisory Board, National Diabetes Advisory Board, and National Commission on Digestive Diseases.

1977   *Rural Health Clinics Act (Public Law 95-210)*—Established rural health clinics in underserved sections of the country.
Health Services and Extension Act of 1977 (Public Law 95-83)—Mandated the development of standards for community preventive health services over a 2-year period.

1978   *Public Health Amendments (Public Law 95-622)*—Biomedical and behavioral research amendments. Established the President's Commission for the Study of Ethical Problems in Medicine and Biomedical and Behavioral Research.
Health Services Research, Health Statistics, and Health Care Technology Act of 1978 (Public Law 95-623)—Established a National Center for Health Care Technology.

1979   *Health Planning and Resources Development Amendments (Public Law 96-79)*—Addressed the rising cost of health care and cost containment by establishing national health priorities and by eliminating inappropriate placement of people in institutions for the mentally ill and mentally retarded, and increasing the quality of care in those institutions for people who needed it. This amendment also placed increased emphasis on community mental health centers utilizing outpatient rather than inpatient treatment. In addition, it developed a certificate of need program for health care facilities seeking federal funds, in order to minimize duplication of services and unnecessary services.

1980   *Health Planning Amendments (Public Law 96-538)*—Revised and extended the act. Deleted the National Commission on Diabetes and formulated the Diabetes Mellitus Interagency Coordinating Committee. Established the Diabetes, Arthritis, and Digestive Diseases Advisory Boards and the Information and Education Center on Digestive Diseases.

1981   *Omnibus Budget Reconciliation Act (Public Law 97-35)*—Enacted many budget and program cuts under the Public Health Service Act. It revised health planning policy; eliminated Public Health Service Hospitals as of the end of fiscal year 1981; consolidated many categorical programs of the Public Health Service Act into block grants to states, but left in place categorical funding for immunization, tuberculosis, venereal disease, family planning, and migrant health programs.

1982   *Tax Equity and Fiscal Responsibility Act of 1982 (Public Law 97-248)*—Authorized massive federal spending cutbacks that had an impact on public health.

1983   *Alcohol and Drug Abuse Amendments (Public Law 98-24)*—Established the National Institute on Alcohol Abuse and Alcoholism and the National Institute on Drug Abuse. Mandated Drug Abuse Strategy Reports on a yearly basis, which represented a continued federal effort to combat the problems of alcoholism and drug abuse. It also represented increased effort to disseminate information and research findings to the states, to provide technical assistance to research and service personnel, and to develop preventive programs designed to reduce alcohol and drug abuse problems. It encouraged the development of effective occupational prevention and treatment programs and private sector programs.

National Organ Transplant Act (Public Law 98-507)—Provided for the establishment of the Task Force on Organ Transplantation and the Organ Procurement and Transplantation Network.

1985 *Nurse Education Amendments of 1985 (Public Law 99-92)*—Extended the programs of assistance for nurse education through fiscal year 1988. Appropriated $9,500,000 yearly for 1986 through 1988.

Health Research Extension Act of 1985 (Public Law 99-158)—Created the National Center for Nursing Research and the National Institute of Arthritis and Musculoskeletal and Skin Diseases.

1986 *Health Services Amendments Act of 1986 (Public Law 99-280)*—Revised and extended the community and migrant health centers programs for 2 fiscal years and repealed the Primary Care Block Grant authority.

Safe Drinking Water Act Amendments of 1986 (Public Law 99-339)—Amended Title XIV of the Public Health Service Act, the Safe Drinking Water Act, to authorize EPA to establish national drinking water regulations and to determine maximum allowable water contaminant levels. Mandated that public water systems increase their monitoring for unregulated contaminants. Increased fines and sentences for tampering with public water systems, and prohibited the use of lead pipes and solder in public water systems.

Health Programs (Public Law 99-660)—Amended the Public Health Service Act to include the National Commission to Prevent Infant Mortality Act of 1986, National Childhood Vaccine Injury Act of 1986, Health Care Quality Improvement Act of 1986, Health Maintenance Organization Amendments of 1986, and the Alzheimer's Disease and Related Dementias Services Research Act of 1986. Repealed Title XV: Health Planning; revised and extended the health maintenance organization program through 1989; established an authority within the Public Health Service under which states can apply for grants for the development of state comprehensive mental health plans and under which grants may be awarded for the training of health professionals in geriatric medicine; established a National Commission to Prevent Infant Mortality; encouraged profes-

sional peer review as a deterrent to malpractice and incompetence in health care; and established a Council on Alzheimer's Disease. The National Vaccine Program was given the responsibility for vaccine research, development, safety, and efficacy testing; licensing of vaccine manufacturers and vaccines; production and procurement of vaccines; evaluating the need for, effectiveness of, and adverse effects of vaccines; and coordinating government and nongovernmental vaccine activities. Established a National Vaccine Injury Compensation Program.

Public Health Service Act Amendments of 1987 (Public Law 100-177)—Amended the Public Health Service Act to extend the authorizations for the National Center for Health Services Research, National Center for Health Statistics, National Health Service Corps, and preventive health programs relating to immunizations and tuberculosis control. Established a Loan Repayment Program for the National Health Service Corps.

1988 *Family Health Services Amendments of 1988 (Public Law 100-386)*—Amended Title III of the Public Health Service Act to revise and extend the community and migrant health centers programs and the program of health services for the homeless.

Grants for Purchase of Drugs Used in the Treatment of AIDS (Public Law 100-471)—Provided for the awarding of grants for the purchase of drugs used in treatment of AIDS. $15,000,000 was appropriated to be used through March 31, 1989.

National Deafness and Other Communication Disorders Act of 1988 (Public Law 100-553)—Amended the Public Health Service Act to establish within the National Institutes of Health a National Institute on Deafness and Other Communication Disorders. The general purpose of the Institute is to conduct and support research and training, disseminate health information, and sponsor other programs with respect to disorders of hearing and other communication processes, including diseases affecting hearing, balance, voice, speech, language, taste, and smell. Established a National Deafness and Other Communication Disorders Data System, and a National Deafness and Other Communication Disorders Information Clearinghouse.

Lead Contamination Control Act of 1988 (Public Law 100-572)—Amended Title XIV of the Public Health Service Act, the Safe Drinking Water Act, to eliminate the use of lead-lined watercoolers.

Clinical Laboratory Improvement Amendments of 1988 (Public Law 100-578)—Amended the Public Health Service Act to revise the authority for the regulation of clinical laboratories. Provided for uniform standards for the certification of clinical laboratories.

Native Hawaiian Health Care Act of 1988 (Public Law 100-579)—Intended to improve the health status of native Hawaiians. Provided for grants and contracts with Papa Ola Lokahi for the purpose of developing native Hawaiian comprehensive health care master plan to promote comprehensive health promotion and disease prevention services, to maintain and improve the health status of native Hawaiians, and to provide for the establishment of native Hawaiian health centers.

Health Omnibus Programs Extension of 1988 (Public Law 100-607)—Amended the Public Health Service Act to include National Institute on Deafness and Other Communication Disorders and Health Research Extension Act of 1988, Organ Transplant Amendments of 1988, AIDS Amendments of 1988, and Health Professions Reauthorization Act of 1988. The amendments extended Public Health Service Act authorities for the Preventive Health Block Grant; sexually transmitted diseases prevention and control grants; health professions education; and nurse training. Established the National Center for Biotechnology Information, the National Commission on Sleep Disorders, and the National Deafness and Other Communication Disorders Program. Created Title XXIV—Health Services with respect to acquired immune deficiency syndrome that provided comprehensive AIDS services including formula grants to states for home and community-based health services for AIDS patients. Required an annual comprehensive report to Congress each year on AIDS expenditures by the Secretary of Health and Human Services, and mandated the Secretary to expedite AIDS grants and research monies. Mandated Clinical Evaluation Units at the National Cancer Institute and the National Institute of Allergy and Infectious Diseases to evaluate AIDS treatment. Mandated support of international AIDS efforts with special emphasis being placed on cooperation with World Health Organization and Panamerican Health Organization AIDS efforts. Established a public information program with respect to AIDS research, treatment, and prevention activities including a toll-free hotline number, data bank on research information, and data bank on clinical trials and treatments. Provided grant monies for the establishment of projects to develop model protocols for the clinical care of individuals infected with the AIDS virus. Established the National Blood Resource Education Program to increase public awareness that giving blood is safe and other aspects of blood donation. Established the Office of AIDS Research within the National Institutes of Health. Provided for ongoing data collection on the national prevalence of AIDS, long-term AIDS research, and social sciences AIDS research. Estab-

lished fellowships and training programs, to be conducted by the Centers for Disease Control, to train individuals to develop skills in epidemiology, surveillance testing, counseling, education, information, and laboratory analysis relating to AIDS. Established projects to promote cooperation between public and private sector AIDS programs and research.

Indian Health Care Amendments of 1988 (Public Law 100-713)—Reauthorized and amended the Indian Health Care Improvement Act.

Health Maintenance Organization Amendments of 1988 (Public Law 100-715)—Allowed insurance companies and other entities to sponsor HMOs.

1990 *Home Health Care and Alzheimer's Disease Amendments of 1990 (Public Law 101-557)*—Authorized demonstration projects for home health care services, funded research on Alzheimer's Disease, renamed Centers of Geriatric Research and Training to Claude D. Pepper Older American Independence Centers, established the Task Force on Aging Research to implement research on the aging process and on diagnosis and treatment of diseases, disorder, and disability related to aging to assist the aged individual in retaining independence.

Transplant Amendments Act of 1990 (Public Law 101-616)—Established the National Bone Marrow Donor Registry and offered assistance for organ procurement organizations.

Vaccine and Immunization Amendment Act of 1990 (Public Law 101-502)—Expanded vaccine-preventable disease programs. Authorized demonstration projects for children 2 years old or younger in low-income areas to provide immunizations, casefinding, and parent education.

Year 2000 Health Objectives Planning Act (Public Law 101-582)—Established a program of grants to States for the development of State plans for meeting the objectives established by *Healthy People 2000*.

Ryan White Comprehensive AIDS Resources Emergency Act of 1990 (Public Law 101-381)—Provided emergency assistance to localities that were disproportionately affected by the HIV epidemic. Gave financial assistance to states and other public or private nonprofit entities to provide for the development, organization, coordination, and operation of more effective and cost-efficient systems for the delivery of essential services to individuals and families with HIV infection. Established HIV Care Grants and demonstration grants for research and services for pediatric patients with HIV. Provided for early intervention services. Established partner notification guidelines and the requirement that states receiving federal monies under the act have laws against intentional infection.

1991　*Health Information, Health Promotion and Vaccine Injury Compensation Amendments of 1991 (Public Law 102-168)*—Provided for health information and health promotion programs with an emphasis on disease prevention. Established the Office of Disease Prevention and Health Promotion.

1992　*DES Education and Research Amendments of 1992 (Public Law 102-409)*—Provided for research on the drug known as diethylstilbestrol to educate health professional and the public on the drug and to provide for longitudinal studies regarding individuals who have been exposed to the drug.

Cancer Registries Amendments Act (Public Law 102-515)—An Act to assist in cancer prevention, early detection, and compilation of morbidity and mortality statistics. Established a national program of state cancer registries. Each state is eligible for a grant and technical assistance from the federal government to operate a registry in which demographic data, industrial and occupational history information, pathological data, and date of diagnosis would be recorded. Authorized the "Breast Cancer Study" in a number of East Coast states with high incidence of breast cancer.

Preventive Health Amendments of 1992 (Public Law 102-531)—This placed major emphasis by the federal government on preventive health and primary prevention activities. Established the National Foundation for the Centers for Disease Control and Prevention (NFCDCP). It changed the name of Centers for Disease Control to Centers for Disease Control and Prevention (CDC). The NFCDCP is organized on a nonprofit basis. Its purpose is to support and implement activities for the prevention and control of diseases, disorders, injuries, and disabilities and for promotion of public health. The act included provisions for programs on injury control; lead poisoning prevention; preventable infertility from sexually transmitted diseases; vaccine services; screening for breast, cervical and prostate cancer; and international cooperation in preventive health measures. It provided for more comprehensive services to Migrant Health Centers in the areas of maternal and child health and community education. NFCDCP activities included (1) programs of fellowships for state and local public health officials to work and study in association with CDC, (2) international exchange programs for public health officials from the United States and abroad who are interested in working in a foreign country, (3) studies, projects, and research on prevention, (4) forums for government officials and private entities to exchange information, (5) meetings, conferences, courses, and training workshops, (6) programs to improve the collection and analysis of data on the health status of various populations, and (7) programs for writing, editing, printing, and publishing books and materials.

Mammography Quality Standards Act of 1992 (Public Law 102-539)—Under this act every facility that performs mammographies must receive certification from the Department of Health and Human Services as of October 1, 1994. These facilities must have appropriate equipment and qualified personnel to perform the radiological imaging and results must be interpreted solely by qualified radiologists. Certification can be for a period of up to three years. If certification is revoked there is a two year period before the facility can own or operate a mammography program again. Authorized Breast Cancer Screening Surveillance Research Grants to look at effectiveness of breast cancer screening programs in the United States.

Health Professions Education Extension Amendments of 1992 (Public Law 102-408)—Revised and extended certain programs relating to the education of individuals as health professionals. Included extensive provisions for nursing education such as advanced nurse education, nurse practitioner and nurse midwife programs, nurse anesthetists, and traineeships.

References

American Cancer Society: *Cancer facts and figures—1993,* New York, 1993, The Society.

American Nurses Association: *Nursing's agenda for health care reform,* Kansas City, Mo., 1991, The Association.

Bretz J: Medicare, *Social Sec Bull* 54(3):45-48, 1991.

Clancy CM, Himmelstein DU, and Woolhandler S: Questions and answers about managed competition, *Health/PAC Bulletin* 23:30-32, 1993.

Coll BD: *Perspectives in public welfare: a history,* Washington, D.C., 1969, U.S. Government Printing Office.

Davis K: Will managed competition work (congressional testimony), *Health/PAC Bulletin* 23:25-26, 1993.

Forgotson E: 1965: the turning point in public health law—1966 reflections, *Am J Public Health* 57(6):934-946, 1967.

Frisof K: Change the health care system? How UHCAN! *Health/PAC Bulletin* 23:40-42, 1993.

Harrington C: A national health care program: has its time come? *Nurs Outlook* 36:214-216, 225, 1989.

Health Care Financing Administration-Office of Public Affairs: *The Medicare handbook, 1993,* Washington, D.C., 1993, U.S. Government Printing Office.

Health Insurance Association of America: *Source book of health insurance data: 1977-78,* Washington, D.C., 1978, The Association.

Health Insurance Association of America: *Source book of health insurance data: 1983-84,* Washington, D.C., 1983, The Association.

Health Insurance Association of America: *Source book of health insurance data: 1992,* Washington, D.C., 1992, The Association.

Himmelstein DU and Woolhandler S: *The national health program chartbook,* Cambridge, Mass., 1992, The Center for National Health Program Studies, Harvard Medical School/Cambridge Hospital.

Institute of Gerontology: *Social Security: the first thirty-five years,* Ann Arbor, 1970, University of Michigan Press.

Institute of Medicine-Committee for the Study of the Future of Public Health: *The future of public health,* Washington, D.C., 1988, National Academy Press.

Kerns WL: General assistance, *Social Sec Bull* 54(9):76, 1991.

Kerns WL: Private social welfare expenditures, 1972-90, *Social Sec Bull* 55(3):59-66, 1992.

Kerns WL and Glanz MP: Private social welfare expenditures, 1972-88, *Social Sec Bull* 54(2):2-11, 1991.

Kotelchuck R: Managed competition: a guide to the thicket, *Health/PAC Bulletin* 23:4-12, 1993.

Loeff J: Supplemental food program for women, infants and children, *Social Sec Bull* 54(9):74, 1991.

McKenzie N: Managed competition and public health: let's do the right thing, *Health/PAC Bulletin* 23:33-36, 1993.

Metropolitan Life Insurance Company: *Brief history of Metropolitan Life's health and safety activities, 1871-1983,* New York, 1983, The Company.

National Center for Health Statistics (NCHS). *Health, United States, and Prevention Profile 1991,* Washington, D.C., 1992, United States Public Health Service.

Nelson WJ: Workers' compensation, *Social Sec Bull* 54(9):28-37, 1991.

Nelson WJ: Workers' compensation coverage, benefits and costs, 1982, *Social Sec Bull* 55(1):51-62, 1992.

Origin of the term "Social Security," *Social Sec Bull* 55(1):63-64, 1992.

Pickett G and Hanlon JJ: *Public health administration and practice,* ed 9, St. Louis, 1990, Mosby.

Richardson BW: *The health of nations, a review of the works of Edwin Chadwick,* vol 2, London, 1887, Longmans, Green & Co.

Schmulowitz J and Bretz JS: Unemployment insurance, *Social Sec Bull* 54(9):20-28, 1991.

Schwartz D and Grundmann H: Social Security programs in the United States—Old Age Survivors, and Disability Insurance, *Social Sec Bull* 52(7):6-19, 1991.

Shattuck L: *Report of the Sanitary Commission of Massachusetts,* Cambridge, Mass., 1948, Harvard University Press (originally published by Dutton & Wentworth in 1850).

Silver GA: *Family medical care: a design for health maintenance,* Cambridge, Mass., 1974, Ballinger.

Smolensky J: *Principles of community health,* ed 4, Philadelphia, 1977, Saunders.

Social Security Administration: *Annual statistical supplement to the Social Security Bulletin, 1992,* Washington, D.C., 1993, The Administration.

Social Security Administration: *Annual statistical supplement to the Social Security Bulletin, 1993,* Washington, D.C., 1993, The Administration.

Social Security Administration: *Understanding Social Security,* Washington, D.C., 1993, The Administration (SSA Publication No. 05-10024).

Social Security Administration: *Fast facts on Social Security,* Washington, D.C., 1993, The Administration.

Tropman EF and Tropman JE: Voluntary agencies. In Minihan A, ed-in-chief: *Encyclopedia of social work,* ed 18, Silver Spring, Md., 1987, National Association of Social Workers, pp. 825-842.

USDHHS: *Healthy people 2000. National health promotion and disease prevention objectives, full report,* Washington, D.C., 1991, U.S. Government Printing Office.

United States Statutes-at-Large, selected years.

Waid MO: Medicaid, *Social Sec Bull* 54(9):49-56, 1991.

Wilner DM, Walkley RP, and O'Neill EJ: *Introduction to public health,* ed 7, New York, 1978, Macmillan.

Wilson FA and Neuhauser D: *Health services in the United States,* ed 2, revised, Cambridge, Mass., 1985, Ballinger.

Selected Bibliography

American Association for Retired Persons: *Health care America. Meeting America's health care needs,* Washington, D.C., 1992, The Association.

American Public Health Association: *A national health program for all of us. The American Public Health Association's Guide to the Health Care Reform Debate,* Washington, D.C., undated, The Association.

Bernstein NR: *APHA, the first one hundred years,* Washington, D.C., 1972, American Public Health Association.

Corning PA: *The evolution of Medicare . . . from idea to law,* Research Report No. 29, Washington, D.C., 1969, U.S. Department of Health, Education, and Welfare, Social Security Administration, Office of Research and Statistics.

Eliot MM: The Children's Bureau, fifty years of public responsibility for action in behalf of children, *Am J Public Health* 52(4):576-591, 1962.

Furman B: A profile of the United States Public Health Service, 1798-1948, Washington, D.C., 1973, National Library of Medicine.

Hanlon JJ, Rogers F, and Rosen G: A bookshelf on the history and philosophy of public health, *Am J Public Health* 50(4):445-458, 1960.

Health Resources Administration: Health in America: 1776-1976, Washington, D.C., 1976, United States Public Health Service.

Kerns WL: Aid to families with dependent children, *Social Sec Bull* 54(9):68-70, 1991.

Loeff J: Food stamps, *Soc Sec Bull* 54(9):71-73, 1991.

Ravenel MP: *A half century of public health. Jubilee historical volume of the American Public Health Association,* New York, 1921, American Public Health Association.

Rosenberg CE: *Origins of public health in America. Selected essays 1820-1855,* New York, 1972, Arno Press.

Schmulowitz J: Supplemental security income, *Soc Sec Bull* 54(9):64-67, 1991.

Smillie WG: The National Board of Health, 1879-1883, *Am J Public Health* 33(8):925-930, 1943.

Social Security Administration: The social security handbook, Washington, D.C., 1993, U.S. Government Printing Office.

Trattner W: *From poor law to welfare state,* ed 3, New York, 1984, Free Press.

Winslow C-EA: *The evolution and significance of the modern public health campaign,* New Haven, 1984, Yale University Press (originally published in 1923).

Organization of United States Health and Welfare Resources

OBJECTIVES

Upon completion of this chapter, the reader should be able to:

1. State the "levels" and "sectors" into which health care is organized and delivered in the United States.
2. Discuss the *Healthy People* initiative.
3. List the three major national goals of *Healthy People 2000*.
4. Explain the core public health functions of local, state, and federal government.
5. Discuss the major divisions of the U.S. Department of Health and Human Services (USDHHS).

6. Describe patterns of organizational structure between state health authorities (SHAs) and local health departments (LHDs).
7. Discuss service functions of SHAs and LHDs.
8. Discuss federal, state, and local governmental welfare organization.
9. Identify private health and welfare resources on the federal, state, and local level.

The intent of this chapter is to assist the nurse in becoming familiar with the *Healthy People* initiative, year 2000 national health objectives, and the organization and functions of health and welfare resources in the United States. Since 1980 the United States has had national health objectives. Across the nation individuals, health and welfare resources, and all levels of government are working to meet these objectives.

The United States has a wealth of health and welfare resources, the scope of which is not seen elsewhere in the world. A brief look at the complicated organization of these resources shows that they are organized in two sectors; public (governmental) and private; and on three levels: federal, state, and local (refer to Chapter 4). This diversity of resources and organization makes the United States notable among the countries of the world for its complicated policy relationships between levels of government and its interweaving of private and public sector activity to maintain the public's health (Institute of Medicine, 1988, p. 37).

In the governmental sector public health functions are usually carried out by the federal Department of Health and Human Services, state health authorities (SHAs), and local health departments (LHDs). Under the Constitution, the individual states have primary responsibility for ensuring the public health. Welfare functions in the governmental sector are largely carried out by the federal Department of Health and Human Services, state departments of human or social services, and their local affiliates. Private sector health and welfare resources are classified as either nonprofit or profit. Private sector resources vary greatly from one locality to another.

HEALTHY PEOPLE 2000: PROVIDING FOR THE PUBLIC'S HEALTH

The word *health* was left out of the U.S. Constitution. The federal government bases its involvement in health and welfare activities on the Preamble to the Constitution, which charges the federal government to provide for the general welfare of the people. Public health has historically been the responsibility of the individual states. It is provided for through state constitutions, legislation, and public health codes.

In 1988 the Institute of Medicine's (IOM) Committee for the Study of the Future of Public Health

published a classic report on public health in the United States called *The Future of Public Health*. This report examined the status of public health in the United States and provided a futuristic view for the public health system. The Committee broadly defined the mission of public health to be the measures that we as a society take collectively to provide the conditions that ensure the people's health (Institute of Medicine, 1988, p. 17).

After careful study of our public health system the IOM committee concluded that the nation had lost sight of its public health goals and that the public health system was in disarray and a threat to the health of the public (Institute of Medicine, 1988, p. 191). This committee found that decision-making in public health is frequently driven by crises and the concerns of organized interest groups rather than by comprehensive analysis or the objective of enhancing the quality of life (Institute of Medicine, p. 5). Some barriers to promoting public health include the lack of consensus on the mission of public health, inequities in public health services, problems in relationships among the several levels of government, the poor public image of public health, and fragmented decision-making (Institute of Medicine, p. 108). In fact, public health resources have become so fragmented and diverse that deliberate action is often difficult if not impossible (Institute of Medicine, p. 1).

The committee stated that an impossible responsibility has been placed on America's public health resources "to serve the basic health needs of entire populations, while at the same time averting impending disasters, providing personal health care to those rejected by the rest of the health system; and to take on the new public health problems while confronting the old" (Institute of Medicine, 1988, pp. 2, 138). According to the committee, public health in the United States requires that continuing and emerging threats to the public health be successfully countered, including immediate crises such as the AIDS epidemic and access to health and welfare services for the indigent; enduring problems such as injuries, chronic illness, teen pregnancy, control of high blood pressure, smoking, and substance abuse; and growing challenges such as the aging of the population, homelessness, and environmental health (Institute of Medicine, pp. 19-30).

The committee also concluded that the American public has come to take the successes of public health for granted and has sometimes become lax in public health practices. The committee stated that it is no wonder the American public health system is in trouble—the wonder is that the system has done so much, for so long, with so little (Institute of Medicine, 1988, p. 2).

The Healthy People Initiative

In 1979, under the presidency of Jimmy Carter, the Surgeon General of the United States issued a landmark report that has shaped public health policy for the past decade: *Healthy People: The Surgeon General's Report on Health Promotion and Disease Prevention,* often referred to as *Healthy People.* This report analyzed the leading causes of death in the United States and suggested that many of these deaths are preventable. It estimated that approximately one half of all U.S. mortality was due to unhealthful behavior, one fifth to environmental hazards, one fifth to human biological factors, and one tenth to inadequacies in the health care system. *Healthy People* was the first in a series of documents developed by the U.S. Department of Health and Human Services (USDHHS) that outlined U.S. public health goals, objectives, services, and standards. These documents are discussed in this chapter, and are listed in the box at right.

Healthy People established broad national health goals targeted for achievement in 1990, and issued a challenge to the nation to accomplish them. It launched an unprecedented initiative to promote healthful lifestyles and improve the health of Americans, and called on all levels of government, professionals, and lay people to undertake a venture that promised to reduce preventable death and disability across the lifespan (USDHHS, 1986, p. v). The goals and subgoals were listed under the areas of healthy infants, healthy children, healthy adolescents and young adults, healthy adults, and healthy older adults.

Healthy People established three target areas: preventive health services (priority areas: family planning, pregnancy and infant care, immunizations, sexually transmissible diseases, and blood pressure control); health protection (priority areas: toxic agent control, occupational safety and health, accidental injury control, fluoridation of community water supplies, and infectious agents control); and health promotion (priority areas: smoking cessation, reducing the misuse of alcohol and drugs, improving nutrition, exercise and fitness, and stress control). *Promoting Health/Preventing Disease: Objectives for the*

◀ *Significant Documents* ▶ *Related to the Healthy People Initiative*

USDHEW: *Healthy people: the Surgeon General's report on health promotion and disease prevention,* Washington, D.C., 1979, U.S. Government Printing Office.

USDHHS: *Promoting health/preventing disease: objectives for the nation,* Washington, D.C., 1980, U.S. Government Printing Office.

USDHHS: *The 1990 objectives for the nation: a midcourse review,* Washington, D.C., 1986, U.S. Government Printing Office.

USDHHS: *Healthy People 2000: national health promotion and disease prevention objectives,* Washington, D.C., 1991, U.S. Government Printing Office.

Related Documents

Public Health Foundation: *Status report: state progress on 1990 health objectives for the nation,* Washington, D.C., 1988, The Foundation.

American Public Health Association: *Healthy communities 2000: model standards. Guidelines for community attainment of the year 2000 national health objectives,* ed 3, Washington, D.C., 1991, The Association.

Nation was published in 1980. It set forth 226 specific and quantifiable objectives necessary for the attainment of the broad national goals established in *Healthy People.* Objectives were established for each of the 15 priority areas and became the national health objectives for 1990.

The 1990 Health Objectives for the Nation: A Midcourse Review was published in 1986. This midcourse review was meant to provide Americans with an assessment of how the nation was doing in its decade-long quest to improve health status. Because of the different data gathering and reporting mechanisms in individual states, it was often difficult to obtain information on how well each state was doing in meeting these objectives.

The midcourse review showed that the nation was on its way to achieving nearly half of the 226 objectives, that about one fourth were unlikely to be achieved, and that in eight cases the trend was away from reaching the 1990 targets (USDHHS, 1986, p. iii). The midcourse review found reductions in both

◀ *Healthy People 2000:* ▶
National Health Goals

- Increase the span of healthy life for Americans
- Reduce health disparities among Americans
- Achieve access to preventive services for all Americans

From USDHHS: *Healthy people 2000: national health promotion and disease prevention objectives, full report, with commentary,* Washington, D.C., 1991, U.S. Government Printing Office, p. 43.

◀ *Healthy People 2000:* ▶
Age Related Objectives

Healthy Infants and Children

Reduce the death rate for children by 15 percent to no more than 28 per 100,000 children aged 1 through 14, and for infants by approximately 30 percent to no more than 7 per 1,000 live births. (Baseline: 33 per 100,000 for children in 1987 and 10.1 per 1,000 live births for infants in 1987)

Healthy Adolescents and Young Adults

Reduce the death rate for adolescents and young adults by 15 percent to no more than 85 per 100,000 people aged 15 through 24. (Baseline: 99.4 per 100,000 in 1987)

Healthy Adults

Reduce the death rate for adults by 20 percent to no more than 340 per 100,000 people aged 25 through 64. (Baseline 423 per 100,000 in 1987)

Healthy Older Adults

Reduce to no more than 90 per 1,000 people the proportion of all people aged 65 and older who have difficulty in performing two or more personal care activities (a reduction of about 19 percent), thereby preserving independence. (Baseline: 111 per 1,000 in 1984-85)

From USDHHS: *Healthy people 2000: national health promotion and disease prevention objectives, full report, with commentary,* Washington, D.C., 1991, U.S. Government Printing Office, pp. 562, 571, 579, and 587.

smoking and per capital alcohol consumption, increased use of automobile seat belts, and reduced death rates from strokes, cirrhosis, and traffic accidents. The review showed that Americans still needed work on the health areas of weight control, illicit drug use, control of violent behavior, teenage pregnancy, infant health, family planning, physical fitness and exercise, and control of sexually transmitted diseases.

Status Report: State Progress on 1990 Health Objectives for the Nation was published in 1988 by the Public Health Foundation. This report reviewed the individual states' progress toward 29 of the 226 national objectives set forth in *Promoting Health/Preventing Disease: Objectives for the Nation,* and served as a resource for state health planning and evaluation activities for the 1990 objectives. The report found that states did not always have the information necessary to evaluate their progress toward the 1990 objectives.

Healthy People 2000: National Health Promotion and Disease Prevention Objectives (1991) continued the efforts started by the federal government in 1979 with *Healthy People.* It is the product of a national effort involving almost 300 national organizations, all the state health authorities, the Institute of Medicine, the National Academy of Sciences, and the U.S. Public Health Service (USDHHS, 1991). It is the focal point of the Healthy People initiative and outlines broad national health goals, age-related objectives, almost 300 national health objectives under 22 priority areas, and objectives for special population groups that address the needs of low-income families, ethnic minority groups, and people with disabilities. The boxes on pp. 142 and 143 give an overview of the national goals, age-related objectives, and priority areas of *Healthy People 2000. Healthy People 2000* will shape the direction of health care in this country for the remainder of

the decade. The Year 2000 Health Objectives Planning Act (Public Law 101-582) established a program of grants to states for the development of state plans for assisting communities in meeting the objectives of *Healthy People 2000.*

Healthy Communities 2000: Model Standards was developed by the American Public Health Association, National Association of County Health Officials, Centers for Disease Control and Prevention, and the Association for State and Territorial Health Officials. The Health Services Extension Act of 1977 (Public Law 95-83) mandated the development of model standards for community preventive health services in American communities. *Healthy Communities 2000* assists communities in establishing achievable community

◀ *Healthy People 2000: Priority Areas with Responsible Agencies* ▶

Health Promotion

1. Physical activity and fitness
   - President's Council on Physical Fitness and Sports
2. Nutrition
   - National Institutes of Health
   - Food and Drug Administration
3. Tobacco
   - Centers for Disease Control and Prevention
4. Alcohol and other drugs
   - Alcohol, Drug Abuse, and Mental Health Administration
5. Family planning
   - Office of Population Affairs
6. Mental health and mental disorders
   - Alcohol, Drug Abuse, and Mental Health Administration
7. Violent and abusive behavior
   - Centers for Disease Control and Prevention
8. Educational and community-based programs
   - Centers for Disease Control and Prevention
   - Health Resources Services Administration

Health Protection

9. Unintentional injuries
   - Centers for Disease Control and Prevention
10. Occupational safety and health
    - Centers for Disease Control and Prevention
11. Environmental health
    - National Institutes of Health
    - Centers for Disease Control and Prevention

12. Food and drug safety
    - Food and Drug Administration
13. Oral health
    - National Institutes of Health
    - Centers for Disease Control and Prevention

Preventive Services

14. Maternal and infant health
    - Health Resources and Services Administration
15. Heart disease and stroke
    - National Institutes of Health
16. Cancer
    - National Institutes of Health
17. Diabetes and chronic disabling conditions
    - National Institutes of Health
    - Centers for Disease Control and Prevention
18. HIV infection
    - National AIDS Program Office
19. Sexually transmitted diseases
    - Centers for Disease Control and Prevention
20. Immunization and infectious diseases
    - Centers for Disease Control and Prevention
21. Clinical preventive services
    - Health Resources and Services Administration
    - Centers for Disease Control and Prevention

Surveillance and Data Systems

22. Surveillance and data systems
    - Centers for Disease Control and Prevention

From USDHHS: *Healthy people 2000: National health promotion and disease prevention objectives, full report, with commentary,* Washington, D.C., 1991, U.S. Government Printing Office, p. 659.

health objectives in conjunction with *Healthy People 2000* (APHA, 1991, p. ix). Its standards encompass all of the priority areas, age groups, and national objectives in *Healthy People 2000.* To date the federal government has not mandated nationwide implementation of the standards, but it does encourage state health authorities (SHAs) and local health departments (LHDs) to use them.

Core Public Health Functions

In *The Future of Public Health* the Committee for the Study of the Future of Public Health (CSFPH) stated that core functions in ensuring public health exist at all levels of government and that these functions are *assessment, policy development,* and *assurance* (Institute of Medicine, 1988, pp. 7-8, 41-42, 141-142). The government's role in ensuring these core functions includes (Institute of Medicine, pp. 141-142):

- *Assessment.* Regularly and systematically collect, assemble, analyze, and make available information on the health of the community, including statistics on health status, community health needs, and epidemiological and other studies of health problems. This is a governmental function that cannot be delegated.
- *Policy development.* Exercise responsibility to

serve the public interest in the development of comprehensive public health policies by promoting use of the scientific knowledge base in decision-making about public health and by leading in the development of public health policy. Agencies must take a strategic approach, developed on the basis of a positive appreciation for the democratic political process.

- *Assurance.* Ensure constituents that services necessary to achieve agreed-upon goals are provided, either by encouraging actions by other entities (private or public sector), by requiring such action through regulation, or by providing services directly. Involve the general public and key policymakers in determining a set of high-priority personal and communitywide health services that governments will guarantee to every member of the community. This guarantee should include subsidization or direct provision of high-priority personal health services for those unable to afford them.

FEDERAL GOVERNMENT: HEALTH AND WELFARE FUNCTIONS AND ORGANIZATION

In addition to these core functions, the committee assigned unique responsibilities to each level of government. The committee recommended the following as additional federal government public health functions (Institute of Medicine, 1988, p. 9):

- Support knowledge development and dissemination through data gathering, research, and information exchange
- Establish nationwide health objectives and priorities, and stimulate debate on interstate and national public health issues
- Provide technical assistance to help states and localities determine their own objectives and to carry out action on national and regional objectives
- Provide funds to states to strengthen state capacity for services, especially to achieve an adequate minimum capacity, and to achieve national objectives
- Ensure actions and services that are in the public interest of the entire nation, such as control of AIDS and similar communicable diseases, interstate environmental actions, and food and drug inspection

Table 5-1 delineates some of the major categories of functions of the federal government in relation to public health and welfare. Federal patterns of organization for carrying out these functions are diverse, and health and welfare programs and services are carried out in many federal agencies. The U.S. Department of Health and Human Services is presented first, since it is the single most important federal agency in matters of health and welfare. Most of the health and welfare functions of the federal government are coordinated and administered through this department.

U.S. DEPARTMENT OF HEALTH AND HUMAN SERVICES (USDHHS)

This department assumed a cabinet-level position on April 11, 1953, as the Department of Health, Education, and Welfare (DHEW), with a charge to safeguard the health and welfare of the nation. In 1980 the DHEW split and became the Department of Health and Human Services (DHHS) and the Department of Education. The DHHS is the department most involved with the nation's human resources and concerns, and it touches the lives of more Americans than any other federal agency. The secretary of the department advises the President on health, welfare, and income security issues. Figure 5-1 depicts the organization of the DHHS.

Several important health and welfare programs are administered through this department, including Old Age, Survivors and Disability Insurance (OASDI), Medicare, Medicaid, Supplemental Security Income (SSI), Aid to Families with Dependent Children (AFDC), and many programs of the Public Health Service Act and Occupational Safety and Health Act. Major components of this department are discussed here, using information from the *U.S. Government Manual.*

Social Security Administration (SSA)

This administration was established on July 16, 1946 when its predecessor, the Social Security Board, was abolished. It guides and directs all of the cash benefit programs of the Social Security Act of 1935. The SSA includes 10 regional offices and over 1300 local offices across the country, and is the major federal agency dealing with social welfare programs for specific population groups. Local offices have responsibility for informing people about SSA programs, assist-

5-1 Federal Government Health and Welfare Functions

Categories of functions	Examples of programs and services
Assessment and planning	Includes a number of ongoing national health assessments. An important service is the collection of national health and welfare statistics. Health planning activities include setting national health objectives and model standards, developing strategies for implementation, and assisting states in implementation. The Health Resources and Services Administration of the U.S. Public Health Service is actively involved in assessment and planning activities.
Assurance	Involves periodic evaluation of progress toward national health objectives and monitoring of the quality and effectiveness of national public health programs and activities. Ensures that actions and services are in the public interest. The Health Resources and Services Administration of the U.S. Public Health Service is actively involved in ensurance activities.
Policy development	Includes enacting the necessary health and welfare legislation and making adequate appropriations for implementing legislative mandates. The Agency for Health Care Policy and Research is actively involved in obtaining suggestions for national health policy.
Personal and community health	Carries out extensive personal and community health services under the mandates of the Social Security Act of 1935, Public Health Service Act of 1944, Occupational Safety and Health Act of 1970, and other legislative acts. Sponsors services in the *Healthy People 2000* priority areas, and provides direct services to special population groups (e.g., American Indians, Native Hawaiians, military personnel, and migrant workers). The Social Security Administration and numerous branches of the U.S. Public Health Service provide many personal and community health and welfare services.
International health and welfare	Is a member of and supports international health and welfare organizations including the United Nations, WHO, and the Peace Corps. Participates in international disaster relief, foreign aid, international pollution control, and world peace activities.
Education and training	Involves promotion of programs preparing health and welfare professionals through such activities as training grants and loans, grants-in-aid to training programs, and continuing education. It also involves federal health education activities and public health publications. Maintains numerous national clearinghouses to distribute informational and educational materials and maintains the U.S. Government Printing Office. Has numerous health publications available at low or no cost to the general public.
Research	Subsidizes research for the advancement of public health and welfare. The National Institutes of Health conduct rigorous research programs and collaborate on international research. The Agency for Health Care Policy and Research is actively involved in obtaining suggestions for national health policy.

ing in filing and processing claims, and helping claimants file appeals.

U.S. Public Health Service (USPHS)

The U.S. Public Health Service is the oldest of the department's component agencies. It was established in 1798 as the Marine Hospital Service and became the USPHS in 1912. Under the direction of the Surgeon General it carries out the mandates of the Public Health Act of 1944 and is charged with protecting and advancing the nation's physical and mental health.

The USPHS collects and disseminates national

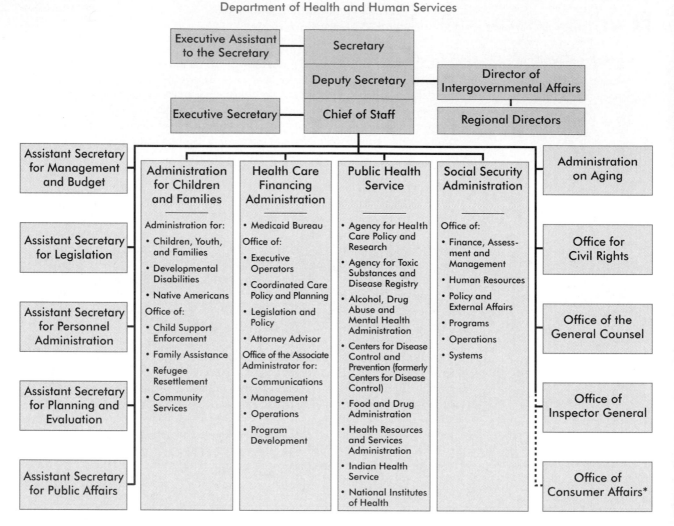

Department of Health and Human Services

* Located administratively in HHS, but reports to the President.

Figure 5-1   Organization of the U.S. Department of Health and Human Service. (From Office of the Federal Registry: *United States government manual 1992/93,* Washington, D.C., 1992, U.S. Government Printing Office, p. 303.)

health statistics, provides laboratory services, works with states to set and implement health policy congruent with national health policy, generates and upholds international health agreements, sponsors and administers programs for the development of health resources, assumes responsibility for the prevention and control of communicable and chronic diseases and conditions, and provides resources and consultation to public and private agencies for planning and implementing public health activities. It is also involved in health care research, including AIDS research. Additionally, it provides grants-in-aid to schools of public health and funding for the training of health care professionals. The USPHS enforces public health laws. The National Center for Health Statistics is a part of the USPHS. The major components of the USPHS are listed in Table 5-2 on pp. 148-149.

Health Care Financing Administration (HCFA)

The Health Care Financing Administration was created by the Department of Health, Education, and

Welfare reorganization of March 8, 1977, and oversees the administration of Medicare, Medicaid, and federal quality control measures designed to improve the delivery of health care services. Chapters 4, 13, and 20 address issues handled by this agency.

Administration on Aging

The Administration on Aging is the principal agency designated to implement programs of the Older Americans Act of 1969. It develops policies, plans programs to promote the health and welfare of older Americans, and administers grants to states to establish state and community programs for older persons.

Administration for Children and Families

The Administration for Children and Families was created April 15, 1991. It administers state grant programs, Head Start services, services for wayward youth, Child Abuse Prevention and Treatment Act provisions, developmental disabilities activities, Child Support Enforcement Act provisions, and refugee resettlement.

OTHER FEDERAL INVOLVEMENT IN HEALTH AND WELFARE

All cabinet level departments in the United States have functions that relate to the improvement of health and welfare conditions in our nation or foreign countries. These departments do not have the scope of public health responsibilities that DHHS has, but they provide essential services that enhance the health status and quality of life of Americans. Briefly summarized are some of the health and welfare functions carried out by other federal departments, as presented in the *U.S. Government Manual.*

Cabinet-Level Involvement

- *Department of Agriculture.* Carries out environmental health activities in the areas of food safety and inspection, sanitation, and assessment of plant and animal disease. Operates programs to protect and develop the nation's natural resources, coordinates rural development programs, and maintains the National Agricultural Library, which houses almost 2 million volumes. Conducts agricultural research and operates cooperative extension services out of the land grant universities, and also operates international food assistance and information exchange programs. Through its food and nutrition programs works to minimize poverty, hunger, and malnutrition in the United States. These programs include food stamps, National School Lunch Program, School Breakfast Program, Special School Milk Program, senior citizen nutrition programs, and Supplemental Food for Women, Infants, and Children program (WIC). WIC is one of the department's largest, most successful, and best-known programs. WIC is discussed more extensively in Chapters 4 and 14.
- *Department of Commerce.* Seeks to promote an understanding of the earth's physical environment and oceanic life. Promotes economic development and encourages technological advancements. Its Bureau of the Census collects and disseminates data about the economy of the country and the characteristics of population groups; census information is discussed more thoroughly in Chapter 12. Its National Institute of Standards and Technology maintains a national measurement system.
- *Department of Defense.* Provides the military forces necessary to deter war and to protect the national security. Administers the health and medical care services for military forces as well as civilian dependents of service personnel. This department also operates the National Civil Defense Program.
- *Department of Education.* Safeguards the nation's educational system. Oversees bilingual education, educational civil rights, education of the handicapped, vocational and adult education, special education and rehabilitative services, and elementary, secondary, and post-secondary education.
- *Department of Energy.* Provides the framework for a comprehensive national energy plan. Is responsible for energy conservation, energy regulatory programs and nuclear energy and weapons. Is involved in environmental restoration, nuclear safety, conservation and renewal of energy, and waste management. Ensures that departmental programs are in compliance with environmental safety and health regulations.
- *Department of Housing and Urban Development* (HUD). Is the principal agency concerned with national housing needs, fair housing opportunities,

5-2 Major Components of the U.S. Public Health Service

Agency	Structure and purpose
Centers for Disease Control and Prevention (CDC)	Established in 1973 as the Center for Disease Control and more recently re-named Centers for Disease Control. In 1992 its name was changed to Centers for Disease Control and Prevention. It is the federal agency charged with pro-tecting the public's health. The agency administers national programs for the prevention and control of communicable and vector-borne diseases and other preventable conditions. It includes nine operating agencies: (1) Epidemiology Program Office, (2) International Health Program Office, (3) Public Health Practice Program Office, (4) National Center for Prevention Services, (5) National Center for Environmental Health and Injury Control, (6) National Institute for Occupational Safety and Health (NIOSH), (7) National Center for Chronic Disease Prevention and Health Promotion, (8) National Center for Infectious Diseases, and (9) National Center for Health Statistics. Some major program components focus on communicable disease prevention and control, health promotion, chronic disease prevention, occupational safety and health, public health emergencies, and international health. NIOSH develops occupational safety and health standards. The centers also coordinate the use of rare therapeutic and immunoprophylactic agents, collect and disseminate health statistics, and direct and enforce national quarantine measures.
National Institutes of Health (NIH)	NIH is the principal biomedical research agency of the federal government. The goal of NIH is to improve the health of the nation through increasing the understanding of processes affecting human health, disability, and disease; advancing knowledge concerning the health effects of interactions between man and the environment; developing methods of preventing, diagnosing, and treating disease; and disseminating research findings. NIH supports biomedical training programs. Institutes in NIH include: (1) National Cancer Institute, (2) National Heart, Lung, and Blood Institute, (3) National Institute of Diabetes and Digestive and Kidney Disease, (4) National Institute of Allergy and Infectious Diseases, (5) National Institute of Child Health and Human Development, (6) National Institute on Deafness and other Communicative Disorders, (7) National Institute of Dental Research, (8) National Institute of Environmental Health Science, (9) National Institute of Neurological Disorders and Stroke, (10) National Eye Institute, (11) National Institute on Aging, (12) National Institute of Arthritis and Musculoskeletal and Skin Diseases; and (13) National Institute of Nursing Research. NIH also includes the National Library of Medicine, National Center for Research Resources, National Center for Human Genome Research, Clinical Center, Division of Computer Research and Technology, and Fogarty International Center.
Food and Drug Administration (FDA)	The FDA was formally established in 1931. Its activities are directed toward protecting the health of the nation against impure and unsafe food, drugs, and cosmetics. Major divisions include (1) Office of Operations, (2) Center for Drug Evaluation and Research, (3) Center for Biologic Evaluation and Research, (4) Center for Food Safety and Applied Nutrition, (5) Center for Veterinary Medicine, (6) National Center for Devices and Radiological Health, (7) National Center for Toxicological Research, (8) Regional Operations, (9) Office of Policy, (10) Office of External Affairs, and (11) Office of Management and Systems.

5-2 Major Components of the U.S. Public Health Service—cont'd

Agency	Structure and purpose
Health Resources and Services Administration (HRSA)	The HRSA was established in 1982. It has leadership responsibility for issues relating to access, equity, quality, and cost of health care. The administration supports states and communities in their efforts to plan and deliver health care, especially to underserved populations. It funds AIDS demonstration projects, administers the National Organ Transplant Act, and processes claims submitted under the National Vaccine Injury Compensation Program. It tracks the supply and requirements of health care professionals and provides leadership to improve the training and utilization of health care personnel. It monitors rural health issues. HRSA provides direct, personal health service for Hansen's disease patients. Major components of the administration include the Bureau of Health Care Delivery and Assistance, Bureau of Health Resources Development, and Maternal and Child Health Bureau.
Indian Health Service (IHS)	In cooperation with Indian tribes, the IHS provides a comprehensive system of health care to American Indians and Alaskan Natives. Its goal is to raise the health status of American Indians and Alaskan natives to the highest level possible. The Service assists Native Americans in developing their health programs by providing health management assistance, training, and health planning activities.
Alcohol, Drug Abuse, and Mental Health Administration (ADAMHA)	The mission of ADAMHA is to find scientifically based solutions to alcohol, drug abuse, and mental health problems. It promotes the federal effort to increase knowledge and effective strategies for control of alcohol and drug abuse and mental illness. The administration conducts and supports research, gathers and analyzes data, and provides public information services. It supports training of scientists to conduct research related to alcoholism, drug abuse, and mental health and administers the alcohol, drug abuse, and mental health services block grant. Major components are National Institute on Alcohol Abuse and Alcoholism, National Institute on Drug Abuse, National Institute of Mental Health, Office for Substance Abuse Prevention, and Office for Treatment Improvement.
Agency for Toxic Substances and Disease Registry (ATSDR)	The ATSDR was established on April 9, 1983. ATSDR provides leadership and direction to activities designed to protect public and worker health from the adverse effects of hazardous substance exposures and transporting accidents. ATSDR collects and disseminates information relating to serious disease and mortality from human exposure to toxic substances or hazardous waste substances. It establishes registries and assists the EPA in identifying hazardous waste substances that need to be regulated. It carries out the health related responsibilities of the Comprehensive Environmental Response, Compensation and Liability Act of 1980, the Resource Conservation and Recovery Act, and provisions of the Solid Waste Disposal Act.
Agency for Health Care Policy and Research (AHCPR)	The AHCPR was established in 1989. It promotes health care research that will help to assure improvements in clinical practice and patient outcomes, improvements in the financing and delivery of health care, increased access to care, and the development of practice guidelines and standardized measures of quality of care for health care providers. It promotes the use and dissemination of health care research findings.

Modified from the Office of the Federal Register: *United States government manual 1992/93*, Washington, D.C., 1992, U.S. Government Printing Office.

and improvement of the nation's communities, especially for low-income families. Provides assistance for low-income housing, the development and modernization of impoverished communities, the establishment of new communities, and oversees emergency shelter grants.

- *Department of the Interior.* Is the custodian of the nation's natural resources; is the nation's major conservation agency. Is responsible for protecting natural resources and preserving the environment and cultural values of national parks. Has jurisdiction over 500 million acres of federal land, oversees the use of land and water resources, and is involved in the reclamation of arid lands and management of hydroelectric power systems. Oversees conservation of fish and wildlife, national parks and lands, and water and minerals resources. Its Bureau of Indian Affairs promotes improvement of health and welfare conditions for Native Americans. The department implements policies for the protection of the environment pursuant to the National Environmental Protection Act of 1969, develops environmental impact statements, and enforces laws concerning flood plains, wetlands, and endangered species. The department places emphasis on assisting communities in environmental land use, and management. It sponsors research and health education programs to improve ecological conditions in the United States, and has numerous publications available.

- *Department of Justice.* Protects the health and welfare of the American public by enforcing federal laws. Is instrumental in protecting civil rights, prosecutes high-level narcotic and drug offenders, and is involved in programs to help reduce homicide, violence, and drug addiction in the United States. The department's Bureau of Prisons is responsible for all health, food and sanitation services in federal prisons. The Environmental and Natural Resources Division represents the United States in litigation involving public lands and natural resources, environmental quality, Indian lands, wildlife resources, hazardous chemical waste, clean air and water laws, and EPA issues.

- *Department of Labor.* Promotes the health and welfare of workers and strives to improve working conditions of Americans. Administers provisions of a variety of federal labor laws, including the Occupational Safety and Health Act of 1970, Job Training and Partnership Act of 1982, and the Em-

ployment Retirement Income Security Act of 1974. It coordinates federal compensation and unemployment programs and enforces safety standards and fair employment practices. Activities of the department's Occupational Safety and Health Administration and the Mine Safety and Health Administration focus on promoting worker health and safety. Through the Bureau of Labor Statistics this department compiles statistics about the American work force.

- *Department of State.* Assists the President in formulating foreign policy, carries out foreign aid and trade agreements, assists in improving the quality of life in underdeveloped countries, and is an advocate of international human rights. Is responsible for refugee programs, international travel, passports, and representing our country abroad. Its Office of Medical Services develops, administers, and staffs a worldwide primary health care system for department employees and their eligible dependents residing abroad.

- *Department of Transportation.* Enforces certain air, land, and water standards in relation to interstate transport. Its U.S. Coast Guard is responsible for promoting boating safety and enforcing the federal Water Pollution Control Act and other laws relating to protection of the marine environment. Its National Highway Safety Traffic Administration is charged with reducing morbidity and mortality on U.S. highways, and conducts programs aimed at reducing traffic accidents. Its Office of Hazardous Materials sets and enforces regulations for the safe transportation of hazardous materials.

- *Department of the Treasury.* Assists other government agencies in preventing illegal drug traffic, illegal possession of firearms, alcoholic beverages, and tobacco products through the U.S. Customs Service and the Bureau of Alcohol, Tobacco, and Firearms.

Besides federal departments, numerous other agencies on the federal level have significant health and welfare functions. The *Veterans' Administration* provides hospital, nursing home, and outpatient medical and dental care to eligible veterans of military service. This agency is also responsible for coordinating compensation, pension, and assistance programs; rehabilitation training for disabled veterans; and life insurance programs and burial services for veterans. In addition, the federal government sponsors the Endangered Species Committee, United States Information Agency, Architectural and Transportation Barriers Compliance Board, Commission on Civil Rights, the Tennessee Valley Authority, National Council on Handicapped, President's Committee on Employment of People with Disabilities, and the Prospective Payment Commission, to name a few.

Two very important governmental agencies that do not have cabinet status are the Environmental Protection Agency (EPA) and ACTION. The EPA is discussed in Chapter 6.

ACTION

ACTION was created as an independent agency in 1971. It is the principal agency in the federal government administering volunteer service programs. Its purpose is to mobilize Americans for voluntary service in the United States through programs which help meet basic needs and support self-help efforts of low-income people and communities. Some of its major programs include Foster Grandparents Program, Retired Senior Volunteer Program, Senior Companion Programs, Volunteers in Service to America (VISTA), and student community service projects. It has 9 regional offices and 45 state offices and is headquartered in Washington, D.C.

International Involvement

Every nation has its own health and welfare policies. However, there is international cooperation and coordination on these issues. The United States is involved with a number of agencies, groups, and governments on an international level to maintain and improve health, welfare, and environmental conditions throughout the world. Several intergovernmental agreements, especially in relation to disease control, trade, immigration, world peace, and respect for basic human rights, have been developed to enhance the well-being of all people.

United Nations (UN)

The United States is extensively involved in international health and welfare issues through the United Nations. This international assembly is dedicated to promoting welfare, peace, and health. Two major United Nations–sponsored groups with which the United States works are the World Health Organization (WHO) and the United Nations' Children's Fund (UNICEF).

World Health Organization (WHO)

Efforts to organize international health activities took place between 1851 and 1909, when a series of meetings known as the International Sanitary Conferences occurred. These meetings were the precursor to the International Office of Public Health in 1909 (Pickett and Hanlon, 1990, p. 74). The primary focus of most international health activity is the control of communicable disease.

In 1948 the World Health Organization was created and became a part of the United Nations (WHO, 1988). The World Health Organization is concerned with standardizing international health activities and regulations, providing statistical and health educational services, promoting research, training health workers, promoting maternal-child health, and controlling communicable diseases. Any nation can belong to WHO without being a member of the United Nations.

A major goal of the World Health Organization is to prevent the spread of disease from one continent to another and to achieve international cooperation for better health throughout the world. To achieve this goal, the WHO publishes international health statistics, recommendations, and documents; has committees to work on the standardization of therapeutic substances, atomic energy, and health laboratory methods; and documents worldwide outbreaks of disease. It sets international quarantine measures and collects and disseminates epidemiological data. WHO is a world clearinghouse for health care information and sets worldwide health standards and practices. WHO is actively involved in coordinating international AIDS research and information. The world headquarters of WHO is located in Geneva, Switzerland.

United Nations' Children's Fund (UNICEF)

UNICEF attempts to meet the emergency and ongoing needs of children, particularly children in developing countries. It has improved maternal and child health and welfare conditions by combating malnutrition (food programs), preventing and controlling communicable diseases (immunization and treatment programs), compiling statistics, supporting research, and providing shelter and other basic welfare needs. The World Health Organization and UNICEF work closely together to promote services for at-risk mothers and children throughout the world.

Peace Corps

The Peace Corps was established in 1961 and was made an independent agency by the International Security and Development Act of 1981. The Corps is charged with promoting world peace and friendship by helping to meet the needs of other countries for trained labor and by promoting a better understanding of the American people. Corps members serve in a volunteer capacity. Main headquarters are in Washington, D.C., with three regional recruitment centers, 16 area recruitment offices, and services in over 90 countries.

Men and women of all ages and from all walks of life serve as volunteers in the Peace Corps. Thousands of Corps volunteers serve in Latin America, Africa, the Near East, Asia, and the Pacific. Volunteers often work in the areas of rural development and agriculture, small business assistance, health, natural resources conservation, and education. The Peace Corps serves as the sponsor for U.S. citizens who serve in the United Nations Volunteer Program. Its World Wise Schools Program in U.S. elementary, junior, and senior high schools helps to increase international understanding and cooperation. It provides opportunities for civic groups, neighborhood, and youth organizations in the United States to sponsor assistance to overseas communities.

STATE AND LOCAL GOVERNMENT: PUBLIC HEALTH SERVICES RELATIONSHIP

Each state is responsible for providing for the health of its residents. Each state has a public health code that authorizes public health activities, and an agency, a state authority, to deal with health. In this text the terms *state health authority (SHA)* and *local health department (LHD)* refer to official government health departments. These agencies are supported by general tax revenues and provide health services at reasonable cost to the general public. The services they offer are discussed later in this chapter; they vary greatly from state to state and community to community.

Each state health authority has local affiliates. State public health codes establish what type of relationship will evolve between SHAs and LHDs.

Patterns of Organizational Structure

Historically three organizational patterns have characterized the administrative relationships be-

tween state and local health departments (Miller, Brooks, DeFriese, Gilbert, Jain, and Kavaler, 1977, p. 932):

1. *Centralized organization.* A state health authority of public health or a state board of health operates local health units that function directly under the state's authority, sometimes through regional administration.
2. *Decentralized organization.* The local government (geopolitical unit of a city, township, county, or some combination) operates a health department. The state health authority offers consultation and advice to the local agency.
3. *Shared organizational control.* State health authorities and local health departments share public health responsibilities, and the state may retain appointive and line authority over local health officers (who are also responsible to local boards or commissions). Sometimes the local departments must submit programs, plans, and budgets to the state health department in order to qualify for federal or state funds.

The relationships between state and local health departments are seldom explicit. Authority for the promulgation of health rules and regulations is often shared by state and local health departments. State health departments usually share in the cost of local health department services, but the cost-sharing ratio varies greatly. Services provided by state and local health departments vary. Some common service areas are discussed here.

Service Functions

An overall goal of state health authorities and local health departments is to enhance personal and community health. This is done through provision of public health services in the following categories:

1. Administrative
2. Communicable disease control
3. Personal health (maternal-child health and adult health)
4. Environmental health and safety
5. Occupational health
6. Vital statistics
7. Laboratory
8. Health education and training
9. Research
10. Emergency and special medical

Public health services are established in the state's public health code, and will vary from state to state.

STATE HEALTH AUTHORITY (SHA)

The U.S. Constitution empowers state governments to protect the health and welfare of their citizens. States are the central authorities in the nation's public health system and have the primary public sector responsibility for public health (Institute of Medicine, 1988, p. 8). The state health authority (SHA) is the agency or department headed by the state health official.

The Institute of Medicine's Committee for the Study of the Future of Public Health recommended that, in addition to the core functions of assessment, policy development, and assurance previously discussed, the public health duties of states should include (Institute of Medicine, 1988, p. 12):

- Assessment of health needs in the state based on statewide data collection
- Assurance of an adequate statutory base for health activities in the state
- Establishment of statewide health objectives, delegating power to local health departments (LHDs) as necessary and holding them accountable
- Ensuring statewide efforts to develop and maintain essential personal, educational, and environmental health services, provision of access to necessary services, and problem-solving for public health
- Guaranteeing a minimum set of essential health services
- Supporting local service capacity, especially when disparities in local ability to raise revenue and/or administer programs exist

In 1970 an amendment to the Public Health Service Act mandated a comprehensive, uniform national reporting system on state and territorial health authorities programs, services, and expenditures. Responsibility for the reporting system was delegated to the Association of State and Territorial Health Officials (ASTHO), which in turn established the Public Health Foundation (PHF) to collect and publish the data. Each year the PHF publishes *Public Health Agencies: An Inventory of Programs and Block Grant Expenditures, Public Health Chartbook,* and *Prevention Block Grant Chartbook.* These three excellent publications provide public health information on every state and territory.

There are 55 state and territorial health agencies (PHF, 1991, Public health agencies, p. 3). Thirty-seven states have an independent state health authority (SHA). Figure 5-2 depicts which states have an independent SHA. Other states have gone to a superagency approach where health, welfare, environmental health, and/or mental health responsibilities are combined into one agency. Fifteen SHAs are also designated as the state mental health agency, and ten as the state environmental health agency. Forty-one SHAs are the designated state crippled children's agency, and ten are the state Medicaid agency (PHF, 1991, Public health chartbook, Figure 1).

A major drawback to superagencies is the blending of health, welfare, and sometimes environmental health services in one agency with the possibility of one detracting from another, and with little emphasis being placed on health issues. The Institute of Medicine's Committee for the Study of the Future of Public Health (1988, p. 152) recommended that public health and income maintenance be organizationally separate agencies that maintain close and cooperative ties.

The chief executive of a SHA is often called the "health officer" or "director." The impact of politics is clearly evident with these positions; state health officers are frequently political appointees with an average term of 2 years (Institute of Medicine, 1988, p. 148). Greater continuity of professional leadership in such positions is needed. Most SHA health officers are physicians, but less than half have had public health training or experience (Institute of Medicine, p. 174). Some states are now requiring that the SHA health officer have public health education on the graduate level. Health professionals from various disciplines with training or experience in public health administration hold SHA health officer positions in some states. In these states physicians have positions as SHA medical directors.

Each state authorizes specific public health services through its public health code, and all of these codes include policies on communicable disease control and the collection of vital statistics. The SHA can delegate authority and responsibility for certain health activities to local health departments (LHDs), but ultimate responsibility for the activity rests with the state. The structure of SHAs differs from state to state. Figure 5-3 is an organization chart depicting how a SHA might be organized.

SHAs spend almost $10 billion each year (Public Health Foundation [PHF], 1991, Public health agencies, p. 3). Although this sounds like a lot of money, it

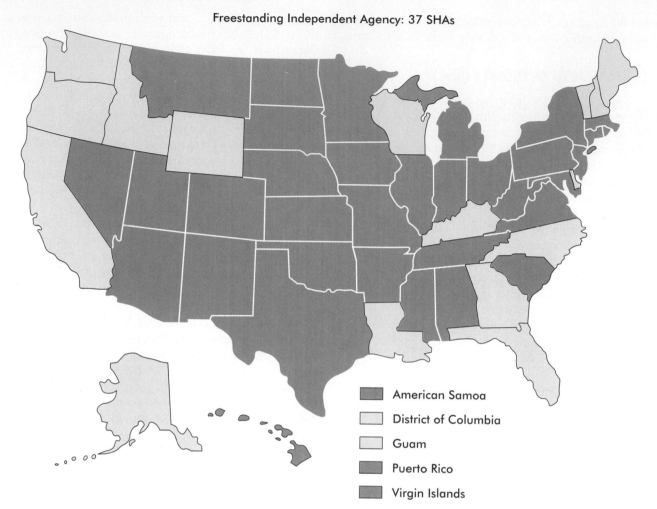

Freestanding Independent Agency: 37 SHAs

■ American Samoa
□ District of Columbia
□ Guam
■ Puerto Rico
■ Virgin Islands

Figure 5-2 State health authorities (SHAs) that are organized as a freestanding independent agency. (From Public Health Foundation: *1991 public health chartbook,* Washington, D.C., 1991, The Foundation, Figure 1.)

amounts to less than $40 per state resident each year on public health. SHA spending is financed primarily from state and federal funds. The amount of monies generated by SHAs from fee-for-service has increased in recent years (PHF, 1989, Public health agencies, p. 1). SHA expenditures by source of funds is in Figure 5-4, and SHA amount of spending by type of program is in Figure 5-5.

Recently states have not been a stable source of funding for SHAs (PHF, 1992, Budget woes, p. 1). Faced with deteriorating fiscal conditions and decreases in state funding, many SHAs are trimming their budgets and cutting back on services offered (PHF, 1992, Budget woes, p. 1). A comparison of how SHAs were funded from 1982 to 1992 is shown in Figure 5-6.

Service Functions

The state health authority is charged with furnishing the leadership and funding to meet state public health needs. It carries out this charge through the service functions described in the following sections.

Administrative

Assessment, policy development, and *assurance* are core functions of SHAs. States provide the legal, statutory

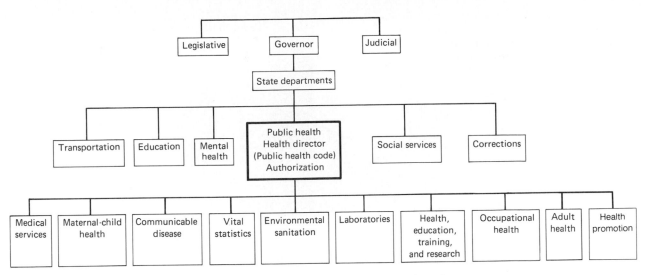

Figure 5-3 Organizational chart of a state health authority.

basis for public health practice. They set legally enforceable health standards, regulations, and policies. Activities include assessment of state health needs, program development, ongoing program evaluation, and quality assurance. States may delegate enforcement of public health law and regulations to local health agencies, but this function is overwhelmingly assigned to states in the public health codes. The state health department may take action against a local health department that is not adhering to state health policies. State health departments also develop standardized forms for statewide use in obtaining statistical information on births, marriages, and morbidity and mortality events.

Health planning activities are carried out in conjunction with the federal government and local communities to promote community health and meet *Healthy People 2000* objectives.

Working with local health departments to promote comprehensive, coordinated services in accordance with state health policy is extremely important. The state health department advises local health departments on health planning, programming and enforcement, budget review, and personnel policies. It can assist them in obtaining staff members and may approve their plan of organization and function. In some states the state health department establishes the qualifications for local health officers.

Consultation services are provided to local health departments and other health agencies. Consultants are available in such fields as maternal-child health, nutrition, epidemiology, community health nursing, mental health, occupational health, and environmental health. These consultant activities are usually well utilized and are a major state health department service.

Administration of federally aided programs is an important function of state health authorities. The federal government provides funding for health programs, many through the Prevention Block Grant. Through this grant, monies are provided for programs and services in areas such as health education/risk reduction, cardiovascular disease, emergency medical services, sex offenses, rodent control, epidemiology, sanitation, and immunizations. Prevention Block Grant monies provide funding for important public health services. Areas frequently funded by these grants are chronic disease, health education/risk reduction, emergency medical services, communicable disease, and environmental health (PHF, 1991, Public health chartbook). Figure 5-7 illustrates how Prevention Block Grant monies are spent.

Coordination of federal, state, and local health programs and services is another function assumed by the SHA. Data are compiled on available health resources and services offered throughout the state.

Legislation for health is promulgated and enforced at the state level. Representatives of the SHA meet regularly with state legislators, congressmen, politicians, health professionals, and community action

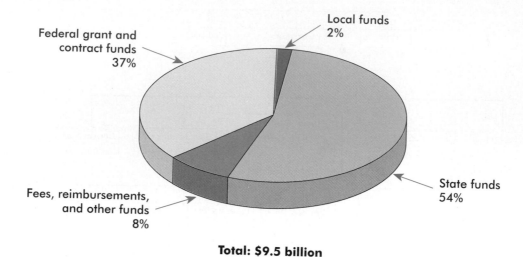

Total: $9.5 billion

Figure 5-4   State health authority (SHA) expenditures by sources of funds. (From Public Health Foundation: *Public health agencies 1991: an inventory of programs and block grant expenditures,* Washington, D.C., 1991, The Foundation, p. 4.)

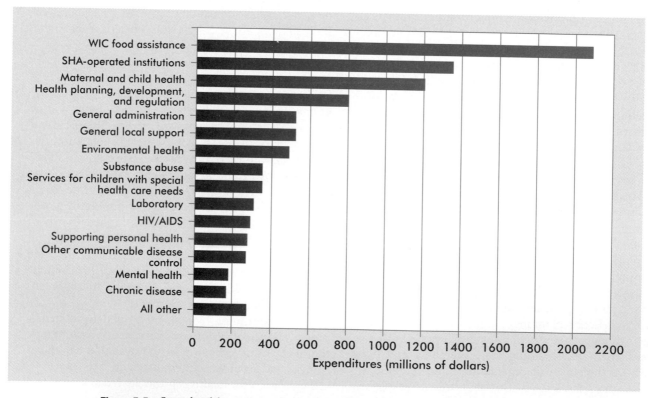

Figure 5-5   State health authority (SHA) spending by type of program. (From Public Health Foundation: *1991 Public health chartbook,* Washington, D.C., 1991, The Foundation, Figure 13.)

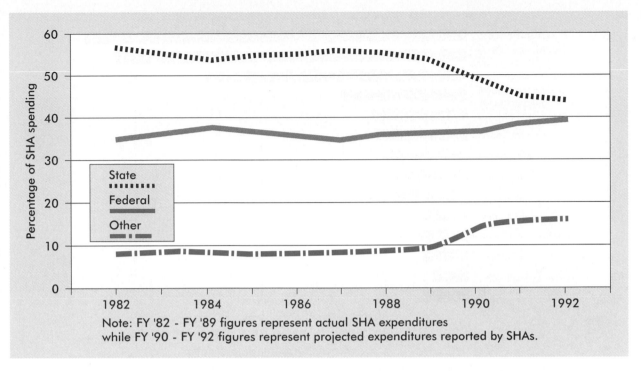

Figure 5-6   State, federal, and other funds as a percentage of total state health agency spending, fiscal year 1982 to fiscal year 1992. (From Public Health Foundation: Budget woes force SHAs to make cuts, *Public Health Macroview* 5(1):2, 1992.)

groups to develop public health legislation representative of the needs of people of the state.

Personnel policies, including hiring and promotional guides, job descriptions, grievance procedures, and personnel manuals, are developed by the SHA. A roster of available health personnel may be kept to assist local health departments to recruit additional staff.

Control of Communicable Disease

Communicable disease control is a major service function of SHAs. The state establishes immunization schedules, quarantine measures, and communicable disease policies. It often provides laboratory diagnostic services and supplies local health departments with biologics such as vaccines. Recent major outbreaks of immunizable childhood communicable diseases such as measles, a rise in cases of tuberculosis, and the AIDS epidemic dramatically illustrate the importance of communicable disease control as a function of SHAs. States cannot afford to become lax in this area. Con-

tinuous, comprehensive efforts are needed to control communicable disease in our nation's communities.

Personal Health Services

Personal health services are all services delivered to individuals, except those related to environmental health. The state is usually not heavily involved in direct provision of personal health services. Local health departments are generally the service providers in this area. Generally the state's role in personal health involves the administration of federal Prevention Block Grant monies and consultation and evaluation services. In some states the SHA provides services to special populations such as migrants, workers (occupational health services), and crippled children. In a few states there are no local health departments, so the SHA is the direct service provider to the community.

SHAs are often involved in setting and enforcing state environmental health standards. Increasingly it is being recognized that there are major environmental

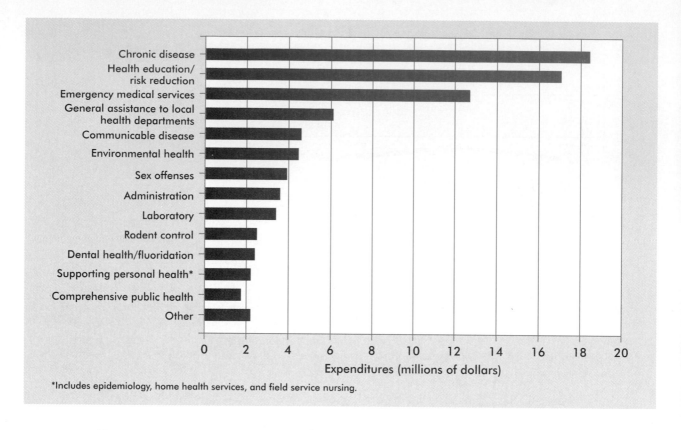

*Includes epidemiology, home health services, and field service nursing.

Figure 5-7 Prevention block grant spending by type of service. (From Public Health Foundation (PHF): *1991 Public health chartbook,* Washington, D.C., 1991, The Foundation, Figure 19.)

health concerns in the United States and the world that must be addressed. Chapter 6 provides information on environmental health.

Occupational Health

State health officials are assuming a more prominent role in occupational health and safety. However, SHAs are the lead agency for occupational health in only five states: New Jersey, New Mexico, North Dakota, Rhode Island, and Texas (PHF, 1991, Public health chartbook, Figure 2B). State occupational safety and health standards must be equal to or exceed federal standards. A number of states code occupational information on death certificates; some states collect data about parental occupation on birth certificates to help pinpoint causes of congenital malformations and disorders; and a few states have registries for occupational diseases (PHF, 1988, SHAs expand, p. 2). Chapter 17 provides information on occupational health in the United States.

Vital Statistics

Vital statistics are collected and disseminated by the SHA. Thirty-one SHAs have centers for health statistics (Institute of Medicine, 1988, p. 176). The state develops standardized forms, including certificates of birth, death, fetal death, marriage, and divorce; licenses for marriage; and epidemiological reporting forms. The state also disseminates statistical information to individuals and agencies, including the National Center for Health Statistics. The state health department has an abundance of statistical information about the health status of its population and the health work force and resources within the state. This is valuable information and available to the general public on request.

Laboratory Services

Laboratory services are operated by most SHAs. Specimens are sent there for analysis; the diagnostic services rendered are primarily in relation to communicable disease control and environmental sanitation. Local health departments and private physicians often use these services on behalf of clients. There is usually no fee, or a minimal fee, to the public for laboratory analysis of reportable communicable diseases. The laboratory also certifies vaccines and other biologics.

Health Education and Training

Education, training, and research are carried out by the SHA. The state promotes the development of new health knowledge through the support of state colleges and universities and research agencies; the development of training and inservice programs for state and local health department personnel; and involvement in research activities. Local health departments find SHAs to be valuable resources when health information and audiovisual media are needed.

The state also promotes community health education activities through the dissemination of health information to the general public. This is usually in the form of printed materials, classes, videos, and public service media announcements. Recently some states have expanded these health education activities to include paid advertising. California, Michigan, and Minnesota were the first SHAs to use paid advertising to present health messages to the general public in the form of radio, TV, and billboards (PHF, 1991, Paid advertising, p. 3). According to the PHF, when using radio and TV the SHAs have tried to have ads air when target groups were watching or listening. The ad campaigns have primarily addressed tobacco use and AIDS and have been effective. In Minnesota 55% of the target group members recalled at least one billboard, 70% recalled at least one radio ad, and more than 95% recalled at least one TV ad; in California the recall rate was approximately 70-75% (PHF, Paid advertising, p. 3). The U.S. Public Health Service is now recommending that more SHAs investigate the possibility of using paid advertising to address public health issues (PHF, Paid advertising, p. 3).

Research

State health departments promote the development of new health care research. They carry out research studies and subsidize research activities. Health policies of the future are influenced by this research. Research funds need to be advocated for and carefully guarded; however, these funds are often the first monies included in budget cuts.

Emergency and Special Medical Services

Special medical services include the provision of hospital and institutional services for chronic or long-term conditions such as mental retardation, mental illness, and tuberculosis. In the event of emergencies such as epidemics and natural disasters, emergency services ensure that the necessary public health care is made available to the community in need.

Staff

The state health department is headed by a chief executive (health officer or other title) who is usually appointed by the governor; this person is traditionally a physician. Other staff members include administrators, clerical workers, and consultants in fields such as community health nursing, occupational health, mental health, epidemiology, statistics, maternal-child health, health education, and nutrition. State health departments have legal counsel available to them, often through the state attorney general's office. States may have regional directors who serve as intermediaries between their regions and the state department. Most state health department personnel, except for the chief executive, are civil service employees.

Community health nurses are a valuable part of state health department staffs. They are hired on a consultant basis and help to establish state health policies, particularly in relation to maternal-child health and adult health services. They work closely with local health departments to improve the quality of care delivered to individuals, families, and aggregates at risk. Generally, community health nurses who work for state health departments are prepared at the master's or doctoral level and have past community health nursing experience.

LOCAL HEALTH DEPARTMENT (LHD)

The Public Health Foundation's definition of a local health department (LHD) is displayed in the box on p. 160. There are nearly 3000 local health departments in the United States (PHF, 1991, Public health agencies, p. 1). According to the PHF definition, no local health departments exist in five states: Arkansas, Delaware, Rhode Island, Vermont, and Virginia (PHF, Public health agencies, p. 142). Where local health departments do not exist , public health services are offered through the state or territorial health authority.

The Institute of Medicine's Committee for the

◀ ***Definition of a Local Health Department*** ▶

Local health department (LHD): an official (governmental) public health agency which is, in whole or in part, responsible to a substate governmental entity or entities. An entity may be a city, county, city-county, federation of counties, borough, township, or any other type of substate governmental entity. A local health department must:

- Have a staff of one or more full-time professional public health employees (e.g., public health nurse, sanitarian);
- Deliver public health services;
- Serve a definable geographic area; and
- Have identifiable expenditures and/or budget in the political subdivision(s) it serves.

From Public Health Foundation: *Public health agencies 1991: an inventory of programs and block grant expenditures,* Washington, D.C., 1991, The Foundation, p. 143.

Study of the Future of Public Health recommends that, in addition to the core public health functions (refer to the section on federal government functions in this chapter), LHDs also be responsible for the following activities (Institute of Medicine, 1988, pp. 9-10):

- Assessment, monitoring, and surveillance of local health problems and needs and resources for dealing with them.
- Policy development and leadership fostering local involvement and a sense of ownership, emphasizing local needs, and advocating equitable distribution of public resources; and complementary private activities commensurate with community needs.
- Assurance that high-quality services, including personal health services, needed for the protection of public health in the community are available and accessible to all persons; that the community receives proper consideration in the allocation of federal, state, and local resources for public health; and that the community is informed about how to obtain public health, including personal health, services, or how to comply with public health regulations.

The local health department is the basic unit for the delivery of public health services. It has responsibility for a specific jurisdiction, often a geopolitical jurisdiction such as a city, town, or county. In the United States many LHDs are organized on either a county or city level. Most Americans benefit directly or indirectly from LHD services.

Local health departments receive their funding from a number of sources, with the largest percentage coming from local tax dollars. Refer to Figure 5-8 for local health department spending by source of funds. LHDs spend over $4.1 billion nationwide (PHF, 1991, Public health agencies, p. 3), providing a number of health services at reasonable cost to the general public.

Many people in the community are not aware of the services available at their LHD. A major role of the community health nurse is to familiarize the public with LHD programs and services. The people of the community support the LHD with their tax dollars, and some people may be more willing to use LHD services when this is brought to their attention.

LHDs usually have a board of health and a health officer. An example of an organizational structure for a local health department is given in Figure 5-9. Each LHD will establish its own organizational pattern.

Just as each LHD establishes its own organization, each determines its own services and methods of service provision. Services offered by LHDs across the nation vary greatly. Table 5-3 presents an overview of the LHD program areas and expenditures in those areas. Under personal health, local health departments have traditionally offered immunization services; services for tuberculosis, sexually transmitted diseases, and other communicable disease; maternal and child health programs; school health; chronic disease programs; family planning; home care; and mental health services.

Traditionally most LHDs have not actively engaged in the provision of ongoing, primary care services. Many people in this country are medically underserved and could benefit from primary care services being provided at reasonable cost through local health departments. The provision of direct patient care services is more popular in the southeastern part of the country. Many LHDs in this area are establishing clinic services to address the growing need for ongoing primary care services for disadvantaged populations. (PHF, 1989, Survey shows).

It will be interesting to note the future role played by LHDs in the provision of primary health care services. The Institute of Medicine's Committee for the Study of the Future of Public Health (CSFPH) cautions us that provision of such service may drain

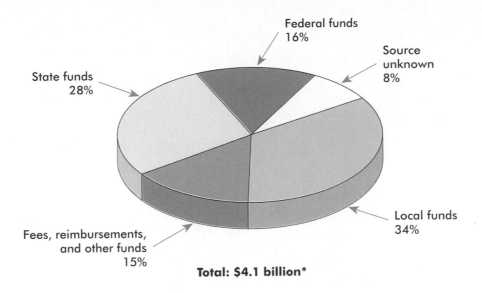

Total: $4.1 billion*

*Includes $1.8 billion in intergovernmental transfers from state health agencies.

Figure 5-8   Local health department spending by source of funds. (From Public Health Foundation: *1991 Public health chartbook,* Washington, D.C., 1991, The Foundation, Figure 7.)

TABLE 5-3   Local Health Department Expenditures by Program Area

Program area	Number of states with LHDs reporting programs	Expenditures* Amount (millions of dollars)	Expenditures* Percentage of total
Total	**44**	**$4,059.9**	**100.0%**
Personal health	39	2,347.4	57.8
Environmental health	34	379.0	9.3
Health resources	20	304.5	7.5
Laboratory	15	34.9	0.9
General administration	20	156.0	3.8
Funds not allocated to program areas	33	838.2	20.6

*Includes $1.8 billion in SHA intergovernmental transfers to LHDs.
From Public Health Foundation: *Public health agencies 1991: an inventory of programs and block grant expenditures,* Washington, D.C., 1991, The Foundation, p. 4.

vital resources away from population-wide services, that the U.S. public health system is inadequately equipped to address these needs, and that this provision of care may pose a threat to the maintenance of crucial disease prevention and health promotion efforts (Institute of Medicine, 1988, pp. 13, 152-153). The committee endorsed the idea that the ultimate responsibility for ensuring equitable access to health care for all rests with the federal government. However, until this federal government responsibility is fulfilled, LHDs are helping to fill a gap in our health care system. Significant changes in the delivery of primary health care services in this country could occur under Clinton's Health Care Reform Mandate.

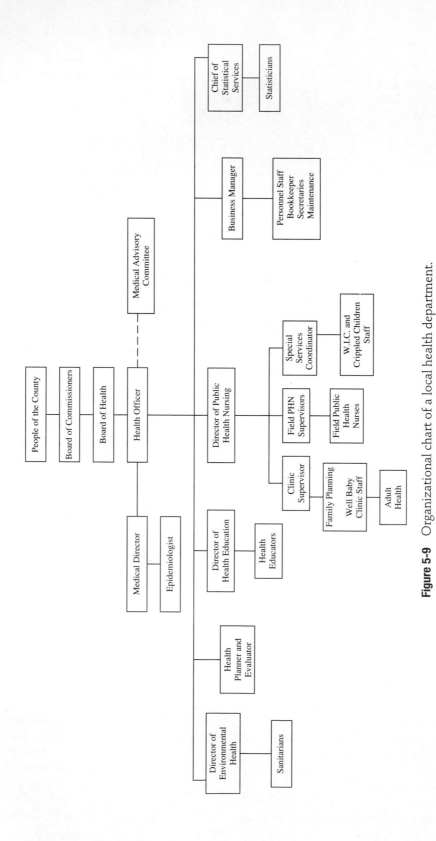

Figure 5-9   Organizational chart of a local health department.

Service Functions

Local health departments have functions similar to those carried out by the state health department, but the services they provide are more direct. Direct services offered by local health departments are extensive.

Administrative

The administrative functions of the local health department are identical in coverage to those implemented by the state health department, but the specific services vary.

Assessment, policy development, and *assurance* are core functions of LHDs. These functions involves the promulgation and enforcement of local health standards, regulations and policies. The standards established by a LHD usually relate to public food handling, storage, preparation, and disposal and to public water supplies, including wells, septic systems, and pools or lakes at recreational facilities. LHDs also supervise and license local health facilities such as hospitals, nursing homes, and restaurants, and carry out ongoing programs.

Extensive health data are collected by LHDs and used for health planning purposes. *Health planning* activities within the LHD include analyzing and determining the public health needs of the people within its jurisdiction and planning health action strategies to meet these needs (refer to Chapter 13). With the current focus on integration of health and welfare services, cooperative planning between community agencies is increasing. The LHD also participates in statewide health planning activities.

Working cooperatively with local health agencies is an important role of the LHD. With today's mounting health concerns and costs, coordinating the activities of private and official health care resources is becoming increasingly important. This coordination helps to minimize duplication of services, eliminate unnecessary services, facilitate case management, and aid in the provision of the greatest number of services at the least amount of cost and community effort. Interagency planning is essential in providing coordinated, comprehensive community health programs and services.

Consultation services are offered by the LHD to groups, organizations, and individuals. These activities usually involve consulting services from community health nurses, environmental engineers, nutritionists, and epidemiologists. Consultation in relation to state and local health policy, environmental safety,

communicable disease control, and personal health services is offered in a variety of community settings including schools, industry, hospitals, nursing homes, and community service groups within the health department's jurisdiction.

Coordination of health services with other community agencies directly relates to working cooperatively with local health agencies that have already been discussed. Coordination is an important function of the LHD. Often the health department provides leadership for resource coordination and development with the local community. Community involvement is encouraged, and consumers are involved in looking at the provision of health services. Consumer participation is discussed in Chapter 13.

Legislation is guided and influenced by the LHD, often in the form of local ordinances and codes. LHDs make their communities public health needs known to the state legislature and influence state public health legislation. It is imperative that local health departments assume leadership in the formulation of public health policy, because they are the direct service providers and have first-hand knowledge of client needs. If local health departments do not become involved in policy making, important preventive health care services may be lacking in a community.

Personnel policies, promotion guides, position descriptions, grievance policies, and manuals are developed by local health departments to facilitate effective personnel management. Staff turnover and job satisfaction are often related to how well an organization is managed (refer to Chapter 22). Some position descriptions and qualifications, such as health officer, may be determined by the SHA, and some health departments use state services to recruit qualified personnel. Many local health department employees are civil service employees, and personnel policies will reflect civil service guidelines.

Control of Communicable Disease

Communicable disease control is a major emphasis of the LHD. Each local health authority, in conformity with regulations of higher authority (state, national, and international), will determine what diseases are to be routinely and regularly reported, who is responsible for reporting, the nature of the reports, and the manner in which the reports are to be forwarded (Benenson, 1990, p. xxiv). Reportable communicable diseases that are required by international health regulations are cholera, plague, smallpox, yellow fever, and those diseases under surveillance by WHO: louse-borne typhus fever and relapsing fever, paralytic poliomyelitis, viral influenza, and malaria (Benenson, 1990, p. xxv).

Communicable diseases reportable to the LHD will vary, and their selection is often dependent on the severity and frequency of the disease. Some communicable diseases will be reported on the basis of individual cases and some only if epidemics occur. Some commonly reportable individual cases of communicable diseases are viral hepatitis, infectious hepatitis, rubella, salmonellosis, venereal syphilis, diphtheria, gonorrhea, leprosy, rubeola, meningococcal meningitis, Q fever, rabies, shigellosis, tetanus, tuberculosis, typhoid, and whooping cough.

The communicable disease services of LHDs include prevention, case finding, early diagnosis, and treatment. Many LHDs operate sexually transmitted disease, tuberculosis, and immunization clinics. These services are provided at little or no cost to the general public. Biologics for immunizations are often distributed to private physicians by the health department. The department also makes epidemiological studies of suspected or reported cases of communicable disease, and the community health nurse is actively involved in this follow-up (refer to Chapter 11).

The health department provides other communicable disease measures, such as enforcing quarantines; conducting public food, water, and refuse disposal inspections; controlling rabies; and maintaining communicable disease statistics. The environmental health division is extensively involved in these measures. Continuing surveillance and prevention of communicable diseases should be stressed (Benenson, 1990, p. xxii). It is too easy to become lax about this surveillance when there has been no recent outbreak of disease.

Personal Health Services

Personal health services are a major component of LHD services. They include both maternal-child health and adult health activities. To carry out these activities the health department offers an extensive array of clinics, classes, and home visit services.

School health is a major component of maternal-child health services on the local level. Community health nurses employed by the health department often function in schools to provide health education, counseling, and direct care services to pupils. They may conduct screening programs, such as for hearing and vision problems and scoliosis, to identify children who have health needs. School health services and the role of the school nurse are discussed in Chapter 15.

Many other maternal-child health services are provided by the LHD. Clinic services include family planning, immunization, sexually transmitted disease control, well-child check-ups, and Early, Periodic Screening, Diagnosis, and Treatment (EPSDT). A variety of other services are offered, including classes for expectant and new parents and home visits to follow up on antepartal and postpartum clients, crippled children, and high-risk infants and mothers. Counseling and health teaching in relation to immunizations, growth and development, and community resources are a few examples of the types of services provided by community health nurses when they make home visits. In addition, programs such as the nutrition program for Women, Infants, and Children (WIC), dental health, and hearing-vision conservation are often provided by the LHD. SHA consultants are often available to facilitate implementation of these services.

Adult health services also involve clinics, classes, and home visit services by the community health nurse. Community health nurses frequently visit adults to provide information about health conditions, including chronic conditions such as heart disease, diabetes, cancer, epilepsy, arthritis, stroke, alcoholism, and drug abuse. In work with clients who have chronic conditions interventions should focus on prevention, detection, treatment, and rehabilitation in an attempt to fend off the need for long-term institutional care and to encourage development of community support services. The community health nurse's major goal when working with adult clients is to enhance their self-care capabilities.

Classes in relation to such conditions as diabetes and hypertension are also conducted by the community health nurse or other health department personnel. In addition, clinics for sexually transmitted disease, family planning, immunization, blood pressure screening, breast cancer screening, and geriatric multiphasic screening are offered to promote wellness in adults. Programs in dental health, substance abuse, accident prevention, and nutrition are essential to an effective program of personal health services (Pickett and Hanlon, 1990). The community health nurse works closely with community resources to assist the adult in meeting health care needs.

Environmental Health

Many of the public health successes we have had in the past in controlling communicable disease have come about as a result of effective environmental health practices (e.g., safe water management, safe sewage disposal). Traditionally health departments have been involved in environmental health as it relates to air and water quality, land use, environmental safety, building codes and safety, noise pollution, waste management, sanitation, food quality and protection, and vector and animal control. Environmental concerns dealing with radiation control and toxic and hazardous substances have recently emerged. Environmental health is further discussed in Chapter 6.

Occupational Health

Occupational health services are not often carried out by LHDs. The Occupational Safety and Health Act of 1970 allows states to establish their own occupational safety and health administrations, but occupational health activities are largely conducted on the state and local level. Some industries are contracting with local health departments to route workers through health department diagnostic and screening programs. Some occupational health nurses, especially those in small industries, are seeking consultation from the nursing staff in the local health department for the development of health policies and procedures and the management of clinic facilities. Although this would seem to be a natural area for LHDs, there has been little involvement by them in the past.

Vital Statistics

Vital statistics in relation to the population that the health department serves are collected and disseminated to individuals, interested groups, and the SHA. The LHD keeps statistics on births, deaths, and reportable communicable diseases, maintains registers of individuals known to have specific communicable diseases where carrier states exist (typhoid), conducts morbidity and mortality surveys as necessary, and maintains records on jurisdictional health facilities.

Laboratory Services

Laboratory services are provided by the LHD. However, many do not have their own laboratories and use state facilities. Laboratory services may be extended to hospitals, clinics, and private practitioners on a contractual, fee-for-service basis. Laboratory services include water analysis, serology, urology, parasitology, identification of microorganisms, x-ray services for tuberculosis control, sanitation laboratory services, and metabolic and genetic screening for conditions such as phenylketonuria (PKU) and sickle cell anemia. These services are essential for communicable disease control and environmental sanitation and safety, as well as for the treatment of genetic and metabolic disorders and genetic counseling related to these conditions.

Health Education and Training

Education and training are a part of LHD services. The LHD provides health education services directly to individual clients, develops and carries out community health education programs, distributes health education materials, provides classes, and serves as a health information center. Health educators with Master's degrees are often hired by LHDs to coordinate health education activities.

Training activities largely involve staff in-service and continuing education programs. Some health departments offer tuition reimbursement for employees who take university course work in public health or related fields as a staff benefit.

Research

Research is engaged in by LHDs to promote the health of aggregates at risk and the community and to strengthen the health care delivery system. Research is carried out by a variety of staff members and can be done in conjunction with program evaluation studies.

Research activities often include morbidity, mortality, and program evaluation studies. State health departments are usually more actively involved in research, but increasingly LHDs are recognizing the need for such activity. Research studies related to service effectiveness and cost containment are especially emphasized at the local level. Staff should be encouraged to engage in research, and research activities should be an ongoing function of the agency.

Emergency and Special Medical Services

Special and emergency medical services offered by the LHD usually involve catastrophic medical care during a natural disaster or an epidemic, compulsory hospitalization through judicial admissions for acute communicable diseases such as tuberculosis, and care for those involved in serious environmental accidents (e.g., hazardous chemical spills or contamination). Health department personnel are also involved in health planning activities designed to meet the emergency needs of community citizens. In order to carry out these diverse functions and meet emergency and special needs, LHDs employ staff members from a variety of disciplines.

Staff

Staff will vary from one LHD to another. The minimum staff includes (1) a health officer, (2) a community health nurse, (3) an environmental engineer (sanitarian), and (4) a clerk. Additional personnel include statistician, epidemiologist, health educator, physical therapist, occupational health specialist, nutritionist, dentist, dental hygienist, veterinarian, and social worker. To provide comprehensive community health services, a basic, multidisciplinary staff is necessary. Historically, the following staff-to-community population ratio was recommended (Hanlon and McHose, 1971, p. 56):

Staff	Population
Health officer/medical personnel	1:50,000
Sanitarians (environmental engineers)	1:15,000
Community health nurses	1:5,000
Office personnel (clerk)	1:15,000

These ratios often are not achieved in many local communities. However, estimating the number of community health personnel needed in a local area is not as simple as previously thought. Multiple factors, such as current health problems in the community and the type and supply of health professionals in an area, influence workforce planning. Staffing needs are based on service delivery needs and as available community resources. LHDs must establish staffing priorities based on available resources and needs.

Health Officer

Traditionally a health officer was a physician with public health training who was licensed to practice in the state. Today the majority of health officers are still physicians, but the field is opening up to other health professionals such as nurses and public health administrators. If the health officer is not a physician, a medical director is hired to provide medical direction and consultation for LHD programs. The health officer administers the agency; prepares and submits bud-

gets; appoints and hires personnel; takes part in program planning, implementation, and evaluation; and serves as a consultant to health department staff and community agencies. The health officer is responsible for seeing that all divisions in the local health department are run efficiently and in a cost-effective manner.

Community Health Nurse

Community health nurses carry out a variety of health activities, which are discussed throughout this text. Community health nurses use a synthesis of nursing and public health theory to promote community health. They are the backbone of the personal health services of the health department and are extensively involved in most health department programs. The types of services offered by the nursing division in a LHD vary, depending on the work force available and other community resources that have been developed to meet the health care needs of community citizens.

If the LHD has a home care program the community health nurse will provide skilled nursing care in the home. Community health nurses are extensively involved in health education activities and conduct a variety of classes (e.g., expectant parent classes, diabetic classes, and family planning information sessions). Professionals in the field recommend baccalaureate preparation for entry-level positions in community health (Anderson and Meyer, 1985; Jones, Davis, and Davis, 1987), because baccalaureate-prepared nurses have more community health nursing content during their educational preparation than other beginning levels of nursing education.

Environmental Engineer

The environmental engineer (sanitarian) is responsible for the elimination or reduction of hazards in the environment. Environmental engineers apply principles of public health, toxicology, health, education, law enforcement, and industrial health, and use practical and technical measures to eliminate or control environmental health problems. They have historically been members of LHD staffs; their efforts have facilitated communicable disease control and promoted a safe and healthy environment.

Clerk

The clerk is responsible for the clerical and secretarial aspects of maintaining the health department. These services are invaluable. It is extremely important to keep in mind that the clerical staff may need to be increased as new programs are developed in the health department. Without an adequate clerical staff it is extremely difficult to effectively and efficiently manage health department services.

STATE AND LOCAL GOVERNMENT WELFARE ORGANIZATION

The provision of welfare assistance and insurance programs in every state and locality is legally mandated as a result of the Social Security Act of 1935 and other legislation. The specific services provided under the Social Security Act are discussed in Chapter 4.

The primary purpose of official governmental welfare agencies is to assist indigent individuals in meeting their basic needs of food, shelter, and clothing. Benefits provided by these agencies are either cash or service (food and shelter).

Official welfare services are organized in much the same manner as official health services. There is usually a department, such as the state department of social or human services, to establish rules and regulations, to set guidelines for service provision, and to administer services, and local branches of the state department of social services to provide direct services to clients. Local departments of social services administer state-subsidized programs such as Aid to Families with Dependent Children, food stamps, General Assistance, and Medicaid. Protective services for children and adults are often administered through departments of social service. Old Age, Survivors & Disability Insurance (OASDI) and Supplemental Security Income (SSI) are administered by the federal government through local Social Security Administration offices. For further discussion of state and local governmental welfare programs refer to Chapter 4.

PRIVATE HEALTH AND WELFARE ORGANIZATION

The United States abounds in private health and welfare resources. These resources can be classified as either profit or nonprofit. Historically there has been limited coordination between these and governmental resources. In addition, there is no central coordination of all private health and welfare resources. Both profit and nonprofit resources exist in the private health and welfare sectors.

Private profit health and welfare services include an increasing number of hospitals, a large percentage of nursing homes, health and welfare professionals in private practice, pharmacies, health business companies (medical equipment companies, hospital supplies), and proprietary social service agencies. These services are available on a fee-for-service basis and are organized primarily as companies and independent businesses.

Private nonprofit resources are often voluntary resources. They are not mandated by any law and provide services on a nonprofit basis. They are represented by individuals, professional societies, service organizations, agencies, and facilities. Their services augment official (government) services. Voluntary resources are uniquely American. Individual voluntary efforts (volunteerism) have likely been with us since this country was founded.

Voluntary efforts have aided the development of American health and welfare resources, provided services that otherwise may not have been possible, and advocated health and welfare reform. The box on p. 168 briefly summarizes the characteristics of voluntary resources that exist in the United States. Figure 5-10 depicts one voluntary agency, the American Red Cross. Refer to Chapters 1 and 4 for additional discussion of voluntary agencies.

The functions of voluntary, nonprofit health agencies were studied in the classic Gunn-Platt Report. The functions of these agencies were described as pioneering and include exploration of and surveying for unmet needs, demonstration, education, supplementation of official activities, guarding of citizens' interest in health, promotion of health legislation, planning and coordination, and development of well-balanced community health programs (Gunn and Platt, 1945). These functions have not altered over time and are becoming increasingly more significant in this era of federal cost containment.

Millions of Americans volunteer their services to assist health and welfare programs each year. Operating funds for voluntary resources come largely from individual contributions, fees for service, membership dues, investment earnings, sales of goods and publications, bequests, grants, contracts for service, and tax funds. Fund-raising is of vital importance to these organizations, and monies are often raised through donation campaigns. One voluntary service agency,

◀ *Voluntary Resources:* ▶
Characteristics, Classifications,
and Examples

Characteristics

Voluntarily organized

Governed by a board of directors which includes lay
and/or professional members

Have no legal powers

Receive support primarily from voluntary contributions, fees for service, third party payers, and grants

Usually provide services to a defined geographical
location

Classifications

Professional Societies

American Nurses Association (ANA), American Public Health Association (APHA)

Service Agencies

Visiting Nurse Association (VNA), American Cancer
Society, American Red Cross, Alcoholics Anony-
mous, Rockefeller Foundation, United Community
Services

Facilities

Universities, public museums, and libraries

Individuals

Modified from Black L: *Community health administration,* Ann Arbor,
1977, University of Michigan School of Nursing.

the United Way, represents a large number of local
voluntary resources with a central fund-raising campaign. Giving to the United Way campaign means
giving to many voluntary resources with one donation. The federal government has encouraged private
philanthropic giving to voluntary organizations by
permitting contributions to be deducted from personal and corporate income tax.

There are usually many private sector resources in
local communities. The Visiting Nurse Association
and home health care programs are discussed in the
next section, because home health care is becoming
one of the major responsibilities of nurses in the
community setting (refer to Chapter 20). Limiting
discussion to these types of private health and welfare
organizations is not meant to imply that other private
agencies do not provide a valuable service to the
community.

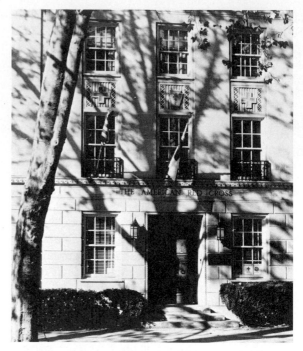

Figure 5-10 For over 100 years the American Red
Cross, a voluntary, nonprofit organization, has initiated
the development and provision of health and welfare
services. Established originally to assist and support
military men and their families during times of war and
to aid victims of disasters, this agency continues to
make significant public health contributions. Some of
its current efforts include the promotion of health education through formal classes and publications, the
collection and distribution of whole blood products,
and the provision of selected health and welfare
services based on community need. Friendly visiting to
senior citizens, the provision of transportation for
medical appointments, and the donation of clothing for
needy families are examples of such services. In addition, the American Red Cross continues to provide
relief for disaster victims and to serve military families.
Local chapters of this organization can be found in
most major cities across the United States. (Courtesy
Henry Parks, photographer.)

Home health care agencies are often administered
by an executive director or chief executive officer
(CEO) who operates under a board of directors if it is
a VNA, or owners of the company if it is a proprietary
agency. Both VNAs and home health care agencies are
primarily staffed and administered by nurses. An
organization chart of a VNA is given in Figure 5-11.
Chapter 20 discusses the organization of all types of
home health care agencies.

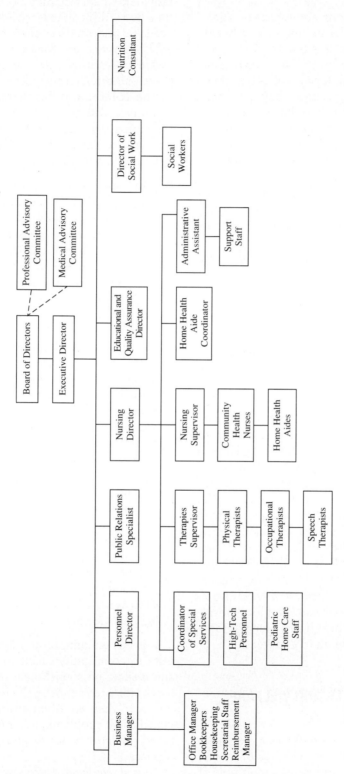

Figure 5-11　Organizational chart of a visiting nurse association.

Visiting Nurse Associations (VNAs)

Visiting Nurse Associations are especially significant voluntary organizations in community health. VNAs began with the Women's Branch of the New York City Mission, organized in 1877 to teach hygiene in the homes of the disadvantaged. VNAs have been discussed in Chapter 1. Historically they have been organized as private, nonprofit, voluntary agencies. VNAs primarily make home visits to people who are in need of skilled nursing, and augment the health education and clinic services of the LHD. Over the years there has been coordination and cooperation between VNAs and LHDs, and in some instances combined agencies were formed. Combination agencies consolidate a LHD and VNA under one administrative structure.

In contrast to the health department, the program emphasis of the VNA is usually on secondary and tertiary preventive activities rather than on primary prevention. However, staff nurses do engage in primary prevention counseling as they provide skilled nursing care. For example, they discuss accident prevention when they assist clients with mobility.

Home Health Care Agencies

These agencies are organized in both the private for-profit and nonprofit sectors. The organization of home health agencies differs from that of local health departments. As with VNAs, they deliver skilled nursing services to individuals in their homes. Shortened length of hospital stays have rapidly increased the need for such agencies, with people being discharged into the community still in need of nursing care. Clients who use the services of home health care agencies are often elderly, disabled, or recently discharged from a hospital setting. These programs are rapidly growing in numbers, largely in the private, for-profit sector. An emerging trend is for local hospitals to start their own home health care agency. Home health care is discussed in depth in Chapter 20.

COORDINATION OF HEALTH AND WELFARE RESOURCES

The diversity of health and welfare resources in the United States has been presented. The lack of coordination between these services presents a multitude of problems for both providers and recipients of service.

Providers of service may become frustrated because they find it difficult to learn about the many resources available and to effect change in the system. Recipients of service are frustrated because they are not aware of resources, do not understand how to use them, and often receive fragmented care. A major role of the community health nurse is to explain and coordinate community services. Lack of resource coordination can adversely affect the quality of care delivered to clients. This is demonstrated in the following case situation.

▶ John Falta, age 19, was in a motorcycle accident that necessitated an amputation below the right knee. He was hospitalized for 6 weeks and upon discharge was referred to a local VNA for skilled nursing services, the Office of Vocational Rehabilitation for rehabilitation training, and the Department of Social Services for assistance with his medical expenses. In addition, a physical therapist from the hospital saw John on a weekly basis at home, and a volunteer from a local amputee self-help group visited him regularly to help him adapt to the changes that had occurred in his life. Each of these health and welfare resources provided a valuable service, but because they were not initially coordinated John found it difficult to understand why so many people were involved in his care. He told the visiting nurse that he was confused and depressed about the onslaught of so many "helping agencies" and the different goals that had been set for him. The nurse suggested that a conference be arranged between John, his family, and the involved resources; John agreed that this was necessary. The conference helped to coordinate John's care and stimulated John's involvement in the rehabilitation process. Because he had a clearer picture of what was happening, his depression decreased and he actively participated in establishing goals for his future.

It is not uncommon to encounter clients like John Falta in community health nursing practice. Health and welfare personnel meet too infrequently to plan for coordinated service delivery. When such meetings do occur, they are often arranged to deal with individual client problems rather than to plan for coordinated preventive health and welfare resources and services.

Lack of coordination occurs between health and welfare resources. A classic example of lack of coordination between health and welfare systems in this country is the administration of the government health insurance program of Medicare and the health assistance program of Medicaid. These programs are locally administered by agencies that are traditionally not considered to be health agencies: the Social Security Administration and state departments of social service. Official and private health agencies have little input into, control over, or administration of these two major governmental health programs. The case situation of John Falta also evidenced such lack of coordination; health care and welfare professionals were not communicating with one another or with professionals from other systems.

Lack of coordination of services has been evident in all sectors of our health and welfare systems for decades. The National Commission on Community Health Services (1966, p. 132) identified minimal coordination between official (government) and private health care agencies. The National Health Planning and Resource Development Act of 1974 (Public Law 93-641) was passed to improve the delivery and coordination of government health care services to all segments of the population. However, in 1981 the Omnibus Budget Reconciliation Act was passed, which ended the federal mandate for Public Law 93-641 planning. It is now hoped that federal block grant program funding will improve the coordination of services (refer to Chapter 13).

Community health nurses are in a unique position to influence coordination of care on both an individual level with clients and a community level with health planners. On an individual level community health nurses are frequently the primary providers in the home setting. At this level one of their major functions is coordination of community resources for the families they visit. The John Falta case illustrates this. On a community level, community health nurses are currently writing grants to obtain block grant funding for community health services. The holistic philosophy of community health nurses provides them with the skills needed to integrate service delivery issues.

Summary

The Institute of Medicine's Committee for the Study of the Future of Public Health found that public health is a vital function that is in trouble in the United States. Public health agencies have many challenges to face, including AIDS, chronic disease, an aging population, leadership, financing, policy development, and funding.

The federal government has taken a leadership role in establishing national health objectives and supporting model public health standards. States need resources and better reporting mechanisms to implement and evaluate these standards. The nation as a whole needs to make a concerted effort to ensure the stability of the public health system. Public health can no longer be taken for granted. Americans must not be lax in their public health practices, or attempt to divest themselves of public health issues. The Clinton administration is now looking at the organization of public health services across the nation, and organizational change appears imminent.

The community health nurse needs to be aware of national health objectives, model standards, and health care reform activities as discussed in this chapter. The nurse must understand how health and welfare resources are organized to enhance service delivery and to familiarize clients with the service delivery system. Nurses must be able to work with communities to promote public health and to help instill in communities the belief that public health is too important a function to be neglected or taken for granted.

◀ *An Exercise in Critical Thinking* ▶

Local health departments (LHDs) all over the United States have historically provided public health services to local communities, and as national health care reform emerges these agencies could play a major role in service provision. Envision new and innovative ways for these LHDs to provide services to the community. How could existing LHD services be enlarged? What new services could LHDs provide? What services do they need to provide to facilitate meeting the *Healthy People 2000* goals and objectives, and how could these services be funded? How do you see the nursing role(s) in community health service delivery?

References

American Public Health Association: *Healthy communities 2000: model standards. Guidelines for community attainment of the year 2000 national health objectives,* ed 3, Washington, D.C., 1991, The Association.

Anderson E and Meyer AT: *Consensus conference on the essentials of public health nursing practice and education,* Rockville, Md., 1985, USDHHS, Public Health Service.

Benenson AS, ed: *Control of communicable diseases in man,* ed 15, Washington, D.C., 1990, American Public Health Association.

Black L: *Community health administration,* Ann Arbor, 1977, University of Michigan School of Nursing.

Gunn SM and Platt PS: *Voluntary health agencies: an interpretative study,* New York, 1945, Ronald Press.

Hanlon JJ and McHose F: *Design for health,* ed 2, Philadelphia, 1971, Lea & Febiger.

Institute of Medicine—Committee for the Study of the Future of Public Health: *The future of public health,* Washington, D.C., 1988, National Academy Press.

Jones DC, Davis JA, and Davis MC: *Public health nursing education and practice* (Accession number HRP-0909092), Springfield, Va., 1987, National Technical Information.

Miller CA, Brooks EF, DeFriese GH, Gilbert B, Jain SC, and Kavaler F: A survey of local public health departments and their directors, *Am J Publ Health* 67:931-939, 1977.

Miller CA, Gilbert B, Warren DG, Brooks EF, DeFriese GH, Jain SC, and Kavaler F: Statutory authorizations for the work of local health departments, *Am J Publ Health* 67:940-945; 1977.

National Commission on Community Health Services: *Health is a community affair,* Cambridge, Mass., 1966, Harvard University Press.

Office of the Federal Register: *United States government manual, 1992-93,* Washington, D.C., 1992, U.S. Government Printing Office.

Pickett G and Hanlon JJ: *Public health administration and practice,* ed 9, St. Louis, 1990, Mosby.

Public Health Foundation (PHF): *Public health chart book,* Washington, D.C., 1988, The Foundation.

Public Health Foundation: SHAs expand occupational role, *Public Health Macroview* 1(4):2, 1988.

Public Health Foundation: *Status report: state progress on 1990 health objectives for the nation,* Washington, D.C., 1988, The Foundation.

Public Health Foundation: Fee income: a small but growing source of support for SHAs, *Public Health Macroview* 2(3):1, 1989.

Public Health Foundation: *Public health agencies 1989: an inventory of programs and block grant expenditures,* Washington, D.C., 1989, The Foundation.

Public Health Foundation: Survey shows wide variation in LHD reporting, *Public Health Macroview* 2(3):2, 1989.

Public Health Foundation: *1991 Public health chartbook,* Washington, D.C., 1991, The Foundation.

Public Health Foundation: Paid advertising—a powerful tool for SHAs, *Public Health Macroview* 4(2):3, 1991.

Public Health Foundation: *Public health agencies 1991: an inventory of programs and block grant expenditures,* Washington, D.C., 1991, The Foundation.

Public Health Foundation: Budget woes force SHAs to make cuts, *Public Health Macroview* 5(1):2, 1992.

U.S. Department of Health, Education, and Welfare: *Healthy people: the Surgeon General's report on health promotion and disease prevention,* Washington, D.C., 1979, U.S. Government Printing Office.

U.S. Department of Health and Human Services (USDHHS): *Promoting health/preventing disease: objectives for the nation,* Washington, D.C., 1980, U.S. Government Printing Office.

USDHHS: *The 1990 health objectives for the nation: a midcourse review,* Washington, D.C., 1986, U.S. Government Printing Office.

USDHHS: *Healthy people 2000: national health promotion and disease prevention objectives, full report, with commentary,* Washington, D.C., 1991, U.S. Government Printing Office.

World Health Organization (WHO): *Four decades of achievement: highlights of the work of WHO,* Geneva, Switzerland, 1988, The Organization.

Selected Bibliography

Cohen WJ: Current problems in health care, *N Engl J Med* 281:193-197, 1969.

Elders MJ: Macroviewpoint: prescription for America's youth, *Public Health Macroview* 5(1):6, 1992.

Harmon RG: Macroviewpoint: partners for the 1990s—public health and primary care, *Public Health Macroview* 4(1):6, 1991.

Houle CO: *Governing boards,* San Francisco, 1989, Jossey-Bass Publishers.

Kennedy EM: *In critical condition: the crisis in American health care,* New York, 1973, Pocket Books.

Larsen BL: Macroviewpoint: Chronic disease control in the '90s—making prevention count, *Public Health Macroview* 4(2):6, 1991.

Lorsch RL: *State and local politics: the entanglement,* Englewood Cliffs, N.J., 1983, Prentice-Hall.

Miller CA, Gilbert B, Warren DG, Brooks EF, DeFriese GH, Jain SC, and Kavaler F: A survey of local public health departments and their directors, *Am J Publ Health* 67:931-939, 1977.

Public Health Foundation: SHA staffing declines 8% from 1979-1985, *Public Health Macroview* 1(4):5, 1988.

Public Health Foundation: Progress on the Healthy People 2000 objectives: alcohol and other drugs, *Public Health Macroview* 3(5):4-5, 1990.

Public Health Foundation: Progress on the Healthy People 2000 objectives: healthy children, *Public Health Macroview* 4(1):4-5, 1991.

Public Health Foundation: Progress on the Healthy People 2000 objectives: nutrition, *Public Health Macroview* 4(2):4-5, 1991.

Public Health Foundation: Progress on the Healthy People 2000 objectives: HIV/AIDS, *Public Health Macroview* 5(1):4-5, 1992.

Remington RD: The future of public health—two years of progress, *Public Health Macroview* 3(5):6, 1990.

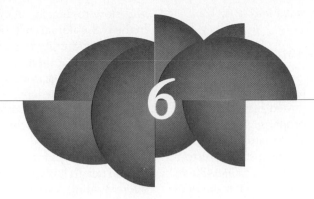

The Nurse and Environmental Health

OBJECTIVES

Upon completion of this chapter, the reader should be able to:

1. Discuss environmental health as a public health concern.
2. Discuss the origins of environmental health in the United States.
3. State four areas addressed in the *Healthy People 2000* national health objectives that relate to environmental health.
4. Describe the nurse's role in environmental health.

5. Name three major pieces of environmental health legislation in the United States.
6. Discuss the role of federal, state, and local governments in environmental health.
7. Discuss selected environmental diseases.
8. Discuss four areas of environmental concern.
9. Understand the health implications of environmental disasters.

We did not inherit the earth from our ancestors. We borrow it from our children.

OLD PENNSYLVANIA DUTCH SAYING

Environmental health has been one of the earliest public health concerns in recorded history. Maintenance of safe food and water, proper sewage disposal, and interment of the dead became matters of law and custom in many societies. Archaeologists and historians have indicated that the Minoans (3000-1430 BC) and the Myceneans (1430-1150 BC) built drainage systems, toilets, and water-flushing systems (Pickett and Hanlon, 1990, p. 21). About 1500 BC the Hebrews had a written hygienic code with environmental practices, Athenians of 1000-400 BC had elaborate environmental sanitation measures, and early Egyptians constructed drainage systems and earth privies for sewage (Pickett and Hanlon, p. 21).

During the Middle Ages, AD 500 to 1500, many of these earlier environmental health practices were ignored, and epidemics of leprosy, typhus, and bubonic plague ravaged the civilized world (Kalisch and Kalisch, 1978, p. 12). In the mid-1300s bubonic plague, known as the Black Death, killed as many as 60 million people (Kalisch and Kalisch, p. 13). Bubonic plague is spread by rodents and their fleas, when left untreated has a case fatality rate of about 50%, and has significant environmental health implications (Benenson, 1990, p. 324).

Environmental health continues to be a primary public health concern. Environmental health is "the systematic development, promotion and conduct of measures that modify or otherwise control those external factors in the indoor and outdoor environment which might cause illness, disability or discomfort through interaction with the human system" (US-DHHS, 1988, p. 11). It has biological, chemical, physical, and sociological components, and includes the immediate and future conditions in which people live.

ENVIRONMENTAL HEALTH IN THE UNITED STATES

The United States based many of its health practices on European tradition (refer to Chapter 4) and was slow to develop environmental health practices. In the U.S. colonial era (1607-1797) little attention was paid to community hygiene and sanitation, and there was almost a complete lack of community organization for health services (Smillie, 1955, pp. 15, 72). During this time epidemics of cholera, smallpox, yellow fever, measles, dysentery, influenza, pneumonia, scarlet fever, diphtheria, malaria, and syphilis continually recurred (Smillie, 1955, pp. 21-60). Although such epidemics were attributed to environmental health hazards such as inadequate ventilation, overcrowding, impure water, and inadequate housing, little was done to improve these conditions (Clark, 1972, p. 30-36).

Early regulations that had an impact on environmental health were enacted. A Virginia law in 1610 stated that no man or woman dare throw out water or suds from foul clothes into the open street, clean pots or kettles within twenty feet of a well or pump, or do the necessities of nature within a quarter mile of the town (Smillie, 1955, p. 61). Those who violated the law could be whipped and punished (Smillie, p. 61). Early environmental measures were often more concerned with the aesthetics of the environment than with related health consequences, and environmental practices frequently were directed at keeping the environment "sightly" and controlling "ill airs."

Early measures to control contagious disease in the United States often involved the use of isolation and quarantine (Smillie, 1955, p. 62). Sanitary police enforced quarantine measures and special "quarantine" physicians were employed to visit those in quarantine (Clark, 1972, 8-10). Quarantine and sanitation reform were accepted by the general public as legitimate governmental functions (Hill, 1976, p. 9). As early as 1796 the federal government enacted a quarantine act to enforce health and quarantine regulations at U.S. ports of entry.

The beginnings of organized environmental health activities in the United States started with the Shattuck Report in 1850 (refer to Chapter 4). This report made numerous public health recommendations, including the formation of state boards of health and the collection of vital statistics. Regarding environmental sanitation, the report emphasized the need for controlling overcrowded housing and providing safe fac-

---

We would like to acknowledge Ellie Brooks, doctoral candidate at the University of Tennessee, Knoxville, College of Nursing for her help in developing this chapter.

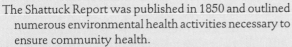

Selected U.S. Environmental Health Activities

The Shattuck Report was published in 1850 and outlined numerous environmental health activities necessary to ensure community health.

In 1872 the American Public Health Association was founded and became an advocate for environmental health activities.

On September 10, 1875, the first U.S. conservation organization, the American Forestry Association, was established. This organization remains active today.

On September 25, 1890, Yosemite Park was established by the U.S. Congress in an effort to preserve our natural lands and forests.

The Wilderness Society was founded on January 21, 1935. It remains an important conservation policy group that works primarily on issues involving federal public lands (national forests, national parks, national wildlife refuges). The group was instrumental in persuading Congress to create a national wilderness system.

The National Wildlife Federation was founded on February 5, 1936, and has the largest membership of any U.S. conservation organization. Its publications include *National Wildlife, International Wildlife,* and the children's magazines *Your Big Backyard* and *Ranger Rick.*

Rachel Carson published the environmental classic *Silent Spring* in 1962. This book about the effects of pesticide use is considered by many to have provided the impetus for the modern environmental movement in the United States.

In 1964 America's first permanent national wilderness system was established.

In 1970 the first annual Earth Day was held. On Earth Day professionals and the lay public focus on activities to promote an awareness of the environment, address environmental health issues, and develop strategies to preserve the environment.

On December 2, 1970, the Environmental Protection Agency (EPA) was established.

In 1979 *Healthy People* assessed environmental health in the United States, and national health objectives relating to environmental health were written in 1980.

In 1989 *50 Simple Things You Can Do To Save the Earth* was published. It sold more than 1.5 million copies. A sequel has now been published.

In 1990 more than 200 million people around the world celebrated the 20th anniversary of Earth Day.

In 1991 *Healthy People 2000* established environmental health as a national health priority area and set national environmental health objectives.

---

tories and buildings, food and water sanitation, and vaccinations against disease (Smillie, 1955, p. 252). The majority of recommendations from this 150-year-old report have been incorporated into contemporary public health practice. Early environmental sanitation activities in the United States included safeguarding community water supplies; proper sewage disposal, refuse, and waste disposal; food and milk sanitation; disinfection and fumigation during epidemics; pest and vector control; and building safety. These activities became functions of state and local boards of health (Smillie, pp. 340-375).

In 1872 the American Public Health Association (APHA) was founded. At that time only 3 states (California, Massachusetts, and Virginia) and the District of Columbia had established boards of health. When APHA was founded, Pasteur and others were in the process of revolutionizing knowledge about disease etiology and treatment and were establishing a strong basis for environmental health activities. Dr. Stephen Smith, a founder of APHA and its first presi-

dent, wrote *The City That Was,* a shocking description of the unsanitary conditions prevailing in New York City. He was a staunch supporter of environmental health activities (Ravenel, 1921, p. 32). The United States had a short-lived National Board of Health (1879-1883) that instituted many environmental health activities in an effort to control epidemics and communicable disease (Shannon, 1976, p. 90).

In this century environmental health activities have expanded from a focus on controlling communicable disease and implementing sanitation activities to protecting and preserving the environment in which we live. This change was facilitated by the community sanitation achieved in the early 1900s, the strides made in reducing conventional pollutants in air and water (Rabe, 1990, Environmental health policy, p. 318), and the development of immunizations and antibiotics. Numerous conservation efforts by the American people have helped to preserve the environment, including establishment of state and national park systems and efforts to protect our nation's endangered wildlife. Extensive environmental health legislation has been passed in this century and is discussed later in this chapter. Some U.S. environmental health activities are listed in the box on p. 175.

ENVIRONMENTAL HEALTH AND THE *HEALTHY PEOPLE 2000* NATIONAL HEALTH OBJECTIVES

National objectives for environmental health were established in 1980. These objectives were based on data presented in the nation's classic public health publication, *Healthy People* (USDHEW, 1979), and were projected to be achieved by 1990. Progress toward achieving them was mixed. It is important to note that progress toward almost 75% of the 1990 environmental health objectives could not be measured because states did not have adequate environmental surveillance and monitoring systems (USDHHS, 1992, pp. 68, 103).

Progress was made with some of the objectives— for instance, in implementing assessments of nationally prioritized hazardous wastes sites. By 1990 92% of these sites (1000 sites) were assessed (USDHHS, 1992, p. 66). Additionally, a 24-hour notification system was established for emergency environmental hazards (404-639-0615). Following notification, a team could be on-site anywhere within the continental United States within 6 to 8 hours (USDHHS, pp. 67-68).

The nation regressed in its attempt to provide safe drinking water for the nation's communities (USDHHS, 1992, p. 66). The United States went from 90% of the population having safe drinking water in 1980 to 80% in 1990, not coming close to meeting the 95% rate that had been set (USDHHS, p. 66). The sequel to *Healthy People, Healthy People 2000,* listed environmental health as one of 22 separate priority areas in the document and reestablished national environmental health objectives. The *Healthy People 2000* environmental health objectives are given in the box on p. 177. They offer significant challenges to the nation in promoting environmental health and preserving the global environment.

Improving state-based environmental surveillance and monitoring systems that define and track environmental disease in the United States is a major environmental health objective. Additional objectives are directed toward providing safe water supplies, reducing human exposure to toxic agents, improving the environment by effective solid waste disposal, eliminating immediate risks from hazardous waste sites, and improving household management of recyclable materials and toxic waste.

According to *Healthy People 2000,* some of the most difficult challenges for environmental health pertain to uncertainties regarding the toxic and ecological effects of fossil fuels and synthetic chemicals. More than 80% of major industrial chemicals have not been tested for their toxic properties and links to diseases. Exposure to lead, air pollutants, and radon are also addressed in *Healthy People 2000.*

THE NURSE AND ENVIRONMENTAL HEALTH

The environment has been a major concept in the domain of nursing since the days of Florence Nightingale. Nightingale's regard for the patient's environment is traced to her work with soldiers in the Crimea. She attributed their sickness and death in part to unsanitary environmental conditions (Reed and Zurakowski, 1989, p. 37). Nightingale identified five factors for nurses to consider in optimizing the physical environment of the ill person: (1) pure air, (2) pure water, (3) efficient drainage, (4) cleanliness, and (5) light (Reed and Zurakowski, p. 37). As the *Healthy People 2000* objectives show, these factors are considered important today.

Since Nightingale, the environment as a domain in nursing has not been well developed. However, the impact of the environment on health is an important aspect of nursing practice and research. Lillian Wald, the founder of public health nursing, was well aware of environmental health issues and the impact they had on community health. She regularly admonished anyone who did not observe city sewage and sanitation laws and was instrumental in the establishment of milk stations to provide safe milk for infants and children (Coss, 1993, pp. 134, 137).

A review of the nursing research literature on the environment from 1961 to 1990 showed only 53 articles that addressed the environment (Kleffel, 1991, p. 43). These articles frequently focused on institutional environments in hospitals and long-term care facilities; only one study addressed the social, economic, and political aspects of the environment (Kleffel, p. 43). This study used an ecological approach to explore environmental variables related to acute infections in children. The study concluded that child health could not be improved independent of changes in the environment (Kleffel, p. 43; McFarland, 1985).

1. Reduce asthma morbidity, as measured by reduction in asthma hospitalizations to no more than 160 per 100,000 people.
2. Reduce the prevalence of serious mental retardation among school-aged children to no more than 2 per 1,000 children by reducing environmental factors such as lead poisoning which causes mental retardation.
3. Reduce outbreaks of waterborne disease from infectious agents and chemical poisoning to no more than 11 per year.
4. Reduce the prevalence of blood lead levels exceeding 15 μg/dL and 25 μg/dL among children aged 6 months through 5 years to no more than 500,000 and zero respectively.
5. Reduce human exposure to criteria air pollutants, as measured by an increase to at least 85 percent in the proportion of people who live in counties that have not exceeded any Environmental Protection Agency standard for air quality in the previous 12 months.
6. Increase to at least 40 percent the proportion of homes in which homeowners/occupants have tested for radon concentrations and that have either been found to pose minimal risk or have been modified to reduce risk to health.
7. Reduce human exposure to toxic agents by confining total pounds of toxic agents released into the air, water, and soil each year to no more than:
   - 0.24 billion pounds of those toxic agents included on the Department of Health and Human Services list of carcinogens.
   - 2.6 billion pounds of those toxic agents included on the Agency for Toxic Substances and Disease Registry list of the most toxic chemicals.
8. Reduce human exposure to solid waste–related water, air, and soil contamination, as measured by a reduction in average pounds of municipal solid waste produced per person each day to no more 3.6 pounds.
9. Increase to at least 85 percent the proportion of people who receive a supply of drinking water that meets the safe drinking water standards established by the Environmental Protection Agency.
10. Reduce potential risks to human health from surface water, as measured by a decrease to no more than 15 percent in the proportion of assessed rivers, lakes, and estuaries that do not support beneficial uses, such as fishing and swimming.
11. Perform testing for lead-based paint in at least 50 percent of homes built before 1950.
12. Expand to at least 35 the number of states in which at least 75 percent of local jurisdictions have adopted construction standards and techniques that minimize elevated indoor radon levels in those new building areas locally determined to have elevated radon levels.
13. Increase to at least 30 the number of states requiring that prospective buyers be informed of the presence of lead-based paint and radon concentrations in all buildings offered for sale.
14. Eliminate significant health risks from National Priority List hazardous waste sites, as measured by performance of clean-up at these sites sufficient to eliminate immediate and significant health threats as specified in health assessments completed at all sites.
15. Establish programs for recyclable materials and household hazardous waste in at least 75 percent of counties.
16. Establish and monitor in at least 35 states plans to define and track sentinel environmental diseases *(sentinel environmental disease include lead poisoning, other heavy metal poisoning, pesticide poisoning, carbon monoxide poisoning, heatstroke, hypothermia, acute chemical poisoning, methemoglobinemia, and respiratory diseases triggered by environmental factors).*

Related National Health Objectives: Food Safety

1. Reduce infections caused by key foodborne pathogens to incidences of no more than:

Salmonella species	16/100,000
Campylobacter jejuni	25/100,000
Escherichia coli	4/100,000
Listeria monocytogenes	0.5/100,000

2. Reduce outbreaks of infections due to *Salmonella enteritidis* to fewer than 25 outbreaks yearly.
3. Increase to at least 75 percent the proportion of households in which principal food preparers routinely refrain from leaving perishable food out of the refrigerator for over 2 hours and wash cutting boards and utensils with soap after contact with raw meat and poultry.
4. Extend to at least 70 percent the proportion of states and territories that have implemented model food codes for institutional food operations and to at least 70 percent the proportion that have adopted the new uniform food protection code ("Unicode") that sets recommended standards for regulation of all food operations.

From USDHHS: *Healthy People 2000: national health promotion and disease prevention objectives, full report, with commentary,* Washington, D.C., 1991, U.S. Government Printing Office, pp. 317-332, 341-343.

Modern nursing scholars consider the concept of environment to be central to the development of nursing knowledge and maintenance of health. Actions of nurses are directed toward promoting health by reducing environmental risks and preserving the earth's environment. Nurses and nursing organizations are becoming more aware of the importance of the environment to health. Nurses frequently care for clients with conditions that originate in the environment, including injuries from hazards at home and work; illnesses and conditions due to exposure to toxic wastes and chemicals and water and air pollution; malnutrition; and communicable diseases (Kleffel, 1991, p. 40). A major focus in community health nursing is placed on examining the interrelationship of environment, health, and disease.

The Role of the Nurse in Environmental Health

Nurses are involved in environmental health activities as professionals and as concerned citizens. An organization, the Nurses' Environmental Health Watch (NEHW), is dedicated to educating nurses and the public about actual and potential threats to human and environmental health. Membership in the organization includes a subscription to the *Health Watch* newsletter. NEHW can be contacted at 181 Marshall Street, Duxbury, Mass., 02332.

The American Holistic Nurses Association has developed a position statement in support of a healthful environment (Schuster, 1990, p. 27), and the International Council of Nurses (ICN) has developed a position statement that delineates the nurse's role in safeguarding the environment. The ICN position statement is given in the box on p. 179. The ICN has addressed the need for the nurse to assist in environmental health education activities, environmental surveillance, multidisciplinary environmental health activities, collaborative community relationships for environmental health, and to become actively involved in environmental health research. Nurses have a major role in safeguarding environmental health.

ENVIRONMENTAL HEALTH LEGISLATION

The Social Security Act of 1935 serves as umbrella legislation, consolidating U.S. social welfare legislation under one law; the Public Health Service Act of 1944 does the same for public health legislation. However, there is no umbrella legislation for environmental health, and numerous environmental health laws exist. The scope of this legislation, coupled with its lack of consolidation, makes it difficult and time-consuming to locate.

Federal, state, and local governments were slow to become involved in environmental health. Environmental legislation has tended to be reactive and responsive to the demands and crises of the moment rather than preventive (Rabe, 1990, Environmental health policy, p. 320). The environmental awareness that evolved in the United States in the 1960s marked the advent of numerous pieces of environmental legislation. In 1969 legislation authorized establishment of the Environmental Protection Agency (EPA). Since then more than a dozen major environmental laws have been passed (Sexton and Perlin, 1990, p. 913).

An overview of selected environmental health legislation in the United States is given in Appendix 6-1. This legislation is diverse and encompasses areas such as the Superfund (the environmental fund created to finance the cleanup of hazardous substances), water and air quality, toxic substances in the environment, pesticides, soil conservation, solid waste disposal, radiation, ocean dumping, environmental research, noise pollution, endangered species, and nuclear waste. The National Environmental Policy Act (Public Law 91-190) of 1969 is one of the most significant, and best-known, pieces of U.S. environmental health legislation. It was from this act that the EPA evolved.

THE ROLE OF FEDERAL, STATE, AND LOCAL AGENCIES IN ENVIRONMENTAL HEALTH

Many of the public health successes that have occurred in relation to communicable disease control, improving the quality of life, and reducing mortality across the lifespan (especially infant mortality), have come about as a result of environmental health practices. The private sector has been involved in environmental health activities, often from the standpoint of serving as an advocate for safeguarding and preserving the nation's lands and wildlife. Public sector involvement has occurred at all three levels of government. Traditionally the federal government has enacted national environmental health legislation, while state health authorities (SHAs) and local health departments (LHDs) have been involved in direct provision of environmental health services and establishing state and local environmental policies and regulations. The activities of federal, state, and local

The Nurse's Role in Safeguarding the Human Environment

The preservation and improvement of the human environment has become increasingly important for humankind's survival and well-being. The vastness and urgency of the task places on every individual and every professional group the responsibility to participate in the efforts to safeguard humankind's environment, and to conserve the world's resources, to study how their use affects humankind and how adverse effects can be avoided.

The Nurse's Role Is to:

Help detect ill effects of the environment on the health of man, and vice-versa.

The nurse should:

- apply observational skills for the detection of ill effects of environment on the individual;
- observe individuals in all settings for effects of pollutants in order to advise on protective and/or curative measures;
- record and analyze observations made of ill effects of environment and/or pollutants on individuals;
- be informed and report observations of the ecological consequences of pollutants and their adverse effects on the human being.

Be informed and apply knowledge in daily work with individuals, families and/or community groups as to the data available on potential health hazards and ways to prevent and/or reduce them.

The nurse should be informed about:

- the studies and identification of the environmental problems at local, national, and international level;
- their effects on man;
- the standards for the protection of the human organism, especially from pollutants;
- ways to prevent and/or reduce health hazards.

Be informed and teach preventive measures about health hazards due to environmental factors as well as about conservation of environmental resources to the individual, families and/or community groups.

The nurse can:

- request and attend continuing education programs about the study of the environment and the application of this knowledge in daily life and work;
- provide health education for both the general public and health personnel in order to create awareness of environmental issues and to involve the public with environmental management and control;
- apply knowledge in areas where nursing intervention may prevent or reduce health hazards;

- report on steps taken to control the significant environmental problems of the area.

Work with health authorities in pointing out health care aspects and health hazards in existing human settlements and in the planning of new settlements.

Nurses can:

- participate in exchange of information and experience about similar environmental problems with authorities in other areas;
- cooperate with health authorities in the preparation of programs to enable national and local authorities to influence their own environments;
- participate in the promotion of legislation to improve health care and reduce/prevent health hazards, and encourage the enforcement of such legislation where/ when appropriate;
- participate in national/local pre-disaster planning; and cooperate in international programs in case of disasters in other countries.

Assist communities in their action on environmental health problems.

The nurse can assist communities in programs to:

- reduce harmful pollutants (chemical, biological or physical, e.g. noise) in air, soil, water and food by industries or other human efforts;
- improve nutrition;
- encourage family planning;
- assess environmental factors in work situations and pursue activities for the elimination or reduction of hazards;
- educate the general public and all levels of nursing personnel in environmental and other health hazards, especially those related to unacceptable levels of contamination.

Participate in research providing data for early warning and prevention of deterious effects of the various environmental agents to which man is increasingly exposed; and research conducive to discovering ways and means of improving living and working conditions.

The nurse, as principal investigator or in collaboration with other nurses or related professions, can carry out epidemiological and experimental research designed to provide data for:

- early warning for prevention of health hazards;
- improving living and working conditions;
- monitoring the environmental levels of pollutants;
- measuring the impact of nursing intervention on environmental hazards.

From International Council of Nurses: *The nurse's role in safeguarding the human environment: position statement,* Geneva, Switzerland, 1986, The Council. Used with permission of the International Council of Nurses, Executive Director, Constance Holleran.

government are discussed to assist the reader in understanding the scope and organization of environmental health resources and services in the United States.

Federal Government and Environmental Health

The federal government is involved in promoting environmental health, often through legislation that protects national and international environmental resources. It is involved in protecting the public from the adverse consequences of exposure to harmful environmental agents (Sexton and Perlin, 1990, p. 913). The federal government is the single largest employer of environmental health professionals in the United States (Sexton and Perlin, p. 913). However, direct provision of environmental health services to local communities is usually carried out through state health authorities (SHAs) and local health departments (LHDs). The federal government's primary environmental health agency is the *Environmental Protection Agency (EPA)*.

The EPA was created on December 2, 1970. It is well-known for its efforts to protect and enhance the American environment to the fullest extent possible under the laws enacted by Congress. It is our nation's foremost environmental agency and serves as the nation's advocate for a livable environment. It has 10 regional offices across the nation.

The EPA works to control and abate pollution in the areas of air, water, solid waste, noise, radiation, and toxic substances, and manages the Superfund toxic waste cleanup program. It is mandated to mount an integrated, coordinated attack on environmental pollution in cooperation with state and local governments. The EPA coordinates and supports research and antipollution activities and also develops and disseminates information on safeguarding the environment. An organizational chart for the EPA is given in Figure 6-1. Executive branch and other federal agency involvement in environmental health activities is described in Appendix 6-2.

State Government and Environmental Health

State health authorities (SHAs) have historically been involved in environmental health activities. Recently there has been a trend toward removing this

authority from SHAs and placing it within other state agencies. This has led to diffuse patterns of responsibility, lack of coordination, and inadequate handling of environmental problems (Institute of Medicine, 1988, p. 150). State public health authorities must strengthen their capacities for identification, understanding, and control of environmental problems as health hazards (Institute of Medicine, pp. 150-151). Some SHAs administer federal environmental health legislation. The Clean Air Act is administered by 10 SHAs, the Clean Water Act by 9, the Safe Drinking Water Act by 27, the Resource Conservation and Recovery Act by 11, Superfund legislation by 11, and the Superfund by 11 (Public Health Foundation, 1991, Figure 2A). The SHA is the lead environmental agency in 10 states (Public Health Foundation, Figure 1). In the other 40 states a separate state level agency, such as the Department of Environment, is the lead environmental agency. Figure 6-2 depicts states in which the lead environmental agency is the SHA.

Local Government and Environmental Health

Local health departments (LHDs) have traditionally offered numerous health services that have a direct impact on the environmental health of the community. These local services are usually offered through environmental engineers or sanitarians, and, community health nurses often work cooperatively with these public health professionals.

On a local level environmental health personnel work to prevent, eliminate, and control environmental hazards (USDHHS, 1988, p. 3). In order to do this they are involved in many different environmental health programs, which Table 6-1 illustrates. LHDs are often responsible for testing community water and air, overseeing solid and hazardous waste disposal, performing food and restaurant inspections, monitoring noise pollution, assuring sanitation of public swimming and recreational facilities, implementing vector (e.g. skunk, rat, and mosquito) control measures, and ensuring safe housing.

THE ENVIRONMENTAL HEALTH WORKFORCE

Almost 80% of all environmental health practitioners are employed by governmental agencies at the federal, state, and local levels (USDHHS, 1988, p. 3). As previously mentioned, the federal government is the largest single employer of environmental health

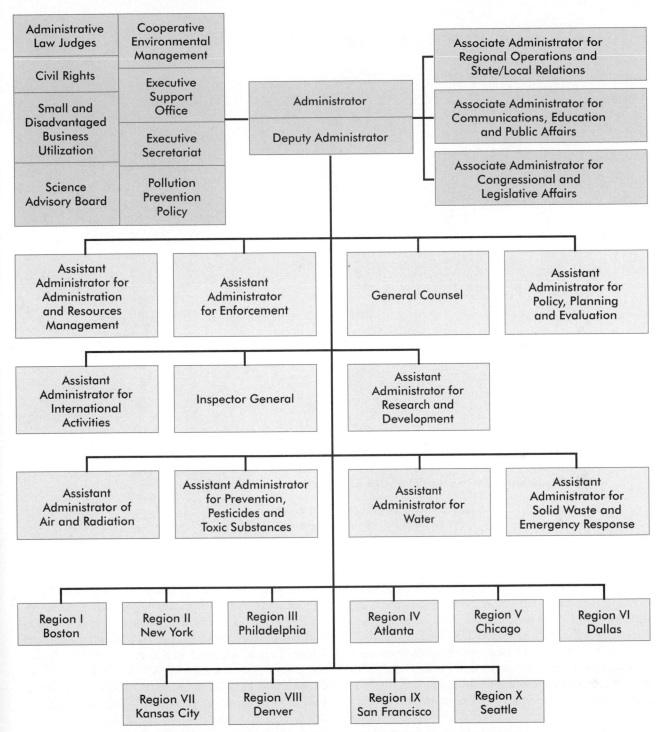

Figure 6-1 Environmental Protection Agency organizational chart. (From *U.S. Government Manual,* Washington, D.C., 1993, U.S. Government Printing Office, p. 565.)

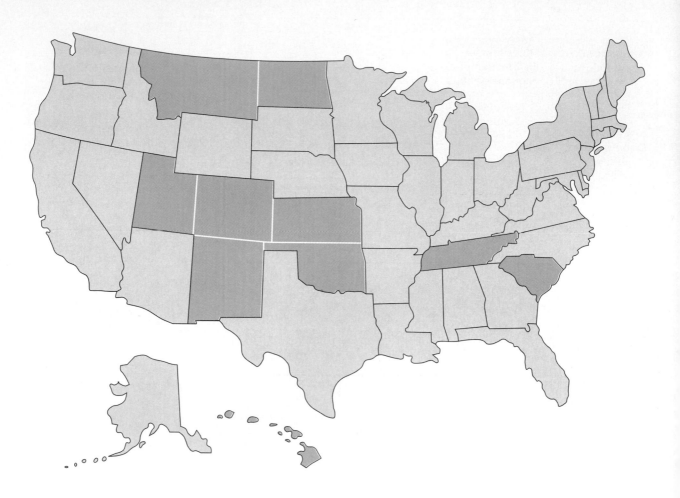

Note: States shown in color have SHAs as the lead environmental agency for the state.

Figure 6-2 SHAs as lead environmental agency. (Redrawn from Public Health Foundation: *1991 Public health chartbook,* Washington, D.C., 1991, The Foundation, Figure 1).

professionals in the United States (Sexton and Perlin, 1990, p. 913). Environmental health professionals are also employed in the private sector, and in recent years this employment has increased (USDHHS, 1988, p. 3).

For half a century the title *sanitarian* has been used to describe the environmental health practitioner who applies technical knowledge obtained from the biological and chemical sciences to promote and protect environmental health (USDHHS, 1988, p. 3). Today more contemporary titles include environmental engineer, environmental health specialist, and environmentalist. Many local health departments across the country employ sanitarians to implement environmental health programs.

Environmental health practitioners are educated to control, preserve, and improve the environment. Although there is continued debate over the actual number of environmental health professionals in the United States, a report to Congress estimated that there are approximately 82,000 (USDHHS, 1988, p. 8). Included in this number are 58,000 occupational health professionals, of which 24,000 are occupational health nurses; when these figures are subtracted there are only 20,000 sanitarians in the U.S. workforce (USDHHS, p. 8). It is estimated that more than 120,000 additional environmental health specialists are needed to meet the nation's demands (Gordon, 1990, p. 904).

6-1 Environmental Health Programs within Local Health Departments (LHDs)

Categories of environmental concern	Programs	Program purpose
Air	Air quality management	To ensure a community air resource conducive to good health, that will not injure plant or animal life or property, and that will be esthetically desirable
Water	Water supply sanitation	To ensure the provision of safe public and private water supplies, adequate in quantity and quality for every person
	Water pollution control	To ensure the cooperation with state water pollution control agencies and that surface and subsurface water supplies meet all state and local standards and regulations for water quality
Waste	Solid waste management	To ensure that all solid wastes are stored, collected, transported, and disposed of in a manner that does not create health, safety, or esthetic problems
	Liquid waste management	To ensure the treatment of liquid wastes in such a manner as to prevent problems of sanitation, public health nuisances, or pollution
	Toxic and hazardous waste management	To ensure that toxic and hazardous wastes are stored, collected, transported, and disposed of in a manner that does not create health or safety problems.
Food	Food protection	To ensure that all people are adequately protected from unhealthful or unsafe food or food products. This necessitates a comprehensive food protection program covering every facility where food or food products are stored, transported, processed, packaged, served, or vended, and regulating sanitation, wholesomeness, adulteration, advertising, labeling weights and measures, and fill-of-containers
Recreational areas	Swimming pool sanitation and safety	To ensure the safety and sanitation of public, semipublic, and private swimming pools
	Recreational sanitation	To ensure that all public recreational areas are operated so as to prevent health and safety problems
Product safety	Consumer product safety	To ensure that all people are adequately protected from unhealthful or unsafe substances or products in the home, business, and industry
Radiation	Radiation control	To prevent unnecessary or hazardous radiation exposure from the transportation, use, or disposal of all types of radiation-producing devices and products
Occupational	Occupational health and safety	To ensure, in cooperation with state officials, the health and safety of workers in places of employment, through controlling relevant environmental factors
Vectors	Vector control	To control all insects, rodents, and other animals which adversely affect health, safety, or comfort
Noise	Noise pollution control	To prevent hazardous or annoying noise levels in residential, business, industrial, and recreational structures and areas
Accidents	Environmental injury prevention	To influence or regulate planning, design, and construction in such a manner as to reduce the possibility of accidents through proper management of the environment.

Modified from American Public Health Association: Position paper on the role of official local health agencies, *Am J Public Health* 65:189-193, 1975; and USDHHS: *Evaluating the environmental health workforce* (HRP#0907160), Rockville, Md., 1988, USDHHS, p. 3.

Continued

TABLE **6-1**	Environmental Health Programs within Local Health Departments (LHDs)—cont'd	
Categories of environmental concern	**Programs**	**Program purpose**
Buildings	Housing sanitation, safety, and rehabilitation	To ensure programs that will provide decent, safe, and healthful housing for all people
	Institutional sanitation, safety, and rehabilitation	To ensure that institutions such as hospitals, schools, nurseries, jails, and prisons are operated so as to prevent sanitation and safety problems

Environmental Health Teamwork

Community health nurses work cooperatively with other health professionals on environmental health concerns. For example, interdisciplinary teams of personnel including nurses, sanitarians, and health educators work together to combat lead poisoning in children. On such a team the nurse might teach about lead poisoning prevention, complete risk assessments on targeted aggregates, do lead screenings in well-baby, WIC, and EPSDT clinics, and participate in community education activities at a local health fair. The environmental health sanitarian may make joint home visits with the community health nurse to conduct an environmental assessment, complete mapping programs to identify clusters of cases within a local community, enforce housing codes to eliminate lead in the home environment, and participate in community education activities. The health educator may organize community education activities and write grants to obtain funds for program development. Another example of a cooperative interaction between nurses and environmental health personnel is their collaboration in conducting epidemiological investigations of serious outbreaks of foodborne diseases such as botulism and salmonella. During these investigations both disciplines interview affected persons, investigate sources of contamination, and may conduct house-to-house surveys to identify ill people.

SELECTED ENVIRONMENTAL DISEASES

Most environmental illnesses and injuries are caused by physical, chemical, biological, or sociological hazards. Many of these environmental diseases are highly preventable (Landrigan, 1992, p. 941). Physical hazards include radiation, dust, vibration, noise, heat, and cold. Chemical hazards include toxicants, irritants, asphyxiants, poisons, carcinogens, mutagens, and teratogens. Biological hazards include infectious agents such as bacteria, viruses and protozoa, plants, insects, fungi, and molds. Sociological hazards include stress, violence, and inadequate housing. Many of these hazards enter the environment through direct discharge into air or water, inadequate landfills, and dumping sites (Blumenthal, 1985, p. 11-12).

Environmental etiology is evident in numerous diseases and conditions including cancer, genetic damage, birth defects, neurological effects, psychological disorders, liver disease, infectious diseases, injuries, and lung disease (Rabe, 1990, Environmental health policy, p. 318). In this century significant strides have been made in controlling environmentally linked diseases such as malaria, yellow fever, typhoid fever, cholera, dysenteries, and milkborne and foodborne diseases. However, waterborne, foodborne, soilborne, and vectorborne diseases, lead poisoning, lung diseases, and cancer are still prevalent.

To aid in determining environmental etiology an environmental health history should be routinely taken by the nurse as part of a client's health history. This environmental history should include the information in the box on p. 185.

Waterborne Diseases

The provision of safe water is a major environmental health challenge. Waterborne diseases are a result of water that is biologically and/or chemically polluted (water pollution is discussed later in this chapter). Waterborne diseases include typhoid, cholera, polio, hepatitis, and bacterial dysentery. Agents responsible for waterborne diseases include parasites such as protozoa, bacteria such as *Salmonella* and *Shigella,* viruses, and chemicals. People living in rural areas, or areas where untreated well water is used, are at greater risk for contracting waterborne diseases than persons using city water.

A waterborne disease outbreak is an incident in which two or more people experience a similar illness after consumption or use of water intended for drinking and in which there is epidemiological evidence that implicates water as the source of the illness (USDHHS, Full report, 1991, p. 318). The most frequent conditions caused by waterborne pathogens are gastroenteritis, giardiasis, and chemical poisoning (USDHHS, p. 318). Control of waterborne disease is addressed in *Healthy People 2000.*

Improvements made in this century in the treatment of water, effective disposal of human wastes, and activities to preserve the integrity of the water supply have greatly diminished the prevalence of waterborne diseases. However, over 20,000 cases of waterborne diseases are reported in the United States each year and the majority of cases go unreported (Blumenthal, 1985, pp. 4, 24). Worldwide morbidity and mortality from waterborne diseases involves millions of people each year (Nadakavukaren, 1990, p. 411). It is estimated that 20% of the U.S. population do not have safe drinking water (USDHHS, 1992, p. 66), and that 30,000 rural communities in this country do not have safe water to drink (Blumenthal, p. 24). Most outbreaks of waterborne disease in the United States involve semipublic water systems during the summer months (Blumenthal, p. 26).

Foodborne Diseases

More than 10,000 cases of acute foodborne illnesses are reported each year in the United States (Blumenthal, 1985, pp. 3-4). However, the majority of cases go unreported, and the number of actual cases in the United States may be as high as a million each year (Blumenthal, p. 30). Foodborne diseases are very prevalent in developing countries.

Factors that may be implicated in outbreaks of foodborne illness include improper holding temperatures for food, inadequate cooking, contaminated equipment, contaminated food, and infected food

> ◀ *Selected Environmental* ▶
> *History Information*
>
> Occupation of family members
> Building materials used and stored in the home (e.g. asbestos)
> Source of water
> Source of fresh fruits and vegetables
> Home heating system
> Home pesticide use
> Contact with pets
> Hobbies (especially hobbies that might increase exposure to chemicals, sunlight, or waste products)
> Types of industry in the neighborhood
> Known exposures to lead or other chemicals
> Vector exposure
> Exposure to known or suspected sources of contaminated air, soil, or water

handlers (Blumenthal, 1985, p. 31). The etiology of many foodborne outbreaks is unknown, but for those of known etiology two thirds are bacterial in origin, about one fifth are chemical, and the remainder are viral or parasitic (Blumenthal, p. 32-33). There are more than 200 known causes of foodborne illness (Bryan, 1975).

Contributors to foodborne disease are *food contaminants.* These contaminants include dirt, hairs, animal feces, fungi, insect fragments, pesticide residues, and traces of chemical substances (Nadakavukaren, 1990, p. 241). Growth hormones in meat and poultry and pesticide residues on fruits and vegetables are well-known food contaminants. According to a report by the National Research Council, tomatoes, beef, potatoes, oranges and, lettuce top the list of dietary sources for public exposure to cancer-causing pesticide residues (Nadakavukaren, p. 245). The Food and Drug Administration (FDA) has established "Defect Action Levels" that specify the maximum limit of contamination the agency permits before legal action is taken to remove the product from the market (Nadakavukaren, p. 242). Some examples of these levels are given in Table 6-2.

Soilborne Diseases

Soilborne parasitic diseases are the most common infectious diseases in the world and are primarily

TABLE 6-2   Examples of FDA Food Defect Action Levels

Product	Defect	Action level
Apricots, canned	Insect filth	Average of 2% or more by count insect-infested or insect-damaged
Beets, canned	Rot	Exceeds average of 5% by weight of pieces with dry rot
Broccoli, frozen	Insects and mites	Average of 60 aphids, thrips, and/or mites per 100 grams
Cherries, maraschino	Insect filth	Average of over 5% rejects due to maggots
Corn, canned	Insect larvae (corn ear worms, corn borers)	Two or more 3 mm or longer larvae, cast skins or cast skin fragments of corn ear worm or corn borer, the aggregate length exceeding 12 mm in 24 pounds
Curry powder	Insect filth	Average of more than 100 insect fragments per 25 grams
	Rodent filth	Average of more than 4 rodent hairs per 25 grams
Olives, pitted	Pits	Average of more than 1.3% by count of olives with whole pits and/or pit fragments 2 mm or longer measured in the longest dimension
Peanut butter	Insect filth	Average of 30 or more insect fragments per 100 grams
	Rodent filth	Average of 1 or more rodent hairs per 100 grams
	Grit	Gritty taste and water-insoluble inorganic residue is more than 25 mg per 100 grams
Tomatoes, canned	*Drosophila* fly	Average 10 fly eggs per 500 grams; or 5 fly eggs and 1 maggot per 500 grams; or 2 maggots per 500 grams

Modified from Nadakavukaren A: *Man and environment: a health perspective*, ed. 3, Prospect Heights, Ill., 1990, Waveland Press, p. 242. Used with permission.

transmitted by the fecal-oral route (Blumenthal, 1985, p. 41). One quarter of the world's population (more than 650 million people) is infected with the large roundworm *Ascaris lumbricoides* (Blumenthal, p. 42). In tropical climates one half of the population may actually be infected with *Ascaris lumbricoides* (Benenson, 1990, p. 50). Prevalence of this large roundworm infection is greatest in children 3 to 8 years old (Benenson, p. 50). A single female *Ascaris* can produce 200,000 eggs per day (Blumenthal, p. 42).

Almost 450 million persons are infected with hookworm worldwide (Beck and Davies, 1981). Pinworm is the most common worm infection in the United States, with prevalence highest in school-age children (Benenson, 1990, p. 157). Climate helps to make these infections more prevalent in the southeastern United States. Community health nurses regularly assess for exposure to soilborne diseases when working with children.

Vectorborne Diseases

A *vector* is a nonhuman carrier of disease organisms that can transmit these organisms directly to humans (Blumenthal, 1985, p. 34). Vector transmission is an indirect form of biological or mechanical disease transmission.

Mechanical transmission includes the disease spread by a crawling or flying insect (e.g., mosquitoes, ticks, and houseflies) that does not require multiplication or development of the transmitted organism (Benenson, 1990, p. 508). *Biological transmission* involves multiplication or development of the organism before the vector can transmit the infective agent (Benenson, p. 508). As with waterborne and foodborne disease, vectorborne illness has a higher prevalence in developing nations. Malaria and yellow fever are two of the most well-known vectorborne diseases. Malaria is endemic throughout most of the nonindustrialized world; it is estimated that over 200 million people are

TABLE 6-3 Some Insect Vectors and Diseases Transmitted by Them

Vector	Disease	Pathogen
Mosquitoes		
Anopheles sp.	Malaria	*Plasmodium* sp. (protozoa)
Culex sp.	Filariasis	*Wucheraria bancrofti* and *Brugia malayi* (nematodes)
Culex sp.	Encephalitis	arbovirus
Aedes aegypti	Yellow fever	arbovirus
Aedes aegypti	Dengue	arbovirus
Biting Flies		
Deer fly	Filariasis	*Loa loa* (nematode)
Black fly	River blindness	*Onchocerca volvulus* (nematode)
Tsetse fly	Sleeping sickness	*Trypanosoma gambiense* and *rhodesiense* (protozoa)
Sandfly	Kala-azar	*Leishmania donovani*
	Tropical ulcer	*Leishmania tropica*
	Cutaneous leishmaniasis	*Leishmania mexicana*
	Espundia	*Leishmania braziliensis* (protozoa)
	Phlebotomus fever	arbovirus
Other Insects		
Gnats	Filariasis	*Mansonella ozzardi* (nematode)
Rat flea	Plague	*Yersinia pestis* (bacteria)
	Murine typhus	*Rickettsia mooseri*
Body louse	Epidemic typhus	*Rickettsia prowazekii*
	Trench fever	*Rickettsia quintana*
Tick	Rocky Mountain spotted fever	*Rickettsia rickettsii*
Tick	Colorado tick fever	arbovirus
Mite	Rickettsialpox	*Rickettsia akari*

Modified from Blumenthal DS, ed: *An introduction to environmental health*, New York, 1985, Springer, p. 35. Used with permission.

infected with malaria worldwide (Blumenthal, 1985, p. 37). Yellow fever was prevalent in the United States until the early 1900s. An epidemic of this disease originating in the port of New Orleans precipitated the formation of a National Board of Health from 1879 to 1883. Vector control measures are important in limiting and eradicating these diseases. Some insect vectors and the diseases transmitted by them are given in Table 6-3.

Lead Poisoning

Lead poisoning is a major environmental health concern and one of our society's most urgent health problems (Murdock, 1991, p. 28). A strong national effort is in place to reduce lead in American homes and eradicate childhood lead poisoning (USDHHS, 1991, Full report, p. 66).

Lead poisoning has been documented throughout history, and some historians theorize that it was one of the conditions leading to the fall of the Roman Empire. Many wealthy and influential Romans could afford to have water piped to their homes and to eat from expensive glazed dishes. These water pipes often contained lead, as did the finishes and glazes used on dishes and tableware. It is hypothesized that the effects of this exposure could have resulted in children of the ruling class being unable to meet their full mental potential and suffering from other forms of neurotoxicity, and in adults evidencing neurotoxicity, bizarre behavior, and sterility (Blumenthal, 1985, p. 51).

Lead poisoning was a serious problem in the early days of the auto industry in this country because many auto workers placed lead in the doors and frames of automobiles. They inhaled lead throughout the day and also ingested lead when they sat around the assembly line to eat their meals. Research studies on lead poisoning in the auto industry, done by Dr. Carey P. McCord of the University of Michigan, resulted in regulations to protect workers from lead inhalation, protective measures for workers, and the first lunchrooms and cafeterias in industry—places for workers to eat that were free from lead particles (McCord, 1976).

Lead can be inhaled, ingested, or transmitted in utero. It is an extremely toxic substance to the cardiovascular, renal, reproductive, and neurological systems (Preventing lead poisoning, 1992, p. 1). Exposure to high levels of lead is potentially fatal. Symptoms of lead poisoning include listlessness, pallor, loss of appetite, irritability, behavioral changes, and developmental or growth delays (refer to Chapter 14). Even low levels of exposure can cause central nervous system damage, hearing impairments, and growth deficits (USDHHS, 1991, p. 14; Lead, 1988, p. 2).

Lead poisoning is an epidemic among young children in the United States (Landrigan, 1992, p. 941), with almost 3 million children younger than 6 years of age (17% of all U.S. children in this age group) having elevated blood lead levels (Agency for Toxic Substances and Disease Registry, 1988; Bourgoin, Evans, Cornett, Lingard, and Quattrone, 1993, p. 1155). Children absorb more than 50% of the lead they ingest, and young children are especially vulnerable to the effects of lead (Preventing lead poisoning, 1992, p. 1). If a calcium or iron deficiency exists, even more lead will be absorbed from the gastrointestinal tract (Preventing lead poisoning, p. 1).

Lead poisoning in children is often contracted from lead in paint, ducts, water, gas fumes, and soil. It is especially prevalent in inner-city areas where high concentrations of lead exist in soil and air near heavily travelled roadways, and in old buildings that may have been painted with lead paint before 1950. The Agency for Toxic Substances and Disease Registry estimates that about 400,000 children are at risk of being born with lead poisoning each year because their mothers have elevated blood lead levels (Nadakavukaren, 1990, p. 28).

Strides have been made in recent years to reduce the incidence of lead poisoning. In 1971 Congress passed the Lead-Based Paint Poisoning Prevention Act, which banned the usage of lead-based paint in interior paints and on furniture and toys. There have been major gains in understanding and treating lead poisoning, and from 1982 to 1988 the average amount of lead ingested daily by U.S. children actually decreased, from 30 µg to 5 µg (Bourgoin, Evans, Cornett, Lingard, and Quattrone, 1993, p. 1155). Finding sources of lead poisoning in the home and community can be a challenge for the nurse. Control of lead poisoning is addressed in *Healthy People 2000*.

Lung Diseases

Environmental pollutants in the air contribute to numerous lung diseases, including bronchial asthma, acute respiratory conditions and irritations, pneumoconiosis, allergic alveolitis, and lung cancer. Reducing human exposure to air pollutants such as ozone, carbon monoxide, nitrogen dioxide, sulfur dioxide, and particulates is important in reducing the incidence of environmentally linked lung diseases.

Asthma affects approximately 10 million Americans (USDHHS, Full report, 1991, p. 317). Childhood asthma is a major health problem that has had increasing rates of morbidity and mortality in recent years. It has been linked to passive inhalation of smoke and other environmental pollutants. Its incidence rises in the summertime, with peak levels of atmospheric ozone, and with year-round increase in nitrogen oxides in the air (Landrigan, 1992, p. 942). In inner cities asthma is the leading cause of hospital admissions for children 5 to 15 years old, with asthma rates highest among black and Hispanic children (Landrigan, p. 942).

Although air quality has improved significantly in recent years, fewer than 50% of Americans live in counties that meet all the EPA standards for air quality (Environmental Protection Agency, 1990). Although significant gains have been made in reducing air pollution from motor vehicles and other sources, additional gains are needed.

Cancer

Although the etiology of many cancers is unknown, there have been definite links of cancer to environmental agents. The relationships between smoking and lung cancer, radon and lung cancer, exposure to the sun and skin cancer, asbestos and malignant mesothelioma, and numerous chemicals and occupational cancers (refer to Chapter 17) are well known. Tobacco has been estimated to account for 30% of all cancers in the United States (USDHHS, 1991, Full report, p. 72). By the year 2000 an estimated 300,000 American workers will have died of diseases caused by asbestos-related lung cancer and malignant mesothelioma (Landrigan, 1992, p. 941). An increasing risk with asbestos is the number of school children exposed to it as a result of insulation in older school buildings. The Environmental Protection Agency estimates that approximately 20,000 cases of lung cancer each year occur as a result of radon exposure (USDHHS, Full report, p. 322). Carcinogenic environmental exposures are often preventable.

PRESERVING THE ENVIRONMENT

People have added to the destruction of the global environment; however, they are becoming increasingly concerned about the global environmental conditions and the ability of the planet to maintain future generations. Recent polls have put environmental issues at the top of Americans' concerns, along with AIDS, crime, and drugs (Schuster, 1990, p. 26). Environmental issues are a part of every major political campaign, and Americans are demanding ecologically sound products, legislation, and activities. Some significant environmental concerns that illustrate what is happening today in this area are given in the box on this page. A discussion of these concerns and their impact on health follows.

Greenhouse Effect

Citizens of the world are in the process of changing the earth's atmosphere. Natural greenhouse gases in the atmosphere form a blanket around the earth and keep the planet warm. These natural gases are predominantly carbon dioxide, methane, and nitrous oxide. When technological gases (especially carbon dioxide) thicken this blanket, they trap more heat around the earth and result in global warming. Eventually the temperature of the earth's surface will warm enough to cause climatic and environmental changes that can be detrimental to health.

Scientists estimate that by 2050 the earth's temperature could increase by as much as four degrees

> ◀ *What Is Happening Today* ▶
> *with the Environment*
>
> Greenhouse effect
> Air pollution
> Ozone depletion
> Water pollution
> Hazardous waste accumulation
> Acid rain
> Loss of biological diversity
> Garbage/solid waste overaccumulation
> Desertification
> Deforestation
> Wetlands depletion
> Energy depletion
> Overpopulation

centigrade (Wittkopf and Kegley, 1990, p. 33). This would be as great a change as the drop of four degrees centigrade that caused the last Ice Age (Doll, 1992, p. 939). Many scientists fear that rising temperatures will melt polar ice caps, raise ocean levels, flood and destroy coastal areas and wetlands, alter weather patterns and change rain distribution, increase the frequency of droughts, and create deserts. Climate changes resulting from global warming can result in "habitats on the move" for humans, plants, and animals, and the creation of conditions more conducive to the spread of many communicable diseases. In addition, climate changes can result in dramatic changes in global patterns of food production and trade (Wittkopf and Kegley, p. 33). In relation to health, global warming can result in food shortages; the extension of areas favorable to vectorborne and parasitic diseases; an increase in communicable diseases; increased incidence of skin cancer, heat stroke, and exhaustion; and patterns of human migration that can result in overcrowding and other unfavorable social conditions.

Air Pollution

Air pollution results when one or more chemicals is in high enough concentrations in the air to harm plants, animals, or humans (Miller, 1992). Particulate matter and excess heat and noise are considered to be air pollutants also.

Is Radon Gas Hiding in Your Home?

When Stanley Watras walked into the Limerick nuclear power plant near Philadelphia on a December morning in 1984 he started radiation-detection alarms ringing. It was determined that the radioactive contamination on Watras had come from outside the nuclear facility, and Watras' home was checked for possible sources of radiation contamination.

To everyone's amazement, tests revealed that the Watras home had levels of radon gas approximately 1000 times higher than normal. Investigators estimated that the Watras family was receiving radiation exposure equivalent to 455,000 chest x-rays a year just by living in their house. The Watras family had been unaware of the radon in their home.

Further investigation showed that radon was "hiding" in thousands of American homes. It was determined that large sections of eastern Pennsylvania, New Jersey, and New York, which are underlain by a uranium geological formation, had thousands of homes where elevated levels of radon existed. Is radon gas hiding in your home?

Modified from Nadakavukaren A: *Man and environment: a health perspective,* ed 3, Prospect Heights, Ill., 1990, Waveland Press, p. 357. Used with permission.

Air pollution has always occurred through natural occurrences in the environment, including volcanoes, pollination, and swamp gas (Blumenthal and Greene, 1985, p. 117). Historically, concern for the effects of air pollution on public health dates back to at least the thirteenth century when government commissions were established in England to investigate sources of air pollution and the fouling of air (Blumenthal and Greene, p. 117). The Industrial Revolution greatly added to the problem of air pollution, and gas-powered vehicles, power plants, and industry continue to contribute to this problem today. Early community efforts to minimize air pollution in the United States included local regulations to control unpleasant "airs," limiting outdoor burning, and controlling smoke. The Clean Air Acts of 1970, 1977, and 1990 (refer to Appendix 6-1) have worked to reduce air pollution in the United States and mandated establishment of national ambient air quality standards for suspended particulates, sulfur oxides, carbon monoxide, nitrogen oxide, man-made ozone, hydrocarbons, and lead.

The American Lung Association sponsors Clean Air Week each year in May and tries to educate the American public about the importance of clean air and lung health. However, according to the Environmental Protection Agency 164 million Americans (66% of the U.S. population) live in areas where the Clean Air Standard is exceeded (Centers for Disease Control and Prevention, 1993, p. 302). *Healthy People 2000* addresses the need for more American cities to comply with these standards. The Centers for Disease Control and Prevention (CDC) recognize that, in order for this to occur, additional educational methods focused on air pollution control and improved coordination between health and environmental agencies is needed (CDC, p. 303). Air pollution is often classified as indoor or outdoor.

Indoor air pollution is a significant concern, and appears to pose a greater risk to human health than does outdoor air pollution. As many as 150 hazardous chemicals can be found in the average American home at concentrations up to 40 times greater than they are found outdoors (Miller, 1992, p. 578). Indoor air pollution is often caused by radon, tobacco smoke, infectious agents, allergens, combustion smoke (e.g., furnaces, fireplaces, woodstoves), household chemicals, pesticides, and building materials (e.g., asbestos, formaldehyde treated products). It has been estimated that up to one third of all U.S. buildings, including the EPA headquarters, suffer from indoor air pollution (Miller, p. 578).

Radon is the second leading cause of lung cancer in the United States (Murdock, 1991, p. 12) and the federal government is trying to educate the American public to its dangers. Radon particles are carried deep into the lung where they release small bursts of energy and damage lung tissue, resulting in possible lung damage, lung disease, and lung cancer. The EPA has ranked radon as one of the most dangerous cancer risks in the environment.

Since the 1980s radon has been recognized as a serious form of indoor air pollution. The box on this page illustrates how radon can hide undetected in the American home. Radon is a colorless, odorless gas formed by radioactive decay of radium and uranium that is found in the natural soil. It enters a building silently and relatively unnoticed through cracks in basement walls, floors, and foundations; joints between walls and floors; well water; and openings around pipes and sump pumps. Radon quietly seeps into millions of American homes, schools, and businesses with no early warning symptoms. The Environmental Protection Agency (EPA) estimates that 7% of American homes (4 million) have elevated radon levels (Murdock, 1991, p. 11). A recent EPA survey found radon in unexpectedly high concentrations in homes in 17 states and recommended that homeowners across the nation test their homes for radon (Nadakavukaren, 1990, p. 359). Although elevated radon levels in buildings pose health threats, these threats can be attenuated by remedial action. The EPA has numerous publications on radon and how to prevent or remove it in buildings.

Tobacco smoke is another major indoor air pollutant and health risk. Bronchitis, pneumonia, asthma, and acute respiratory infections occur up to twice as often as normal during the first two years of life in children of parents who smoke. The more smoking in the home, the higher the prevalence of respiratory symptoms (Murdock, 1991, p. 12).

Research conducted by the National Aeronautics and Space Administration (NASA) has indicated that the use of houseplants can actually help to absorb contaminants in the air; they plan to use plants as part of the biological life support system aboard future orbiting space stations (Why clean, 1990, 1F). NASA found that plants help to remove benzene, formaldehyde, and carbon monoxide and put oxygen back into the environment. Indoor air pollutants frequently cause acute and chronic respiratory infections and conditions, allergic reactions, headaches, and cancer. They pose serious threats to human health.

Outdoor air pollution, or ambient air pollution, is prevalent in the United States. Major ambient air pollutants are carbon oxides, sulfur oxides, nitrogen oxides, volatile organic compounds (e.g., methane, benzene, formaldehyde), suspended particles, photochemical oxidants (e.g., ozone, hydrogen peroxide), radioactive substances, heat, and noise (Miller, 1992, pp. 575-576).

Smog is a major form of outdoor air pollution. All major American cities suffer from some level of smog. It is more prevalent in industrial areas with dense population, large numbers of motor vehicles, and a sunny, dry climate. The word *smog* originated as a combination of the words smoke and fog. Smog harms plants, animals, and people. It has been blamed for numerous outbreaks of respiratory illness and distress in addition to crop losses and deforestation

(pine trees are very susceptible). Outdoor air pollution can result in such health conditions as lung cancer, bronchial asthma, acute respiratory illnesses/ conditions, and skin and eye conditions. Lung damage from polluted air is a risk for millions of Americans. Air pollution also damages agriculture, vegetation, and property, creates aesthetic problems, and affects the economy in terms of property damage and loss, morbidity, mortality, and absenteeism from work.

Ozone Depletion

An invisible layer of natural ozone shields and protects the earth's surface against ultraviolet radiation. People are destroying this natural ozone shield by use of chlorofluorocarbons (CFCs) and other manmade chemicals. CFCs are compounds made up of carbon, chlorine, and fluorine. They are routinely used in refrigeration and air conditioning (e.g. freon), aerosol sprays, and cleaning agents; 750,000 metric tons of chloroflurocarbons are used annually worldwide (Elmer-Dewitt, 1992, p. 64). CFCs deplete the ozone layer when they rise into the stratosphere and their chlorine atoms react with ozone. International agreements have been put in place to phase out CFC use by the year 2000; the United States may cease its production as early as 1996 (Lemonick, 1992, p. 60).

Sherwood Rowland, at the University of California at Irvine, issued the first ozone depletion alert in 1974 (Lemonick, 1992, p. 62). A hole in the ozone layer over Antarctica was confirmed in 1985 (Lemonick, p. 60). Recently, researchers have found the first signs of ozone depletion in North America (Snider, 1993, A1). Ozone levels have declined from 4% to 8% over the last decade (Lemonick, p. 60). Holes in the ozone layer deplete our natural protection from the sun, making it increasingly important to wear sunglasses, protective clothing, and sunscreen when exposed to the sun for prolonged periods. It is crucial to minimize the time spent in the sun during the peak period of 10 AM to 3 PM, minimize sunbathing, and avoid being in the sun for long periods of time. Ozone depletion is a health hazard. It is expected to result in increased incidence of skin cancer and accelerated skin aging, eye cataracts, mutations in DNA, immune-system weakening, depletion of food crops by interference with the process of photosynthesis, and phytoplankton depletion (phytoplankton is important in the ocean food chain). Scientists are also concerned about the possible effects of ozone depletion on climate.

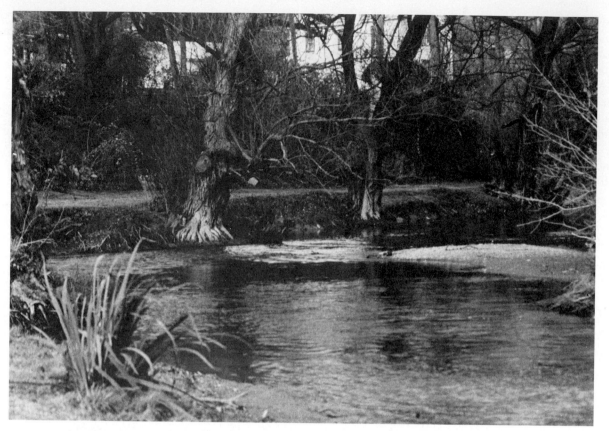

Figure 6-3 Safeguarding our natural resources is a major public health need. Despite all our modern technology, our nation has not been effective in controlling disease outbreaks related to environmental pollutants. In recent years there has been a dramatic rise in the number of disease outbreaks from contaminated water. (Courtesy Henry Parks, photographer.)

Water Pollution

The human body's dependence on a regular intake of water is second only to its need for oxygen (Nadakavukaren, 1990, p. 391). As amazing as it may seem, only 3% of the Earth's water is fresh and only 1% of this water is suitable for drinking. Americans use almost 100 billion gallons of fresh water every day, much more than other countries (Loehr, 1989, p. 26). Water is a renewable resource, but in the near future water supply could become a serious crisis in many areas of the United States.

Water resources in the United States are not evenly distributed. Areas in the Pacific Northwest receive about 80 inches of rainfall annually, whereas the driest state, Nevada, receives only 9 inches annually (Nadakavukaren, 1990, p. 391). Droughts in the Midwest and flooding along the Mississippi help to illus-

trate rainfall and water discrepancies in the United States. Existing U.S. water supplies are rapidly being polluted and depleted. Even where there are abundant sources of water, serious problems result if that water is unfit for human consumption. We need to conserve and protect our nation's water supplies (refer to Figure 6-3).

Sources of potential water pollution are construction activities, industrial wastes, human and animal wastes, landfill waste, accidental spills, mining operations, leaking underground storage tanks, agricultural waste and runoff, fallout of airborne pollutants, urban street runoff, fertilizers, and pesticides. Homeowners add to groundwater contamination by dumping household chemicals down the drain or on the ground and through the use of septic tanks. Further, household septic tanks are used by almost 30% of the U.S.

population, account for 3.5 billion gallons of waste being introduced into the soil each day, and have the potential to add to water pollution (Loehr, 1989, p. 26).

In less-developed countries millions of people do not have access to safe drinking water. Each year millions of people worldwide become ill and die from preventable waterborne diseases such as polio, typhoid, cholera, hepatitis, and bacterial dysentery. The United States has set a goal that 95% of the population will have safe drinking water by the year 2000 (USDHHS, 1992, p. 66).

Hazardous Waste

Hazardous wastes pose serious health problems. A hazardous waste has been defined as "any material that is of no further use and cannot be disposed of safely by allowing it to enter the environment in its original form in an uncontrolled manner" (Carden, 1985, p. 179). Such wastes have properties that make them especially hazardous to human health, including flammability, acute or chronic toxicity, radioactivity, the presence of pathogens, explosiveness, or a tendency to react rapidly with other materials to produce flammable or toxic gases and excessive heat (Carden, p. 180). Hazardous wastes are often divided into the categories of radioactive, infective, and chemical (Carden, p. 181).

Hazardous wastes pollute water, air, soil, and food, and accumulate in the natural food chain. They produce birth defects, poisoning, and tumors. It has been estimated that each year one metric ton of hazardous waste is produced for every U.S. citizen, and that only a small percentage of this waste is disposed of properly (Loehr, 1989, p. 27). Improper disposal of hazardous industrial waste has lead to Superfund legislation, numerous health problems, and communities being evacuated and relocated. Disposal of hazardous household waste is becoming a problem. Today there are more chemicals in the average American home than were in a chemical laboratory at the turn of the century.

Recently an environmentally sound process called bioremediation has been used to devour waste products and unwanted hazardous waste materials. In bioremediation special bacteria are utilized to break down hazardous waste into nonhazardous compounds. Such safe, innovative methods to deal with hazardous waste materials need to be developed and encouraged. Hazardous and toxic wastes have been linked to acute and chronic illness, cancer, birth defects, blindness, and sterility.

Acid Rain

Sulfur dioxide is the primary component of acid rain. Electric utilities are responsible for the majority of sulfur dioxide emissions in the United States. Sulfur dioxide and nitrogen oxides mix in the atmosphere and are changed chemically into sulfuric acid and nitric acid that fall back to earth in the form of acid rain or snow. Areas along the Appalachian Mountains have rain that has the acidic content of lemon juice. In lakes, rivers, and streams this acidic content can upset the ecological balance needed to sustain fish, plant, and animal life. It is estimated that the effects of acid rain in the United States cost up to $10 billion a year (Miller, 1992, p. 586). You can help prevent acid rain by conserving energy. Acid rain harms building and car finishes, kills aquatic life, can result in crop depletion, harms human and animal health, and results in the loss of plant and animal diversity. It is thought to be responsible for certain dermatological conditions.

Loss of Biological Diversity

Extinction is forever! Once a plant, animal, or insect species is gone we can never get it back. Unfortunately, we are living through the greatest extinction event of the last 65 million years. For the first time in millions of years species are vanishing more rapidly than new ones are evolving (Nadakavukaren, 1990, p. 142).

Since the Pilgrims landed in 1620, more than 500 species and varieties of U.S. plants and animals have become extinct (U.S. Department of the Interior, 1992). The American passenger pigeon became extinct in this century, the American peregrine falcon and the California condor are on the brink of extinction, and the American eagle is endangered.

To protect endangered species, the Endangered Species Act of 1973 was passed. It gave the United States one of the most far-reaching laws ever enacted by any country to prevent the extinction of imperiled animals and plants. As of April 1990 more than 560 native mammals, birds, reptiles, crustaceans, plants, and other life forms were officially protected. In addition, more than 500 foreign species are now protected under the act. The U.S. Department of the Interior (U.S. Fish and Wildlife Service) is charged with protecting American wildlife and endangered species.

Number of species

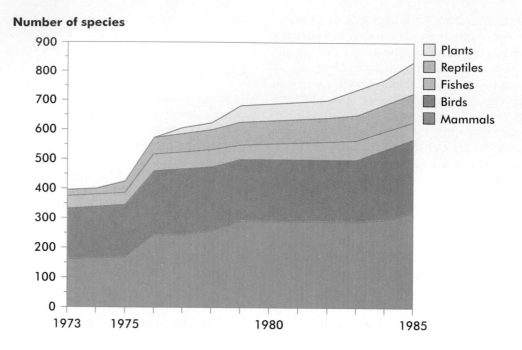

Number of species

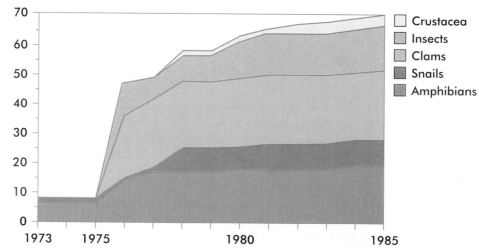

Figure 6-4   Listed endangered and threatened species, 1973-1985. (From Nadakavukaren A: *Man and environment: a health perspective,* ed 3, Prospect Heights, Ill., 1990, Waveland Press, p. 141. Used with permission.)

Each year several thousand species of plants and animals become extinct worldwide (Miller, 1992, p. 414). If poaching, animal exploitation, environmental pollution, and destruction of critical habitats continues at the present rate, within the next few decades one half of the world's plant, animal, and insect species could be lost forever (Miller, p. 414). A look at how the number of endangered and threatened species has grown is given in Figure 6-4.

We need to remember that everything in nature is

interlinked. Species diversity is a major determinant of ecological stability and survival. As we lose plant and animal species we increase the risk of our own extinction. With the loss of each plant species we could possibly be losing a cure for AIDS, cancer, or numerous other diseases or conditions.

Garbage and Solid Waste Disposal

The first city dump appears to have been established in Athens, Greece around 500 BC (Nadakavukaren, 1990, p. 458). Athenians also banned throwing garbage into the streets and allowed no waste to be dumped closer than one mile from the city walls (Nadakavukaren, p. 458).

The United States has the dubious distinction of being the world's biggest solid waste producer. With only 4.5% of the world's population, Americans produce 33% of the world's solid wastes—11 billion tons each year (Miller, 1992, p. 519). Trash and solid waste have become major national problems. Americans throw away 185 million tons of garbage a year (Miller, p. 519), or almost 4 pounds per person each day. Much of this solid waste is placed in landfills or burned. More than two thirds of the nation's landfills have closed since the late 1970s and most of those remaining will be full and forced to close by 1995 (Beck, Hager, King, Hutchinson, Robins, and Gordon, 1989, p. 67).

In 1992 the state of Tennessee picked up 26,658 tons of trash along its highways at a cost of more than $5 million (Tennessee Department of Environment and Conservation, 1993, p. 1). Adding to the problem are agricultural and mining waste, household trash, industrial/business trash, and yard waste. Over 2 billion tons of mineral wastes are produced annually by the mining industry alone (Nadakavukaren, 1990, p. 459). Together, agricultural and mining wastes account for 91% of the total waste generated in the United States (Nadakavukaren, p. 460). Trash, landfills, piles of refuse, and unsightly, unsanitary conditions are becoming a regular part of the American landscape; "America the beautiful" may soon be a phrase from the past.

Today the three Rs of waste control are *Reuse, Recycle,* and *Reduce.* Americans need to practice the three Rs more. Recycling is becoming more popular in the United States, but less than 11% of U.S. solid waste is recycled (Beck, Hager, King, Hutchinson, Robins, and Gordon, 1989, p. 67). In support of

recycling and preserving the environment, this text is printed on recycled paper.

Reusing "reusables" and reducing the amount of garbage and solid waste has been slower to gain momentum than recycling; just look at how disposable items are used in everyday life and health care settings. The best way to manage garbage and waste is not to produce it in the first place. Some information on the extent of U.S. garbage is presented in the box on p. 196. Garbage and solid waste produce health risks such as the possibility of soil and water pollution, spread of communicable disease, and accidental illness and injury.

Desertification

Most desertification occurs naturally at the edges of existing desert due to dehydration of the top layers of soil, but desertification can also occur due to overgrazing, improper soil management and utilization of water resources, and deforestation (Miller, 1992, p. 320). Two billion acres (an area the size of Brazil or 12 times the size of Texas) have become desert during the past 50 years, each year 15 million acres become desert (an area the size of West Virginia), and an estimated 63% of rangelands and 60% of rainfed cropland are threatened by desertification (Miller, p. 320). In the American Southwest overgrazing is largely responsible for the formation of Arizona's Sonoran Desert (Nadakavukaren, 1990, p. 138).

Once land has become desert it is difficult to reclaim. Restoration efforts often involve reforestation. Loss of land previously used for food production has a direct impact on nutrition and quality of human life. Also, migration of people and animals due to "habitats on the move" can result in overcrowding and other undesirable social conditions.

Wetlands Destruction

U.S. wetlands are rapidly being depleted and destroyed. These wetlands include swamps, marshes, ponds, river bottoms, flood plains, and ponds. Until recently many wetland areas were seen as nuisances because of water accumulation and insects, and many wetlands were drained for agricultural, industrial, and residential purposes. However, environmentalists and the general public are now recognizing their value and legislation has been passed to preserve and protect remaining wetlands.

◀ *A Look at U.S. Trash* ▶

Existing U.S. landfill capacity will be exhausted in approximately 10 years; by 1995 more than ½ of all American cities will exhaust their existing landfills.

U.S. cities collect and dispose of 150 to 180 million tons of wastes annually.

We generate 158 tons of waste each year in the United States, approximately 1300 pounds of solid waste per person. The average American family produces 100 pounds of trash each week or about 4 pounds per person per day.

We generate enough waste each year in the United States to fill the New Orleans Superdome from top to bottom twice a day, every day of the year. Only about half of this trash is recyclable.

Americans throw away 18 billion disposable diapers a year and these diapers can take up to 500 years to decompose in a landfill (cotton diapers decompose in 1 to 6 months). These diapers have the potential for the presence of over 100 intestinal pathogens. Some states are considering banning the use of disposable diapers.

Americans throw away enough iron and steel each year to supply all American automakers continuously. Every three months Americans throw away enough aluminum to rebuild our entire commercial airfleet (Note: 1 discarded aluminum can will still be trash 500 years from now.)

American schools can spend as much money disposing of trash as they do on textbooks.

It is estimated that each American uses about 190 pounds of plastic each year. Much of this plastic is used for wrapping and is discarded soon after we use it (e.g., fast food wrappings, food packaging materials).

Modified from The Earthworks Group: *Simple things you can do to save the earth: 1991 tip-a-day calendar,* New York, 1990; Andrews and McNeel, and Nadakavukaren A: *Man and environment: a health perspective,* ed 3, Prospect Heights, Ill., 1990, Waveland Press.

We have built on wetland flood plains in this country and have made many cities vulnerable to flooding. Recent flooding along the Mississippi River has shown this to be true and demonstrated the serious loss of life and property destruction that can occur in floods. In relation to health, wetlands serve as living filters for purifying contaminated surface waters (Nadakavukaren, 1990, p. 139) and, when left intact, serve as natural floodplains.

Deforestation

Our forests are rapidly being depleted. An area the size of Austria is deforested each year (Wittkopf and Kegley, 1990, p. 32). In many underdeveloped countries forests are being cleared and burned to make way for farms and industry. In the United States it takes over 500,000 trees to supply Americans with their Sunday papers each week (The Earthworks Group, 1990). Although trees are a renewable resource, they are renewable at a slow rate.

Carbon dioxide is removed from the atmosphere by green plants during photosynthesis. Cutting down forests destroys the natural process of removing carbon dioxide from the atmosphere. Deforestation accelerates global warming and results in "habitats on the move" and loss of plant and animal life (Wittkopf and Kegley, 1990, p. 32).

Rainforests are forests that receive at least 100 inches of rain each year (Rainforests, 1990, p. 3). Tropical rainforests are located in a narrow region near the equator in Africa, South and Central America, and Asia. Once there were more than 5 billion acres of rainforest; today there is less than half that amount (Rainforests, p. 3).

Although rainforests make up only 6% to 7% of the Earth's surface, over half of the world's plant, animal and insect species live in them (Myers, 1992, p. 282). If the current rate of rainforest destruction continues, at least 1 million species of plants, animals, and insects will become prematurely extinct in the next 15 years (Miller, 1992, p. 258). One in four pharmaceuticals has components from a rainforest plant. Seventy percent of the plants identified by the National Cancer Institute as being helpful in the treatment of cancer are found only in the rainforests.

Energy Depletion

The United States has the distinction of being the world's largest energy user and waster (Miller, 1992, p. 441). At least 43% of all energy used in the United States is unnecessarily wasted, and this waste equals all the energy consumed by two thirds of the world's population (Miller, p. 441). Major sources of U.S. energy are the nonrenewable resources of petroleum, coal, and natural gas. Other sources are nuclear and hydroelectric power.

The largest users of energy in the United States are energy-inefficient buildings, factories, and vehicles. Unnecessarily wasted energy in the United States has been estimated to cost about twice as much as the annual federal budget deficit or more than the entire military budget. Energy costs in the United States could be greatly reduced if energy was used as efficiently as in countries such as Japan and Sweden. Every winter the energy equivalent of all the oil that flows through the Alaskan pipeline in a year leaks through American windows (The Earthworks Group, 1990).

Overpopulation

Overpopulation contributes to depletion of natural resources and increased sewage and solid wastes. In 1991 the world population was 5.4 billion and it is expected to reach 7 billion by the year 2006 (Miller, 1992, p. 5-6). Already 1 of 5 people in the world is hungry or malnourished and lacks safe drinking water (Miller, p. 4). Overpopulation places a strain on world food supplies and causes overcrowding and unsafe health conditions. Population growth is already outstripping food production in areas where 2 billion people live (Miller, p. 366). Poverty, malnutrition, overcrowding, increased susceptibility to disease, and shortened life span are all health-related conditions that are affected by overpopulation.

ENVIRONMENTAL DISASTERS

Throughout history natural and man-made disasters have disrupted food and water supplies and sanitation, causing communicable disease, injury, illness, and death. Recent media coverage of disaster events such as 1992's Hurricane Andrew, considered one of the worst hurricanes of the century, and the 1993 flooding of the Midwest along the upper Mississippi River regions has clearly shown the devastating environmental health effects that disasters impose on human life and property. The definition that Congress uses to identify a major disaster is given in the box on this page.

Legislation has been enacted to provide federal assistance to individuals and communities to recover from the devastation caused by disasters to human life and property. The Disaster Relief Act of 1966 (Public Law 89-769) was a landmark piece of legislation that affected disaster relief efforts. In addition to providing disaster funds this law mandated a Disaster Assistance Study. In response to this study the Disaster Relief Act of 1970 (Public Law 91-606) was passed. This act repealed previous disaster relief legislation with the exception of Section 302 of the 1966 act, which

---

◀ *Defining Emergency and* ▶
Major Disaster

Emergency

Any hurricane, tornado, storm, flood, high water, wind-driven water, tidal wave, tsunami, earthquake, volcanic eruption, landslide, mudslide, snowstorm, drought, fire, explosion, or other catastrophe in any part of the United States which requires Federal emergency assistance to supplement State and local efforts to save lives and protect property, public health and safety or to avert or lessen the threat of a disaster.

Major Disaster

Any hurricane, tornado, storm, flood, high water, wind-driven water, tidal wave, tsunami, earthquake, volcanic eruption, landslide, mudslide, snowstorm, drought, fire, explosion, or other catastrophe in any part of the United States which in the determination of the President, causes damage of sufficient severity above and beyond emergency services by the Federal Government, to supplement the efforts and available resources of States, local governments, and disaster relief organizations in alleviating the damage, loss, hardship, or suffering caused thereby.

From U.S. Congress: *Disaster Relief Act Amendments of 1974* (Public Law 93-288), Section 102.

---

pertained to providing disaster assistance to public educational facilities.

The Disaster Relief Act of 1970 defined *disaster* and provided direction for coordinating disaster assistance, ranging from early disaster warnings to relocation. The Disaster Relief Act Amendments of 1974 (Public Law 93-288) distinguished between the terms *disaster* and *emergency*. These definitions still provide the basis on which a catastrophic environmental event is declared a disaster.

The Amendments of 1974 expanded the scope of coverage under the act, further clarified the administration of disaster relief efforts, mandated federal disaster assistance programs for immediate relief, and provided assistance for long-term economic recovery for disaster areas. Although little can be done to prevent natural disasters, much can be done to reduce the impact through disaster preparedness, activities that minimize the potential environmental threats to food, water, and sanitation, and implementation of measures to prevent man-made disasters. "The most

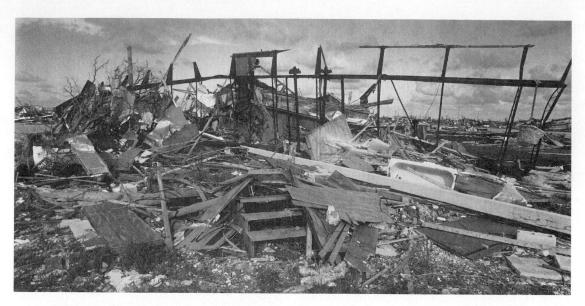

Figure 6-5 Hurricanes and other environmental disasters cause many community-wide health problems. (Courtesy U.S. Department of Agriculture.)

important community resource in a disaster is individual preparedness" (Garcia, 1985, p. 229).

Nurses have functioned in key leadership roles during disaster preparation and response and have contributed to the alleviation of the physical and emotional stress of disaster victims (Komnenich and Feller, 1991). The American Nurses Association is currently working with federal agencies, specialty nursing organizations, the American Red Cross, and military and civilian experts to develop a national disaster preparedness plan for nurses (Turner, 1993, p. 3). Recent meetings of the ANA with the American Red Cross have shown an immediate need for 500 specialty prepared nurses to be added to the American Red Cross disaster relief program (Turner, p. 3). It has been recommended that educational institutions and employers of nurses provide education on disaster preparedness for nurses (Turner, p. 3).

During a disaster many major environmental health problems emerge (Figure 6-5). On a personal level families can become homeless, food and water supplies can become contaminated, breadwinners can lose their jobs, families can lose their loved ones, and communicable disease and other conditions such as domestic violence and depression can become rampant. Community health nurses have unique skills for assisting communities in planning for disaster relief efforts and addressing problems that occur

during a disaster (Figure 6-6). Community health nurses' knowledge of community resources, community assessment and organization, epidemiology, health planning, and family health promotion provides a background for organizing and participating in community relief efforts. An in-depth discussion of these skills is provided in Chapters 12 and 13. Nurses can reduce the impact of potential disaster effects through participation in community disaster preparedness programs; local, state, and federal activities designed to reduce risks for man-made disasters; in community disaster planning; and by actively promoting public and personal awareness for individual, family, and community safety in the event of a disaster.

Summary

Environmental health is a primary public health concern. Environmental health problems exist worldwide and cause problems such as communicable disease, respiratory conditions, cancer, poverty, and ecological disturbances in the environment. Major manmade and natural disasters in recent years have caused tremendous economic instability and extensive personal suffering in many communities across the United States and the world. *Health People 2000* has directed attention toward dealing with environmental concerns in the United States by establishing specific

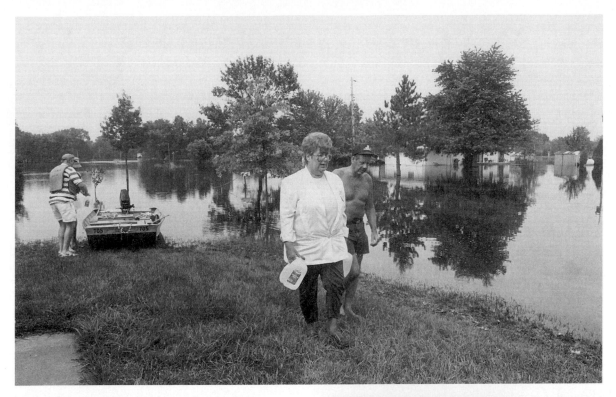

Figure 6-6 A nurse/disaster planner boats out to flooded areas and assists an 86-year-old widow who refused to leave her home until conditions became extremely severe. Nurses functioning in situations such as these need to use crisis intervention skills to help individuals and families cope with the stresses they are experiencing. (Courtesy Kathy Kuper.)

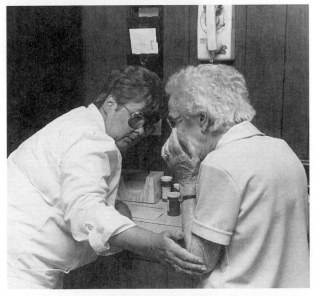

environmental health objectives. Worldwide, nurses are being encouraged to safeguard the human environment. Specific environmental health roles for nurses have been identified and were shared in this chapter. Community health nurses have unique skills to deal with environmental health issues. Environmental health legislation supports public health professionals in their efforts to resolve environmental health problems.

Florence Nightingale was aware of the importance of the environment in nursing, and nurse scholars today reinforce this importance. The environment cannot be overlooked in the provision of nursing care. Nurses need to look beyond the historical role of environmental health activities in preventing commu-

nicable disease and be concerned about preserving the integrity of the global environment. They need to focus on preserving and protecting that which we cannot create. Remember that pollution is not only unhealthy, it is difficult to eradicate and extinction is forever!

◀ *An Exercise in Critical Thinking* ▶

Examine the local community in which you live. What types of environmental hazards exist? What types of environmental disasters have occurred or have the potential to occur in this community? What are some of the agencies that have responded or would respond to a disaster? What disaster provisions has the community made? Describe some of the activities you see nurses being responsible for in a disaster. What actions could the nurse take to promote environmental health?

APPENDIX 6-1
Selected U.S. Environmental Health Legislation

1948 *Water Pollution Control Act (Public Law 80-845)*—Authorized the Public Health Service to help states develop water pollution control programs and to aid in the planning of sewage treatment plants.

1955 *Air Pollution Control Act (Public Law 84-159)*—Provided aid to states and localities to protect air quality. Forerunner of the Clean Air Act of 1963. Emphasized state responsibility for prevention and control of air pollution.

1956 *Federal Water Pollution Control Act (Public Law 84-600)*—Expanded the 1948 law to deal more aggressively with water pollution.

1963 *Clean Air Act (Public Law 88-206)*—Authorized direct grants to states and localities for air pollution control; provided for federal enforcement of interstate air pollution; directed major research efforts for control of motor vehicle exhaust, removal of sulfur from fuel, and the development of air quality criteria.

1964 *Water Resources Research Act (Public Law 88-404)*—Authorized research to protect U.S. water resources.

1965 *Solid Waste Disposal Act (Public Law 89-272)*—Established a program of grants to states to develop solid waste disposal programs.
Land and Water Conservation Act (Public Law 88-578)—Established a land and water conservation fund to assist state and federal agencies in meeting present and future outdoor recreation needs of the American people.
Water Resources Planning Act (Public Law 89-90)—Authorized further planning for water resources and water pollution control programs.

1966 *Disaster Relief Act of 1966 (Public Law 89-769)*—Authorized assistance to U.S. communities suffering a major natural disaster.

1969 *National Environmental Policy Act (Public Law 91-190)*—One of the best-known and most significant pieces of U.S. environmental health legislation. Established national environmental policy and authorized formation of the Environmental Protection Agency (EPA).

1970 *Resource Recovery Act (Public Law 91-512)*—Shifted the emphasis from solid waste disposal to overall problems of control, recovery, and recycling of wastes.
Environmental Education Act (Public Law 91-516)—Authorized the establishment of education programs to encourage public understanding of policies and environmental activities designed to enhance environmental quality. Established the Office of Environmental Education.
Environmental Quality Act (Public Law 91-224)—Attempted to limit the effects of pollution on the environment and enhance environmental quality. Included provisions to increase water quality in the United States including Great Lakes demonstration projects and undergraduate scholarships for the study of water treatment and pollution control. Authorized the Office of Environmental Quality.
Disaster Relief Act (Public Law 91-606)—Revised and expanded Federal programs for aid, assistance, emergency welfare services, and the reconstruction and rehabilitation of areas in the United States devastated by the effects of major natural disasters.
Lead-Based Paint Poisoning Prevention Act (Public Law 91-695)—Provided federal assistance to help cities and communities combat lead-based paint poisoning. Established demonstration and research projects.
Clean Air Act Amendments (Public Law 91-604)—Strengthened and expanded air pollution control activities; granted broad regulatory responsibilities to the Environmental Protection Agency. Emphasized research, training, and control. Addressed the problem of motor vehicle emissions and aircraft emission. Established a new Title IV: Noise Pollution.

1972 *Water Pollution Control Act (Public Law 92-500)*—Almost totally revised the Clean Water Act of 1948 and the federal water program. Congress overrode President Nixon's veto to pass this act. Shifted efforts from water preservation to pollution control and water quality. It established water pollution control standards for industry. Set as a goal the elimination of pollutant discharges from navigable waters.

Federal Environmental Pesticide Control Act (Public Law 92-516)—Established national monitoring of pesticide residues in water and food and strengthened existing provisions for product labeling and registration.

Marine Mammal Protection Act (Public Law 92-522)—Developed to protect marine mammals from extinction. Established the Marine Mammal Commission, international programs and research grants.

Noise Control Act (Public Law 92-574)—Authorized broad federal mandates to coordinate noise research and control activities, established noise standards and improved public education and information.

1973 *Endangered Species Act (Public Law 93-205)*—The first federal law to protect endangered and threatened species of U.S. fish, wildlife, and plants.

1974 *Safe Drinking Water Act (Public Law 93-523)*—Amended the Public Health Service Act to require the Environmental Protection Agency to set national drinking water standards and to aid states and localities in enforcement.

1976 *Toxic Substances Control Act (Public Law 94-469)*—Regulated toxic chemicals already in existence and tried to prevent new hazardous chemicals from entering the market. Required EPA to test existing hazardous chemicals, gather and disseminate information about these chemicals, and prevent future chemical risks by premarket screening and tracking. An overall goal of the act was to prevent unreasonable injury to health or the harm to the environment associated with the manufacture, processing, distribution, use, or disposal of hazardous chemical substances.

1977 *Clean Air Act Amendments (Public Law 95-95)*—A major overhaul of the Clean Air Act. It established a National Commission on Air Quality and a Task Force on Environmental Cancer and Heart and Lung Disease.

Soil and Water Resources Conservation Act (Public Law 95-192)—Provided for furthering the conservation, protection, and enhancement of the nation's soil, water, and related resources to enhance sustained use. Authorized public participation and mandated certain programs throughout the Department of Agriculture.

Clean Water Act of 1977 (Public Law 95-217)—Amended the Federal Water Pollution Control Act. Authorized grants to municipalities for research, demonstration projects and training.

1978 *National Ocean Pollution Research, Development and Monitoring Planning Act of 1978 (Public Law 95-273)*—Established a program of ocean pollution research and monitoring.

Water Research and Development Act (Public Law 95-467)—Promoted a more comprehensive and responsive national program of water research and development of water resources. Established centers for cataloging research and mandated interagency coordination and EPA consultation.

1980 *Asbestos School Hazard Detection and Control Act (Public Law 96-270)*—Established a program for the inspection of schools to detect the presence of hazardous asbestos materials; provided for loans to states or local educational agencies to contain or remove hazardous asbestos materials from schools and replace such materials with suitable building materials.

Solid Waste Disposal Act Amendments (Public Law 96-482)—Required 5-year action plans for federal resource conservation and recovery activities that were to be coordinated and nonduplicated. Established the Interagency Coordinating Committee on Federal Resource Conservation and Recovery Activities.

Comprehensive Environmental Response, Compensation and Liability Act of 1980 (Public Law 96-510)—Known as the Superfund, this act provided for liability, compensation, cleanup, and emergency response for hazardous substances released into the environment, and cleanup of inactive hazardous waste disposal sites. EPA was to oversee the programs of the act. It established the Agency for Toxic Substances and Disease Registry and the Hazardous Substance Response Trust Fund.

1982 *Nuclear Waste Policy Act (Public Law 97-425)*—Provided for the development of repositories for the disposal of high level radioactive waste and spent nuclear fuel. Established a program of research and demonstration projects on the disposal of these products.

1983 *International Environmental Protection Act (Public Law 98-164)*—Title VII of the Department of State Authorization Act. It increased U.S. involvement in international environmental protection activities, especially in relation to endangered species and wildlife conservation.

1984 *Water Resources Research Act (Public Law 98-242)*—Preceded by an act in 1964. Authorized an ongoing program of water resources and research. Acknowledged the need for a water supply of high quality and quantity. Grant programs were established.

1986 *Safe Drinking Water Act Amendments of 1986 (Public Law 99-339)*—The most significant amendments to the Safe Drinking Water Act to date. Authorized EPA to set national drinking water standards and determine maximum allowable water contaminant levels. Set a 3-year deadline for EPA to establish standards for 83 contaminants. Required EPA to promulgate requirements for disinfection and filtration of public water and provide technical assistance on these practices. Mandated that public water systems increase their monitoring of unregulated contaminants. Increased fines and sentences for tampering with public water systems and required EPA to take enforcement action in cases in which drinking water was tampered with and the state did not take action. Established grants to state and local authorities to develop groundwater protection programs. Prohibited the use of lead pipes and solder in public water systems.

Federal Lands Cleanup Act of 1986 (Public Law 99-402)—Provided for a program of cleanup and maintenance on federal lands. A public lands cleanup day was designated as the first Saturday after Labor Day each year (states may select another day if the designated day is not climatically or otherwise appropriate).

Superfund Amendments and Reauthorization Act of 1986 (Public Law 99-499)—Directed the administrator of EPA to identify and assess locations and levels of radon gas in naturally occurring deposits of uranium in residences and structures. Amended and extended the Comprehensive Environmental Response, Compensation, and Liability Act of 1980 through 1988.

Asbestos Hazard Emergency Response Act of 1986 (Public Law 99-519)—Amended the toxic Substances Control Act to require EPA to promulgate regulations and issue rules requiring inspection and reinspection of the nation's schools for asbestos. Required development of asbestos management plans for the nation's schools.

Emergency Wetlands Resources Act of 1986 (Public Law 99-645)—Promoted the conservation of migratory waterfowl, the conservation of wetlands, and improvement and rehabilitation of the nation's water resources.

Water Resources Development Act of 1986 (Public Law 99-662)—Provided for the conservation, development, improvement, and rehabilitation of the nation's water resources.

1987 *Water Quality Act of 1987 (Public Law 100-4)*—Amended the Water Pollution Act (1948) to further safeguard the quality of the nation's water supply.

Toxic Substances Control Act Amendment—School Asbestos Management (Public Law 100-368)—Amended the provisions of the Toxic Substances Control Act, related to asbestos in the nation's schools, by making adequate time provisions for education agencies to submit and implement asbestos management plans.

1990 *National Park System Resources Damage Act (Public Law 101-337)*—Aimed at preventing and minimizing destruction, loss or injury to national park resources. Provided for making people liable for damages to parks. Improved the ability of the Secretary of the Interior to protect and manage park resources.

Oil Pollution Act (Public Law 101-380)—Established limitations on liability for damages resulting from oil pollution. Established a fund for the payment of compensation for oil pollution damages and authorized an oil pollution research program.

Clean Air Act Amendments (Public Law 101-549)—Amended the Clean Air Act to provide for the attainment of national air quality standards that promoted health, especially in relation to carbon monoxide, ozone, sulfur oxides, nitrogen dioxide, and lead.

Pollution Prosecution Act of 1990 (Public Law 101-593)—Title II of the act established the National Enforcement Training Institute to train federal, state and local lawyers, inspectors, criminal investigators and technical experts in enforcement of the nation's environmental laws. Increased the number of civil investigators assigned to assist EPA's Office of Enforcement.

Global Change Research Act of 1990 (Public Law 101-606)—Required the establishment of a United States Global Change Research program aimed at understanding and responding to global change. Encouraged international discussion toward protocols in global change research.

Environmental Research Geographic Local Information Act (Public Law 101-617)—Provided a method of locating private and governmental research on environmental issues by specific geographic locations. EPA will identify major environmental research relating to a specific geographical area, compile and maintain the research, and make it available to the public. EPA is authorized to enter into contractual agreements to obtain the data.

America the Beautiful Act of 1990 (Public Law 101-624)—This act was Title XII, Subtitle C of the Food, Agriculture, Conservation and Trade Act of 1990. Authorized the President to designate a private nonprofit foundation to be eligible for a grant to be used to create public awareness and a spirit of volunteerism in relation to tree planting projects in U.S. communities and urban areas.

Global Climate Change Prevention Act of 1990 (Public Law 101-624)—This act was Title XIV of the Food, Agriculture, Conservation and Trade Act of 1990. Established, within the Department of Agriculture, a global climate change program to coordinate all issues and activities relating to climate change including policy analysis and research.

1992 *Community Environmental Response Facilitation Act (Public Law 102-426)*—Amended the Comprehensive Environmental Response, Compensation and Liability

Act of 1980 to require the federal government, before termination of federal activities on any federal property, to identify that no hazardous substance was stored, released, or disposed of improperly. Made the federal government responsible for conducting any corrective action necessary to protect human health and environment at the time of property transfer.

Energy Policy Act of 1992 (Public Law 102-486)—Established a national energy policy. Encouraged the use of vehicles that use alternative energy supplies; promoted the conservation and efficient use of energy by consumers; developed standard plans for the construction of new power plants; and encouraged the use and production of alternate fuels.

Oceans Act of 1992 (Public Law 102-587)—Protected the marine environment and reauthorized and amended the Marine Mammal Protection Act. Established a partnership among the U.S. Fish and Wildlife Service, state agencies, and private organizations to conserve fish and wildlife. Established international fishing agreements.

From *U.S. Statues-at-Large* (selected years) and U.S. Department of Health, Education, and Welfare: *Health in America 1776-1976,* Washington, D.C., 1977, U.S. Government Printing Office.

APPENDIX 6-2

Selected Federal Agencies Involved in Environmental Health: United States

Department of Agriculture
- U.S. Forest Service
- Soil conservation

Department of Commerce
- Ocean research and monitoring

Department of Defense
- Pollution control in defense facilities

Department of Energy
- Energy policy
- Nuclear energy

Department of Health and Human Services
- National Institute of Environmental Health Services (publishes *Environmental Health Perspective*)
- *Healthy People* documents
- National Institute of Occupational Safety and Health
- Agency for Toxic Substances and Disease Registry
- Food and Drug Administration

Department of Housing and Urban Development
- Public housing
- Urban parks
- Urban planning

Department of the Interior
- U.S. Fish and Wildlife Service
- National Wildlife Refuge System
- Public lands
- National parks

Department of Justice
- Environmental litigation

Department of Labor
- Occupational Safety and Health Administration

Department of State
- International environmental health policy

Department of Transportation
- Monitors airplane noise
- Monitors oil pollution

Council on Environmental Quality
- Coordinates environmental policy
- Monitors environmental quality

Environmental Protection Agency
- Primary agency in charge of protecting and enhancing the U.S. natural environment
- Enforces U.S. environmental health legislation
- Controls U.S. environmental pollution
- Implements environmental research

Nuclear Regulatory Commission
- Licensing and regulation of nuclear energy and power

Tennessee Valley Authority
- Electric power

National Library of Medicine
- Toxicology Data Network (TOXNET). A computerized system available 24 hours a day, seven days a week, which includes:

  Hazardous Substance Data Bank
  Toxic Chemical Release Inventory
  Integrated Risk Information System
  Registry of Toxic Effects of Chemical Substances
  Chemical Carcinogenesis Research Information System
  Genetic Toxicology
  Developmental and Reproductive Toxicology
  Environmental Teratology Information Center Backfile
  Environmental Mutagen Information Center Backfile

Modified from Sexton K and Perlin SA: The federal environmental health workforce in the United States, *Am J Publ Health* 80(8):913-920, 1990; and Council on Environmental Quality: *Environmental Quality, 16th annual report of the Council on Environmental Quality,* Washington, D.C., 1985, The Council.

References

Agency for Toxic Substances and Disease Registry: *The nature and extent of lead poisoning in children in the United States: a report to Congress,* Washington, D.C., 1988, USDHHS.

American Public Health Association: Position paper on the role of official local health agencies, *Am J Public Health* 65:189-193, 1975.

Beck JW and Davies JE: *Medical parasitology,* ed 3, St. Louis, 1981, Mosby.

Beck M, Hager M, King P, Hutchinson S, Robins K, and Gordon J: Buried alive, *Newsweek* November 27, 1989, pp. 66-76.

Benenson AS: *Control of communicable diseases in man* ed 15, Washington, D.C., 1990, American Public Health Association.

Blumenthal DS, ed: *An introduction to environmental health,* New York, 1985, Springer.

Blumenthal DS and Greene M: Air pollution. In Blumenthal DS, ed: *An introduction to environmental health,* New York, 1985, Springer, pp. 117-144.

Bourgoin BP, Evans DR, Cornett JR, Lingard SM, and Quattrone AJ: Lead content in 70 brands of dietary calcium supplements, *Am J Public Health* 83(8):1155-1160, 1993.

Bryan FA: *Disease transmitted by foods,* Atlanta, 1975, USDHEW [CDC 75-8237].

Carden JL: Hazardous waste management. In Blumenthal DS, ed: *An introduction to environmental health,* New York, 1985, Springer, pp. 179-205.

Centers for Disease Control and Prevention: Populations at risk from air pollution—United States, 1991, *Morbidity and Mortality Weekly Report* 42(16):301-304, 1993.

Clark HG: Origins of public health in America: superiority of sanitary measures over quarantines. An address delivered before the Suffolk District Medical Society at its third Anniversary meeting, Boston, Mass., April 24, 1852. In Rosenberg CE, ed: *Medicine and society in America,* New York, 1972, Arno Press.

Coss C: Lillian D. Wald: progressive activist, *Public Health Nurs* 10(3):134-138, 1993.

Council on Environmental Quality: *Environmental quality, 16th annual report of the Council on Environmental Quality,* Washington, D.C., 1985, The Council.

Doll R: Health and the environment in the 1990s, *Am J Public Health* 82(7):923-941, 1992.

Dolphins, *Kids for Saving Earth News,* Fall 1990, p. 2.

Elmer-Dewitt P: How do you patch a hole in the sky that could be as big as Alaska? *Time* 139(7):64-65, February 17, 1992.

Environmental Protection Agency: *National air quality and emissions trends report, 1988,* EPA-450/4-90-002. Washington, D.C., 1990, EPA.

Garcia LM: *Disaster nursing. Planning, assessment and intervention,* Rockville, Md., 1985, Aspen.

Gordon LJ: Who will manage the environment? *Am J Public Health* 80(8):904-905, 1990.

Hill L: Health in America: a personal perspective. In U.S. Department of Health, Education, and Welfare: *Health in America 1776-1976,* DHEW Pub. No (HRA) 76-616, Washington, D.C., 1976, U.S. Government Printing Office, pp. 3-15.

Institute of Medicine (Committee for the Study of the Future of Public Health): *The future of public health,* Washington, D.C., 1988, National Academy Press.

International Council of Nurses: *The nurse's role in safeguarding the human environment: position statement,* Geneva, Switzerland, 1986, The Council.

Kalisch PA and Kalisch BJ: *The advance of American nursing,* Boston, 1978, Little, Brown.

Kleffel D: Rethinking the environment as a domain of nursing knowledge, *Advances in Nursing Science* 14(1):40-51, 1991.

Komnenich P and Feller C: Disaster nursing. In Fitzpatrick JJ, Taunton RL, and Jacox AK: *Annual Review of Nursing Research,* volume 9, New York, 1991, Springer, pp. 123-134.

Landrigan R: Commentary: environmental diseases—a preventable epidemic, *Am J Public Health* 82(7):941-943, 1992.

Lead: assessing its health hazards, *Health and Environment Digest* 2(6):1-5, 1988.

Lemonick MD: The ozone vanishes, *Time* 139(7):60-63, February 17, 1992.

Loehr RC: Groundwater contamination—the problem and potential solutions, *National Forum* 69(1):26-28, 1989.

McCord CP: Conversation with author regarding industrial lead poisoning, Ann Arbor, Mi., 1976, University of Michigan.

McFarland J: Use of an ecologic model to identify children at risk for infection and to quantify the expected impact of the risk factors, *Public Health Nurs* 2(1):1-22, 1985.

Miller GT: *An introduction to environmental science. Living in the environment,* ed 7, Belmont, Calif., 1992, Wadsworth.

Murdock BS, ed: *Environmental issues in primary care,* Minneapolis, Minn., 1991, Minneapolis Department of Health.

Myers N: Guest essay: tropical forests and their species, going, going . . . ? In Miller GT: *An introduction to environmental science. Living in the environment,* ed 7, Belmont, Calif., 1992, Wadsworth.

Nadakavukaren A: *Man and environment: a health perspective,* ed 3, Prospect Heights, Ill., 1990, Waveland Press.

Pickett G and Hanlon JJ: *Public health administration and practice,* ed 9, St. Louis, 1990, Mosby.

Preventing lead poisoning, *Health Watch* 12(1):1-3, 1992.

Public Health Foundation: *1991 Public health chartbook,* Washington, D.C., 1991, The Foundation.

Rabe B: Environmental health policy. In Pickett G and Hanlon JJ: *Public health administration and practice,* ed 9, St. Louis, 1990, Mosby, pp. 317-330.

Rabe B: Environmental control. In Pickett G and Hanlon JJ: *Public health administration and practice,* ed 9, St. Louis, 1990, Mosby, pp. 330-342.

Rainforests, *Kids for Saving Earth News,* Fall 1990, p. 3.

Ravenel MP: *A half century of public health. Jubilee historical volume of the American Public Health Association,* New York, 1921, American Public Health Association.

Reed PG and Zurakowski TL: Nightingale revisited: a visionary model for nursing. In Fitzpatrick JJ and Whall AL: *Conceptual models of nursing,* ed 2, Norwalk, Conn., 1989, Appleton and Lange, pp. 33-47.

Schuster EA: Earth caring, *Advances in Nursing Science* 13(1): 25-30, 1990.

Sexton K and Perlin SA: The federal environmental health workforce in the United States, *Am J Public Health* 80(8):913-920, 1990.

Shannon JA: The American experience with biomedical science. In U.S. Department of Health, Education, and Welfare, *Health in America 1776-1976,* DHEW Pub. No. (HRA) 76-616, Washington, D.C., 1976, U.S. Government Printing Office, pp. 89-107.

Smillie WG: *Public health: its promise for the future,* New York, 1955, Macmillan.

Snider M: Ozone loss measured over North America, *USA Today* April 22, 1993, A1.

Tennessee Department of Environment and Conservation: $5 million to $7 million dollars a year for Tennessee trash, *The Tennessee Conservationist* (Student Edition) 4(3):1, May 1993.

The Earthworks Group: *Simple things you can do to save the earth. 1991 tip a day calendar,* New York, 1990, Andrews and McNeel.

Turner UA: ANA, Red Cross cite need for more RNs to be trained for disaster relief, *The American Nurse* September 1993, p. 3.

USDHEW: *Health in America 1776-1976,* Washington, D.C., 1977, U.S. Government Printing Office.

USDHEW: *Healthy People,* Washington, D.C., 1979, U.S. Government Printing Office.

USDHHS: *Evaluating the environmental health workforce* [HRP 0907160], Rockville, Md., 1988, USDHHS.

USDHHS: *Healthy People 2000: health promotion and disease prevention objectives for the nation, summary report,* Washington, D.C., 1990, U.S. Government Printing Office.

USDHHS: *Healthy People 2000: national health promotion and disease prevention objectives for the nation, full report, with commentary,* Washington, D.C., 1991, U.S. Government Printing Office.

USDHHS: *Health United States 1991 and prevention profile,* Washington, D.C., 1992, U.S. Government Printing Office.

United States Department of Interior: *Why save endangered species?,* 1992, The Department.

U.S. Government Manual, Washington, D.C., 1993, U.S. Government Printing Office.

Why clean air lovers are becoming indoor-houseplant lovers, *USA Today* January 26, 1990, p. 1F.

Wittkopf ER and Kegley CW: Our imperiled environment. Impediments to a global response, *National Forum* 70(1):32-35, 1990.

Selected Bibliography

Affigne AD: International impacts of ecological crisis, *National Forum* 70(1):26-29, 1990.

Brown L: Six pressing environmental concerns, *National Forum* 70(1):8-11, 1990.

Cleveland H: Introducing the global commons, *National Forum* 70(1):4-7, 1990.

Environmental Protection Agency: *Environmental progress and challenges:* EPA's update, Washington, D.C., 1988, EPA.

Freudenberg N: Citizen action for environmental health: report on a survey of community organizations, *Am J Public Health* 74(5):444-448, 1984.

History of a marine mammal/fishery interaction, *Marine Conservation News* 5(3):12, 1993.

Hodge TD and Steele JE: A conceptual framework for community-based environmental health information systems: a viewpoint, *Can J Public Health* 79(1):49-52, 1988.

Koren H: *Handbook of environmental health and safety: principles and practices,* ed 2, vols I and II, Chelsea, Mich., 1991, Lewis.

Mancino D: The future and environmental health nursing, *IMPRINT* 32(3):42-45, 1985.

Nightingale F: *The art of nursing,* London, 1946, Claude Morris Books. (Original work published in 1859).

Norwood C: *At highest risk,* New York, 1980, Penguin Books.

Pringle L: *Water: the next great resource battle,* New York, 1982, MacMillan Publishing Co.

Public health and the global environment (Editorial), *Can J Public Health* 81(1):3-4, 1990.

Rycroft RW: Acid rain: air quality, global change, or what? *National Forum* 70(1):40-42, 1990.

The marine mammal exemption program: what it does, what it does not, *Marine Conservation News* 5(3):12, Autumn 1993.

Udall JR: Global warming, *National Forum* 70(1):36-39, 1990.

Wilson JG: *The environment and birth defects,* New York, 1973, Academic Press.

Unit Three

Family-Centered Approach to Community Health Nursing Practice

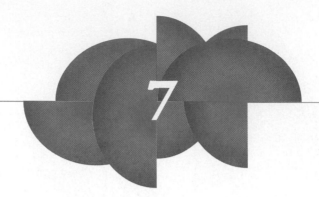

Family Assessment and Cultural Diversity: Tools and Concepts

OBJECTIVES

Upon completion of this chapter, the reader should be able to:

1. Construct a personal definition for the term *family*.
2. Identify variations in family structure in the United States.
3. Describe the cultural diversity among American families.
4. Discuss the meaning of the phrase *the family is the unit of service*.
5. Explain how theoretical frameworks for family study enhance family-focused community health nursing practice.
6. Discuss the structural and process parameters for family assessment and their relevance to community health nursing practice.
7. Discuss how cultural factors influence health and health behaviors.
8. Formulate guidelines for completing a cultural assessment.
9. Describe tools used to facilitate the family assessment process.

The ancient trinity of father, mother, and child has survived more vicissitudes than any other relationship. It is the bedrock underlying all other family structures. Although more elaborate family patterns can be broken from without or may even collapse of their own weight, the rock remains. In the Götterdämmerung which otherwise science and overfoolish statesmanship are preparing for us, the last man will spend his last hours searching for his wife and child.

LINTON *(1959, p. 52)*

Despite the fact that major social, demographical, and economic changes have altered traditional family structures and lifestyles in the past three decades, families remain one of the central institutions in the United States (Fine, 1992). Even though traditional family forms have changed due to such events as divorce, single parenthood, and a growing number of mothers in the work force (refer to box on p. 210), the family is still the basic social unit in society. The family continues to play a vital role in fulfilling the emotional support and nurturing needs required by all human beings; bureaucratic organizations of society cannot fulfill these needs.

It has long been recognized that "families are America's most precious resource and most important institution. Families have the most fundamental, powerful, and lasting influence on our lives. The strength of our families is the key determinate of the health and well-being of our nation, of our communities, and of our lives as individuals" (White House Conference on Families, 1978, p. 286). Families in this country are durable and resilient; despite difficulties and challenges, they tend to function well and remain the basic institution in which individuals aggregate socially (Fine, 1992, p. 430).

THE AMERICAN FAMILY: CULTURALLY AND STRUCTURALLY DIVERSE

Diversity and *change* are the terms that best describe today's American family. Cultural backgrounds, socioeconomic levels, and family structures differ throughout the nation. The two-parent nuclear family unit—mother, father, and children—established through the legal sanction of marriage is less prevalent, and alternative family forms are more common and more accepted (Fine, 1992). Table 7-1 illustrates some

variations in family lifestyles in the United States.

Household composition has changed significantly in the past two decades. In 1992 there were 95.7 million households in our nation. Of these, 70% were family households, which was an 11% drop from 1970 (refer to Figure 7-1). Between 1970 and 1992 there was a phenomenal change in the type of family households: the proportion of all family groups with children accounted for by single parents rose from 13% in 1970 to 30% in 1992. The box on p. 212 illustrates that small households have also become more common. Households composed of only one or two persons increased from 44% in 1970 to 57% in 1992. One-person households had the highest rate of increase, but data reflect that household size has stabilized since 1989 (U.S. Bureau of the Census, 1993, pp. 16-17).

The wide variety of ethnic and racial groups enriches the diversity of family life in the United States (refer to Figure 7-2 on p. 213). It is projected that the U.S. population will become more diverse by race and Hispanic origin. By the middle of the twenty-first century it is anticipated that the black population will almost double, the Asian and Pacific Islander population will increase to more than five times its current size, and the Hispanic-origin population will triple its current size. After 1995 it is predicted that the Hispanic-origin population will add more people to the nation than any other cultural group (U.S. Bureau of the Census, 1993, p. 5).

Future fertility and immigration will significantly influence the country's population characteristics in the next 60 years. It is projected that births will slowly decline until the year 2000, but after the year 2015 there will be more births every year than ever before in American history. Since 1980 approximately 27% to 29% of the nation's population growth has been due to net international migration and it is anticipated that immigration will be higher in the future (U.S. Bureau of the Census, 1993, pp. 3, 5). Between 1980 and 1990 the foreign-born in the United States increased by 40.4%, from 14.1 million to 19.8 million persons. The number of foreign-born persons in the United States in 1990 was the largest number of foreign-born individuals in the history of the United States. Between 1980 and 1990, European immigration decreased and Latin American and Asian immigration increased significantly (refer to Table 7-2 on p. 212).

With increasing diversity and change, new opportunities and challenges have emerged for families and

Text continues on p. 213

◀   *Select Trends That Have Recently Altered Traditional Family Patterns*   ▶

Increase in Divorce*

- Number of currently divorced persons more than tripled, from 4.3 million in 1970 to 15.8 million in 1991.
- Nine percent of all adults ages 18 and over were divorced in 1991.
- Rise in percentage divorced differed by race between 1970 and 1991: the proportion of white adults rose from approximately 3% to 8%; black adults divorced rose from about 4% to 11%; Hispanic adults divorced rose from about 4% to 7%.

Later Marriages and Increase in Never-Married

- The median age for women at first marriage rose only about 1 year—from 20.2 years to 21.1 years between 1955 and 1975—but climbed 3 full years, to 24.1 years, between 1975 and 1991.
- The median age for men at first marriage exhibited a pattern similar to women between 1955 and 1975 (from 22.6 to 23.5 years) and 1975 and 1991 (from 23.5 to 26.3 years).
- Number of never-married persons nearly doubled between 1970 and 1991, from 21 to 41 million.

Rise in Mother-Child Families

- The proportion of children living with one parent more than doubled, from 12% to 26%, between 1970 and 1991.
- The majority (88%) of children in a one-parent home live with the mother.
- Children of divorced (37%) and children of never-married (33%) made up the largest proportion of one-parent children in 1991.

- Black children (58%) are more likely to be living with one parent than white children (20%) and children of Hispanic origin (30%).
- Demographers estimate that half of all children will live in mother-child families at some time in their lives as a result of divorce, separation, widowhood, or unwed parenthood.

Growing Number of Mothers in the Labor Force

- The percentage of mothers with children younger than 18 working in the civilian labor force rose from 47% in 1975 to 67% in 1991.
- Fifty-three percent of women with an infant younger than 1 were in the labor force in 1991.
- Most families need more than one income because income has not kept up with inflation.
- Sixty percent of married-couple families with children under 18 years had both parents working in 1990.

Longer Average Lifespan

- An American baby born in 1988 can be expected to live, on the average, nearly 75 years, which is a significant improvement over the 47-year life expectancy of persons born in 1900.
- The average lifespan varies considerably for different population groups. For example, among both blacks and whites the life expectancy of females exceeds that for males, with the discrepancy between the sexes greater for blacks than whites.

*The number divorced is a count of currently divorced and not yet remarried.

Data from Children's Defense Fund: *The state of America's children 1992,* Washington, D.C., 1992, The Fund; Levitan SA and Conway EA: *Families in flux: new approaches to meeting workforce challenges for child, elder, and health care in the 1990s,* Washington, D.C., 1990, The Bureau of National Affairs; U.S. Bureau of the Census: *Population profile of the United States: 1991,* current population reports, series P-23, No. 173, Washington, D.C., 1991, U.S. Government Printing Office; U.S. Bureau of the Census: *Marital status and living arrangements: March 1991,* current population reports, Series P-20, No. 461, Washington, D.C., 1992, U.S. Government Printing Office; and U.S. Department of Health and Human Services: *Health status of minorities and low-income groups,* ed 3, Washington, D.C., 1991, U.S. Government Printing Office.

TABLE 7-1 Variations in Family Lifestyles in the United States

Traditional family structures	Emerging experimental family structures

Traditional family structures

1. *Nuclear family*—husband, wife, and offspring living in a common household, established through the legal sanction of marriage
   a. Single career
      (1) Husband breadwinner, wife at home
      (2) Wife breadwinner, husband at home (usually this pattern is accepted by society only if the husband is ill, is obtaining advanced education, or is unemployed and looking for employment)
   b. Dual career
      (1) Both spouses gainfully employed from the outset of the marriage
      (2) Wife's career interrupted due to child-rearing responsibilities
      (3) Wife starts career after children enter school
2. *Reconstituted nuclear family*—remarried men and women, living in a common household with children from both previous marriages, children from one previous marriage, or children from previous marriages and children from current marriage
   a. Single career
   b. Dual career
3. *Dyadic nuclear family*—childless husband and wife; one or both partners gainfully employed
4. *Single-parent family*—one parent, as a consequence of divorce, abandonment, or separation (with financial aid rarely coming from the second parent), and usually including preschool or school-age children or both
   a. Parent working
   b. Parent not working, supported by government funds (welfare or social security), family or life insurance, and savings
5. *Single adult*—living alone, usually with a career, who may or may not desire to marry
6. *Three-generation family*—three generations or more living in a household
7. *Middle-aged or aging couple*—husband as provider, wife at home (children have been "launched" into college, career, or marriage)
8. *Kin network*—nuclear households or unmarried members living in close geographical proximity and operating within a reciprocal system of exchange of goods and services
9. *Second-career family*—wife entering the work force when the children are in school or have left the parental home
10. *Institutional family*—children in orphanages, residential schools, or correctional institutions

Emerging experimental family structures

1. *Binuclear family*—divorced parents assuming joint custody and coparenting responsibilities for a minor child; the child is part of a family system consisting of two nuclear households
2. *Commune family*
   a. Monogamous—household of more than one monogamous couple with children, sharing common facilities, resources, and appliances; socialization of the child is a group activity
   b. Group marriage—household of adults and offspring known as one family, where all individuals are married to each other and all are parents to the children; usually develops a status system with leaders believed to have charisma
3. *Unmarried-parent-and-child family*—usually mother and child, where marriage is not desired or possible
4. *Unmarried-couple-and-child family*—usually a commonlaw marriage with the child their biological issue or informally adopted
5. *Dyadic nuclear family*—husband and wife who have voluntarily chosen not to have children (national support groups are forming to help these couples maintain their position); one or both partners gainfully employed
6. *Homosexual families*—a homosexual couple, male or female, living together with or without children; children may be informally or legally adopted
7. *Cohabiting retired couple*—an unmarried retired couple living together, usually because financial hardship would result if they married (retirement benefits would decrease)

Modified from Sussman MB, chairperson: *Changing families in a changing society, 1970 White House Conference on Children, Forum 14 report*, Washington, D.C., 1971, U.S. Government Printing Office, pp. 228-229; Ahrons CR: The binuclear family: two households, one family, *Alternative Lifestyles* 2:449-515, 1979.

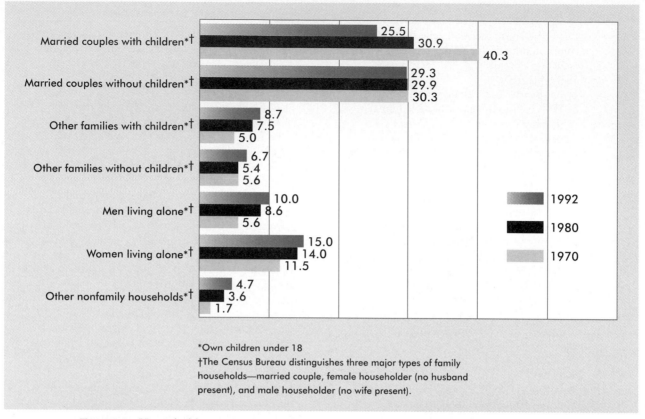

*Own children under 18

†The Census Bureau distinguishes three major types of family households—married couple, female householder (no husband present), and male householder (no wife present).

Figure 7-1   Household composition in the United States: 1970 to 1992. (From U.S. Bureau of the Census: *Population profile of the United States: 1993,* current population reports, series P23-185, Washington, D.C., 1993, U.S. Government Printing Office, p. 16.)

Number of Households and Size of Households in the United States: 1970 to 1992

Households in—

1970	63.4 million
1980	80.8 million
1990	93.3 million
1992	95.7 million

Persons per household in—

1970	3.14
1980	2.76
1990	2.63
1992	2.62

From U.S. Bureau of the Census: *Population profile of the United States: 1993,* current population reports, series P23-185, Washington, D.C., 1993, U.S. Government Printing Office, p. 16.

TABLE 7-2   National Origins of the Foreign-Born Population in the United States: 1980 and 1990

Of the 14.1 million foreign-born in the United States in 1980 and the 19.8 million foreign-born in 1990—

Foreign-born	1980	1990
European	36.6%	22.0%
Asian	18.0%	25.2%
Mexican	15.6%	21.7%
Caribbean	8.9%	9.8%
Central American	2.5%	5.7%
South American	4.0%	5.2%
African	1.4%	1.8%
Other countries	13.0%	8.6%

From U.S. Bureau of the Census: *Population profile of the United States: 1993,* current population reports, series P23-185, Washington, D.C., 1993, U.S. Government Printing Office, p. 40.

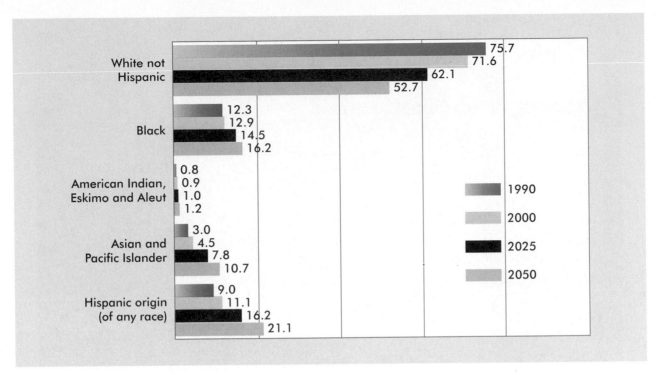

Figure 7-2   Race and Hispanic origin populations in the United States, percent of the total population: 1990, 2000, 2025, 2050. (From U.S. Bureau of the Census, *Population profile of the United States: 1993,* current population reports, series P23-185, Washington, D.C., 1993, U.S. Government Printing Office, p. 5.)

society. For example, men are increasingly enjoying the opportunities associated with parenthood (see Figure 7-3) and women are valuing the career options available to them in the job market. However, as women move into the workforce, families often need to deal with complicated child care and elder care arrangements and have to coordinate family and work roles and intergenerational relationships. This is occurring because the institutions that make up the American society have been slow to adapt to the changing needs of families (Levitan and Conway, 1990). In the coming years, society must address child care and elder care concerns as well as issues such as increasing poverty, the dramatic rise in premarital childbearing, out-of-control health care costs, and maintaining the viability of social support organizations as volunteer workers become less available (Levitan and Conway; Spanier, 1989; Bengtson and Dannefer, 1987). Social policy must take into consideration the needs of varying family forms and lifestyles, because the American family is changing.

Defining the Family

It is obvious from reviewing Table 7-1 and data related to the demographic characteristics of the population that what actually constitutes a family is no longer easy to define. Various family organizational structures have made the concept of the family an elusive one, open to numerous definitions depending on one's value system. The traditional definition of this term—a group of two or more persons related by blood, marriage, or adoption who reside together—is no longer adequate for understanding and studying the needs of the American family. A much broader definition is needed to portray the significant commitments individuals can make to each other, even though they choose an alternative family form (e.g., a cohabiting or homosexual relationship) outside of the bonds of marriage. A family in its broadest sense is a group of two or more persons related by blood, marriage, adoption, or emotional commitment who have a permanent relationship and who work together to meet life goals and needs.

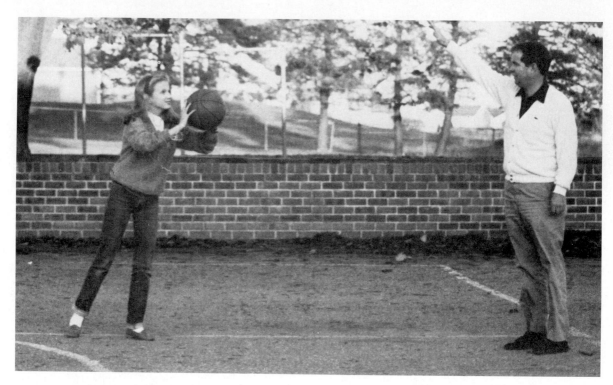

Figure 7-3   Increasingly, fathers are becoming more involved in parenting and are significantly influencing a child's socialization. (Courtesy Henry Parks, photographer.)

It is extremely important that practitioners in the helping professions remain flexible in their interpretation of the word *family* so that social policies that enhance the growth of all types of families are developed. Families who are not legally bound together by marriage have the same needs as families who are. They need financial resources, social and educational opportunities, and health services to meet their basic needs. Denying them options to strengthen their family life does not strengthen our nation and is not sensitive to their needs.

In addition to reexamining the definition of the word *family,* community health nurses must also carefully identify their attitudes and values about family life. Although community health nurses may not choose a particular mode of living for themselves, their personal preferences should not influence their clinical judgments about the adequacy of family functioning when they work with families whose lifestyles differ from theirs. Data collected from the family should be the key factor the community health nurse uses to determine family strengths and needs. A single-parent

mother, for instance, may be meeting the needs of her child much more appropriately than a married couple who are having conflicts in their marriage. Assumptions about how well a family is providing for its members should not be made solely on the basis of the family's organizational structure.

THE FAMILY AS A UNIT OF SERVICE

Despite the changing nature of the American family, community health nurses still subscribe to the philosophy that the family is the basic unit of service in community health nursing practice. They recognize that the family, as the major socializing unit of society, determines how its individual members relate and act in our culture. They believe that the family greatly influences the beliefs, values, attitudes, and health behaviors of its members and realize that the health of individual family members affects the health of the entire family unit. They see that the family provides support and encouragement at times of stress and joy. They value the role the family has in facilitating the physical and psychosocial growth of its members.

Ronald Peterson (1978) put into very simple but impressive terms the significance of the family in promoting the growth of its individual members when he presented the following concept of the family at a national conference on the chronic mentally ill client:

A family is a place where I think a lot of things go on. You really don't feel you're being "raised," that people are doing things to you, to raise you. Your life seems "real" and most of the time, almost everything that happens to you, you talk about it. Sometimes you have good news, sometimes you have bad news. But most of the time, it's just talking about what is going on.

It's a place you go from, to the doctor or to the hospital or the dentist, or school, or to the movies or to a job. But it's a place where you belong, where you somehow learn a lot. You change I'm sure, but usually without knowing it. And you certainly are not looked at as a patient or one who is being rehabilitated. You don't get discharged or terminated, and even when you grow up and get a job of your own and move away, it's a place you keep in touch with and visit. There's always an interest, and that's what makes the difference.

Community health nurses have found, like Peterson, that families do make a difference; families provide supportive and nurturing services in a way no other social institution does. Families influence health beliefs and attitudes even when they are not physically present. They often extend themselves much further in providing assistance than would friends or health care professionals. It is for these reasons that community health nurses believe in the family-centered approach to nursing care.

Historically the family-centered approach to community health nursing practice grew out of the recognition that the physical care of an individual client could not be divorced from all other aspects of a client's functioning. Innovative community health nursing leaders of the early 1900s recognized that a preventive, holistic approach to the delivery of nursing services was essential if the health of an individual, the family, and the community was to be maintained and enhanced. They saw the need to work with the family and the community in order to achieve their goals with individual clients.

The concept of family-centered care has evolved over time. Initially focus was placed on analyzing how the family could assist its members to achieve health and well-being. Gradually the enhancement of the health and well-being of the entire *family unit* became the primary objective for community health nursing visits, with emphasis placed on analyzing family dynamics and identifying the health status of all family members.

Clinical practice and research has sufficiently demonstrated, over a considerable period, the value of the family-centered approach to community health nursing practice. "The family constitutes perhaps the most important social context within which illness occurs and is resolved. It consequently serves as a primary unit in health and medical care" (Litman, 1974, p. 495). The family influences the development of health behavior, the use of health services, and health outcomes for individuals (Danielson, Hamel-Bissell, and Winstead-Fry, 1993; Litman, 1974; Loveland-Cherry, 1989; Pratt, 1976; Schor, Starfield, Stidley, and Hankin, 1987).

Although the family-centered approach to nursing care is valued, it is not fully realized in the clinical setting. Lack of knowledge regarding family processes, federal legislation that financially supports individual services, insufficient criteria for judging family health, and heavy caseload demands impede nurses' efforts to implement family care. However, a renewed focus on the family is emerging as service provision in the home setting grows rapidly.

Community health nursing leaders of the past were truly creative and innovative. They were far ahead of their time when they subscribed to the belief that family care was a key principle in community health nursing practice. It was not until the 1950s that most professional disciplines actually began to focus attention on working with families rather than with individual clients. It was only at this time that social scientists initiated systematic theory building in relation to family processes. Thus it is no wonder that the family-centered approach to nursing care is not fully operational in the practice setting. Theoretical knowledge to guide clinical judgments, and the support for its use, are needed before a particular nursing care approach can be fully implemented.

Knowledge gained about family functioning since the 1950s has made it easier for nurses to analyze family strengths and needs and to intervene appropriately with families. Selected theoretical frameworks currently being used to study the family are briefly summarized below. These frameworks help nurses to organize the family assessment process systematically and to identify the range of variables essential for understanding family relationships. They do not, however, ensure that family-centered care will be implemented. The community health nurse must internalize the belief that working with the family as a unit is important; otherwise the goal of family-centered practice will be compromised.

THEORETICAL FRAMEWORKS FOR FAMILY NURSING

Use of a theoretical framework for guiding the family assessment process is essential in the clinical setting. A theory—"a set of relatively specific and concrete concepts and propositions that describe, explain, or predict something of interest" (Whall and Fawcett, 1991, p. 4)—helps the practitioner to assess family structure and process in an organized and logical fashion. Theories provide boundaries to consider when collecting data about client situations and facilitate the synthesis of data so family strengths, needs, and interventions can be identified. When a theoretical framework is lacking, it is difficult to group data and to identify relationships between all of the variables that influence family health.

The family can be analyzed from multiple perspectives. Duvall and Miller (1985), who partially listed the kinds of family studies currently being conducted, identified 16 disciplines (e.g., anthropology, demography, history, law, and public health) involved in family study. Burr and Leigh (1983) found at least 19 disciplines, including nursing, that shared an interest in developing a knowledge base related to the family. The field of family study has had an interdisciplinary focus since its origin. An interdisciplinary focus adds depth to family study because concepts about several facets of family life are synthesized.

Theory-building in relation to the family is a relatively new phenomenon. It was only four decades ago that family scholars developed an interest in theory construction. At that time a much greater emphasis was placed on scientific study to discover relationships between family concepts that could be generalized across cultures and to identify how cultural variables affected family dynamics (Christensen, 1964, p. 10).

Between 1950 and 1990, literature on the family in nursing and other disciplines increased dramatically (Berardo, 1980; Broderick, 1971; Holman and Burr, 1980; Whall and Fawcett, 1991). During the 1970s the field of family research and theory-building experienced phenomenal growth as new areas of family research such as domestic violence, teenage parenthood, and family stress and coping emerged (Berardo; Holman and Burr). An increasing interest in family-focused research among nurses also occurred during this time (Barnard, 1984; Feetham, 1984; Gilliss, 1983; Murphy, 1986). The Family Nursing Continuing Education Project, a 3-year project begun in 1987, was designed to foster a nationwide network of family nurses who hoped to achieve a common knowledge and research base for their practice (Krentz, 1989, p. 4).

It is important for practitioners to have an awareness of trends and developments in family research and theory-building because, as research becomes more refined, conceptual frameworks for clinical practice emerge. Research on family stress and coping has, for example, provided a conceptual framework that assists practitioners in identifying families who are having difficulty coping and the factors involved in successful crisis resolution (refer to Chapter 8).

"The development of *explicit* family nursing theory is just beginning" (Artinian, 1991, p. 53). The original thrust of the major nursing theorists, when examining the concept of person, was centered on the individual. Recent expansion of some of the major conceptual models of nursing (King, 1983; Neuman, 1983; Rogers, 1983; Roy, 1983) to include a focus on the family is evident and is providing an explicit impetus for formal family nursing theory development (Whall and Fawcett, 1991).

Historically family theorists used five major conceptual frameworks to study the family: interactional, structural-functional, situational, institutional, and developmental. These were first outlined by Hill and Hansen in their landmark 1960 article, "The Identification of Conceptual Frameworks Utilized in Family Study." In 1964 Christensen devoted several chapters in his book, *Handbook of Marriage and the Family,* to the analysis of these frameworks. Both of these writings are now considered classics in the field of family study, because they had a tremendous influence on the development of family theory in the 1960s.

Broderick (1971, p. 141), after an extensive review of marriage and family living literature, concluded that three of the five original frameworks survived in the 1960s. These were interactional, structural-functional, and developmental. In addition, he saw several new conceptual frameworks for family analysis emerging:

balance theory, game theory, exchange theory, and general systems theory.

Holman and Burr (1980), upon reviewing the growth of family theories in the 1970s, found that symbolic interaction theory, exchange theory, and systems theory emerged as the major schools of thought. The interactionist approach was the most influential framework in the 1970s and its use remains steady over time. Although some work was done on the developmental framework during this period, major study to expand and refine it did not occur (Holman and Burr, pp. 731-732).

Following is a brief overview of some of the theoretical frameworks that have guided clinical practice in recent years. Practitioners generally find that an eclectic approach, or one that integrates concepts from several frameworks, best meets their needs when completing a family assessment.

Structural-Functional Approach

The structural-functional framework was developed by social scientists from sociology and social anthropology. It views the family as a social system that interacts with other social systems within society. It focuses on the analysis of family interplay between collateral systems, such as school, work, or health care worlds, and the transactions between the family and its subsystems (husband-wife dyad, sibling cliques, and personality systems of individual family members). With this approach emphasis is placed on examining the functions society performs for the family, as well as the functions the family performs for society and its individual family members. In addition, this framework looks at how the structure (organization) of systems affects their functioning (Hill and Hansen, 1960, pp. 303-304).

The family in the structural-functional approach is seen as open to outside influences and transactions, but both the family and its individual family members are considered to be reactive, passive elements of systems rather than active agents of change. This framework deals poorly with social change processes and dynamics. It handles well the relationships between the family and other social systems (Hill and Hansen, 1960, pp. 303-304).

Although the structural-functional approach is no longer considered a major research framework in the field of family studies, it continues to be a meaningful framework for guiding family assessment in the clinical setting. The broad scope of this framework allows for the analysis of the multiple environmental forces that influence family functioning in addition to family interactions and transactions (Aldous, 1978, p. 14). The changing nature of the American family makes it increasingly critical for the practitioner to examine the interplay between the family and its external environment. Many functions once assumed primarily by the family system, such as child-rearing responsibilities, are now being shared by collateral systems in the community.

Interactional Approach

Frequently labeled as the *symbolic* interactional frame of reference, this approach comes from sociology and social psychology. The interactionalist views the family as a unity of interacting personalities within which individual family members occupy a position or positions, such as husband-father, wife-mother, and daughter-sister. A cluster of roles—such as provider, homemaker, companion, and sex partner—are assigned to each of these positions, and a set of social norms or behavioral role expectations is perceived for each of these roles by the individual fulfilling them. Perceptions about role expectations emerge from an individual's self-concept and from an individual's reference group. As each individual carries out the various roles, role expectations are retained, modified, or discarded based upon the reactions of others within the family environment (Aldous, 1978, pp. 10, 14).

Interactionalists view the family as being relatively closed to outside systems. Family members are seen as actors and reactors who interact with their environment through symbolic communication. As a reactor, an individual does not simply respond to stimuli from the external environment. Symbolic communication evolving from the self and the environment helps individuals interpret and select the environment to which they respond. Based on this assumption, interactionalists stress that investigators or clinicians must see the world from the point of view of the individual (Stryker, 1964, pp. 134-135).

The interactional framework emphasizes analysis of the internal aspects of family functioning but neglects the family's relationships with other social systems. This framework identifies how relationships with others affect an individual's functioning. In addition to role analysis, interactionalists examine communication, decision-making and problem-solving processes, conflict, reactions to stress, and other family situations—such as divorce and domestic violence—that are influenced by family interactions and interactive processes (Aldous, 1978, p. 14; Hill and Hansen, 1960, pp. 302-303).

Developmental Approach

Concepts from various disciplines and approaches (rural sociology, child psychology, human development, sociology, and structural-functional and interactional approaches) were synthesized to create the developmental approach to family study. This approach looks at family development throughout its generational life cycle. It examines developmental tasks and role expectations for children, parents, and the family as a unit and traces how they change throughout family life (Hill and Hansen, 1960, pp. 307-308).

Duvall and Miller (1985) summarize the key features of the developmental approach to family study as follows. The developmental approach:

1. Keeps the family in focus throughout its history.
2. Sees each family member in interaction with all other members.
3. Watches the ways in which individuals and the family unit influence one another.
4. Recognizes what a given family is going through at any particular time.
5. Highlights critical periods of personal and family growth and development.
6. Views both the universals and the variations among families.
7. Beams in on the ways in which culture and families influence each other.
8. Provides a basis for forecasting what a given family will be going through at any period in its life span.

The developmental approach identifies specific tasks to be accomplished during a series of stages throughout the traditionally defined family life cycle. In this approach the stages in the family life span begin with marriage before the conception of children and end with aging and the adjustment to retirement. The developmental approach helps practitioners examine family change and functioning over time when families have a traditional family structure. It is less effective in analyzing change in the nontraditional family system.

General Systems Theory

First introduced by biologist Ludwig von Bertalanffy (1968, p. 11), systems theory is currently being used in many disciplines. General systems theory is a science of wholeness. "Its subject matter is the formulation of principles that are valid for 'systems' in general, whatever the nature of their component elements and the relations or 'forces' between them" (von Bertalanffy, p. 37). The goal of general systems study is to develop a theory that unites scientific thinking across disciplines and provides a framework for analyzing the "whole" of any given system.

Von Bertalanffy (1968, p. 83) defines a system as "a complex of elements in interaction." Although the definition of systems varies slightly from author to author, several commonalities emerge. It is generally agreed that a system consists of two or more connected elements that form an organized whole and that interact with each other.

Churchman (1968, p. 29) proposed five basic considerations that must be kept in mind when thinking about the meaning of a system:

1. The total system objectives and, more specifically, the performance measures of the whole system
2. The system's environment: the fixed constraints
3. The resources of the system
4. The components (elements or subsystems) of the system, their activities, goals, and measures of performance
5. The management of the system

Churchman, like many system scientists, uses an input-process-output-feedback model to depict the structural relationships of a system. An example of this type of model is shown in Figure 7-4. In simplistic terms, this model illustrates that all systems have *inputs* or resources which, when *processed,* help the system to achieve its goals or *outputs.* It further shows that a system has interdependency characteristics; change in any part of the system will change all parts. *Feedback* and information processing mechanisms within the system or from the environment provide data that a system needs to determine progress in meeting its goals.

When analyzing any system it is extremely important to recognize that all systems have fixed environmental constraints and choices that can be made about how the system will use its resources (inputs). Families, for example, must send their children to school after they reach a certain age. This is a *legal constraint,* not easily altered by a family system. To change this constraint would require consensus action by multiple systems. A family system does have some choice, however, about where the children will attend school. If a family does not like a particular public school district, this family may decide to move to another school district or to enroll the children in a private school.

No system can function in a vacuum. The environment of any system greatly affects how the system is able to function. Families' choices of educational opportunities for their children vividly illustrate this point. Some families may want to send the children to private school but are unable to do so because of *educational constraints* placed on them from the environment; in some settings private schools are unavailable. Other families may not be able to choose private school education because of *economic constraints* placed on them from the environment; their incomes may be insufficient to meet the financial requirements of a private educational system.

The processing of inputs (resources) received from the environment requires a series of dynamic, interrelated transactions. These transactions link together the environment, the system inputs, and the system outputs.

Processes are simply "the actions needed to get the job done" (Clemen, 1974, p. 26). Different types of processes are needed to accomplish particular tasks. Those processes of special interest to community health nurses are discussed throughout this text. Processes used by families to maintain healthy family functioning are discussed in a later section of this chapter. Presented in Chapter 9 (nursing process) and Chapter 10 (referral process and discharge planning) are the dynamic actions used by community health nurses to enhance client growth. Examined in Chapter 11 (epidemiological process), Chapter 12 (community diagnosis process), and Chapter 13 (planning process) are the dynamic actions integrated by community health nurses to plan and implement services for aggregates at risk. Covered in Chapter 22 (management process) and Chapter 23 (quality processes) are the dynamic actions carried out by community health nurses to ensure effective and efficient use of nursing time and delivery of quality care.

The feedback mechanism is the most significant aspect of a system. It assists the system in identifying

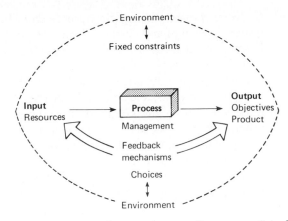

Figure 7-4 Structural arrangements of a system. (Modified from Clemen SJ: *Introduction to health care facility: food services administration,* University Park, Penn., 1974, Pennsylvania State University Press, p. 24.)

its strengths and needs and in evaluating how well it is accomplishing its goals. Feedback provides data essential for effective adaptation to internal and external system changes. It provides information that helps the system to select corrective actions when problems exist.

A system needs a mechanism that facilitates the sharing of both positive and negative feedback. A family system that discourages negative input often remains static or develops dysfunctional patterns. This can lead to disorganization, confusion, or chaos. Lack of positive feedback, however, can also lead to dysfunctional behavior. Positive feedback helps families to maintain healthy patterns of functioning and to stimulate creative ideas. If members of a family system receive only negative feedback, they become discouraged and find it difficult to use their creative talents.

In addition to the input-process-output-feedback element, all systems have several other characteristics. The following list briefly summarizes some of the more significant ones:

1. *Boundaries.* Every system has filtering mechanisms, or boundaries, that regulate the flow of energy to and from other systems. Boundaries in a system are not physical barriers. Rather, they are abstract entities such as norms, values, attitudes, and rules that inhibit or facilitate human transactional processes between systems.

2. *Exchange of energy.* Energy transport is crucial to the survival of any system. Without it, dysfunction results. An effectively functioning system uses energy to obtain resources (inputs) from the outside, to process resources to achieve its goals, and to release outputs into the environment. Energy that promotes order in a system is labeled *negentropy.* Energy that results in chaos or disorganization is termed *entropy* (von Bertalanffy, 1968; Wiener, 1968). All living systems contain entropy and negentropy. A system becomes distressed if extreme entropy exists for a considerable length of time. Family systems that are ineffectively dealing with crisis situations may reflect the concept of entropy. These families frequently lack energy to carry out their normal patterns of functioning and thus chaos or disorganization results.

3. *Hierarchical order.* In all systems there is order and patterning. Von Bertalanffy (1968, p. 27) noted that fundamental to general systems theory is the concept of hierarchical order in structure (order of parts) and function (order of processes). This implies that all systems are interconnected through a complex array of processes with other systems (external interacting systems), their subsystems (relationships among family members), and suprasystems (community/reference groups) and that there is a logical relationship among the parts of all systems. Both a family's internal and external environment influences family functioning and, thus, both need to be assessed during the clinical process. Most families interact with multiple systems in their environment, such as the health care system and educational institutions. Internally, "the family is a system of interacting personalities intricately organized into positions, roles, and norms which are further organized into subsystems within the family" (Friedman, 1986, p. 86). The nuclear family with more than one child differentiates and carries out its functions through at least three subsystems: the spouse subsystem, the parent-child subsystem, and the sibling subsystem. It may also have other subsystems such as a grandparent-grandchild or an aunt-nephew subsystem (Friedman, p. 86).

4. *Open or closed systems. Open* and *closed* are terms used in general systems theory to describe how a system interfaces with its environment. A system that isolates itself from others is viewed as a closed system. A system that exchanges energy and resources with other systems is an open system. All living systems are open systems. The degree of their openness varies, however, depending on how well they transport energy to maintain themselves.

5. *Self-regulation.* An open system, through its feedback mechanism or its information processing element, obtains data needed to adjust to its environment. The circular nature of its input-process-output-feedback unit helps a system to adapt the flow of inputs and outputs so that it can achieve a balance between what is taken from the environment and what is released into the environment. It helps the system to maintain homeostasis or equilibrium (von Bertalanffy, 1968, pp. 160-163). "The term equilibrium utilized as an optimal state may or may not account for growth needs" (Whall, 1991, p. 321). If this concept is interpreted to mean sameness or calmness, change and growth is negated (Whall); a more positive connotation is necessary when working with families. Families need to grow and change throughout their life cycle to achieve goals important to the family unit.

Increasingly, health care professionals and family scholars are applying the concepts, principles, and models of system theory to the study of the family. General systems theory provides a conceptual framework that is consistent with the holistic nature of humankind and professional practice. It offers a logical way to integrate all the factors that make an impact on family functioning and link the family together into a meaningful whole. It provides the basis for a humanistic philosophy of professional practice. The reason it does so is that family analysis from a systems perspective examines the family as a whole, rather than from isolated cause-and-effect relationships. Functional and dysfunctional patterns of behavior are considered to be products of system functioning. Family structure, functions, and processes are analyzed to determine why adaptive or maladaptive behavior is occurring within the family. This, in turn, negates individual blame and focuses attention on how the system must change in order to achieve productive functioning.

Use of Theoretical Frameworks in the Practice Setting

Table 7-3 summarizes select characteristics of the four family theories just discussed. Since only an introductory description was presented, the reader will find it useful to explore the literature in depth when selecting a conceptual framework for guiding practice. Of particular interest is literature that helps readers to examine the application of concepts in nursing practice (Bomar, 1989; Friedman, 1986; Whall, 1991).

It is important to remember that no one theoretical framework focuses attention on all aspects of family functioning. An example is a situation in which a nurse visits a young married couple in their twenties who have just had their first child. Using a developmental framework, the nurse would direct his or her evaluation of family health on how well the family and individual members were accomplishing stage-specific development tasks. On the other hand, systems-oriented nurses would focus their analysis on how the change in the family system (the addition of a new family member) has affected system functioning as a whole (e.g., its resources and goals, family processes, subsystems—especially the spouse relationships—and the family's interactions with its external environment).

Community health nurses generally use a combination of several theoretical frameworks to guide the family assessment process. This is appropriate because client situations vary and because no one framework explains all family phenomena. In the clinical setting it is essential for the nurse to examine the multiple aspects of family functioning, including the family's relationships with other social systems and its interactions with the environment; an effective management plan can only be developed after all of these areas have been assessed.

PARAMETERS TO CONSIDER DURING THE FAMILY ASSESSMENT PROCESS

In terms of the family, parameters related to both family structure and process should be considered during the family assessment process. This is true no matter what conceptual framework or combination of frameworks is selected to guide community health nursing practice. These parameters assist the nurse in obtaining a holistic view of the family, helping the nurse to identify who the family is and how family members interact to carry out their family functions.

Structural Parameters for Family Assessment

Structural components of a family are those variables that provide organization for the family system. They assist the family in coordinating their activities so that family and individual needs are met. Briar (1964, pp. 251-254), in his classic article on family organization, identified eight major structural characteristics of families: (1) division of labor, (2) distribution of power and authority, (3) communication, (4) boundaries of the family's world, (5) relations with other groups and systems, (6) ways of obtaining and giving emotional support, (7) rituals and symbols, and (8) a set of personal roles. These, as well as cultural values and attitudes and religious beliefs, are described below. Briar's delineation of the structural components of a family continues to be consistent with recent notions about the structural parameters of family life.

Division of Labor

Families allocate leadership responsibilities for maintaining their household in a variety of ways. Some follow traditional norms, with the man assuming major responsibility for the provider role and the woman for the homemaker role, regardless of the other role responsibilities each person has in the partnership. Some divide tasks according to their likes and dislikes or the level of competence each person has in relation to a particular task. Others share responsibilities equally, based on the demands each person has from other role positions.

Cultural background is an important variable to consider when the nurse examines family role performance. Ethnicity significantly influences the development of attitudes about the division of labor within the family unit. For example, within the traditional nuclear family, it is common for Navajo Indian (Hanley, 1991) and Italian (Bowen, 1991) women to be responsible for the domestic duties associated within the home and for the men from these ethnic groups to be responsible for any outside work needed to maintain the family and its home. However, intracultural diversity also exists, and individuals may not practice or possess all the characteristics of the ethnic group with which they identify (Fong, 1985).

Families who rigidly define either the provider or homemaker role tend to experience more stress when family members are unable to perform their expected tasks than do families who have a flexible division of labor (Beavers, 1977; Lewis, Beavers, Gossett, and Phillips, 1976; Otto, 1963; Pratt, 1976). It is also extremely difficult for families with rigid patterns of

TABLE 7-3 Select Characteristics of Four Family Theories

Theory	Focus of analysis	Advantages	Disadvantages
Structural-functional	Family interplay between collateral systems. Transactions between the family and its subsystems.	Allows for analysis of the multiple forces that influence family functioning. Handles well family interactions and transactions.	Family and its individual family members are considered to be reactive, passive elements of systems. Deals poorly with social change processes and dynamics.
Interactional	Internal aspects of family functioning, including role analysis, communication, decision-making, problem-solving and conflict resolution processes, reactions to stress and other family dynamics (e.g., divorce and domestic violence) influenced by family interactions.	Views family members as having control over their environment (e.g., family members interpret and select the environment to which they respond). Focuses on seeing the world from the client's perspective.	Neglects family relationships with other systems.
Developmental	Accomplishment of individual and family developmental tasks throughout the generational life cycle. Change in the family system over time.	Highlights critical periods of family growth and development. Keeps the traditionally defined family in focus throughout its life span. Recognizes and helps to predict what a given family is experiencing at any particular time.	Does not define critical stages and developmental tasks for nontraditional families.
Systems	Analysis of the family as a whole. Interdependence of the various parts of the family system and change. Interactions of the family system and its external environment.	Unites scientific thinking across disciplines. Provides a holistic perspective for analyzing family functioning that negates blame. Allows for analysis of family relationships with other systems and environmental influences on health. Examines family change and adaptation processes.	Complex theory can make it difficult for an inexperienced practitioner to fit all family dynamics into the specific categories defined within the system.

functioning to mobilize new coping mechanisms when experiencing a crisis. Health care professionals, for instance, often observe confusion and disorganization when a spouse dies. This confusion is heightened if the man or woman has not been prepared to deal with the demands of daily living. Assuming responsibilities for tasks one is not accustomed to performing is difficult at any time, but especially when one is experiencing a crisis.

Identifying how the division of labor is handled by

a family helps the community health nurse to understand the stresses family members are experiencing when changes have occurred. Role strain results when families do not take into consideration that role responsibilities change over time. Mothers, for example, are often confronted with excessive role demands after the birth of a child. This is especially true if husbands do not share the responsibility for housekeeping and child care tasks. Role strain also occurs when family members are unable to perform the activities related to a given role. This is particularly noticeable when role modifications are needed because of the prolonged absence of one family member. Absences that are a result of illness, divorce, separation, or vocational responsibilities frequently require drastic modifications in a family's division of labor and result in role strain.

All family members can experience role strain. Children may be required to assume adult responsibilities excessive for their age and level of growth and development. This most often occurs during times of crisis or when parents have not assumed adult leadership responsibilities required to maintain their household. Role-reversal behavior between parents and children is often present when child abuse occurs (Flanzraich and Dunsavage, 1977, p. 13). It is important for community health nurses to recognize that children do experience role strain when they assume parental functions, and to avoid reinforcing role-reversal patterns. It is easy to praise a child who is functioning beyond his or her chronological age. This praise, however, may support the continuance of family patterns that are unhealthy and that adversely affect a child's emotional growth and development.

Distribution of Power and Authority

Power was conceptualized by Bredemeir and Stephenson (1965, p. 50) as "the capacity to carry out, by whatever means, a desired course of action despite the resistance of others and without having to take into consideration their needs. When power is institutionalized through respect, fear, esteem, or position, it is referred to as authority."

Several variables affect who will have power in the family system. The position of power can be *culturally* prescribed, usually with the father being in a position of authority by virtue of his role as a male. This is frequently seen in Spanish-American and Asian cultures, where male dominance is the norm. Power can also be *situationally* prescribed when family members do not necessarily follow cultural norms but develop a power structure based on their circumstances and personal interactions. The continuum of family power based on cultural and situational variables ranges from complete dominance to complete absence of power, both of which can produce dysfunctional family patterns. Complete dominance by one family member poses a threat to the self-esteem of other family members and makes it difficult for individuals to resolve the independence-dependence conflicts that arise during adolescence and young adulthood. Complete absence of power in a family system tends to produce confusion, disorganization, and chaos. Dysfunctional families frequently exhibit power structures on either end of the continuum. Healthy families usually fall in the middle of the continuum, where power is shared by adult members but children are involved in the decision-making process.

Exchange theory helps to explain why an equal or unequal distribution of power evolves in a family system. Sharing of power is more likely to occur when all family members perceive that they have resources to contribute that enhance the family's ability to achieve its goals and to meet the needs of individual family members. Family members who do not value their contributions or whose contributions are not valued by other family members will probably not have power within the family system.

Understanding the relationship between issues of power and decision-making is essential to effect permanent changes within a family system. If the power and authority structure of a family is ignored, nursing interventions are often inappropriate and place additional stress on family members who lack the power to make decisions about needed health actions. Family members who have power must be consulted if changes in health behavior are to occur. One community health nurse, for instance, realized after several home visits to a Spanish-American family that the only way she would influence the family to obtain needed surgery for their 4-year-old preschooler was to talk with the child's father. Although the mother stated frequently that she felt it was important for her son to have surgery, no action was taken. When the mother was finally asked how her husband felt about this matter, the nurse discovered that he felt surgery was unnecessary and that he was the one who made the final decision about needed health care.

In situations where the dominant family member is temporarily immobilized, it is extremely important for the community health nurse to recognize that the family may reassign the dominant position to the nurse. Because of the nurse's professional status, families under stress may initially allow a nurse to assume a position of authority within the family structure. They may follow the nurse's suggestions to relieve the anxiety they are experiencing at the time. These suggestions may not necessarily be appropriate for the family, but the family may follow through on them because its anxiety level is so high. A family under stress will frequently try anything to reduce its level of discomfort. Nurses must recognize that this does happen, because when families are experiencing pain it is easier at times to do things for them than to foster family decision-making. Taking over decision-making for a family is not therapeutic.

Communication Patterns

Verbal and nonverbal interactions within a family usually display significant regularities or patterns. Norms involving what is shared and not shared with whom are implicitly, if not explicitly, known by all family members. Messages are provided in a variety of ways to let family members know how to communicate within and outside the family system.

The ability to communicate accurately and effectively is essential to all aspects of family functioning because communication is an integral part of daily living. It helps the family to carry out its functions, to meet the needs of individual family members, and to move toward achieving its goals.

Communication is an extremely complex process, involving not only what is said but also how it is said and the *behavioral interactions* that occur during the course of a conversation. An individual can communicate even when verbal information is not shared. Watzlawick, Beavin, and Jackson (1967, pp. 48-49) noted that because all behavior in an interactional situation has message value, it is impossible for a person not to communicate. They believe that "activity or inactivity, words or silence, all have message value which influence others; others, in turn, cannot avoid responding to these communications and are thus, themselves communicating." Even silence conveys a message to an individual who is sharing thoughts, ideas, or feelings.

Communication-oriented theorists believe that family communication patterns need to be analyzed along several dimensions (Haley, 1971; Jackson, 1968; Satir, 1972; Watzlawick, Beavin, and Jackson, 1967). Verbal, nonverbal, and behavioral processes should be observed to identify the following aspects of a family's communication patterns.

1. *Content.* What actually is conveyed is known as the content of communication. Observations should be made to determine what is being shared and what is not. It is not unusual for individuals to feel uncomfortable about sharing information concerning personal topics such as sexuality, finances, and troubled relationships with significant others. A health care professional needs to "listen between the lines" in order to help clients verbalize areas of concern beyond those that are explicitly expressed.

2. *How content is shared.* The sharing of content does not necessarily convey to the receiver accurate knowledge, facts, or ideas, or help the receiver to understand the message a person is attempting to share. Content becomes functional when there is clarity of thought, organization of ideas, and accuracy and completeness of facts. It is difficult for the receiver to understand what is being said when information is being withheld, when an overabundance of data is being shared, or when conflicting messages are being conveyed. These problems tend to distort reality and confuse the listener. They can lead to a lack of responsiveness or hostile interchange.

3. *Behavioral interactions.* How an individual responds, either verbally or nonverbally, during a conversation provides clues to others about how this individual views what is being said or how he or she regards the sender. Body mannerisms, eye contact, silence or responsiveness to content, vocal characteristics, and ways of eliciting information all provide behavioral messages that guide the course of a conversation. Behavioral messages are often far more meaningful in a positive or negative sense than verbal content. They may provide "double-level messages, with the voice saying one thing and the rest of the person saying something else" (Satir, 1972, p. 60). Healthy families tend to share fewer "double-level" messages than nonhealthy families.

4. *Interpretation of content and behavioral interactions.* How information and interactions are interpreted varies from one individual to another. Perceptions about messages being conveyed are influenced by several factors, including

things such as previous experiences when communicating with others, the motivations of persons involved in a conversation, feelings about oneself, and current stresses being experienced. For example, families who have low self-esteem frequently find it difficult to interpret messages positively; praise is often not heard or is negated. The interpretation of messages is a key factor that determines the difference between healthy and pathological communication. When assessing family communication patterns it is extremely important to note whether real-life events and the feelings and thoughts of others are accurately perceived. When healthy communication patterns exist, clarification is sought if individuals do not understand what is being said. Feelings such as sadness, joy, or anger are not attributed to others without validation.

5. *Ways of communicating.* Satir (1975, pp. 141-149) noted that individuals use five major transactional modes to communicate when they are under stress. These are placating, blaming, superreasonable, irrelevant, and congruent modes.

   a. *Placating* refers to a mode of communication that entails agreeing with what is being said, even when one does not inwardly desire to do so. The placater is trying to please others and does not share personal feelings and reactions. Placating may occur if an individual does not wish to engage in a conversation.

   b. *Blaming* patterns of behavior result when an individual has a need to prove that he or she is strong. Techniques such as fault-finding, dictatorship, or cutting remarks are used to demonstrate that one has power. Individuals who use blaming techniques are usually very insecure. Often they exert control over others in order to achieve a sense of security through power.

   c. *Superreasonable* communication occurs when a person intellectualizes and avoids the sharing of feelings and emotions. Individuals who are afraid to deal with feelings and emotions frequently do not recognize the need to make constructive changes in their lives; they suppress feelings of anxiety that are needed to motivate them

to examine dysfunctional patterns of behavior.

   d. *Irrelevant* transactions are illogical from the perspective of what is happening in an individual's environment. Irrelevant communication patterns affect the flow of a conversation, as well as problem-solving and decision-making processes.

   e. *Congruent* interactions result when feelings and content are integrated and information sharing is logical in relation to what is happening in the environment. When using congruent communication, an individual is "real"; that is, there is a consistency between what the individual outwardly shares and what is inwardly felt. This is the most functional way to interact with others. Satir (1975, p. 48) has found that when the other transactional modes of communication become patterned, psychosomatic and other illnesses often result.

6. *Linguistic characteristics.* Families have varying dialects or language differences depending on their cultural background, their socialization process, and their geographical location. It is important for a community health nurse to note these differences because they can interfere with communication, especially when a family's or a nurse's dialect is incongruent with the dialect of others in their environment. Generally clients are more than willing to help healthcare professionals understand language differences if the health care professional shows an interest in learning about them.

Cultural differences among families are reflected in all aspects of verbal and nonverbal communications. Gestures, posture, facial expression, eye contact, touch, vocabulary, grammatical structure, voice qualities, and silence all send important messages to members of a specific ethnic group. For example, in some cultures (Mexican and some American Indian) touch is considered magical and healing; in other cultures, such as the Vietnamese, touch produces anxiety because it is believed that the soul can leave the body on physical contact (Roccereto, 1981; Giger and Davidhizar, 1991). During the family assessment process it is important to determine if there are cultural behaviors or styles of communication that the client practices. The bowing of the head to show respect in the traditional Japanese culture and speaking softly in the

Southeast Asian culture are examples of these behaviors (Fong, 1985).

The primary goal of observing family communication patterns is to determine if the patterns established by a particular family are functional; that is, do they help the family to carry out its functions, to relate effectively to the environment, to meet the needs of individual family members, and to achieve its goals? It is important to remember that ways of achieving functional communication between family members can vary from one family to another. In recent professional and lay literature there has been a tendency to idealize frank, honest self-disclosure. Frankness may not always be functional, however; stating what one thinks without taking into consideration another person's feelings can be irresponsible. Honest interchanges in communication can occur without frank disclosure. Being honest is saying only what you mean, not everything (Hacker, 1985).

Hacker (1985), a health educator who specializes in sexuality counseling, has found that both clients and health care professionals are often afraid of handling sensitive topics because they are confused about the difference between honesty and self-disclosure. To her, an honest individual is one who says what he or she means and is comfortable with what is not shared. Self-disclosure is the frank sharing of one's private feelings, thoughts, and actions, often without evaluating the appropriateness of doing so in one's current situation. Hacker has found that self-disclosure is not necessarily the key to the successful handling of sexuality issues. Rather, she believes that one needs to be honest with oneself about personal sexuality concerns. Only then will one be able to deal with value issues and feelings. Shakespeare was wise when he said in *Hamlet,* "This above all: to thine own self be true,/ And it must follow, as the night the day,/ Thou canst not then be false to any man" (*Hamlet,* act 1, scene 3).

Boundaries of Family World

Boundary development and maintenance is essential for family survival and growth. Families must have effective filtering mechanisms so that the exchange of energies corresponds to the needs of the family. Energy exchanges that occur too rapidly or too slowly can be disruptive to the family system. Families need to bring inputs into their system and release outputs into the environment so that they can carry out their functions. However, they also need to limit the amount of input from the environment to prevent system overload and to limit the release of outputs to prevent energy depletion.

The rate of energy flow between the family and the environment must vary in order for the family to maintain the integrity of its system. Families who do not adjust their energy flow to correspond to their current circumstances have difficulty handling stress and change. In times of family stress and change, limiting the exchange of inputs and outputs conserves energy needed to carry out activities of daily living. A new mother or father, for instance, may need to reduce working hours (output) in order to conserve energy for child care activities and to provide emotional support for others in the family system.

It is not uncommon for community health nurses to work with families who are having difficulty adjusting energy flow to and from their family system. Some of the most frequent difficulties in relation to boundary maintenance issues which will be encountered in clinical practice are summarized below:

1. *Boundaries too loose.* Disorganized, multiproblem, and crisis-prone families tend to take little control over what enters or exits their environment. They have numerous outsiders (inputs), such as health care professionals or legal authorities, working with them, and often they do not set rules about how and when family members should interact outside the family system. These families usually come to the attention of health care professionals because their outputs are not acceptable to the suprasystem (community). It is not unusual for such families to be referred to the community health nurse when their children enter school, because they lack the energy to fulfill the health requirements (immunizations and physical examinations) mandated by the educational system for school entry. In these situations, families' energies are often used to deal with outsiders or crises rather than to take care of the needs of individual family members.

2. *Boundaries too rigid.* Some families allow few inputs to cross their boundaries. They isolate themselves from the larger community and may not obtain the resources needed for family growth. Families from differing cultural backgrounds or families who have members with a mental or physical handicap may limit

inputs from the environment because they are afraid that the larger society will not accept their differences. Conflicts between these families and their environment arise when they do not release outputs (do not send their children to school) or when their outputs are inadequate (children not prepared to handle environmental demands and pressures).

3. *Boundaries not agreed upon.* At times community health nurses find a discrepancy between the views of one family member and another regarding boundary maintenance. Families may have some boundaries that are well defined and others that are unclearly defined. They may, for example, use community resources appropriately but may not agree on how often and when they should interface with friends and the extended family. Lack of agreement on boundary maintenance issues can lead to conflict, disequilibrium, and system disintegration.

Relations with Other Groups and Systems

The development of relationships with other groups, such as extended kin or neighbors, and other systems, such as church, school, or health care agencies, is directly related to the way the family handles its boundary maintenance functions. Family boundaries can facilitate or inhibit the establishment and maintenance of interpersonal relationships with others outside the family system. Families with rigid boundaries have few contacts with persons outside their family system; families with flexible boundaries tend to encourage close interactions with others.

When assessing family relationships outside the family system, it is important to look at the *type* of relationships they have as well as the contact allowed. Interaction with numerous people does not necessarily mean that the family is meeting their support, companionship, and growth needs. Some families develop relationships that involve more giving than receiving. In these situations, family energies are devoted to helping others but the family receives very little support in return. In other families individual family members are allowed to interact with anyone, even though their interactions may not be positive. Children, for example, may encounter legal difficulties because there are no controls placed on their relationships with people who are engaging in illegal activities.

Ways of Obtaining and Giving Emotional Support

Families need to achieve a balance between their relationship with others and their relationship with family members. If the family excludes itself from its external environment, there may be a lack of support from others during times of stress and crisis. If, on the other hand, the family devotes all its energy to helping others, it is highly unlikely that the family will be able to meet the emotional needs of individual family members.

Families meet their emotional needs in a variety of ways. They develop norms that regulate sources of support, provide guidelines for giving support, and define when support will be given. When assessing the ways a family obtains and gives emotional support, the following factors should be considered:

1. *Distribution of support.* All family members need support, encouragement, and praise. If support is not evenly distributed, family members who are not receiving what they need may seek support from their environment and isolate themselves from the family system, or they may withdraw and limit contact with others outside the family, as well as within the family system.

2. *When support is given.* Some families provide support only during times of stress and crisis. Others are supportive during times of stress but also during normal functioning periods. The sharing of love, attention, and affection only when family members are distressed can be dysfunctional in that it may reinforce such behaviors as illness, truancy, and other destructive activities. All human beings need emotional care and nurturing. If they are unable to obtain emotional support without manifesting symptoms of distress, they may develop physical or psychosocial difficulties in order to receive the attention needed for emotional survival. Often such individuals are unaware that they are doing this.

3. *Acceptance of family members.* How an individual family member is viewed by other family members greatly affects the amount of emotional support the individual will receive. Family goals that define desired achievements, norms that regulate acceptable and unacceptable behavior, and the emotional maturity of the family all influence how well individual family members will be accepted by other

family members. Individuals within the family who do not conform to family norms and goals usually receive less support than those who do. Illustrating this is the teenager from a family with high educational aspirations who does not share these aspirations and decides not to go to college. This teenager very quickly receives a message from other family members that this is an inappropriate decision. If she or he does not alter these views, family members may withdraw support and encouragement even if the family member succeeds outside the educational environment.

4. *How support is given.* Families use both verbal and nonverbal communication to provide support for their members. Some share support spontaneously, whereas others are more reserved and do not give support until it is elicited from them. Individuals from families who spontaneously share with each other may sense a lack of support if they marry individuals from families who were reserved in their interactions with others. This can also occur when individual family members observe how their friends' families provide support for their members. Children, for instance, may perceive that they are not loved by their parents if they observe spontaneous sharing in the homes of their friends.

Set of Personal Roles

Every family has the task of organizing its roles in a way that helps the family to achieve its goals and to carry out its functions. There is no one role-allocation pattern that works for all families. Families must allocate and differentiate roles in a manner which facilitates their functioning.

Personal roles as well as family roles evolve when families organize their role structure. Some common examples of personal roles are "the 'baby' in the family; the 'good' child; the 'bad' child; the scapegoat; the strict parent; and the 'sickest' member of the family. Such roles, even when they emerge fortuitously, can become patterned very quickly. As a result, the person may be 'locked' in the role, with important consequences for how others will treat him and what they will expect of him" (Briar, 1964, p. 254). When assessing family dynamics it is extremely important to identify how personal role allocation has influenced the behavior of all family members. The "sick" mem-

ber of the family, for example, is often not allowed to do things that he or she is capable of doing. Frequently family members "take care" of this person so well that he or she never learns how to function independently.

Rituals and Symbols

Family rituals and symbols come from two major sources. First, some are adopted from the culture as a whole or a subculture within the wider culture. Second, they develop from human transactional processes that have occurred within the family system (Briar, 1964, pp. 253-254).

Family rituals and symbols develop around multiple aspects of family life. They help family members and outsiders to identify what the family views as important. They provide structure for activities of daily living and for special occasions.

Examples of the types of rituals and symbols that develop in family systems follow. Although some of the rituals within a family appear very similar to societal ones, family rituals usually have some very specific, unique characteristics.

1. Mealtimes: designating times for meals, seating arrangements during meals, and conversation sharing.
2. Family names: giving nicknames to all family members or naming children for specific family members.
3. Holidays: serving specific types of food or carrying out certain kinds of activities (refer to Figures 7-5 and 7-6).
4. Religious observances: saying prayers at mealtime or bedtime or engaging in specific activities when a family member has died.

Family rituals and symbols are extremely significant and are usually valued highly by families. They are often continued even when individual family members do not view them as important. Frequently pressure is placed on family members to conform to family rituals and symbols until the entire family unit alters its views about them.

Cultural Values and Attitudes

Numerous factors influence the biological, psychosocial, and spiritual development of all human beings. Human growth and development begins with genetic characteristics inherited from parents but then branches off in different directions as one interacts with one's environment. Within this environment, caring and nurturing by significant others greatly

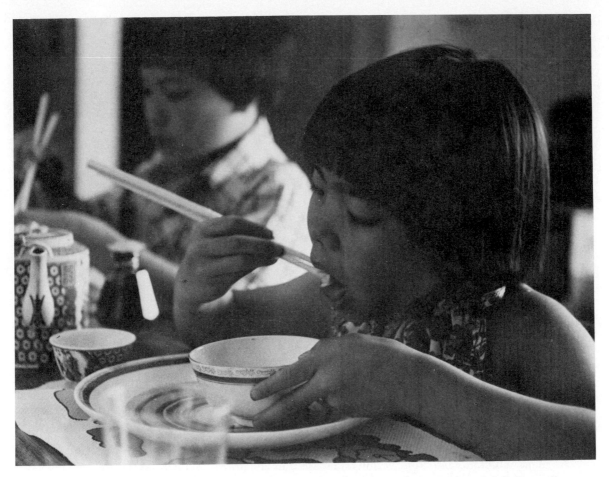

Figure 7-5   Cultural values and attitudes provide a foundation for activities of daily living.

affects how growth progresses and what decisions are made about handling activities of daily living. Through environmental conditioning people learn patterns of behavior that influence how they relate to others, how they act in social situations, and how they make decisions about significant issues. Because these patterns of behavior provide stability and security, they are not easily altered; they continuously influence the direction of one's life. They shape beliefs and values that provide a foundation for future decision making.

Culture is the term used to describe the values, attitudes, and patterns of behavior that are transmitted to all individuals in a particular social environment. Social scientists have defined culture in many ways, but most of these definitions have three central themes: (1) beliefs, values, and patterns of behavior are

learned and passed on from one generation to the next; (2) culture provides a prescription for daily living and decision-making; and (3) the components of a culture are valued by members of the culture and are considered to be right and not open to questioning.

Every culture has a schema, composed of specific components, that shapes such things as family structure, dietary habits, religious practices, the development of art, music, and drama, ways of communicating, dress, and health behavior (refer to Figures 7-5 and 7-6). A culture schema, for instance, affects how one perceives health and illness and when and from whom one seeks health care. Because the Jewish culture values the sacredness of human life and health, members of this particular cultural group have traditionally respected health care providers and have engaged in activities, regardless of the expense, to restore health.

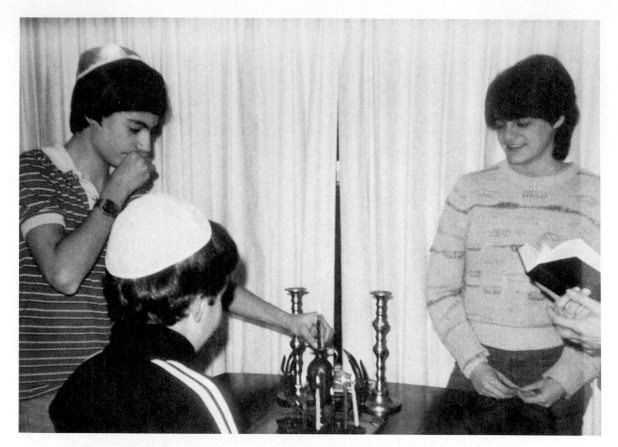

Figure 7-6 For centuries religious systems have significantly influenced the development of customs and rituals within family systems and have preserved and transmitted these traditions from one generation to another. Hanukkah, a festive Jewish holiday lasting for 8 days in early December, has been celebrated for centuries in memory of the rededication of the temple of Jerusalem under the Maccabees in 164 BC. Hanukkah is a celebration of freedom: freedom to practice one's own religion. It is a joyous time that includes a symbolic lighting of candles, the sharing of gifts, and the serving of special foods.

The value the Jewish culture places on health is reflected in a favorite Yiddish parting phrase, *Sei gesund,* "be well" (Kensky, 1977, p. 197). In contrast to the health values held by the Jewish culture are the beliefs and values transmitted by the Mexican-American culture. Many individuals from this culture are influenced by a folk system that encourages the use of folk medicine and supports the belief that one has very little control over one's life; it is felt that supernatural forces cause disease and that one can do very little to prevent illness. Mexican healers, *curanderos(as),* rather than health care professionals are used by some Mexican-American families when health care services are needed (Baca, 1973; Prattes, 1973; Samora, 1978).

A rich diversity of cultural values and attitudes exists in our nation. In community health nursing practice, encountering clients who have beliefs that differ from those of the health care professional is a common occurrence. In order for community health nurses to work effectively with such clients, they must develop an appreciation for the inherent worth of different cultural patterns. This involves a process that not only increases one's knowledge about various cultural schemata but also increases one's acceptance of all human beings and their cultures.

Developing cultural sensitivity in clinical practice enriches and broadens the nurse's approach to diverse families and can lead to a more effective delivery of care. Crucial to this process is being aware of one's own cultural background. Health care professionals, like clients, are influenced by their own social conditioning, which has a long-lasting effect on everything they do. It is often difficult to recognize the effects of earlier influences, because patterns of functioning derived from social conditioning become a way of life. These patterns subtly influence behavior even when they are no longer recognized on a conscious level. Hence, health care professionals need to examine carefully how their values and attitudes are affecting their clinical judgments. This process can be painful, especially when it is identified that one's interventions are not therapeutic because the client's health beliefs have been discounted. If this happens, remember that all practitioners have at one time or another experienced professional situations in which they have not been effective because of value conflicts. Being able to identify that one's behavior is adversely affecting professional interactions and to take action to alter nontherapeutic intervention is one of the characteristics of a sensitive professional.

Select characteristics of some ethnic and racial groups are presented in Table 7-4. They illustrate cultural variations in relation to health beliefs and practices, family relationships, and communication processes. However, nurses must understand that there are also intracultural variations based on generational differences within groups (Fong, 1985).

When learning about specific cultural beliefs it is best to seek information from members of the particular culture being studied. Many cultural patterns are not written or recorded. Most, in fact, are transmitted from one generation to another through oral communication and behavioral transactions. When receiving input from individuals who represent a given cultural group, it is extremely important to remember that not all individuals within a cultural group have similar characteristics. Knowledge about cultural values and attitudes helps identify factors to consider when collecting data about family functioning. This knowledge, however, *never* replaces the need to obtain specific data from individual families during the assessment process. When working with families in the community setting, a cultural assessment should be done to determine their unique characteristics and needs.

Cultural assessments assist nurses in individualizing family care. When conducting a cultural assessment, community health nurses need to focus on collecting basic cultural data that identify major family values, beliefs, customs, and behaviors that influence and relate to health needs, health care practices, and

family attitudes about health and illness, health care providers, and health care systems (Orque, Bloch, and Monrroy, 1983, p. 55; Tripp-Reimer, Brink, and Saunders, 1984, p. 79). According to Tripp-Reimer, Brink, and Saunders (p. 79), "basic cultural data include: ethnic affiliation, religious preference, family patterns, food patterns, and ethnic health care practices."

Appendix 7-1 displays a cultural assessment tool developed by Bloch (1983) to facilitate cultural assessments in the clinical setting. This tool identifies content areas such as race, language and communication processes, and nutritional variables to be considered when making a cultural assessment. In their text *Ethnic Nursing Care,* Orque, Bloch, and Monrroy examine specific factors to consider when providing nursing care for Black, Raza/Latina, Filipino American, Chinese American, Japanese American, South Vietnamese, and American Indian clients. Referring to this text and other writings (Giger and Davidhizar, 1991) will help the reader to plan appropriate nursing interventions when working with families from these ethnic minority groups.

When using Bloch's cultural assessment guide, remember that a barrage of questions related to the cultural content areas on this tool is inappropriate. This type of interviewing inhibits communication and adversely affects the nurse-client relationship. When collecting any type of information during the assessment phase of the nursing process the community health nurse must focus on building a therapeutic relationship in addition to obtaining data (refer to Chapter 9). The Giger and Davidhizar (1991) textbook provides some valuable guidelines to consider when collecting cultural data.

Religious Beliefs

Cultural values and attitudes are often shaped and maintained by religious systems. From earliest times religious systems have preserved and transmitted traditions from one generation to another, and have greatly influenced the development of norms for social behavior. Spiritual beliefs valued by these systems have provided a foundation for moral behavior in societies; they have also helped to maintain order and cohesiveness in social groups.

Despite major changes in religious systems in the past two decades, spiritual beliefs still affect the lives of most individuals. They influence such things as contraceptive practices, dietary habits, developmental transitions through rites of passage, selection of marriage partners, reactions to health and illness, and

Text continues on p. 240

TABLE 7-4 Cultural Characteristics Related to Health Care of Children and Families

Cultural group	Health beliefs	Health and diet practices
Asian Americans		
Chinese	A healthy body viewed as gift from parents and ancestors and must be cared for Health is one of the results of balance between the forces of *yin* (cold) and *yang* (hot), energy forces that rule the world Illness caused by imbalance Believe blood is source of life and is not regenerated *Chi* is innate energy Lack of *chi* and blood results in deficiency that produces fatigue, poor constitution, and long illness	Goal of therapy is to restore balance of *yin* and *yang* Acupuncturist applies needles to appropriate meridians identified in terms of *yin* and *yang* Acupressure and *tai chi* replacing acupuncture in some areas Moxibustion is application of heat to skin over specific meridians Wide use of medicinal herbs procured and applied in prescribed ways Folk healers are herbalist, spiritual healer, temple healer, fortune healer Meals may or may not be planned to balance hot and cold Milk intolerance relatively common Use of condiments, e.g., monosodium glutamate and soy sauce, may create difficulty with some diet regimens, e.g., low-salt diets

Japanese	Three major belief systems:
	  Shinto religious influence
	    Humans inherently good
	    Evil caused by outside spirits
	    Illness caused by contact with polluting agents, e.g., blood, corpses, skin diseases
	  Chinese and Korean influence
	    Health achieved through harmony and balance between self and society
	    Disease caused by disharmony with society and not caring for body
	  Portuguese influence
	    Upholds germ theory of disease
		Believe evil removed by purification
		
		Energy restored by means of acupuncture, acupressure, massage, and moxibustion along affected meridians
		
		Kampō medicine—use of natural herbs
		
		Believe in removal of diseased parts
		
		Trend is to use both Western and Oriental healing methods
		
		Care for disabled viewed as family's responsibility
		
		Take pride in child's good health
		
		Seek preventive care, medical care for illness
		
		Older persons avoid some food combinations (e.g., milk and cherries, watermelon and crab) and believe pickled plums to have special properties

References: Bloch, 1983; Char, 1981; Chen-Louie, 1983; Chow, 1976; Ehling, 1981; Greathouse and Miller, 1981; Hashizume and Takano, 1983; Holland and Sweeney, 1985; Hollingsworth, Brown, and Brooten, 1980; Jacques, 1976; Lacay, 1981; Monrroy, 1983; Orque, 1983a, 1983b; Sodetaini-Shebata, 1981.
From Whaley LF and Wong DL: *Nursing care of infants and children,* ed 4, St. Louis, 1991, Mosby, pp. 54-59.

Family relationships	Communication	Comments
Extended family pattern common Strong concept of loyalty of young to old Respect for elders taught at early age—acceptance without questioning or talking back Children's behavior a reflection on family Family and individual honor and "face" important Self-reliance and self-restraint highly valued; self-expression repressed Males valued more highly than females; women submissive to men in family	Open expression of emotions unacceptable Often smile when do not comprehend	Do not react well to painful diagnostic workup; are especially upset by drawing of blood Deep respect for their bodies and believe it best to die with bodies intact; therefore may refuse surgery Believe in reincarnation Older members fear hospitals; often believe hospital is a place to go to die Children sometimes breast-fed for up to 4 or 5 years*
Close intergenerational relationships Family provides anchor Family tends to keep problems to self Value self-control and self-sufficiency Concept of *haji* (shame) imposes strong control; unacceptable behavior of children reflects on family Many adopt practices of contemporary middle class Concern for child's missing school may result in sending to school before fully recovered from illness	*Issei*—born in Japan; usually speak Japanese only *Nisei, Sansei,* and *Yonsei* have few language difficulties New immigrants able to read and write English better than to speak or understand it Make significant use of nonverbal communication with subtle gestures and facial expression Tend to suppress emotions Will often wait silently	Generational categories: *Issei*—1st generation to live in U.S. *Nisei*—2nd generation *Sansei*—3rd generation *Yonsei*—4th generation *Issei* and *Nisei*—tolerant and permissive childrearing until 5 or 6, then emphasis on emotional reserve and control Cleanliness highly valued Time considered valuable and used wisely Tendency to practice emotional control may make assessment of pain more difficult

*Most Asian cultures consider the child 1 year old at the time of birth. Traditional Chinese custom adds 1 year on January 1 regardless of the birthday—a child born in December is 2 years old the next January.

Continued

7-4 Cultural Characteristics Related to Health Care of Children and Families—cont'd

Cultural group	Health beliefs	Health and diet practices
Vietnamese	Good health considered to be balance between *yin* (cold) and *yang* (hot) Believe person's life has been predisposed toward certain phenomena by cosmic forces Health believed to be result of harmony with existing universal order, harmony attained by pleasing good spirits and avoiding evil ones Belief in *am duc*, the amount of good deeds accumulated by ancestors Many use rituals to prevent illness Practice some restrictions to prevent incurring wrath of evil spirits	Family uses all means possible before using outside agencies for health care Fortune-tellers determine event that caused disturbance May visit temple to procure divine instruction Use astrologer to calculate cyclical changes and forces Regard health as family responsibility; outside aid sought when resources run out Certain illnesses considered only temporary (such as pustules, open wounds) and ignored Seek generalist health healers May use special diets to prevent illness and promote health Lactose intolerance prevalent
Filipino	Believe God's will and supernatural forces govern universe Illness, accidents, and other misfortunes are God's punishment for violations of His will Widely accept "hot" and "cold" balance and imbalance as cause of health and illness	Some use amulets as a shield from witchcraft or as good luck pieces Catholics substitute religious medals and other items

American black	Illness classified as:
	  Natural—affected by forces of nature without adequate protection, e.g., cold air, pollution, food and water
	  Unnatural—evil influences, e.g., witchcraft, voodoo, hoodoo, hex, fix, rootwork; symptoms often associated with eating
	Believe serious illness sent by God as punishment, e.g., parents punished by illness or death of child
	Believe serious illness can be avoided
	May resist health care because illness is "will of God"
		Self-care and folk medicine very prevalent
		Folk therapies usually religious in origin
		Attempt home remedies first; poorer people do not seek help until illness serious
		Usually seek help from:
		  "Old lady"—woman in community with a common knowledge of herbs; consults regarding pediatric care
		  Spiritualist—has received gift from God for healing incurable diseases or solving personal problems; strongly based in Christianity
		  Priest (voodoo priest/priestess)—most powerful healer
		  Root doctor—meets need for herbs, oils, candles, and ointments
		Prayer is common means for prevention and treatment

Family relationships	Communication	Comments
Family is revered institution Multigenerational families Family is chief social network Children highly valued Individual needs and interests are subordinate to those of family group Father is main decision maker Women taught submission to men Parents expect respect and obedience from children	Many immigrants are not proficient in speaking and understanding English May hesitate to ask questions Questioning authority is sign of disrespect: asking questions considered impolite Use indirectness rather than forthrightness in expressing disagreement May avoid eye contact with health professionals as a sign of respect	Consider status more important than money Children taught emotional control Time concept more relaxed—consider punctuality less significant than other values, i.e., propriety Place high value on social harmony
Family is highly valued with strong family ties Multigenerational family structure common, often with collateral members as well Personal interests are subordinated to family interests and needs Members avoid any behavior that would bring shame on the family	Immigrants and older persons may not be able to speak or understand English	Tend to have a fatalistic outlook on life Believe time and providence will solve all
Strong kinship bonds in extended family; members come to aid of others in crisis Less likely to view illness as a burden Augmented families common (unrelated persons living in same household) Place strong emphasis on work and ambition Sex-role sharing among parents	Alert to any evidence of discrimination Place importance on nonverbal behavior May use nonstandard English or "black English" Use "testing" behaviors to assess personnel in health care situations before seeking active care Best to use simple, direct, but caring approach	High level of caution and distrust of majority group Social anxiety related to tradition of humiliation, oppression, and loss of dignity Will elect to retain dignity rather than seek care if values are compromised Strong sense of peoplehood High incidence of poverty Black minister a strong influence in black community Visits by family minister are sought, expected, and valued in helping to cope with illness and suffering

Continued

7-4   Cultural Characteristics Related to Health Care of Children and Families—cont'd

Cultural group	Health beliefs	Health and diet practices

Haitian*	Illnesses have a supernatural or natural origin
	
	Supernatural illness are caused by angry voodoo spirits, enemies, or the dead, especially deceased ancestors
	
	Natural illnesses are based on conceptions of natural causation:
	  Irregularities of blood volume, flow, purity, viscosity, color and/or temperature (hot/cold)
	  Gas (*gaz*)
	  Movement and consistency of mother's milk
	  Hot/cold imbalance in the body
	  Bone displacement
	  Movement of diseases
	Health is maintained by good dietary and hygienic habits
		Health is a personal responsibility
		Foods have properties of "hot"/"cold" and "light"/"heavy" and must be in harmony with one's life cycle and bodily states
		Natural illnesses are treated by home remedies first
		Supernatural illness treated by healers: voodoo priest (*houngan*) or priestess (*mambo*), midwife (*fam saj*), and herbalist or leaf doctor (*dokte fey*)
		Amulets and prayer used to protect against illness due to curses or willed by evil people

Hispanic-American, Mexican-American (Latino, Chicano, Raza-Latino)	Health beliefs have strong religious association Believe in body imbalance as a cause of illness, especially imbalance between *caliente* (hot) and *frio* (cold) or "wet" and "dry" Some maintain good health is a result of "good luck"—a reward for good behavior Illness prevented by performing properly, eating proper foods, and working proper amount of time; accomplished through prayer, wearing religious medals or amulets, and sleeping with relics at home Illness is a punishment from God for wrongdoing, forces of nature, and the supernatural	Seek help from *curandero* or *curandera*, especially in rural areas Curandero(a) receives his/her position by birth, apprenticeship, or a "calling" via dream or vision Treatments involve use of herbs, rituals, and religious artifacts Practice for severe illness—make promises, visit shrines, offer medals and candles, offer prayers Adhere to "hot" and "cold" food prescriptions and prohibitions for prevention and treatment of illness

*This section was written by Lydia DeSantis, Ph.D., R.N.

Family relationships	Communication	Comments
Maintenance of family reputation is paramount	Recent immigrants and older persons may speak only Haitian creole	Will use biomedical and ethnomedical (folk) systems simultaneously
Lineal authority supreme; children in a subordinate position in family hierarchy	May prefer family/friends to act as translators and confidants	Resistant to dietary and work restrictions
Children valued for parental social security in old age and expected to contribute to family welfare at an early age	Often smile and nod in agreement when do not understand	Adherence to prescribed treatments directly related to perceived severity of illness
Children viewed as "gifts from god" and treated with indulgence and affection	Quiet and gentle communication style and lack of assertiveness lead health care providers to falsely believe they comprehend health teaching and are compliant	
	Will not ask questions if health care provider is busy or rushed	
Traditionally men considered breadwinners, women homemakers	May use nonstandard English	High degree of modesty—often a deterrent to seeking medical care
Males are considered big and strong (*macho*)	Most bilingual; many only speak Spanish	Youngsters often reluctant to share communal showers in schools
Strong kinship; extended families include *compadres* (godparents) established by ritual kinship	May have a strong preference for native language and revert to it in times of stress	Relaxed concept of time—may be late for appointments
Children valued highly and desired, taken everywhere with family		Magicoreligious practices common
Many homes contain shrines with statues and pictures of saints		May view hospital as place to go to die

Continued

7-4 Cultural Characteristics Related to Health Care of Children and Families—cont'd

Cultural group	Health beliefs	Health and diet practices
Puerto Rican	Subscribe to the "hot-cold" theory of causation of illness Believe some illness caused by evil spirits and forces	Infrequent use of health care systems Seek folk healers—use of herbs, rituals Consult spiritualist medium for mental disorders *Santeria* is system and practitioners are called *santeros* Treatments classified as "hot" or "cold"
Cuban-American†	Prevention and good nutrition are related to good health	Diligent users of the medical model, in part because of aggressive public health practices on the island prior to and after the revolution Eclectic health-seeking practices, including preventive measures, extensive use of the medical model, and, in some instances, folk medicine of both religious and nonreligious origins; home remedies; in many instances seek assistance of *santeros* (Afro-Cuban healers) and spiritualists to complement medical treatment Nutrition is important; parents show overconcern with eating habits of their children and spend a considerable part of the budget on food; traditional Cuban diet is rich in meat and starch; consumption of fresh vegetables added in U.S.
Native American (numerous tribes)	Believe health is state of harmony with nature and universe Respect of bodies through proper management All disorders believed to have aspects of supernatural Violation of a restriction or prohibition thought to cause illness Fear of witchcraft May carry objects believed to guard against witchcraft Theology and medicine strongly interwoven	Medicine persons: Altruistic persons who must use powers in purely positive ways Persons capable of both good and evil—perform negative acts against enemies Diviner-diagnosticians—diagnose but do not have powers or skill to implement medical treatment Specialists—use herbs and curative but nonsacred medical procedures Medicine persons—use herbs and ritual Singers—cure by the power of their song obtained from supernatural beings, effect cures by laying on of hands

†This section was written by Mercedes Sandaval, Ph.D.

Family relationships	Communication	Comments
Family usually large and home-centered—the core of existence	May use nonstandard English	Relaxed sense of time
Father has complete authority in family—family provider and decision-maker	Spanish speaking or bilingual	Pay little attention to *exact* time of day
Wife and children subordinate to father	Strong sense of family privacy—may view questions regarding family as impudent	Suspicious and fearful of hospitals
Children valued—seen as a gift from God		
Children taught to obey and respect parents; corporal punishment to ensure obedience		
Strong family ties with mother and father kinships	Most are bilingual (English/Spanish) except for segments of the senior population	In less than 30 years Cubans have been able to obtain a higher standard of living than other Hispanic groups in U.S.
Children supported and assisted by parents long after becoming adults		Have been able to retain many of their former social institutions: bilingual and private schools, clinics, social clubs, the family as an extended network of support, etc.
Elderly cared for at home		Many do not feel discriminated against nor harbor feelings of inferiority with respect to Anglo-Americans or "mainstream" population
Extended family structure — usually includes relatives from both sides of family	Most continue to speak their Indian language as well as English	Time orientation—present
Elder members assume leadership roles	Nonverbal communication	Respect for age
		Going to hospital associated with illness or disease; therefore may not seek prenatal care since pregnancy viewed as natural process

the development of customs and rituals (refer to Figure 7-6).

Spiritual beliefs of clients are often not addressed in the clinical setting. This is unfortunate because these beliefs frequently comfort distressed individuals and help them cope with illness and crisis. Involving spiritual leaders in a client's care and allowing clients to verbalize their feelings about their religious values can strengthen the relationships between health care professionals and clients and can promote effective decision-making about needed health care services.

Process Parameters for Family Assessment

Basic to the understanding of family functioning is the analysis of family processes. Family processes are methods used by families to determine how their structure evolves, how decisions are made, and how the family carries out its functions to maintain stability and to promote growth within the family unit.

There are several parameters to consider when assessing family processes:

1. How the family integrates its role relationships
2. How the family uses information from the environment
3. How the family adapts to changes within the family system and its environment
4. How the family makes and implements decisions
5. How the family deals with conflict or disagreement
6. How the family maintains the integrity of the family unit and the personal autonomy of family members

Family health is a function of process rather than outcome. It is family process that helps the family manage stress, survive crises, deal with conflict, and organize itself so that it can achieve its goals. Usually, however, a family comes to the attention of the health care professional because its outputs are inadequate or because the family perceives difficulty in meeting its goals. When assessing family functioning it is extremely important to examine process variables as well as outcomes desired by a family; family processes frequently need to be altered before desired outcomes can be reached.

Direct observation of the family system is the best way to gain an understanding of family processes. This is especially true during times of crisis, because it is during these periods that functional or dysfunctional behaviors become more evident. Decision-making and communication patterns should be analyzed carefully in an assessment of family processes. Chapter 8 presents the concepts of stress and crisis and examines some of the factors that affect decision-making when people are distressed. Parameters to observe when looking at family communication patterns have been discussed previously in this chapter. Publications by Ackerman (1959, 1970), Bowen (1973), Haley (1971), Jackson (1968), Minuchin (1974), Satir (1972), and Watzlawick, Beavin, and Jackson (1967) provide an in-depth analysis of family processes and are very useful references for practitioners who view the family as their unit of service.

Table 7-5 presents characteristics that reflect dysfunctional processes in a family unit. These behaviors were identified by the North American Nursing Diagnosis Association, a national organization established to develop standard nursing diagnoses for the profession. Having an understanding of these behaviors assists the community health nurse in identifying families who need nursing intervention.

TOOLS THAT FACILITATE THE FAMILY ASSESSMENT PROCESS

A community health nurse can use a variety of tools to facilitate family assessment. Some of these tools are discussed below. They are designed to help the practitioner elicit data about certain aspects of family structure, function, and process and to aid the health professional in determining major family concerns, needs, and strengths. Assessment tools, however, are only guides, and before using them one needs to have an understanding of family theory and of communication processes that enhance effective nurse-client relationships.

Family Assessment Guides

Many community health agencies have developed family assessment guides so that staff members can focus attention on family functioning in addition to the health status of individual family members. Appendix 7-1 is an example of such a tool. When completed it provides a quick visual summary of family strengths, family behaviors that need to be altered, and anticipated guidance needs.

7-5　The North American Nursing Diagnosis Association: Altered Family Processes

Diagnostic label	Definition	Etiology/related factors	Defining characteristics
Altered family processes	Inability of family system (household members) to meet needs of members, carry out family functions, or maintain communications for mutual growth and maturation	Situational crisis or transition Developmental crisis or transition	Inability of family members to relate to each other for mutual growth and maturation Failure to send and receive clear messages Poorly communicated family rules, rituals, symbols; unexamined myths Unhealthy family decision-making processes Inability of family members to express and accept wide range of feelings Inability to accept and receive help Does not demonstrate respect for individuality and autonomy of members Rigidity in functions and roles Fails to accomplish current (or past) family developmental tasks Inappropriate (nonproductive) boundary maintenance Inability to adapt to change Inability to deal with traumatic or crisis experience constructively Parents do not demonstrate respect for each other's views on child-rearing practices Inappropriate (nonproductive) level and direction of energy Inability to meet needs of members (physical, security, emotional, spiritual) Family uninvolved in community activities

From Gordon M: *Manual of nursing diagnosis 1993-1994*, St. Louis, 1993, Mosby, pp. 307, 309.

Generally, family assessment guides examine both the family's relationships with its environment and its internal functioning. It is extremely important when designing guides to facilitate the data collection process to take into consideration the need to identify both functional and dysfunctional behaviors within a family system. It is very easy to focus only on family problems. When this is done, areas of family dysfunctioning may be overemphasized. This can have a devastating affect on the family and the nurse and lead to frustration, discouragement, and a feeling of hopelessness for all. Nurses who are unable to see family strengths "burn out" quickly; families who never receive positive feedback for what they are handling well question their ability to adequately maintain themselves and often become dependent on others for decision-making.

Before constructing a family assessment guide, an agency needs to make a careful analysis of its philosophy of nursing practice so that it is reflected in the assessment tool being developed. For instance, a belief in preventive health behavior would be operationalized if staff members were encouraged to discern anticipatory guidance needs and then to plan nursing intervention strategies that might prevent future health problems. Perhaps hazards in the environment have not yet caused an accident; however, if hazards, such as medications left where small children can reach them, are not eliminated a serious health problem may result. Health counseling assists parents in realizing how much of a threat medication might be to small children, and it may be the impetus that influences preventive health changes in a family's environment.

The community health nurse should be allowed to use a variety of assessment methodologies when implementing an agency's philosophy of practice. If a tool interferes with a practitioner's clinical style it is highly unlikely to be used. Or, if the practitioner does attempt to use it even though it does not relate to the practitioner's frame of reference, the nurse-client relationship may be distorted. Family assessment tools should be used to provide guidelines for data collection only. They should not tie a nurse into a particular interactive style or theoretical framework for family assessment.

A family assessment tool must be easily used by the practitioner. Tools that take a minimal amount of time to complete and that provide a composite picture of family strengths and needs are most beneficial. Many community health nurses have heavy caseload demands and become frustrated if asked to fill out a lengthy assessment form.

Family assessment tools are useful only when the practitioner has the theoretical background to handle them. Knowledge of role theory, cultural values and attitudes, family decision-making, and concepts of stress and crisis is essential for effective use of an assessment guide. Assessment tools can never replace a genuine understanding of theories that analyze family functioning or that describe how nurse-client interactions affect the therapeutic process.

Genograms

A genogram is a tool that aids the community health nurse in collecting generational information about family structure and processes. It visually portrays to the nurse and the family how the family has evolved. It very quickly helps the community health nurse to identify the relationships between significant family members, the health status of individual family members, and the family's reactions to sociocultural and spiritual variables that have affected their lives.

Figure 7-7 is a partial genogram constructed by a community health nurse during her sixth home visit to the Z. family. Before doing the genogram the nurse had been helping the family members deal with their feelings about the son's recent diagnosis of allergies. She identified a discrepancy in how each parent viewed the son's health status. Wondering whether this was related to previous life experiences, the nurse completed a genogram with the family. By doing this the nurse was able to trace each parent's attitudes about health and illness. She was also able to identify that the family lacked a significant support system, that both parents had had an unhappy childhood, and that they were afraid that they were "going to raise their son wrong." In addition, she discovered that the family was having difficulty adjusting to recent role changes and that all family members had unresolved feelings about the death of two children in the family. The community health nurse who constructed the genogram shown in Figure 7-7 found that this tool helped both her and the family to focus more clearly on current significant events and gain an appreciation for how past happenings were influencing present health behavior. The development of the genogram provided structure for the interviewing process and helped the community health nurse obtain an extensive family history very rapidly.

Genograms schematically depict a family tree. Geneticists, physicians, and nurse clinicians have used them to trace genetic disorders in families. They are now being used by health care professionals to integrate health and sociocultural data. A family tree drawn by a professional differs from one drawn by a family in that the professional uses theory as a basis to elicit data about family structure, function, and process. Normally a family tree done by a layperson illustrates only structural information.

The interview process is the most critical component to consider when completing a genogram. If information concerning child-rearing practices, health beliefs and attitudes, significant social data, and traditions passed on from one generation to another is not obtained, the genogram has very little meaning. Completing the actual drawing of a genogram takes minimal skill; focusing the conversation on relevant aspects of family functioning requires not only interviewing skill but also knowledge of family dynamics.

Eco-Map

An eco-map is another tool used by health care professionals that schematically portrays factual data about family relationships. It helps the family and the nurse to visually analyze a family's interactions with its external environment. Presented in Figure 7-8 is an eco-map developed by Dr. Ann Hartman for workers in a child welfare practice (Hartman, 1978, p. 466). Based on a systems theoretical framework, Hartman's tool examines boundary-maintenance aspects of fam-

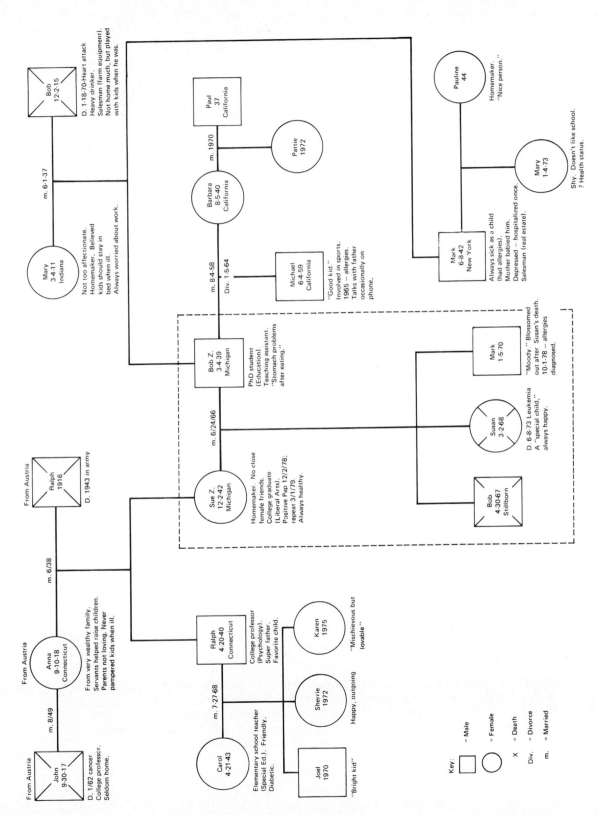

Figure 7-7 Sample genogram of the Z. family.

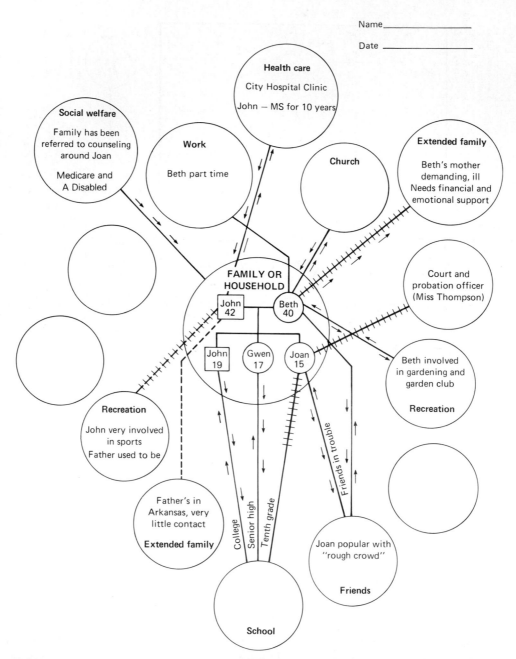

Figure 7-8   Eco-map. Fill in connections where they exist. Indicate nature of connections with a descriptive word or by drawing different kinds of lines: _____ for strong; - - - - for tenuous; ++++ for stressful. Draw arrows along lines to signify flow of energy, resources, etc. (→→→). Identify significant people and fill in empty circles as needed. (From Hartman A: Diagrammatic assessment of family relationships, *Social Casework* 59:470, 1978.)

ily functioning. It dramatically illustrates the amount of energy used by a family to maintain its system, as well as the presence or absence of situational supports and other family resources. By using this tool, for example, families can identify that their energies are being used to handle stressful encounters with external systems rather than to enhance positive, supportive relationships with others. For instance, if a family's flow of energy as depicted on the eco-map reflects only an outward directional process (→→→), the family may recognize why its goals are not being achieved.

Community health nurses have found the use of the eco-map beneficial because they are frequently involved with clients who have encounters with numerous health and welfare agencies, who have few support systems, or who "lack energy" to maintain their family system. An eco-map assists families in visualizing how their relationships with external systems are affecting their state of well-being. One community health nurse decided to use this tool with a family because its multiple relationships with agencies were unclear and because the family members were having difficulty verbalizing their feelings about their "hopeless" family situation. "We have tried everything, and still our situation gets worse." The use of the eco-map increased the family's involvement in the therapeutic process and gave them something concrete to do, which relieved at least some of their anxiety about their "hopeless" state of affairs. When the eco-map was completed it was obvious to both the nurse and the family that there were numerous stressors affecting the family's feelings about itself. The family was allowing health and social agencies to take over its affairs, extended-family members gave only negative feedback, friends seldom visited, and the family had few leisure activities. The eco-map pointed out to the family the multiple problems they were encountering and assisted the nurse in planning her intervention strategies as well.

It is impossible to function effectively in the community health setting without looking at how the family interfaces with its external environment. The eco-map enhances the community health nurse's ability to gain this type of information. It is an especially useful tool because it summarizes on one page family strengths, conflicts, and stresses in relation to its interactions with individuals and agencies outside the family system.

Family-Life Chronology

Community health nurses may encounter families who are experiencing relationship problems, a situation that makes it difficult for them to concentrate on health concerns or to take needed health actions. These families can find it hard to examine objectively what is happening in their relationships or to make a decision about seeking counseling. Satir's (1967, p. 135) family-life chronology model (Figure 7-9) helps the community health nurse and the family to identify interactive processes that have evolved. Stresses are often related only to current family changes, such as a chronic health problem, an additional family member, or financial difficulties. Helping a family's members to look at how successful they have been in handling interpersonal interactions up to this point may provide the positive reinforcement they need to examine how they can alter their current behavior to reduce existing stresses. Sometimes, however, it will be found that a family has had long-standing relationship problems. Helping family members to identify the chronic nature of their current difficulties may assist them in seeing the need for psychosocial counseling.

The process for collecting a family-life chronology is discussed in Satir's book, *Conjoint Family Therapy: A Guide to Theory and Technique* (1967). Community health nurse practitioners have found this book to be a valuable reference that helps them work more effectively with families experiencing distress in their relationships.

A community health nurse cannot ignore relationship problems when working with families in their homes. Such difficulties can disrupt all parameters of family functioning and are often the key factor in preventing a family from taking needed health action. If these difficulties are not addressed, nursing intervention strategies can be ineffective. Dealing with the symptoms of distress such as physical health problems, complaints about lack of time for leisure activities, or feelings of depression, rather than with the relationship difficulties themselves will not alter a family's functioning in any lasting way. One mother, for example, complained to the community health nurse that she had no time for herself and that she found caring for three children, 4, 6, and 8 years old, very restrictive. Suggestions by the community health nurse on how she might care for her children and still have time for leisure activities were ignored. The mother finally shared with the nurse that her husband

To mates

Asks about how they met, when they decided to marry, etc.

To wife	**To husband**
Asks how she saw her parents, her sibs, her family life	Asks how he saw his parents, his sibs, his family life
Brings chronology back to when she met her husband	Brings chronology back to when he met his wife
Asks about her expectations of marriage	Asks about his expectations of marriage

To mates
Asks about early married life; comments on influence of past

To mates as parents
Asks about their expectations of parenting; comments on the influence of the past

To child
Asks about the child's views of the parents, how he or she sees them having fun, disagreeing, etc.

To family as a whole
Reassures family that it is safe to comment; stresses need for clear communication; gives closure, points to next meeting, gives hope

Figure 7-9   Main flow of family-life chronology. (From Satir V: *Conjoint family therapy: a guide to theory and technique,* Palo Alto, Calif., 1967, Science and Behavior Books, p. 135.)

felt that "a woman's place was in the home. Even if I enrolled my 4-year-old son in a nursery school, I still could not get out of the house. My husband gets very upset if I am gone from home without him." This woman was depressed and discouraged. She loved her children but also wanted to explore adult interests; the only way she was able to accomplish this was to deal with the conflicts between herself and her husband.

The preceding situation illustrates that, in working with individual family members, a nurse must determine how other members of the family view the issues being raised. Otherwise significant data will be missed and interventions will be planned that are inappropriate to the needs of the family. It is best to obtain the ideas and opinions of all family members by seeing them together. If this cannot be arranged, asking questions such as "How does your husband react when you talk about getting a job?" provides clues about family interactions and differing value systems. It must be emphasized that family meetings can be arranged more frequently than they are; often nurses do not suggest this strategy because they do not feel comfortable dealing with family dynamics.

Recent Experience Life Change Questionnaires

Research since the early sixties has documented that significant life changes can adversely affect the health status of individuals (Rahe, 1972). The Life Change Questionnaire (refer to Table 7-6), developed by Holmes, Rahe, Masuda, and others, has been used throughout the United States and in foreign countries to demonstrate the relationships between a cluster of events requiring life changes and illness. It has been shown that individuals whose life change units (LCU) are greater than the value of 150 in a year's time are more susceptible to illness than individuals whose life change units are below this value. Studies conducted by Rahe while at the University of Washington in Seattle, for instance, demonstrated that 50% of the individuals whose life change units ranged from 150 to 300 LCU had an illness within the following year. In addition, 70% of those individuals whose LCU values exceeded 300 had an illness the following year (Rahe, 1972).

Practitioners as well as researchers have used the Life Change Questionnaire to identify persons at risk

TABLE 7-6	Life Change Events

Events	LCU values	Events	LCU values
Family		Changing to a new school	20
Death of spouse	100	Change in residence	20
Divorce	73	Major change in recreation	19
Marital separation	65	Major change in church activities	19
Death of a close family member	63	Major change in sleeping habits	16
Marriage	50	Major change in eating habits	15
Marital reconciliation	45	Vacation	13
Major change in health of family	44	Christmas	12
Pregnancy	40	Minor violations of the law	11
Addition of new family member	39		
Major change in arguments with wife	35	**Work**	
Son or daughter leaving home	29	Being fired from work	47
In-law troubles	29	Retirement from work	45
Wife starting or ending work	26	Major business adjustment	39
Major change in family get-togethers	15	Changing to different line of work	36
		Major change in work responsibilities	29
Personal		Trouble with boss	23
Detention in jail	63	Major change in working conditions	20
Major personal injury or illness	53		
Sexual difficulties	39	**Financial**	
Death of a close friend	37	Major change in financial state	38
Outstanding personal achievement	28	Mortgage or loan over $10,000	31
Start or end of formal schooling	26	Mortgage foreclosure	30
Major change in living conditions	25	Mortgage or loan less than $10,000	17
Major revision of personal habits	24		

From Rahe RH: Subjects' recent life changes and their near-future illness reports, *Ann Clin Res* 4:250-265, 1972. This study report was supported by the Bureau of Medicine and Surgery, Department of the Navy, under Research Work Unit MF51.524.002-5011-DD5G (Report No. 72-31). Opinions expressed are those of the author and are not to be construed as necessarily reflecting the official view or endorsement of the Department of the Navy.

for illness. When they discover individuals who have high LCU values, they discuss the impact of several life changes on one's health status and the importance of not making other major life changes at this time.

Increasingly, based on the recognition that the types of life-change events that produce stress vary across the life span, research is being conducted to increase the relevance of the life event questionnaire for a particular developmental age group or for specific population groups. Norbeck (1984) has modified the life event questionnaire to address the needs of adult females of childbearing age. Norbeck's modified tool deals with significant concerns of women such as having difficulties with contraception, changing child care arrangements, being the victim of violent acts (rape, assault, and so on), and parenting conflicts (Norbeck, p. 64).

Barnard's (1988) Difficult Life Circumstance (DLC) scale was designed to ascertain the existence of chronic family problems among high-risk families dealing with pregnancy. The items on the DLC scale address such things as domestic violence, child abuse, long-term illness, and problems with alcohol and drug use. Barnard found that families with a high DLC score (a score reflecting the existence of several difficult life circumstances) had less favorable maternal and family outcomes than families with a low DLC score.

Beall and Schmidt (1984) have developed a tool for

- ☐ Graduation (.57)
- ☐ Pet dies (.55)
- ☐ Fights with parents (.67)
- ☐ Getting pressure about having sex (.63)
- ☐ Caught cheating or lying repeatedly (.73)
- ☐ Getting a major illness/injury/car accident (.81)
- ☐ Becoming religious or giving up religion (.63)
- ☐ Referral to the principal's office (.47)
- ☐ Getting acne/warts (.45)
- ☐ Trouble getting a date when it was not a problem before (.61)
- ☐ Problems developed with teachers/employers (.59)
- ☐ Making career decisions (college, majors training, etc.) (.64)
- ☐ Starting to go to weekend parties/rock concerts (.35)
- ☐ First day of school (.37)
- ☐ Going on first date/starting to date (.53)
- ☐ Death of a parent/guardian (.95)
- ☐ Not getting promoted to next grade (.76)
- ☐ Getting caught using drugs (.86)
- ☐ Getting attacked/raped/beat up (.84)
- ☐ Getting a ticket or other minor problems with law (.58)
- ☐ Parents getting a divorce/separation (.83)
- ☐ Getting expelled/suspended (.71)
- ☐ Fad pressure (.43)
- ☐ Breaking up with boy/girlfriend (.57)
- ☐ Getting minor illness (cold, flu, etc.) (.30)
- ☐ Arguments with peers/brothers/sisters (.46)
- ☐ Starting to perform (speeches, presentations, musical or drama performances) (.60)
- ☐ Getting a bad report card (.59)

- ☐ Getting fired from a job (.63)
- ☐ Going into debt (.72)
- ☐ Being stereotyped/discriminated/having bad rumors spread about you (.70)
- ☐ Death of a close family member (.94)
- ☐ Death of a boy/girlfriend/close friend (.94)
- ☐ Getting V.D. (.86)
- ☐ Getting someone pregnant/getting pregnant (.92)
- ☐ Taking finals/SAT test (.61)
- ☐ Moving to a different town/school/making new friends (.67)
- ☐ Getting a car (.35)
- ☐ Trying to get a job/job interview (.49)
- ☐ Getting an award, office, etc. (.36)
- ☐ Making a team (drill, athletic, debate) (.44)
- ☐ Getting married (.73)
- ☐ Getting beat up by parents (.86)
- ☐ Taking the driver license test (.55)
- ☐ Getting a new addition to the family (.45)
- ☐ Going to the dentist or doctor (.37)
- ☐ Going to jail/reform school (.88)
- ☐ Starting to use drugs (.82)
- ☐ Getting braces (.45)
- ☐ Going on a diet (.41)
- ☐ Losing or gaining weight (.49)
- ☐ Changing exercise habits (.21)
- ☐ Pressure to take drugs (.71)
- ☐ Moving out of the house (.56)
- ☐ Falling in love (.66)
- ☐ Getting a bad haircut (.57)
- ☐ Getting glasses (.49)
- ☐ Family member moving out (.47)

Figure 7-10 Youth adaptation rating scale. The number after each item is the ratio value or degree of severity. This ratio value was determined by dividing the total value for each item by the highest possible score. Events with a high ratio value produce greater stress and require a greater degree of adaptation than do events with a lower ratio value. (From Beall S and Schmidt G: Development of a youth adaptation rating scale, *J School Health* 54(5):197-200, 1984. Copyright 1984, American School Health Association, Kent, Ohio 44240.)

use with adolescents (refer to Figure 7-10). The Youth Adaptation Rating Scale is not designed to be used as a predictor of illness. Rather, it was developed "to measure the causes of adolescent adaptation and to provide parents, teachers, and adolescents with a clearer perception of events that may cause stress during the adolescent years" (Beall and Schmidt, p. 197). This tool was tested in a variety of settings and by six ethnic groups. Adolescents were asked to rank each item on the tool using a five-point descriptive scale with a zero indicating that the event was not stressful at all and the number five reflecting a very stressful event that would require a major change in one's life. No significant differences existed between the ethnic groups or the adolescents from communities of different sizes. It was found, however, that the need for adaptation or the recognition of that need becomes more evident as the adolescent grows older and matures (Beall and Schmidt, pp. 199-200).

The Life Change Questionnaire and the developmental and aggregate specific tools such as those developed by Barnard, Norbeck, and Beall and Schmidt can be used to facilitate nursing assessment as well as teaching or learning processes. Use of these tools can help community health nurses quickly discern individuals who are experiencing multiple stressors. These tools can also assist community health nurses in teaching about normative life events, which contribute to stress during a specific developmental stage, and coping strategies for dealing with stress.

Clinically it has been found that clients who have encountered several major life changes frequently do not recognize that this has happened. Life change questionnaires can help clients to visualize the relationship between their feelings of distress and the events that have been occurring in their lives. This recognition often promotes the development of effective stress management techniques.

Videotaping

Videotaping is another tool which has helped the community health nurse to identify family dynamics. It has been used in some community health nursing settings to assess family interactions when a handicapped child is performing activities of daily living. Community health nurses have used videotaping in these situations to observe simultaneously the inter-

actions of a child and family, as well as the functional capabilities of the client being assessed. It is important to observe both the client and significant others during a functional assessment, because behavior of significant others either inhibits or enhances functional capabilities.

Videotaping provides specific data about family dynamics and a child's functional abilities that are often missed during a home visit. It is easy to overlook small accomplishments of a child when other things are occurring in the environment. It is equally easy to miss nurse or family behaviors that negatively affect a child's performance. For instance, use of videotaping enabled one nurse to identify that she had not given the 4-year-old child she was assessing sufficient time to complete the tasks she asked him to perform. A repeat assessment on her next home visit provided her with more accurate data in relation to the child's level of functioning. Without videotaping, this child's level of performance would have been assessed inappropriately.

Families are usually receptive to videotaping, especially when the community health nurse explains that a more accurate evaluation of a child's abilities may be obtained through the use of this tool. Assuring them that confidentiality will be maintained also relieves their anxiety.

A videotaped child assessment can be very motivating to families because it dramatically illustrates a child's strengths and needs. Videotaping helps a family to identify positive and negative behaviors that are promoting or inhibiting a child's growth. The impact of seeing actual behaviors is not quickly forgotten.

Summary

Despite its changing nature, the family is still considered the basic unit of service in community health nursing settings. Historical evidence from clinical practice and research has sufficiently demonstrated that family-centered nursing services more effectively meet the needs of individuals, families, and communities than do services delivered only to individual clients. Viewing the family from the traditional perspective, however, is no longer appropriate because alternative family life-styles and culturally diverse family forms are becoming more evident in our society. The nuclear family unit is no longer the only acceptable form of family life.

It is essential for community health nurses to have an understanding of family theory in order to implement a family-centered preventive health approach to nursing care. Theory helps the practitioner to assess family structure, function, and process in an organized and logical fashion. It provides parameters to consider when one is collecting data about client situations. It assists in explaining the phenomena that are occurring within a family, which in turn helps one to plan effective intervention strategies.

Tools such as the genogram, the eco-map, and the Life Change Questionnaire are available for facilitating the family assessment process. These tools do not, however, take the place of a genuine understanding of family dynamics. They only provide guidelines for the organization and collection of data.

◀ *An Exercise in Critical Thinking* ▶

Given the following case situations, discuss how a nursing assessment from a holistic family perspective would differ from a nursing assessment directed toward the identified client (Sally Huling/Cissy Jones).

You are visiting Sally Huling, a 16-year-old teenager recently referred to the Visiting Nurse Association following her hospitalization for regulation of an unstable diabetic condition. Sally lives with her parents, a 10-year-old brother, and a 5-year-old sister in a four-bedroom, well-kept home in a middle-class neighborhood. While she was hospitalized both Sally and her family expressed anxiety about Sally's diabetic condition.

You are visiting Cissy Jones, age 2, who was referred for community health nurse follow-up by the nurse in the well-child clinic because of notable strabismus, and her family. The Jones family's income is minimal. They have inadequate furniture and clothing for their son, age one month. Although Mrs. Jones appears tired upon your first home visit, she is anxious to talk about resources for obtaining eye care for Cissy.

APPENDIX 7-1
Bloch's Ethnic/Cultural Assessment Guide

Categories	Guideline questions/instructions	Data collected
Cultural		
Ethnic origin	Does the patient identify with a particular ethnic group (e.g., Puerto Rican, African)?	
Race	What is the patient's racial background (e.g., Black, Filipino, American Indian)?	
Place of birth	Where was the patient born?	
Relocations	Where has he lived (country, city)? During what years did patient live there and for how long? Has he moved recently?	
Habits, customs, values, and beliefs	Describe habits, customs, values, and beliefs patient holds or practices that affect his attitude toward birth, life, death, health and illness, time orientation, and health care system and health care providers. What is degree of belief and adherence by patient to his overall cultural system?	
Behaviors valued by culture	How does patient value privacy, courtesy, respect for elders, behaviors related to family roles and sex roles, and work ethics?	
Cultural sanctions and restrictions	*Sanctions*—What is accepted behavior by patient's cultural group regarding expression of emotions and feelings, religious expressions, and response to illness and death?	

Bloch's Ethnic/Cultural Assessment Guide—cont'd

Categories	Guideline questions/instructions	Data collected
Language and communication processes: Language(s) and/or dialect(s) spoken Language barriers	*Restrictions*—Does patient have any restrictions related to sexual matters, exposure of body parts, certain types of surgery (e.g., hysterectomy), discussion of dead relatives, and discussion of fears related to the unknown? What are some overall cultural characteristics of patient's language and communication process? Which language(s) and/or dialect(s) does patient speak most frequently? Where? At home or at work? Which language does patient predominantly use in thinking? Does patient need bilingual interpreter in nurse-patient interactions? Is patient non–English-speaking or limited English-speaking? Is patient able to read and/or write in English?	
Communication process	What are rules (linguistics) and modes (style) of communication process (e.g., "honorific" concept of showing "respect or deference" to others using words only common to specific ethnic/cultural group)? Is there need for variation in technique of communicating and interviewing to accommodate patient's cultural background (e.g., tempo of conversation, eye/body contact, topic restrictions, norms of confidentiality, and style of explanation)? Are there any conflicts in verbal and nonverbal interactions between patient and nurse? How does patient's nonverbal communication process compare with other ethnic/cultural groups, and how does it affect patient's response to nursing and medical care? Are there any variations between patient's interethnic and interracial communication process or intracultural and intraracial communication process [e.g., ethnic minority patient and White middle-class nurse, ethnic minority patient and ethnic minority nurse; beliefs, attitudes, values, role variations, stereotyping (perceptions and prejudice]?	
Healing beliefs and practices Cultural healing system	What cultural healing system does the patient predominantly adhere to (e.g., Asian healing system, Raza/Latina Curanderismo)? What religious healing system does the patient predominantly adhere to (e.g., Seventh Day Adventist, West African voodoo, Fundamentalist sect, Pentacostal)?	
Cultural health beliefs	Is illness explained by the germ theory or cause-effect relationship, presence of evil spirits, imbalance between "hot" and "cold" (yang and yin in Chinese culture), or disequilibrium between nature and man? Is good health related to success, ability to work or fulfill roles, reward from God, or balance with nature?	
Cultural health practices	What types of cultural healing practices does person from ethnic/cultural group adhere to? Does he use healing remedies to cure *natural* illnesses caused by the external environment [e.g., massage to cure *empacho* (a ball of food clinging to stomach wall), wearing of talismans or charms for protection against illness]?	

Continued

Bloch's Ethnic/Cultural Assessment Guide—cont'd

Categories	Guideline questions/instructions	Data collected
Cultural healers	Does patient rely on cultural healers [e.g., medicine men forAmerican Indian, Curandero for Raza/Latina, Chinese herbalist, hougan (voodoo priest), spiritualist, or minister for Black American]?	
Nutritional variables or factors	What nutritional variables or factors are influenced by the patient's ethnic/cultural background?	
Characteristics of food preparation and consumption	What types of food preferences and restrictions, meaning of foods, style of food preparation and consumption, frequency of eating, time of eating, and eating utensils are culturally determined for patient? Are there any religious influences on food preparation and consumption?	
Influences from external environment	What modifications if any did the ethnic group patient identifies with have to make in its food practices in White dominant American society? Are there any adaptations of food customs and beliefs from rural setting to urban setting?	
Patient education needs	What are some implications of diet planning and teaching to patient who adheres to cultural practices concerning foods?	
Sociological		
Economic status	Who is principal wage earner in patient's family? What is total annual income (approximately) of family? What impact does economic status have on life-style, place of residence, living conditions, and ability to obtain health services?	
Educational status	What is highest educational level obtained? Does patient's educational background influence his ability to understand how to seek health services, literature on health care, patient teaching experiences, and any written material patient is exposed to in health care setting (e.g., admission forms, patient care forms, teaching literature, and lab test forms)?	
	Does patient's educational background cause him to feel inferior or superior to health care personnel in health care setting?	
Social network	What is patient's social network (kinship, peer, and cultural healing networks)? How do they influence health or illness status of patient?	
Family as supportive group	Does patient's family feel need for continuous presence in patient's clinical setting (is this an ethnic/cultural characteristic)? How is family valued during illness or death?	
	How does family participate in patient's nursing care process (e.g., giving baths, feeding, using touch as support [cultural meaning], supportive presence)?	
	How does ethnic/cultural family structure influence patient response to health or illness (e.g., roles, beliefs, strengths, weaknesses, and social class)?	
	Are there any key family roles characteristic of a specific ethnic/cultural group (e.g., grandmother in Black and some American Indian families), and can these key persons be a resource for health personnel?	
	What role does family play in health promotion or cause of illness (e.g., would family be intermediary group in patient interactions with health personnel and making decisions regarding his care)?	

APPENDIX 7-1
Bloch's Ethnic/Cultural Assessment Guide—cont'd

Categories	Guideline questions/instructions	Data collected
Supportive institutions in ethnic/cultural community	What influence do ethnic/cultural institutions have on patient receiving health services (i.e., institutions such as Organization of Migrant Workers, NAACP, Black Political Caucus, churches, schools, Urban League, community clinics)?	
Institutional racism	How does institutional racism in health facilities influence patient's response to receiving health care?	
Psychological		
Self-concept (identity)	Does patient show strong racial/cultural identity? How does this compare to that of other racial/cultural groups or to members of dominant society? What factors in patient's development helped to shape his self-concept (e.g., family, peers, society labels, external environment, institutions, racism)? How does patient deal with stereotypical behavior from health professionals? What is impact of racism on patient from distinct ethnic/cultural group (e.g., social anxiety, noncompliance to health care process in clinical settings, avoidance of utilizing or participating in health care institutions)? Does ethnic/cultural background have impact on how patient relates to body image change resulting from illness or surgery (e.g., importance to appearance and roles in cultural group)? Any adherence or identification with ethnic/cultural "group" identity? (e.g., solidarity, "we" concept)?	
Mental and behavioral processes and characteristics of ethnic/cultural group	How does patient relate to his external environment in clinical setting (e.g., fears, stress, and adaptive mechanisms characteristic of a specific ethnic/cultural group)? Any variations based on the life span? What is patient's ability to relate to persons outside of his ethnic/cultural group (health personnel)? Is he withdrawn, verbally or nonverbally expressive, negative or positive, feeling mentally or physically inferior or superior? How does patient deal with feelings of loss of dignity and respect in clinical setting?	
Religious influences on psychological effects of health/illness	Does patient's religion have a strong impact on how he relates to health/illness influences or outcomes (e.g., death/chronic illness, cause and effect of illness, or adherence to nursing/medical practices)? Do religious beliefs, sacred practices, and talismans play a role in treatment of disease? What is role of significant religious persons during health/illness (e.g., Black ministers, Catholic priests, Buddhist monks, Islamic imams)?	
Psychological/cultural response to stress and discomfort of illness	Based on ethnic/cultural background, does patient exhibit any variations in psychological response to pain or physical disability of disease processes?	

Continued

APPENDIX 7-1

Bloch's Ethnic/Cultural Assessment Guide—cont'd

Categories	Guidelines questions/instructions	Data collected
Biological/Physiological (Consideration of *norms* for different ethnic/cultural groups)		
Racial-anatomical characteristics	Does patient have any distinct racial characteristics (e.g., skin color, hair texture and color, color of mucous membranes)? Does patient have any variations in anatomical characteristics (e.g., body structure [height and weight] more prevalent for ethnic/cultural group, skeletal formation [pelvic shape, especially for obstetrical evaluation], facial shape and structure [nose, eye shape, facial contour], upper and lower extremities)? How do patient's racial and anatomical characteristics affect his self-concept and the way others relate to him? Does variation in racial-anatomical characteristics affect physical evaluations and physical care, skin assessment based on color, and variations in hair care and hygienic practices?	
Growth and development patterns	Are there any distinct growth and development characteristics that vary with patient's ethnic/cultural background (e.g., bone, density, fatfolds, motor ability)? What factors are important for nutritional assessment, neurological and motor assessment, assessment of bone deterioration in disease process or injury, evaluation of newborns, evaluation of intellectual status, or capacity in relationship to motor/sensory development in children? How do these differ in ethnic/cultural groups?	
Variations in body systems	Are there any variations in body systems for patient from distinct ethnic/cultural group (e.g., gastrointestinal disturbance with lactose intolerance in Blacks, nutritional intake of cultural foods causing adverse effects on gastrointestinal tract and fluid and electrolyte system, and variations in chemical and hematological systems [certain blood types prevalent in particular ethnic/cultural groups])?	
Skin and hair physiology, mucous membranes	How does skin color variation influence assessment of skin color changes (e.g., jaundice, cyanosis, ecchymosis, erythema, and its relationship to disease processes)? What are methods of assessing skin color changes (comparing variations and similarities between different ethnic groups)? Are there conditions of hypopigmentation and hyperpigmentation (e.g., vitiligo, mongolian spots, albinism, discoloration caused by trauma)? Why would these be more striking in some ethnic groups? Are there any skin conditions more prevalent in a distinct ethnic group (e.g., keloids in Blacks)? Is there any correlation between oral and skin pigmentation and their variations among distinct racial groups when doing assessment of oral cavity (e.g., leukoedema is normal occurrence in Blacks)?	

APPENDIX 7-1
Bloch's Ethnic/Cultural Assessment Guide—cont'd

Categories	Guidelines questions/instructions	Data collected
Diseases more prevalent among ethnic/cultural group	What are variations in hair texture and color among racially different groups? Ask patient about preferred hair care methods or any racial/cultural restrictions (e.g., not washing "hot-combed" hair while in clinical setting, not cutting very long hair of Raza/Latina patients). Are there any variations in skin care methods (e.g., using Vaseline on Black skin)? Are there any specific diseases or conditions that are more prevalent for a specific ethnic/cultural group (e.g., hypertension, sickle cell anemia, G6-PD, lactose intolerance)? Does patient have any socioenvironmental diseases common among ethnic/cultural groups [e.g., lead paint poisoning, poor nutrition, overcrowding (prone to tuberculosis), alcoholism resulting from psychological despair and alienation from dominant society, rat bites, poor sanitation]?	
Diseases ethnic/cultural group has increased resistance to	Are there any diseases that patient has increased resistance to because of racial/cultural background (e.g., skin cancer in Blacks)?	

From Bloch B: Bloch's assessment guide for ethnic/cultural variations. In Orque MS, Bloch B, and Monrroy LSA, eds: *Ethnic nursing care: a multicultural approach*, St Louis, 1983, Mosby, pp. 63-69.

APPENDIX 7-2
Family Assessment Guide

Family name _____ Family ID no. _____

Source of referral _____

Reason for referral _____

Occupational status _____

Health insurance _____

Medical emergency plan _____

Preventive health care _____

Family composition: Map family constellation; include health problems of individual members.

Date		Assessment parameters	Rating		Significant data
1st	2d		1st	2d	
		1. *Structural characteristics* a. Financial resources b. Educational experiences c. Allocation of family and personal roles d. Division of labor e. Distribution of power and authority			

Continued

Family Assessment Guide—cont'd

Date		Assessment parameters	Rating		Significant data
1st	2d		1st	2d	
		f. Cultural influences			
		(1) Health beliefs and attitudes			
		(2) Family goals			
		(3) Norms for social behavior			
		(4) Spiritual beliefs			
		(5) Beliefs about folk diseases and medicine			
		g. Activities of daily living			
		(1) Dietary habits			
		(2) Child-rearing practices			
		(3) Housekeeping			
		(4) Sleeping arrangements			
		(5) Laundry facilities			
		(6) Transportation			
		(7) Care of ill family members			
		(8) Knowledge of health problems			
		(9) Understanding of health promotion practices			
		2. *Process characteristics*			
		a. Atmosphere of home			
		b. Communication patterns			
		c. Decision-making processes			
		(1) How decisions made			
		(2) How decisions implemented			
		d. Conflict negotiation			
		e. Achievement of developmental tasks			
		f. Adaptation to change			
		g. Autonomy of individual family members			
		3. *Relationships with external systems*			
		a. How family boundaries established			
		b. Use of information from environment			
		c. Contact with extended families			
		d. Interactions with friends and neighbors			
		e. Attitudes about community systems			
		(1) Health			
		(2) Welfare			
		(3) Educational			
		(4) Others (describe)			
		f. Use of the referral process			
		(1) Ability to seek assistance			
		(2) Level of independence			
		4. *Environmental characteristics*			
		a. Neighborhood			
		(1) Accessibility of facilities to meet basic needs			
		(2) Availability of recreational, educational, religious, and other resources			

APPENDIX 7-2
Family Assessment Guide—cont'd

Date			Rating		
1st	**2d**	**Assessment parameters**	**1st**	**2d**	**Significant data**

		(3) Safety (physical and psychosocial)
		b. Housing
		   (1) Suitability in relation to family needs
		   (2) Condition of structural components
		   (3) Suitability of home furnishings
		   (4) Sanitation (water source and sewage and garbage disposal and housekeeping practices)
		   (5) Accident hazards
		   (6) Barriers to family mobility			

Professionals and volunteers working with family (identify person and agency)

Summary of family strengths (based on categories rated No. 1)

Description of family priorities and assistance desired

Specific factors to consider when developing and implementing a management plan

Assessor _____ Date _____
Assessor _____ Date _____
Assessor _____ Date _____

Note: Code for recording assessment data—use a different color ink for the first and second assessment or rating (generally it takes several home visits to complete a family assessment). Rating scale: 1 = strength; 2 = problem; 3 = anticipatory guidance warranted; 4 = problem—family does not wish to change this area of functioning at this time; 5 = not applicable. Family functioning should be rated every 4 months to assist in evaluating family progress and nursing intervention strategies.

References

Ackerman NW, ed: *The psychodynamics of family life: diagnosis and treatment of family relationships,* New York, 1959, Basic Books.

Ackerman NW, ed: *Family process,* New York, 1970, Basic Books.

Ahrons CR: The binuclear family: two households, one family, *Alternative Lifestyles* 2:449-515, 1979.

Aldous J: *Family careers: developmental change in families,* New York, 1978, Wiley.

Artinian NT: Philosophy of science and family nursing theory development. In Whall AL and Fawcett J: *Family theory development in nursing: state of the science and art,* Philadelphia, 1991, FA. Davis, pp. 43-54.

Baca JE: Some health beliefs of the Spanish speaking. In Reinhardt A and Quinn M, eds: *Family-centered community nursing: a sociocultural framework,* St. Louis, 1973, Mosby.

Bane MJ: *Here to stay—American families in the twentieth century,* New York, 1976, Basic Books.

Barnard KE: MCN keys to research: the family as a unit of measurement, *MCN* 9:21, 1984.

Barnard KE: Difficult life circumstances (DLC). In Krentz LG, ed: *Nursing and the promotion/protection of family health: workshop proceedings,* Portland, Ore., September 1988, Oregon Health Sciences University.

Beall S and Schmidt G: Development of a youth adaptation rating scale, *J School Health* 54:197-200, 1984.

Beavers WR: *Psychotherapy and growth: a family systems perspective,* New York, 1977, Brunner/Mazel.

Bengtson UL and Dannefer D: Families, work, and aging: implications of disordered cohort flow for the twenty-first century. In Ward RA and Tobin SS, eds: *Health in aging: sociological issues and policy directions,* New York, 1987, Springer.

Berardo FM: Decade preview: some trends and directions for family research and theory in the 1980s, *J Marriage Family* 42:723-728, 1980.

Bernard J: The adjustments of married mates. In Christensen HT, ed: *Handbook of marriage and the family,* Chicago, 1964, Rand McNally, pp. 675-739.

Bloch B: Bloch's assessment guide for ethnic/cultural variations. In Orque MS, Bloch B, and Monrroy LSA, eds: *Ethnic nursing care: a multicultural approach,* St. Louis, 1983, Mosby, pp. 49-75.

Bloch B: Nursing care of Black patients. In Orque MS, Bloch B, and Monrroy LSA, eds: *Ethnic nursing care: a multicultural approach,* St. Louis, 1983, Mosby, pp. 81-114.

Bomar PJ, ed: *Nurses and family health promotion: concepts, assessment, and interventions,* Baltimore, 1989, Williams & Wilkins.

Bowen M: Toward the differentiation of a self in one's own family. In Framo JL, ed: *Family interaction: a dialogue between family researchers and family therapists.* New York, 1973, Springer.

Bowen M: Italian Americans. In Giger JV and Davidhizar RE: *Transcultural nursing: assessment and intervention,* St. Louis, 1991, Mosby, pp. 293-314.

Bredemeir HC and Stephenson RN: *The analysis of social systems,* New York, 1965, Holt.

Briar S: The family as an organization: an approach to family diagnosis and treatment, *Soc Service Rev* 38:247-255, 1964.

Broderick CB: Beyond the five conceptual frameworks: a decade of development in family theory, *J Marriage Family* 33:139-159, 1971.

Brownlee AT: *Community, culture and care: a cross-cultural guide for health workers,* St. Louis, 1978, Mosby.

Burr WR and Leigh GK: Famology: a new discipline, *J Marriage Family* 45:467-480, 1983.

Castles MR: Game theory as a conceptual framework for nursing practice. In Hymovich DP and Barnard MU, eds: *Family health care,* New York, 1973, McGraw-Hill.

Char EL: The Chinese American. In Clark AL, ed: *Culture and child bearing,* Philadelphia, 1981, F.A. Davis.

Chen-Louie T: Nursing care of Chinese American patients. In Orque MS, Bloch B, and Monrroy LSA, eds: *Ethnic nursing care: a multicultural approach,* St. Louis, 1983, Mosby, pp. 183-218.

Children's Defense Fund: *The state of America's children 1992,* Washington, D.C., 1992, The Fund.

Chow E: Cultural health traditions: Asian perspectives. In Branch MF and Paxton PP, eds: *Providing safe nursing care for ethnic people of color,* New York, 1976, Appleton-Century-Crofts, pp. 99-114.

Christensen HT, ed: *Handbook of marriage and the family,* Chicago, 1964, Rand McNally.

Churchman CW: *The systems approach,* New York, 1968, Dell.

Clemen SJ: *Introduction to health care facility: food services administration,* University Park, Penn., 1974, Pennsylvania State University Press.

Danielson CB, Hamel-Bissell, and Winstead-Fry: *Families, health and illness: perspectives on coping and intervention,* St. Louis, 1993, Mosby.

Duvall EM and Miller BC: *Marriage and family development,* ed 6, New York, 1985, Harper & Row.

Ehling MB: The Mexican American (El Chicano). In Clark AL, ed: *Culture and childbearing,* Philadelphia, 1981, F.A. Davis.

Eshleman JR and Clarke JN: *Intimacy, commitments, and marriage: development of relationships.* Boston, 1978, Allyn and Bacon.

Feetham SL: Family research: issues and directions for nursing. In Werley HH and Fitzpatrick JJ, eds: *Annual review of nursing research,* vol 1, New York, 1984, Springer, pp. 3-25.

Fine MA: Families in the United States: their current status and future prospects, *Family Relations* 41:430-434, 1992.

Flanzraich M and Dunsavage I: Role reversal in abused/neglected families, *Children Today* 6:13-15, 1977.

Fong CM: Ethnicity and nursing practice, *TCN* 7:1-10, 1985.

Friedman MF: *Family nursing: theory and assessment,* ed 2, Norwalk, Conn., 1986, Appleton-Century-Crofts.

Giger JN and Davidhizar RE: *Transcultural nursing: assessment and intervention,* St. Louis, 1991, Mosby.

Gilliss CL: The family as a unit of analysis: strategies for the nurse researcher, *Adv Nurs Sci* 5(3):50-59, 1983.

Gordon M: Manual of nursing diagnosis 1993-1994, St. Louis, 1993, Mosby.

Greathouse B and Miller UG: The Black American. In Clark AL, ed: *Culture and childbearing,* Philadelphia, 1981, F.A. Davis.

Hacker S: The primary task of the health professional in dealing with adolescent sexuality, *Int J Adolescent Med Health* 1(1,2):73-80, 1985.

Haley J, ed: *Changing families,* New York, 1971, Grune & Stratton.

Hanley CH: Navajo Indians. In Giger JN and Davidhizar RE: *Transcultural nursing: assessment and intervention,* St. Louis, 1991, Mosby, pp. 215-240.

Hanson SM: Family nursing: past, present and future. In Krentz LG, ed: *Nursing of families in transition,* Portland, Ore., 1987, Oregon Health Sciences University.

Hartman A: Diagrammatic assessment of family relationships, *Soc Casework* 59:465-476, 1978.

Hashizume S and Takano J: Nursing care of South Vietnamese patients. In Orque MS, Block B, and Monrroy LSA, eds: *Ethnic nursing care: a multicultural approach,* St. Louis, 1983, Mosby, pp. 219-244.

Hill R and Hansen DA: The identification of conceptual frameworks utilized in family study, *Marriage Family Living* 22:299-311, 1960.

Holland S and Sweeney E: *Vietnamese children and families: the impact of culture,* Washington, D.C., 1985, Association for Care of Children's Health.

Hollingsworth AO, Brown LP, and Brooten DA: The refugees and childbearing: what to expect, *RN* 43:45-48, 1980.

Holman TB and Burr WR: Beyond the beyond: the growth of family theories in the 1970s, *J Marriage Family* 42:729-741, 1980.

Jackson DD, ed: *Communication, family and marriage,* vol 1, Palo Alto, Ca, 1968, Science and Behavior Books.

Jacques G: Cultural traditions: a Black perspective. In Branch MF and Paxton PP: *Providing safe nursing care for ethnic people of color,* New York, 1976, Appleton-Century-Crofts, pp. 115-124.

Kensky AD: Cultural influences on the Jewish patient. In Clemen SA and Will M, eds: *Family and community health nursing: a workbook,* Ann Arbor, 1977, University of Michigan Press.

King IM: King's theory of nursing. In Clements IW and Roberts FB: *Family health: a theoretical approach to nursing care,* New York, 1983, Wiley, pp. 177-188.

Krentz LG: *Nursing of families and the health care delivery system: workshop proceedings,* Portland, Ore., 1989, Oregon Health Sciences University.

Lacay G: The Puerto Rican in mainland America. In Clark AL, ed: *Culture and childbearing,* Philadelphia, 1981, F.A. Davis Co.

Levitan SA and Conway EA: *Families in flux: new approaches to meeting workforce challenges for child, elder, and health care in the 1990s,* Washington, D.C., 1990, The Bureau of National Affairs.

Lewis J, Beavers R, Gossett JT, and Phillips VA: *No single thread: psychological health in family systems,* New York, 1976, Brunner/Mazel.

Linton R: The natural history of the family. In Anshen RN, ed: *The family: its function and destiny,* revised ed, New York, 1959, Harper & Row.

Litman TJ: The family as a basic unit in health and medical care: a social-behavioral overview, *Soc Sci Med* 8:495-519, 1974.

Loveland-Cherry CJ: Family health promotion and health protection. In Bomar PJ: *Nurses and family health promotion: concepts, assessment and interventions,* Baltimore, 1989, Williams & Wilkins, pp. 13-25.

Minuchin S: *Families and family therapy,* Cambridge, Mass., 1974, Harvard University Press.

Monrroy LSA: Nursing care of Raza/Latina patients. In Orque MS, Bloch B, and Monrroy LSA: *Ethnic nursing care: a multicultural approach,* St. Louis, 1983, Mosby, pp. 115-148.

Murphy S: Family study and nursing research, *Image: J Nurs Scholar* 18(4):170-174, 1986.

Neuman B: Family interventions using the Betty Neuman health-care systems model. In Clements IW and Roberts FB: *Family health: a theoretical approach to nursing care,* New York, 1983, Wiley, pp. 177-188.

Norbeck J: Modification of life event questionnaires for use with female respondents, *Res Nurs Health* 7:61-71, 1984.

Nye FI: *Role structure and analysis of the family,* Beverly Hills, 1976, Sage.

Orque MS, Bloch B, and Monrroy LSA: *Ethnic nursing care: a multicultural approach,* St. Louis, 1983, Mosby.

Orque MS: Nursing care of Filipino American patients. In Orque MS, Bloch B, and Monrroy LSA: *Ethnic nursing care: a multicultural approach,* St. Louis, 1983a, Mosby, pp. 149-182.

Orque MS: Nursing care of South Vietnamese patient. In Orque MS, Bloch B, and Monrroy LSA: *Ethnic nursing care: a multicultural approach,* St. Louis, 1983b, Mosby, pp. 245-270.

Otto H: Criteria for assessing family strengths, *Family Process* 2:329-338, 1963.

Peterson R: *What are the needs of the chronic mental patients?* Presented at the APA Conference on the Chronic Mental Patient, Washington, D.C., January 11-14, 1978.

Pratt L: *Family structure and effective health behavior: the energized family,* Boston, 1976, Houghton Mifflin.

Prattes O: Beliefs of the Mexican-American family. In Hymovich D and Barnard M, eds: *Family health care,* New York, 1973, McGraw-Hill.

Rahe RH: Subjects' recent life changes and their near-future illness reports, *Ann Clin Res* 4:250-265, 1972.

Roccereto L: Selected health beliefs of Vietnamese refugees, *J School Health* 51:63-64, 1981.

Rogers ME: Science of unitary human beings: a paradigm for nursing. In Clements IW and Roberts FB: *Family health: a theoretical approach to nursing care,* New York, 1983, Wiley, pp. 219-228.

Roy C: Roy adaptation model. In Clements IW and Roberts FB: *Family health: a theoretical approach to nursing care,* New York, 1983, Wiley, pp. 255-278.

Samora J: Conceptions of health and disease among Spanish-Americans. In Martinez RH, ed: *Hispanic culture and health care: fact, fiction, folklore,* St. Louis, 1978, Mosby.

Satir V: *Conjoint family therapy: a guide to theory and technique,* Palo Alto, Calif., 1967, Science and Behavior Books.

Satir V: *Peoplemaking,* Palo Alto, Calif., 1972, Science and Behavior Books.

Satir V: You as a change agent in helping families to change. In Satir V, Stachowiak J, and Taskman H, eds: *Helping families to change,* New York, 1975, Jason Aronson.

Schor E, Starfield B, Stidley C, and Hankin J: Family health: utilization and effects of family membership, *Med Care* 25(7):616-625, 1987.

Sodetaini-Shebata AE: The Japanese American. In Clark AL, ed: *Culture and childbearing,* Philadelphia, 1981, F.A. Davis.

Spanier GB: Bequeathing family continuity, *J Marriage Family* 51(2):3-13, 1989.

Stryker SL: The interactional and situational approaches. In Christensen HT, ed: *Handbook of marriage and the family,* Chicago, 1964, Rand McNally, pp. 125-170.

Sussman MB, chairperson: *Changing families in a changing society, 1970 White House conference on Children, Forum 14 report,* Washington, D.C., 1971, U.S. Government Printing Office.

Tripp-Reimer T, Brink PJ, and Saunders JM: Cultural assessment: content and process, *Nurs Outlook* 32:78-82, 1984.

U.S. Bureau of the Census: *Marital status and living arrangements: March 1991,* current population reports, series P-20, No. 461, Washington, D.C., 1992, U.S. Government Printing Office.

U.S. Bureau of the Census: *Population profile of the United States: 1991,* current population reports, series P-23, No. 173, Washington, D.C., 1991, U.S. Government Printing Office.

U.S. Bureau of the Census: *Population profile of the United States: 1993,* current population reports, series P23-185, Washington, D.C., 1993, U.S. Government Printing Office.

U.S. Department of Health and Human Services: *Health status of minorities and low-income groups,* ed 3, Washington, D.C., 1991, U.S. Government Printing Office.

USDHHS, Maternal and Child Health Bureau: *Child health USA '91,* DHHS Pub No. (HNS-MCH 91-12, Washington, D.C., 1991, U.S. Government Printing Office.

von Bertalanffy L: *General systems theory,* New York, 1968, George Braziller.

Watzlawick P, Beavin JH, and Jackson DD: *Pragmatics of human communication: a study of interactional patterns, pathologies, and paradoxes,* New York, 1967, Norton.

Whaley LF and Wong DL: *Nursing care of infants and children,* ed 4, St. Louis, 1991, Mosby.

Whall AL: Family system theory: relationship to nursing conceptual models. In Whall AL and Fawcett J: *Family theory development in nursing: state of the science and art,* Philadelphia, 1991, F.A. Davis.

Whall AL and Fawcett J: *Family theory development in nursing: state of the science and art,* Philadelphia, 1991, F.A. Davis.

White House Conference on Families, 1978, Joint hearings before the subcommittee on Child and Human Development of the Committee on Human Resources, U.S. Senate and the Subcommittee on Select Education of the Committee on Education and Labor, House of Representatives, Ninety-fifth Congress, Washington, D.C., 1978, U.S. Government Printing Office.

Wiener N: Cybernetics in history. In Buckley W, ed: *Modern systems research for the behavioral scientist,* Chicago, 1968, Aldine.

Selected Bibliography

Allen ML, Brown P and Finlay B: *Helping children by strengthening families: a look at family,* Washington, D.C., 1992, Children's Defense Fund.

Burr WR, Hill R, Nye FI, and Reiss IL, eds: *Contemporary theories about the family, vol 2, General theories/theoretical orientations,* New York, 1979, Free Press.

Burr WR, Hill R, Nye FI, and Reiss IL, eds: *Contemporary theories about the family, vol 1: research-based theories,* New York, 1979, Free Press.

Clements IW and Roberts FB: *Family health: a theoretical approach to nursing care,* New York, 1983, Wiley.

Egan MG: A family assessment challenge: refugee youth and foster family adaptation, *TCN* 7:64-69, 1985.

Frederick RF and Herrick J: Family rules: family life styles, *Am J Orthopsychiatry* 44:61-69, 1974.

Germain CP: Cultural care: a bridge between sickness, illness, and disease, *Holistic Nurse Pract* 6:1-9, 1992.

Gilliss CL, Highley BL, Roberts BM, and Martinson IM: *Toward a science of family nursing,* Menlo Park, Calif., 1989, Addison-Wesley.

Handel G, ed: *The psycho-social interior of the family,* Chicago, 1967, Aldine-Atherton.

Hareven TR, ed: *Transitions: the family and the life course in historical perspective,* New York, 1978, Academic Press.

Hill RA: *The strengths of black families,* New York, 1972, Emerson Hall.

Hitchcock JM and Wilson HS: Personal risking: Lesbian self disclosure of sexual orientation to professional health care providers, *Nursing Research* 41:178-183, 1992.

Krause HD: "Family values" and family law reform, *J Contemporary Health Law and Policy* 9:109-128, 1993.

Lapp CA, Diemert CA, and Enestvedt R: Family-based practice: discussion of a tool merging assessment with intervention, *Family Community Health* 12:21-28, 1990.

Lino M: Families with children: changes in economic status and expenditures on children over time, *Family Economics Review,* 6:9-17, 1993.

Martin M and Henry M: Cultural relativity and poverty, *Public Health Nurs* 6:28-34, 1989.

Nye FI: Fifty years of family research, 1937-1987, *J Marriage Family* 50:305-316, 1988.

Speer JJ and Sachs B: Selecting the appropriate family assessment tool, *Pediatr Nurs* 11:349-355, 1985.

U.S. Bureau of the Census: *Exploring alternative race-ethnic comparison groups in current population surveys,* current population reports, P23-182, Washington, D.C., 1992, U.S. Government Printing Office.

U.S. Bureau of the Census: *The Black population in the United States: March 1991,* current population reports, P20-464, Washington, D.C., 1992, U.S. Government Printing Office.

U.S. Bureau of the Census: *The Hispanic population in the United States: March 1991,* current population reports, series P-20, No. 455, Washington, D.C., 1991, U.S. Government Printing Office.

Whall AL: The family as the unit of care in nursing: a historical review, *Public Health Nurs* 3:240-249, 1986.

Whall AL: *Family therapy theory for nursing: four approaches,* Norwalk, Conn., 1987, Appleton-Century-Crofts.

Foundations for Family Intervention: Families under Stress

OBJECTIVES

Upon completion of this chapter, the reader should be able to:

1. Discuss the concepts of stress and crisis as they relate to family functioning.
2. Describe factors that affect the outcome of a family crisis.
3. Identify characteristics that signal ineffective individual or family coping during periods of stress and crisis.
4. Differentiate between developmental and situational crises and give examples of each type of crisis.
5. Describe general principles that the community health nurse should apply when giving constructive assistance to families in crisis.
6. Explain nursing intervention strategies used by community health nurses to promote effective family functioning during periods of stress and crisis.
7. Describe how culture influences perceptions of stress and crisis.

Accept me as I am so I may learn what I can become.

A major preventive responsibility of the community health nurse is to help individuals and families handle stressful life events so that their energies can be used to achieve self-fulfillment and to develop a capacity to extend themselves to others. Some stress is normal and essential for life and growth. Stress provides the stimulus needed to adapt to the ever-changing conditions of life. Too much stress, however, prevents people from seeing what "they can become."

Selye (1976, p. xv) has found that any emotion or activity, whether it produces joy or sadness, causes stress. He believes that stressful life events (refer to Table 7-4) will more likely result in disease and unhappiness when individuals and families are not prepared to deal with them. Persons who are not prepared to handle the pressures and experiences encountered throughout life often do not recognize signals of distress that reflect a need to mobilize different coping mechanisms.

Community health nurses are in a key position to help individuals and families adapt to new or threatening life changes. In their work in the home and other settings they encounter clients who are experiencing various degrees of stress. Many times these clients have not had life experiences or exposure to knowledge that would assist them in altering patterns of functioning that intensify stress. Most parents, for instance, have not been prepared to handle children whose growth and development significantly deviate from normal patterns of functioning. Hence, they experience heightened distress and are frequently open to professional intervention. Illustrative of this is the situation encountered by a community health nurse when she visited the Slavovi family for the first time:

▌ The Slavovi family was referred to the community health nurse for health supervision follow-up after the birth of their fourth child, Stephanie, who had multiple handicaps. Even though this was the family's first exposure to community health nursing service, Mr. and Mrs. Slavovi talked freely when the nurse visited. Both manifested high levels of anxiety and confusion about how to care for their newborn infant. Angel and Maria Slavovi had always taken great pride in being good parents. Stephanie's physical and mental handicaps were particularly distressing to them: "We don't know how to help her. She continues to cry even when we hold her and seems to hurt all the time. Children need loving. Why doesn't Stephanie want us to hold her? We must be doing something wrong."

Having an understanding of the concept of stress helps the community health nurse to intervene more effectively with clients like the Slavovis. Stress theory provides the foundation for identifying signs and symptoms of distress and for recognizing potential stressors. It also provides clues about how to bring about change when a client's usual methods of coping are no longer effective.

For at least 50 years the concept of stress has been discussed in the literature (Knapp, 1988). Several authors have written extensively about this concept, including Cannon (1929, 1935); Cassel (1974, Psychiatric; 1974, Psychosocial); Figley and McCubbin (1983); Hill (1949); Lazarus (1966, 1981); Lazarus and Folkman (1984); McCubbin, Cauble, and Patterson (1982); McCubbin and Figley (1983); and Selye (1976). Since only a very brief overview of the concept of stress will be presented in this text, the reader may wish to refer to the writings of these authors for further study.

THE STRESS PHENOMENON

Selye (1976, p. 1) has defined stress as "the nonspecific response of the body to any demand." It is a dynamic state triggered by stressors which help to maintain an internal balance within human systems. Stressors are "anything which produce stress" (Selye, p. 78).

Stress theory is based on the concepts of homeostasis (state of physiological balance) and adaptation. Because stress is an inherent and integral part of life, individuals and families must constantly readjust to maintain themselves. A state of balance is maintained when a person learns to recognize the signals of distress and then adapts or changes functioning to meet the demands of the stress encountered. *Distress,* as defined by Selye, "is unpleasant or disease-producing stress" (Selye, 1976, p. 465). In contrast, *eustress* "is seen as good, pleasant, or curative stress" (Selye, p. 466).

Physiological responses (Figure 8-1) in the nervous and endocrine systems alert individuals to the occurrence of distress or eustress. These responses produce feelings such as joy, fatigue, or uneasiness. They help individuals to identify that their steady state is being threatened.

The physiological changes that occur in response to stress are nonspecific. They produce changes that affect a person's entire body and that happen any time an individual is experiencing stress, no matter what the cause. According to Selye (1976, p. 163), the nonspecific responses to stress evolve in three stages, which he has labeled the *general adaptation syndrome* (GAS):

1. The *alarm reaction,* during which defense mechanisms are mobilized.
2. The *stage of resistance,* when adaptation is acquired because optimum channels of defense were developed.
3. The *stage of exhaustion,* which reflects a depletion of adaptation energy necessary to cope with prolonged and intensified stress.

Although stress is essential for life and growth, every individual has limits beyond which stress is no longer healthy. When these limits are reached, individuals and families become exhausted and the energies needed to deal with activities of daily living become depleted. Our bodies provide numerous physiological and psychological signals that reflect energy depletion and disruption of homeostasis. Examples of these signals are presented in the box on p. 264.

In terms of the family, stress is manifested by ineffective family patterns, as well as by the occurrence of signs and symptoms of stress in its individual family members. Child abuse and neglect, domestic violence, strained communication patterns, and decision-making conflicts are a few such ineffective patterns that may result when a family is under stress. Others are shared in Table 7-2.

All individuals and families have the capacity to deal with distress. However, in order to do so they need to learn the boundaries of stress that they can tolerate and the nurturing, coping, and adaptive resources that promote growth and homeostasis. Complex and dynamic interactions between multiple variables influence a family's abilities to effectively mobilize resources to prevent crisis. Hill (1949, p. 9; 1965) illustrated this complexity in his classic ABCX model of family stress. He proposed that the interactions between the following factors influence whether or not a family under stress experiences a crisis:

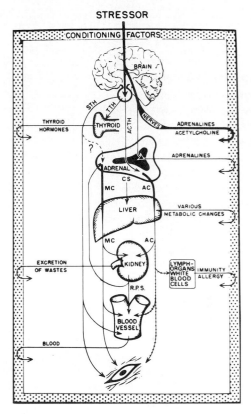

Figure 8-1 Physiological responses to stress. (From Selye H: *The stress of life,* New York, 1976, McGraw-Hill, p. 151.)

A (the event and associated hardships) → interacting with **B** (the family's crisis-meeting resources, its role structure, flexibility, and previous history with crisis) → interacting with **C** (the definition the family makes of the event) → produces **X** (crisis).

According to Hill, a crisis-prone family is one that experiences stressor events (A) with great frequency and severity, defines these events (C) more frequently as crisis-provoking, has meager crisis-meeting resources (B), and has failed to learn from past experience with crises (Hill, 1965, p. 40).

Most family stress theorists have built on the work of Reuben Hill and confirm and expand on his theories of the dynamic and complex nature of family stress and crisis (Boss, 1987; Lazarus, 1974; McCubbin and McCubbin, 1987, 1993; McCubbin and Patterson, 1983a, 1983b). For example, McCubbin and Patterson

◀ *Examples of Physiological and* ▶
Psychological Signals of Stress

Physiological Signals

Pounding of the heart
Dryness of the throat and mouth
Sweating
Frequent need to urinate
Diarrhea, indigestion, vomiting
Migraine headaches
Missed menstrual period
Loss of or excessive appetite
Increased smoking and alcohol and drug use
Increased use of legally prescribed drugs (e.g., tran-
   quilizers or amphetamines)
Pain in neck or lower back

Psychological Signals

General irritability, hyperexcitation or depression
Impulsive behavior, emotional instability
Overpowering urge to cry or run and hide
Inability to concentrate, flight of thoughts, and gen-
   eral disorientation
Floating anxiety
Trembling, nervous tics
Nightmares
Neurotic or psychotic behavior
Accident proneness

From Selye H: *The stress of life,* New York, 1976, McGraw-Hill, pp.
174-177.

(1983b) and McCubbin and McCubbin (1993) have put forth the notion of the "pile up of stressors," believing that families are seldom dealing with a single stressor during crisis. Family vulnerability to stress, "ranging from high to low, is determined by (1) the accumulation, or pile up, of demands on or within the family unit, such as financial debts, poor health status of relatives, and changes in a parent's work role or work environment, and (2) the trials and tribulations associated with the family's particular life-cycle stage with all of its demands and changes" (McCubbin and McCubbin, 1993, p. 28). The box on p. 265 summarizes some major reasons for family stress in our nation and provides data which help the community health nurse to identify families who are at risk for crises. At-risk families across the life span are discussed in Chapters 14 through 20.

Since an extensive discussion of family stress models is beyond the scope of this book, readers are encouraged to expand their knowledge through review of the original writings of family stress theorists identified in the previous paragraph. Here it is important to recognize that, during the clinical family assessment process, the needs and coping strategies of a family should be comprehensively addressed. A complex array of internal and external factors make a family vulnerable to crisis during times of stress, and family coping strategies dynamically change across the life cycle as families respond to the demands of daily living.

EFFECTS OF CULTURE ON PERCEPTIONS OF STRESS AND CRISIS

Cultural patterns of the family must be considered when assessing client situations during periods of stress. Cultural characteristics of families influence their perceptions about the causes of sickness and stress, the meaning and treatment of illness, appropriate coping behaviors, self-care activities, relationships with health care providers and significant others, and expression of stress and discomfort (Ailinger, 1985; Capers, 1985; Davitz, Sameshima, and Davitz, 1976; Germain, 1992; Kleinman, Eisenberg, and Good, 1978; Lewis, Messner, and McDowell, 1985; Ross, 1981; Snow, 1974; Sobralske, 1985; Villarruel and Ortiz de Montellano, 1992). When considering the effects of culture on perceptions of stress and crisis, it is important to remember that scientists and anthropologists recently have distinguished between the terms *illness* and *disease* to aid them in explaining why health professionals and clients can differ in their views of a hazardous event. Illness does not necessarily correlate with the biomedical interpretation of disease. In Western culture, what an individual/family feels and expresses in terms of stress and discomfort is labeled *illness. Disease,* on the other hand, is a physician-diagnosed condition that deviates from clearly defined norms. In terms of these culturally defined definitions, illness can occur in the absence of disease and vice versa (Giger and Davidhizar, 1991; Twaddle, 1981). It is important to differentiate between these concepts because "where only disease is treated, care will be less satisfactory to the patient and less clinically effective than where both disease and illness are treated to-

◀ *America's Families Under Stress* ▶

Declining Family Income

- Between 1973 and 1990, the median income of young families with children (those headed by someone younger than 30) plunged by nearly one-third—32 percent—after adjusting for inflation.
- Forty percent of all children in young families were living in poverty in 1990.
- Full-time, year-round work at the minimum wage of $4.25 an hour gives a family of three an income that equals only 80 percent of the 1991 poverty level.

More Births to Teens

- In 1989 there were 517,989 births to women younger than 20. Roughly two-thirds of these births were to unmarried teenagers, and about one-quarter of the total were repeat births.
- The 1989 teen birth rate of 58.1 births per 1,000 teenagers was the highest teen birth rate since 1970.

Lack of Access to Health Care

- Forty percent of all children lacked employer health coverage in 1990, even though more than 85 percent of all children lived in working families. The gaps in Medicaid and private insurance left 8.4 million children with no health insurance at all.
- In 1989 only about one-quarter of all infants were born to mothers who received early prenatal care, the lowest proportion since 1978. The proportion of infants born to mothers who received late or no prenatal care (6.4 percent) was higher than in any year since 1973.
- In nine major cities, only 10 to 42 percent of children starting school in 1991 had received appropriate preschool vaccinations on time.

Growing Hunger and Homelessness

- About 5.5 million children younger than 12 (one in eight) don't regularly get enough to eat.
- An estimated 100,000 children go to sleep homeless each night.

More Children and Families in Crisis

- More than 4.5 million women of childbearing age were current users of illegal drugs in 1990.
- At the peak of the crack crisis, as many as 375,000 infants were estimated to be born drug-exposed each year.
- An estimated 2.7 million children were reported abused or neglected in 1991, up from 1.1 million in 1980. Neglect cases accounted for about half of all reports.
- In 1990 an estimated 407,000 children were in foster care, an increase of almost 50 percent since 1986. Infants comprise a growing percentage of children entering care in some states.

From Allen ML, Brown P, and Finlay B: *Helping children by strengthening families: a look at family support programs,* Washington, D.C., 1992, Children's Defense Fund, pp. 9, 10-12.

gether" (Kleinman, Eisenberg, and Good, p. 256).

Kleinman, Eisenberg, and Good (1978, p. 252) believe that illness is culturally shaped in the sense that it is individually perceived—that is, how individuals and families experience and cope with disease is based on their explanations of sickness. In clinical practice it is not uncommon to encounter a wide variation in families' and individuals' explanations of sickness. Community health nurses encounter clients whose beliefs are consistent with the Western biomedical model, which focuses on scientific explanations for disease and illness occurrence, but community health nurses also work with many families whose beliefs about health and illness have evolved from the folk medicine system.

Snow (1974), in his classic article on folk medical beliefs, noted that these beliefs promote both natural and unnatural explanations for illness. According to Snow, *natural* explanations emphasize that there is a direct connection between the body and the forces of nature, and that there is safety in harmony and balance and danger in anything that is done to interfere with natural processes. Natural illnesses occur when the individual is inadequately protected against the forces of nature such as cold air and impurities in food, water, and air, or when there is an imbalance between natural forces (Snow, 1974). Community health nurses find that families holding these beliefs will take measures to protect themselves against dangerous elements in nature. For example, Chinese families frequently overdress their infants to prevent cold air from entering into their bodies (Chen-Louie, 1983).

A commonly held natural imbalance supported by the Hispanic, Filipino, and Arab cultures is that which exists between "cold" and "hot," or yin (cold) and yang (hot) in the Chinese culture (Chang, 1991; Whaley and Wong, 1991). This belief classifies illnesses, foods, areas of the body, and medicines according to intrinsic hot and cold properties (Snow, 1974). These properties can both cause illnesses and treat them and must be kept in balance to maintain health. Persons holding those beliefs will eat yin/cold foods such as honey, vegetables, and fruits when they have a disease with excessive yang/hot forces such as infections, fever, and hypertension (Ludman and Newman, 1984). Crucial to these beliefs are the implications they hold for nursing practice, because community health nurses who respect cultural differences work with families within the context of their cultural perspectives. They may, for instance, assist families in maintaining the harmony of nature by planning a balanced diet with them that avoids hot or cold food at given times.

Not all illnesses have folk explanations involving the disruption of forces in nature. Some result when individuals fall out of favor with the Lord and an evil influence or the devil takes over. Others are caused by witchcraft. "Witchcraft is based on the belief that there are individuals with the ability to mobilize unusual powers for good or evil" (Snow, 1974, p. 85). Snow found that belief in witchcraft as a cause of illness is widespread among Haitians, Trinidadians, Puerto Rican Americans, American blacks, and Mexican-Americans.

Illnesses that result from supernatural evil influences or forces beyond nature have been labeled *unnatural* by Snow (1974). Evil forces can cause all types of physical and mental health stresses that are frightening to families because they cannot be cured by natural remedies or health personnel. A common health belief found among people from Latin America, South Asian, Near Eastern, and some African societies is the belief in the evil eye (Pasquale, 1984). This phenomenon involves the belief that the gaze of the human eye can bring illness and misfortune to people. "Envy is the pivotal emotion that activates people's ability to cause harm and misfortune to others" (Pasquale, p. 32). According to Pasquale, the evil eye phenomenon is a cluster of beliefs that associates people's internal strength-weakness states with the power of the evil eye. When these states are in balance

individuals are not likely to cast or fall victim to the evil eye. However, when people have an excess of envy their strength increases and they are capable of casting the evil eye intentionally or unintentionally. Children are particularly vulnerable to the gaze of the evil eye because their internal strength-weakness states are immature. People exposed to the evil eye often have a sudden onset of illness and may have a variety of symptoms such as fever, nausea, diarrhea, and nervousness. Preventive and treatment measures for the evil eye phenomenon usually involve supernatural rituals carried out by the client or approved healers (Pasquale). For example, Hindus paint a spot of lampblack on children's foreheads as a precautionary measure against the evil eye (Maloney, 1976).

A knowledge of folk health beliefs can assist the community health nurse in understanding clients from the client's perspective and may prevent a client from being labeled noncompliant. This knowledge can also help the nurse to avoid unintentional involvement in spell-casting, such as giving the evil eye when admiring a new baby during a home visit. Lack of understanding can create barriers to therapeutic nursing intervention. When visiting clients from differing cultures it is important to remember that folk explanations for sickness are not limited to the poor and uneducated. Clients from all socioeconomic levels believe in folk explanations for illness (Pasquale, 1984). It is also important to remember that there is significant intracultural variation in relation to health beliefs and practices. As families from different cultures assimilate Western beliefs, some of their traditions are relinquished and others are retained (Louie, 1985). However, folk medical beliefs continue to be documented in the client–health care professional relationship (Eckholm, 1990; Kay and Yoder, 1987).

It should be obvious at this point that similar stressful events can be variously interpreted by clients based on the differing explanatory models of health and illness used by them: a serious infection may be blamed on germs, on evil influences, on impurities in the water, on the entry of cold air into the body of a susceptible individual, or on divine punishment. This in turn affects clients' perceptions about the seriousness of the infection, needed treatment regimens, and acceptance of therapeutic interventions. Illustrative of this are the beliefs held by many Spanish-speaking people. Often they view illness and pain as punishment from God for evil deeds and believe they must accept suffering to atone for their sins. As a result they may refuse pain relievers and nursing care and may engage in various types of penance (Ross, 1981).

Since the meaning of illness and stress is individually perceived within a person's cultural context and self-concept, serious stressful events may or may not evolve into a crisis. Individuals and families who interpret these events as challenges to accomplish significant life goals are often able to develop coping mechanisms to effectively deal with their distress. However, if they perceive stressful events as the will of God, a spirit possession, or events out of their control, a crisis may emerge.

THE CRISIS PHENOMENON

Crisis, like stress, is an elusive concept that can be identified only by recognizing the manifestations or characteristic signs and symptoms of the crisis state. That is why it is so important for nurses to have a firm understanding of the crisis sequence. Concepts of crisis help the practitioner to quickly recognize clients who need to adjust their coping mechanisms. It is especially critical for community health nurses to be well-grounded in crisis theory because they frequently encounter clients, such as the Slavovi family, in the home environment who are dealing with new, different, or threatening stressful events. Early identification of those clients who are having difficulty coping with these events could prevent an intensified crisis state.

A preventive health philosophy stimulated the development of crisis theory and intervention. Erich Lindemann (1944), in his classic study of grief reactions, identified the need for preventive counseling with clients experiencing loss through death or separation. After investigating the responses of clients who had lost a relative in the famous Coconut Grove fire in Boston, he concluded that appropriate psychiatric intervention with clients who were experiencing grief could prevent prolonged and serious social maladjustment (Lindemann, p. 147). He further concluded, after observing clients who experienced an "anticipatory grief reaction," that prophylactic counseling could prevent family crisis (Lindemann, p. 148). Anticipatory grief reactions occur when there is a threat of death, such as when soldiers engage in war activities. Clients in these situations go through all the stages of grief. It has been found in some cases that wives of soldiers in the war handled the grief process so effectively that they emancipated themselves from their spouses. This pre-

cipitated a crisis if husbands returned from the war, because their wives needed to reestablish marital relationships before they could express feelings of love and caring. Husbands in these situations felt that their wives no longer loved them and frequently asked for a divorce (Lindemann, pp. 147-148).

Crisis reactions such as those described by Lindemann can be predicted and often prevented. Lindemann, Caplan, and other crisis theorists have delineated a sequence of events that occur when a client is experiencing a crisis, as well as factors that intensify the crisis state. In addition, these theorists have identified situations that frequently precipitate a crisis during the developmental life cycle of a family. They also discovered therapeutic processes that have a positive influence on client functioning when the family is experiencing a crisis.

The Crisis Sequence

Gerald Caplan (1961, p. 18), the father of preventive psychiatry, describes *crisis* as a state

provoked when a person faces an obstacle to important life goals that is, for a time, insurmountable through the utilization of customary methods of problem solving. A period of disorganization ensues, a period of upset, during which many different abortive attempts at solution are made. Eventually some kind of adaptation is achieved, which may or may not be in the best interests of that person and his fellows.

When describing the normal sequence of events that occur during a crisis, Caplan (1964, pp. 40-41) identifies four characteristic phases:

1. An initial phase when an individual's tension rises as he or she uses habitual problem-solving responses to achieve emotional homeostasis.
2. A second stage, in which tension increases and the individual becomes ineffective and upset because normal coping mechanisms were not effective in resolving the state of crisis.
3. A third threshold when tension mounts and stimulates the mobilization of new and emergency problem-solving mechanisms. The problem may be resolved if an individual can redefine the situation in order to cope with it and can adjust to role changes that have occurred.

TABLE 8-1 The North American Nursing Diagnosis Association: Family Coping: Potential for Growth

Diagnostic label	Definition	Etiology	Defining characteristics
Family coping: Potential for growth	Family member has effectively managed adaptive tasks involved with the client's health challenge and is exhibiting desire and readiness for enhanced health and growth in regard to self and in relation to the client.	Readiness for seeking self-actualization	Family member attempts to describe growth impact of crisis on his or her own values, priorities, goals, or relationships Family member is moving in direction of health-promoting and enriching lifestyle which supports and monitors maturational processes, audits and negotiates treatment programs, and generally chooses experiences which optimize wellness Individual expresses interest in making contact on a one-to-one basis or on a mutual-aid group basis with another person who has experienced a similar situation

From Gordon M: *Manual of nursing diagnosis, 1993-1994*, St. Louis, 1993, Mosby, p. 369.

4. A final phase when tension mounts beyond the limits an individual can tolerate; major disorganization results.

Inherent in Caplan's description of a crisis are several key ideas: (1) change that threatens an individual's ability to meet life goals disrupts the individual's homeostasis; (2) crisis results when an individual's customary methods of adaptation are ineffective in handling change; (3) disorganization occurs during the crisis state; (4) crisis is self-limiting, with a subsequent reduction of emotional tension (adaptation); (5) biopsychosocial homeostasis following a crisis may be at a level the same as, better than, or worse than the precrisis level. The goal of crisis intervention is to help the client to maintain a level of functioning equal to or better than the precrisis level.

It is not uncommon for community health nurses to work with families who have been unable to return successfully to their precrisis level of functioning after experiencing a crisis. When first encountered by the community health nurse these families often present multiple difficulties, ineffective problem-solving methods, and feelings of helplessness and hopelessness.

Community health nurses also encounter families who not only return to precrisis levels of functioning but, in addition, experience growth during crisis situations. Many families develop new methods of coping that provide alternative ways for them to handle future stresses and crises. Many also develop a cohesive family unity that increases the supportive and nurturing aspects of their family lifestyle and that encourages risk-taking. Risk-taking may expose individuals and families to other growth-producing opportunities. Characteristics of families who show potential for growth during crisis are delineated in Table 8-1.

Multiple factors affect how well a family handles stress and deals with crises. Community health nurses who understand these variables are better able to help families achieve successful resolution and growth during a crisis state.

Factors Affecting the Outcome of a Crisis

Aguilera (1994, p. 31) contends that there are three balancing factors that relate to the precipitation and successful resolution of a crisis. These are *perception of the event, available situational supports,* and *adequate coping mechanisms.* Figure 8-2 on p. 272 presents the paradigm developed by Aguilera (p. 32) to study the influence of these balancing factors during times of stress. It illustrates that clients must achieve a realistic perception of the event, develop adequate situational supports, and mobilize coping mechanisms to achieve successful adaptation during periods of disequilibrium.

Aguilera's paradigm provides a logical and useful model for analyzing a client's ability to adjust when experiencing stress. The paradigm provides a framework for identifying significant parameters to assess when working with individuals and families who have encountered threatening life events. A data base relative to each of Aguilera's balancing factors should be obtained when working with such persons. In her text, *Crisis Intervention: Theory and Methodology,* Aguilera has shared several case situations that illustrate the significant influence these balancing factors have during times of stress.

Perception of the Event

Crisis is the emotional reaction that occurs in relation to a new, different, or threatening event, not the event itself. Basically, the extent of this emotional reaction is determined by how the client (individual, family, aggregate) defines his or her particular circumstances (Aguilera, 1994; Burr, 1973; Caplan, 1964; Hansen and Hill, 1964; Rahe, 1974).

Perception of a hazardous event is a multidimensional phenomenon. McCubbin and McCubbin (1993) noted that "the assessments families make include many components of the stressor, such as the intensity, the degree of controllability of the situation, the amount of change expected of the family system, and whether or not the family is capable of responding to the situation" (p. 50). During the clinical family assessment process it is important to guide the interview to obtain data about the multiple variables that influence how a client perceives a hazardous situation. The box on this page identifies factors to be considered when assessing a client's response to current stressors. In Chapter 7 information about the structural and process parameters of family functioning was presented. This information helps the practitioner to

> ◄ *Factors Influencing a Family's Perception of a Stressful Event* ►
>
> - Number of stressors family is experiencing
> - Family's past experiences in handling current stressor(s)
> - Biopsychosocial status of the client before encountering stressful event(s)
> - Duration of exposure to current stressor(s)
> - Magnitude or seriousness of current event(s)
> - Suddenness of the event
> - Family's understanding of the stressor event(s)
> - Impact of event on family structure and process
> - Family's perceptions about its ability to manage the demands of the stressful event

examine the impact of the stressful situation on the family system. For example, it would be important to assess how the family was handling its division of labor when a family member is ill and unable to carry out his or her normal patterns of functioning.

Even though the responses of individuals and families to hazardous events are highly variable, there is evidence that supports the theory that distress increases when one encounters multiple stressors (McCubbin and McCubbin, 1993; McCubbin and Patterson, 1983, Family Stress; Rahe, 1974); experiences the stressor or stressors for a prolonged length of time (Selye, 1976); is exposed to a stressor with little or no time for anticipating problem-solving (Hansen and Hill, 1964); faces an event that is highly ambiguous (McHugh, 1968); or encounters a situation that presents hardship or has serious consequences such as death (Hill, 1949). When distress heightens, clients are more likely to have a distorted view of the current stressor. They may experience such feelings as helplessness, hopelessness, anxiety, fatigue, or depression. It must be emphasized, however, that even when one or more of the above factors exist in stressful occurrences, the perceived meaning of occurrences varies from one individual to another. The above factors only place individuals more at risk for developing crisis.

Caplan (1964, pp. 42-43), in his classic work on family crisis, has found that for a stressor to become problematic "it must be perceived as a threat or loss to need satisfaction or as a challenge." He believes that two major variables, personality and sociocultural factors, significantly affect how one perceives life events. These variables determine the type of life experiences one has, prescribe the limits of acceptable behavior when dealing with stress, and influence how one feels about one's abilities to handle changes in life. Case situations can best illustrate how the variables of personality and sociocultural influences affect one's perception of an event.

▶ **Mrs. Farias was 34 years old and left with two sons, 8 and 10 years old, and one daughter, age 14, when her husband was killed in a car accident. The community health nurse had encountered the Farias family before Mr. Farias's death because Carmelina, their 14-year-old daughter, needed orthopedic follow-up for a scoliosis problem discovered through health screening at her high school. During a home visit 8 months after Mr. Farias's death, the community health nurse became concerned about Mrs. Farias's physical and psychological health. She looked uncared for, her home was untidy, and she had no interest in talking about Carmelina's health problems. Weeping, Mrs. Farias shared with the nurse that "nothing was going right lately; the children don't obey, I can't get my husband's life insurance, and my friends haven't visited lately." She became particularly distressed when she talked about how she was going to feed her family in the future. "Our savings are almost gone. I can't get a job. What will I do? I have never worked, because Julio thought that a wife should stay at home. My folks thought that girls should marry and raise a family. I never was good at much except maybe cooking, housekeeping, and loving the kids. My family thinks it is wrong to take money from the welfare department. They say they will help me until I remarry, but I know they don't have anything extra. Besides, I am too old to remarry. Most men I know want their own children, not someone else's. You can't meet men when you are my age."**

Another case situation illustrates different family reactions to the death of its male provider.

▶ **Mrs. Ulisses was a 33-year-old widow with two daughters, 2 and 6 years of age, and two sons, ages 8 and 11. Her husband was killed while hunting. The community health nurse started visiting Mrs. Ulisses after she brought her 2-year-old to the well-baby clinic 6 weeks after her husband's death. At that time she expressed a desire to obtain information about day-care centers. The nurse visited regularly for a year to help Mrs. Ulisses sort out what she would like to do in the future. She and her husband were never able to save much, so Mrs. Ulisses applied for financial assistance from the Department of Social Service. She did not like receiving Aid to Families with Dependent Children funds but felt that she needed time to make child-care arrangements before she went back to work. Seven and a half months after her husband's death, Mrs. Ulisses enrolled in college. "I know I can find a job, because I have worked off and on since age 15. If I had some training, however, I would be more secure in the future. I am still not sure if I want to get married again, so I better prepare myself to care for my family."**

Both Mrs. Farias and Mrs. Ulisses were facing similar situations. They experienced the loss of a significant other who had assumed the provider role in their family system when he was living. Mrs. Farias, however, was more threatened by her circumstances because past and current cultural influences affected her ability to be flexible when role changes were needed. In addition, Mrs. Farias lacked confidence (personality factor) in her abilities to succeed in work and social settings. Her life experiences were focused on preparing her for traditional female roles only.

Mrs. Ulisses, on the other hand, was discouraged at times but was actively involved in planning for a future career. She was better prepared to assume the provider role, having worked off and on since her teenage years, and felt more confident about her abilities to succeed outside the home setting. Her life experiences provided her with a different perception of her female role.

Situational Supports

It has long been recognized that meaningful human relationships can assist individuals to cope with the stresses of life (Cobb, 1976; Kaplan, Cassel, and Gore, 1977). It has been demonstrated that presence of social support can play a significant role in "modifying the deleterious health effects of stress, in influencing the use of health services, and in affecting other aspects of health behavior such as compliance with medical regimens" (Hamburg and Killilea, 1979, p. 256). A review of studies related to social support, stress, and health and illness outcomes by Hamburg and Killilea (pp. 256-257) shows that social supports can:

1. Reduce the number of complications of pregnancy for women under high life stress (Nuckolls, Cassel, and Kaplan, 1972)
2. Help prevent posthospital psychological reactions in children after a tonsillectomy (Jessner, Blom, and Waldfogel, 1952)
3. Aid recovery from surgery (Egbert, Battib, Welch, and Bartlett, 1964)
4. Aid recovery from illness (Chambers and Reiser, 1953; Chen and Cobb, 1960; Mather, 1974)
5. Reduce the need for steroids in adult asthmatics in periods of stress (deAraujo, Van Arsdel, Holmes, and Dudley, 1973)
6. Protect against clinical depression in the face of adverse events (Brown, Bhrolchain, and Harris, 1975)
7. Reduce psychological distress and physiologic symptoms following job loss and bereavement (Burch, 1972; Cobb, 1974; Gore, 1973; Maddison and Walther, 1967; Parkes, Benjamin, and Fitzgerald, 1969)
8. Protect against the development of emotional problems that can be associated with aging (Blau, 1973; Lowenthal and Haven, 1968)
9. Reduce the physiological symptomatology in those working in highly stressful job environments (Cobb, 1974; Cobb, Kasl, French, and Norstebo, 1969)
10. Help patients to continue needed medical treatment and promote adherence to needed medical regimens (Bakeland and Lundwall, 1975; Caplan, Robinson, French Jr., Caldwell, and Shinn, 1976; Haynes and Sackett, 1974).

Social supports can have a positive effect on health. They can provide a buffer against the effects of high stress and have a mediating effect that stimulates the development of coping strategies and promotes mastery. Lack of social supports can exacerbate the impact of stressful life events (Cassel, 1976; Cobb, 1976; Hamburg and Killilea, 1979; Pilisuk and Parks, 1983).

Although it has been shown that social support can positively influence the outcome of a stressful event or crisis, research has also demonstrated that the *type* of social support is significant to consider when evaluating this variable during the family assessment process (Gottlieb, 1983; Krause, 1986). Thus it is important to ascertain from families their perceptions about the *quality of the interactions* they have with others, as well as the *amount of contact* they have with social supports.

Use of a genogram and/or an eco-map (refer to Chapter 7) often helps the practitioner to assess clients' perceptions about the quality of their internal and external social resources.

During periods of disequilibrium persons need supportive relationships that allow them to verbalize feelings and encourage them to sort out the realities of their situation. Clients also need assistance with problem-solving. In addition, concrete help is frequently needed to facilitate their ability to obtain resources such as financial assistance from their environment (refer to Chapter 10). Behaviors that support a client's distorted perception of the event are not helpful. A friend, for example, who reinforces a client's blaming behaviors inhibits client growth and successful resolution of a crisis; this type of behavior supports the client's current ineffective coping style, which in turn prevents the client from mobilizing more effective coping mechanisms.

When working with clients who are experiencing a crisis, it is extremely important to remember that their significant others may also be in crisis. Often the practitioner finds that others in a client's social network are experiencing as much or more distress than the client. Thus they are unable to provide the assistance needed by the client to achieve healthy adaptation and may, in fact, be reinforcing maladaptive behaviors. Because of this, significant others are often included in the therapeutic process so that they do not inhibit a client's growth and so that they receive the help they themselves need to cope with the stressful changes being experienced.

Adequate Coping Mechanisms

The stress-crisis sequence evolves when an individual's usual coping mechanisms or ways of reducing stress are inadequate to deal with the threatening event(s) being encountered. If the client becomes immobilized, he or she will probably emerge from the crisis functioning at a level lower than the precrisis state. On the other hand, if the client is able to mobilize untapped inner strengths or resources, positive outcomes may result; the client could resolve problem(s) and learn new ways of coping with stress in the future. The client could also experience growth.

During the crisis sequence clients generally experience heightened anxiety, which often results in two types of behavior. First, the client will attempt, sometimes frantically, to use previously learned patterns of coping to alleviate discomfort. Clients usually cling to

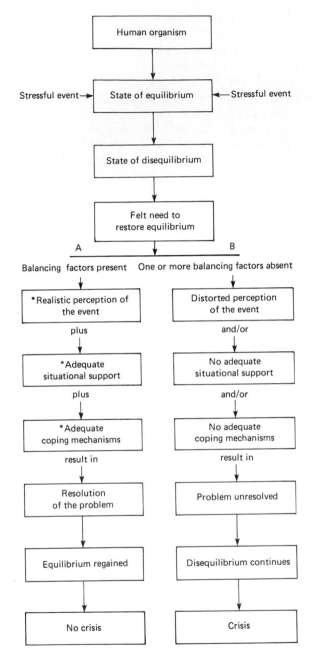

Figure 8-2 Paradigm: effect of balancing factors in a stressful event; * = balancing factors. (From Aguilera DC: *Crisis intervention: theory and methodology,* ed 7, St. Louis, 1994, Mosby, p. 32.)

the familiar during a state of anxiety because it provides a sense of stability, even if real stability does not exist. Second, because a high level of anxiety is accompanied by feelings of helplessness and hopelessness, clients are frequently more amenable to outside

influence and assistance. This is especially true during the period of disequilibrium. When reorganization and equilibrium begin to occur and new adaptive or maladaptive defense patterns evolve, this is less true. That is why crisis theorists stress the importance of high-quality therapeutic intervention during the time the family in crisis is establishing new coping mechanisms. Caplan (1964, p. 53) has found that intervention at this time can be the critical balancing factor in helping clients to achieve positive outcomes during crisis states.

One major task for a family that is experiencing a crisis is to recognize that customary coping mechanisms are ineffective and that new patterns for coping must be established. Some clients, particularly those who have adequate situational supports and who have been flexible in the past, are able to accomplish this task with little or no assistance. Other clients, especially those who have few or no situational supports, who rigidly define role patterns, and who lack maturity because of past experiences, will need help from others in developing new ways for handling stress. These persons are frequently unable to identify the nature of the stress they are experiencing or why their patterns of functioning are ineffective.

Changing patterns of family functioning in times of crisis requires the family to reexamine its structural and process parameters of family functioning. As new ways of handling the demands of the stressors (e.g., hardships associated with caring for a disabled family member) emerge, families may need to change their goals and expectations for the family unit. Take, for example, the Slavovi family discussed in the beginning of this chapter. Angel and Maria were working hard so that their children could have a better life than they had. They focused on the children doing well in school, believing that they needed a good education to succeed in later life. As Angel and Maria became more comfortable with handling Stephanie's basic care needs they began to realize that her physical and mental handicaps would make it difficult for her to deal with educational demands in a regular school setting. This realization was stressful for Angel and Maria because they feared for Stephanie's future. Situations like these are distressing to families because they must compromise or accept a less than perfect solution in order to successfully adapt (McCubbin and McCubbin, 1993).

It should be obvious at this point that the balancing forces in Aguilera's paradigm (Figure 8-2) are interrelated and must be viewed as a composite of forces rather than as isolated elements. If this view is not taken, nursing interventions may be inappropriate to meet the needs of the client. Ms. Himes's case situation is a good example. She called the county health department and requested nursing service for her mother. Without emotion she stated that "someone needs to show me how to care for her. I don't know what to do any longer."

> Sally Himes was a 50-year-old single woman. She lived with her 85-year-old mother, who had had a CVA 15 years ago that left her paralyzed and unable to speak. Before her father's death Ms. Himes had promised him that she would always take care of her mother. When the community health nurse arrived at the Himes home, Sally immediately took her into the bedroom to see her mother, who appeared very comfortable in her current surroundings. Sally insisted, however, that the nurse check her over. "I am doing something that is not right. The doctor needs to visit more frequently to give mother shots for water in her lungs." The nurse examined Sally's mother carefully and, finding nothing seriously wrong, decided to spend the rest of the visit talking with Sally.
>
> After the nurse provided positive reinforcement for how well Sally was caring for her mother, Sally replied, "The mailman came today." It took several probing questions like, "Was there something special about the mailman's visit?" before Sally identified that she had received an invitation to her niece's wedding. She was distressed because her mother had not also been invited. "They don't care about her anymore." Further interviewing revealed that for the past 2 years Sally had isolated herself from family and friends because she felt her mother's condition was deteriorating and that significant others were too busy. "I can't leave her. No one else knows what to do. Besides, my family has lots of other responsibilities. I always thought they cared about mother, but now I wonder. If they really cared, they would have invited her to Sue's wedding. Sometimes I really get discouraged. I wonder if my family and friends care about me."

The invitation Sally had received from her family challenged her thought processes. It brought to a conscious level feelings of noncaring, which was fortunate because Sally had been coping with these feelings by withdrawing. She was no longer able to ask for assistance from her family and friends and increasingly limited most of her social contacts. With the help of the community health nurse she was able to identify why she had become so upset when the invitation was delivered. She was also able to recognize that she needed to make changes in her situation so that her own needs and expectations could be met. One nursing intervention strategy, arranging a conference with the entire family, resulted in a plan in which all family members would share the responsibility for the care of Sally's mother. This would not have happened if the community health nurse had focused only on helping Sally to see that her perceptions about how well she was caring for her mother were distorted. Changes in Sally's situation would also not have occurred if emphasis had been placed on examining only Sally's feelings about who was invited to Sue's wedding. Helping Sally to recognize that she needed quality situational supports and needed to reexamine patterns of family functioning was critical to the successful resolution of her crisis.

When nurses work with clients who are experiencing heightened stress, they find that a *triggering event* (e.g., the invitation to Sue's wedding) stimulates the development of a crisis. This event produces a "pile up" of stress to the point where the client is no longer able to adapt. The triggering event must be recognized as a signal of distress; otherwise clients will not be helped to develop new ways of coping. At times it is easy to miss these symptoms because the triggering event is often a minor occurrence. For example, a child who comes sobbing into the health clinic at school because of a shove by peers on the playground could need just a little extra attention. On the other hand, if this child perceives the push to mean that he or she is not liked, the child may be having difficulty developing social relationships. The sobbing could be a cry for help. Taking time to collect sufficient data helps a nurse to discriminate between simple and serious difficulties such as those described above. It is usually wise for a community health nurse to obtain information about the client's daily functioning, support systems, and recent life changes when she or he believes that an emotional reaction to an event is disproportionate to what one would expect. Family assessment tools and life change questionnaires, like those presented in Chapter 7, can facilitate collection of such information.

It will also be found when working with clients, particularly those who tend to perceive all difficulties as crises, that problems from the past are reactivated during the crisis state. This happens because these clients have been unsuccessful in dealing with these

8-2 The North American Nursing Diagnosis Association: Ineffective Individual Coping Diagnostic Category

Diagnostic label	Definition	Etiology	Defining characteristics
Ineffective coping: Individual	Impairment of adaptive behaviors and problem-solving abilities for meeting life's demands and roles. Methods of handling stressful life situations are insufficient to control anxiety, fear, or anger.	Situational crises (specify type) Maturational crises (specify type) Personal vulnerability Knowledge deficit (specify) Problem-solving skills deficit	*Verbalization of inability to cope *Inability to ask for help Inability to solve problem effectively Anxiety, fear, anger, irritability, tension Presence of life stress Inability to meet role expectations Inability to meet basic needs Alteration in societal participation Destructive behavior toward self and others Inappropriate or ineffective use of defense mechanisms Change in usual communication patterns High rate of accidents Verbal manipulation Excess food intake, alcohol consumption; smoking Digestive, bowel, appetite disturbance; chronic fatigue or sleep pattern disturbance

*Denotes critical or major defining characteristics.
From Gordon M: *Manual of nursing diagnosis, 1993-1994*, St. Louis, 1993, Mosby, p. 355.

problems and thus have developed ineffective coping mechanisms (Caplan, 1964, p. 41). This can compound the effects of the current threatening event but can also provide an opportunity for growth. Clients can be helped to resolve old as well as new problems during times of crisis and can learn coping strategies that promote growth.

Having an awareness of behaviors that are commonly observed when individuals and families have developed ineffective coping mechanisms enhances the community health nurse's ability to quickly identify clients who are experiencing distress, crisis, or dysfunctional family dynamics. The North American Nursing Diagnosis Association identified characteristics of individuals and families who have ineffective coping patterns when it accepted "individual and family coping" as appropriate nursing diagnostic categories. These characteristics are displayed in Tables 8-2 and 8-3, and can assist community health nurses in

determining when individuals and families are having difficulty handling stress. The ineffective behaviors presented in Table 8-3 are primarily identified in terms of how a family relates to a client with an identified problem. During times of distress and crisis families may also develop dysfunctional patterns of functioning that affect the entire family unit. Deceptive, confused, or secretive communication, inability to meet basic needs of family life (e.g., impaired home management), inappropriate or lack of decision-making and problem solving, and family interactions characterized by constant conflict, are a few examples of such patterns. Others are shared in Table 7-2.

Types of Crises

Although crisis is basically an individual perceptual matter, certain life events have frequently been found to produce or increase the potential for crisis.

TABLE 8-3 The North American Nursing Diagnosis Association: Ineffective Family Coping Diagnostic Categories

Diagnostic label	Definition	Etiology	Defining characteristics
Ineffective family coping: Compromised	Usually supportive primary person (family member or close friend) providing insufficient, ineffective, or compromised support, comfort, assistance, or encouragement which may be needed by client to manage or master adaptive tasks related to health challenge	Knowledge deficit Emotional conflicts Exhaustion of supportive capacity Role changes (family) Temporary family disorganization Developmental or situational crises	Client expresses concern or complaint about significant other's response to his/her health problem Significant person describes preoccupation with personal reactions (e.g., fear, guilt, anticipatory grief, anxiety) to client's illness, disability, or other situational or developmental crises Significant person describes or confirms inadequate understanding of knowledge base which interferes with effective assistive or supportive behaviors Significant person attempts assistive or supportive behaviors with less than satisfactory results Significant person withdraws or enters into limited or temporary personal communication with client at time of need Significant person displays protective behavior disproportionate (too little or too much) to client's abilities or need for autonomy
Ineffective family coping: Disabling	Behavior of significant person (family member or primary person) disables own capacities and client's capacities to effectively address tasks essential to either person's adaptation to the health challenge	Chronically unexpressed guilt/anxiety/hostility/etc. (significant other) Dissonant discrepancy of coping styles (for dealing with adaptive tasks by the significant person and client or among significant people) Highly ambivalent family relationships Arbitrary handling of family's resistance to treatment (which tends to solidify defensiveness as it fails to deal adequately with underlying anxiety)	Neglectful care of client in regard to basic human needs and/or illness treatment Distortion of reality regarding client's health problem including extreme denial about existence or severity Intolerance Rejection Abandonment Desertion Carrying on usual routines disregarding client's needs Psychosomaticism Taking on illness signs of the client Decisions and actions by family which are detrimental to economic or social well-being Agitation, depression, aggression, hostility Impaired restructuring of a meaningful life for self, impaired individuation, prolonged overconcern for client Neglectful relationships with other family members Client's development of helpless, inactive dependence

From Gordon M: *Manual of nursing diagnosis, 1993-1994*, St. Louis, 1993, Mosby, pp. 371, 373, 375, 377.

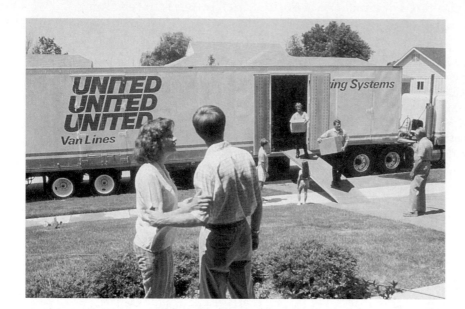

Figure 8-3 Moving is a normal transition event, but it can cause a great deal of stress. (Courtesy United Van Lines.)

These events are viewed as developmental, situational, or a combination of the two. They encompass change, either internally or externally produced, that necessitates altering one's thinking, feelings, and coping style.

Developmental or maturational crises occur across the life spectrum. They relate to critical transition points in the course of normal human development that involve many physical, psychological, and social changes. These transition stages, such as entry into school, puberty, starting a career, leaving home, moving (refer to Figure 8-3), marriage, parenthood, middlescence, retirement, and facing one's own death and that of others because of aging, require many role changes and produce heightened stress. The role changes that occur during these anticipated crises are discussed in Chapters 14 through 19.

Situational crises also occur across the lifespan, but they are usually not anticipated and do not relate to normal maturational processes. They are precipitated by such things as divorce, illness, accidents, changes in social status, cultural relocation, and early death of a significant other. Since situational crises are frequently sudden and unexpected, an individual or family faces this type of crisis situation without benefit of anticipatory problem solving. This puts the individual or family more at risk for developing distress, because they are unprepared to deal with the changes that accompany these life events.

Sometimes situational and developmental crises occur simultaneously. When this happens an individu-al's or a family's adaptive energies are seriously overtaxed. Multiple stressors make it more difficult for these persons to evaluate realistically the changes that are occurring and to adjust their coping style to accommodate them. For example, a 5-year-old child who has recently changed cultural settings must deal with stresses related to school entry in addition to those related to living in a new environment. School entry is in itself often very traumatic. This, coupled with the pressures that result from relocation such as learning a different language, developing all new friendships, and adjusting to an unfamiliar lifestyle, can be overwhelming.

Several developmental and situational crises such as teenage parenthood, changing careers, and a newly diagnosed chronic illness are discussed in Chapters 14 through 19. When community health nurses work with families who are experiencing such crises, each family member's level of stress should be assessed. A system's framework (refer to Chapter 7) can be especially helpful in identifying the impact of a crisis on the entire family unit. Both structural and process parameters of family functioning, as well as the biopsychosocial components of individual functioning, should be examined during times of stress. During the assessment process it is important to focus on what is occurring and how the family is handling its feelings and the activities of daily living. At times individuals and families attempt to establish blame elsewhere to relieve anxiety. Blaming behavior does not lead to healthy coping.

Because community health nurses are frequently present when crisis-producing events are occurring, they are in a favorable position to initiate supportive interventions that will enhance a client's ability to adapt. In order to do so they must know about life events that can precipitate crisis, must recognize signs and symptoms that signal distress, and must develop skill in using several types of intervention strategies with clients who are experiencing stress or crisis.

PRINCIPLES OF FAMILY SUPPORT

When intervening with families, it is important to keep in mind several principles of family support. Allen, Brown, and Finlay (1992) have highlighted these principles as presented in the box on this page. Essentially these authors advocate a holistic approach to family stress management that respects cultural differences, individual family variations, and a family's right of self-determination. It is also important that families have system resources that enhance their abilities to deal with stressful events.

NURSING INTERVENTION STRATEGIES

Community health nurses use a variety of intervention approaches to facilitate adaptation during times of stress and to enhance successful resolution of crisis. Some of these approaches will be briefly summarized under three major categories: *supportive, educative* and *problem-solving.* Separating strategies into categories is an artificial technique that is used here only to focus discussion about ways to effect client change. In reality community health nurses find that often they must integrate several intervention approaches in order to intervene effectively with clients.

Establishing rapport and collecting adequate data to identify the task to be accomplished are the essential first steps in any intervention process. These steps are discussed in Chapters 7 and 9 and are not repeated here. They should, however, be kept in mind when selecting a particular intervention modality.

Supportive Approach

The multiple symptoms that clients experience when dealing with stressful events and/or crises were previously discussed in this chapter. These symptoms can be very unpleasant and can create great discomfort because they are difficult for clients to understand. Some clients, when experiencing these symptoms,

---

◀ **Principles of Family Support** ▶

- Emphasize the family unit
- Build on family strengths
- Make participation voluntary
- Address family needs comprehensively
- Develop parenting skills (if appropriate to needs of family)
- Provide nurturing connections with others
- Respond to individual and community needs
- Work to prevent crises
- Respect individual and cultural differences
- Coordinate and cooperate with other agencies

From Allen ML, Brown P, and Finlay B: *Helping children by strengthening families: a look at family support programs,* Washington, D.C., 1992, Children's Defense Fund, pp. 8, 10-12.

---

fear that something is seriously wrong with them, and this tends to increase their anxieties and fears.

Clients who are experiencing symptoms of distress need to reduce these symptoms before they can actively engage in activities that will lead to problem resolution. Supportive intervention by significant others (family, friends, and professionals) can assist clients in dealing with symptoms of distress. Two types of support are especially helpful: (1) providing an opportunity for the client to share feelings with persons who are accepting and nonjudgmental and (2) assisting the client with concrete daily tasks, such as home management and keeping health appointments. Community health nurses frequently help clients who are experiencing crisis with concrete tasks by making referrals for homemakers or home health aides or by helping the client to mobilize family resources. At times they also provide this assistance themselves during home visits. They may, for example, feed an infant while talking to a distressed mother.

It is important to remember that clients who are experiencing distress often need time to deal with their feelings and to sort out realities before they can engage in problem-solving and in learning new knowledge. Ignoring the feeling levels of clients during these times can disrupt the therapeutic relationship and may result in the client withdrawing or becoming increasingly distressed. Following the principles of crisis intervention delineated by Caplan (discussed later in this chapter) helps to develop a caring, trusting, professional relationship with clients in crisis.

TABLE 8-4   Relationship of Teaching Process to Nursing Process

Assessment	Diagnosis	Goals	Intervention	Evaluation
Nursing Process				
General screening questions to detect patient's need to learn; if positive, use teaching process	One of the problem statements may be a need to learn or a nursing diagnosis	Learning goals are a subset of the goals	Teaching intervention may be delivered with other intervention	Evaluating whether the nursing care outcome was met
Teaching Process				
Refined assessment of need to learn and readiness	Learning diagnosis	Setting of learning goals	Teaching	Evaluating learning

From Redman BK: *The process of patient education*, ed. 7, St. Louis, 1993, Mosby, p. 13.

Educative Approach

Health education has traditionally been a function of the community health nurse. Lillian Wald cared for the sick in the home and also provided instruction so that families were better equipped to assist their ill members. Lina Rodgers taught personal hygiene to school-age children and their families and as a result the spread of disease was reduced and wellness was promoted. Funds were made available through Federal Maternal and Child Health Grants in the 1920s and 1930s so that community health nurses could be hired to provide health teaching in relation to child care, nutrition, and family-life education. Monies were also allocated at this time for preventive health teaching services aimed at combating communicable diseases such as tuberculosis and childhood illnesses.

The health education function of nurses in the community setting has remained viable over the years. It is still a major focus of all community health nurses, regardless of the setting in which they practice, because practitioners in the field have clearly demonstrated the value of this activity.

Health beliefs and behavior are the targets of teaching or the educative approach in nursing practice (Redman, 1993). Health education activities are designed to promote wellness and to prevent illness. They are used to prepare clients to deal with maturational and situational events that produce stress. They are also used to promote personal habits that foster

optimal health, including obtaining immunizations to prevent communicable disease, eating balanced meals, and seeking medical care when ill. Psychosocial and physical aspects of health and disease are taken into consideration when the community health nurse uses this intervention strategy.

The teaching-learning or educative process as delineated by Redman (1993, p. 12) is summarized as follows:

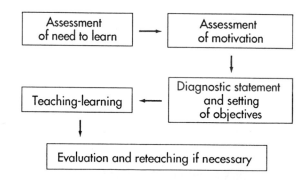

The steps in this process parallel the steps of the nursing process (refer to Table 8-4). The client's knowledge base and motivation or readiness for learning are assessed, diagnostic statement(s) about client need are developed, specific teaching goals/objectives are established, and teaching-learning plans are implemented and evaluated.

The educative strategy has two major components: (1) increasing the learner's understanding of new events and his or her healthy functioning through the acquisition of knowledge and (2) helping the learner to apply the new information. Need to learn and readiness of the learner must be assessed and established before either of these components can be implemented successfully. Sharing information the client does not wish to assimilate does not increase client understanding. In fact, when this happens clients frequently do not concentrate on what is being shared.

The concept of learner readiness or motivation is a complex, multidimensional phenomenon. It involves the interaction between multiple interrelated variables such as clients' perceptions of health and illness, family patterns of health care, and availability and accessibility of resources. Various models have been proposed by social scientists and nurses to explain why clients are or are not motivated to engage in health behaviors (Cox, 1982; Fishbein and Ajzen, 1975; Kulbok, 1985; Pender, 1987, Health promotion in practice; Rosenstock, 1966, 1974; Rotter, 1966). One of the most widely used models, the *Health Belief Model,* examines why individuals engage in diagnostic and other disease-prevention activities (Rosenstock, 1974). In the mid-1960s Rosenstock stimulated significant interest among health professionals in the use of this model when he examined in the literature why people use health services (Rosenstock, 1966). The Health Belief Model, developed by a group of social scientists, advances the idea that readiness to take health action is dependent on several variables including (1) perceived susceptibility to a specific condition, (2) perceived seriousness of a given health problem, (3) perceived benefits and barriers to taking action, and (4) cues to action such as knowledge that someone else has become affected by the condition. The Health Belief Model emphasizes that the beliefs that define readiness have both cognitive and emotional components and the motivational variables that promote disease-oriented, preventive health action are individually defined (Rosenstock, 1966).

The Health Belief Model is useful in explaining health-promoting behaviors that are triggered by an interest in preventing disease occurrence. Other conceptual models have been developed to examine health-promoting behaviors that are wellness-oriented rather than disease-focused. An example of such a model is the Health Promotion Model developed by Pender (1987, Health and health promotion). In this model

cognitive-perceptual factors are considered to be the primary determinants of behavior and are identified as (1) importance of health; (2) perceived control of health; (3) perceived self-efficacy; (4) definition of health; (5) perceived health status; (6) perceived benefits of health-promoting behaviors; and (7) perceived barriers to health-promoting behaviors. Demographic characteristics, biologic characteristics, interpersonal influences, situational factors and behavioral factors are hypothesized as influencing health behaviors through cognitive-perceptual processes. As in the Health Belief Model, cues to action are considered important in the initiation of health actions. (Pender, 1987, Health and health promotion, pp. 13-14)

An in-depth discussion of this model can be found in Pender's (1987) book *Health Promotion in Nursing Practice.*

Health behavior models such as those just discussed emphasize the importance of assessing more than cognitive understanding or knowledge when determining learner readiness. Often underlying psychosocial factors are the key variables that influence why people do or do not engage in positive health action. If that is the case, these factors must be dealt with before the health professional initiates cognitive teaching strategies.

Use of the nursing process (refer to Chapter 9) combined with an understanding of the principles of teaching and learning aids the community health nurse in assessing learner readiness. These factors also help to individualize educational plans based on client needs and circumstances. Writings by Brill (1978), Lorig (1992), Pohl (1978), and Redman (1993) are valuable resources if one wants to review or expand knowledge in relation to the principles of teaching and learning.

After community health nurses establish learner readiness, they and their clients mutually develop teaching and learning goals. Together they also select from a variety of alternative intervention options a teaching strategy that best fits the client's needs and circumstances. Frequently a combination of two or more teaching methods is used. For example, a community health nurse might combine discussion, demonstration, and use of pamphlets to teach new parents how to bathe a baby. Or the nurse might use group process, audiovisual aids, self-instructional materials, and a baby bath demonstration to teach this same procedure. Whatever techniques are selected, the learner should have the opportunity to obtain new knowledge and to apply the knowledge gained. For instance, understanding how to bathe a baby does not always increase a new parent's level of comfort when doing so. Being allowed to demonstrate what has been learned when assistance is available is more likely to promote ease with such a procedure.

Developing specific, measurable, client-centered goals for the teaching and learning process is essential for several reasons. Specific goals help to determine what content or information is needed by the client. They also aid in developing and implementing teaching techniques relevant to the client's needs. In addition, they facilitate evaluation of the learning process because they define what the client desires to learn. A global goal such as "learning about growth and development" does none of these things. It does not define what information parents need in order to handle the developmental needs of their child more effectively. A goal which states that "Jean will verbally identify the developmental tasks of a 1-year-old" is much clearer.

Individualizing teaching and learning plans is crucial because client needs vary even when different people encounter similar situations. Some parents understand normal growth-and-development processes very well but have difficulty handling the physical aspects of child care. Others are at ease with feeding, bathing, and clothing their infant but become frustrated when the child does not achieve developmental tasks, even if it is too soon for him or her to accomplish them. Differences like these are not uncommon among clients who are experiencing similar situations.

Opportunities to use the educative strategy in the community health setting are endless. Teaching a child at school how to prevent infection when hurt, discussing sexuality issues with a mother who has preadolescent children, and sharing information about the hereditary aspects of diabetes when a family history reflects a need are a few examples of when a community health nurse uses the educative strategy. Education is not always needed, however, and can be misused. This happens particularly when the nurse makes an assumption about what the client needs to learn without first assessing the situation, or when the nurse imposes information on the client because of value conflicts. Some parents who have several children, for example, desire to have more. Continuing to teach about family planning after demonstration that the parents know how to prevent pregnancy and understand the pros and cons of increasing their family

size is meeting the nurse's needs, not the family's needs.

Problem-Solving Approach

In the community health setting, nurses encounter clients who are having difficulty making decisions about a variety of personal life events. Specifically, community health nurses help clients to make decisions about such things as career choices, maintaining or establishing intimate relationships with others, when and where to obtain preventive and curative health care services, how to deal with family conflicts, how to handle financial crises, or how to provide needed care for aging family members. At times clients dealing with situations such as these have difficulty identifying why they cannot make a decision about what to do. They know that something is wrong because symptoms of anxiety are present, but they are unable to take action to reduce their stress.

There are various reasons why clients are unable to alter their behavior in ways to help them resolve their stress appropriately. Examples are illustrated in the case situations that follow.

▶ **CLIENT HAS NOT SPECIFICALLY IDENTIFIED THE NATURE OF THE PROBLEM**
Barb Lehi, a 28-year-old wife and the mother of two children, returned to work when her youngest child entered school. Her family adjusted well to her role change because joint decision-making occurred prior to Barb's employment. Barb was enjoying what she was doing but began to have tension headaches 2 months after she started her new job. She felt her headaches were related to the adjustments she had to make in her daily routine, and assumed that they would go away shortly. They did not, however, until she was able to identify that she was having guilt feelings about being a working mother and its effect on her family.

▶ **CLIENT HAS A VESTED INTEREST IN NOT IDENTIFYING THE PROBLEM**
Mrs. Jackson, a 68-year-old widow living by herself, kept finding reasons why she should not see a physician after she started having "fainting spells." Her family became frustrated and worried and asked the community health nurse to visit. Referral for medical evaluation was successfully implemented only when Mrs. Jackson was able to verbalize that being ill was the only way she could get attention from her family. Her family visited very

sporadically when she was well but daily when she was ill.

CLIENT IS UNABLE TO ACKNOWLEDGE FEELINGS

Gail Hayes, a 31-year-old mother and wife, provided no stimulation for her 2-year-old daughter who was retarded due to rubella exposure in utero. The community health nurse became involved after hearing from a neighbor that Gail left her daughter alone in the house when she visited friends and neighbors. After several home visits, the nurse discovered that Gail did so because "I can't stand to be with her. She is such a fussy child and wants attention all of the time. I hate seeing her so deformed and feel guilty because if I hadn't gotten measles while pregnant she would be all right." Gail had never before acknowledged these feelings. When she did, she was able to use the help offered by others and to relate more effectively to her daughter.

CLIENT DOES NOT ASSUME ACCOUNTABILITY FOR FEELINGS

Bob Woodrow, a 40-year-old construction worker, was referred to the health department for rehabilitative services after a myocardial infarction. Because of the strenuous nature of construction work it was recommended that he seek other employment. He verbalized an interest in obtaining job training through the Division of Vocational Rehabilitation but took no action. When the community health nurse questioned why, he responded by placing the blame on others. "My wife thinks it is too soon and nags me about not going back to work. I am not sure if my physician thinks I should, because he is always so vague about what is happening with my heart. My car needs fixing before I can use it regularly, and we don't have the money to get it fixed." It took several months for Bob to see that he was not taking action because of his own fears about having another heart attack and about not being able to succeed in a new line of work.

CLIENT CANNOT DISTINGUISH BETWEEN FEELINGS AND FACTS

Carol Strang, a 17-year-old junior, repeatedly visited the school nurse for minor physical concerns. Assessments made by the nurse revealed that this occurred when Carol felt that she was not performing well academically. In reality Carol was very successful in her schoolwork, ranking in the top 5% of her class. In addition, she had several close friends who provided praise for her academic achievements. Carol, however, perceived that she was achieving satisfactorily only when she received straight As. When she received anything less than an A, she expressed feelings associated with failure.

CLIENT LACKS EXPERIENCE WITH PROBLEM-SOLVING

Mrs. Raabe, a 71-year-old widow, became confused and severely upset after her husband's death. All her life she had been cared for by others. Her parents and her brothers anticipated her needs because she was the "baby" of the family and "helpless." Because her husband assumed the same role as her family, Mrs. Raabe felt lost when he died. She found managing her finances particularly stressful since she had never taken care of the family budget. She needed help with such basics as writing a check, depositing money in the bank, and balancing her income and expenses.

CLIENT HAS UNDETECTED PHYSICAL OR PERCEPTUAL PROBLEMS

Mrs. La Rosa, a 37-year-old divorced mother of six children, was referred to the health department by her caseworker from the Department of Social Service. Her caseworker believed that Mrs. La Rosa was neglecting her children and felt that environmental conditions were dangerous to the family's health. Mrs. La Rosa told the community health nurse that "I know I should keep my home more tidy, but I am just too tired to keep up with things that need to be done around the house. Sometimes all I want to do is sleep." The community health nurse assisted her in obtaining a medical evaluation. It was found during this evaluation that Mrs. La Rosa had hypertension and diabetes. When both of these conditions were under control, home management and child care skills improved.

CLIENT MISSED ESSENTIAL STEPS IN SKILL DEVELOPMENT

Mr. and Mrs. Lueck were extremely upset when their 10-year-old retarded son was sent home from camp because he could not handle activities of daily living such as bathing and toileting. "Tommie always does these things at home. They just don't know how to work with retarded kids." Upon talking with the Luecks, the community health nurse discovered Tommie did wash himself when bathing at home, but that family members helped him with most of the activities necessary for completing a bath. For example, the family ran his bath water for him; assembled the materials he needed to take a bath, including soap, washcloth, and towel; and selected the clothing he would wear afterward. It was obvious to the nurse but not the parents that Tommie never really learned how to handle his personal hygiene needs. He had skill in washing body parts, but lacked decision-making skill about how and when to carry out these activities.

▶ CLIENT IS UNABLE TO GENERATE ALTERNATIVE OPTIONS DURING PROBLEM-SOLVING OR FEARS THE CONSEQUENCES OF A NEWLY GENERATED ALTERNATIVE

Amy Schmidt, wife and mother of two preschoolers, was physically abused by her husband regularly and expressed a desire to leave him. She found it difficult to take this action because she thought that it was impossible for her to do so. She felt trapped because she had no job skills and her family and friends were unable to assist her financially. In addition, she felt that the abuse would not stop even if she left home because her husband could always find her. The community health nurse assisted Mrs. Schmidt in identifying ways to obtain financial aid and legal assistance to control her husband's behavior. Mrs. Schmidt was also helped to see that living alone could be less frightening for her and her children than being physically abused.

The situations presented above are far more complex than indicated by the discussion. They are briefly summarized to illustrate that there are many reasons why established problem-solving patterns are ineffective during times of stress and crisis. Identifying the specific reason(s) for each client's stress is the essential first step when the community health nurse uses the problem-solving approach to enhance client growth.

A community health nurse has two major goals when using the problem-solving approach: (1) to assist the client in solving immediate problem(s) and (2) to help the client increase independent problem-solving abilities. Implicit in these goals is the belief that clients can learn skills that will help them to make decisions wisely and to alter behavior accordingly. A community health nurse who has difficulty internalizing this belief will find it hard to move a client toward independence. This nurse is more likely *to do for* the client than *to work with* the client.

A variety of nursing interventions can be used to help a client enhance his or her problem-solving abilities, including such things as individual counseling, group work, role modeling, referral to community resources, client contracting, and behavioral modification. When using any one of these techniques the community health nurse should focus on helping the client to identify the nature of the problem(s), to discover alternative options for problem solving, to make decisions about which option is most appropriate, and to take action to resolve the problem(s). The community health nurse should not assume that the client will take action after making a decision about the most appropriate option and prematurely close the family to service. Taking action is often the most difficult step in the problem-solving process because it is at this point that the client is giving up the secure familiar for the threatening unknown.

Clients must be allowed to make decisions and to take action for themselves before they are able to achieve independent problem-solving abilities. It is natural to want to "rescue" clients when they are experiencing pain. *Rescue behavior,* such as giving advice and doing for the client, reduces anxiety only temporarily, because the client is not prepared to handle stress in the future. It can be helpful for the community health nurse to share alternative ways for handling stresses, but the client should be encouraged to evaluate suggestions in terms of his or her own circumstances. The client should be given the message that no one way is being advocated but that these options have worked with others in the past.

When clients are experiencing crisis they often desperately want others to make decisions for them. Cadden (1964, pp. 293-296) has delineated several principles of crisis intervention that help a community health nurse avoid rescue activities and provide constructive aid to the family. These are:

1. *Help the client confront the crisis* by supporting expression of feelings and emotions such as fear, guilt, and crying.
2. *Help the client confront the crisis in manageable doses* without dampening the impact of the crisis to a point where the client no longer recognizes the need to alter coping mechanisms. Drugs and diversional activities are helpful when they are used to decrease unmanageable stress. They are harmful when they prevent the client from looking at the realities of his or her situation.
3. *Help the client to find the facts* because truth is

less frightening than the unknown. Clients may need frequent visits during periods of crisis because they may not have the energy to analyze all the stresses they are experiencing during one home visit.

4. *Do not give the client false reassurance* because this leads to mistrust and maladaptive coping behaviors. To succeed in resolving a crisis, a client needs reassurance that supports his or her ability to handle the crisis situation.

5. *Do not encourage the client to blame others* because blaming only reduces tension momentarily and can help the client to suppress feelings. This can result in maladaptive behaviors that decrease the client's level of functioning after crisis resolution.

6. *Help the client to accept help* because some clients avoid confronting a crisis by denying that they need help and that a problem exists. If the client does not face the crisis, he or she will not mobilize coping mechanisms that will enhance growth.

7. *Help the client with everyday tasks* in a manner that reflects kindness and thoughtfulness rather than one that gives a message that the client is weak or incompetent. Clients need help with everyday tasks because it takes considerable energy to resolve a crisis; thus clients often lack sufficient energy to handle daily activities as well.

Problem-solving takes time. Both the client and the community health nurse must guard against expecting change too rapidly. When progress is slow a client may question if the nurse can really help, and the nurse often begins to wonder whether or not the client really wants to change. At times both of these feelings are justified. More frequently, however, the need is for the client and nurse to recognize that well-established patterns of behavior cannot be changed immediately.

Community health nurses cannot help all clients to learn to make decisions wisely. Some situations are beyond their competence and must be referred to others who are better qualified. Because competence varies from one community health nurse to another as a result of differences in academic preparation and work experiences, nurses must learn how to discriminate between situations that they can and cannot handle. Peer and supervisory conferences will assist a new nurse to objectively evaluate her or his skills.

Underestimating one's ability to help a client, rather than overestimating competency, is often more of a problem when nurses begin practice in the community health setting. Most clients experiencing stress and crisis do not need psychotherapy. Instead, they need someone who cares and who will provide supportive guidance and positive reinforcement for the strength they have.

Summary

The community health nurse is often the primary source of assistance when an individual or a family is experiencing stress. Stress is a normal human phenomenon necessary for survival and growth. It triggers the general adaptation syndrome that helps people adapt to the demands and pressures of life. Although stress is essential for survival and growth, every individual has limits beyond which stress is no longer tolerated. Prolonged and intensified stress results in crisis, especially when an individual's coping mechanisms are inadequate to reduce disequilibrium.

A person in crisis experiences disorganization and heightened stress. Crisis is self-limiting but biopsychosocial homeostasis following a crisis may be at a level equal to, better than, or lower than the precrisis level. Timely supportive intervention may be the critical factor that determines if an individual or family has a positive or negative outcome during periods of crisis.

◀   *An Exercise in Critical Thinking*   ▶

You are the community health nurse visiting the Slavovi family described on p. 262 of this chapter. Shortly after arriving at their home for your first home visit, it becomes obvious that Angel and Maria want you to tell them "the right way to do things with Stephanie" and that they are hoping to find someone who can "cure her." (Hospital personnel had shared with the family that Stephanie has cerebral palsy and needs long-term health and educational follow-up.) Considering the factors that influence the outcome of a crisis, discuss with a peer the type of assessment data you would collect on your first home visit and how you would apply the principles of crisis intervention in this situation.

References

Ailinger RL: Beliefs about treatment of hypertension among Hispanic older persons, *TCN* 7:26-31, 1985.

Allen ML, Brown P, and Finlay B: *Helping children by strengthening families: a look at family support programs,* Washington, D.C., 1992, Children's Defense Fund.

Aguilera DC: *Crisis intervention: theory and methodology,* ed 7, St. Louis, 1994, Mosby.

Bakeland F and Lundwall L: *Dropping out of treatment: a critical review,* *Psychol Bull* 82:738-783, 1975.

Blau ZS: *Old age in a changing society,* New York, 1973, New Viewpoints.

Boss PG: Family stress. In Sussman M and Steinmetz S, eds: *Handbook on marriage and the family,* New York, 1987, Plenum, pp. 445-450.

Brill NI: *Working with people: the helping process,* Philadelphia, 1978, Lippincott.

Brown GW, Bhrolchain MN, and Harris TO: Social class and psychiatric disturbance among women in an urban population, *Sociology* 9:225-231, 1975.

Burch J: Recent bereavement in relation to suicide, *J Psychosom Med* 16:361-366, 1972.

Burr WR: *Theory construction and the sociology of the family,* New York, 1973, Wiley.

Cadden V: Crisis in the family. In Caplan G, ed: *Principles of preventive psychiatry,* New York, 1964, Basic Books, pp. 228-296.

Cannon WB: *Bodily changes in pain, hunger, fear, and rage,* New York, 1929, Appleton.

Cannon WB: Stresses and strains of homeostasis, *Am J Med Sci* 189:1-14, 1935.

Capers CF: Nursing and the Afro-American client, *ICN* 7:11-17, 1985.

Caplan G: *An approach to community mental health,* New York, 1961, Grune and Stratton.

Caplan G: *Principles of preventive psychiatry,* New York, 1964, Basic Books.

Caplan RD, Robinson EAR, French JRP Jr., Caldwell JR, and Shinn MB: *Adhering to medical regimens: pilot experiments in patient education and social support,* Ann Arbor, 1976, University of Michigan, Institute for Social Research.

Cassel JC: The contribution of the social environment to host resistance, *American Journal of Epidemiology* 104:107-123, 1976.

Cassel JC: Psychiatric epidemiology. In Caplan G, ed: *American handbook of psychiatry, vol 2,* New York, 1974, Basic Books.

Cassel JC: Psychosocial processes and stress: theoretical formulation, *Int J Health Serv* 4:471-482, 1974.

Chambers WN and Reiser MF: Emotional stress in the precipitation of congestive heart failure, *Psychosom Med* 15:38-60, 1953.

Chang K: Chinese Americans. In Giger JN and Davidhizar RE: *Transcultural nursing: assessment and intervention,* St. Louis, 1991, Mosby.

Chen E and Cobb S: Family structure in relation to health and disease, *J Chron Dis* 12:544-567, 1960.

Chen-Louie T: Nursing care of Chinese American patients. In Orque MS, Bloch B, and Monrroy LSA: *Ethnic nursing care,* St. Louis, 1983, Mosby.

Cobb S: Physiological changes in men whose jobs were abolished, *J Psychosom Res* 18:245-258, 1974.

Cobb S: Social support as a moderator of life stress, *Psychosomatic Medicine* 38:300-314, 1976.

Cobb S, Kasl SV, French JRP, and Norstebo G: The intrafamilial transmission of rheumatoid arthritis VII. Why wives with rheumatoid arthritis have husbands with peptic ulcers, *J Chron Dis* 22:279-293, 1969.

Cox C: An interaction model of client health behavior: theoretical prescription for nursing, *Adv Nurs Sci* 5:41-56, 1982.

Davitz LJ, Sameshima Y, and Davitz J: Suffering as viewed in six different cultures, *AJN* 76:1296-1297, 1976.

de Araujo G, Van Arsdel PP, Holmes TH, and Dudley DL: Life change, coping ability and chronic intrinsic asthma, *J Psychosom Res* 17:359-363, 1973.

Eckholm E: AIDS and folk healing, a Zimbabwe encounter, *New York Times* October 5, 1990, pp. 1-2.

Egbert LD, Battib GE, Welch CE, and Bartlett MK: Reduction of post-operative pain by encouragement and instruction of patients, *N Engl J Med* 270:825-827, 1964.

Figley CR and McCubbin HI: *Stress and the family, vol II. Coping with catastrophe,* New York, 1983, Brunner/Mazel.

Fishbein M and Ajzen I: *Belief, attitude, intention and behavior: an introduction to theory research,* Reading, Mass., 1975, Addison-Wesley.

Germain CP: Cultural care: a bridge between sickness, illness, and disease, *Holistic Nurse Pract* 6:1-9, 1992.

Giger JN and Davidhizar RE: *Transcultural nursing: assessment and intervention,* St. Louis, 1991, Mosby.

Gore S: *The influence of social support and related variables in ameliorating the consequence of job loss,* Doctoral dissertation, Philadelphia, 1973, University of Pennsylvania.

Gordon M: *Manual of nursing diagnosis, 1993-1994,* St. Louis, 1993, Mosby.

Gottlieb BH: *Social support strategies: guidelines for mental health practice,* Beverly Hills, Calif., 1983, Sage.

Hamburg A and Killilea M: Relation of social support, stress, illness, and use of health services. In Hamburg D, ed: *Healthy people: the Surgeon General's report on health promotion and disease prevention,* DHEW PHS Pub. No. 79-55071A, Washington, D.C., 1979, U.S. Department of Health, Education, and Welfare.

Hansen DA and Hill R: Families under stress. In Christensen HT, ed: *Handbook of marriage and the family,* Chicago, 1964, Rand McNally, pp. 783-819.

Haynes RB and Sackett DL: *A working symposium: compliance with therapeutic regimens, annotated bibliography,* Hamilton, Ont., 1974, McMaster University Medical Center, Department of Epidemiology and Biostatics.

Hill R: *Families under stress: adjustment to the crises of war separation and reunion,* New York, 1949, Harper.

Hill R: Generic features of families under stress. In Parad HJ, ed: *Crisis intervention: selected readings,* New York, 1965, Family Service Association of America, pp. 32-74.

Jessner L, Blom GE, and Waldfogel S: Emotional implications of tonsillectomy and adenoidectomy on children, *Psychoanal Study Child* 7:126-169, 1952.

Kaplan BH, Cassel JC, and Gore S: Social support and health, *Med Care* 15(5):47-58, 1977.

Kay M and Yoder M: Hot and cold in women's ethnotherapeutics: the American Mexican west, *Soc Sci Med* 25:347-355, 1987.

Kleinman A, Eisenberg L, and Good B: Culture, illness, and care: clinical lessons from anthropologic and cross-cultural research, *Annals of Internal Medicine* 88:251-258, 1978.

Knapp TR: Stress versus strain: methodological critique, *Nurs Res* 37:181-184, 1988.

Krause N: Social support, stress and well-being among older adults, *J Gerontol* 41:512-519, 1986.

Kulbok PP: Social resources, health resources, and preventive health behavior: patterns and predictions, *Public Health Nurs* 2:67-81, 1985.

Lazarus RS: *Psychological stress and the coping process,* New York, 1966, McGraw-Hill.

Lazarus RS: Psychological stress and coping in adaptation and illness, *International Journal of Psychiatry in Medicine* 5:321-333, 1974.

Lazarus RS: The stress and coping paradigm. In Eisdorfer C, Cohen D, Kleinman A, and Masim P, eds: *Models for clinical psychopathology,* New York, 1981, Spectrum, pp. 177-214.

Lazarus RS and Folkman S: *Stress, appraisal and coping,* New York, 1984, Springer.

Lewis S, Messner R, and McDowell WA: An unchanging culture, *J Gerontol Nurs* 11:21-26, 1985.

Lindemann E: Symptomatology and management of acute grief, *Am J Psychiatry* 101:141-148, 1944.

Lorig K: *Patient education: a practical approach,* St. Louis, 1992, Mosby.

Louie KB: Providing health care to Chinese clients, *ICN* 7:18-25, 1985.

Lowenthal MF and Haven C: Interaction and adoption intimacy: a critical variable, *Am Sociol Rev* 33:20, 1968.

Ludman EK and Newman JM: The health-related food practices of three Chinese groups, *J Nutrition Education* 16:4, 1984.

Maddison DC and Walther WL: Factors affecting the outcome of conjugal bereavement, *Br J Psychiatry* 113:1057-1067, 1967.

Maloney C: Don't say "pretty baby" lest you zap it with your eye—the evil eye in South Asia. In Maloney C, ed: *The evil eye,* New York, 1976, Columbia University Press, pp. 102-248.

Mather HG: Intensive care, *Br Med J* 2:322, 1974.

Mather HG, Pearson NG, Read KLQ, Shaw DB, Steed GR, Thorne MG, Jones S, Guerrier CJ, Eraut CD, McHugh PM, Chowdhury NF, Jafary MH, and Wallace TJ: Acute myocardial infarction: home and hospital treatment, *Br Med J* 3:334-338, 1971.

McCubbin H, Cauble E, and Patterson J, eds: *Family stress in coping, and social support,* Springfield, Ill., 1982, Charles C. Thomas.

McCubbin H and Figley CR: *Stress and the family, vol I: coping with normative transitions,* New York, 1983, Brunner/Mazel.

McCubbin MA and McCubbin HI: Family stress theory and assessment: The T-Double ABCX Model of Family Adjustment and Adaptation. In McCubbin HI and Thompson A, eds: *Family assessment inventories for research and practice,* Madison, Wisc., 1987, University of Wisconsin-Madison, pp. 3-32.

McCubbin MA and McCubbin HI: Families coping with illness: The Resiliency Model of Family Stress, Adjustment, and Adaptation. In Danielson CB, Hamel-Bissell BP, and Winstead-Fry P, eds: *Families, health, and illness: perspectives on coping and interventions,* St. Louis, 1993, Mosby, pp. 21-63.

McCubbin HI and Patterson JM: Family transitions: adaptation to stress. In McCubbin HI and Figley CR, eds: *Stress and the family, vol 1: coping with normative transitions,* New York, 1983a, Brunner/ Mazel.

McCubbin HI and Patterson JM: Family stress adaptation to crises: a double ABCX model of family behavior. In Olson DH & Miller BC, eds: *Family studies review year book vol 1,* Beverly Hills, 1983b, Sage, pp. 87-106.

McHugh P: *Defining the situation: the organization of meaning in social interactions,* Indianapolis, 1968, Bobbs-Merrill.

Nuckolls KB, Cassel JC, and Kaplan BH: Psycho-social assets, life crisis and prognosis of pregnancy, *Am J Epidemiol* 95:431-441, 1972.

Parkes CM, Benjamin B, and Fitzgerald RE: Broken heart: a study of increased mortality among widowers, *Br Med J* 1:740, 1969.

Parkes CM: *Bereavement studies of grief in adult life,* New York, 1972, International Universities Press.

Parsons T: On becoming a patient. In Folta JR and Beck ES, eds: *A sociological framework for patient care,* New York, 1966, John Wiley.

Pasquale EA: The evil eye phenomenon: its implications for community health nursing, *Home Healthcare Nurse* 2:32-37, 1984.

Pender NJ: Health and health promotion: conceptual dilemmas. In Duffy ME and Pender NJ, eds: *Conceptual issues in health promotion: report of proceedings of a wingspread conference,* Indianapolis, 1987, Sigma Theta Tau, pp. 7-23.

Pender NJ: *Health promotion in nursing practice,* Norwalk, Conn., 1987, Appleton-Century-Crofts.

Pilisuk M and Parks S: Social support and family stress. In McCubbin H, Sussman M, and Patterson J, eds: *Social stress and the family: advances and developments in family stress theory and research,* New York, 1983, Haworth, pp. 137-156.

Pohl ML: *The teaching function of the nursing practitioner,* Dubuque, 1978, Brown.

Rahe RH: The pathway between subjects' recent life changes and their near-future illness reports: representative results and methodological issues. In Dohrenwend BS and Dohrenwend BP, eds: *Stressful life events,* New York, 1974, Wiley.

Redman BK: *The process of patient education,* ed 7, St. Louis, 1993, Mosby.

Rosenstock IM: Why people use health services, *Milbank Q* 44:94-127, 1966.

Rosenstock IM: Historical origins of the health belief model, *Health Education Monograph* 2(4):328-335, 1974.

Ross HM: Societal/cultural views regarding death and dying, *TCN* 3:1-15, 1981.

Rotter JB: Internal versus external control of reinforcement, *Psychological Monograph* 80(1), 1966.

Selye H: *The stress of life,* New York, 1976, McGraw-Hill.

Snow LF: Folk medical beliefs and their implications for care of patients: a review based on studies among Black Americans, *Annals of Internal Medicine* 81:82-96, 1974.

Sobralske MC: Perceptions of health: Navajo Indians, *ICN* 7:32-39, 1985.

Twaddle AC: Sickness and the sickness career: some implications. In Eisenberg L and Kleinman A, eds: *The relevance of social science for medicine,* Dordrecht, Holland, 1981, D Reidel Publishing.

Villarruel AM and Ortiz de Montellano B: Culture and pain: a Mesoamerican perspective, *Adv Nurs Sci* 15:21-32, 1992.

Whaley LF and Wong DL: *Nursing care of infants and children,* ed 4, St. Louis, 1991, Mosby.

Selected Bibliography

Allan JD: Identification of health risks in a young adult population, *J Commun Health Nurs* 4:223-233, 1987.

Antonousky A: *Health, stress, and coping,* San Francisco, 1979, Jossey-Bass.

Bushy A: Rural women: lifestyle and health status, *Nurs Clinics of North America* 28:187-197, 1993.

Craft MJ and Willadsen JA: Interventions related to family, *Nurs Clinics of North America* 27:371-396, 1992.

Family Nursing Continuing Education Project: *Nursing of families in transition: workshop proceedings,* Portland, Ore., 1987, Oregon Health Sciences University.

Family Nursing Continuing Education Project: *Nursing of families with acute or chronic illness: workshop proceedings,* Portland, Ore., 1988, Oregon Health Sciences University.

Hyman RB and Woog P: Stressful life events and illness onset: a review of crucial variables, *Res Nurs Health* 5:155-163, 1982.

Johnson JE and Lauver DR: Alternative explanations of coping with stressful experiences associated with physical illness, *Adv Nurs Sci* 11(2):39-52, 1989.

Krentz LG, ed: *Nursing and the promotion/protection of family health: workshop proceedings,* Portland, Ore., 1988, Oregon Health Sciences University.

Laffrey SC, Loveland-Cherry CJ and Winkler SJ: Health behavior: evolution of two paradigms, *Public Health Nurs* 3:92-100, 1986.

Manfredi C and Pickett M: Perceived stressful situations and coping strategies utilized by the elderly, *J Commun Health Nurs* 4:99-110, 1987.

McHatton M: A theory of timely teaching, *Am J Nurs* 7:798, 1985.

Pugh LC and Milligan R: A framework for the study of childbearing fatigue, ANS 15:60-70, 1993.

Rakel BA: Interventions related to patient teaching, *Nurs Clinics of North America* 27:397-424, 1992.

Simons MR: Interventions related to compliance, *Nurs Clinics of North America* 27:477-494, 1992.

Wismont JM and Reame NE: The lesbian childbearing experience: assessing developmental tasks, *Image: J Nurs Scholarship* 21:137-141, 1989.

Wright LM and Leahey M: *Families and chronic illness,* Springhouse, Penn., 1987, Springhouse Corporation.

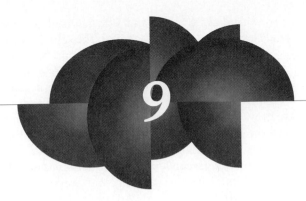

9

Use of Family-Centered Nursing Process with Culturally Diverse Clients

OBJECTIVES

Upon completion of this chapter, the reader should be able to:

1. Discuss four key elements inherent in the definition of the family-centered nursing process.
2. Distinguish between the phases of the family-centered nursing process.
3. Describe the relationship between the phases of the family-centered nursing process.
4. Compare and contrast the family-centered nursing process and the individual-focused nursing process.
5. Identify the importance of applying theoretical concepts as a basis for decision-making in practice and theory bases applicable to community health nursing.
6. Discuss cultural phenomena that influence nursing practice.

7. Summarize the nursing responsibilities related to a home visit and the importance of each to the development of a therapeutic nurse-family relationship.
8. Describe client rights and related agency obligations throughout the provider/client relationship.
9. Formulate criteria for assessing healthy and ineffective family behaviors.
10. Construct examples of family-centered nursing diagnoses, interventions, and evaluation statements.
11. Discuss the philosophy underlying the use of contracting as a community health nursing intervention strategy and provide examples of contracting with families.

For a green plant to survive, it must reach sunlight. So nature provides that if the plant's growth is blocked in one direction, it can grow in another.

CONOCO OIL COMPANY

People, like green plants, can grow in multiple directions. Stumbling blocks along the way do not necessarily stop growth (refer to Figure 9-1). Caring, support, and assistance from significant others can help humanity to change the course of its development when barriers are inhibiting the growth process. Persons can grow, change and develop within the family unit (Whall, 1991, p. 321). Although human growth follows a predictable pattern, all families and their individual members are still unique. As they develop, they make choices about pathways to take to reach sunlight and to achieve happiness. Although physiological, psychosocial, cultural, and spiritual forces influence family decision-making about what brings a rich and satisfying life, every family also needs the opportunity to define which pathways lead to personal growth and self-fulfillment. Families and health care providers who encourage others to make independent decisions about life choices are more likely to facilitate growth than those who impose on others their beliefs about appropriate life pathways.

Community health nurses can facilitate the family growth process. They work to develop trusting, supportive relationships so that clients can reach out and use their help when needed. Some clients will not seek assistance from community health nurses because they have found other support systems more relevant to them. However, when a client does accept the help offered by a community health nurse, it is extremely important for the nurse to recognize that her or his role is to help the client determine which pathways to brightness are appropriate for that family. The nurse cannot know what is best for other human beings. Taking away a family's independence leads to darkness, not light.

Increasingly, nurses and other health care professionals have accepted the client's right of self-determination in relation to decision making and change. They have identified that doing *for* the client instead of working *with* him or her can result in client dependence and limits on behavioral action. Clients must internalize the need for change before they will alter their behavior. An example is a family who had one of its members hospitalized for cardiac problems

and was advised to modify the family diet. In the hospital the client was served low-sodium, low-cholesterol food and did not have the option to eat other types of foods. The client's physician has ordered this diet to be ongoing. If the family does not understand the reason for the recommended diet, or finds it difficult to adapt current food patterns, it is highly unlikely that this diet will be used at home. Families in their own environment make decisions about what they will eat. A nurse can influence family change but only families can alter their behavior.

At times the concept of individual self-determination is difficult to operationalize, because a professional's personal feelings can influence the interactions between that person and the client. It is easy for a nurse to feel like a failure when a client does not alter health actions, especially when this behavior is adversely affecting the client's health status. Viewing oneself as a client often helps. Stop and think for a while how you make changes in your lifestyle. For most people, being ordered to change produces feelings of resentment and increases resistance. People want to believe that they are capable of making decisions about their lives, and they want the freedom to make choices even if the choices have negative consequences. Depending on the situation, clients may want or need varying degrees of guidance and support, but at all times they should be given the message that they are capable of independent decision-making.

To function effectively in the community setting, a nurse must accept the fact that clients are responsible for their health behavior, even when they choose a plan of action that the nurse would not choose. Nurse-defined goals for clients are seldom achieved. Goals defined by the client are more frequently accomplished. The nurse who takes over for clients quickly becomes frustrated with the lack of client response and may "burn out."

The nursing process helps the community health nurse facilitate client goal setting. This therapeutic process is used by nurses in all settings. However, it is labeled the *family-centered nursing process* in the community health setting because community health nurses use it to analyze family functioning and to extend services to the family as a whole. This focus is based on the belief that the family is the basic unit for nursing service: family functioning affects the health of all family members by inhibiting or facilitating the growth process, by influencing when family members

Figure 9-1 Nature doesn't explore just one path to reach a goal. Neither should man. (Courtesy Conoco Oil Company.)

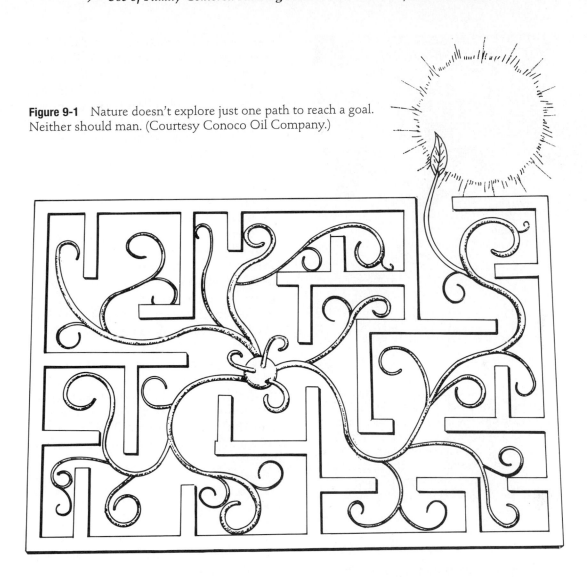

will accept help from community systems, and by establishing values, attitudes, and beliefs (refer to Figure 9-2).

FAMILY-CENTERED NURSING PROCESS DEFINED

The family-centered nursing process is a systematic approach to scientific problem solving, involving a series of circular dynamic actions—assessing, analyzing, planning, implementing, evaluating, and terminating—for the purpose of facilitating optimum client functioning. There are four key elements in this definition:

- *Systematic approach.* This process enables the community health nurse to function in an orderly, logical manner. The nurse plans her or his actions to achieve specific goals and recognizes that time and efforts are often wasted if a "hit-or-miss" approach is used.
- *Scientific problem-solving.* Decisions made about client needs and appropriate nursing interventions are based on scientific principles. The problem-solving approach is used in everyday life. The nursing process differs from simple problem solving: scientific knowledge gained from advanced study assists the nurse in refining the data analysis process in relation to health, illness, and prevention, and in expand-

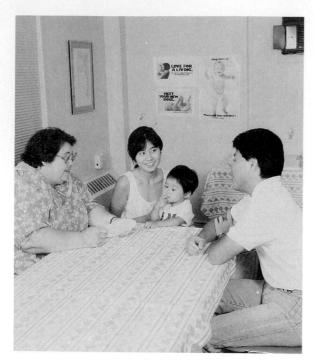

Figure 9-2 The family-centered approach to nursing care focuses on the family as the unit of service. When utilizing the nursing process in the community setting, nurses assess family dynamics as well as individual functioning and establish client-centered goals relevant to the needs of the entire family unit. (From Barkauskas VH, Stoltenberg-Allen C, Baumann LC, and Darling-Fisher C: *Health and physical assessment,* St. Louis, 1994, Mosby).

ing intervention options that aid clients in maximizing their self-care capabilities. McCain (1965, p. 82), in her classic article on the nursing process, stressed that this process helps nurses function in a deliberative rather than an intuitive way. This notion has been supported in recent literature (Carpenito, 1989; Gordon, 1994, 1993; Weber, 1991).

• *Series of circular, dynamic actions.* No one action alone helps the community health nurse to enhance client growth. All phases of the nursing process must be carried out in order for sound decision-making and effective nursing intervention to occur. *Dynamic* implies that care plans are revised when assessment and evaluation data reflect needed change. The nursing process is circular in nature because each phase provides data that either validate or alter original nursing diagnoses, goals, and plans.

• *Purpose of facilitating optimum client functioning.* Nursing interventions should help the client resolve his or her health care needs and achieve specific, client-defined goals and objectives. A helping interactive process whereby the client and the nurse share data for the purpose of identifying ways to make things less difficult for the client facilitates this process. To effectively facilitate client functioning, the nurse must individualize nursing actions, since clients define optimum functioning differently.

An effective community health nurse learns that, by using a systematic process, more satisfying results can be obtained. The nurse knows that it is necessary to base his or her practice on scientific knowledge consistent with the standards of the profession. This knowledge guides the data collection and analysis processes which, in turn, provide the foundation for establishing nursing diagnoses, specific client goals, nursing interventions, and evaluation criteria. Illustrative of this are the factors the nurse takes into consideration when working with a family who has a child with juvenile diabetes. Based on scientific information, the nurse knows that this child needs such things as:

• Adequate nutrition
• Proper hygiene
• Insulin injections
• Regular blood glucose testing
• Adequate exercise
• Socializing experiences, such as interactions with peers

Teaching about these needs may be inappropriate or ineffective unless the nurse considers the following:

• Family's financial situation
• Family's daily living patterns and how these patterns may need to be altered to provide adequate nutrition, proper hygiene, and appropriate medication for the child
• Family's perceptions of the child's health and knowledge about his or her health status
• Child's emotional reaction to the diabetic condition and knowledge about his or her health status
• Health of the family unit

In order to achieve desired goals in a family situation the nurse must recognize that having knowledge only about a disease process is inadequate to address the impact of illness on the family system. Intervention strategies are often ineffective until the nurse identifies the family's perception of the situation and coping strategies currently being used. One community health nurse, for instance, visited intensively the family of a 6-year-old child who had brittle diabetes. The child did not follow her prescribed diabetic regimen and one consequence was frequent hospitalizations for treatment of diabetic coma. When the nurse finally questioned the parents about their perceptions of their child's health condition, she discovered that they were not ready to accept the diagnosis as permanent. Denying the diagnosis was their way of coping with it. The nurse had to help the parents handle their feelings of guilt and anger before she could discuss treatment plans with them.

The family-centered nursing process facilitates the analysis of psychosocial influences in addition to physiological ones. Looking more closely at the nursing process, the reader will find that it consists of the following six phases:

- Assessing
- Analyzing
- Planning
- Implementing
- Evaluating
- Terminating

Although each phase is discussed separately, it should be remembered that they interrelate and overlap. The interdependent nature of these phases, along with nursing activities during each phase, is presented in Table 9-1. When examining Table 9-1 it is important to remember that a comprehensive family assessment evaluates multiple components of family health (refer to figure 9-3) and that the family should be the central focus throughout the nursing process. Collected data should always be validated with the family before nursing diagnoses, goals, and intervention strategies are formulated. The family-centered nursing process is a client-oriented, not a nurse-oriented, process.

THEORY GUIDES PRACTICE

The ANA (1986) standards of community health nursing practice specify that "the nurse applies theoretical concepts as a basis for decisions in practice" (p. 5). In order to function effectively in community health the nurse must integrate skills and knowledge relevant to both nursing and public health (ANA, p. 1). Public health knowledge includes concepts from epi-

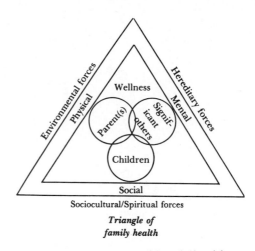

Figure 9-3 Triangle of family health.

demiology, biostatistics, environmental health, social sciences, and public health administration. Core concepts from the epidemiological model (host, agent, and environment) and levels of prevention (primary, secondary, and tertiary) guide public health practice.

Historically the major focus of epidemiology was on the investigation of epidemics or disease outbreaks. Today public health professionals examine variables that keep people healthy, as well as factors that cause the occurrence of disease and unhealthy conditions. Concepts from epidemiology help the nurse to identify at-risk clients (individuals, families, and aggregates) for the purposes of identifying or preventing disease and rehabilitating clients with active disease or disability. During the assessment phase of the nursing process nurses complete a health risk appraisal. As previously discussed, a *health risk appraisal* is a process whereby data are collected and analyzed to identify characteristics that may make clients vulnerable to illness, premature death, or unhealthy conditions (e.g., hereditary links to disease such as sickle cell anemia; behaviors which increase the potential for disease occurrence or premature death; and risk factors related to unhealthy conditions such as child maltreatment). Once a risk profile is established nurses initiate educational strategies to help clients acquire knowledge about ways to reduce health risks. The at-risk concept and other epidemiological concepts are discussed extensively in Chapter 11.

Nursing conceptualizations focus on four essential concepts—person, environment, health, and nursing (Fawcett, 1984, The Metaparadigm; Flaskerudt and

TABLE 9-1 Relationships among the Phases of the Family-Centered Nursing Process

Assessing →	Analyzing →	Planning →	Implementing →	Evaluating →	Terminating →
Process for obtaining a data base	A cognitive data-ordering process for the purpose of identifying nursing diagnoses	Formulation of desired family outcomes (goals) and identification of actions (intervention strategies) to achieve goals	A systematic approach to action used by the family and nurse to achieve desired family outcomes	A continuous, concurrent process used to critique each component of the nursing process	A therapeutic process that helps the client and the nurse to end their relationship

Assessing	Analyzing	Planning	Implementing	Evaluating	Terminating
1. Develop a trusting relationship: a. Explain purpose of community health nursing visit b. Describe what community health nurse has to offer c. Facilitate the sharing of thoughts, feelings, and data d. Set time parameters for evaluation and frequency and length of visits 2. Collect data in variety of ways: a. Observation b. Interview c. Inspection d. Physical assessment	1. Make differential conclusions about family needs by: a. Using theoretical knowledge to identify significant signs and symptoms b. Grouping data to show relationships between assessment categories and to identify *patterns* of behavior c. Relating family data to relevant clinical and research findings d. Comparing nursing diagnoses with diagnoses of other health	1. Consider three key principles: a. Individualization of client care plans b. Active client participation c. Client's right of self-determination 2. Formulate client centered goals and objectives: a. Establish realistic goals consistent with the data base and nursing diagnoses b. State goals and objectives in specific, achievable, and measurable terms c. Develop goals and objectives	1. Base nursing actions on data obtained during the assessment phase; family needs, knowledge receptivity, and level of understanding: a. Demonstrate awareness of proper timing when carrying out intervention activities b. Adapt or modify intervention strategies when client situation changes c. Modify activities to accommodate factors in the home 2. Recognize social, cultural, economic	1. Elicit ongoing feedback from client to determine if goals, plans, and interventions are appropriate 2. Identify the results of intervention activities taken by: a. Client b. Community health nurse c. Other health care professionals 3. Determine why intervention activities have been ineffective, if warranted 4. Modify the management plan when appropriate 5. Use a variety of methods to evaluate:	1. Deal with feelings associated with termination 2. Review client achievements 3. Discuss what the therapeutic process has meant 4. Plan carefully the termination of visits 5. Share with client how to reestablish contact if needed 6. Discuss with client self-care requirements upon discharge

e. Contact with secondary sources
f. Review of records
3. Assess all parameters of family functioning:
   a. Family dynamics
   b. Health status—individual family members
   c. Physiological data
   d. Psychosocial data
   e. Sociocultural data
   f. Environmental data
   g. Preventive health practices
4. Obtain data from multiple sources:
   a. Client, family
   b. Health team members
   c. Community agencies
   d. Significant others
   e. Relevant records
5. Use standards of care to focus the interviewing process (refer to Chapter 23)

professionals
2. Formulate specific nursing diagnoses:
   a. Base diagnoses on a strong data base
   b. Identify the functional aspects of a client's current health status
   c. Determine various levels of family functioning
      (1) Strengths
      (2) Needs
      (3) Anticipatory guidance warranted
   d. Identify when data are insufficient to make a nursing diagnosis

in collaboration with the family (contracting)
d. Identify family as well as individual goals and objectives
e. Formulate cognitive, affective, and psychomotor objectives when appropriate
f. Distinguish between nurse-focused goals and client-focused goals
3. Identify alternative intervention strategies:
   a. Identify various intervention activities based on assessment data, nursing diagnoses, and client goals and objectives
   b. Determine activities that the client, the nurse, and other health professionals might carry out to help the client achieve desired goals and objectives

and environmental barriers, and work within these limitations (refer to Chapter 10)
3. Carry through with planned interventions
   a. Performing nursing care activities
   b. Engaging the family in the referral process
   c. Implementing teaching, learning plans
   d. Helping family to problem solve
   e. Providing supportive intervention
   f. Keeping appointments with the family
4. Base intervention activities on scientific principles and knowledge:
   a. Review literature to obtain knowledge in relation to content being taught or situation being encountered
   b. Consult with peers, supervisor, and other health care

a. Obtain feedback from client
b. Consult with peers, supervisors, and other health care professionals
c. Summarize records
d. Conduct nursing audits (refer to Chapter 23)

Continued

TABLE 9-1 Relationships among the Phases of the Family-Centered Nursing Process—cont'd

Assessing	Analyzing	Planning	Implementing	Evaluating	Terminating
		c. Identify pros and cons of each intervention strategy d. Assist the client in identifying alternative courses of action and in making decisions about actions to be implemented 4. Establish priorities in relation to client goals and intervention strategies: a. Differentiate between problems that need immediate action and those that can wait b. Consider the health and safety of the client c. Use theory and the family data base to identify potential crisis situations 5. Identify criteria for evaluating goal attainment	professionals to expand knowledge and to evaluate appropriateness of nursing interventions		

Halloran, 1980; Whall and Fawcett, 1991). Nursing models specify the nursing perspective related to these concepts and their interrelatedness. A nursing "conceptual model comprises abstract, general concepts, and statements that describe and link the concepts. Each conceptual model of nursing represents a particular frame of reference within which patients (persons/clients), their environments and health states, and nursing activities are viewed, and thus it presents a comprehensive holistic view of nursing care" (Fawcett and Carino, 1989, p. 2).

Several nursing models have been developed in an attempt to capture a comprehensive, holistic view of nursing care. They have met with varying degrees of success. Examples of such models include Johnson's Behavioral System Model, King's Conceptual Framework of Nursing, Neuman's Health Care Systems, Orem's Self-Care Framework, Rogers' Science of Unitary Human Beings, Roy's Adaptation Model, White's Model for Public Health Nursing Practice (refer to Chapter 2) and Anderson's Community as Client Model (refer to Chapter 3). Although most of the nursing models focus on the individual as the unit of analysis, rather than the family and the community, some concepts being advanced by nurse theorists can be applied in the community health nursing arena (refer to Table 9-2). Recent work has begun to provide an understanding of conceptual nursing models as

---

TABLE 9-2 Examples of Nursing Theory Bases Applicable to Community Health Nursing

Applicable content	Name of nursing theory base	Primary author	Nursing examples
Client's self-care ability changing with state of health	Self-Care Framework	Orem, 1971, 1980, 1985, 1991; Orem and Taylor, 1986	Blazek and McCaellen, 1983; Bliss-Holtz, 1988; Campbell, 1986; Chang, Uman, Linn, Ware, and Kane, 1985; Galli, 1984; Hanchett, 1988; Harper, 1984; Kearney and Fleisher, 1979; Kruger, Shawver, and Jones, 1980; Maunz and Woods, 1988; Michael and Sewall, 1980; Nunn and Marriner-Tomey, 1989; Pridham, 1971; Walborn, 1980
Maintaining stressors within client's adaptation Interdependence and role function modes of person in family	Adaptation Model	Roy, 1970, 1976, 1983, 1984, 1987, 1988; Roy and Roberts, 1981	Fawcett, 1981; Hanchett, 1988; Kehoe, 1981; Limandri, 1986; Schmitz, 1980; Wagner, 1976
Primary, secondary, tertiary prevention Lines of defense	Health Care Systems Model	Neuman, 1972, 1980, 1982, 1989	Beitler, Tkachuck, and Aamodt, 1980; Benedict and Sproles, 1982; Bigbee, 1984; Buchanan, 1987; Hoch, 1987; Pinkerton, 1974; Story and Ross, 1986; West, 1984
Holistic health Time perception	Science of Unitary Human Beings	Rogers, 1970, 1980, 1983, 1986, 1989, 1990	Boyd, 1985; Fawcett, 1977; Hanchett, 1979, 1988; Laffrey, 1985; Levine, 1976; Rawnsley, 1977; Whall, 1981; Wood and Kekahbah, 1985

Developed by J. Atwood, Professor and Director, NRSA Pre- and Post-Doctoral Institutional Instrumentation Fellowship Program, College of Nursing and Cancer Prevention and Control, Behavioral Sciences Coordinator, Arizona Cancer Center, University of Arizona, Tucson, Ariz., 1990.

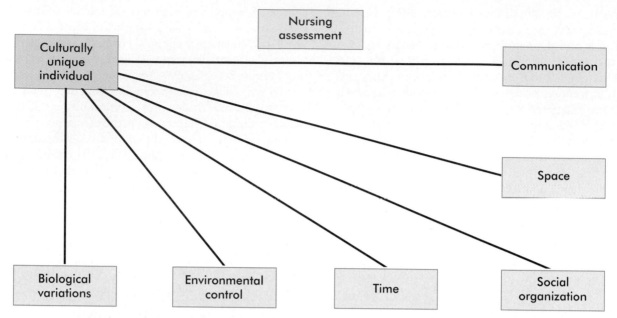

Figure 9-4   Application of cultural phenomena to nursing care and nursing practice. (Fom Giger JN and Davidhizar RE: Transcultural nursing: assessment and intervention, St. Louis, 1991, Mosby, p. 5.)

they relate to the community as client (Hanchett, 1988) and the family as client (Chin, 1985; Clements and Roberts, 1983; Gonot, 1986; Hanson, 1984; Johnston, 1986; Riehl-Sisca, 1985; Whall, 1981, 1986; Whall and Fawcett, 1991). Friedemann (1989a; 1989b) is concentrating her scholarly efforts on developing a new conceptual model of nursing that focuses exclusively on the family.

Community health nursing focuses on the three levels of prevention (primary, secondary, and tertiary), values the holistic nature of humankind, and recognizes the importance of increasing a client's self-care capabilities to promote independence. Community health nurses use a variety of assessment strategies to obtain a holistic perspective about an individual's health status and family dynamics, including a family's role functions and interdependence behaviors (refer to Chapter 7). Based on assessment data, community health nurses implement intervention strategies that assist clients in maintaining stress at a functional level (within a client's adaptation zone or lines of defense). For example, they coordinate resources for clients who are experiencing stress to decrease the input clients must handle.

Since a comprehensive discussion about nursing theory is beyond the scope of this text, the reader is encouraged to examine writings by the primary au-

thor to obtain an accurate understanding of the theoretical and conceptual bases in each nursing model. Examining how others have discussed the application of these models in practice, research and education can also be beneficial. Table 9-2 provides nursing examples related to community health nursing practice that have applied nursing theory.

CULTURAL FACTORS INFLUENCE PRACTICE

As significant demographic changes have altered the ethnic and racial composition of our nation's population (refer to Chapter 7), an increased appreciation for cultural diversity has emerged. "The concept of the melting pot, now outmoded, has been replaced by the recognition that this diversity lends strength and uniqueness to the fabric of our society . . . and that greater efforts at understanding and valuing our differences as well as our similarities are needed" (Randall-David, 1989, p. 1). Using an assimilation model that views all clients from the nurse's own cultural perspective negates the value of cultural differences and leads to ineffective nursing practice. It has been well documented that clients bring to the helping relationship values, attitudes, beliefs, and priorities that have developed over generations and that influence health beliefs and practices. In fact, cultural

---

◀ *Cultural Phenomena to Be Considered throughout the Nursing Process* ▶

Communication

Communication includes all verbal and nonverbal behavior between people, including things such as vocabulary, grammatical structure, silence, touch, facial expressions, eye and body movements, and expression of warmth and humor.

Space

Providing culturally competent care involves examining how families use and control their interpersonal space, including objects in the environment and spatial behavior. Families control their environment to protect them from harm, to maintain privacy, to control what occurs in their interpersonal space, and to promote self-identity.

Social Organization

A variety of social organizations (e.g., family, religious groups, ethnic and racial groups, kinship groups, and special interest groups) in a client's environment influence the patterning of cultural behaviors. All of these organizations develop structural and process characteristics that promote specific values, attitudes, beliefs, and norms about growth and development processes, health practices, life goals, and family functioning (refer to Chapter 7).

Time

Both clock time (an interval of time) and social time influence family behavior. Clock time directs regularity in our lives. Social time refers to patterns and orientations (e.g., past, present, future) that relate to social processes and to the conceptualization and ordering of social life.

Environmental Control

This term refers to the ability of a family from a particular cultural group to plan activities that control nature or to direct factors in the environment. Health practices and actions taken by families when a family member is ill are affected by how the environment is viewed. Families' views about the environment are influenced by things such as their beliefs about locus of control (internal or external), causes of health and illness (natural or unnatural), and people-to-nature orientation (dominate nature, live in harmony with nature, or subjugate to nature). Views about the environment are also influenced by families' relationships with systems in their environment (e.g., folk medicine or religious system).

Biological Variations

This phenomena involves examining norms for different cultural/ethnic groups in relation to anatomical characteristics, skin and hair physiology, growth and development patterns, susceptibility and resistance to disease, variations in body systems, and nutritional preferences and deficiencies.

Modified from Giger JN and Davidhizar RE: *Transcultural nursing: assessment and intervention,* St. Louis, 1991, Mosby.

---

patterning influences families' decision about when to obtain care and whom they should consult when care is needed.

Nurses in the community health setting are privileged to enter the homes and lives of culturally diverse families in very intimate ways. They show respect for this privilege by seeking information that increases their awareness of a family's situation from its perspective. The effective community health nurse takes into account cultural factors throughout the helping process. Giger and Davidhizar (1991) have identified six cultural phenomena (refer to Figure 9-4) that "are evidenced among all cultural groups but which vary with application and use across cul-

tures" (p. 5). These concepts, discussed briefly in the box above, are explored in depth in Giger and Davidhizar's book, *Transcultural Nursing: Assessment and Intervention.*

Table 7-2 provided specific examples of how cultural phenomena vary across cultures. These variations influence the use of the nursing process throughout all of its stages. For example, ethnic differences have been found in how members of a specific culture communicate symptoms such as pain and how they respond to these symptoms. The Navajo Indians, for instance, have very few words for describing the nature of pain and their value system supports bearing pain in silence (Simons, 1985). This can lead to an

◀ *Examples of Disparity in Health Beliefs* ▶

Example #1

Carlos is a 15 year old from a poor urban area where drugs proliferate and many young men trade sex for drugs or money. You are fairly certain that Carlos does not use IV drugs, but know that he often has sex with men for money. Carlos believes that only homosexual men are at risk for AIDS. Because he considers his prostitution a job, not a sexual identity, he does not think of himself as being at risk for AIDS.

Ethnocentric Solutions:

1. Convince Carlos that he is gay because he has sex with men; therefore he is at risk for AIDS.
2. Diagnose Carlos as "noncompliant" because he does not alter his behavior after you inform him of the risks.

Ethnorelative Solutions:

3. Respect Carlos's beliefs and try to teach him about risky behaviors without discussing sexual identities or applying a label to his behavior.

Example #2

Harold and Sarah are expecting their first child. Sarah comes to a prenatal clinic for her first visit. The nurse notes that Sarah is 26 years old, well-educated, and healthy. Sarah is informed that she has no unusual risks for her pregnancy. The baby is born healthy, but 10 months later, the clinic is being sued because the baby has Tay-Sachs disease and Harold and Sarah were not told that they, as Ashkenazi Jews, were at risk.

Ethnocentric Solutions:

1. Blame Sarah for not informing the clinic, because she did not "look Jewish."
2. Blame the clinic administrators, who did not include "Jewish" as a racial identity as well as a religion.

Ethnorelative Solutions:

3. Alter clinic health assessment records to ensure reporting of racial/ethnic identity. Educate staff on health and risk for illness factors that differ by race or ethnicity.

Example #3

June, a 35-year-old surgical nurse, grew up in a fundamentalist religion, although she rarely attends church now. June admits a middle-aged female patient who is to undergo major surgery the next day. The patient, Barbara, insists that her companion, Alicia, be present for the preop teaching and any discussions of her health. June explains that only spouses or biologic family members will be allowed to visit Barbara in the recovery room or the ICU after surgery. When Barbara explains that she considers Alicia her spouse, June leaves the room. Later she comments to coworkers, "It wouldn't be so bad if she didn't throw her homosexuality in my face like that! It really bothers me when those people flaunt their sexuality!" She avoids Barbara's room for the rest of the shift.

Ethnocentric Solutions:

1. Uphold hospital policy and do not allow Alicia to visit or make decisions with Barbara.
2. Refuse to care for Barbara, or if giving her care, avoid any discussion of her sexual identity.

Ethnorelative Solutions:

3. Reconsider hospital policies. Must "significant others" be so narrowly defined? What are the purposes of the restrictions?
4. Examine personal beliefs. How did June come to be so negative about lesbians? Does her religious background—much of which she has already rejected—affect her current views?
5. Find out more information about the health care needs of lesbians. Ask Barbara about her wishes and include Alicia in her care.

Example #4

Tammi is a 75-year-old woman who was born in China and immigrated to the United States when she was 40. She lives in a predominantly Chinese neighborhood and maintains her traditional values and customs. Although the nurse introduced himself as Tony several times and has asked Tammi to call him by his first name, she continues to call him "doctor." Whenever Tony calls her Tammi, she looks away, but does not say anything about it. Tony is finding it increasingly difficult to communicate with Tammi. Later Tony learns from Tammi's daughter that it is not proper to call strangers by their first name, and it is disrespectful for 25-year-old Tony to call an elder by her first name. It is also not considered polite to make demands upon authority figures, but to take what they offer.

◀   *Examples of Disparity in Health Beliefs—cont'd*   ▶

Ethnocentric Solutions:

1. Diagnose an alteration in communication or lack of assertiveness because Tammi failed to inform Tony of her wishes.
2. Tell Tammi that in this country, we call people by their first names.

Ethnorelative Solutions:

3. Ask her how she would like to be addressed. Offer your whole name and she can choose how to address you.
4. Offer her choices instead of asking open-ended questions.

Example #5

   Clara is an 82-year-old African-American woman from a small rural community. She has arthritis and congestive heart failure. She has experienced considerable knee pain recently, and Ruth is following up on her prescription for

an antiinflammatory. Ruth, a community health nurse, discovers that Clara never filled the prescription, but is using a "mustard plaster" made of various greens from her garden. She states that the pain is gone and she has no need for expensive pills.

Ethnocentric Solutions:

1. Label her as "noncompliant" and encourage her to fill the prescription.
2. Try to persuade her that the greens have no therapeutic value. She should use "real" medicine.

Ethnorelative Solutions:

3. Try to determine whether there are other reasons for her rejecting the medication, such as not being able to afford the prescription.
4. Believe her when she says she has no pain and encourage her to continue the mustard plaster treatments.

From Eliason MS: Ethics and transcultural nursing care, *Nurs Outlook* 41(5):227-228, 1993.

inaccurate assessment and diagnosis regarding the severity of a client's pain, which in turn can influence the nature of interventions (e.g., amount of pain medication given) and evaluation (e.g., relief of pain) of the client's status.

   The box on pp. 298-299 describes other situations that illustrate how disparity in health beliefs can adversely affect the therapeutic process. In these situations Eliason (1993) identifies how *ethnocentrism,* "an individual's belief that his or her own cultural group's beliefs and values are the best or the only acceptable beliefs" (p. 226), can adversely influence clients' acceptance of the health care professional and health teaching. Eliason has also identified ethnorelative solutions for reducing cultural barriers to the therapeutic process in the case examples shared in this box. "*Ethnorelativity* is the ability to conceive of alternative viewpoints and to respect the beliefs of another culture even though they are different from one's own (Eliason, p. 226).

   Even though specific incidents can be provided that illustrate how cultural patterning differs across ethnic and racial groups, *it is critically important to mention again*

that intracultural variations exist and that an individualized assessment is necessary to identify family values, attitudes, beliefs, and norms. However, having an awareness of cultural differences helps the practitioner to focus the assessment process.

PHASES OF THE FAMILY-CENTERED NURSING PROCESS

   It may be found that phases and terms within the nursing process are labeled differently from what the reader has seen before. There are hundreds of books and articles written on the nursing process, and terminology varies from one author to another. The dispute over terminology serves to confuse practitioners and makes it difficult to recognize that it is the *process,* not the terminology, that is significant. Focusing on the process aspects of the phases as they are discussed will allow the reader to effectively implement the family-centered nursing process regardless of the terminology used in different practice settings.

Assessing

The assessment phase involves a systematic data collection process which provides the foundation for making nursing diagnoses. During this phase the community health nurse places emphasis on collecting specific data about client (family) functioning so that objective conclusions regarding the client's health status can be made. Inferences about a client's level of functioning should be made only after a sufficient data base has been obtained.

The primary responsibilities of the community health nurse during the assessment phase are threefold: (1) developing a trusting, therapeutic relationship; (2) using a variety of data collection methods to obtain client information from all available resources; and (3) assessing all parameters of family health, including family dynamics, family resources, health status of individual family members, and environmental factors that influence family health. Careful attention given to all three of these activities helps the community health nurse to clearly delineate client needs and goals and intervention strategies that may enhance client growth.

First Home Visits

Home visiting is a long-established method for promoting family health at all levels of prevention (GAO, 1990; National Commission to Prevent Infant Mortality, 1989). Despite a recent trend emphasizing aggregate-based interventions such as group-work and clinic or school services, home visiting continues to be a significant component of community health nursing practice. In the home health care setting, it is the principal means by which community health nurses provide services for clients and their families. Recent laws, in particular those dealing with Medicaid prenatal care expansions and services to developmentally delayed and at-risk infants and toddlers and their families, include provisions that provide a new impetus for home visiting (GAO, p. 24).

Making first home visits to families can be stressful, especially for a nurse entering an unknown environment controlled by the client rather than the health care professional. First home visits can also be challenging, particularly if the nurse recognizes that he or she is providing a valuable service. In general families are receptive and interested in the services community health nurses have to offer. There may be times, however, when a family prefers to handle its health care needs within the family unit without assistance

from "outsiders." If this is the preferred family pattern of functioning, the community health nurse must accept the family's decision and not view this as a personal failure. Sometimes families do not appear interested in home visits because they are unaware of how a community health nurse may assist them.

Educating a family about community health nursing services may provide the family with the information needed to make an informed decision regarding continued visits. When supplying this data the nurse should focus on issues pertinent to the family. For example, when a community health nurse receives antepartum referrals for families having difficulty paying for care, he or she frequently helps these families to identify community resources that would be helpful to them. Or, if the community health nurse receives a referral for an elderly family needing home health care, the nurse would focus attention on home care services relevant to the family's needs, including where to obtain supplies and equipment, the role of the home health aide, and resources in the community that will deliver meals or help with family home maintenance activities.

First home visits can influence families' receptivity to future home visits. Carefully planned first visits can facilitate relationship building and assist nurses to demonstrate the contributions they can make in helping families to deal with current health needs. Table 9-3 outlines how to prepare for a first home visit, tasks to initiate during the visit, and postvisit activities. The goals for the first visit should be to establish a positive client/nurse working relationship, obtain baseline data on the family situation, and address the immediate concerns of the family. The extent to which the nurse carries out the tasks identified in Table 9-3 during the initial visit will vary depending on the family's circumstances. Some tasks will not be done at all because they are not appropriate for the client's situation. For example, doctor's orders are not required for families receiving only health promotion services. On the other hand, nurses do not provide home health or care of the sick services without a doctor's order. It is critical to remember that the assessment phase of the nursing process is ongoing and should extend throughout the length of the nurse/client relationship. *It is not feasible or appropriate to obtain all needed data during the initial contact.*

Community health nurses encounter a variety of situations on first home visits, such as families who want parenting education or elderly couples who have

TABLE 9-3 First Home Visits: Responsibilities and Tasks

Responsibility	Tasks
I. Previsit preparation	Review available family data including referral information and previous family records.
	Clarify data with others if unclear (e.g., contact family physician and/or other referral sources or talk with intake nurse).
	Establish a plan for the visit.
	Consider appropriate community resources.
	Review theory related to identified family problems.
	Prepare for a safe visit (e.g., identify exact location of home, consider safety issues in relation to the neighborhood being visited, and request escort or shared visit services if needed).
II. Establish contact with family	Contact family via the phone, if available.
	Identify self, including name and agency you are representing.
	Explain who referred family to agency and purpose of referal.
	Discuss briefly services CHN can provide such as sharing data about available community resources.
	Identify family's need for CHN services and willingness to have nurse visits.
	Schedule home visit at a time convenient for family.
III. Home visit intervention	
A. Relationship-building period	Introduce self and role.
	Introduce agency, agency obligations, and programs and services.
	Explain purpose of home visit.
	Build a nurse/client relationship.
	Discuss client rights and responsibilities.
	Assess safety of care plan: is a primary caregiver present and available if needed?
	Consider safety issues for the health care provider (e.g., park near the home, don't enter the house if the client is not home, and dress professionally, avoiding expensive jewelry and suggestive clothing).
B. Intervention period	Carry out a client assessment.
	Carry out a family assessment.
	Carry out an environmental assessment, especially in relation to client safety and health needs.
	Elicit family's perceptions of how a CHN can assist.
	Assess doctor's orders and need for changes if appropriate.
	Assess appropriateness of stated third-party reimbursement.
	Assess need for other services such as physical therapy or referral to a community agency for parenting classes.
	Assess need for equipment and supplies.
	Confirm medication orders, dosages, and client knowledge of medications.
	Identify client's knowledge base related to identified problems (e.g., disease process or care of infant).
	Discuss estimated length of service.
C. Closing period	Summarize visit activities with family.
	Together decide what the client/family will be doing between now and the next visit.
	Inform client/family how to reach nurse between visits.
	Set time for next visit.
IV. Postvisit activities	Begin the nursing care plan.
	Document visit.
	Make contacts on behalf of client/family if needed (e.g., initiate other services, contact physician regarding needed change in order, or inform vendors about needed equipment and supplies).
	Complete agency reporting forms and paperwork for third-party reimbursement.
	Evaluate visit progress.

requested assistance with care of an ill family member. While the major focus on these visits may vary from care of the sick to health teaching, the provision of health promotion services is a primary component of all community health nursing visits. Health promotion activities should not be neglected during care of the sick visits. Examples of health promotion interventions implemented during these type of visits are teaching to increase the client's self-care capabilities, environmental assessment to prevent home accidents, and referral for respite services to prevent caregiver burnout.

As in any situation, it is important to consider issues of environmental safety when visiting in an unfamiliar area. Statistical data reflect that crime is on the rise in all socioeconomic neighborhoods and in a variety of health and welfare organizations. Although reports of crime involving community health nurses are unusual, take precautions to avoid unsafe or potentially unsafe situations. Most community health agencies have safety guidelines to follow including refusing rides from strangers, dressing professionally, not wearing expensive jewelry and suggestive clothing, planning ahead to avoid appearing lost, leaving an established visit plan in the agency, and not entering an environment where safety is questionable. Families being visited may also provide the nurse with safety guidelines such as where to park one's car in the neighborhood and best times during the day to visit.

Some nurses find that they have fears about all aspects of the environment because they are in surroundings entirely different from what they have previously experienced. If this is the case, the nurse will find it helpful to discuss her or his fears with a colleague who can help objectively analyze the situation. On the whole nurses have found that the community is an exciting and challenging environment that is open to caring professionals.

Relationship Building

The type of relationship established during the assessment phase can be the critical factor in helping the client determine whether or not to accept the assistance offered by the community health nurse. It is natural for clients to evaluate their interactions with community health nurses during the assessment phase. Most people take time to assess how others respond to them before they develop a trusting relationship that allows disclosure of personal thoughts, feelings, and problems.

Explaining the purpose of community health nursing visits, describing services the community health nurse can provide, and fostering a nonthreatening atmosphere that allows the client to share data at his or her own pace often promote trust between the nurse and the client. Clarifying why the community health nurse is visiting is essential. When clients do not understand the purpose of nursing visits it is hard for them to become involved in the therapeutic process. Lack of clarity in the therapeutic relationship can result in frustration and mistrust and inhibit the expression of thoughts, feelings, and data. Clients usually do not share information freely until they understand why the information is needed.

Sharing with clients their rights and responsibilities and agency obligations can help to clarify the purpose of home visits. All clients have the right to be active participants in the care process, including continuity of care decisions, and to have their privacy and property respected. They also have the right to voice complaints without fear of reprisal. Table 9-4 delineates specific client rights and responsibilities and related agency obligations as defined by the Health Care Financing Administration (HCFA) and the National Association for Home Care (NAHC).

Clients are more likely to develop a trusting relationship with professionals who are open and honest and who show a genuine concern for their welfare than with professionals who do not demonstrate these characteristics. An interview style that reflects sensitivity, a nonjudgmental, accepting attitude, and a respect for the client's rights facilitates the development of a trusting relationship. A skillful interviewer avoids barriers to communication such as false reassurance, advice-giving, excessive talking, and the showing of approval or disapproval. At times this is not easy. For example, families under stress may press for advice. Frequently a family member will say, "What would you do if you were me?" An empathic interviewer responds to the family's feelings of distress but supports its ability to make its own decisions. Advice-giving can lead to an unhealthy dependency.

The community health nurse needs to be careful not to foster inappropriate dependency. However, it is important to realize that interdependency is not negative and that clients may request assistance with problem solving. A mature adult recognizes and acts on the need for support, caring, and assistance from others while maintaining independent decision-making. Sometimes a professional's fear of depen-

TABLE 9-4   Client Rights and Responsibilities and Related Agency Obligations

Rights/obligations	Client rights	Agency obligations
Notice of rights	To be fully informed of all his or her rights and responsibilities	Provide client with a written notice of rights in advance of initiating care Obtain signed verification from client or client's caregiver that they have received written notice of rights
Exercise of rights and respect for property and person	Have property treated with respect Voice grievances and suggest change in service without fear of reprisal or discrimination Have family or guardian voice grievances when judged incompetent Right to privacy	Investigate complaints made by client or client's family or guardian Document existence of complaint and resolution of complaint
To be informed and to participate in planning care and treatment	Receive appropriate and professional care related to physician orders Choice of care provided Receive information necessary to give informed consent before the start of any care Know how to reach agency staff 24 hours a day, 7 days a week, and what to do in an emergency Refuse treatment within the confines of the law and be informed of the consequences of this action Reasonable continuity of care To be informed in reasonable time of anticipated termination of service and plans for transfer to another agency	Admit client for service only if the agency has the ability to provide safe professional care at the level of intensity needed Share with client physician orders Advise client in advance of care, the disciplines that will furnish care and the frequency of visits Advise client in advance of any changes in care Involve client in the planning of care Inform client of agency policies and procedures
Confidentiality of medical record	Agency maintains confidentiality of the clinical records	Advise client of agency's policies and procedures regarding disclosure of information in clinical records
Liability for payment	Receive information regarding changes for services, the client's potential liability for these charges, and client's eligibility for third party reimbursements Right of referral if service denied solely on the inability to pay for service	Inform client orally and in writing and in advance of care the extent to which third party reimbursement may pay for care and charges client may have to pay Notify client orally and in writing changes in eligibility for services from third party reimbursement
Home health hotline	Know about the availability of a toll-free home health hotline in the state to voice complaints about agency services or to have questions answered about home care	Inform client in writing how to reach the home health hotline

Data from Health Care Financing Administration (HCFA): *Conditions of participation: home health agencies*, 42CFR Part 484, Sections 484.1 through 484.52, Washington, D.C., October 1989, U.S. Department of Health and Human Services; Health Care Financing Administration (HCFA): Medicare Program: home health agencies: conditions of participation, *Federal Register* 56:32967—32975, July 18, 1991; and National Association for Home Care (NAHC): *Code of ethics*, Washington, D.C., 1982, The Association, pp. 1-2.

dency can be detrimental to the client-professional relationship. It can prevent the professional from demonstrating to clients a genuine interest in helping.

Numerous books discuss interviewing techniques that promote a therapeutic relationship. Readers are encouraged to examine various theoretical viewpoints of counseling in order to determine which style fits their needs. Whatever interviewing or counseling style is used, however, it must be individualized for each unique client. For example, some individuals do not verbalize spontaneously: they share what they feel is important to share and then are silent until further information is requested. A nurse who firmly believes in a nondirective approach would have difficulty relating to such clients if he or she did not adjust the interviewing style.

Family Interviews

Working with families presents special interviewing challenges for the community health nurse because families are composed of several unique individuals who have varying needs, concerns, and communication styles. Since the goal of community health nursing service is to help the family as a whole rather than to help each individual family member separately, it is important to interview the family unit together if possible. The nurse facilitates effective interaction between all family members in order to promote the family's nurturing and decision-making processes. At times this can be difficult, especially when conflicting interests need to be negotiated between family members.

When a nurse is allowed to cross the family boundaries and is accepted by the family system, the influences the nurse has on that system must be examined carefully. The nurse needs to watch closely her or his own interactions between individual family members and avoid taking sides in family decision-making. For instance, a nurse who firmly believes that all women need a career outside the home may strongly support a female client's desires to work without allowing her husband or significant other to verbalize his concerns. In situations like these the nurse needs to help the family evaluate the pros and cons of taking a certain action, and then encourage joint decision-making between the couple.

It is particularly easy for community health nurses to support one family member's view over another because they are not always able to see the entire family unit at one time. Remembering that taking sides is not therapeutic and that it can lead to or reinforce ineffective family patterns can help a nurse take action that supports effective communication within the family unit.

The values, attitudes, and beliefs held by the community health nurse can also disrupt the nurse/family interview. Professionals bring to the therapeutic process cultural patterning that influences thinking about variables such as how roles should be implemented, how a home should be managed, and how children should be raised. The nurse may unconsciously label family behavior as ineffective if it is not consistent with her or his beliefs. Use of peer collaboration and supervision helps the professional nurse to identify when personal beliefs are affecting the therapeutic process.

The guidelines presented in the box on p. 305 can assist the nurse in avoiding barriers to therapeutic communication and in establishing an effective client/nurse relationship in varying cultural situations.

Sources and Methods for Collecting Data

During the assessment phase both primary and secondary data are collected from all available sources to determine how well the family is coping with the encountered stressors. Primary data are those data which the community health nurse actually obtains from the client or sees, hears, feels, or smells in the client's environment. An astute community health nurse carefully notes observations and verbal information received from the client. Significant clues about a client's level of functioning can be obtained by observing how the client interacts within the environment. It is not unusual for the community health nurse to discern a child discipline problem by repeatedly watching parents interact with their children during home visits. When a nurse observes client functioning, it is important to remember that inferences about client problems should be based on *patterns* of behavior rather than isolated incidents of behavior. Labeling behavior ineffective after one observation is a dangerous practice and can adversely affect the nurse-family relationship.

In the community health setting, secondary data are obtained from a variety of sources such as significant others, personnel from health and social agencies, the family's physician, spiritual leaders, and health records. When these data are recorded the source of the information should also be indicated. Generally the community health nurse receives either verbal or

Guidelines for Establishing a Therapeutic Relationship with Clients from Other Cultures

1. **Assess Personal Beliefs Surrounding Persons from Different Cultures**
   - Gain an awareness of your personal beliefs and past experiences
   - Identify how your personal beliefs and experiences could influence the therapeutic process
   - Set aside personal values, biases, ideas, and attitudes that are judgmental and may negatively affect nursing care

2. **Assess Communication Variables from a Cultural Perspective**
   - Identify client's ethnic identity, including generation in America (e.g., first or second generation)
   - Use client as the primary informant when assessing client's ideas, attitudes, beliefs, and values
   - Determine cultural factors (e.g., beliefs about eye contact) that could influence the therapeutic process and respond appropriately

3. **Plan Care Based on the Communicated Needs and Cultural Background**
   - Seek knowledge about the client's cultural customs and beliefs
   - Encourage client to communicate cultural interpretations of health, illness, and health care
   - Identify sources of discrepancy between the client's and your conceptions of health and illness
   - Determine cultural idiosyncrasies that influence communication patterns (e.g., avoiding questions about income and neighbors in some cultures)
   - Evaluate the effectiveness of nursing interventions and modify plan of care if necessary

4. **Modify Communication Approaches to Meet Cultures Needs**
   - Recognize that illness and stress can influence the client's ability to communicate
   - Be attentive to signs of anxiety, confusion, and fear and respond in a therapeutic manner
   - Recognize that in some cultures (e.g., Navajo Indian) it is believed to be ethically wrong to speak for another person

5. **Understand that Respect for the Client and Communication Needs is Central to the Therapeutic Relationship**
   - Identify the client's cultural patterns related to the concept of respect

   - Demonstrate respect through use of a kind and attentive approach and active listening
   - Modify your communication patterns based on cultural assessment data

6. **Communicate in a Nonthreatening Manner**
   - Adhere to the client's social and cultural amenities
   - Avoid the appearance of being too busy and hurried
   - Allow time for relationship-building before personal matters are discussed with clients from some cultures
   - Determine the need for changes in your therapeutic approach (e.g., direct versus indirect)

7. **Use Validating Techniques in Communication**
   - Use restating and validating interviewing techniques to identify the client's understanding
   - Do not assume that the meaning has been transmitted without distortion, even if an interpreter is used

8. **Be Considerate of Reluctance to Talk when the Subject Involves Sexual Matters**
   - Recognize that in some cultures (e.g., Spanish-speaking or Arabic) sexuality issues are addressed more freely with persons of the same sex
   - Adhere to cultural norms in relation to sexuality discussions

9. **Adopt Special Approaches when the Client Speaks a Different Language**
   - Use a caring tone and facial expressions to alleviate the client's fears and anxieties
   - Talk slowly but not loudly, enunciating words
   - Keep messages simple
   - Use gestures, pictures, actions, and drawings to facilitate client understanding
   - Avoid using medical terms and jargon
   - Use an appropriate bilingual language dictionary

10. **Use Interpreters to Improve Communication**
    - Select an interpreter who has transcultural sensitivity and understands how to be a client advocate
    - Have interpreter translate message into understandable terms
    - Obtain feedback to validate client understanding

Modified from Giger JN and Davidhizar RE: *Transcultural nursing: assessment and intervention,* St. Louis, 1991, Mosby, pp. 22-26.

written permission from the client before making contact with secondary sources of data outside the family system. This practice not only protects the client's right of privacy but also promotes honesty and trust in the therapeutic relationship. In addition, seeking a client's permission to obtain information from others demonstrates to the client that the nurse respects the client's right of self-determination.

When using secondary data the nurse must recognize that it may not accurately reflect clients' perceptions of themselves or their needs. Instead, secondary data may reflect what others perceive about clients' situations. This point is particularly significant for a community health nurse to keep in mind, because frequently secondary data about the problems of family members are obtained when these individuals are not present. When this occurs the community health nurse often finds it necessary to make arrangements to obtain primary data. For example, she or he may visit a child in school or schedule a home visit after school hours in order to identify how this child is reacting to a newly diagnosed health problem.

Various assessment methodologies should be used to collect primary and secondary data. Interview, observation, direct examination (auscultation, percussion, palpation, inspection, and measurement), contact with secondary sources of data, and review of relevant records are methods used by the community health nurse to obtain an accurate and complete profile of a family's situation. These methods are used to identify client strengths as well as client needs.

The significance of using a variety of methods to collect data about family functioning cannot be overstated. No one data collection method provides the community health nurse with all the information needed to formulate accurate nursing diagnoses. The Daniels family case situation that follows illustrates this fact by showing the difference between the type of data one nurse obtained from interview and from direct observation.

▶ **Following hospitalization of Mr. Daniels for an acute exacerbation episode of multiple sclerosis, the Daniels family was referred to the health department for health supervision follow-up. Ms. Garitt, hospital social worker, requested that a community health nurse assess this family's needs in relation to its understanding of multiple sclerosis, its ability to handle activities of daily living, its knowledge of community resources, and the im-**

pact of Mr. Daniels' illness on family functioning. While Jane Mathews, CHN, was interviewing the family and collecting data on the entire family situation, she asked Mr. and Mrs. Daniels how they were managing Mr. Daniels' exercises. Both related that they were doing them regularly. Mrs. Daniels accurately described how the exercises should be done and verbalized that she felt comfortable handling them, since she was instructed how to do so by hospital staff. While Mrs. Daniels was demonstrating what she had learned it was found that she did have an understanding about the proper exercises for her husband. However, her body mechanics were inappropriate, and this caused severe backache that she failed to mention during the interviewing process. In addition to Mrs. Daniels' poor body mechanics, the nurse also discovered that Mr. Daniels was very demanding of his wife, expecting her to do exercises for him that he could do independently. Further exploration revealed that Mr. Daniels was doing very little for himself. Before his illness he had been the "man of the house. Now I can't do anything." Through demonstration and return demonstration the nurse showed Mr. Daniels that he was not helpless and assisted Mrs. Daniels in learning how to position herself appropriately when helping her husband. The nurse also helped the family identify family patterns that were fostering dependency.

If the community health nurse in the above situation had not observed Mr. and Mrs. Daniels's functioning, it could have taken her a considerable length of time to collect the data needed to accurately identify the real concerns in this family situation. Observing family interactions provided this nurse with data about family functioning that were not obtained through interview.

Assessing All Parameters of Family Health

The family-centered approach to nursing care focuses on the family as a unit rather than a collection of individual family members. This implies that the family is viewed as a system in which the actions and health status of one family member always affect the behavior and health status of all other family members. Thus, when community health nurses assess family health they not only examine the health status of individual family members but look at family dynamics as well (refer to Figure 9-5). Chapter 7 presents guidelines for examining family dynamics and includes a family assessment tool (refer to Appendix 7-2) that facilitates the collection of family functioning data. Gordon (1993) has developed a family assessment guide based on the eleven functional health pattern areas that practitioners have found useful.

Family Dynamics

To discern functional and ineffective characteristics of family dynamics, a community health nurse must establish criteria for evaluating family health to use for comparison purposes. In addition, a community health nurse must identify what types of data are needed for analyzing family functioning in order to focus assessment procedures. As previously mentioned, a conceptual framework should be used to organize the collection of family functioning data. It is also important to remember that if major emphasis is placed on the biological aspects of a family's health status during the beginning phase of a relationship, it may be difficult to refocus the family when the nurse wants to assess other parameters of family functioning. Explaining early in the therapeutic process why data about family dynamics are needed facilitates the collection of this type of information.

Identifying criteria for evaluating family health involves a process wherein one examines one's conceptual beliefs about health and about people and then delineates specific behaviors that reflect healthy functioning in relation to the family. Throughout this text emphasis has been placed on viewing health "not merely as the absence of disease, but as a state of complete physical, mental, and social well-being" (WHO, 1947). Dunn (1961), in his classic writings, focused on wellness when discussing the concept of complete well-being. He believed that implicit in this concept is the idea of high-level wellness, which he defines as "an integrated method of functioning which is oriented toward maximizing the potential of which the individual is capable, within the environment where he is functioning." He saw wellness as being influenced by variables that are both internal and external to individual systems. "Well being both in body and mind and within the family and within community life should be interrelated in order for the individual to achieve a zest for life." Wellness, according to Dunn, is a dynamic state, "ever-changing in its characteristics. . . . What is complete today, may be incomplete tomorrow" (pp. 2-4). This implies that one

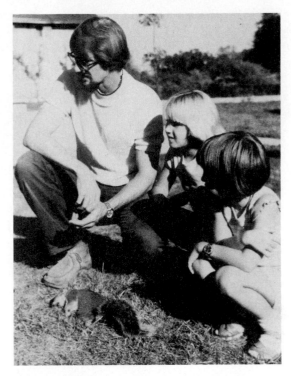

Figure 9-5 Family dynamics influence how well individual family members handle critical life events. The ability to provide support and security during times of stress (exposure to death) is a family strength that should be reinforced.

always has the potential for growth, a philosophy that promotes a humanistic or caring approach to all humankind. We believe that all clients should be approached in this way.

Inherent in Dunn's concept of "high-level wellness" for an individual is a conceptualization of family health. He saw the individual being influenced by his "inner and outer [family] worlds" (Dunn, 1961, p. 25). Because families are responsible for meeting the needs of their individual members, as well as for maintaining a functional family unit, family health can be defined as "an integrated method of functioning which is oriented toward maximizing the potential" (Dunn, p. 4) of individual family members throughout the lifespan while maintaining the integrity of the family as a system. To be useful for comparison purposes this global definition of family health must be translated into criteria that identify growth-producing family behaviors. Potential for growth is unique for each individual and each family unit. Client behavior must

TABLE 9-5   Criteria to Consider when Assessing "Healthy" Family Functioning: Three Authors' Viewpoints

Assessment parameters	Authors		
	Otto (1963): Family strengths	Pratt (1976): Family structure and health behavior characterizing the energized family	Curran (1983): Traits of a healthy family
Adaptive abilities	The ability to provide for the physical, emotional, and spiritual needs of a family The ability to use a crisis or seemingly injurious experience as a means of growth Ability for self-help, and ability to accept help when appropriate An ability to perform family roles flexibly The ability to communicate effectively	Combined health behaviors of all family members are energized; all family members tend to care for their health Actively and energetically attempt to cope with life's problems and issues Flexible division of tasks and activities	The healthy family admits to and seeks help with problems The healthy family communicates and listens
Atmosphere and affect	The ability to be sensitive to the needs of family members The ability to provide support, security, and encouragement	Responsive to the particular interests and needs of individual family members Regular and varied interaction among family members	The healthy family teaches respect for others The healthy family has a sense of play and humor The healthy family shares leisure time The healthy family fosters table time and conversation
Individual autonomy and integrity of family system	Mutual respect for the individuality of family members A concern for family unity, loyalty, and interfamily cooperation	Egalitarian distribution of power Provide autonomy for individual family members	The healthy family respects the privacy of individual members The healthy family affirms and supports individual members The healthy family maintains a balance of interaction among members The healthy family has a strong sense of family in which rituals and traditions abound The healthy family exhibits a sense of shared responsibility The healthy family develops a sense of trust The healthy family has a shared religious core

| | TABLE 9-5 | Criteria to Consider when Assessing "Healthy" Family Functioning: Three Authors' Viewpoints—cont'd | |

		Authors	
Assessment parameters	Otto (1963): Family strengths	Pratt (1976): Family structure and health behavior characterizing the energized family	Curran (1983): Traits of a healthy family
Relation-ships with others	The ability to initiate and maintain growth-producing relationships and experiences within and without the family The capacity to maintain and create constructive and responsible relationships in the neighborhood, school, town, and local and state government	Provide regular links with the broader community through active partici-pation in community activities	The healthy family values service to others The healthy family teaches a sense of right and wrong

Modified from Otto H: Criteria for assessing family strength, *Family Process,* 2:333-336, 1963; Pratt L: *Family structure and effective health behavior: the energized family,* Boston, 1976, Houghton Mifflin, pp 84-92; Curran D: *Traits of a healthy family,* copyright by Doris Curran, Minneapolis, Mn, 1983, Winston Press, pp 23-24. All rights reserved. Used with permission.

be analyzed from the client's perspective because ineffective or maladaptive behavior in one family can be functional or adaptive in another. The family's perceptions about how well it is functioning must be the key factor that helps a nurse determine whether or not a family is reaching its potential. If the family's perceptions are not understood, the community health nurse cannot influence a family to alter these perceptions.

Reviewing writings by Beavers (1977), Curran (1983), Lewis, Beavers, Gossett, and Phillips (1976), Otto (1963), and Pratt (1976), and examining the Family Coping Index, a tool developed by the Richmond-Hopkins Cooperative Nursing Study (Free-man and Lowe, 1964), will help the reader to delineate criteria for evaluating family health. The similarities between these authors' findings are striking. Flexible role patterns, responsiveness to the needs of indi-vidual members, active problem-solving mechanisms, ability to accept help, open communication patterns, and the provision of a warm, caring atmosphere were some of the main commonalities found in healthy families in these authors' studies. Table 9-5 presents an outline of the specific variables identified by Otto, Pratt, and Curran. Although these variables are not

intended to be normative, they do provide guidelines for data comparison purposes.

Since culture affects how a person perceives health and illness and the manner in which clients seek health care, it is important to examine the family's cultural beliefs, values, and practices when assessing family functioning. "Cultural assessments are performed to identify patterns that may assist or interfere with a nursing intervention or treatment regimen" (Tripp-Reimer, Brink, and Saunders, 1984, p. 81). Cultural assessments help the community health nurse to individualize the nursing care plan for each family. Chapter 7 provides guidelines for completing a cul-tural assessment.

Individual Functioning

The purpose of a family health assessment is to obtain pertinent data about the functioning of indi-vidual family members as well as the family system. In keeping with the view of health presented above, family members are viewed from an integrated, holis-tic, individual perspective. Biological, psychological, sociocultural, spiritual, developmental, and environ-mental parameters of functioning are assessed in order to determine the client's perception of his or her health

◀   *Select Cultural and Biopsychosocial Characteristics of an Individual*   ▶

Physical Appearance (Body)

Age and developmental stage
Sex and gender identity
Size, height, weight
Skin color
Hair color, configuration, presence/absence
Race (self-identified, perceived by others)
Posture, facial expression
Grooming, personal hygiene
Dress: style, condition
Presence of physical disability
Other characteristics not listed above

Mental Characteristics. Psychological Orientation (Mind)

Cognitive ability, intelligence
Level of consciousness
Emotional disposition, temperament
Aptitude, ability
Sensory acuity (visual, auditory)
Personal traits
Mental health
Other characteristics not listed above

External Influences (Social and Physical Environment)

Family history, ancestry, geographical origin
Strength of family unit, lines of authority
Role in family, birth order
Languages, communication patterns
Expectations and behavioral norms for age, sex, role
Format (rituals) for major life events (birth, marriage, illness, death)

Economic and work opportunities, access to resources
Housing, living arrangements
Dominant religion, other religions
Theories of disease causation
Availability, quality, variety of health care services
Political, governmental structure
Dietary customs, access to food
Community resources in education, art, music, recreation
Geographical and climatic features
Other influences not listed above

Internal Synthesis of Body, Mind, and Environment (Self)

Self-concept, self-perception, expectations of self
Beliefs, values, spirituality, religious affiliation
Affect, mood, congruity between words and affect
Attitudes toward health and self care: health history, use of health services
Personal goals, short- and long-term
Work role, economic contribution to self, others
Areas of accomplishment, achievement, sources of pride
Knowledge base, use of educational opportunities
Response to stress, coping strategies, ability to adapt
Language usage: formal, slang, dialect
Food preferences, dietary restrictions
Interests in applied and fine arts, crafts, hobbies, music, literature
Reading ability and preferences
Other characteristics not listed above

Modified from Sibley BJ: Cultural influences on health and illness. In Long BC, Phipps WJ, and Cassmeyer VL: *Medical-Surgical Nursing,* ed 3, St. Louis, 1992, Mosby, p. 32.

status. Select cultural and biopsychosocial characteristics to consider when completing an individual health assessment are presented in the box above.

In general, clients do not think systematically about all of the variables that affect their health. A major role of the community health nurse when completing an individual health assessment is to increase the client's awareness of all the factors that influence healthy functioning. A health assessment should be purposeful, meaningful, and goal-directed and should provide the client with an opportunity to identify both per-

sonal strengths and needs in relation to the individual's current level of functioning. Data about preventive health practices and healthy aspects of coping, along with information about ways in which the client handles illness, should be elicited.

The vehicles used for organizing an individual functional assessment are the health history and the physical examination. Exploring the techniques of physical appraisal is beyond the scope of this text. Writings by Barkauskas, Stoltenberg-Allen, Baumann, and Darling-Fisher (1994); Bowers and Thompson

(1992); Fox (1981); and Guzzetta, Bunton, Prinkey, Sherer, and Seifert (1989) discuss extensively the physical examination process. It is essential for community health nurses to have skill in completing a gross physical appraisal, since clients may not have a regular source of medical care even though they may have health problems. Community health nurses must have the ability to distinguish between *abnormal* and *normal* health findings. Price and Wilson (1992) provide a theoretical basis for analyzing health assessment findings. In addition, community health nurses need skill in the use of the referral process (refer to Chapter 10) in order to help clients obtain needed health care services when abnormal findings are identified.

"A nursing health history differs from a medical health history in that it focuses on the meaning of illness and hospitalization [health care] to the patient [client] and his family as a basis for planning nursing care. The medical history is taken to determine whether pathology is present as a basis for planning medical care" (McPhetridge, 1968, p. 68). When completing a health history, the community health nurse explores carefully the client's perceptions of his or her health status and how current stressors are affecting functioning; emphasis is placed on identifying the client as a unique individual rather than as a person who has a specific disease process.

Components included in a health history vary slightly from one author to another. Basically the goal of a health history is to determine how well the client is meeting health needs and how activities of daily living have been altered to meet these needs. A comprehensive review of the client's past and current health status is elicited to identify an accurate and complete composite of the client's health functioning. With this information the client and the nurse can explore ways for increasing the client's self-care capabilities.

Mahoney, Verdisco, and Shortridge (1982, pp. 6-7) identified the following seven components of an individual health history, which are still valid:

1. *Reason for contact.* Why the client is seeking help at this time
2. *Biographical data.* Structural variables common to all clients such as name, age, sex, marital status, religious preference, ethnic background, educational level, occupational status, health insurance, and social security information
3. *Current health status.* The client's perceptions of his or her health, with a specific delineation

of current complaints and activities of daily living
4. *Past health history.* Data relative to the previous health or illness state of the client and contact with health care professionals, including a description of developmental accomplishments, health practices, known illnesses, allergies, restorative treatment, and social activities such as foreign travel which might be related to the client's current health status
5. *Family history.* A description of the current health status of each family member, relationships among family members, and a genetic history in relation to health and illness
6. *Social history.* An accounting of intrapersonal and interpersonal factors which influence the client's social adjustment, including environmental stressors which may be increasing or decreasing the client's vulnerability to crisis during times of stress
7. *Review of systems.* A systematic assessment of biological functioning from head to toe

When completing a health history it is extremely important to elicit the client's expectations of the health care provider. If the client's and the professional's expectations are inconsistent, frustration results for all parties involved. For instance, a client who has diabetes and is expecting a cure will likely have difficulty working with a health care professional whose goal is to help the client live a normal life within the limitations of his or her condition. If the discrepancy between these two goals is not resolved, neither of these goals will be reached.

Every nurse must decide on a format which will facilitate data collection. Although formats may vary, it is crucial to collect data in an orderly fashion on all parameters of client functioning before a nursing care plan is developed. There are times when a crisis situation warrants dealing with the immediate concerns of the client before all data are collected. In order to intervene effectively during times of crisis, the health care professional needs an adequate data base. Without this data base, it is impossible to help the client to make appropriate choices about solutions for resolving current health stress.

Assessment guides can help the community health nurse collect health data in an orderly fashion. Assessment tools designed to collect information about the health status of individual family members should help the nurse to examine multiple aspects of a client's functioning. Appendices 9-1 and 9-2 are examples of assessment forms that help community health nurses organize this beginning phase of the nursing process. These tools aid the nurse in identifying psychosocial as well as physical components of a client's health status. In addition, they help a nurse to integrate individual and family functioning data by raising issues pertinent to the needs of all family members. Other examples of assessment guides, based on the 11 functional health pattern areas, can be found in Gordon's (1993), *Manual of Nursing Diagnosis, 1993-1994.*

Assessment tools have limitations and must be used only as guides to focus a nurse's attention on significant parameters to assess during the health interview and the physical examination process. Spontaneous interchange between the nurse and the client must always be allowed so that the client can fully express needs and can determine priorities that relate to her or his lifestyle. A barrage of questions from an assessment form stifles communication.

Analyzing

Once individual and family data are collected the analysis phase of the nursing process begins. This phase encompasses a cognitive data ordering process, which results in the formation of nursing diagnoses. Nursing diagnoses are inferences made about "the individual's, the family's, or the community's health problem/condition and the primary etiological or related factor(s) contributing to the problem/condition that is the focus of nursing treatment" (Gordon, 1989, p. xiii).

Nursing diagnoses are based on *patterns* reflected in assessment data and identify actual or potential client problems amenable to nursing interventions (Gordon, 1989). They also delineate client strengths that should be reinforced when the nurse is helping the client to enhance his or her self-care capabilities. In the community health setting, nursing diagnoses examine the needs and strengths of family units in addition to the needs and strengths of individual clients. If the identified needs of a family or individual clients are not amenable to nursing intervention, the community health nurse makes a referral to an appropriate care provider (refer to Chapter 10).

In order to formulate nursing diagnoses the community health nurse must group data so that relationships between assessment categories can be analyzed and patterns of behavior can be identified. Establishing relationships between assessment categories involves looking at all parameters of individual and family functioning. It requires a synthesis of data to determine the unique combination of biological, psychosocial, developmental, spiritual, and environmental factors that are making an impact on a specific family unit. It is important to synthesize data collected from a family, as client needs vary even when clients are experiencing similar situations. For example, one community health nurse was visiting two families who were both expressing concern about a child who cried when preparing to leave for school. In one family situation the nurse's diagnosis of this behavior was anticipatory anxiety (Susie was distressed as a result of family illness). Assessment data revealed that (1) Susie had enjoyed school until her father had a heart attack; (2) Susie's father had his heart attack while she was at school; and (3) Susie had been asking lately if her father was going to die. In the other family situation the nursing diagnosis in relation to the child's crying was quite different. This diagnosis was altered growth and development, social skills (Bonnie's dependency on her mother was inhibiting her psychosocial development). The community health nurse came to this conclusion after the parents shared that (1) Bonnie started school a year late because she was "immature" for her developmental age; (2) Bonnie had never enjoyed school; (3) Bonnie spent most of her free time with her mother, even when children her own age were around; and (4) Bonnie would cling to her mother when babysitters came to the house.

Nursing diagnoses must be based on strong data validated by the client; this data must be synthesized before nursing diagnoses are established. Formulating diagnoses without adequate information, or in relation to fragmented pieces of data, leads to invalid diagnoses and inappropriate client goals and nursing interventions. A nursing diagnosis that is based only on environmental observations (fragmented data) and that focuses on "unsafe housekeeping practices" provides very little direction for client and nursing intervention. Unsafe housekeeping practices can result from several factors, including lack of home management skill, energy depletion due to maturational and situational crises, and differing values about environmental safety. How a community health nurse would intervene when unsafe housekeeping practices are encountered is greatly influenced by the data base obtained and the nursing diagnosis developed. For example, an educative strategy is used when a client lacks home management skill, whereas a crisis intervention approach is initiated when a client's energies are depleted because of crisis.

Use of scientific knowledge such as Maslow's hierarchy of needs, theories of growth and development, family theories, and concepts of stress and crisis enhances a community health nurse's ability to synthesize data and to formulate an appropriate nursing diagnosis. Scientific knowledge helps a nurse to identify significant signs and symptoms of distress and to organize collected data into a meaningful whole. Grouping the symptoms presented by a client and then comparing them to clinical and research findings such as those presented in Chapter 8 aids the nurse in determining when a client may be in a state of crisis or vulnerable to crisis.

When comparing collected data with relevant clinical and research findings, it is important to identify nursing diagnoses in relation to client strengths as well as client needs. Discerning client strengths helps the community health nurse to reinforce self-sufficiency skills, which in turn aids the nurse in avoiding dependency-building nursing activities. In the community health nurse setting, special emphasis is placed on identifying nursing diagnoses that relate to situations or potential problems that warrant anticipatory guidance counseling. This emphasis is based on the belief that primary prevention should be a major focus in community health nursing practice. Situations throughout the life span that warrant anticipatory guidance are covered in Chapters 14 through 20.

Synthesizing data and formulating nursing diagnoses can be difficult when the nurse works with clients in the community health setting because data about several individuals and family dynamics must be integrated. Peer consultation, supervised clinical practice, and comparison of nursing diagnoses with diagnoses of other health professionals can help practitioners to increase their diagnostic abilities. Knowing when to seek assistance from others is one earmark of a professional nurse.

Nursing Classification Systems

Use of nursing classification systems can also help practitioners to refine their diagnostic skills and to document the effectiveness of nursing interventions. In addition, these systems can facilitate the collection of assessment data and can assist in organizing these data. Two such systems, one developed by The North American Nursing Diagnosis Association and the other by the Visiting Nurse Association of Omaha, Nebraska, are being used by nurses across the country. Other nursing classification systems are shared in Chapter 23.

The North American Nursing Diagnosis Association was established in St. Louis, Missouri, in 1973 for the purpose of developing a standard nomenclature for describing health problems amenable to treatment by nurses (Kim and Moritz, 1982, p. xvii). Since its inception this association has sponsored several National Nursing Diagnosis Conferences, which have resulted in the identification of appropriate *nursing* diagnostic categories for practitioners. Currently there are 131 nursing diagnoses that have been accepted for clinical testing by the North American Nursing Diagnosis Association (refer to Table 9-6). These diagnoses are grouped under 11 diagnostic categories that were derived from significant functional health patterns. These functional health patterns provide a format for an admission assessment and a data base for nursing diagnosis (Gordon, 1993). Gordon, in *Manual of Nursing Diagnosis, 1993-1994,* explicates in more detail how to use the classification system and the functional health patterns to facilitate nursing assessments and the identification of nursing diagnoses. As previously mentioned functional health patterns assessment tools that can be used to guide the nursing assessment process are found in Gordon's book. Gordon stresses that the nursing diagnoses accepted for clinical testing by the North American Nursing Diagnosis Association are in the process of development and need to be refined. All professional nurses are encouraged to submit refinements of accepted diagnoses to the North American Nursing Diagnosis Association, 1211 Locust Street, Philadelphia, Pennsylvania 19107.

The classification system developed by the Visiting Nurse Association of Omaha was designed to provide an organizing framework for client problems diagnosed by nurses in the community health setting. This classification scheme, based upon the ANA definition of community health nursing, is an orderly arrangement of a nonexhaustive list of client problems that are grouped into four major domains: environmental, psychosocial, physiological, and health behaviors. Definitions for each of these domains are as follows (Simmons, 1980, pp. 6, 8):

1. *Environmental*—Refers to the material resources and physical surroundings of the home, neighborhood, and broader community in which the client lives. This domain focuses on factors

TABLE

9-6 The North American Nursing Diagnosis Association: Nursing Diagnostic Categories and Diagnoses Accepted for Clinical Testing, 1990*

Diagnostic categories	Nursing diagnoses
Health perception—health management pattern	**Altered health maintenance**
	Ineffective management of therapeutic regimen
	Total health management deficit
	Health management deficit (specify)
	Noncompliance (specify)
	High risk for noncompliance (specify)
	Health-seeking behaviors (specify)
	High risk for infection
	High risk for injury (trauma)
	High risk for poisoning
	High risk for suffocation
	Altered protection
Nutritional-metabolic pattern	**Altered nutrition: High risk for more than body requirements** or high risk for obesity
	Altered nutrition: More than body requirements or exogenous obesity
	Altered nutrition: Less than body requirements or nutritional deficit (specify)
	Ineffective breastfeeding
	Effective breastfeeding
	Interrupted breastfeeding
	Ineffective infant feeding pattern
	High risk for aspiration
	Impaired swallowing or uncompensated swallowing impairment
	Altered oral mucous membrane
	High risk for fluid volume deficit
	Fluid volume deficit
	Fluid volume excess
	High risk for impaired skin integrity or high risk for skin breakdown
	Impaired skin integrity
	Pressure ulcer (specify stage)
	Impaired tissue integrity (specify type)
	High risk for altered body temperature
	Ineffective thermoregulation
	Hyperthermia
	Hypothermia
Elimination pattern	**Constipation** or intermittent constipation pattern
	Colonic constipation
	Perceived constipation
	Diarrhea
	Bowel incontinence
	Altered urinary elimination pattern
	Functional incontinence
	Reflex incontinence
	Stress incontinence
	Urge incontinence
	Total incontinence
	Urinary retention

*Diagnoses accepted by the North American Nursing Diagnosis Association appear in boldface type. Diagnoses found to be useful in clinical practice but not yet accepted are in roman type.
From Gordon M: *Manual of nursing diagnosis, 1993-1994*, St. Louis, 1993, Mosby, pp. iv-ix.

9-6 The North American Nursing Diagnosis Association: Nursing Diagnostic
Categories and Diagnoses Accepted for Clinical Testing, 1990—cont'd

Diagnostic categories	Nursing diagnoses
Activity-exercise pattern	**High risk for activity intolerance**
	Activity intolerance (specify level)
	Fatigue
	Impaired physical mobility (specify level)
	High risk for disuse syndrome
	High risk for joint contractures
	Total self-care deficit (specify level)
	Self bathing-hygiene deficit (specify level)
	Self dressing-rooming deficit (specify level)
	Self feeding deficit (specify level)
	Self toileting deficit (specify level)
	Altered growth and development: self-care skills (specify level)
	Diversional activity deficit
	Impaired home maintenance management
	Dysfunctional ventilatory weaning response (DVWR)
	Inability to sustain spontaneous ventilation
	Ineffective airway clearance
	Ineffective breathing pattern
	Impaired gas exchange
	Decreased cardiac output
	Altered tissue perfusion (specify)
	Dysreflexia
	High risk for peripheral neurovascular dysfunction
	Altered growth and development
Sleep-rest pattern	**Sleep-pattern disturbance**
Cognitive-perceptual pattern	**Pain**
	Chronic pain
	Pain self-management deficit (acute, chronic)
	Uncompensated sensory deficit (specify)
	Sensory-perceptual alterations: input deficit or sensory deprivation
	Sensory-perceptual alterations: input excess or sensory overload
	Unilateral neglect
	Knowledge deficit (specify)
	Impaired thought processes
	Uncompensated short-term memory deficit
	High risk for cognitive impairment
	Decisional conflict (specify)
Self-perception-self-concept pattern	**Fear (specify focus)**
	Anxiety
	Mild anxiety
	Moderate anxiety
	Severe anxiety (panic)
	Anticipatory anxiety (mild, moderate, severe)
	Reactive depression (situational)
	Hopelessness

Continued

9-6 The North American Nursing Diagnosis Association: Nursing Diagnostic Categories and Diagnoses Accepted for Clinical Testing, 1990—cont'd

Diagnostic categories	Nursing diagnoses
Role-relationship pattern	**Powerlessness (severe, low, moderate)**
	Self-esteem disturbance
	Chronic low self-esteem
	Situational low self-esteem
	Body image disturbance
	High risk for self-mutilation
	Personal identity disturbance
	Anticipatory grieving
	Dysfunctional grieving
	Disturbance in role performance
	Unresolved independence-dependence conflict
	Social isolation
	Social isolation or social rejection
	Impaired social interaction
	Altered growth and development: social skills (specify)
	Relocation stress syndrome (or relocation syndrome)
	Altered family processes
	High risk for altered parenting
	Altered parenting
	Parental role conflict
	Parent-infant separation
	Weak mother-infant attachment or parent-infant attachment
	Caregiver role strain
	High risk for caregiver role strain
	Impaired verbal communication
	Altered growth and development: communication skills (specify)
	High risk for violence
Sexuality-reproductive pattern	**Sexual dysfunction**
	Altered sexuality patterns
	Rape-trauma syndrome
	Rape-trauma syndrome: compound reaction
	Rape-trauma syndrome: silent reaction
Coping—stress-tolerance pattern	**Ineffective coping (individual)**
	Avoidance coping
	Defensive coping
	Ineffective denial or denial
	Impaired adjustment
	Post-trauma response
	Family coping: potential for growth
	Ineffective family coping: compromised
	Ineffective family coping: disabling
Value-belief pattern	**Spiritual distress (distress of human spirit)**

external to the client that affect the health or illness of that client.

2. *Psychosocial*—Refers to patterns of behavior, communication, relationship, and development. This domain includes problems that address the relationships of the client as an individual or the family with other persons. These persons may be immediate or extended family members, significant others, neighbors, acquaintances, or community workers. Thus, this group of problems often reflects inability of the individual or family to interact positively with persons inside or outside the family unit.

3. *Physiological*—Refers to the functional status of processes that maintain life. Because of the focus of the problems in this domain, the labels tend to be referenced to the client as an individual rather than to the client as a family unit.

4. *Health behaviors*—Refers to activities that maintain or promote wellness, promote recovery, or maximize rehabilitation. The problems address health-seeking behaviors that have the potential to improve the quality of the client's life. Personal motivation on the part of the client is especially critical in resolving this group of problems since he or she must change health behavior appropriately, often without rapid or visible benefits.

Within each of these domains are the names of identified problems that may be actual or potential, modifiers of these problems, and signs or symptoms of the problems. The signs and symptoms are general statements that condense more specific information about a client. Additionally, problems may be referenced to either an individual or to a family. Presented in Table 9-7 are examples of how the classification scheme developed by the Visiting Nurse Service of Omaha is organized according to domain, problem label, modifier, and sign or symptom.

Directly related to the problem classification scheme and the nursing process is a problem-rating scale that helps nurses to evaluate client outcomes at regular time intervals and a nursing intervention scheme consisting of nursing activities aimed at addressing specific nursing problems (Simmons, Martin, Crews, and Scheet, 1986).

The structure of the Omaha classification scheme easily adapts to a computerized system of record keeping (Simmons, Martin, Crews, and Scheet, 1986). Data can be efficiently stored and retrieved and each client problem can be identified by a numerical code. Computerized management information systems are becoming the norm across the country (refer to Chapters 22 and 23).

Planning

After nursing diagnoses are established and validated with the client, the community health nurse and the client move into the planning phase of the nursing process. Two major activities occur during this phase: (1) client-centered goals and objectives (criteria) for evaluating goal attainment are formulated and (2) alternative interventions are identified and evaluated. A *goal* is a broad desired outcome toward which behavior is directed, such as "the family will value preventive health care services." An *objective* delineates client behaviors that reflect when a goal has been reached. "The family will obtain a regular source of medical care by September" might be one objective established to determine if the above goal has been accomplished. *Alternative interventions* are activities that may be implemented by the client, the nurse, and other health care professionals to help the client achieve the desired goals. For example, in relation to the above objective, the nurse might discuss with the client the services of all the available medical resources in the community and assist the client in obtaining transportation if necessary.

All goals and objectives should be stated in specific and realistic terms and relate to the nursing diagnoses that have been established. They should not include expectations that are beyond the professional's or client's resources or capabilities. A goal of a severely retarded child achieving normal growth and development is extremely unrealistic. It is very appropriate to work toward maximizing this child's potential but inappropriate to expect that this child will reach normal growth and development parameters. Expecting that the family of this child will continue to function exactly as they did before the child's birth is also unrealistic. During times of stress and crisis change is necessary and unavoidable. A goal statement that focuses on the family demonstrating constructive

TABLE 9-7   The Visiting Nurse Service of Omaha, Nebraska: Organization of Classification Scheme for Client Problems in Community Health Nursing: Selected Examples

Domain	Problem label	Modifier	Sign or symptom
Environmental	Income	Deficit	Low/no income
			Uninsured medical expenses
			Inadequate money management
			Able to buy only necessities
			Difficulty buying necessities
			Other (specify)
Psychosocial	Communication with community resources	Impairment	Unfamiliar with options/procedures for obtaining services
			Difficulty understanding roles/regulations of service provider
			Dissatisfaction with services
			Language barrier
			Inadequate/unavailable resources
			Other (specify)
Physiological	Hearing	Impairment	Difficulty hearing normal speech tones
			Absent/abnormal response to sound
			Abnormal results of hearing screening test
			Other (specify)
Health-related behaviors	Nutrition	Impairment	Weighs 10 percent more than average
			Weighs 10 percent less than average
			Lacks established standards for daily caloric/fluid intake
			Unbalanced diet
			Improper feeding schedule for age
			Nonadherence to prescribed diet
			Other (specify)

From Simmons DA, Martin KS, Crews CC, and Scheet NJ: *Client management information system for community health nursing agencies*, NTIS Accession No HRP-0907023, Springfield, Va, 1986, National Technical Information Service, pp. 60, 61, 64, 68.

behavior to reduce stressors related to the care of their developmentally disabled child is more appropriate.

Goal statements and objectives that are written in positive terms provide direction for nursing interventions more effectively than those that have a negative orientation. Negative goal statements such as "parents will not use harsh disciplinary measures with their children" tend to focus on family weaknesses rather than on family strengths, which can be mobilized to reduce current stresses. Positive goal statements, such as "parents will talk with their children when the children act out," lead to the development of more positive interventions for achieving goals.

The nurse may find that, after client-centered goals are developed, the client finds it impossible to work on all of them immediately. When this happens the nurse and the client should work together to differentiate between problems that require immediate action and those that are of less concern to the client. When establishing priorities in relation to client goals the nurse must keep in mind that the client has the right to make the final decision about goals on which to focus. The nurse does have a responsibility to share concerns when she or he believes that client actions are unsafe or are precipitating a crisis situation.

After client-centered, positively stated goals have been established and priorities determined, behavioral objectives that can be measured should be written. The importance of formulating specific objectives for evaluating goal attainment must be stressed. Broad, general goals do not provide sufficient direction for planning intervention strategies. "Maximizing the potential" of a child who has a developmental lag, for example, does not specifically identify needed areas of improvement. Objectives such as those listed below more appropriately facilitate the development of intervention strategies because they focus on specific developmental needs of the child and the family.

- Joel will achieve daytime bladder and bowel control by December.
- Joel will eat solid foods by October.
- Joel's family will share their feelings about Joel's condition.
- Joel's family will verbally identify how their feelings about Joel's condition positively or adversely affect his growth and development.
- Joel's family will identify strategies to reduce the stress associated with his care.
- Joel's parents will share ways to maintain a healthy spouse relationship.

Interventions, like objectives, should be specific and based on sound scientific knowledge. "Teaching about growth and development" or "provide support to the family" are not specifically stated interventions. They are extremely global and do not take into account the individual needs of a particular family. A community health nurse might better prepare for family visits if the above interventions were stated as follows: "discuss various ways to achieve daytime bladder and bowel control" and "teach caregiver stress management techniques." Currently, research is being conducted at the University of Iowa to develop a classification of nursing interventions, including interventions related to the family (Bulechek and McCloskey, 1992; Craft and Willadsen, 1992). This research will help the practitioner to define and validate nursing interventions.

When delineating a plan for intervention both family and nurse activities should be identified. If only nursing actions are established, the client cannot be an active participant in the therapeutic process. Unfortunately, family resources are frequently overlooked when intervention strategies are developed. For instance, plans are too often made to involve community resources in the client's care even though friends or family members are available and would be more than willing to assist the client in achieving goals.

When intervention strategies are discussed it may be found that referral to other health care professionals can best help the client to meet his or her needs. In these instances the community health nurse should discuss with the family how essential data about their situation can be shared. The family's permission should be obtained before releasing any information to other health care agencies. The client has the right to determine what data, shared in confidence with the nurse, should or should not be shared with others. Indiscriminate exchange of client information among professionals violates the client's right to confidentiality and usually promotes mistrust and resistance to professional intervention. The principle of confidentiality is most often violated when goals are not mutually established and the nurse shares or seeks data to validate nurse-focused goals.

Interdisciplinary collaboration is appropriate and often essential. However, the family must support the need for such an approach before it can be fully successful. Application of the principles of the referral process which are discussed in Chapter 10 usually help a nurse to reduce resistance to interdisciplinary collaboration.

Three key principles must be taken into consideration during all phases of the planning process. These are (1) individualization of family care plans; (2) active family participation; and (3) the family's right of self-determination. The family-centered nursing process is a scientific process designed to meet the needs of *clients*. Inherent in this concept is the belief that clients have unique needs and, thus, care cannot be standardized. Unique needs of clients can be discovered only by actively involving the client in the therapeutic process. Active client participation also promotes client commitment to goal attainment and decreases resistance to change. Taking over for a client may reinforce a client's feelings of inadequacy or increase the client's resentment of authority figures. These types of feelings can foster dependency or rejection of aid offered by the community health nurse.

For clients to fully participate in the therapeutic process they must have the right to refuse any course of action they deem inappropriate for them. The community health nurse can help a client to examine the pros and cons of certain health actions or the consequences of continuing a particular pattern of functioning. The nurse should not make decisions for the client or expect the client to make decisions in the way the nurse would make them. This is not meant to imply that the nurse should reinforce behavior which could be harmful to the client. Rather, it emphasizes that clients are responsible for the decisions they make and that they should not be rejected (e.g., viewed as "hopeless" or "resistant to change") if they do not make decisions in the way the health care professional would make them. Occasionally the community health nurse does intervene without a client's consent because the client is a threat to others (e.g., child abuse, spread of communicable disease) or to herself or himself (suicidal). Even in these situations the community health nurse works with the client, if possible, to help reduce the distress being experienced and to develop new patterns of coping.

To effectively apply the principles of individualization, active participation, and self-determination, the community health nurse must *internalize* the belief that all clients are unique and capable of making decisions about health care issues. Nurses must also consistently examine how personal attitudes, beliefs, motivations, and conditioning are influencing their professional relationships. Personal biases can and do subtly influence how professionals interact with clients. One community health nurse, for instance, found it difficult to maintain a therapeutic relationship with families when the male provider in the family had a "drinking problem." She would support the female's viewpoints without helping her to analyze how she might be reinforcing her husband's ineffective behavior. The nurse recognized that this was happening and was able to verbalize that she felt her sister died prematurely as a result of stress associated with her husband's drinking problem. When the nurse was conscious of her feelings she was able to deal with them and to better assist clients in these situations.

Professional Contracting

Contracting with families is one way of consistently monitoring professional biases and applying the principles of individualization, active participation, and self-determination. A contract—a mutual agreement between two or more persons for a specific purpose—provides a framework for evaluating the interactions that are occurring between people. It does so because a contract clearly identifies what each person in the relationship can expect from the other person in the relationship.

Contracts are used for a variety of reasons. They may be formal, legally binding, long-term agreements, such as when a couple buys a home, or they may be casual, short-term commitments, such as when a friend consents to dog-sit while the dog's owner is gone on vacation. Contracts are also being used effectively by health care professionals to encourage their clients to participate more actively in dealing with their own health care needs. In these situations the contract assumes a different purpose. It becomes a method of professional intervention that facilitates the helping relationship with clients. Contracting has been used by health care professionals more frequently in recent years because there is a growing interest in promoting a philosophy of professional practice that supports the client's self-care capabilities. Increased use of contracting has also occurred because it has been found that clients who are actively involved in identifying their own health needs and in formulating health care goals are more likely to change their health behaviors than clients who have no voice in these decisions.

A professional contract may be defined very simply as a mutually agreed-upon working understanding that relates to the terms of treatment and is continuously negotiable between the nurse and the family (Boehm, 1989; Maluccio and Marlow, 1974; Seabury, 1976). The contract may be either written or oral, but it must be clear and explicit to all parties involved. When methods for reinforcing clients' actions are explicitly spelled out the contract is labeled a *contingency contract*. The contingency contracting process is based on theories of behavior modification, which postulate that reinforcers or rewards increase the probability that a desired response will occur. Before implementing contingency contracting the professional should have a firm understanding of the principles of behavior modification.

The professional using the contracting method of intervention must feel comfortable with the philosophy that all individuals have the potential for growth and that they are capable of effective decision-making. The professional must also believe that the client has the right to determine which course of action will best meet his or her health care needs. In essence, contracting is a philosophy of practice that governs how the community health nurse implements the family-centered nursing process. The nurse who believes in contracting involves the client in all aspects of care. She or he makes an agreement with the client that spells out explicitly the responsibilities of both nurse and client in achieving mutually defined, client-centered goals. The quality of explicitness implies that terms of intervention are known to both the client and the nurse. When contracting occurs, all involved parties have a mutual understanding about:

1. Purpose of client-nurse interactions
2. Nursing diagnoses

3. Desired outcomes (goals) toward which behavior is directed
4. Priority needs in relation to client goals
5. Methods of intervention
6. Specific activities each party will carry out to achieve stated goals
7. Established time parameters for evaluation and the frequency and length of visits

Contracting increases the clarity in nurse-client interactions. Specific commitments are made orally so that each party is aware of its role in the therapeutic process. Increased clarity often enhances the therapeutic relationship. This is especially true when clients have multiple problems or are unable to identify the nature of their problems. A case situation can best illustrate this point.

▸ The Beech family, two parents with five children, had been visited by community health nurses for years. The family folder reflected many problems: marital stress, financial difficulties, poor nutrition, lack of preventive health care for family members, irregular school attendance, and frequent childhood infections were the primary problems with which the family was dealing. Infrequent visits were made by the community health nurse because the family continually failed to deal actively with health care needs. Because they moved frequently, the Beech family never had consistent contact with one nurse for any length of time. Finally the community health nurse decided to talk with Mrs. Beech about terminating nursing service because she believed that the family did not desire assistance. To her surprise, Mrs. Beech verbalized that her family did need help and that she really wanted the nurse to continue visiting. She further shared that she had difficulty concentrating on anything because the family had so many problems to handle. The nurse agreed with Mrs. Beech that it was an impossible task to solve all the family problems at once. She proposed that it might be helpful if the family and the nurse could work together to resolve the one health problem Mrs. Beech felt was most distressing at that time. Mrs. Beech had trouble focusing on one particular concern because she had never before attempted to do so. Because she spent a considerable amount of time talking about Mary, her 10-year-old who had recently failed a hearing test at school, the nurse asked if Mrs. Beech might want to explore ways to resolve this health care problem. The nurse also suggested that it might be helpful to order the family's health problems from most significant to least significant. Since these suggestions were acceptable to Mrs. Beech, the following contract was established:

- *Purpose of client-nurse interactions:* **The community health nurse will help the family to establish priorities in relation to their health problems and to handle their problems in manageable doses.**
- *Priority need:* **Mary's failure of hearing test at school.**
- *Mutual goal:* **Mary's hearing problem will be evaluated by a physician.**
- *Method of intervention:* **Family will take Mary to the hearing specialist she had seen before. (This decision was made after the nurse discussed all the possible resources where Mary could obtain care and Mrs. Beech shared that Mary had had hearing problems in the past.)**
- *Responsibilities of family:* **(1) Make appointment with the doctor; (2) arrange for child care for the two preschoolers for the afternoon of the appointment; (3) arrange for transportation; and (4) together with the nurse, make list of questions to ask the doctor during the visit.**
- *Responsibilities of nurse:* **Contact the physician to share the results of Mary's hearing test and Mrs. Beech's fears about health care professionals. (Mrs. Beech had been frequently criticized by health care professionals in the past for waiting too long before she sought medical help.) Visit weekly to evaluate how plans for Mary's care are progressing and to help the family establish priorities for health care action.**
- *Time limits:* **Mary to see the physician by the end of the month.**

Mary saw the physician within the appropriate time frame; it was determined that she would need ear surgery. Since the contracting method of intervention helped Mrs. Beech to achieve her first goal, Mrs. Beech and the nurse agreed to renegotiate for follow-up based on the doctor's recommendation. Many other contracts were made before this family case record was closed. Accomplishing resolution of one problem helped family members to see that their situation was not hopeless. Setting priorities in relation to goal attainment decreased the family's anxiety about all the problems they had to handle.

Contracting is a dynamic, complex process that gradually evolves as the therapeutic relationship is strengthened. It should not be viewed as a simple procedure, involving only a discussion about goals, intervention strategies, and time limits. To successfully engage a family in the contracting process the community health nurse must help the family to gain a clear understanding of its needs. The nurse must also explain the nature of a therapeutic relationship and explore with the client the range of alternative interventions that are available.

When thinking about contracting with clients, it is important to remember that clients may not know about all the resources available to them. They also may not know why they are experiencing distress at this time. An elderly woman, for instance, may recognize that she is concerned about the physical aspects of caring for her ill husband, but she may not realize that some of her stress is related to role changes as a result of her caregiver responsibilities.

Initially a contract may be very general and include only an agreement to explore the nature of the client's problems and the meaning of a therapeutic relationship. The terms of a contract become more inclusive as specific data are obtained. Establishing time parameters is important even when a general contract is developed, because they emphasize the need for reviewing progress made in relation to goal attainment.

Contracting is an effective way to involve families in their own health care. Contracting can reinforce ineffective family patterns, however, if the nurse does not analyze carefully family dynamics. When a contract supports unhealthy family functioning it is labeled a *corrupt contract* (Beall, 1972, p. 77). A corrupt contract might evolve, for instance, when a community health nurse is working with a family who would like their aging parents to move to a nursing home. Sometimes families push for nursing home placement to meet their own needs rather than the needs of their aging parents. If the community health nurse supports the family's decision and encourages the parents to move without talking to them about their needs and desires, he or she is violating the rights of the aging parents and the principles of contracting.

During the contracting process a community health nurse may identify problems, such as lack of protection against communicable diseases or inadequate dental care, that do not seem to be of concern to the family. In these situations a nurse-centered goal rather than a client-centered goal is formulated. A nurse-centered goal should be stated as such and should not emphasize family action like the "family will make an appointment at the immunization clinic." Instead it should focus on increasing the family's awareness of the problem and be stated in such terms as "the family will verbalize an understanding of immunizations." Distinguishing carefully between nurse goals and family goals helps the community health nurse to prevent imposing personal values on clients and helps the nurse to focus on the problems and goals important to the family. Generally, families do not explore problems identified by the nurse that they do not see as problems until they have achieved their own client-centered goals.

Throughout the contracting process the community health nurse must clearly document on the family record assessment data, goals, objectives, intervention strategies, and evaluation findings. Written data are retrievable, whereas oral information can be easily lost or misinterpreted. The family service record should provide concrete data organized in a manner that can be easily analyzed. Lack of documentation discourages effective evaluation of nursing care and client goal attainment. It is often indicative of inadequate data analysis and insufficient planning. In Chapter 23 the significance of accurate recording in relation to the development of a sound quality improvement program is discussed. The record system used in the community health setting is extremely important, and a variety of formats can be effectively used to document all aspects of the nursing process.

It is crucial that the record format represents and shows the flow between all aspects of the nursing process presented in Table 9-1. This is not an easy task, but it must be addressed. The quality of the record system will affect the quality of care given to a client, especially in relation to continuity of care. It is often helpful to place diagnoses, goals, plans, interventions, and evaluation findings on one sheet in the record so that the relationship between each phase and the next one can be easily identified. If the phases of the nursing process are on different pages of the record, it is difficult to coordinate diagnoses, goals, plans, interventions, and evaluation findings.

Implementing

The implementation phase of the nursing process deals specifically with how activities are carried out to achieve client goals. Together, the client and the nurse select and test intervention strategies to determine their appropriateness in helping the client move toward problem resolution. Priorities concerning when actions will be taken are established so that the client can deal with his or her problems in manageable doses. If needed, other resources are mobilized to help the client handle the change process.

Because change is often threatening, a warm, caring, supportive atmosphere that reinforces client accomplishments should be fostered. Focusing on what remains to be accomplished rather than emphasizing positive results that have already occurred serves only to discourage the client. Honest, positive feedback can be the motivating factor that promotes client involvement in the therapeutic process. Positive feedback can also help to increase clients' self-esteem and confidence in their ability to assume responsibility for maintaining and promoting their health status.

The community health nurse uses a variety of intervention strategies to help clients alter those aspects of life they desire to change. Some of these are discussed in Chapter 8, where the supportive, educative, and problem-solving strategies were explored. Nursing actions should be based on sound scientific principles and knowledge. If a planned intervention, for instance, is to increase the client's understanding of how to prepare nutritious meals, the teaching methodology chosen should take into consideration specific client characteristics such as financial resources, demands on the homemaker's time, nutritional needs of all family members, and cultural preferences in relation to food likes and dislikes. It should also reflect current knowledge about nutritional requirements and appropriate application of the principles of teaching and learning.

All other phases of the nursing process are usually carried out during the implementation phase. While clients are actively participating in the intervention process they share data verbally or nonverbally through action taken or not taken. The community health nurse must analyze these new data carefully to determine if care plans need to be revised. Nursing care plans should never be static. Rather, they should be continuously open to renegotiation as the client's situation changes or new data are discovered.

The community health nurse must be flexible when implementing intervention strategies, since new data are often generated that alter original nursing diagnoses and client goals. Some clients are unable to

identify the nature of their problems until they attempt to change their behavior and find that change does not relieve their discomfort. This was illustrated in Chapter 8, when Mrs. Lehi discovered that her headaches were related to guilt feelings about being a working mother rather than to excessive demands on her time. In this situation the nurse and Mrs. Lehi revised their original goal, "Mrs. Lehi will discover ways to adjust her daily schedule to reduce stress," to "Mrs. Lehi will identify ways to achieve her self-fulfillment needs and maintain the integrity of the family unit without distress." Intervention strategies were altered accordingly. Instead of discussing Mrs. Lehi's daily activities and support systems, the nurse and Mrs. Lehi explored issues such as Mrs. Lehi's feelings about motherhood, the needs of school-age children, an individual's need for self-fulfillment, and how a family can grow as its subsystems grow.

Both the client and the nurse should have responsibilities to meet when interventions are planned and mutually agreed upon. If either the client or nurse is unable to meet these responsibilities, this must be discussed and interventions revised as necessary. The family-centered nursing process is a collaborative process and the client must be involved in its implementation. A nurse who assumes responsibilities that the client can independently handle instead of talking about why planned interventions are not being implemented is not helping the client to move toward goal achievement.

During the implementation phase it is not unusual to discover that clients do not wish to pursue a particular goal, even though they expressed a desire to do so during the planning phase. Sometimes clients verbalize an *awareness* that a problem exists but are not ready to change their behavior in the way necessary to resolve that problem. Clients may not recognize the difference between awareness and readiness until concrete plans have been made to alter their current situation. If this happens, it can be difficult for these clients to verbally convey to the nurse that they are not ready for change. Frequently they share this message nonverbally by not taking action. That is why it is so important for the community health nurse to find out why clients are not meeting commitments that had been mutually agreed upon. Goals and plans should be modified if clients are not ready to alter their behavior.

Some clients are resistant to change because all their alternatives for change have negative consequences. A woman, for example, who has limited financial resources, no preparation for a job, and few support systems may be very hesitant to divorce her husband even though their marital relationship is destructive to her emotional health. The fear of not being able to support herself and being alone might be far more stressful to her than the emotional pain she is experiencing in the marital relationship. When community health nurses encounter such a situation, they must remain empathic and guard against feeling that the woman has no options. Community health nurses do find it difficult to handle situations when all the alternatives for change have some negative consequences. However, clients in these situations can be assisted by helping them to identify their strengths, obtain needed resources to achieve their goals, and recognize that they can achieve control over their lives.

Evaluating

Evaluation is the continuous critiquing of each aspect of the nursing process. Although it is discussed as a separate phase, it must take place concurrently with all phases of the nursing process. Ongoing feedback should be elicited from the client to determine whether goals, plans, and intervention strategies are appropriately focused. When objectives are established, defining how they will be evaluated is a necessity. A well-written objective will contain the potential for evaluation. For example, "John will learn how to give his own insulin injection by the end of the month" is a concise statement that can be used to determine whether John has achieved a desired goal.

Evaluation criteria, which help the family and the nurse to determine if expected client outcomes or family goals and objectives are being reached, should be established after the first nurse/client interaction. Developing evaluation criteria early in the helping relationship validates the importance of evaluation and provides direction for client and nurse actions. Presented in Table 9-8 is a care plan for the Lopez family (refer to the box below) that illustrates how one community health nurse initially established evaluation criteria to determine whether expected out-

◀ *The Lopez Family* ▶

The Lopez family consists of Juan, age 35, Elena, his 30-year-old wife, five children, and Mr. Lopez's mother, Teresa. The family is second generation Mexican-American from Texas, representative of a stream of Spanish-speaking families who yearly migrate north to harvest a variety of crops. Six months ago the family decided to stay in a northern midwest community when Mr. Lopez was offered a permanent job as a farmhand, because they felt the children could have a better education and life than the parents had experienced. Spanish is spoken in the home. Mr. Lopez speaks some English but is unable to read or write it. Mrs. Lopez has limited comprehension of English and has had no education beyond the fourth grade. Mr. Lopez's mother speaks only Spanish. The children speak English but are behind in school achievement due to frequent family moves.

The family lives in a five-room house that is on the farm property. Although housekeeping practices are adequate, the home is in poor condition, in need of paint and repairs. It has running water, the source of which is a well. A septic system is used for sewage disposal. There is electricity for lighting and heating and bottled gas is used for cooking.

The family lives rent-free in the house, which is provided by the owner of the farm; utilities are also provided by the owner. Family income is limited to Mr. Lopez's income of $100 per week and his mother's income of $65 per month from SSI. Only Grandmother Lopez has health insurance, on the basis of SSI. The tenant farm on which the family lives is ten miles from the nearest town. Mr. Lopez has a pickup truck that the family uses for transportation when necessary. However, Mr. Lopez finds it difficult to get off work during daytime hours to take the family in for medical care.

Health problems are evident in the family. Mr. Lopez is in need of dentures and all of the school-age children are in need of dental care, as reported by their teachers. Juanita, age 7, was recently referred for ophthalmological examination following vision screening at school. Francesca, age 3, is in need of medical care for a draining ear. All of the children are behind in their immunizations; the adults in the family do not know which "shots" they have had. Mrs. Lopez is in her seventh month of pregnancy and has had no medical care. The family expresses a desire to obtain care for their children but "we have no extra money to pay a doctor. We can hardly afford to buy food and clothing for the kids."

9-8 Lopez Family: Initial Care Plan

Assessment data	Nursing diagnoses	Expected client outcomes	Nursing interventions	Evaluation criteria
Children behind in school achievement due to frequent family moves. Family moved north so "children could have a better education."	Family coping, potential for growth as evidenced by family's desire to obtain a better education and life for their children.	Children will succeed in the educational system.	1. Verbally, positively reinforce the family's decision to obtain an education for its children. 2. Identify barriers to successful school achievement. 3. Provide family with information about school policies and procedures.	1. All children will attend school regularly. 2. Children will report satisfying school experiences. 3. Children obtain passing grades in school.
Family has no regular source of medical care. Family cannot afford to go to the doctor. Family members have obvious health needs. Difficult for family to obtain medical care during daytime hours. Family expresses a desire to follow up on the children's health needs.	Health maintenance, altered, due to limited financial resources and access problems.	Family will obtain the resources needed to follow up on family members' health needs. Family will obtain a regular source of medical and preventive health care.	1. Discuss family's beliefs about health and illness and health care. 2. Share with family resources in community to assist them in meeting their health needs (e.g., Lions' Club and MSS). 3. Discuss barriers to the utilization of the referral process. 4. Discern family's interest in obtaining a regular source of care. 5. Advocate for the family if needed. 6. Provide opportunities for breadwinner to meet work responsibilities while obtaining health care for the family.	1. Family members' health needs will be corrected: a. Mr. Lopez will obtain dentures. b. Mrs. Lopez will obtain prenatal care. c. Juanita will obtain an eye examination. d. Francesca will obtain medical care for her ear infection. e. All of the children will obtain dental care. f. All family members' immunization will be up-to-date.

Continued

TABLE 9-8   Lopez Family: Initial Care Plan—cont'd

Assessment data	Nursing diagnoses	Expected client outcomes	Nursing interventions	Evaluation criteria
Only grandmother has health insurance. Children have limited clothing for school. Total family income is $465/month.	Income deficit as evidenced by uninsured medical needs and difficulty buying necessities.	Family will be able to obtain the necessities of life.	1. Discuss with the family expectations regarding their needs. 2. Share with family community resources that could help to expand the family income (e.g., food stamps, health department immunization clinic, and clothing closet). 3. Provide assistance in meeting basic family needs.	1. Family will have adequate food and clothing. 2. Family obtains needed medical care. 3. Family is able to maintain its home.
Mr. Lopez speaks some English but is unable to read or write. Mrs. Lopez has limited comprehension of English, as does the grandmother.	Communication with community systems impaired, related to foreign language barriers.	Family will be able to communicate basic needs with health care providers.	1. Use culturally appropriate visual aids to facilitate family understanding. 2. Seek a translator to discuss critical health issues. 3. Show respect for the family's cultural differences (e.g., seek information about family customs, traditions, and health beliefs). 4. Keep language simple and talk slowly. 5. Involve the father in the conversation. 6. Show respect to all family members. 7. Use nonverbal communication (e.g., pictures, drawings, or gestures) to clarify situations with the family.	1. Family obtains adequate food and clothing. 2. Family expresses satisfaction with their encounters in the community.

TABLE 9-8		Lopez Family: Initial Care Plan—cont'd		
Assessment data	**Nursing diagnoses**	**Expected client outcomes**	**Nursing interventions**	**Evaluation criteria**
Home in need of repairs and painting. Nitrates in well water potentially harmful to a new infant.	Environment impaired, due to presence of lead paint and well water.	Lead paint will be removed from the environment. Family will know if well water is safe, especially for a new infant.	1. Elicit the family's understanding of lead poisoning and its effects. 2. Assist family in obtaining community resources for repair of home if desired. 3. Help the family to obtain testing to discern safety of water for all family members.	1. Well water is tested. 2. Family verbalizes an understanding of lead poisoning. 3. Family takes action to protect children from lead poisoning.

comes were achieved. When reviewing these criteria, note how they relate to each stage of the nursing process.

Although evaluation is one of the most significant aspects of the nursing process, it is the one most frequently neglected or haphazardly done. When developing the nursing care plan, intervals should be established for the systematic review of all aspects of the nursing process. Some community health agencies have a policy stating that all records should be summarized and analyzed after a given number of visits have been made or when the family case is being transferred to another nurse. Even if such a policy does not exist, summarization of records must be done on a regular basis because it facilitates evaluation of client services and outcomes. A well-written summary helps the community health nurse synthesize data and vividly identify what has or has not been accomplished in a specified period of time.

Summarizing records is one way to ensure that a systematic evaluation of family progress is done. Consulting with peers, supervisors, and other health care professionals can also help a community health nurse review progress or lack of progress in family situations. Evaluation is absolutely essential and it must be carefully planned; lack of evaluation often prolongs the therapeutic process.

When evaluating the effectiveness of intervention strategies implemented by the client, the nurse, and other health care professionals, it is not sufficient just to identify that the family is participating in the therapeutic process. The *outcome* of actions taken by the family and health care professionals must also be examined. Noting only that the family has kept an appointment at a clinic provides very little data about the effectiveness of this intervention strategy. Identifying what happened when the family went to the clinic and what motivated them to do so is far more significant. This type of data provides the key for future interventions. Finding out, for instance, if the family was satisfied with the care they received or if the family understood the recommendations for follow-up can help the nurse to identify barriers to the utilization of health care services. Data obtained from these types of questions can also assist the nurse in planning interventions specific to the current needs of the family.

When evaluating the effectiveness of intervention strategies, the nurse may find that clients are not reaching their goals. This happens for a variety of reasons that are not always obvious to either the client or the nurse. Outlined below are some factors for the nurse to consider as guidelines when examining why client goals have not been achieved:

1. Data base inadequate to identify the actual needs of the family
2. Goals and objectives too broad and general
3. Goals and objectives not mutually established; nurse's goals being imposed on the family
4. Family priorities in relation to goals and objectives not ascertained
5. Family attempting to deal with too many problems at once
6. Family energies depleted as a result of maturational and situational crises
7. Barriers to care not identified because follow-up on client and nurse actions is neglected
8. Nursing diagnoses, goals, and objectives not revised as the family situation changes
9. Intervention strategies inappropriate
10. Family lacks the support they need to reduce anxiety during the change process
11. Coordination of care among all health professionals being neglected; family receiving inconsistent messages about appropriate intervention actions; gaps in services

The coordination of services among all professionals is crucial. It should not be assumed that particular services will be provided by an agency when a client is referred to that agency. When multiple agencies are working with a family, clearly defined mechanisms for deciding who will do what and for evaluating the quality of the care being delivered by the health team should be established. The client must be involved in determining how interdisciplinary collaboration and coordination will evolve. Generally clients are more than willing to consent to an interdisciplinary approach to the delivery of health care when they understand why it is important and how it will help them.

When an interdisciplinary approach is used to provide services for clients, the community health nurse must carefully evaluate when nursing services are and are not needed. Referring a client to another community agency does not necessarily mean that all of the client's needs will be met by that agency. The community health nurse still has a responsibility to evaluate the effectiveness of the referrals that have been made (refer to Chapter 10) and to discern if the client has other needs that are amenable to nursing interventions. After the referral has been implemented successfully, it may be found that nursing ser-vices are no longer needed; the client is then prepared for termination and the family case is closed to service.

Use of the evaluation process helps the community health nurse to provide care to clients more effectively. It assists the nurse in determining which goals have been accomplished, either completely or partially, and helps the nurse to modify intervention strategies if goals are not being reached. It also aids the nurse in making sound decisions about when to terminate nursing services.

Terminating

Terminating is seldom identified as a separate phase in the nursing process. It is alluded to during the evaluation phase, but very little attention is devoted to discussing what impact termination has on the nurse and the client in the community health setting. Frequently, feelings associated with the separation process are not handled by the client or the nurse. To effectively intervene with clients in the community health setting, a nurse must become *involved*. The inability to deal with feelings associated with the termination process can stifle the development of close, caring professional relationships. For this reason we label terminating as a separate phase in the family-centered nursing process.

Terminating is the period when the client and nurse deal with feelings associated with separation and when they distance themselves (Kelly, 1969, p. 2381). Ending a meaningful relationship with a client should be carefully planned. Clients, as well as nurses, need time to deal with the strong emotions that are often evoked by separation. Anger, sadness, denial, and rejection are some normal feelings experienced by both the client and the nurse during the termination phase. The type of reaction that occurs depends, to a great extent, on how the nurse and the client have dealt with separation in the past. In social situations the sense of sadness is verbalized when friends are leaving, but "denial, suppression and repression of feelings are encouraged" (Sene, 1969, p. 39). Because of this type of socialization process, clients and nurses alike have not learned how to talk freely about what separation means to them.

In the community health setting the nurse encounters termination issues frequently. Some clients are seen on a short-term basis, in three or four visits, whereas long-term relationships are established with other clients who have multiple problems to resolve. It is not uncommon to have a client move abruptly or to have a staff nurse's district changed. Clients who have experienced frequent changes in the nurse assigned to their case may have trouble becoming closely involved with any nurse. Talking about what these changes mean to the client and the nurse can be a learning process for both. A nurse who uses denial to cope with feelings associated with termination will be unable to help the client deal with these feelings.

Our clinical experiences have demonstrated that the issue of termination is too often neglected in the community health setting. Family case situations are closed without prior notice to the family, or a nurse's district is changed without providing sufficient time for the nurse to handle the termination process with clients. At times cases are not closed because the client regresses when it is discovered that the nurse believes her or his services are no longer needed. The client may verbalize the same belief but still regress because he or she is not given the opportunity to explore feelings associated with loss. One 40-year-old client who had multiple sclerosis abruptly stopped doing his exercises when the nurse remarked how well he was progressing. He finally verbalized that he was afraid the nurse would no longer visit when he was able to care for himself. At other times the nurse does not close a family case to service because of difficulty in ending the relationship with the family. The nurse may only visit monthly "just to see how they are doing," not recognizing that she or he is having difficulty ending a meaningful relationship.

The need to handle separation issues when terminating a nurse-client relationship is essential. Termination may not be an easy process, especially when the nurse and the client have had a long-term relationship. Clients need a supportive atmosphere that encourages them to express feelings and emotions. Often the nurse must initiate discussion about termination before the client will feel free to share feelings about this issue. This was dramatically illustrated when one of the authors ended a long-term relationship with a family because they were moving.

▶ **The Grostics had been visited weekly for approximately a year because they were dealing with both developmental and situational crises. Child neglect had been evident when the family case was first opened, but a year later both children were happy, thriving youngsters. Upon moving, Mrs. G. felt that the family still needed nursing services, so plans were made to refer the family for community health nursing follow-up in their new community. Both the client and nurse had shared positive feelings throughout their relationship, but neither verbalized these feelings when plans for referral were discussed. Mrs. G.'s mother altered this situation. She saw the nurse in the immunization clinic prior to the nurse's last visit to the family and stated that Mrs. G. was very upset about having a new nurse. "No one could be like you." Finally, during the last visit both the nurse and Mrs. G. hugged each other and openly discussed what they were feeling. The nurse felt even better when she heard that the family was doing well in their new location.**

A client helped the nurse in this situation see the value of dealing with feelings associated with termination and the rewards of involvement. Although termination may be difficult, it is a learning and growing experience for both nurse and client. When properly implemented, both are able to see what has and has not been accomplished in the therapeutic process and the reason(s) for the termination. Often termination occurs because all the goals established for the relationship have been reached and there is no further need for nursing service. The client should be informed that, if health needs arise in the future, the community health nurse can be contacted again. Keeping records open just for the sake of keeping them open when no health goals are being actively worked on is not a good use of nursing time, nor does it project a realistic picture to the client of what nursing services are about.

Summary

The family-centered nursing process is a systematic approach to scientific problem solving, involving a series of circular, dynamic actions—assessing, analyzing, planning, implementing, evaluating, and terminating—for the purpose of facilitating optimum client functioning. Nurses in all settings use this process in order to practice in an orderly, logical manner. It enables the nurse to individualize care for each client.

The principles of individualization, active participation, self-determination, and confidentiality must be applied in all phases of the nursing process. Contracting is increasingly used with clients because health care professionals experience more positive results when they encourage it. *Contracting* is a term used to denote a process that involves the establishment of mutually defined goals and intervention strategies. It is a working agreement between client and nurse, explicitly stated, in which all parties involved are working together to achieve a common goal.

Use of the family-centered nursing process is rewarding and challenging. The family-centered nursing process assists the nurse in helping clients from diverse cultural and ethnic backgrounds to mobilize personal strengths that will enhance their self-care capabilities. It provides the nurse with a framework for facilitating client decision-making about health care matters. It also enables the nurse to become truly involved with other human beings in a supportive, therapeutic way.

◀ *An Exercise in Critical Thinking* ▶

Based on the data provided below, develop an initial care plan for the Athen family, using the following format:

Assess-ment data	Nursing diagnoses	Expected outcomes/ goals	Nursing interven-tions/ actions	Evalua-tion criteria

The Athen Family

You are the public health nurse from the Pottsville County Health Department and are visiting Mr. and Mrs. Athen, an elderly couple (89 and 85 respectively) who were referred by their family physician for monitoring of Mr. Athen's leg ulcers. Mr. Athen wears glasses and a hearing aid but is in good health considering his age. He has leg ulcers on both ankles, which he dresses himself, but is concerned because they are not healing well. Mr. Athen is the primary caregiver for his wife and caretaker of the household. Mrs. Athen has left-sided hemiplegia from a CVA 8 years ago. She uses a wheelchair for mobility and a guard rail for walking and range of motion exercises. The family lives in a well-kept ranch-style home, which is wheelchair accessible. Their daughter and her husband live 30 miles away and are available for emergency help and specific projects. However, they do not visit often due to caregiver responsibilities for their 40-year-old son, who is severely disabled from cerebral palsy. The Athens are devoted to each other and will do everything they can to stay out of a nursing home. They are concerned about what will happen to their grandson should his parents die or become unable to care for him.

APPENDIX 9-1

King County Health Department, Seattle, Washington, Nursing Assessment Guide: Antepartum

Patient's name _____

EDC _____ GRAV _____ PARA _____ ABORT _____ DATE MED. CARE STARTED _____

M.D. _____ HOSP. _____ SIGNIFICANT MEDICAL HISTORY OF PREGNANCIES _____

Mother's opinion of previous pregnancy, delivery, and newborn (NB) _____

Current pregnancy	Yes	No	First assessment, comments Trimester 1 2 3 Date _____	Yes	No	Second assessment, comments Trimester 1 2 3 Date _____
Medical Supervision						
Medical appointments made						
Plans to keep						
Dental appointments made						
Plans to keep						
M&I dental care completed						

Pt understanding of doctor's orders is:

_____

Signs and Symptoms

Nausea						
Vomiting						
Heartburn						
Spotting						
Bleeding						
Edema						
Leg cramps						
Varicosities						
Backache						
Dyspnea						
Constipation						
Hemorrhoids						
Dysuria						
Frequency						

Continued

APPENDIX 9-1

APPENDIX 9-1
King County Health Department, Seattle, Washington, Nursing Assessment Guide: Antepartum—cont'd

Nursing assessment—Antepartum—Part 2

Current pregnancy	Yes	No	First assessment, comments Trimester 1 2 3 Date _____	Yes	No	Second assessment, comments Trimester 1 2 3 Date _____
Fetal Movements						
Braxton Hicks						
Other						
Personal Management Weight gain						
Normal						

Diet—type _____
   Breakfast
   Lunch
   Dinner
   Snacks
   Dislikes
   Fluid intake pattern
   Comments						

Sleep—No. of hours						
Naps						
Physical activity						
Very active						
Moderately active						
Limited activity						
Clothing						
Supportive						

King County Health Department, Seattle, Washington, Nursing Assessment Guide: Antepartum—cont'd

Nursing assessment—Antepartum—Page 3   Patient's name _____
Current pregnancy
Emotional (complete with patient's feelings towards)

	First assessment, comments	Second assessment, comments
	Trimester 1 2 3 Date _____	Trimester 1 2 3 Date _____
Pregnancy		
Motherhood		
Changes in self-image		
Mood swings		
Pregnancy and parenthood affecting personal family goals		
Husband-wife social and sexual relationships		
Stresses created by emotional and physical changes of this pregnancy		
Anxiety re: labor and delivery		
Social and financial family stability re: future plans for NB		
Past and present personality difficulties		
Fetus		
Father's awareness of, interest and attitude		

Continued

King County Health Department, Seattle, Washington, Nursing Assessment Guide: Antepartum—cont'd

Nursing assessment—Antepartum—Page 4   Patient's name _____

	Yes	No	Trimester 1 2 3 Date _____	Yes	No	Trimester 1 2 3 Date _____
Plans for Delivery						
Made plans for hospitalization						
Make arrangements for care of family at home						
Knows what to expect of hospital routine						
Knows signs of labor						
Knows what to expect during labor and delivery						
Knows what to expect PP						
Plans for Newborn						
Plans to breast feed						
Plans to bottle feed						
Adequate layette and equipment						
Plans to have help PP						
Knows what to expect of NB						
Family Planning						
Knows methods of birth control						
Wants information on family planning						

What kind of help does family want from CHN?   What kind of help does family want from CHN?

_____   _____

_____   _____

_____   _____

Printed with permission from the Nursing Division, King County Health Department, 1000 Public Safety Building, Seattle, Washington.

APPENDIX 9-2

King County Health Department, Seattle, Washington, Nursing Assessment Guide: Postpartum

Patient's name _____

GRAV _____ PARA _____ M.D. _____

HOSPITAL _____ SIGNIFICANT MEDICAL HISTORY OF PREGNANCIES _____

Check items which best describe patient or complete with notation.

Postpartum exam	First assessment date _____				Second assessment date _____	
	Yes	No			Yes	No
Temp _____						

Breasts

Physical appearance:

Normal						
Engorgement						
Soreness						
Soft						
Cracked						
Redness						
Caked						
Inverted						
Lactation: Leaking						
Filling						
Nursing						
Not nursing						
"Dry up" pills						

Abdomen

Fundus (firmness, position)						
C-section (incision)						

Rectovaginal

Laceration						
Episiotomy: None						
Clean						
Healing						
Painful						
Hemorrhoids						
Other						

Continued

APPENDIX 9-2

King County Health Department, Seattle, Wash., Nursing Assessment Guide: Postpartum—cont'd

Check items which best describe patient or complete with notation.

Postpartum exam	First assessment date _____ Yes	No	Second assessment date _____ Yes	No
Lochia				
Rubra				
Serosa				
Alba				
Clots				
No. pads per day				
Voiding				
No difficulty				
Anuria				
Dysuria				
Frequency				
Burning				
Bowels				
Constipated				
No difficulty				
Other				

First assessment date _____   Second assessment date _____

Personal Health Practices (Describe what the patient is doing about the following.)

A. Care

   Bathing _____

   Peri-care _____

   Breast care _____

B. Rest _____

   Sleep _____

   Recreation _____

   Exercise and activity _____

C. Foundation garment _____

D. Diet—Type _____

   Breakfast _____

   Lunch _____

   Dinner _____

APPENDIX 9-2
King County Health Department, Seattle, Wash., Nursing Assessment Guide: Postpartum—cont'd

Snacks _____

Dislikes _____

Fluid intake _____

   Comments _____

_____

E. Sexual relations _____

Psychosocial (Describe mother's feeling or reaction to the following.)

Pregnancy _____

_____

Labor _____

_____

Delivery _____

_____

Newborn _____

_____

Motherhood _____

_____

Family's reaction to labor, delivery, NB _____

_____

Other _____

_____

Medical Supervision	Yes	No		Yes	No
Medical appointments made					
Plan to keep					
Dental care up to date					

Patient's understanding of
doctor's orders is _____

Family Planning

Future family plans (method, problems) _____

What kind of help does family want from CHN? _____

_____

_____

_____

_____

Printed with permission from the Nursing Division, King County Health Department, 1000 Public Safety Building, Seattle, Washington.

References

American Nurses Association: *Standards of community health nursing practice,* Kansas City, Mo, 1986, The Association.

Barkauskas VH, Stoltenberg-Allen C, Baumann LC, and Darling-Fisher C: *Health and physical assessment,* St. Louis, 1994, Mosby.

Beall L: The corrupt contract: problems in conjoint therapy with parents and children, *Am J Orthopsychiatry* 42(1):77-81, 1972.

Beavers WR: *Psychotherapy and growth: a family systems perspective,* New York, 1977, Brunner/Mazel.

Beitler B, Tkachuck B, and Aamodt D: The Newman model applied to mental health, community health, and medical-surgical nursing. In Riehl JP and Roy C, eds: *Conceptual models for nursing practice,* ed 2, New York, 1980, Appleton-Century-Crofts.

Benedict MB and Sproles JB: Application of the Neuman model to public health nursing practice. In Neuman B, ed: *The Neuman systems model: application to nursing education and practice,* New York, 1982, Appleton-Century-Crofts, pp. 223-240.

Bigbee J: The changing role of rural women: nursing and health implications, *Health Care Women Int* 5:307-322, 1984.

Blazek B and McCaellen M: The effects of self-care instruction on locus of control in children, *J School Health* 53:554-556, 1983.

Bliss-Holtz UJ: Primiparas' prenatal concern for learning infant care, *Nurs Res* 37:20-24, 1988.

Boehm F: Patient contracting. In Fitzpatrick JJ, Taunton RL, and Benoliel JQ, eds: *Annual review of nursing research,* vol 7, New York, 1989, Springer, pp. 143-153.

Bowers AC and Thompson JN: *Clinical manual of health assessment, ed 4,* St. Louis, 1992, Mosby.

Boyd C: Toward an understanding of mother-daughter identification using concept analysis, *Adv Nurs Sci* 7(3):78-86, 1985.

Buchanan BF: Human-environment interaction: a modification of Neuman Systems Model for aggregates, families, and the community, *Public Health Nurs* 4:52-64, 1987.

Bulechek GM and McCloskey JC: Defining and validating nursing interventions, *Nurs Clinics of North America* 27:289-299, 1992.

Campbell JC: Nursing assessment for risk of homicide with battered women, *Adv Nurs Sci* 8(4):36-51, 1986.

Carpenito LJ: *Nursing diagnosis: application to clinical practice,* Philadelphia, 1989, Lippincott.

Chang BL, Uman GC, Linn LS, Ware JE, and Kane RL: Adherence to health care regimens among elderly women, *Nurs Res* 34(1):27-31, 1985.

Chin S: Can self-care theory be applied to families? In Riehl-Sisca, ed: *The science and art of self-care,* Norwalk, Conn., 1985, Appleton-Century-Crofts, pp. 56-62.

Clements IW and Roberts FB, eds: *Family health: a theoretical approach to nursing care,* New York, 1983, Wiley.

Craft MJ and Willadsen JA: Interventions related to family, *Nurs Clinics of North America* 27:517-540, 1992.

Curran D: *Traits of a healthy family,* Minneapolis, Minn., 1983, Winston Press.

Dunn H: *High level wellness,* Washington, D.C., 1961, Mount Vernon Publishing.

Eliason MS: Ethics and transcultural nursing care, *Nurs Outlook* 41(5):225-228, 1993.

Fawcett J: The relationship between identification and patterns of change in spouses' body images during and after pregnancy, *Int J Nurs Stud* 14:199-213, 1977.

Fawcett J: A framework for analysis and evaluation of conceptual models of nursing, *Nurse Educator* 5(6):10-14, 1980.

Fawcett J: Needs of Cesarean birthparents, *J Obstet Gynecol Neonatal Nurs* 10:371-376, 1981.

Fawcett J: *Analysis and evaluation of conceptual models of nursing,* Philadelphia, 1984, Davis.

Fawcett J: The metaparadigm of nursing: present status and future refinements, *Image: J Nurs Scholarship* 16(3):84-87, 1984.

Fawcett J and Carino C: Hallmarks of success in nursing practice, *Adv Nurs Sci* 11(4):1-8, 1989.

Flaskerudt JH and Halloran EJ: Areas of agreement in nursing theory development, *Adv Nurs Sci* 3:31-42, 1980.

Fox J: *Primary health care of the young,* New York, 1981, McGraw-Hill.

Freeman R and Lowe M, directors, Richmond-Hopkins Cooperative Nursing Study: *The family coping index,* Richmond, Va, 1964, Richmond Instructive Visiting Nurse Association and City Health Department and the Johns Hopkins School of Public Health.

Friedemann ML: Closing the gap between grand theory and mental health practice with families. Part 1: the framework of systemic organization for nursing of families and family members, *Archives of Psychiatric Nursing* 3:10-19, 1989a.

Friedemann ML: Closing the gap between grand theory and mental health practice with families. Part 2: the control-congruence model for mental health nursing of families, *Archives of Psychiatric Nursing* 3:20-28, 1989b.

Galli M: Promoting self-care in hypertensive clients through patient education, *Home Healthcare Nurse* March-April:43-45, 1984.

GAO: *Home visiting: a promising early intervention strategy for at-risk families,* GAO/HRD-90-83, Washington, D.C., 1990, General Accounting Office (GAO).

Giger JN and Davidhizar RE: *Transcultural nursing: assessment and intervention,* St. Louis, 1991, Mosby.

Gonot PW: Family therapy as derived from King's conceptual model. In Whall AL, ed: *Family therapy theory for nursing: four approaches,* Norwalk, Conn., 1986, Appleton-Century-Crofts, pp. 33-48.

Gordon M: *Nursing diagnosis: process and application, ed 3,* St. Louis, 1994, Mosby.

Gordon M: *Manual of nursing diagnosis, 1988-1989,* St. Louis, 1989, Mosby.

Gordon M: *Manual of nursing diagnosis, 1993-1994,* St. Louis, 1993, Mosby.

Guzzetta CE, Bunton SD, Prinkey LA, Sherer AP, and Seifert PC: *Assessment tools for clinical practice: designed for use with nursing diagnosis,* St. Louis, 1989, Mosby.

Hanchett ES: *Community health assessment: a conceptual tool kit,* New York, 1979, Wiley.

Hanchett ES: *Nursing frameworks and community as client: bridging the gap,* Norwalk, Conn., 1988, Appleton-Lange.

Hanson J: The family. In Roy C, ed: *Introduction to nursing: an adaptation model,* ed 2, Englewood Cliffs, N.J., 1984, Prentice-Hall, pp. 519-533.

Harper DC: Application of Orem's theoretical constructs to self-care medication behaviors in the elderly, *Adv Nurs Sci* 6(3):29-46, 1984.

Health Care Financing Administration (HCFA): *Conditions of participation: home health agencies,* 42CFR Part 484, Sections 484.10 through 484.52, Washington, D.C., October 1989, U.S. Department of Health and Human Services.

Health Care Financing Administration (HCFA): Medicare Program: home health agencies—conditions of participation, *Federal Register* 56:32967-32975, July 18, 1991.

Hoch CC: Assessing delivery of nursing care, *J Gerontal Nurs* 13:10-17, 1987.

Johnston RL: Approaching family intervention through Rogers' conceptual model. In Whall AL, ed: *Family therapy theory for nursing: four approaches,* Norwalk, Conn., 1986, Appleton-Century-Crofts, pp. 11-32.

Kearney BY and Fleisher BJ: Development of an instrument to measure exercise of self-care agency, *Res Nurs Health* 2:25-34, 1979.

Kehoe CF: Identifying the nursing needs of the postpartum Cesarean mother. In Kehoe CF, ed: *The Cesarean experience: theoretical and clinical perspectives for nurses,* New York, 1981, Appleton-Century-Crofts.

Kelly HS: The sense of an ending, *Am J Nurs* 69:2378-2381, 1969.

Kim MJ and Moritz DA: *Classification of nursing diagnoses: proceedings of the third and fourth national conferences,* New York, 1982, McGraw-Hill.

Kruger S, Shawver M, and Jones L: Reactions of families to the child with cystic fibrosis, *Image: J Nurs Scholarship* 12:67-72, 1980.

Laffrey SC: Health behavior choice as related to self-actualization and health conception, *West J Nurs Res* 7:279-295, 1985.

Levine NH: A conceptual model for obstetric nursing, *J Obstet Gynecol Neonatal Nurs* 5(2):9-15, 1976.

Lewis J, Beavers R, Gossett JT, and Phillips UA: *No single thread: psychological health in family systems,* New York, 1976, Brunner/Mazel.

Limandri BJ: Research and practice with abused women: use of the Roy adaptation model as an explanatory framework, *Adv Nurs Sci* 8(4):52-61, 1986.

Mahoney EA, Verdisco L, and Shortridge L: *How to collect and record a health history, ed 2,* Philadelphia, 1982, Lippincott.

Maluccio AN and Marlow W: The case for the contract, *Social Work* 19:28-36, 1974.

Maunz ER and Woods NF: Self-care practices among young adult women: influences of symptoms, employment and sex-role orientation, *Health Care Women Int* 9:29-41, 1988.

McCain F: Nursing by assessment—not intuition, *Am J Nurs* 65:82-84, 1965.

McPhetridge LM: Nursing history: one means to personalize care, *Am J Nurs* 68:68-75, 1968.

Michael MM and Sewall KS: Use of the adolescent peer group to increase the self-care agency of adolescent alcohol abusers, *Nurs Clin North Am* 15(1):157-176, 1980.

National Association for Home Care (NAHC): *Code of ethics,* Washington, D.C., 1982, The Association.

National Commission to Prevent Infant Mortality: *Home visiting: opening doors for America's pregnant women and children,* Washington, D.C., 1989, The Association.

Neuman B: The Betty Neuman model: a total person approach to viewing patient problems, *Nurs Res* 21(3):264-269, 1972.

Neuman B: The Betty Neuman health-care systems model: a total person approach to patient problems. In Riehl J and Roy C, eds: *Conceptual models for nursing practice,* ed 2, New York, 1980, Appleton-Century-Crofts.

Neuman B, ed: *The Neuman systems model,* New York, 1982, Appleton-Century-Crofts.

Neuman B: *The Neuman systems model, application to education and practice,* ed 2, Norwalk, Conn., 1989, Appleton-Lange.

Nunn D and Marriner-Tomey A: Applying Orem's model in nursing administration. In Henry B, Arndt O, Di Vincenti M, and Marriner-Tomey A, eds: *Dimensions of nursing administration: theory, research, education, practice,* Boston, 1989, Blackwell Scientific, pp. 63-67.

Orem DE: *Nursing: concepts of practice,* New York, 1971, McGraw-Hill.

Orem DE: *Nursing: concepts of practice,* ed 2, New York, 1980, McGraw-Hill.

Orem DE: *Nursing: concepts of practice,* ed 3, New York, 1985, McGraw-Hill.

Orem DE: *Nursing: concepts of practice,* ed 4, St. Louis, 1991, Mosby.

Orem DE and Taylor SG: Orem's general theory of nursing. In Winstead-Fry P, ed: *Case studies in nursing,* New York, 1986, National League for Nursing, pp. 37-71.

Otto H: Criteria for assessing family strength, *Family Process* 2:329-338, 1963.

Pinkerton A: Use of the Neuman model in a home health-care agency. In Riehl JP and Roy C, eds: *Conceptual models for nursing practice,* New York, 1974, Appleton-Century-Crofts.

Pratt L: *Family structure and effective health behavior: the energized family,* Boston, 1976, Houghton Mifflin.

Price S and Wilson L: *Pathophysiology,* ed 4, St. Louis, 1992, Mosby.

Pridham KF: Instruction of a school-age child with chronic illness for increased responsibility in self-care, using diabetes mellitus as an example, *Int J Nurs Stud* 8:237-246, 1971.

Randall-David E: *Strategies for working with culturally diverse communities and clients,* Bethesda, Md., 1989, The Association for the Care of Children's Health.

Rawnsley MM: *Perceptions of the speed of time in aging and in dying: an empirical investigation of the holistic theory of nursing proposed by Martha Rogers,* doctoral dissertation, Boston, 1977, Boston University.

Riehl-Sisca J, ed: *The science and art of self-care,* Norwalk, Conn., 1985, Appleton-Century-Crofts.

Rogers ME: *An introduction to the theoretical basis of nursing,* Philadelphia, 1970, FA Davis.

Rogers ME: Nursing: a science of unitary man. In Riehl JP and Roy C, eds: *Conceptual models for nursing practice,* ed 2, New York, 1980, Appleton-Century-Crofts, pp. 329-337.

Rogers ME: Science of unitary human beings: a paradigm for nursing. In Clements IW and Roberts FB, eds: *Family health: a theoretical approach to nursing care,* New York, 1983, Wiley, pp. 219-228.

Rogers ME: Science of unitary human beings. In Malinski UM, ed: *Explorations on Martha Rogers' science of unitary human beings,* Norwalk, Conn., 1986, Appleton-Century-Crofts, pp. 3-8.

Rogers ME: Rogers' science of unitary human beings. In Parse RR, ed: *Nursing science: major metaparadigms, theories, and critique,* Philadelphia, 1989, Saunders, pp. 139-146.

Rogers ME: Nursing: science of unitary, irreducible, human beings: update, 1990. In Barrett EAM: *Visions of Rogers' science-based nursing,* New York, 1990, National League for Nursing, pp. 5-11.

Roy C: Adaptation: a conceptual framework for nursing, *Nurs Outlook* 18(3):42-45, 1970.

Roy C: *Introduction to nursing: an adaptation model,* Englewood Cliffs, N.J., 1976, Prentice-Hall.

Roy C: Family in primary care: analysis and application of the Roy adaptation model. In Clements IW and Roberts FB, eds: *Family health: a theoretical approach to nursing care,* New York, 1983, Wiley, pp. 375-378.

Roy C: *Introduction to nursing: an adaptation model,* ed 2, Englewood Cliffs, N.J., 1984, Prentice-Hall.

Roy C: Roy adaptation model. In Parse RR, ed: *Nursing science. Major metaparadigms, theories and critique,* Philadelphia, 1987, Saunders, pp. 35-44.

Roy C: An explication of the philosophical assumptions of the Roy adaptation model, *Nurs Sci Quart* 1(1):26-34, 1988.

Roy C and Roberts SL: *Theory construction in nursing: an adaptation model,* Englewood Cliffs, N.J., 1981, Prentice Hall.

Schmitz M: The Roy adaptation model: application in a community setting. In Riehl JP and Roy C, eds: *Conceptual models for nursing practice,* ed 2, New York, 1980, Appleton-Century-Crofts.

Seabury BA: The contract: uses, abuses and limitations, *Social Work* 21(8):39-45, 1976.

Sene B: Termination in the student-patient relationship, *Perspect Psychiat Care* 8:39-45, 1969.

Sibley BJ: Cultural influences on health and illness. In Long BC, Phipps WJ, and Cassmeyer VL: *Medical-surgical nursing,* ed 3, St. Louis, 1992, Mosby, p. 32.

Simmons DA: *A classification scheme for client problems in community health nursing,* DHHS Pub No HRA 80-16, Hyattsville, Md., 1980, USDHHS.

Simmons DA, Martin KS, Crews CC, and Scheet NJ: *Client management information system for community health nursing agencies,* NTIS Accession No HRP-0907023, Springfield, Va., 1986, National Technical Information Service.

Simons RC: *Understanding human behavior in health and illness,* ed 3, Baltimore, 1985, Williams and Wilkins.

Story EL and Ross MM: Family centered community health nursing and the Betty Neuman systems model, *Nurs Papers* 18(2):77-88, 1986.

Tripp-Reimer T, Brink PJ, and Saunders JN: Cultural assessment: content and process, *Nurs Outlook* 32:78-82, 1984.

Wagner P: Testing the adaptation model in practice, *Nurs Outlook* 24:682-685, 1976.

Walborn KA: A nursing model for the hospice: hospice primary and self care nursing, *Nurs Clin North Am* 15(1):205-217, 1980.

Weber G: Making nursing diagnosis work for you and your client, *Nursing and Health Care* 12:424-430, 1991.

West M: *Patterns of health in mothers of developmentally disabled children,* unpublished master's thesis, University Park, 1984, Pennsylvania State University.

Whall AL: Nursing theory and the assessment of families, *J Psychiatr Nurs Mental Health Serv* 19(1):30-36, 1981.

Whall AL, ed: *Family therapy theory for nursing: four approaches,* Norwalk, Conn., 1986, Appleton-Century-Crofts.

Whall AL: Family system theory: relationship to nursing conceptual models. In Whall AL and Fawcett J: *Family theory development in nursing: state of the science and art,* Philadelphia, 1991, F.A. Davis, pp. 317-342.

Whall AL and Fawcett J: *Family theory development in nursing: state of the science and art,* Philadelphia, 1991, F.A. Davis.

Wood R and Kekahbah J, eds: *Examining the cultural implications of Martha E. Rogers; science of unitary human beings,* Lecompton, Ks., 1985, Wood-Kekahbah Associates.

World Health Organization: Constitution of the World Health Organization, *WHO Chron* 1:29-43, 1947.

Selected Bibliography

Aukamp U and Shaw R: *Nursing care plans for adult health clients: nursing diagnosis and interventions,* Norwalk, Conn., 1990, Appleton-Lange.

Berg CL and Helgeson DM: That first home visit, *Community Health Nurs* 1:207-216, 1984.

Brink P: Value orientations as an assessment tool in cultural diversity, *Nurs Research* 33:198-203, 1983.

Carey R: How values affect the mutual goal setting process, *Community Health Nurs* 6:7-14, 1989.

Dossey BM, Keegan L, Guzzetta CE, and Kolkmeier LG: *Holistic nursing: a handbook for practice,* Rockville, Md., 1988, Aspen.

Fitzpatrick JJ and Whall AL, eds: *Conceptual models of nursing: analysis and application,* ed 2, Norwalk, Conn., 1989, Appleton-Lange.

Gulino C and LaMonica G: Public health nursing: a study of role implementation, *Public Health Nurs* 3:80-91, 1986.

Helgeson DM and Berg CL: Contracting: a method of health promotion, *J Community Health Nurs* 2:199-207, 1985.

Henderson V: The nursing process . . . is the title right? *J Adv Nurs* 7:103-109, 1982.

Houldin AD, Saltstein SW, and Ganley KM: *Nursing diagnoses for wellness: supporting strengths,* Philadelphia, 1987, Lippincott.

Lapp CA, Diemert CA, and Enestvedt R: Family-based practice: discussion of a tool merging assessment with intervention, *Fam Community Health* 12:21-28, 1990.

Martin ME and Henry M: Cultural relativity and poverty, *Public Health Nurs* 6:28-34, 1989.

McCloskey J and Bulechek GM: *Nursing interventions classification (NIC),* St. Louis, 1992, Mosby.

Muecke MA: Community health diagnosis in nursing, *Public Health Nurs* 1:23-35, 1984.

Nettle C, Jones W, and Pifer P: Community nursing diagnosis, *J Community Health Nurs* 6:135-145, 1989.

Porter EJ: Critical analysis of NANDA nursing diagnosis taxonomy I, *Image: J Nurs Scholarship* 13:136-139, 1986.

Putzier DJ & Padrick KP: Nursing diagnosis: a component of nursing process and decision making, *Topics in Clinical Nursing* 5:21-29, 1984.

Rakel BA: Interventions related to patient teaching, *Nurs Clinics of North America* 27:397-423, 1992.

Simons MR: Interventions related to compliance, *Nurs Clinics of North America* 27:477-494, 1992.

Tadych R: Nursing in multiperson units: the family. In Riehl-Sisca, ed: *The science and art of self-care,* Norwalk, Conn., 1985, Appleton-Century-Crofts, pp. 49-55.

Werley H and Lang N: *Identification of the nursing minimum data set,* New York, 1988, Springer.

Wright LM and Leahey M: *Nurses and families: a guide to family assessment and intervention,* Philadelphia, 1994, F.A. Davis.

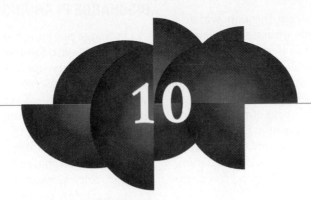

Continuity of Care through Discharge Planning and the Referral Process

OBJECTIVES

Upon completion of this chapter, the reader should be able to:

1. Discuss the concept of continuity of care.
2. Define discharge planning and discuss the characteristics of this concept.
3. Understand the role that legislation has played in the discharge planning process.
4. Discuss the nurse's role in discharge planning and the referral process.

5. Summarize the basic principles that should be considered when making a referral.
6. Analyze the steps of the referral process.
7. Distinguish between the levels of nursing intervention in the referral process.
8. Discuss barriers to the use of the referral process.

Continuity of care is a process through which a client's *ongoing* health care needs are assessed, planned for, coordinated, and met. It provides for appropriate, uninterrupted care along the health continuum (ANA, 1986a, p. 14) and facilitates the client's transition to different settings and levels of health care. The process demands thorough assessment of client needs, multidisciplinary planning and intervention, care management, client and family participation, anticipatory guidance, resource use, follow-up, and evaluation. Continuity of care is important in helping to ensure quality health care.

Traditionally community health nurses have been instrumental in facilitating continuity of care. The significant role of the community health nurse in this process was emphasized by the American Nurses Association (ANA) in both its *Standards of Community Health Nursing Practice* (1986) and *Standards of Home Health Nursing Practice* (1986) (refer to Chapters 2 and 20). In *Standards of Home Health Nursing Practice,* ANA identified a separate standard for continuity of care that charged the nurse with providing for uninterrupted client care through the use of discharge planning, care management, and coordination of community resources (ANA, 1986a, p. 14).

On a daily basis the community health nurse is involved in continuity of care activities such as continuing teaching in the home that was begun in the hospital, referring clients to necessary health care resources in the community, coordinating efforts between community health agencies, assisting clients in planning for ongoing health care needs, and working as a home care coordinator. The nurse often assumes a client advocate role when clients need continuing health and welfare services.

When continuity of care is not planned for, the results can be disastrous to the client and costly to the health care system. An example of such a situation is given in Appendix 10-1, illustrating how an ineffectively planned hospital discharge for a ventilator-dependent child resulted in family stress, hospital readmission, and additional health care costs.

Every client should have the opportunity to reach his or her optimum potential for health and recovery; planning for continuity of care helps to ensure that this occurs. Integral components of continuity of care are *discharge planning,* the *referral process,* and *care management.* The concept of care management is discussed in Chapters 19 and 20.

DISCHARGE PLANNING

Discharge planning has evolved from focusing on a single event—the referral of a client to a community service or facility upon discharge from an acute care setting—to a process that has been expanded to numerous health care settings and whose long-term goal is to ensure continuity of health care (Rorden and Taft, 1990, p. 22). In this text discharge planning is examined from this broader perspective and encompasses client discharge from a variety of health care settings and services including hospitals, mental health facilities, nursing homes, outpatient settings, group health education experiences, home care, and community health nursing service.

Discharge planning facilitates the transition of the client to different settings and levels of care. It also facilitates continuity of care by consolidating the gains made at one level or setting while arranging for the resources necessary to meet the needs of another level or setting. It helps to ensure that health care needs do not go unmet, that health care is coordinated and uninterrupted, and that clients progress along the health continuum. As the process of discharge planning has evolved it has had many definitions. Some definitions in the literature are given in the left box on p. 343.

History of Discharge Planning

Discharge planning efforts are not new. There is evidence of discharge planning in the late 1800s and early 1900s (Shamansky, Boase, and Horn, 1984, p. 15; O'Hare and Terry, 1988, p. 6). Lillian Wald was one of the first to recognize the need for such planning, and nurses have historically been involved in discharge planning efforts. In 1906 Bellevue Hospital in New York City referred to a nurse whose entire time and care was given to befriending those about to be discharged (O'Hare and Terry, p. 6).

The 1960s saw the first official use of the term *discharge planning* (Shamansky, Boase, and Horn, 1984, p. 16). Discharge planning became a part of many hospital programs, and Edith Wensley's (1963) *Nursing Service Without Walls* urged hospitals to emphasize planning for home care services and referral to community services upon discharge. The National League for Nursing urged hospitals, nursing homes, and home nursing care agencies to have a designated staff person to develop plans for the next stage of nursing care, to implement continuity of care activities, and to develop well-defined, clearly written procedures for client

◀ *Some Definitions of* ▶
Discharge Planning

Discharge planning is the vehicle that moves the patient to the proper level of care and/or facility (Bristow, Stickney and Thompson, 1976, p. 5).

Discharge planning is the process of activities that involve the patient and a team of individuals from various disciplines working together to facilitate the transition of that patient from one environment to another (McKeehan, 1981, p. 3).

Centralized, coordinated programs developed by a hospital to ensure that each patient has a planned program for needed continuing or follow-up care (Hartigan and Brown, 1985, p. 101).

Discharge planning is a process made up of several steps or phases whose immediate goal is to anticipate changes in patient care needs and whose long-term goal is to insure continuity of health care (Rorden and Taft, 1990, p. 22).

◀ *Characteristics of* ▶
Discharge Planning

Discharge planning follows the steps of the nursing process.

Discharge planning incorporates the client and family.

Discharge planning is multidisciplinary and involves care management.

Discharge planning involves use of community resources.

Discharge planning takes into consideration the setting in which the client is being placed.

referral (O'Hare and Terry, 1988, p. 7). The passage of Medicaid and Medicare legislation in 1965 placed new emphasis on discharge planning efforts.

In the 1970s discharge planning became inextricably linked with quality assurance. This occurred largely as a result of Medicaid and Medicare legislation in 1972 (Public Law 92-603), which mandated that skilled nursing facilities and hospitals receiving these monies maintain centralized, coordinated programs to ensure that each patient had a planned program of continuing care which met postdischarge needs.

In the 1980s federal legislation again shaped the course of discharge planning. A prospective payment system (PPS), aimed at reducing the length of stay in acute care facilities, was enacted for Medicare in 1982. This legislation was instrumental in the development of discharge planning activities across the nation because it gave hospitals a financial incentive to discharge patients as early as possible. Thus, discharge planning became a method of cost containment (Willihnganz, 1984).

During the 1980s discharge planning became a hospital priority. The American Hospital Association (AHA) developed guidelines for discharge planning that included early identification of patients likely to need posthospital care; patient and family education, assessment, and counseling; discharge plan development, coordination, and implementation; and postdischarge follow-up (AHA, 1984; Corkery, 1989, p. 19).

The Medicare provisions of the Omnibus Budget Reconciliation Act of 1986 also strengthened the need for discharge planning. This act influenced discharge planning by mandating the development of a standardized, uniform needs assessment instrument to evaluate the posthospital needs of Medicare patients (Burlenski, 1989, p. 2; McBroom, 1989, p. 1). This legislation required that hospitals receiving Medicare reimbursement notify patients of their right to discharge planning services (Blaylock and Cason, 1992, p. 5; Corkery, 1989, p. 19). There is no doubt that discharge planning efforts will expand in the future and that nurses will continue to play important roles in the discharge planning process. A major thrust in today's health care system is managed care, which helps to control cost and to facilitate client access to care.

Characteristics of Discharge Planning

Discharge planning has a number of characteristics that are significant for the community health nurse. These characteristics are summarized in the box above and are discussed here.

Discharge planning follows the steps of the nursing process. Discharge planning involves assessment, diagnosis, planning, implementation, and evaluation. These steps are familiar and can be readily conceptualized in relation to discharge planning. The success of discharge planning activities is largely dependent on how accurately discharge needs are assessed and

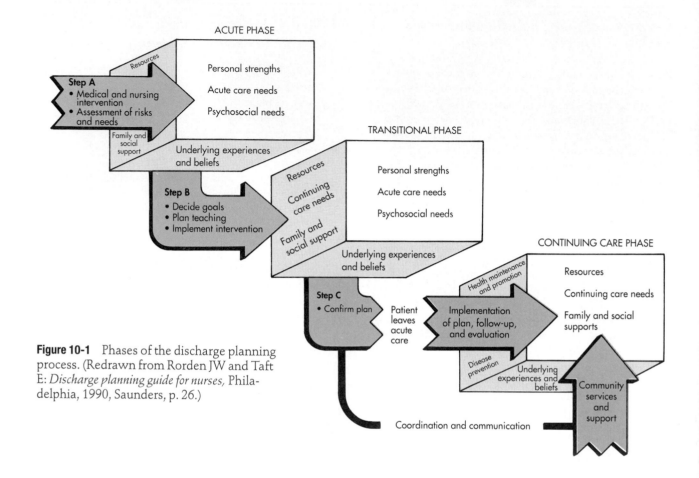

Figure 10-1 Phases of the discharge planning process. (Redrawn from Rorden JW and Taft E: *Discharge planning guide for nurses,* Philadelphia, 1990, Saunders, p. 26.)

diagnosed (Arenth and Mamon, 1985, p. 20). Rorden and Taft (1990, pp. 24-27) have described this process as occurring in three phases: *acute, transitional,* and *continuing care.* According to Rorden and Taft, in the acute phase medical attention dominates discharge planning efforts, whereas in the transitional phase the need for acute care is still present but its urgency is reduced and clients can begin to address and plan for future health care needs. In the continuing care phase the client is able to plan and implement continuing care activities. It is never too early to start discharge planning efforts (Weinberger, 1989, p. 75). A schema for these phases is given in Figure 10-1.

Discharge planning incorporates the client and family. Discharge planning involves the client, family, and caregivers in a collaborative effort to meet discharge planning needs. The client and family should be incorporated from the beginning of discharge planning efforts. The success of discharge planning

activities is largely dependent on the extent to which the client and his and her family participate in the planning process (Arenth and Mamom, 1985, p. 20).

Discharge planning is multidisciplinary and involves care management. The holistic approach necessitated in discharge planning requires multidisciplinary planning efforts and is most effective when a multidisciplinary approach is used (Corkery, 1989, p. 19; DeRienzo, 1985, p. 34; Packard-Helie and Lancaster, 1989, p. 32; Esper, 1988, p. 66. Since numerous health care professionals are involved in delivering services to clients, common goals accepted by all involved parties are established to prevent duplication and fragmentation of services, facilitate development and implementation of intervention strategies, and effectively manage care. Many health care facilities, especially hospitals, have instituted multidisciplinary discharge planning teams that are frequently lead by nurses and social workers (Feather, 1989, p. 3). However, other health care professionals must be involved in discharge planning efforts. A listing of some professionals that frequently work together in discharge planning efforts are given in the box at right.

Discharge planning involves use of community resources. Discharge planning focuses on matching client and family needs with community resources (Arenth and Mamon, 1985, p. 20). It is important to know which community agencies the client is already utilizing so that duplication of efforts and uncoordinated plans of care can be minimized or avoided. The process for facilitating client use of community resources is discussed later in this chapter.

Discharge planning takes into consideration the setting in which the client is being placed. The physical and the psychosocial environment of the setting need to be carefully assessed. Different settings necessitate different interventions; the case of 70-year-old Mrs. Flowers is an example.

> ▶ **Mrs. Flowers' cooking, cleaning, laundry, medical, and personal needs were taken care of while she was in the hospital. Now she is ready to return home, where she is responsible for these activities of daily living but unable to handle all of them by herself. Options to assist her, such as homemaker services, transportation, friendly visitors, Meals-on-Wheels, the local Visiting Nurse Association, the help of a friend or relative, or a more supervised living situation, should be explored and set in place before Mrs. Flowers leaves the hospital setting. Mrs. Flowers' support systems, financial resources, perceptions, and goals should also be evaluated, and the length of time that she will need care should be considered. From the outset she must be involved in establishing and implementing her discharge plan of care.**

Discharge Planning Documentation

Discharge planning efforts need to be supported by systematic documentation (McKeehan, 1981, p. 10). In line with this, many agencies have developed standardized discharge planning policies and forms. Such standardized forms may include information on the client's level of functioning, health care follow-up needs and home adaptation, health education needs, support systems available, and community resources

---

Health Care Professionals Working Together to Facilitate Discharge Planning

Nurses*
Social workers*
Physicians
Health educators
Nutritionists
Physical therapists
Occupational therapists
Speech therapists
Rehabilitation therapists
Psychologists

*Nurses and social workers have historically been at the forefront of discharge planning efforts and client advocacy in discharge planning.

---

recommended or being used (Kromminga and Ostwald, 1987, p. 224).

The discharge questionnaire in Appendix 10-2 is designed to facilitate assessment of clients' needs before their departure from a formal health care setting, but it could be used in various settings. The information assists the nurse in identifying multiple client needs. It examines the psychosocial and the biological aspects of functioning and emphasizes preventive health care practices, in addition to needs for curative care. From the data obtained hospital personnel and community health nurses have baseline information essential for planning continuity of care. Nurses at all levels in the organization play an important role in the discharge planning process.

THE ROLE OF THE NURSE IN DISCHARGE PLANNING

Community health nurses can be proud of the important role they have played in discharge planning efforts. Even before recent legislation mandated these activities community health nurses recognized the need for discharge planning to facilitate continuity of care. In acting on this need community health nurses from local health departments often worked in cooperation with hospitals as *home care coordinators/liaisons* to assess patients' home care needs and to implement discharge planning activities. Today nurses are key members of multidisciplinary discharge planning teams.

The nurse coordinating discharge planning efforts must realize that not all nurses have a complete or adequate understanding of this process. A major role of the nurse involved in discharge planning is to "educate" nurses and students about their responsibilities in providing continuity of care. The nurse as a discharge planner should facilitate collaborative relationships among hospital nurses, community health nurses, and a variety of community agencies.

Nursing Assessment, Diagnosis, and Planning

As mentioned previously, the discharge planning process follows the steps of the nursing process. A thorough *nursing assessment* of client needs begins the discharge planning process and facilitates planning and intervention efforts. Some areas for the nurse to assess to determine client needs upon discharge are identified in Figure 10-2. An example of how a nurse assessed discharge planning needs is presented in Figure 10-3.

The nurse assesses the client's physical health, functional status, and numerous psychosocial variables such as the client's living situation, level of education, financial resources, social support systems, health values and attitudes, cultural and ethnic background, perceptions of the situation, barriers to care, and care preferences. The nurse also assesses resource availability, how the client has used resources in the past, and what community resources the client is presently working with.

Following assessment, client needs are diagnosed and interventions are planned to meet these needs. Discharge planning interventions such as health education, referrals to appropriate community agencies, and planning for appropriate equipment in the home environment are developed, implemented, and evaluated.

Nursing Interventions

Discharge planning interventions focus on assisting clients in achieving the maximum level of functioning. Interventions may be educative, therapeutic, or rehabilitative in nature. In planning interventions the nurse should be aware that as the client moves from one level of care to another or one setting to another

change occurs, and gains that had been made may be lost or curtailed (Reischelt and Newcomb, 1980).

Intervention strategies need to be carefully planned and implemented in order to maximize growth at each level. If this does not occur the resulting situation can become overwhelming for the client. Donnie's case (Appendix 10-1) is an example.

Donnie was a ventilator-dependent child who spent his first 3 years of life in an acute intensive care unit. Donnie's first hospital discharge was ineffectively planned and implemented, and resulted in his readmission to the hospital 2 months later. Donnie's second hospital discharge was successful because the discharge planning teams carefully assessed the services and resources needed by the family to handle Donnie's medical problems in the home. Donnie's parents were trained to handle his ventilator equipment and were helped to obtain financial assistance and supportive community services.

This example illustrates how educating and involving the family, appropriately assessing discharge needs, and coordinating community resources is crucial to successful implementation of discharge goals. Interventions that fail to address the needs of the family unit may not be implemented.

Nursing interventions will involve sharing community resource information with clients, coordinating multidisciplinary planning efforts, making discharge planning referrals, evaluating discharge planning efforts, and alleviating client and family anxiety about continuing care needs. Clients and their families may find it difficult to consider continuing care needs when they are in the acute phase, dealing with an acute care episode. Even in the transitional phase the client and family may respond negatively to the accelerated rate of hospital discharge and may resist discharge planning efforts. The nurse will need to work cooperatively with the client and family, be sensitive to where they are in their readiness to assume care responsibilities, and help them to see how discharge planning efforts will help them more readily reach their goals.

Nursing Evaluation

As with all parts of the nursing process, discharge planning efforts need to be evaluated. Evaluation is ongoing and assesses the effectiveness and outcomes of the process in addition to client satisfaction. (Kromminga and Ostwald, 1987, p. 224; Shamansky, Boase, and Horn, 1984, p. 20; Slevin and Roberts, 1987, p. 50).

Circle all that apply and total. Refer to the risk factor index.*

Age
  0 = 55 years or less
  1 = 56 to 64 years
  2 = 65 to 79 years
  3 = 80+ years

Living situation/social support
  0 = lives only with spouse
  1 = lives with family
  2 = lives alone with family support
  3 = lives alone with friends' support
  4 = lives alone with no support
  5 = nursing home/residential care

Functional status
  0 = independent in activities of daily living and
      instrumental activities of daily living
  Dependent in:
    1 = eating/feeding
    1 = bathing/grooming
    1 = toileting
    1 = transferring
    1 = incontinent of bowel function
    1 = incontinent of bladder function
    1 = meal preparation
    1 = responsible for own medication
        administration
    1 = handling own finances
    1 = grocery shopping
    1 = transportation

Cognition
  0 = oriented
  1 = disoriented to some spheres† some of the time
  2 = disoriented to some spheres all of the time
  3 = disoriented to all spheres some of the time
  4 = disoriented to all spheres all of the time
  5 = comatose

Behavior pattern
  0 = appropriate
  1 = wandering
  1 = agitated
  1 = confused
  1 = other

Mobility
  0 = ambulatory
  1 = ambulatory with mechanical
      assistance
  2 = ambulatory with human assistance
  3 = nonambulatory

Sensory deficits
  0 = none
  1 = visual or hearing deficits
  2 = visual and hearing deficits

Number of previous admissions/
emergency room visits
  0 = none in the last 3 months
  1 = one in the last 3 months
  2 = two in the last 3 months
  3 = more than two in the last 3 months

Number of active medical problems
  0 = three medical problems
  1 = three to five medical problems
  2 = more than five medical problems

Number of drugs
  0 = fewer than three drugs
  1 = three to five drugs
  2 = more than five drugs

Total score:

*Risk factor index: score of 10 = at risk for home care resources; score of 11 to 19 = at risk for extended discharge planning; score greater than 20 = at risk for placement other than home.
If the patient's score is 10 or greater, refer the patient to the discharge planning coordinator or discharge planning team.
†Spheres = person, place, time, and self.
Copyright 1991 Ann Blaylock

Figure 10-2   Blaylock Discharge Planning Risk Assessment Screen. (From Blaylock A and Cason CL: Discharge planning predicting patients' needs, *J Gerontological Nurs* 18(7):8, 1992. Used with permission.)

GOALS: Successful transition of client to home/community setting; healthy growth and development of mother and infant; successful adjustment to parenting

Psychosocial Factors	Health Status	Functional Status	Assessed Discharge Planning Needs
17-year-old unmarried primipara	Uneventful postpartum period	Independent in activities of daily living	Lack of knowledge of infant care
Resides with mother	No known medical/health problems		Lack of knowledge of community resources
No means of financial support	Breastfeeding infant		Potential lack of social/emotional support systems
Unfamiliar with community resources	No source of regular medical follow-up		Need for regular medical follow-up
No means of transportation	Infant healthy, Apgar 9		Disruption in normal growth and development processes (e.g., education and other normal developmental tasks)
11th grade education—plans to return to school			
Has never cared for an infant and requesting help with infant care			
Bonding well with infant			
No recent contact with infant's father			
Requesting home follow-up			

INCORPORATION OF CLIENT/FAMILY INTO PLANNING PROCESS

MULTIDISCIPLINARY PLANNING

POSSIBLE COMMUNITY RESOURCES/REFERRALS

Family   Friends   Work   Neighbors   School   Church

OTHER

(Local Health Department: Nurses, WIC, Clinics; LaLeche League; Young Mothers Support Group; DHHS: AFDC, Medicaid; Child and Family Services; Mom's Day Out Programs; Dial-A-Ride)

Figure 10-3 The nurse as a discharge planner: assessing discharge planning needs. (Modified from Siegel H: Nurses improve hospital efficiency through a risk assessment model at admission, *Nurs Management* 19(10):42, 1988. Used with permission.)

When evaluating, the nurse elicits information from referral agencies and from the client to determine if continuing care needs were met.

Cost-effective and time-efficient discharge planning follow-up and evaluation have been carried out by telephone. Two innovative studies of such follow-up were described by Garland (1992) and North, Meeusen, and Hollinsworth (1991). In Garland's study telephone calls were placed 7 to 10 days after discharge to obtain information such as whether the community health nurse had come as scheduled, if equipment and supplies came as arranged, if outpatient therapies started on schedule, if clients were able to obtain and take medications as prescribed, and if clients had received sufficient discharge planning preparation. In North's study telephone calls were placed 10 to 14 days after discharge, with the nursing summary, discharge assessment, and medication schedule available to aid the nurse in accurate recall and to assist with evaluation. Both studies addressed client and family satisfaction with discharge preparation and identified actual problems after discharge. The studies obtained information useful for staff efforts to improve discharge planning and showed client satisfaction with the discharge planning process.

In evaluating the discharge planning process the nurse should remember that, whatever the discharge planning needs, efforts should focus on facilitating continuity of care, family adaptation and growth, and matching the client with appropriate community resources.

The Community Health Nurse as a Home Care Coordinator

The community health nurse working as a home care coordinator is often part of a hospital or other acute care setting discharge planning team. The term *home care coordinator* naturally evolved around the early focus of discharge planning—moving the client from the hospital setting back to the community.

The nurse working as a home care coordinator is often employed by either the local health department (LHD) or the hospital. With increased emphasis on discharge planning in relation to funding and cost-effectiveness, many hospitals are employing nurses to work as discharge planners and are establishing multidisciplinary discharge planning teams.

THE REFERRAL PROCESS DEFINED

The *referral process* is a systematic problem-solving approach involving a series of actions that help clients use resources for the purpose of resolving needs. Clients may be either individuals or groups who require assistance from others in order to achieve their maximum level of functioning. In a study by Luker and Chalmers (1989) the prime purpose of referring clients to other resources was to provide the client with additional expertise or services. The community health nurse's major goals for initiating a referral are to promote high-level wellness, enhance self-care capabilities, and enhance quality of care.

Referring clients to resources is an important function of community health nurses. Completing a form or telling a client to contact a community agency is only one small aspect of this process. The referral process demands knowledge, skill, and experience to be implemented effectively. It demands knowledge

of community resources, an ability to solve problems and set priorities, and the ability to collaborate and coordinate. It is an integral part of comprehensive, continuous client care and is essential to community health nursing practice (Luker and Chalmers, 1989, p. 173).

The community health nurse will make referrals to and receive referrals from health care resources. Referrals can be categorized according to referral initiator, the extent of client contact made with the resource, the level of difficulty of the process, and the source of the referral. Working through the referral process with a client can be an enriching and rewarding experience. Table 10-1 is a chart illustrating different types of referral.

Basic Principles of Referral

Wolff's (1962) classic article on referral delineated basic principles to take into consideration when helping clients to use the referral process. Others (Combs, 1976; USDHHS, Source book, 1982; Wheeler-Lachowycz, 1983) have reinforced the value of these principles and have expanded on them. These principles are listed here:

1. *There should be merit in the referral.* The referral should meet the needs and objectives of the client and should be necessary. Before referring the client to community resources it is extremely important to assess what resources are available in the client's own environment. Often it will be found that family, friends, and neighbors can do as much as or more than formal community health resources.

2. *The referral should be practical.* The client should be able to use the referral in an efficient, effective manner. The referral should not be a waste of time, money, and effort on behalf of the client, the resource, or the referral facilitator.

3. *The referral should be individualized to the client.* A referral that meets the needs of one client may not meet the needs of another. It is essential to assess the individual needs and concerns of clients before decisions about the appropriateness of a referral are made. For example, some clients can learn very well in a group setting whereas others cannot.

4. *The referral should be timely.* It should come at a time when the client is ready to work on the

TABLE 10-1   Types of Referral by Initiator, Extent of Contact with Resource, Level of Difficulty, and Source

	Type of referral	Example
Initiator	*Primary*: Referral initiated by client, often readily	Client suggesting marriage counseling
	Secondary: Referral initiated by someone other than client	Community health nurse suggesting marriage counseling
Extent of contact with resource	*Formal*: Contact made with a resource on behalf of a client; contact can be made by the client or someone on the client's behalf; contact generally made with client's permission; these referrals are often processed through a system of standardized forms and procedures	Client contacting a local department of social service (DSS) about obtaining food stamps Community health nurse talking about services a family member can provide, which the client subsequently uses or
	Informal: Discussion of a resource between two or more persons without contact being made with the resource; often the initial step toward a formal referral	Client and community health nurse discussing available DSS services (e.g., food stamps, general assistance, Aid for Families with Dependent Children, Medicaid)
Level of difficulty	*Simple*: Referral reaches need resolution on the initial attempt	On initial attempt, client goes to DSS and obtains food stamps
	Complex: Referral does not meet need resolution on the initial attempt; process needs to be reworked (refer to Figure 10-6 for steps in process)	Client goes to DSS seeking food stamps and finds out that she or he is not eligible, but the need for assistance with food budgeting still exists. Other community resources such as the Nutritional Extension Service may be more appropriate
Source	*Interresource*: Referrals made from one resource to another	Community health nurse referring client from the local health department to a neighborhood health clinic
	Intraresource: Referrals made within the resource itself	Community health nurse referring client to local health department sanitarian for water sampling
	Self: Client refers himself to a resource for service; some agencies will not accept these referrals	Client calls local health department to arrange for community health nursing visits

health care need and when it is the appropriate time to work on the need.

5. *The referral should be coordinated with other activities.* The referral should be congruent with other health care activities that are occurring. This aids in maximizing health care interventions, preventing duplication of service, and carrying out contradictory intervention strategies.

6. *The referral should incorporate the client and family into planning and implementation.* It has already been stressed that it is critical for the client and family to be involved in health planning and intervention, and that without this involvement interventions are likely to fail.

7. *The client should have the right to say no to the referral.* This principle acknowledges the client's right to self-determination. A competent cli-

ent has the right to make decisions about health care (ANA, Standards of community health, 1986, p. 3). The client has the right to refuse a referral unless legal authority dictates otherwise. Cases of law are the exception and will vary from state to state. An example of a law that could require the community health nurse to refer a client without his or her consent is a child abuse law that mandates reporting suspected child abuse and neglect cases.

In order to protect this right of self-determination, the client must be aware of the referral. Referrals are sometimes made for clients without their consent, but this is not good referral practice. In following up on a referral the nurse may find that the client was unaware of the referral and does not want it. In such a case the nurse should explain the reason for the referral, the services the nurse can provide, and apologize for any inconvenience to the client. This type of nursing intervention may help the client to see why the referral was made, and even to accept the referral.

At times individuals are referred without their knowledge or consent because the referring agency considers them a threat to their own safety or the safety of others. The client still has the right to refuse a referral unless legal authority dictates otherwise.

The refusal of a referral may be difficult for the nurse to accept, especially if the referral appears to be helpful to the client. However, the client's right to say no must be respected.

Confidentiality and Referral

Confidentiality of client information is an important professional ethic for the nurse to honor. As with self-determination, confidentiality is violated only if laws intervene. Nurses must receive the client's permission to share personal data and the information that is shared should be carefully evaluated. Sharing of information should be in the client's best interest and for purposes of facilitating optimum care. Loosely sharing information about clients among staff members when it does not facilitate client care is not professional or ethical. Many agencies have release-of-information forms for sending and receiving data about clients. It is preferable to obtain written permis-

sion to share data. Maintaining confidentiality is a professional responsibility.

Developing a Referral System

Before referral activities take place a referral system needs to be in place. Developing a referral system involves determining the types of resources necessary to carry out health care activities, locating these resources in the community, collecting information on the resources, developing a referral list, developing a referral protocol, developing a follow-up system, training people to make referrals, and periodically updating the referral and resource information (USDHHS, 1982, Source book, p. 27). These activities are discussed throughout this chapter.

Answering a Referral

Answering referrals is an important part of the referral process and helps to maintain effective communication networks between the client, staff, and resources (Reischelt and Newcomb, 1980). If referrals are not answered or are answered incompletely or tardily, the referral source may become discouraged and not send further referrals. Prompt, complete, and courteous answering of a referral helps to establish and maintain good working relationships and facilitates follow-up and continuity of client care.

Referrals should be answered as soon as possible, ideally within a week after they have been received. The nurse should include in the communication with the referring agency comments on the needs that were recognized by the referring agency, as well as current assessment data, nursing diagnoses, and future actions and plans. If the client and nurse decide that nursing service should be continued, the referring agency should be given this information.

REFERRAL RESOURCES

Once the need for a referral has been established, the appropriate resources must be located in the community. The community health nurse needs to collect information on community resources and be familiar with them (Figure 10-4).

A *resource* is defined as an agency, group, or individual that assists a client in meeting a need. Resources provide multiple services and have varying requirements for usage. The community health nurse needs to be knowledgeable about community resources,

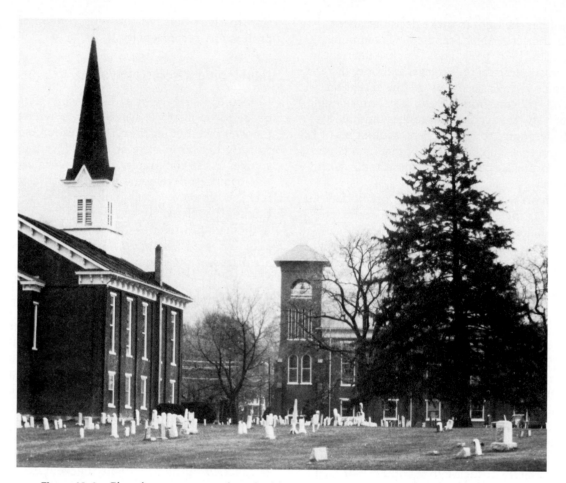

Figure 10-4   Churches are extremely valuable community resources that are often overlooked by health care professionals. Many churches provide community services including temporary food, shelter, and clothing; home visiting to ill and disabled persons; home repair services for elderly church members; and monies to assist needy families who lack essentials of daily living. Community health nurses frequently find that churches will assist them to meet specific client needs, especially when there is no other community resource that can do so. (Courtesy Henry Parks, photographer.)

increase client awareness of resources, and assist the client in resource use.

Health care resources can be described as formal and informal. *Formal* health care resources exist primarily for the provision of health care services. They include, but are not limited to, hospitals, extended-care facilities, skilled nursing homes, health departments, outpatient facilities, and the offices of private health care practitioners.

Informal health care resources provide health services but do not exist primarily for this purpose. These resources can be relatives in the client's home, service

organizations, and self-help groups. They are scattered throughout the community, are minimally coordinated, and are often more difficult to recognize than formal resources. An example of an informal health care resource is the local Lion's Club, which provides free ophthalmological examinations and eyeglasses to children in the community who could not otherwise obtain them. It provides a health care service but its primary function is not health-related. There are many such resources within the community and they are important to the provision of community health services.

Health professionals and local health departments are excellent sources of information on community resources. Developing a network with helping professionals in the community can assist the nurse in compiling resource information and facilitate client care (Meisenhelder, 1982). Frequently, compilations of local resources are done by groups such as United Way Community Services, chambers of commerce, departments of social service, offices on aging, and health departments. Major service organizations, such as associations for retarded citizens, will compile resources specific to the groups they represent. City offices and planning commissions will also have local resource information. Before referring a client, the nurse should independently explore the resource and know whether it is appropriate for the client being referred.

Collecting Information on Referral Resources

When collecting information on referral resources the nurse needs to develop a systematic way of recording and filing information (USDHHS, Source book, 1982, p. 28). Creating an ongoing file with a standard format, such as the one shown in Figure 10-5, can be helpful. Such a file should list resources both alphabetically and by service. In addition to the resource information on file the nurse can also keep resource brochures or other print materials to assist clients in resource selection. Resources that are frequently used, or used with success, may be color-coded or tabbed for easy accessibility. It is necessary that resource information be clear, accurate, and concise.

The following essential information about a resource is readily kept on file cards or in a loose-leaf notebook: (1) name of resource (include address, phone number, and name and title of person in charge or contact person), (2) purpose and services, (3) eligibility (who may use the resource, including special requirements such as age and income), (4) application procedure, (5) fees, (6) office hours and days, and (7) geographical area served. Cards should be dated to aid in file updating (refer to Figure 10-5). Data should also be kept on clients' response to use of the resource.

The nurse should also be aware of specific information that a resource requests of a client when it provides service. Information frequently requested by resources includes the following:

1. Name, address, and telephone number of the client
2. Client age, sex, and marital status
3. Names and birthdates of family members and others living in the household
4. Medical care source and health history
5. Financial status and records
6. Resources with whom the client is presently working
7. Reason for seeking referral

A grid showing frequently used resources can be a very valuable reference when one is visiting clients in the community setting. A grid that includes service areas and specific resources is especially helpful. An example of such a grid is presented in Table 10-2. It is not all-inclusive, and resources will vary from area to area, but it does illustrate how a service resource grid can be organized.

STEPS OF THE REFERRAL PROCESS

The referral process is a systematic, problem-solving approach that involves a number of client and nurse actions (Atwood, 1971; USDHHS, Source book, 1982). Figure 10-6 on p. 356 depicts the steps involved in successful implementation of a referral. It will be found, when helping a client obtain needed assistance from community resources, that the process is circular. That is, as data are obtained in one step, other steps may need to be repeated. It is crucial to remember that these steps are interconnected and interrelated.

The following are the basic steps of the referral process:

1. Establish a working relationship with the client
2. Establish the need for a referral
3. Set objectives for the referral
4. Explore resource availability
5. Client decides to use or not use referral
6. Make referral to resource
7. Facilitate referral
8. Evaluate and follow up

Client participation throughout the process is essential. The community health nurse guides the client through the process by facilitating informed decision-making, assessing client needs and objectives, exploring alternatives for need resolution, assisting the client in using resources, and evaluating the results of the entire process. The client is encouraged to be independent whenever possible.

Figure 10-5 Resource information.

National Foundation—March of Dimes
Payne County Office

Address: 20100 Maplewood, Mio, MI 47236
Phone: 811-2110 (Area 516)
Person in charge: Mrs. Nellie Scott, Director

Purpose and services:	Through referral and direct aid, assistance is provided in the areas of prenatal care, genetic counseling, diagnosis, and treatment. Offers prevention and treatment services for clients who have congenital malformations or birth defects through research, direct patient services, and public education. Sponsors scholarships in related health fields.
Eligibility:	No restrictions.
Application procedure:	Referrals by private physicians, public health clinics, or health departments. Individuals are encouraged to contact the office for further information.
Fees:	None
Office hours:	9 AM to 3 PM, Tuesday-Saturday
Geographical area served:	Payne County Compiled 6/94
Client satisfaction:	Responds immediately to clients' calls. Especially good at obtaining adaptive equipment.

Establish a Working Relationship with the Client

The referral process usually evolves after a working relationship with the client has been established. This relationship involves the formation of trust between the nurse and the client. A trusting relationship is encouraged by nurses when they show respect, empathy, and genuine concern for the client (Rorden and Taft, 1990, p. 46). As a means of building this relationship the nurse focuses on clients' feelings and perceptions of their situations and starts "where clients are at." The nurse needs to be willing to look at the situation from the client's frame of reference and take into consideration cultural variations regarding health practices, resource use, and perceptions of events (refer to Chapters 7, 8, and 9).

Trust may develop almost immediately, but more often evolves over a period of time. While establishing the relationship the nurse is able to assess the situation and gather the data necessary for helping the client to make health decisions. A relationship of trust facilitates communication and cooperation in the nurse-client relationship.

In many cases the referral process will commence as this relationship develops to its potential. If referrals are necessitated early in the relationship, the nurse should proceed with caution to be sure that sufficient data have been collected to determine if the referral is appropriate.

Establish the Need for a Referral

The community health nurse uses the nursing process to help the client identify what health care

TABLE 10-2 Resource Grid

Service needed	Types	Resource
Food	1. Emergency	1. Department of Social Services, Salvation Army, local churches, American Red Cross, Goodfellows
	2. Low-cost or free foods	2. Food stamps, food coops, school lunch programs, WIC
	3. Counseling	3. Expanded nutrition program, Health Department
Financial assistance	1. Emergency and short-term	1. Department of Social Services, Salvation Army, Goodfellows, Lion's Club, Traveler's Aid, Volunteers of America, Kiwanis
	2. Long-term	2. Department of Social Service, Social Security Administration, Veterans Administration
Housing	1. Emergency	1. Catholic Social Services, Jewish Action League, United Way Community Service, Department of Social Service, American Red Cross, Salvation Army, local churches, domestic violence facilities
	2. Public (low-cost)	2. Housing Commission, Department of Socal Service

Modified from the University of Michigan, School of Nursing, Family and Community Health Nursing: *Resource Grid*, Ann Arbor, undated, University of Michigan, School of Nursing.

needs necessitate referral. Clients often require assistance from the community health nurse in diagnosing referral needs. The nurse assists the client in looking at referral alternatives. The client should be asked about preferences and special needs, and information on resources should be shared with the client (USDHHS, Source book, 1982, p. 31).

When establishing a need for referral it is important to discriminate between problems the community health nurse can and cannot handle. For example, some budgeting problems can be dealt with by a community health nurse and others cannot. A community health nurse can help a family to analyze how its members can obtain the most for their food dollars by discussing such things as meal planning, low-cost meals, and inexpensive sources of protein. On the other hand, if the family is having difficulty with creditors, they may need to be referred to a credit-counseling resource.

The nurse should be honest with the client about the client's assessed health needs. The client may not be aware of a need, such as immunizations to prevent communicable disease, or the need for diagnostic and screening procedures for at-risk aggregates, until the nurse discusses the significance of these preventive and diagnostic procedures.

There may be situations in which the nurse finds it difficult to accept perceived client needs. People have differing values and attitudes in relation to health care, and the clients' health care priorities may not be the same as those of the nurse. For example, clients from different cultures may expect that their folk or cultural remedies will provide a cure for their illness (Hoeman, 1989). As a result they may not see a need for Western medical care. Asking clients questions about the type of treatment they think they need, what results they hope to receive from treatment, what they think caused their health problem, and what they have been doing for their condition (e.g., pregnancy, infection, illness) can elicit problem-specific cultural information and data about factors that may influence acceptance of referral (Tripp-Reimer, Brink, and Saunders, 1984, p. 81).

If the clients are using denial as a coping mechanism it can be difficult to have them realistically assess an existing health care need. This can be the case when psychosocial problems such as loss of a loved one, marital crises, budgeting, and childrearing problems occur. Clients must be ready to deal with their problems before they will use a referral resource. Honest confrontation can be very motivating and necessary when clients have difficulty taking action. This is particularly true when a caring relationship has been established between the client and the community

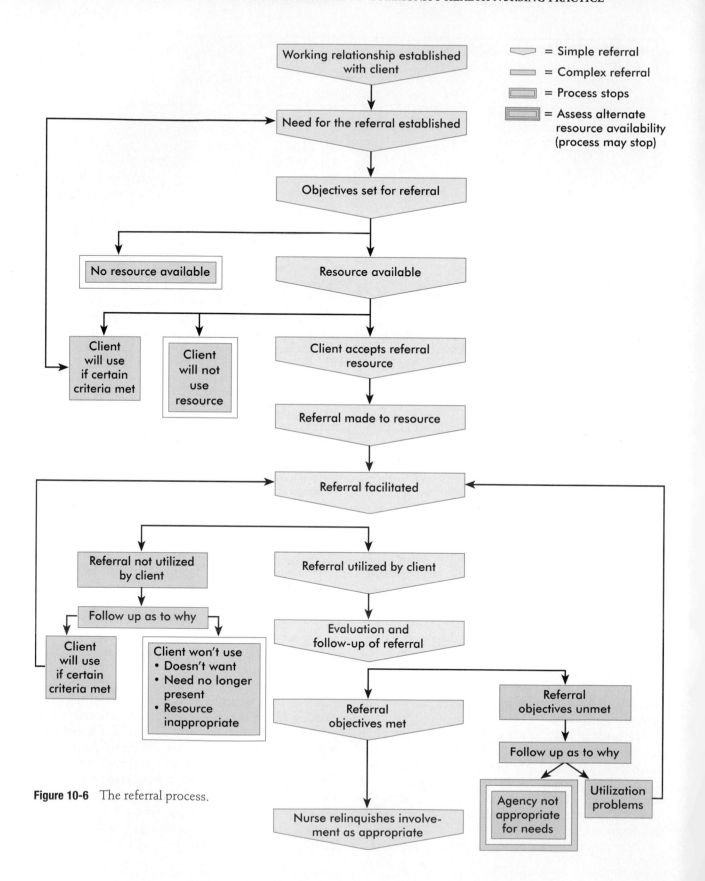

Figure 10-6   The referral process.

health nurse and when the client realizes that the nurse is acting in his or her best interests.

The community health nurse and client should thoroughly assess the need for referral. Unnecessary or unwanted referrals are costly, often strain relationships between referring agencies, and can adversely affect nurse-client relationships. Once the need for a referral has been established the nurse and client should establish objectives for the services required and should look at which resources in the community can best meet the client's needs.

Set Objectives for the Referral

What the client would like to see accomplished, tempered with what is realistically feasible, combine to determine the objectives for the referral. The nurse can help the client to be realistic in resource expectations, but the decision about specific objectives to be achieved should be made by the client. It is often helpful to write out objectives with the client in behavioral terms such as "Mrs. Black will contact the Department of Social Services in regard to obtaining food stamps by March 30." An integral part of setting objectives for the referral is deciding on what services are necessary from the referral source, as well as on a time frame for obtaining these services. The nurse should be careful when setting objectives not to attempt more than what is reasonable to be accomplished within a specified time period.

In this phase of the referral process one may find that the client expects inappropriate interventions. An agency usually does not solve the clients' problems, but instead helps clients to help themselves. For example, Mrs. Quinn, a single mother, wanted counseling only for her 16-year-old daughter, who planned to drop out of school and marry her 21-year-old boyfriend. Mrs. Quinn thought a counseling agency could "talk some sense into her." The community health nurse assisted Mrs. Quinn in seeing that a family counseling agency helps a family to deal with its problems rather than assuming responsibility for them. Joint counseling sessions arranged through the local Family and Neighborhood Counseling Center helped both mother and daughter to communicate together more effectively and to understand each other's concerns and needs. These sessions also helped the family to develop a pattern of functioning that facilitated family problem solving and decision-making.

Explore Resource Availability

A source of aid must be available before a referral can be made. An appropriate resource is one that can meet the client's needs and objectives and is available, acceptable, and accessible to the client. If more than one appropriate resource exists, the client should be allowed to choose between them. If no resource is available the referral objectives may need to be redefined or a resource developed. Many times resources in the community will reconsider the services they provide to clients, especially if the community health nurse acts as an advocate for certain services.

Client Decides to Use or Not Use Referral

The client can say yes, no, or maybe when considering a referral. If the client says yes, the referral process continues. If the client says no or maybe, the nurse should explore with the client the reasons why. If the client does not want the referral under any condition, the right to self-determination must be respected unless legal issues intervene.

The nurse should not become discouraged or believe he or she has failed if the client does not accept a referral. Imposing services on the client does not help; it only causes frustration for the nurse and the client and may adversely affect the client's use and perception of the health care system.

If the client would use a referral if certain criteria were met, the nurse may be able to assist the client in meeting these criteria. For example, a client might say that she would use a referral to the health department immunization clinic for her 2-year-old if transportation to the clinic could be arranged. The nurse may be able to help this client obtain transportation services from other community resources. If a client continues to place conditions on referral use the nurse and client should take a close look at the reasons behind these conditions. It is possible that the client really does not want the referral but fears saying no.

It may be that clients do not want to use one resource to meet a health care need but are willing to use another resource. An example of this is Mrs. Schlosser.

▶ Mrs. Schlosser was an elderly client who was eligible for food stamps but would not apply for them. She viewed food stamps as charity and stated, "I do not accept welfare." The community health nurse was frustrated because Mrs. Schlosser's diet was inadequate, largely for financial reasons. Discussing the food stamp program with Mrs. Schlosser did not change her mind about using food stamps. Thus the nurse explored alternatives with her. Because Mrs. Schlosser wanted to eat better, she was receptive to learning about how to prepare low-cost, nutritious meals at home and was also interested in applying for a reduced-cost, Meals-on-Wheels program in which she would pay for her meals. Mrs. Schlosser had refused a referral for food stamps, but she and the nurse were able to develop alternatives that helped to meet her nutritional needs.

Timing influences how the client responds to the referral. Studies have shown that a referral should occur as soon as possible after detecting a risk; a rapid, well-handled referral often reinforces the importance of taking positive health action to the client (USDHHS, 1982, Source book, p. 27).

Referral Made to a Resource

When the nurse is referring a client to a resource the referral content should be specific and comprehensive and should reflect the client's objectives for the referral (Combs, 1976, p. 126). The appropriate forms should be filled out and procedures followed. A release of information form is obtained. Clients usually do not hesitate to sign an information release form when they have decided that they need a referral. If an appointment is necessary it is made. The client should be encouraged to be as independent as possible in contacting the resource.

Many referrals can be made, at least initially, by telephone. Telephone referrals may be faster and more informative, since the agency can request any additional or specific information that is needed at the time. A written referral can always follow. If the referral is written it will include information such as client and family awareness of the diagnosis and prognosis; complete and detailed orders for medications and treatments; people living with the client; the client's religion, spoken language, and diet; address and phone number; titles such as Doctor, Mrs., Mr.; goals for and estimated length of service; nursing diagnoses; and method of health care financing (Wheeler-Lachowycz, 1983).

An example of a referral form used by one local health department to refer clients to another resource

is presented in Figure 10-7. This form includes essential referral information, such as data about the person making the referral, the individual or family being referred, the reason for the referral, summary of the client's situation, resources being used by the client, a statement on whether or not the client is aware of the referral, and a place for the receiving resource to share information with the referral agency to facilitate follow-up and evaluation.

Often resources request that clients bring certain types of information with them to their first appointment. If clients are not aware of this requirement they may have to return to the resource with the information or may be denied service. Returning to a resource takes additional time, effort, and money. It may present a barrier to the client using the referral.

Facilitate the Referral

Facilitating a referral involves a number of nursing interventions, including preparing the client for the use of community services and identifying and overcoming barriers to the use of these services. It is important to remember that client motivation is critical; if the client is not motivated to make the referral work, the referral process probably will not be successful. Barriers that decrease client motivation are discussed later in this chapter.

Evaluation and Follow-up

As with all aspects of the nursing process, referrals need to be evaluated. Ongoing evaluation and follow-up are probably of most importance in the referral process. Throughout the process the community health nurse evaluates the client's responses to the referral to determine if changes need to be made.

Effective evaluation of the referral process encompasses reviewing how well client needs are being met. Evaluation enhances the nurse's competency in using the process. In evaluating, the nurse must realize that there are times when a referral is not or was not effective. However, this judgment should not be made quickly. Some clients need support and encouragement, especially if their problems are not resolved immediately. The case of Mr. Connant is an example.

▶ **Mr. Connant decided that he was not going back to the mental health clinic for counseling after his** first visit because the clinic counselor "did nothing but talk." In evaluating this situation, the nurse realized that she needed to discuss more specifically with Mr. Connant his expectations of counseling along with the need for him to share his feelings about his first session with the counselor at the clinic. Supportive assistance by the nurse facilitated Mr. Connant's return to the mental health center. Later he expressed gratitude for the nurse's encouragement because counseling was helping him to work through many of the issues that had been troubling him.

During evaluation the client should be helped to understand the referral process and anticipatory guidance should be used in preparing the client to use the process in the future. If a client evidences the same problem over and over the nurse and client should thoroughly assess why this is happening. For example, repeated need for emergency food orders should be a clue that the client is having difficulty managing his or her budget. This could be a result of having a too-limited income or of not knowing how to allocate funds that are available. Emergency food orders will not solve either of these problems on a long-term basis, so the client needs to be assisted in exploring other options.

Probably the hardest part of the evaluation phase is realizing when it is time for the nurse to relinquish involvement with the client. This is an especially difficult task when the client and nurse have developed a strong, positive working relationship, and termination in these situations can provoke uneasy feelings in both the nurse and the client (refer to Chapter 9). Usually clients are ready to function independently when they can identify personal health care needs, take initiative to contact health care resources, and take action to resolve health care problems. If a client does not demonstrate these behaviors or demonstrates them only when the community health nurse is not available, the nurse-client relationship should be closely examined, as it may be fostering an unhealthy dependency.

BARRIERS TO USE OF THE REFERRAL PROCESS

For each resource and each client, the nurse must identify the barriers that adversely affect the use of referral services. Barriers involve individual and resource components. For example, an agency may have high fees for services (a resource barrier), which the client is unable to afford (a client barrier). In this case fees are both a resource barrier and a client barrier. Some common resource and client barriers are briefly described in the following sections.

Resource Barriers
Attitudes of Health Care Professionals

The attitudes and biases of health care professionals have a great impact on whether clients use resource services (Goldstein, 1983). Clients are quick to sense the attitudes of health care personnel, and if they are not treated with respect and courtesy, they are hesitant to return. Abrupt answers to a client's questions, minimal communication with the client, communication in health care jargon, and conveying frustration when clients ask questions are a few examples of behaviors that foster negative reactions to community resources. Although the values and attitudes of the nurse may differ from the client's, the nurse must be open to the opinions of others and maintain a nonjudgmental attitude. A good rule of thumb is to treat clients the way that you would like to be treated.

An attitude that became a barrier to the use of a health care resource is shown in the following example.

▶ **The nurse in charge of an antepartal clinic for low-income mothers refused to make appointments for clinic clients because "these people wouldn't keep appointments anyway." As a result, the clinic operated on a first-come-first-served basis. Since no appointments were available clients had to arrive very early at the clinic to sign in. There were usually long waits to be seen. Clients frequently traveled by bus to get to the clinic and had to make arrangements for child care to be able to come. It was common for clients to leave the clinic before they were seen due to transportation or child care problems. Many became discouraged with the system and did not seek further prenatal care.**

Attitudes and practices such as these do not facilitate clients' use of health care services or promote preventive health action.

OAKLAND COUNTY DEPARTMENT OF HEALTH

1200 North Telegraph Road   27725 Greenfield
Pontiac, Michigan 48053   Southfield, Michigan 48075
Telephone 858-1280   Telephone 424-7000

REFERRAL FORM

TO _____   FROM: _____

ADDRESS _____   ☐ PONTIAC OFFICE

_____   ☐ SOUTHFIELD OFFICE

Attention: _____   Telephone # _____ Date _____

REGARDING _____   Aware of referral? ☐ Yes ☐ No

ADDRESS _____   Telephone # _____

FAMILY ROSTER (Names, birthdate, relationship)

REASON FOR REFERRAL

SITUATION

(over)

KNOWN MEDICAL, AGENCY, COMMUNITY RESOURCES

REPLY REQUESTED: ☐ No ☐ Yes   (see back)

Figure 10-7 Sample referral form. (Used by permission of the Nursing Division, Oakland County Health Department, Pontiac, Mich.)

Continuation of situation:

Agency reply to Oakland County Health Department

_____

(Signature)

Date _____

Figure 10-7, cont'd. For legend, see opposite page.

Physical Accessibility of Resource

Clients are less likely to use resources that are not readily accessible. Once a resource is beyond walking distance, other means of transportation must be found. Public transportation is scarce in this country. Even if a family has a car, it may not be available at the time of the resource appointment. The problem is greatly magnified if the resource is at such a distance that the client must make arrangements for overnight stays in order to use its services. Overnight stays often necessitate making arrangements for the care of small children or other members of the family, and they can be very costly to the client. Community resources such as a Ronald McDonald House have helped to meet this accessibility need.

Cost of Resource Services

How much a client can or is willing to pay for a health service is an individual matter. Any cost at all may be more than clients can pay if their income is minimal. If the service is not absolutely necessary or critical to the client's activities of daily living, the cost may be viewed as too high even when the client has money available for the service. On the other hand, if the client places a high priority on receiving a given service, he or she may not object to paying high fees.

Client Barriers

Priorities

If the need is not of high priority for the client, he or she may not become actively involved in using the referral services. If other needs are considered to be of higher priority, the nurse should assist the client in meeting these needs first. It may be more important for the family to care for an ill family member than to take a child to the well-baby clinic for immunizations; or if the family is having difficulty meeting its basic needs of food, clothing, and shelter, preventive health care services may not be viewed as a priority.

Motivation

If the client is not highly motivated to work on a need, it is not likely that much will be done by the client toward meeting that need. An integral part of client motivation is the concept of *awareness vs. readiness.* The fact that the client is aware of a need does not mean that he or she is ready to act on the need. If a differentiation is not made between awareness and readiness, the nurse may feel responsible for the failure of the client to follow through on a referral. Once it is established that the client is not ready to act on a need, the nurse needs to assist the client in prioritizing the needs upon which he or she is ready to act. A good example of awareness vs. readiness is a client who acknowledges that the house needs to be cleaned but after numerous nursing visits, much discussion, and ample time, the house is still not cleaned. The client is aware of the need but is not ready to act on it.

Previous Experience with Resources

If a client has not had a positive experience in using a resource in the past, she or he may be hesitant to use this resource again or to use other community resources. In these situations it is important to acknowledge the client's feelings and to explain ways to make further contacts with community services more meaningful. *Complaints about resources can be entirely justified.* However, it will be found that some clients were not ready to make needed changes when they used a community service the first time; hence, they have a negative view of the service because of the fact that their problems were not resolved. This is frequently the case when clients are dealing with multiple stressors.

Lack of Knowledge about Available Resources

Clients need to know about resources before they will use them. A key role of the community health nurse is to help clients learn about health care services in the community. Lack of knowledge about resources is a major barrier to the use of health care services.

Lack of Understanding of the Need for a Referral

Clients who do not understand the need for a referral frequently do not take action to obtain referral services. This is often true of families who neglect to have their children immunized. Many people know that children need "baby shots" but do not understand why. These people will be more likely to follow through on a consistent basis in obtaining immunizations if they know the purpose for receiving immunizations and the consequences of not obtaining adequate protection against communicable diseases.

Client Self-Image

If clients do not have a positive self-image, they may be hesitant to seek care and may view themselves as unworthy of such care. The nurse should acknowledge these feelings and develop intervention strategies which will help clients to increase self-esteem.

Cultural Factors

Cultural differences can be a barrier to effective use of the referral process. Language is one of the most obvious cultural barriers. In our health care system, clients who do not speak English can have a difficult time using resources and obtaining appropriate health care.

Every culture has beliefs regarding health care practices. Cultural beliefs about the cause of illness, nutrition, preventive health care, and death and dying vary greatly. The norms and values of a culture can also affect health care practices. For example, in traditional Arab culture women are generally not allowed to leave their homes or immediate neighborhoods without a male escort. Thus health care services are better used by these women if they are located in a neighborhood facility.

In some cultural groups where preventive health services are not routinely sought the nurse may have a difficult time gaining compliance on referrals for immunizations and routine physical examinations. Ethnic and cultural values and attitudes are pervasive in a person's life, and it is important that the nurse identify them in relation to health care practices (Rorden and Taft, 1990, p. 97). However, an effective nurse does *not* use racial, cultural, or ethnic stereotypes in anticipating client preferences and providing client care (Rorden and Taft, p. 98).

Financial

Health care in the United States is expensive. Many clients do not use health care services because they cannot afford them. Chapter 5 discussed methods of health care financing in the United States and the cost of health care. Clients such as the near-poor client, who does not qualify for welfare assistance but may be medically indigent, frequently have difficulty paying for health care. The same is true for families who are uninsured or underinsured. It is a challenge for the nurse to find resources that will assist such clients.

Accessibility

Access, as a barrier to service, has become a national health care concern and is a major barrier to the use of health care services (USDHHS, 1991). In many communities necessary health care services are not readily available. This is becoming increasingly evident in rural communities where hospitals and other acute care facilities are closing or cutting back on services at an alarming rate (refer to Chapter 3).

Lack of access to services because of limited or no transportation is a major barrier to the use of health care services. It has been well documented that clients frequently do not seek health care because they have problems with transportation to health care facilities. If low-cost public transportation is not available, car pooling, the use of volunteer transportation services, or establishing outreach clinic services in the neighborhood may help to reduce transportation barriers. Frequently local churches and departments of human or social services have programs to assist people with transportation needs. Local offices on aging and senior centers frequently have transportation services available for the elderly.

LEVELS OF NURSING INTERVENTION WITH REFERRAL

Clients have varying levels of ability to assume independent functioning when using health care resources, and this necessitates different levels of professional intervention by the community health nurse. Identifying the level at which the client is functioning helps the community health nurse to focus intervention strategies when using the referral process. Levels of nursing intervention are presented here.

Level I: At this level the client is largely dependent on the nurse and will need assistance with all aspects of the referral process. Frequently these clients have not had life experiences that have prepared them to deal adequately with systems external to their family unit, or their energies are depleted by crisis. These clients need considerable support and encouragement and, often, concrete help from the community health nurse before they can follow through on a needed referral. Frequently they assume a passive role. They may sincerely want assistance from others but fail to take action because they lack the energy or knowledge to do so, and basically feel inadequate to handle the referral by themselves. Community health nursing intervention with these clients involves health teaching and counseling so that they can identify health needs that necessitate referral. In addition, supportive assistance is necessary while they are learning how to use health care resources. A major goal when working with these clients is to help them to become more actively involved in taking responsibility for meeting their own health needs. At first the community health nurse may have to assist these clients with making all the arrangements for warranted health care; just keeping an appointment can be a major accomplishment for them. Sometimes it is easier to do for the client than to work with him or her, especially if the client follows through when the nurse makes all the necessary arrangements and decisions. It is important, however, for the community health nurse to work toward helping clients use health resources independently.

Level II: At this level mutual participation is evident. The client does not wait for the community health nurse to initiate discussion about health care needs. Rather, the client actively seeks information to determine what health actions are needed to resolve current health problems or to enhance wellness in the future. Clients at this level may need health teaching to understand the value of preventive health practices, to locate community resources that they can afford,or to learn about community services such as low-cost or free transportation, which will help them to use needed resources. They are more likely, however, to raise challenging questions and to identify when health care resources are inappropriate to meet their needs. At times it may be difficult to recognize when these clients need assistance because they are functioning so well in most aspects of their lives.

Level III: At this level the client can use the referral process independently. The nurse may be used as a resource person but otherwise assumes a passive participant role.

Summary

Community health nurses provide general, comprehensive, and continuous care to clients in the community setting. Through the use of discharge planning and referral processes they ensure continuity of care by coordinating services with other health care providers and by linking clients to health care resources. Several key concepts are inherent in these processes: (1) clients have the basic responsibility for maintaining their health; (2) clients have the right to accept or refuse health care services; (3) planned intervention by professionals can promote full use of resources by community citizens; (4) interdisciplinary collaboration and coordination are essential to ensure continuity of care; and (5) clients can learn to independently use health care services. Effective use of discharge planning and the referral process not only helps clients to resolve their current health needs, but also prepares them to make decisions about how to handle health needs in the future.

There are limitless opportunities for the community health nurse to facilitate continuity of care through discharge planning and the referral process.

◀ *An Exercise in Critical Thinking* ▶

You are a health department nurse who has been assigned to work with a local hospital's discharge planning team. You are trying to familiarize yourself with community resources and the nursing role in the discharge planning process. How would you begin to gather data about community resources? What types of information would you want to obtain about your role with the discharge planning team? What type of criteria would you use to identify clients in need of continuing care upon hospital discharge?

APPENDIX 10-1

THE CHILD AT HOME WITH A CHRONIC ILLNESS

I am Donnie's mother. I am here to present the parents' view. I will describe the implications of a child's chronic illness on the family, the financial issues, and the complex problems encountered by my family. In addition, I will compare experiences reported by other parents in our parents' group.

Donnie, my sixth child, was born with defects that involved the left side of his body including his left lung, which later on had to be removed. At the time of his birth, we were told that Donnie had to undergo immediate surgery because of what is called an omphalocele, which means that his navel and stomach had evolved outside his abdomen. Within 4 hours of birth, he was transported from Joliet Hospital to Children's Memorial Hospital in Chicago, where the first stage of surgery was performed immediately.

For us as parents, the first shock in the delivery room was knowing that our child had multiple birth defects. We were overpowered by fear of losing our child. Later, the fear was intensified by observing our child in the ICU, when his heart stopped 18 times and he had to be resuscitated. Only because of the prompt response from health care personnel, Donnie survived all this without brain damage.

During his first 3 years in an acute intensive care unit, Donnie underwent a total of 20 operations. Most of the time he was breathing with the help of a machine—a ventilator—receiving numerous intravenous infusions and treatments while we were watching as helpless bystanders. We often did not understand what was done, the reason why, and we had no knowledge of the alternatives.

Our main social contacts were other parents of critically ill children in the ICU waiting area who, over a period of months, became like close friends to us. Some were the unlucky ones; their children died. We grieved with them, always thinking that we could be next. After years of this, we shut ourselves off and avoided contacts with those parents—even to the point of being abrupt.

We did not receive professional help to deal with the psychological stress we were under. My husband dealt with it by talking constantly about it, while I tried not to think or talk about it, which caused great problems between us. We lost a lot of our friends. They did not know what to say, so it was easier for them not to see us. Besides, we were no fun to be with, because we were constantly talking about our problem.

During his years in the ICU, attempts were made to wean Donnie off the ventilator. A pediatrician forcefully suggested that we take Donnie home, that is, to die. We took Donnie home. He had a tracheostomy; that is, a hole in his trachea. He was breathing poorly by himself; we thought he would not live much longer. We were not prepared to properly take care of him at home. We did not even know how to regulate oxygen flow. He was home for two months, only to return to the Children's Memorial ICU because of pneumonia and failure to thrive. By then, we had lived through two months of a nightmare with no help, no medical caregivers, no sleep—only worry. We were exhausted and burned out.

We shared this experience years later with other parents who at the time were sent home unprepared, with a child who could not breathe by himself without a mechanical aid. This couple had ventilated their child by hand 24 hours a day, taking turns day and night for months, until the decision was made that the child needed a mechanical ventilator at home.

Our home is in Joliet, Illinois, 60 miles from Children's Memorial Hospital in Chicago. Rather than spend 2 to 4 hours on the road a day, we chose to move into the waiting rooms at Children's Memorial Hospital, where we lived for over a year. We slept on the couch, showered in the basement locker rooms, ate hospital food, and paid parking fees. Our 5 children, ranging in age from 17 to 12 years, were left unattended most of the time. They learned to take care of themselves. After about a year, my husband and I decided that one of us had to stay at home in Joliet because our other children were beginning to feel the effects of our absence. I went to Joliet, returning to the hospital occasionally, and my husband stayed with Donnie. Consequently, he lost his business and to live we had to borrow money from family members. Besides dealing with this stress, there was no money or time to go on vacations with the other children. We haven't had a family vacation for 10 years!

Our insurance covered $100,000 of Donnie's care. After a few months, we were told to apply for financial assistance to Illinois Public Aid and the Division of Services for Crippled Children. Children's Memorial Hospital was very helpful in helping us apply. We qualified because Donnie was born with multiple deformities.

Why is it much easier to get aid if a child is born with defects than if some illness or accident causes defects at a later date? Others in our parent-group had children who had problems getting financial help. One parent was called into the hospital billing department and was presented with an astronomical hospital bill and was asked "How are you going to pay for this?" Some parents were advised to go on unemployment, go on public aid, and even get a divorce.

After spending the better part of 3½ years in an Acute ICU, Donnie was transferred into an intermediate care unit for his long-term care. Repeated attempts to wean him from his breathing machine caused him to be lethargic, puffy, and turn blue. He ceased to grow. The only time he was well was when he was on his ventilator. Then he became a very active, happy child. His many arrests had apparently not damaged his brain. He had become a very precocious child, even inventing his own sign language!

Even though we were at his bedside as much as possible, many of the functions of a parent were taken over by nurses and other health caretakers. Correcting bad behavior or eating habits is hard to accomplish outside of a family setting.

Since Donnie was confined to this unit by being on the ventilator, he lacked opportunity for an education appropriate for a 4-year-old. At this time, he got ½ hour of tutoring a day. Children's Memorial Hospital, being an acute care hospital, was unable to provide additional education for a chronically disabled child.

Then in 1978 a new idea was presented to us by a new staff physician. Give Donnie optimal ventilation so he can grow. Prepare him to go home safely with his ventilator. With our memories of the past experience, the idea horrified us. But after meeting with qualified medical personnel, we were assured that we would be trained and would have medical help to support us. Donnie needed to go home in order not to become socially handicapped. Once while I was talking to him on the phone, I told him I was sitting at the kitchen table. After he hung up, he asked his nurse "What is a kitchen table?" My other children were delighted when we told them that Donnie could come home, and they were anxiously awaiting his arrival.

In 1978 no money was allocated by Federal or State law to care for ventilator-dependent children at home. The State knew how to pay the high costs of intensive care but had no experience in providing funding for less expensive care at home. A long period of negotiation took place. The state officials finally found the solution to pay 100% for ⅔ less expensive medical care at home. We were luckier than others in the parents' group who were faced with the spend-down money (money to be paid according to income by the family to the state).

Some parents in our group had private insurance. The insurance company refused to change their reimbursement policy for home care. The insurance company was willing to pay everything in hospital, but refused payment for home care. As a result, the insurance company rapidly spent the $500,000 in the hospital. This money could have lasted for years at home. They had no incentive to change. Therefore, public funds were needed sooner, because the private insurance money was gone so quickly while the patient remained in the ICU. So the burden was transferred to the State and ultimately to the taxpayer.

Transition

It took nine months from the time the decision was made to send Donnie home before it really happened. During that time we built a specially adapted addition to our house. Regular meetings with the health care team were held. These meetings clearly defined goals acceptable to all, and provided clear objectives and specific plans for action. Each team member had accountability. The home discharge team included the dedicated clinical staff who had cared for Donnie over the years. The coordinator was his nurse; the educator was his respiratory therapist. Both were caregivers who had received him in the ICU shortly after his birth. The team also involved physical and child-life therapists, special service staff, social workers, etc. Initially, several members had to overcome their own fear and negative thinking, but the more educated they became, the more they were able to overcome this barrier.

My husband and I were trained to handle Donnie's ventilator equipment by both classroom teaching and "hands-on" experience. We passed a test and were certified. Nurses we recruited, selected, and hired to provide 24-hour home care were trained with us at the hospital, in the classroom, and at the bedside. Community support services, including a primary physician and emergency room staff in Joliet, were well-informed about their responsibility prior to their consent. Nursing, physical therapy, and respiratory therapy plans and exact procedures were clearly written, and local suppliers of medical equipment were found, motivated, and well-prepared. Funding was finally approved because of highly motivated and responsible actions of the leaders and staff of the Division of Services for Crippled Children, the Illinois Department of Public Health and SSI Disabled Children's Program.

The team work of all these individuals made the home program a reality.

Home

On September 19, 1979, our son came home to stay. It has been a difficult task. We are dealing with a lack of privacy, the ventilator breaking down, lack of service for equipment, and difficulties in getting medical supplies.

However, the benefits of having Donnie at home far outweigh the difficulties.

We are now a normal family, maybe different in some ways, but we are all together, sharing all the experiences of life. We no longer divide our time among our children. Donnie's health has improved; he has grown several inches. His oxygen need has decreased. His social life is no longer limited to the ICU where he never knew the difference between day and night. He is now getting an education, doing average-to-above-average work. He no longer has to regard cardiac arrests in the bed next to him as his only occasion for "social-get-together." Instead he goes to weddings; he was a ring bearer at his brother's wedding where he never missed a dance. Donnie is a joy to be with. He loves his religion. He celebrated his Holy Communion last month. He tolerates being off the ventilator with oxygen longer. He races his race car (recently he placed first in competition), climbs trees, and he even fell and broke his arm at a birthday party. Donnie worries right now whether he will get married one day. He is concerned that it is not much fun to go trick or treating, because no matter how he dresses up, everybody recognizes him by his tracheostomy. His nightly prayer includes: "Dear God, if you are listening, please get rid of my trach so I can play football."

We know we can go back to Children's Memorial Hospital any time we have any problems with Donnie. He will be well taken care of by loving people who know him and care for him and us.

We are deeply grateful to the staff of Children's Memorial Hospital. They never gave up hope. And thank God nobody pulled the plug in the ICU. Thank you.

From USDHHS: *Report of the Surgeon General's Workshop on Children with Handicaps and Their Families,* DHHS Publication No. PHS 83-50194 Washington, D.C., 1982, U.S. Government Printing Office, pp. 27-30.

APPENDIX 10-2
Discharge Questionnaire

The staff on (unit name) wants to make your return to the community as easy for you as possible. The nurse who is primarily responsible for helping you plan your discharge is _____. He or she will help you and your family reach any resources you may need for your health care at home. There are many agencies, including home care, which assist people in the community with health care problems.

Please complete the following questions with your family as soon as you feel able. Your discharge nurse will be in contact with you within a few days of your admission.

Data #1
When you get home
1. With whom will you live? _____
2. Will they be able to help with your care if needed? _____
3. Will you have difficulty getting around your home—stairs, small bathroom, low bed, safety problems, to the telephone, to shower, or bathtub? _____
4. Will you have any problems in getting any of the following—transportation, food, medicine, heat, place to stay, child care, pet care, water supply? _____
5. Will you need any of these to function at home—wheelchair, brace, cane, walker, crutches, special equipment? _____

From Stone M: Discharge planning guide, *Am J Nurs* 79: 1445-1447, 1979.   *Continued*

APPENDIX 10-2

Discharge Questionnaire—cont'd

6. How much of the following will you be able to do? (Please mark appropriate column.)

	Independent	With family	Unable to do
Turning in bed			
Bathing			
Dressing			
Eating			
Sitting			
Standing			
Transfers to tub			
Transfers to toilet			
Walking			

Data #2

1. Have you had a problem with any of these areas recently?
   - a. Eyes/ears
   - b. Mouth/throat/teeth
   - c. Skin
   - d. Lungs/breathing
   - e. Breasts
   - f. Heart/blood vessels
   - g. Stomach/bowel
   - h. Bladder/kidneys/urine
   - i. Genitals
   - j. Mental status
   - k. Nerves/muscles
2. Will you have difficulty getting to your physician, nurse, or therapist often enough to have these checked? _____

Data #3

Please mark any of the following areas that you would like to know more about:
1. Your disease/illness/accident
   - a. What caused it
   - b. What can be done to prevent a repeat
   - c. How to recognize a repeat
   - d. How it will affect you later
2. Your medication
   - a. What it does
   - b. How much to take
   - c. When to take it
   - d. What side effects to be aware of
3. Your treatments, procedures, or exercises
   - a. What they do for you
   - b. How to do them
   - c. How often to do them
   - d. What difficulties to be aware of
4. Supplies or equipment you'll use at home
   - a. What it does
   - b. When to use it
   - c. How to get more or to get repairs

APPENDIX 10-2
Discharge Questionnaire—cont'd

---

5. Your nutrition
   a. How it affects you
   b. Special diets—how much to eat, when to eat, what to avoid
   c. How much and what to drink
6. Preventive health practices
   a. How to examine your breasts
   b. Pap smears
   c. Birth control
   d. Effect of cigarettes
   e. Effect of alcohol and drugs

   f. Dental health
   g. Seat belts
   h. Immunizations (yourself or children)
   i. Exercise
7. Other _____

Data #4

1. Which of these agencies are you involved with?
   a. VNA/Home Health
   b. Senior Citizens
   c. Vocational Rehabilitation
   d. Social Welfare
   e. Planned Parenthood
   f. Mental Health Agency
   g. Diet Club
   h. Alcoholics Anonymous
   i. Cancer Society

   j. Ostomy Club
   k. Meals-on-Wheels
   l. Diabetes Association
   m. Dialysis Association
   n. MS Society
   o. MD Society
   p. Association for the Blind
   q. Other _____
2. Please mark any of the areas that you would especially like to discuss with your discharge nurse.
   a. Finances, jobs
   b. Drugs, alcohol
   c. Caring for children or elderly relatives
   d. Emotional or nerve problem
   e. Sexuality
   f. Family or marital relationships

   g. Grieving
   h. School or work
   i. Problem, retirement
   j. Spiritual needs
   k. Legal problems
   l. Other _____

STOP HERE. YOUR DISCHARGE NURSE WILL HELP YOU COMPLETE THE FORM. Ask to see him or her if you haven't met yet, especially if you think you might go home soon.

Assessments (To be done by RN and patient)
1. Will there be a need for help with physical care at home?
2. Will there be a need for a nurse or therapist at home to assess physical status, disease process, or exercise and therapy?
3. Will the patient or family need more health education about any of the areas above (Data #3), either during hospitalization or at home?
4. Will the patient or family need more information or assistance with any of the psychosocial areas listed in Data #4?

Plan (To be done by patient and nurse together)
Consider the four assessments above. If there are *no* yes responses, proceed to section B and complete. If there are any yes responses, you *must* select either part 1 or part 2 of section A before completing section B.
A. 1. No referral necessary, but must have further education before discharge regarding _____
   2. Refer to: (see above list of agencies)
B. 1. Equipment or supplies to leave with patient _____
   2. Transfer plan _____
   3. Medical follow-up _____
   4. Surgical follow-up _____

References

American Hospital Association: *Guidelines: discharge planning,* Chicago, 1984, The Association.

American Nurses Association: *Standards of home health nursing practice,* Kansas City, Mo., 1986a, The Association.

American Nurses Association: *Standards of community health nursing practice,* Kansas City, Mo., 1986b, The Association.

Arenth LM and Mamon JA: Determining patient needs after discharge, *Nurs Management* 16(9):20-24, 1985.

Atwood J: *Principles of the nursing referral process,* unpublished research project, Ann Arbor, 1971, University of Michigan.

Blaylock A and Cason CL: Discharge planning predicting patients' needs, *J Gerontological Nurs* 18(7):5-10, 1992.

Bristow O, Stickney C, and Thompson S: *Discharge planning for continuity of care,* New York, 1976, National League for Nursing.

Burlenski M: President's message, *Access* 7(1):2, 4, 1989.

Combs PA: A study of the effectiveness of nursing referrals, *Public Health Rep* 91:122-126, 1976.

Corkery E: Discharge planning and home health care: what every staff nurse should know, *Orthopaedic Nurs* 8(6):18-27, 1989.

DeRienzo B: Discharge planning, *Rehabilitation Nurs* 10(4):34-36, 1985.

Esper PS: Discharge planning—a quality assurance approach, *Nurs Management* 19(10):66-68, 1988.

Feather J: J Hospital discharge planning: how has it changed since DRG's, *Next Step* VI(3):1-3, 8, 1989.

Garland M: Discharge follow-up by telephone, *Rehabilitation Nurs* 17(6):339-341, 1992.

Goldstein H: Starting where the client is, *Social Casework* 64:267-275, 1983.

Hartigan EG and Brown J: *Discharge planning for continuity of care,* New York, 1985, National League for Nursing.

Hoeman SP: Cultural assessment in rehabilitation nursing practice, *Nurs Clinics of North America* 24(1): 277-289, 1989.

Kromminga DK and Ostwald SK: The public health nurse as a discharge planner: patient's perceptions of the process, *Public Health Nurs* 4:224-229, 1987.

Luker KA and Chalmers KI: The referral process in health visiting, *Int J Nurs Stud* 26(2):173-185, 1989.

McBroom A: Uniform needs assessment instrument nearing completion, *Access* 7(1):1, 3-4, 1989.

McKeehan KM: *Continuing care: a multidisciplinary approach for discharge planning,* St. Louis, 1981, Mosby.

Meisenhelder JB: Networking and nursing, *Image: J Nurs Scholarship* 14:77-80, 1982.

North M, Meeusen M, and Hollinsworth P: Discharge planning: increasing client and nurse satisfaction, *Rehabilitation Nurs* 16(6):327-329, 1991.

Oakland County Health Department, Nursing Division: *Referral form,* Pontiac, Mich., Oakland County Health Department, undated.

O'Hare P and Terry M: *Discharge planning: strategies for assuring continuity of care,* Rockville, Md., 1988, Aspen.

Packard-Helie MT and Lancaster DB: A vital link in continuity of care, *Nurs Management* 20(8):32-34, 1989.

Reischelt PA and Newcomb J: Organizational factors in discharge planning, *J Nurs Adm* 10(10):36-42, 1980.

Rorden JW and Taft E: *Discharge planning guide for nurses,* Philadelphia, 1990, Saunders.

Shamansky SL, Boase JC, and Horn BM: Discharge planning yesterday, today and tomorrow, *Home Health Care Nurse* 2(13):14-21, 1984.

Siegel H: Nurses improve hospital efficiency through a risk assessment model at admission, *Nurs Management* 19(10):38-40, 42, 44-45, 1988.

Slevin AP and Roberts AS: Discharge planning: a tool for decision making, *Nurs Management* 18(12):47-50, 1987.

Stone M: Discharge planning guide, *Am J Nurs* 79:1445-1447, 1979.

Tripp-Reimer T, Brink PJ, and Saunders JM: Cultural assessment: content and process, *Nurs Outlook* 32(2):78-82, 1984.

United States Department of Health and Human Services (USDHHS): *Source book for health education materials and community resources,* Washington, D.C., 1982, U.S. Government Printing Office.

USDHHS: *Report of the Surgeon General's Workshop on children with handicaps and their families,* DHHS Publication No. PHS 83-50194, Washington, D.C., 1982, U.S. Government Printing Office.

USDHHS: *Healthy people 2000: promoting health and preventing diseases. Objectives for the nation,* Washington, D.C., 1991, USDHHS.

University of Michigan, School of Nursing, Family and Community Health Nursing: *Resource grid,* Ann Arbor, undated, University of Michigan, School of Nursing.

Wensley E: *Nursing service without walls,* New York, 1963, National League for Nursing.

Wheeler-Lachowycz J: How to use your VNA, *Am J Nurs* 83:1164-1167, 1983.

Willihnganz G: The next step: pre-admission planning for discharge needs, *Coordinator* 3:20-21, 1984.

Wolff I: Referral—a process and a skill, *Nurs Outlook* 10:253-256, 1962.

Weinberger B: Discharge planning: the sooner the better, *Nursing 89* 19:75-76, 1989.

Selected Bibliography

Beaudry ML: Effective discharge planning matches patient need and community resources, *Hospital Prog* 56(12):29-30, 1975.

Campbell HW: Nurses' commitment makes a difference in discharge planning, *Kentucky Nurse* 37(3):13-14, 1989.

Crittenden FJ: *Discharge planning for health care facilities,* Bowie, Md., 1983, Robert J. Brady Co.

Danis DM: Discharge referrals, *J Emerg Nurs* 9:44-45, 1983.

Jowett S and Armitage S: Hospital and community liaison links in nursing: the role of the liaison nurse, *J Advanced Nurs* 13:579-587, 1988.

Mackey JF: Lack of referral networks: a parent's perspective, *Birth Defects* 26(2):105-108, 1990.

Mamon J, Steinwachs DM, Fahey M, Bone LR, Oktay J, and Klein L: Impact of hospital discharge planning on meeting patient needs after returning home, *Health Services Research* 27(2):155-175, 1992.

McClelland E, Kelly K, and Buckwalter KC: *Continuity of care: advancing the concept of discharge planning,* New York, 1985, Grune and Stratton.

Pittman L, Morton W, Edwards L, and Holmes D: Patient discharge planning documentation in an Australian multidisciplinary rehabilitation setting, *Rehabilitation Nurs* 17(6):327-331, 1992.

Volland PJ: *Discharge planning: an interdisciplinary approach to continuity of care,* New York, 1988, National Health.

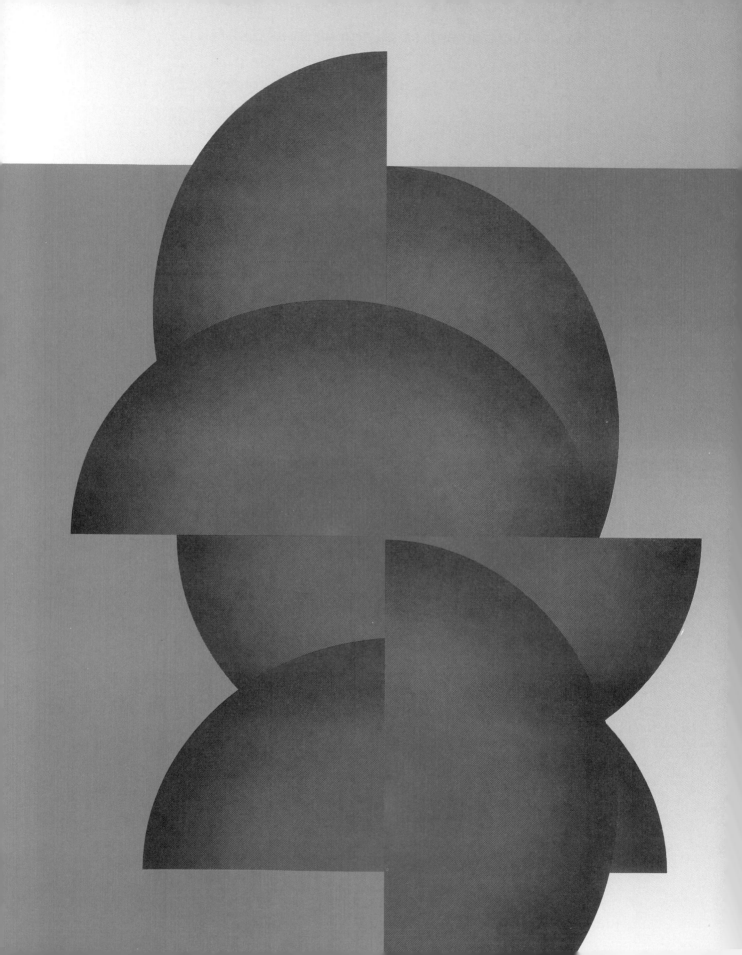

Part Two

PLANNING HEALTH SERVICES FOR AGGREGATES AT RISK

The uniqueness of community health nursing practice lies in the nurse's ability to assess the health needs of a community, to identify aggregates at risk, and to plan, implement, and evaluate intervention strategies that promote community wellness. A variety of approaches can be used to analyze the state of wellness in a community. Because community health nurses work with individuals, families, and populations across the life span, a developmental, age-correlated approach to determining aggregates at risk can be extremely useful. The increasing number of clients across the life span who receive care at home and who have long-term care needs is a growing concern of all health care professionals.

Community health nurses use knowledge from public health and nursing practice in order to fulfill their responsibility to the population as a whole. Part Two explores how knowledge from these fields of practice is synthesized by nurses in the community when they plan health programs for aggregates at risk across the life span. Emphasis is placed on analyzing how nurses use epidemiology, community diagnoses, health planning, management, quality improvement, and nursing principles to deliver high-quality services in various community settings. Achieving the *Healthy People 2000* objectives is a major focus in Part Two.

As we approach the year 2000, *health care reform* is in the forefront of the public mind and is bringing with it many opportunities and challenges for community health nursing. To deal with these challenges nurses must become politically active and more deeply involved in research activities. They must also develop skills to handle management information systems and address the ethical dimension of their practice.

Unit Four

Community Assessment, Diagnosis, Organization, and Health-Planning Activities

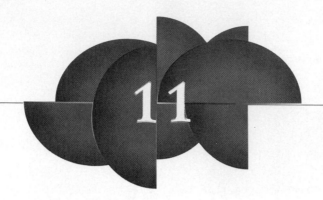

Concepts and Strategies of Epidemiology

OBJECTIVES

Upon completion of this chapter, the reader should be able to:

1. Define the term *epidemiology* and describe how the science of epidemiology has evolved over time.
2. Discuss the basic epidemiological concepts of populations at risk, natural life history of disease, levels of prevention, host-agent-environment relationships, multiple causation, and person-place-time relationships.
3. Summarize the steps of the epidemiological process.
4. Describe how the epidemiological process parallels the nursing process.
5. Discuss barriers to the epidemiological control of disease.
6. Differentiate between the common communicable diseases encountered by community health nurses in the practice setting.
7. Discuss epidemiology as it relates to chronic disease control.
8. Discuss the use of epidemiological concepts in community health nursing practice.
9. Explain the relevance of public health statistics to community health nursing practice.

A hound it was, an enormous coal black hound, but not such a hound as mortal eyes have ever seen. Fire burst from its open mouth, its eyes glowed with a smoldering glare, its muzzle and hackles and dewlap were outlined in flickering flames.

SIR ARTHUR CONAN DOYLE

The quote above is a description of the Hound of the Baskervilles, the object of Sir Arthur Conan Doyle's story based on an actual Devonshire legend and considered the greatest of all Holmesian tales. Sherlock Holmes used his brilliant powers of deduction and keen insight to find out why the demonic howl of this hound had brought fear to the Baskerville family. He was able, with his unique problem-solving abilities, to deduce that the howling of the hound was calculated to cause the death of the rightful heirs of the Baskerville fortune. The inheritance would thus fall into the hand of the bastard son of the villainous Hugo Baskerville.

Professionals in community health function very much like the great detective Sherlock Holmes to promote and protect the health of the community. They use an investigative problem-solving process to study the determinants of health and disease frequencies in populations and to plan and implement health promotion and disease control programs. These persons use knowledge, concepts, and methods of epidemiology to relate causative events (howl of the hound) to given occurrences (death) in order to identify at-risk aggregates (Baskerville heirs).

EPIDEMIOLOGY DEFINED

The word *epidemiology* derives from the Greek word *epidemic.* Literally translated, this means *epi,* "upon," *demos,* "people" (collectively). Historically the major focus of the epidemiologist was on analyzing major disease outbreaks (epidemics) so that ways to control and prevent disease occurrence in populations

We are indebted to Associate Professor Elizabeth Keller Beach and to Edna Jennings, friends and colleagues who helped both faculty and students to increase their understanding of the basic concepts of epidemiology and to recognize the value of applying these concepts in the clinical setting. Their support, assistance, and encouragement facilitated learning. Content and illustrations in this chapter reflect many of the ideas shared by them.

(people, collectively) could be determined. Today the definition of epidemiology has been expanded to include the study of variables that affect health, as well as those that influence disease and condition occurrence.

There are many variations in the definition of the term *epidemiology,* but the meanings are essentially the same. Throughout this chapter the following definition, adapted from MacMahon and Pugh's (1970, p. 1) classic writings, is used:

Epidemiology is the systematic, scientific study of the distribution patterns and determinants of health, disease and condition frequencies in populations, for the purpose of promoting wellness and preventing disease/conditions.

Implicit in this definition are two basic assumptions. The first is that patterns and frequencies of health, disease, and conditions in populations can be identified. The second is that factors determining or contributing to the occurrence of health, disease, or conditions can be discovered through systematic investigation.

Community health nurses use the epidemiological process to carry out their systematic investigation of health, disease, and conditions in populations. This process is graphically depicted in Figure 11-1 and is discussed in detail later in this chapter. Note that the epidemiological process shown in Figure 11-1 is similar to the nursing process. The steps are labeled differently but, in essence, they both involve a series of circular, dynamic problem-solving actions. Table 11-1 illustrates this point. Learning the language of epidemiology gives one a distinct advantage, however, because the terminology of epidemiology is used by all community health professionals; the terminology of the nursing process is not.

History and Scope of Epidemiology

Originally the major focus and scope of epidemiology and public health involved the control of epidemics caused by communicable diseases such as smallpox, plague, diphtheria, whooping cough, cholera, and scarlet fever. The primary goal was to limit the spread of disease and to prevent its recurrence. Although the scope of epidemiology has changed dramatically over time, communicable disease control remains a major priority worldwide. Communicable diseases are still not conquered and new ones such as AIDS are emerging.

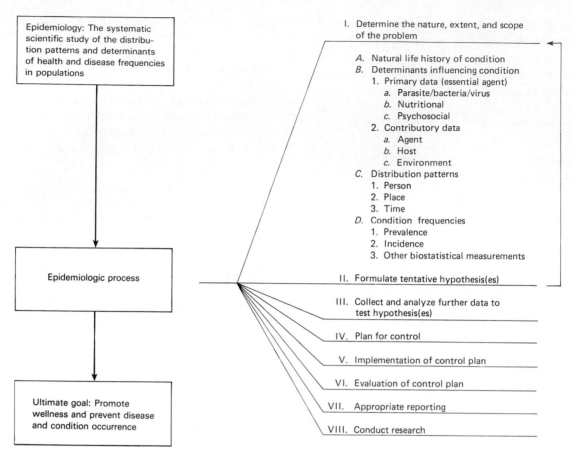

Figure 11-1   Graphical explanation of epidemiology.

Some of the most dramatic examples of communicable disease occurrence in epidemiological history happened when people who had not acquired natural or passive immunity came in contact with the disease. For example, scholars and scientists believe that the small band of Spaniards that conquered the Aztecs would not have been able to do so without the help of smallpox, which, when introduced into the Aztec community, reduced the community's ability to defend itself during war; that Captain Cook was able to make his Hawaiian conquests through the accidental transmission of measles; and that the introduction of diseases such as smallpox, scarlet fever, and tuberculosis made the American Indians vulnerable to conquest. The "Lost Colony," the Roanoke Island settlement founded in 1587 by Sir Walter Raleigh, mysteriously disappeared; many historians believe it succumbed to communicable disease. Lost in the mysterious disappearance was Virginia Dare, the first English child born in North America (Prescott, 1936; Woodward, 1932).

The 19th century brought about innovations that helped control communicable diseases such as the discoveries of Joseph Lister, a British surgeon who pioneered antiseptic surgery; Louis Pasteur, a French microbiologist who originated the germ theory of disease and developed pasteurization; and Robert Koch, a German medical scientist recognized as the father of microbiology. Koch developed pure cultures and discovered the tuberculosis, anthrax, and cholera bacilli, and in 1905 won a Nobel Peace Prize for his work in physiology. In the 20th century the development of elaborate health care technology, along with the discovery of "sulfa" drugs, penicillin, and vaccines, did much to aid in the prevention, control, and treatment of communicable disease.

TABLE 11-1 Comparison of the Nursing Process and the Epidemiological Process

Nursing process	Epidemiological process

Assessing (data collection to determine nature of client problems)	I. Determine the nature, extent, and scope of the problem
	  A. Natural life history of condition
	  B. Determinants influencing condition
	    1. Primary data (essential agent)
	      a. Parasite/bacterium/virus
	      b. Nutritional
	      c. Psychosocial
	    2. Contributory data
	      a. Agent
	      b. Host
	      c. Environment
	  C. Distribution patterns
	    1. Person
	    2. Place
	    3. Time
	  D. Condition frequencies
	    1. Prevalence
	    2. Incidence
	    3. Other biostatistical measurements

Analyzing (formulation of nursing diagnosis or hypothesis)	II. Formulate tentative hypothesis(es) III. Collect and analyze further data to test hypothesis(es)
Planning	IV. Plan for control
Implementing	V. Implement control plan
Evaluating	VI. Evaluate control plan
Revising or terminating	VII. Make appropriate report
Research	VIII. Conduct research

In 1917 the American Public Health Association published *Control of Communicable Diseases in Man.* That handbook is now in its 15th edition (Benenson, 1990) and is a worldwide classic on communicable disease. It should be included in every nurse's library.

Today the scope of epidemiology has broadened to include the study of chronic diseases and conditions in addition to psychosocial concerns and communicable diseases. In 1928, for example, New York City sent out "healthmobiles" to rid the city of one of its most dreaded diseases—diphtheria (refer to Figure 11-2). Today healthmobiles are still being used in many U.S. cities, but they are screening people for chronic conditions such as hypertension, glaucoma, cancer, and diabetes rather than for communicable disease.

Contemporary epidemiologists examine variables that keep people healthy. They analyze the etiology of chronic conditions, accidents, and other health-related phenomena such as child abuse, abortion, domestic violence, and communicable diseases including hepatitis B and AIDS. Epidemiologists are emphasizing the importance of studying *social,* as well as physical, factors that affect distributions of disease. Social epidemiologists investigate ways in which social conditions influence the likelihood that disease will develop. They focus attention on studying diseases and conditions—such as ulcers, heart disease, and alcoholism—that are influenced by social variables.

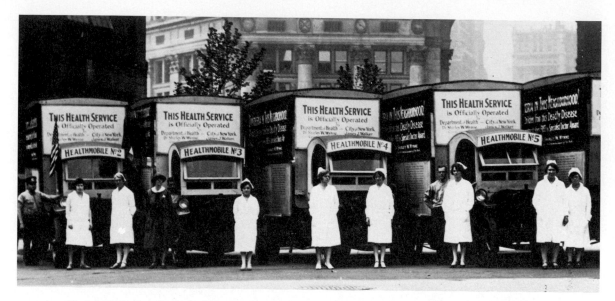

Figure 11-2 Death to diphtheria! Together with the able help of the visiting nurses, Mayor Jimmy Walker and Health Commissioner Hirley T. Wynne waged war on one of America's most dreaded diseases. This 1926 fleet of "healthmobiles" brought trained diphtheria detection teams to every hidden pocket of the city. (From Visiting Nurse Service of New York.)

EPIDEMIOLOGY AND THE COMMUNITY HEALTH NURSE

Effective implementation of the epidemiological process requires a multidisciplinary approach. Nurses, environmental engineers, physicians, laboratory technicians, statisticians, health officers, social workers, laypersons, and others all carry out necessary and essential roles in the investigation and control of disease and the promotion of wellness. Any health professional can and should function as a member of the epidemiological team.

Community health nurses participate on the epidemiological team in a variety of ways. Their contacts with families in the home and with groups in various settings (clinics, schools, and industry) put them in a unique position to carry out many epidemiological activities. They regularly become involved in case finding, health teaching, counseling, and follow-up essential to the prevention of communicable diseases, chronic conditions, and other health-related phenomena. Illustrative of this are the actions taken by the community health nurse in the following case situation to prevent the spread of a streptococcal infection and the occurrence of chronic complications.

▶ While visiting the Wills family, the community health nurse learned that Bobbie had a severe sore throat. Because Bobbie's symptoms were indicative of a streptococcal infection, the nurse stressed the significance of a proper medical evaluation to rule out or confirm a diagnosis of strep throat. The family followed through immediately. Bobbie's throat culture came back positive for streptococcal disease and he was treated with penicillin. The community health nurse, on a follow-up visit, taught the parents about the necessity of continuing the medication for 10 days even if Bobbie had no symptoms; she knew that a 10-day course of penicillin was needed to eliminate the streptococcal organisms. She also knew from theory and experience that if the organisms were not eliminated Bobbie could have serious chronic complications. By using her epidemiological knowledge, this nurse was able to effectively abort rheumatic fever, which can lead to a chronic heart condition or other chronic problems such as kidney disease.

In addition to the activities just described, community health nurses also use epidemiological concepts to carry out research in the community setting. A research team may carry out a study to survey major community needs (refer to Chapter 12) or to identify gaps in knowledge relative to disease causation, prevention, and control. A community health nurse's ongoing, comprehensive contact with the community and its resources allows her or him to make key contributions during these types of studies.

A community health nurse must apply the principles of epidemiology in order to provide preventive health services to aggregates in the community (refer to Chapter 2). The nurse must understand the significance of expanding epidemiological study to investigate health and disease in populations, as well as in individuals. Only in this way will the community health nurse effectively meet the health needs of the community as a whole.

BASIC CONCEPTS OF EPIDEMIOLOGY

To use the epidemiological process effectively, community health nurses need to have an understanding of the basic concepts, tools, and terms of epidemiology. Since epidemiology is operationally defined in terms of disease measurements, an understanding of the biostatistical concepts is essential. Biostatistics helps to describe the extent and distribution of health, illness, and conditions in the community and aids in the identification of specific health problems and community strengths. Biostatistics also facilitates the setting of priorities for program planning.

In addition to biostatistics, there are several basic concepts that guide epidemiological study. These are aggregates at risk, the natural life history of a disease, levels of prevention, host-agent-environment relationships, multiple causation, and person-place-time relationships. In general these concepts provide a foundation for explaining how disease develops and how health is maintained, who is most susceptible to disease, and how disease can be prevented and health promoted.

Study of Aggregates at Risk

A key concept of epidemiology is that the study of disease in populations is more significant than the study of individual cases of disease. Epidemiological research has demonstrated that using large sampling groups is essential for formulating valid conclusions about the distribution patterns and determinants of

health, disease, and condition frequencies in populations. It is by observing large groups that commonalities and differences among people who have or do not have a particular disease or condition can be identified.

The identification of commonalities and differences among groups focuses attention on the essential or contributory factors that produce illness or promote health. For example, it has been found repeatedly, through sampling of large groups, that people who smoke are more likely to develop coronary disease than people who do not smoke. This fact may never have been established if only individual cases had been examined, because some people who develop coronary disease do not smoke.

A preventive health philosophy has led professionals in community health to emphasize the study of groups. The goal of epidemiological study is to identify *aggregates at risk,* so that preventive health measures such as those presented in Table 11-2 can be used to stop the progression of disease or health-related phenomena. As previously defined in Chapter 2, aggregates at high risk are those who engage in certain activities or who have certain characteristics that increase their potential for contracting an illness, injury, or a health problem. For example, parents who were abused as children are at risk for abusing their own children. These activities or characteristics are known as *risk factors.*

Risk Factors

Risk factors are determined by a risk estimate process. Risk estimates are derived by comparing the frequency of deaths, illnesses, or injuries from a specific cause in a group having some specific trait or risk factor, with the frequency in another group not having that trait, or in the population as a whole (Surgeon General, 1979, volume I, p. 2). Risk factors fall under three major categories: (1) inherited biological characteristics; (2) physical, social, family, economic, and environmental factors; and (3) behavioral or lifestyle patterns. These risk factors increase susceptibility to death, illnesses, injuries, or psychosocial conditions. It has been shown, for instance, that "inherited biological characteristics can increase one's risk for some mental disorders, infectious diseases, and common chronic diseases such as certain cancers, heart disease, lung disease, and diabetes. Inherited characteristics also predispose individuals to conditions generally

TABLE 11-2 Epidemiology in Action: Health Measures Needed to Improve the Health of At-Risk Groups at Each Life Stage

Infants	Children	Adolescents and young adults	Adults	Elderly
Education for parenthood	Early comprehensive childhood development programs	Comprehensive injury prevention programs, including roadway safety	Public education about smoking, alcohol, good nutrition, and adequate exercise, including how poor health habits increase risk of disease	Work and social activity for retired persons
Genetic counseling	Special support services to aid families under stress (e.g., child abuse, low income, etc.)	Educational programs about smoking, alcohol, and drug use		Education about adequate exercise and nutrition
Good prenatal care				Preventive multiphasic screening programs
Sound prenatal nutritional guidance and services				
Counseling services to decrease adverse maternal habits that affect fetal development (e.g., smoking, drinking, drugs, exposure to radiation)	Injury reduction education	Nutrition and exercise guidance	Protection from environmental health habits	Education about proper use of medications
	Comprehensive pediatric care	Family planning services	Worksite health and safety programs	Immunizations for influenza
Amniocentesis	Immunizations	Sexually transmissible disease services including education, screening, and treatment	Hypertension prevention, screening, and control programs	Home safety programs
Breast feeding	Lead poisoning screening		Pap smears	Community and home services that facilitate independent living
Regular comprehensive care	Fluoridation of water supplies	Immunizations	Regular breast self-examination	
Immunizations	Dental care	Mental health	Education about cancer signs	
Social services including financial assistance, day care, improved foster and adoption programs, and counseling for families under stress	Nutritional and exercise guidance	Actions to reduce the availability of firearms	Mental health services	
	Education to prevent and eliminate dysfunctional health habits (smoking, alcohol use, drug use, unprotected sexual activity, poor dietary activity and exercise patterns)	Comprehensive violence prevention programs	Dental care	
Newborn screening and follow-up			Comprehensive violence prevention programs	

Data from Surgeon General: *Healthy people: the Surgeon General's report on health promotion and disease prevention*, vol II. Washington, D.C., 1979, U.S. Government Printing Office, pp. 149-155; USDHHS: *Healthy People 2000: national health promotion and disease prevention objectives, full report with commentary*, Washington, D.C., 1991, U.S. Government Printing Office, pp. 9-28.

recognized as inherited, like sickle cell anemia and hemophilia" (Surgeon General, volume I, p. 13).

Although heredity can increase the risk for the occurrence of disease or adverse health conditions, health problems usually result from multiple interacting factors. When these multiple risk factors come together they form an interrelated web of forces that increases their potential for causing harm.

Increasingly it is recognized that *environmental factors* and *lifestyle patterns* are crucial variables in the development of disease and adverse conditions. Many of the leading causes of death could be substantially reduced if persons at risk improved their lifestyle patterns of diet, smoking, exercise, alcohol consumption, and use of antihypertensive medication. It has been stated that approximately 20% of all premature deaths could be eliminated if environmental hazards were controlled (Surgeon General, 1979, vol. I). Anticipatory guidance at each stage across the lifespan can help individuals, families, and aggregates to develop lifestyle patterns that promote health and reduce the risk of disease and adverse health conditions. Table 11-2 summarizes the measures which assist clients at various life stages to improve their state of well-being.

In recent years the importance of socioeconomic and family environmental factors in the development of poor health and disease has been particularly stressed. It has been shown that "health disparities between poor people and those with higher incomes are almost universal for all dimensions of health. Poverty reduces a person's prospects for long life by increasing the chances of infant death, chronic disease and traumatic death; poverty is also associated with significant developmental limitations" (US-DHHS, 1991, *Healthy People 2000,* pp. 29-30). The disadvantaged experience more health risk because they often have inadequate income for good nutrition, safe housing, and adequate acute and preventive health care and are frequently exposed to more physical hazards in the environment (USDHHS, 1991, *Healthy People 2000* and Health status of minorities and low-income groups; Michigan Department of Public Health, 1987, 1988).

Chapters 14 through 19 discuss many health problems related to socioeconomic and family environmental factors such as accidents, child abuse, suicide, domestic violence, alcoholism, and nutritional problems. Appendix 11-2 discusses information about the thirteen most commonly acquired sexually transmitted diseases (STDs). STDs present major health risks for several segments of the population in the United States. Although the agents for STDs are known, we have been unable to control these diseases, and many are reaching epidemic proportions. The spread of STDs dramatically demonstrates that social determinants of disease cannot be ignored. Social situations and behavior patterns promote host exposure to STD agents.

Identifying aggregates at risk assists community health professionals to use available health resources effectively. It also aids in establishing priorities for the allocation of funds and the use of health work force time. In Table 22-1, "Priorities in Community Health Nursing," guidelines for determining priorities for community health nursing services are presented. These guidelines are based on the at-risk concept and the philosophy of prevention.

Natural Life History of Disease

In the search for commonalities that may produce disease and health-related phenomena in specific aggregates, epidemiological study focuses on determining the natural life history of these conditions. Observing the natural life history of disease and health-related phenomena aids in identifying agent-host-environmental factors that influence their development, characteristic signs and symptoms during their different periods of progression, and approaches to preventing and controlling their effects on humans.

In their classic textbook Leavell and Clark (1965, pp. 17-18) identified two distinct periods in the natural life history of any disease: *prepathogenesis* and *pathogenesis.* The combination of the processes involved in both of these stages is termed the *natural life history* of a disease or a condition. In the prepathogenesis period disease has not developed but interactions are occurring between the host, agent, and environment that produce disease stimulus and increase the host's potential for disease. The combination of high serum cholesterol levels and smoking, for example, increases the host's potential for developing coronary heart disease.

The pathogenesis period in the natural life history of disease begins when disease-producing stimuli (smoking or elevated serum cholesterol levels) start to produce changes in the tissues of humans (arteriosclerosis in the coronary vessels). Figure 11-3 shows the interrelationship between the prepathogenesis period and the pathogenesis period and how the latter

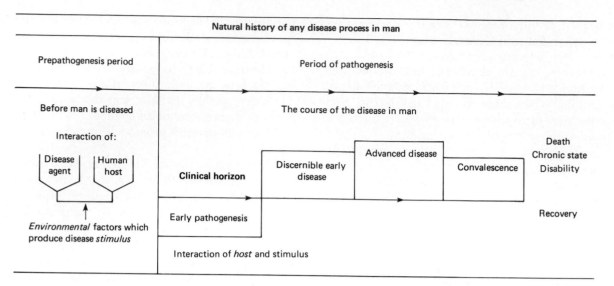

Figure 11-3 Prepathogenesis and pathogenesis periods of natural history. (From Leavell HR and Clark EG: *Preventive medicine for the doctor in his community: an epidemiologic approach,* New York, 1965, McGraw-Hill, p. 18.)

progresses from the presymptomatic stage to advanced, overt disease. It also shows that disease occurs as a result of processes that happen in the *environment*—prepathogenesis—and processes that happen in *humans*—pathogenesis (Leavell and Clark, 1965, p. 18).

Levels of Prevention

The study of the natural life history of disease facilitates the achievement of the ultimate goal of epidemiology—the development of effective methods of preventing and controlling disease or conditions in populations. By identifying significant host-agent-environment relationships that influence the progression of the natural life history of a condition, the epidemiologist can identify aggregates at risk and develop ways to prevent disease occurrence among them.

A continuum of preventive activities is essential for the promotion of health in any community. As previously discussed in Chapter 2, preventive activities can be grouped under three levels: *primary* (health promotion and specific protection), *secondary* (early diagnosis, prompt treatment, and disability limitation), and *tertiary* (rehabilitation). Figure 11-4 presents a schema illustrating how to apply these levels of prevention in

relation to the natural history of any disease. It implies that carrying out preventive activities during both the prepathogenesis and pathogenesis periods can alter the progression of a disease or a health problem. The degree to which preventive activities can be implemented will vary depending on the completeness of knowledge one has about the disease or health problem in question (Leavell and Clark, 1965, p. 20).

Host-Agent-Environment Relationships

When analyzing the natural life history of a disease or a condition and how to apply the three levels of prevention, epidemiological study focuses on the relationship of three variables: host, agent, and environment. These variables are defined as follows:

Agent: An animate or inanimate factor that must be present or lacking for a disease or a condition to occur

Host: Living species (humans or other animals) capable of being infected or affected by an agent

Environment: Everything external to a specific agent and host, including humans and animals

The interaction between host-agent-environment is frequently referred to as the *epidemiological triangle* (Figure 11-5). This triangle illustrates that it is the interactions (depicted by arrows in the model) among

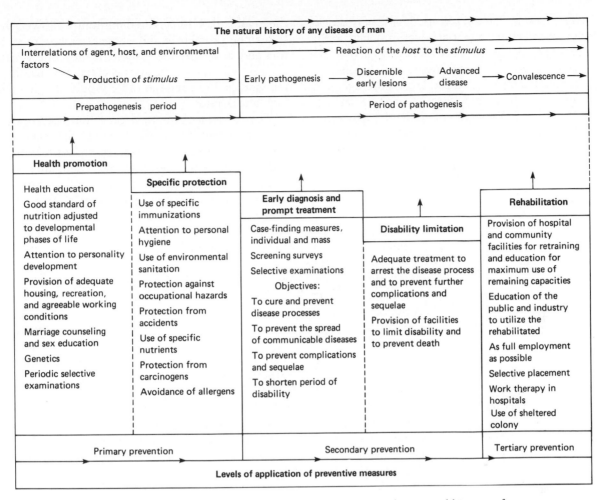

| The natural history of any disease of man | | |

Interrelations of agent, host, and environmental factors → Production of *stimulus* →	Reaction of the *host* to the *stimulus* →
	Early pathogenesis → Discernible early lesions → Advanced disease → Convalescence →
Prepathogenesis period	Period of pathogenesis

Health promotion

Health education

Good standard of nutrition adjusted to developmental phases of life

Attention to personality development

Provision of adequate housing, recreation, and agreeable working conditions

Marriage counseling and sex education

Genetics

Periodic selective examinations

Specific protection

Use of specific immunizations

Attention to personal hygiene

Use of environmental sanitation

Protection against occupational hazards

Protection from accidents

Use of specific nutrients

Protection from carcinogens

Avoidance of allergens

Early diagnosis and prompt treatment

Case-finding measures, individual and mass

Screening surveys

Selective examinations

Objectives:

To cure and prevent disease processes

To prevent the spread of communicable diseases

To prevent complications and sequelae

To shorten period of disability

Disability limitation

Adequate treatment to arrest the disease process and to prevent further complications and sequelae

Provision of facilities to limit disability and to prevent death

Rehabilitation

Provision of hospital and community facilities for retraining and education for maximum use of remaining capacities

Education of the public and industry to utilize the rehabilitated

As full employment as possible

Selective placement

Work therapy in hospitals

Use of sheltered colony

| Primary prevention | Secondary prevention | Tertiary prevention |

Levels of application of preventive measures

Figure 11-4 Levels of application of preventive measures in the natural history of disease. (From Leavell HR and Clark EG: *Preventive medicine for the doctor in his community: an epidemiologic approach,* New York, 1965, McGraw-Hill, p. 21.)

these variables that determine whether there is health or disease/conditions in a community. Health is maintained when the host-agent-environment variables are in a state of equilibrium. Disease or conditions occur when there is a change in any one of the three variables that disturbs the state of equilibrium.

Agents are biological, chemical, or physical and include bacteria, viruses, fungi, pesticides, food additives, ionizing radiation, and speeding objects. The normal habitat in which an infectious (biological) agent lives, multiples, and/or grows is called a *reservoir.* These habitats include humans, animals, and the environment. The capacity of an infectious agent to infect *(infectivity)* and to produce subsequent disease *(patho-*

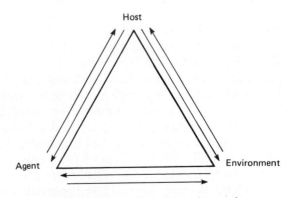

Figure 11-5 Epidemiological triangle.

genicity) is variable. The *virulence* or degree of pathogenicity of an infectious agent also varies (CDC, 1987, Principles of epidemiology: disease, pp. 5-7).

A wide variety of characteristics are classified as host factors. Examples of these factors are age, sex, ethnic group, socioeconomic status, lifestyle, and heredity (CDC, 1987, Principles of epidemiology: agent, p. 5). Four types of environment factors—physical, social, economic, and family—are elaborated on in a later section of this chapter and in Chapter 6.

Multiple Causation

The theory of multiple causation of disease illustrates and confirms that it is the interactions and relationships between host-agent-environment that actually cause a disease or condition—*not* host, agent, or environmental factors alone. The theory of multiple causation is critical to epidemiology. It is only natural to assume that the introduction of a disease agent (e.g., influenza virus) into a community is enough to cause illness among its members. However, in addition to this causative agent there must be a susceptible host and an environment conducive to the interaction of agent and host. Factors such as the level of immunity in the population, individual susceptibility, availability of vectors, and the amount of contact between members of the population will affect disease/condition occurrence. The following example of an influenza outbreak illustrates how these factors influence disease occurrence.

An influenza outbreak that occurred in the United States demonstrates the concept of multiple causation. The agent, the influenza virus A/USSR, was introduced into the population. Outbreaks of this disease occurred in groups of young adults and children in environments of close contact: schools, colleges, and military training camps. Attack rates in these areas were high, ranging from 40% to 70% in most cases. The disease did not usually appear in adults over 25 years of age.

An analysis of this situation illustrates that the proper combination of multiple factors is necessary before disease will result. Outbreaks occurred in young adults and children because there was a virulent agent, susceptible hosts who lacked immunity, and crowded environmental conditions that supported the spread of the agent. The disease usually did not occur in those over 25 because they had been exposed to this virus earlier and had developed acquired immunity to

the organism. This acquired immunity allowed them to maintain a balance in host-agent-environment factors and to escape the disease. If only one variable, such as a virulent agent, was necessary to cause illness, individuals 25 years and older would also have had high attack rates.

The concept of multiple causation becomes even more apparent when one studies the natural life history of noninfectious diseases, chronic conditions, and health-related phenomena. Friedman's (1974, p. 5) classic diagram of the web of causation for myocardial infarction (Figure 11-6) clearly demonstrates that it is the interplay between multiple host-agent-environment characteristics that causes a chronic condition.

Person-Place-Time Relationships

The study of relationships is necessary for the community health professional to formulate valid hypotheses about disease or condition causation. Identification of measurable variables that can facilitate rapid and efficient data collection is essential to this study. In epidemiological study the variables found to be most useful are *person* (who is affected), *place* (where affected), and *time* (when affected). Some of the most frequently analyzed characteristics of these variables are presented in Table 11-3.

Timing is a critical factor in disease diagnosis and control. Immediate reporting of a disease outbreak is crucial since the validity of data is often directly proportional to the time lapse incurred in obtaining the information. If a significant amount of time is lost in reporting, the ability to formulate valid hypotheses is decreased.

When monitoring incidence of infectious disease, the terms used to distinguish relative frequency in time and space include the following:

Sporadic: Presence of occasional cases of the event apparently unrelated in time or space

Endemic: Constant long-term presence of an event at about the frequency expected from the past history of the community

Epidemic: Presence of the event at a much higher frequency than expected from the past history of the community, usually over a short period of time (for example, one case of cholera would be labeled epidemic in a U.S. community; on the other hand, in some foreign countries, several

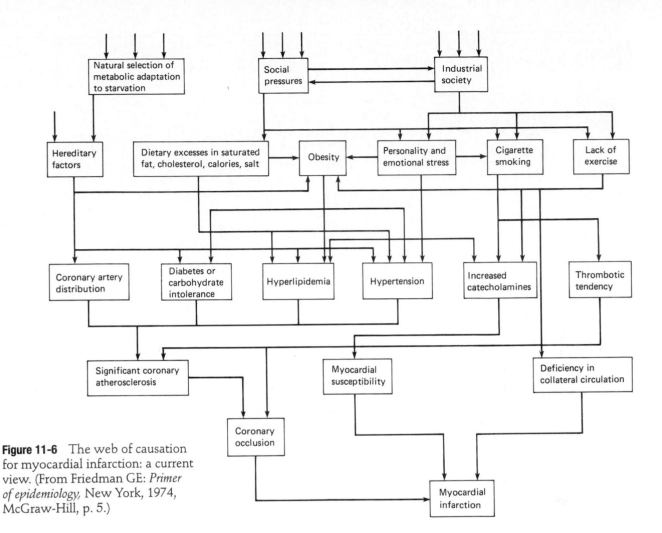

Figure 11-6 The web of causation for myocardial infarction: a current view. (From Friedman GE: *Primer of epidemiology,* New York, 1974, McGraw-Hill, p. 5.)

cases of cholera would be considered an endemic occurrence).

Pandemic: Presence of an event in epidemic proportions, involving many communities and countries in a relatively short period of time.

When the nurse monitors any disease or condition it is important to remember that there are wide variations in the degree of symptoms. These variations range from inapparent infection to severe, pronounced symptomatology. Manifestations of infectious disease relate to the disease progression process or stages of infection (refer to Figure 11-7). The duration of each stage identified in Figure 11-7 and the potential outcomes vary considerably, depending on the infecting agent and host factors (Grimes, 1991, p. 19). Benenson (1990), in his book *Control of Communicable Diseases in Man,* summarizes significant informa-

tion about the stages of infection for the major infectious diseases in the world.

It is the inapparent, or *subclinical,* symptoms that are the most significant in terms of disease transmission or occurrence. If efforts to prevent transmission or progression of a disease or a condition are limited to people with clinical manifestations, a very large proportion of the problem will be missed. The iceberg analogy is frequently used to illustrate the importance of identifying individuals with subclinical symptoms during an epidemiological study. Most of the iceberg, as illustrated in Figure 11-8, is submerged. This unseen section is the most insidious and potentially dangerous portion because often the seafarer takes no action to avoid it. Individuals with subclinical infections or symptoms, like the submerged portion of the iceberg, present the most danger because they do not have

TABLE 11-3 Epidemiological Variables

Variable	Characteristics
Person: delineation of group involved	• Age, sex, race distribution • Socioeconomic status, occupation, education • Health habits and behaviors or lifestyle • Acquired resistance and susceptibility • Health history—natural resistance, hereditary characteristics
Place: geographical distribution in subdivisions of the area affected	• *Physical environment:* weather; climate; geography; radiation; vibration; noise; pressure; animal reservoirs; pollutants; housing facilities; workplace hazards; and sources of air, water, and food contamination • *Social environment:* population density and mobility; community groups; occupations and other roles; beliefs and attitudes; technological developments; transportation; educational practices; and health care delivery system • *Economic environment:* source of income; income level; employment status; job frustrations; and income for nutrition, housing, and other basic needs • *Family environment:* family history; family dynamics; strategies used to handle stress; type, number, and timing of major life changes; home atmosphere; and family health and cultural patterns (refer to Chapters 7 and 8)
Time: chronological distribution of onsets of cases by days, weeks, months	• *Incubation period:* determine life cycle; factors affecting multiplication and virulence of organism • Seasonal trends • Onset of event • Duration of event

Data from MacMahon B and Pugh T: *Epidemiology principles and methods,* Boston, 1970, Little, Brown, pp. 31-32; Surgeon General: *Healthy people: the Surgeon General's report on health promotion and disease prevention,* vol I, Washington, D.C., 1979, U.S. Government Printing Office, pp. 13-14; Centers for Disease Control, Training and Laboratory Program Office: *Principles of epidemiology: agent, host, environment* (self-study course 3030-G, manual 1), Atlanta, Ga., 1987, The Centers, pp. 12-30.

obvious symptoms and are less likely to use preventive measures. An example of this is a female client who has asymptomatic gonorrhea. This person frequently transmits gonorrhea for a considerable length of time before it is known that she has the disease.

Psychosocial phenomena such as substance abuse and domestic violence tend to remain submerged much longer than infectious diseases because the symptoms are not recognized and/or acknowledged. Increasingly it is being recognized that these problems are far more prevalent than statistics reflect. Communities are beginning to conduct epidemiological investigations in order to determine the real magnitude of these problems.

MEASUREMENT OF EPIDEMIOLOGICAL EVENTS

As previously discussed, the relative frequency of an event in time and space is important to monitor to determine health and disease patterns in a community. A variety of methods are used to collect data about these patterns and to identify aggregates at risk in a population. These methods are discussed in Chapter 12 and include such interventions as analyzing all available statistics, carrying out surveys, and interviewing key community informants. Basic statistical concepts used in epidemiology will be emphasized in this chapter. Statistical data helps health professionals to make comparisons over time and between different populations.

In community health several terms are used to describe health or health-related data. These are biostatistics, vital statistics, demographic statistics, and morbidity and mortality statistics.

Biostatistics is the overall broad term used to identify any data that delineate health or health-related events. Health statistics that describe birth, adoption, death, marriage, divorce, separation, and annulment patterns

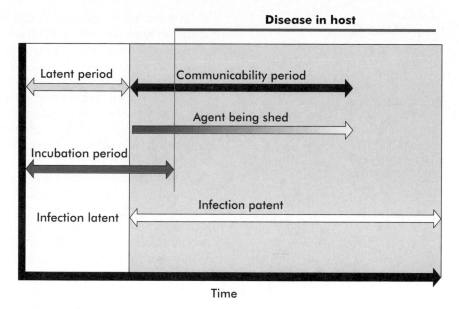

Figure 11-7   Stages of infection. Infection in the host proceeds in identifiable stages; the length of each stage varies with the pathogenic agent and host factors. The **latent period** begins with pathogenic invasion of the body and ends when the agent can be shed (communicability period). The **incubation period** begins with invasion of the agent, during which the organism reproduces, and ends when the disease process begins. The **communicability period** begins when the latent period ends and continues as long as the agent is present. The disease period follows the incubation period and ends at variable times. This stage may be subclinical or produce overt symptoms, and it may resolve completely or become latent. (Redrawn from Grimes DE: *Infectious diseases,* St. Louis, 1991, Mosby, p. 19.)

are labeled *vital statistics.* Because these events must be registered in each state, trends can be ascertained within each state and the country as a whole. Usually at least 5 years' data should be examined to see if significant patterns are occurring over time. Monitoring these significant changes helps the community health nurse to identify health promotion activities needed across the lifespan. For example, major causes of death for each developmental age group (refer to Chapters 14 through 19) are calculated from death registries each year. These death rates assist the health professional in determining key community health problems and in substantiating a need for specific health programs or further epidemiological investigation. The development of programs to prevent accidents and the establishment of screening clinics to identify at-risk persons for hypertension are examples of health activities that have been initiated to reduce the number of preventable deaths in the United States.

Data related to the analysis of death trends are classified as *mortality statistics.*

Infant and maternal death rates or mortality statistics have traditionally been used in community health to make judgments about the health status of a community. Deaths in these two population groups are considered to be preventable and are often associated with poor environmental conditions and inadequate health care. Thus, they may reflect not only unmet health needs but also deficiencies in the health care delivery system which need to be corrected.

Demographic statistics also aid the practitioner in identifying significant characteristics of a population, such as socioeconomic status, which influence the delivery of health care services in a community. Demographic data describe the number, characteristics, and distribution of people in a given area and changes in the population over time. These data are

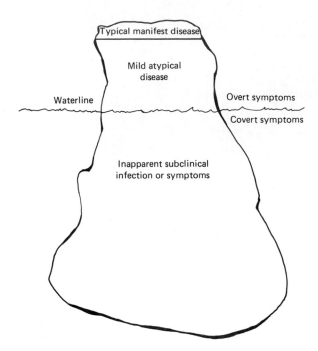

Figure 11-8 Comparison of inapparent infection to an iceberg. (Modified from Beach EK: *Environmental health and communicable disease module,* Ann Arbor, Mich., 1974, The University of Michigan, School of Nursing— Community Health Nursing, p. 183.)

collected by censuses, special surveys, and registration systems (Duncan, 1988). Vital statistics are collected by state registration systems. Special surveys are conducted by local, state, and federal government agencies, voluntary organizations, and private agencies and institutions. Special surveys are carried out to monitor current health problems, attitudes about health issues, or the health status of specific population groups. For example, the University of Michigan's Institute for Social Research annually surveys high school seniors and young adults to determine the prevalence, trends, and attitudes about drug use in this population group. This epidemiological research provides a foundation for determining service programming needs.

Census data provide a wealth of information about a community's population characteristics. Census tracts and census blocks have been established and maintained throughout the country so that social and economic changes can be easily identified from one census to another. For the 1990 census the census tract was a key geographical statistical unit (Robey, 1989).

Census tracts are small areas in large cities that have a population between 3000 to 6000 and fairly homogeneous characteristics with respect to ethnic origin and socioeconomic composition (Mausner and Kramer, 1985). Census blocks are similar to census tracts but are located almost exclusively in nonmetropolitan areas (Robey, 1989). Census tracts and census block boundaries are preserved from one national census to another so that variations in population characteristics can be studied over time.

The first national census was conducted in August 1790; a census has been completed every decade since, for several reasons. Census data are used to establish the number of representatives per state in the House of Representatives. These data are also used when revenue-sharing and other federal and state funds are allocated. In addition, census data assist marketing studies; academic research; federal, state, and local planning; affirmative action programs; and many other demographic, statistical, and epidemiological activities (Robey, 1989).

Similar types of data are collected from one census to another so that trends over time can be analyzed. Some data (e.g., sex, race, age, name, address, marital status, and relationship to head of household) are collected from 100% of the enumerated population. More extensive information such as income, education, housing, and occupation are collected from a sample of the population (National Center for Health Statistics, Health, United States, 1989, p. 194). Although no census has been 100% accurate, extensive efforts are made to reach the greater proportion of the nation's population, including disadvantaged populations such as the homeless. It is, however, more difficult to reach the poor and alienated because they are harder to locate (Robey, 1989). In spite of this limitation, census data are extremely valuable.

Health professionals analyze census data because a significant relationship has been documented between educational background, economic status, and living conditions and the number of health needs in specified populations (USDHHS, 1991, *Healthy People 2000*). This information can be obtained at a nominal cost from the United States Bureau of the Census, Washington, D.C.

In addition to vital and demographic statistics, the community health nurse uses morbidity statistics to assess the health status of the community. *Morbidity data* describe the extent and distribution of illness in a community. These data assist the nurse in identifying specific health problems and in setting priorities for program planning. One midwestern community, for example, used morbidity statistics to support the need for a neighborhood health clinic in one of their inner-city districts. A comprehensive analysis of these statistics revealed that 52% of all new tuberculosis cases, 61% of all new syphilis cases, 72% of all new gonorrhea cases, and 37% of all accidental poisoning cases occurred in one particular section of the city in a given time period. It was evident from this information that the health needs in this district were much greater than in other sections of the city. Special funds were allocated to determine if a new approach to delivering health services could alter the disease trends in this area; significant positive changes were noted within a 3-year time frame. Because morbidity statistics were collected before and during the time the clinic was in existence, state legislators responded favorably to a request for additional funds to keep the clinic open. Health professionals in this situation had documented the need for and the effectiveness of their pilot health clinic. The use of statistics helped these health professionals to establish a neighborhood health center and to keep the center functioning after the trial period.

How to Use Statistical Data*

Usually community health professionals express absolute numbers or actual counts in terms of relative numbers. This is done because relative numbers make it easier to compare results in populations of differing sizes or to visualize what proportion of a given population is affected by a given phenomenon. A *relative number* is one that shows a relationship between two absolute numbers; this relationship is expressed in terms of a round number. A *percentage* is an example of a relative number; 100 is the round number used to show relationships when percentages are calculated.

The value of using relative numbers becomes clearer when the nurse actually works with raw data. For example, stating that 45 teenagers in a mental health institution need foster home placement has very little meaning until this number is related to the total number of teenagers in the institution. If there are only 100 teenagers in this setting, then 45 is a signifi-

*Handout materials distributed by the community health nursing faculty at Michigan State University, East Lansing, Michigan, provided the framework for this section.

cant proportion (45%) of this given population. If, on the other hand, there are 1000 teenagers in this environment, 45 is a relatively small proportion (4.5%) of the total population. The percentages are identified by relating 45 (absolute number) to 100 or 1000 (absolute numbers) and then multiplying the results by 100 (round number).

Raw data from populations of differing sizes cannot be compared unless absolute numbers are converted to relative numbers. For instance, knowing the number of students who received free lunches in 1993 in each school in the county becomes relevant only when one summarizes the percentage of children in each school who received free lunches. The following figures illustrate how deceptive absolute numbers can be when making comparisons from one population to another; even though the number of children (250 vs. 75) receiving free lunches is much higher in the Burns Park High School, the proportion of children needing free lunches in Kent Elementary School is two times greater than the proportion of children needing free lunches in Burns Park High School:

$$\frac{75}{150} \times 100 = 50\% \text{ of the children in Kent Elementary}$$
$$\text{School received free lunches in 1993}$$

$$\frac{250}{1000} \times 100 = 25\% \text{ of the children in Burns Park High}$$
$$\text{School received free lunches in 1993}$$

Besides percentages, two other relative numbers—ratios and rates—are commonly used to analyze health or health-related events. A *ratio* expresses the size of one number in relation to the size of another number. The number of females to males (sex ratio) and per capita expenditure for health care in a given state are examples of ratios. Per capita ratios are obtained by dividing the amount of money spent for health care (event) by the population in a given state (population).

A *rate* is actually a ratio with the additional features of expressing what has happened in terms of a certain unit of time and the population at risk for a given event. It delineates the relationship between the number of times an event has occurred to the size of the population at risk. In demographic and epidemiological study, the unit of time for a rate is usually a year unless otherwise stated.

The formula for a rate is given as follows:

$$\frac{\text{event in a given time}}{\text{pop. at risk in same time period}} \times \text{round no.}$$

The *event* in this formula is the number of times a phenomenon (births, deaths, or disease) has occurred. The *population* is usually the number of persons at risk for a given event. The round number is one that makes the rate above the value of 1. If, for instance, an event such as polio occurs infrequently within a large population at risk, the round number used would be 100,000. On the other hand, when an event such as death occurs frequently within a population at risk, the round number used would be 1000.

Following are examples of how to apply the rate formula. Note particularly the population at risk, which varies depending on the nature of the event. When morbidity rates (incidence and prevalence) are calculated, the total population of the community may be at risk. In determining infant mortality rates, only infants born within a certain time period are at risk.

Incidence Rate

The incidence rate is the number of *new* cases of a disease in a population over a period of time.

Incidence rate = number of "new" cases of a specified disease or condition occurring during a given time period (as during a year) ÷ population at risk during a given time period × 100,000

Bay City, January through December 1993, 50 new cases of diabetes in a population of 75,000.

$$\text{Incidence rate} = \frac{50}{75,000} \times 100,000 = 66.66$$

Incidence rate for diabetes in Bay City 1993: 66.66 new cases of diabetes per 100,000 population.

Prevalence Rate

The prevalence rate is the number of *old* and *new* cases of a specified disease existing at a given time.

Prevalence rate = number of "old *and* new" cases of a specified disease or condition existing at a point ÷ total population at a point × 100,000

Bay City, December 1993, 1200 cases of diabetes in a population of 75,000.

$$\text{Prevalence rate} = \frac{1200}{75,000} \times 100,000 = 1600$$

Prevalence rate for diabetes in Bay City, December 1993: 1600 cases of diabetes per 100,000 population.

Infant Mortality Rate

The infant mortality rate is the number of deaths of infants under 1 year of age per 1000 live births during a given year.

Infant mortality rate = number of deaths under 1 year of age during a given year ÷ number of live births during a given year × 1000 live births

Bay City, 1993, 25 infant deaths.

$$\text{Infant mortality rate} = \frac{25}{1275} \times 1000 = 19.6$$

Infant mortality rate Bay City 1993: 19.6 infant deaths per 1000 live births.

Frequently Calculated Rates and Ratios

In addition to the previous examples several other rates and ratios are used to measure the state of health in a community. The formulas for calculating rates and ratios frequently used in community health nursing practices are presented in Table 11-4. Besides helping to identify the major health problems in a community, these statistics aid in projecting future health service and personnel needs. For example, examining the crude birth rate assists health care professionals in determining the demand for childhood health services over the next 20 years.

Rates, ratios, or percentages are the types of descriptive statistics most commonly used in community health nursing practice. At times, however, there is a need to use other descriptive measures, such as averages, in order to organize and characterize data. This is so when a series of measurements or quantitative data is being analyzed. Generally, in any series of data characteristic values tend to cluster near the center of the distribution. Thus averages are often labeled measures of central tendency.

Measures of Central Tendency

Averages help to identify a value that is most characteristic of a set of raw data. There are several kinds of averages used to summarize quantitative measurements; the most frequently used ones in community health nursing practice are the arithmetic mean, the median, and the mode.

The *mean* is the arithmetic average of a set of observations. It is the value in a series of data equiva-

TABLE 11-4 Formulas for Rates and Ratios Frequently Calculated in Community Health Nursing Practice

Rate or ratio	Formula	Commonly used round number
Mortality Statistics		
Crude death rate	Number of deaths from all causes during a given year ÷ population estimated at midyear	× 1000 population
Age-specific death rate	Number of deaths for a specified age group during a given year ÷ population estimated at midyear for the specified age group	× 1000 population
Cause-specific death rate	Number of deaths from a specific condition during a given year ÷ population estimated at midyear	× 100,000 population
Maternal mortality rate	Number of deaths from puerperal complications during a given year ÷ number of live births during the same year	× 100,000 live births
Infant mortality rate	Number of deaths under 1 year of age during a given year ÷ number of live births during the same year	× 1000 live births
Neonatal mortality rate	Number of deaths under 28 days of age during a given year ÷ number of live births during the same year	× 1000 live births
Fetal mortality rate	Number of fetal deaths 20 weeks gestation or more during a given year ÷ number of live births and fetal deaths during the same year	× 1000 live births and fetal deaths
Birth-death ratio	Number of live births in a specified population ÷ number of deaths in a specified population	× 100
Case fatality ratio	Number of deaths from specified disease or condition ÷ number of reported cases of the specified disease or condition	× 100
Morbidity Statistics		
Incidence rate	Number of "new" cases of a specified disease or condition occurring during a given time period ÷ population at risk during the same time period	× 100,000 population
Prevalence rate	Number of "old" and "new" cases of specified disease or condition existing at a point ÷ total population at a point	× 100,000 population
Vital and Demographic Statistics Other Than Mortality		
Crude birth rate	Number of live births during a given year ÷ population estimated at midyear	× 1000 population
General fertility rate	Number of live births during a given year ÷ population estimated at midyear for females ages 15-44 during the same year	× 1000 female population (15-44 years old)
General marriage rate	Number of marriages during a given year ÷ number of persons 15 years of age and over in the population in the same year	× 1000 persons 15 years of age and over
General divorce rate	Number of divorces during a given year ÷ persons 15 years of age and over in the population in the same year	× 1000 persons 15 years of age and over
Dependency ratio	Persons under 20 years of age and persons 65 years and over ÷ total population ages 20-64	× 100

lent to the sum of the measurements divided by the number of measurements. The formula for calculating the mean is:

$$\text{Arithmetic mean} = \frac{\text{sum of measurements}}{\text{no. of measurements}}$$

A community health nurse who wanted to determine the average weight of children in a second grade classroom would compute the average or mean as follows:

Weight of children in pounds: 51.2, 53.1, 55, 54, 53, 47.5, 48.8, 52.9, 50.5, 51.5, 53, 49.5, 53, 55.1, 49.9

Sum of measurement = 778.3 or 778

Number of measurements = 15

Mean weight = 51.9

$$\text{Arithmetic mean} = \frac{778}{15} = 51.86 \text{ or } 51.9$$

Knowing the mean or "average" value of a series of measurements helps the community health nurse to identify quickly persons who may have health needs or who are at risk for health problems in the future. Persons who fall far below or far above the average should be comprehensively assessed to determine why this is happening.

The *median* is the "middle" value in a series of quantitative data that divides the measurements into two equal parts. That is, 50% of the measurements are less than and 50% are greater than the median value. To calculate the median, the measurements in the distribution must be arranged in order of size. Referring again to the children in the second grade classroom, the median weight of these children would be determined by putting all of their weights in numerical order so that the middle value can be identified. This is illustrated below:

47.5, 48.8, 49.5, 49.9, 50.5, 51.2, 51.5, **52.9** (median), 53, 53, 53 (mode), 53.1, 54, 55, 55.1

The median is 52.9, or the eighth measurement, because 50% of the measurements are less than this value and 50% are greater than this value. If there had been an even number of measurements, the median would be found by dividing the sum of the two middle measurements by two, which is illustrated here.

48.8, 49.5, 49.9, 50.5, 51.2, 51.5, **52.9, 53,** 53, 53, 53.1, 54, 55, 55.1

Middle measurements = $(52.9 + 53.0) \div 2 =$
52.95 (median)

The median is usually computed when there are very high or very low extremes in a series of measurements, because the mean is distorted by very high or low values but the median is not. When census tract data are reported, for instance, median income is usually given because there is such a great variation in family income, ranging from below poverty level to over $50,000. Generally, however, the mean is the most frequently used measure of central tendency in community health practice because it takes into account all measurements in a series and is the most stable.

The *mode* is the measurement that appears most frequently in a series of quantitative data. It is identified by counting the number of times a particular value appears. The measurements do not have to be ordered. Fifty-three pounds is the mode or typical value of the weights of our second-grade classroom children because it occurred more frequently than any other weight. The mode is helpful when one wants to identify an average value very quickly. It is only an estimate, however, and not too reliable; other measurements of central tendencies should be used when refining data analysis.

Relative numbers, including rates, ratios, percentages, and measures of central tendency are computed so that comparisons of health experiences between populations can be made. "All epidemiology depends on comparisons" (Last, 1986, p. 11).

EPIDEMIOLOGICAL PROCESS AND INVESTIGATION

Basic concepts in epidemiology have been discussed to lay a foundation for epidemiological investigation of community health problems. These concepts aid in identifying variables to consider when describing the distribution patterns and determinants of health, disease, and condition frequencies in populations. They help to analyze causal relationships in disease or condition outbreaks. To establish these causal relationships, health professionals use a scientific process known as the epidemiological process.

The *epidemiological process* is a systematic course of action taken to identify (1) who is affected (persons); (2) where the affected persons reside (place); (3)

when the persons were affected (time); (4) causal factors of health and disease occurrence (host-agent-environment determinants); (5) prevalence and incidence of health and disease (frequencies); and (6) prevention and control measures (levels of prevention) in relation to the natural life history of a disease or a condition.

The epidemiological process has eight basic steps, which are graphically illustrated in Figure 11-1. Although each step is discussed separately, it is important to remember that these steps may overlap and may not always follow a sequential pattern. They are interrelated and dependent on each other. For example, data collected in the initial step provide a foundation for all subsequent steps.

Step I: Determine the Nature, Extent, and Possible Significance of the Problem

The primary responsibilities during this initial step are twofold: (1) to verify the diagnosis by data collection from multiple sources, and (2) to determine the extent and possible significance of the verified problem. Data gathering begins when an index case is reported or when there is a noticeable change in the incidence rate for a particular disease or condition. The *index case* is the case that brings a household or other group to the attention of community health personnel. Once this case is known to health professionals, data are collected from a variety of sources in order to determine if a problem really exists.

Clinical observations, laboratory studies, and lay reporting assist the epidemiological team in confirming the homogeneity of the current events. If, for instance, four hospital emergency rooms have reported that several individuals were treated for food poisoning in the last 24 hours, health personnel would want to immediately take the following actions:

1. Interview the affected persons to determine the nature of their symptoms and to identify loci of origin according to person, place, and time.
2. Review laboratory studies to confirm a common causative organism. This process could establish that there are several events occurring at the same time.
3. Interview friends, relatives, and lay acquaintances to discern their description of the

events that led up to the reported illness and to determine if other individuals have symptoms.

It is important to remember that timely, accurate and thorough data collection are critical factors in Step I. Significant data may be destroyed if the data collection process is too slow. In addition, if only the "tip of the iceberg" or the most obvious events are observed, the extent of the problem will not be identified. The health professional needs to be like a detective, beginning by interviewing the affected individual and then branching out into this individual's environment to track down the host-agent-environment factors that influence disease occurrence. As previously discussed, the measurable variables that facilitate rapid and efficient data collection about host-agent-environment factors are person, place, and time.

Analyzing data in terms of person, place, and time helps to establish the magnitude of the problem. Data tell the health professional the proportion of the people affected, the seriousness of the effects on the host and the community, improvement or regression over time, and geographical distribution of the disease or condition. They also help in identifying potential sources of infection and causal relationships.

The use of spot maps (refer to "Analysis of All Available Data" in Chapter 12) facilitates pinpointing the exact geographical location of the disease or condition. This type of map vividly and visually portrays an epidemiological problem very rapidly. If it is used on a regular basis, health personnel can compare current prevalence and incidence with the expected rates and can identify significant departures from normal. As was discussed previously, *incidence* is the number of new cases of a disease in a population over a period of time (cases just starting). *Prevalence* is the number of old and new cases of a specific disease at a given time.

When comparing prevalence and incidence rates, a word of caution is necessary. If there is a distinct departure from normal, it must be ascertained that a problem really exists. It may be that there is only an improvement in reporting, not an actual increase in disease occurrence.

If there has been an actual increase in the incidence of a particular disease or condition, the health professional makes an educated guess as to the nature of the causative agent, based upon the data collected. This formulation of a tentative diagnosis or hypothesis is done in order to enhance further data collection.

Step II: Formulate Tentative Hypothesis(es)

When dealing with infectious diseases a rapid preliminary analysis of data is imperative. This is essential because infectious diseases can spread quickly, can affect a large number of people in a short period of time, and can have great ranges in severity. Usually this analysis results in the formulation of several hypotheses. Explanation of the most probable source of infection is made in terms of (1) the agent causing the problem; (2) the source of infection, including the chain of events leading to the outbreak of the problem; and (3) environmental conditions that allowed it to occur. Tentative hypotheses must be tested and may be found to be inappropriate. Laboratory tests are invaluable in validating hypotheses. An example of how tentative hypotheses are established is provided in the following situation.

▶ **From September 5-8, 1974, the "World's Largest American Indian Fair" was held near Gallup, New Mexico (Horwitz, Pollard, Merson, and Martin, 1977, pp. 1071-1076). An estimated 80,000 persons attended the fair. Beginning on September 6, 1974, and during the next few days, several hundred people with gastrointestinal symptoms sought attention at two hospitals near Gallup. Over 130 of them had stool cultures positive for a *Salmonella* group C organism, *Salmonella newport*. The hospitals immediately reported the apparent outbreak to the health department. Preliminary tentative hypotheses indicated that either the community water supply of the area or food served at a free barbeque that attracted thousands on September 5, 1974, was the vehicle of transmission for the agent *Salmonella newport*. Evidence favoring a water source included a broken water pipe at the fair grounds in an area soiled with animal feces. The barbeque was suspected because food preparation practices were reportedly improper and those who attended the barbeque appeared to have a high illness attack rate.**

Since two possible sources of infection were favored in this situation, health personnel took immediate steps to correct both problem situations and collected and analyzed further data to determine the exact cause of the *Salmonella* outbreak.

Waiting until all data are collected before instituting control measures can amplify the magnitude of the problem. A health professional must be willing to take risks while carrying out an epidemiological investigation.

Step III: Collect and Analyze Further Data to Test Hypothesis(es)

A basic starting point in this step is to identify the group selected for attack by the disease or problem under investigation. Individual epidemiological health histories should be done to classify persons according to their exposure to suspected or causative agents and to identify the clinical data and bacteriological findings needed to substantiate the diagnosis. Significant variation of incidence in contrasted population groups should then be noted. These variations can be identified through study of attack rates.

An *attack rate* is an incidence rate that identifies the number of people at risk who became ill. In studying an outbreak of foodborne disease such as the one at the American Indian Fair, the attack rate for persons who ate certain foods would be compared with the attack rate for persons who did not eat certain foods. This is done in an attempt to identify which food was infected by the causative agent.

Attack rates are calculated in the following manner:

$$\frac{\text{No. of persons affected}}{\text{No. of persons eating food item}} \times 100$$

$$\frac{\text{No. of persons affected}}{\text{No. of persons } not \text{ eating food item}} \times 100$$

Table 11-5 illustrates how attack rates are graphically summarized. The attack rates in this table were calculated when people became ill after a banquet. They show that one food item, custard, was probably the infected food (note the differences between the two attack rate percentages). Generally, the vulnerable food that shows the greatest differences between the two attack rate percentages is the infected food.

It is essential to remember that attack rates do not positively confirm an infective food. Last (1986, pp. 35-36) has identified the following five reasons why the association of illness with a particular food is often difficult:

1. Some individuals are resistant to the agent and do not become ill even though exposed.
2. The definition of an ill person employed may include some who have unrelated illnesses, unless there is a specific test; and even then, if the illness is one that is prevalent, the ill subjects may include some cases not due to the ingestion of the common vehicle.
3. Contamination of one food by traces of another may take place during serving or before.

TABLE 11-5 Attack Rate Table

Vulnerable food	Persons who did eat vulnerable food				Persons who did not eat vulnerable food			
	Sick	Well	Total	Attack rate (%)	Sick	Well	Total	Attack rate (%)
Baked ham	19	56	75	25	30	5	35	86
Custard	45	15	60	**75**	4	46	50	**8**
Jello	20	35	55	36	29	26	55	53
Cole slaw	48	58	106	45	1	3	4	25
Baked beans	45	55	100	45	4	6	10	40
Potato salad	25	45	70	36	24	16	40	60

From Communicable Disease Center: *Food-borne disease investigation: analysis of field data,* Atlanta, Ga., 1964, U.S. Public Health Service, p. 8.

4. Errors in history-taking may occur. These may be unbiased errors, due to memory lapses or misunderstanding; or they may be due to biases, either on the part of the questioner or the subject. Several kinds of biases are possible; the questioner may have a preconceived notion of what food was responsible and press his questions more vigorously with respect to that food in the case of ill persons than non-ill persons; or the subject may have preconceived notions leading to the same result. The subject may have reasons for wishing either to claim or disclaim illness. Biases may affect the accuracy either of food histories or illness histories and produce spurious association.

5. Finally, biased sampling may also lead to spurious results.

All of these factors can affect the validity of an attack rate and thereby the choice of the appropriate infective food. Laboratory studies are necessary to identify the etiological agent and its vector. A *vector* is an animate or inanimate vehicle such as food, clothing, or insects that transports disease from an infected host to a new host. However, identifying the causative agent is not the only step in preventing further spread of disease. Knowing the agent assists in treating ill individuals who seek medical care but does not tell how the disease is being transmitted. If the chain of transmission is not broken, disease will continue to occur.

Since one factor alone never causes a disease or condition, it is not sufficient to identify only a causative agent and the infective food. After the possible agents and the attack group have been identified, the common source(s) to which affected individuals were exposed should be investigated. With foodborne disease the origin, method, and preparation of suspected foods would be primary factors to examine. Concurrently, environmental conditions should be evaluated. These conditions would include such things as the sanitary status of the restaurant, the area where food was served, and the water and dairy supply. Figure 11-9 depicts the type of data that one state collects when enteric infections such as *Salmonella newport* are suspected. Community health nurses are frequently responsible for completing this form during an epidemiological investigation. In some health departments nurses are also responsible for collecting specimens for laboratory analysis. The epidemiological division of the state or local health department will provide information on how to properly collect, preserve, and ship specimens for epidemiological analysis.

Completing an epidemiological case history form provides an opportunity for health teaching and case finding. Often the community health nurse identifies new cases during this process and helps clients to learn about the nature of the disease and how to prevent its spread.

It is important to use a variety of data-collection methods in determining the extent and source of an epidemiological problem because individuals who have only minor symptoms of illness often do not seek treatment. In the Gallup, New Mexico, outbreak, the extent of the problem was determined by a large questionnaire survey conducted from September 19-25, 1974. Using recently made maps of dwellings in the area, 500 dwellings housing 2000 persons were randomly selected for a visit by an interviewer who completed a questionnaire. The interviewer inquired

All other persons in household

	Name	Age	Relation	History of recent illness	Laboratory data
1.					
2.					
3.					
4.					
5.					
6.					
7.					
8.					
9.					
10.					

Visitors to household during past month

	Name	Age	Relation	Address	Laboratory data
1.					
2.					
3.					
4.					
5.					
6.					

Case laboratory data

Specimens				Date	Positive	Negative	Laboratory
Blood	Feces	Urine	Bile				

Informant _____

Investigation by _____

Health Dept. _____

Please use ink in making out histories   Date _____

Figure 11-9   Enteric infections case history. (From Division of Epidemiology, Michigan Department of Public Health, Lansing, Mich.)

ENTERIC INFECTIONS _____ CASE HISTORY
(Insert type)

DIVISION OF EPIDEMIOLOGY
Michigan Department of Public Health   No. _____

Name _____ Birth date _____ Birthplace _____

Address _____

Occupational address _____

Physician _____ Address _____

Health officer _____ Address _____

CLINICAL HISTORY: Date of onset _____ Diarrhea _____

Vomiting _____ Temp. _____ Weight loss _____ Other symptoms _____

_____ Duration of symptoms _____

Present condition _____

Previous pertinent history, if any _____

Source of water: ___ Well   ___ Municipal   ___ Other (specify) _____

Source of milk: ____ Pasteurized (name dairy)_____

                     ____ Unpasteurized (source) _____

Source of food: ____ Restaurant (name) _____

                     ____ Private home, other then given _____

                     ____ Other (specify) _____

Sewage disposal   ____ Privy   ____ Septic tank   ____ Municipal

_____

Additional epidemiological data pertaining to this case:

Figure 11-9, cont'd.   For legend, see opposite page.

about the occurrence and characteristics of diarrheal illnesses, the types and location of the household water supply, the amount of water consumed at the fair, the time of eating at the barbeque, and the types of food eaten. This survey revealed that attendance at the barbeque was highly associated with illness and confirmed laboratory studies that eliminated water as a vehicle of transmission. It also showed that eating potato salad at the barbeque was strongly associated with illness (Horwitz, Pollard, Merson, and Martin, 1977, pp. 1072, 1074).

Often food is strongly associated with gastrointestinal illness, especially when the illness occurs among a large number of people who have attended a social gathering. As was previously discussed, eating custard at a banquet (refer to Table 11-5) was associated with illness.

Tentative hypothesis(es) must be tested. The survey conducted at Gallup, New Mexico, helped to confirm one of the original hypotheses on the source of contamination, the food served at the barbeque, and eliminated another, the contaminated water. At times, however, none of the original hypotheses is appropriate.

Testing hypothesis(es) helps to determine if the initial control measures were sufficient to resolve the current outbreak. It also aids in identifying the natural life history of the disease and where further action is needed.

Step IV: Plan for Control

When planning for control, it is essential to identify preventive activities based on the knowledge of the natural history of the disease in question, which can be used to control the further spread of disease occurrence. Host-agent-environment factors should be analyzed to determine the following:

1. Populations at risk
2. Primary, secondary, and tertiary preventive measures available (refer to Table 11-2) that would
   a. Alter the behavior or susceptibility of the host (health education, casefinding, immunization, treatment, or rehabilitation)
   b. Destroy the agent (heat, drug treatment, or spraying with insecticides)
   c. Eliminate the transmission of the agent (changes in host's health habits or environmental conditions)

3. Feasibility of implementing the control plan, considering such factors as available community resources, time required, cost of control vs. partial or no control, facilities, supplies, and personnel needed
4. Priorities in relation to legal mandates, significance of the problem relative to other community needs, and the feasibility of implementing the control plan

Public Opinion

Public opinion can have a significant impact on the effectiveness of any control plan. In the Gallup outbreak of salmonellosis, one control measure could have been to ban future food preparation and consumption for groups of persons numbering over 100 so that careful attention could be given to details. It is highly unlikely that this plan would be well received, since fairs are a major form of recreation on the Navajo Nation Indian Reservation and the Indians travel considerable distances to attend them. Clearly stating regulations for food preparation, with the mandatory attendance of one environmentalist per 1000 persons to oversee food preparation, would probably be a more realistic control measure for this situation.

Breaking the Chain of Transmission

Control measures are generally directed toward breaking the chain of transmission (refer to Figure 11-10). This includes destroying or treating the reservoir of infection, interrupting the transmission of the agent from the reservoir to the new host, and decreasing the ability of the agent to adapt and multiply within the host. A *reservoir* is a living species or an inanimate object such as soil in which an infectious agent lives and multiplies and upon which it depends for survival and reproduction. When attempting to break the chain of transmission, the concept of multiple causation must be applied.

Referring again to the Gallup outbreak, the major cause of the disease was error in food preparation. There was prolonged storage of precooked ingredients for potato salad, within the 44° to 114° F range in which *Salmonella* have been demonstrated to multiply. The initial source of the *Salmonella* is unknown (Horwitz, Pollard, Merson, and Martin, 1977, p. 1074). As is often the case, the food handlers at this large gathering were laypersons and their work was unsupervised. Large gatherings of people at which food is served should be considered high-risk settings for

TABLE 11-6 Types of Acquired Immunity

Type of immunity	How acquired	Length of resistance
Natural		
Active	Natural contact and infection with the antigen	May be temporary or permanent
Passive	Natural contact with antibody transplacentally or through colostrum and breast milk	Temporary
Artificial		
Active	Inoculation of antigen	May be temporary or permanent
Passive	Inoculation of antibody or antitoxin	Temporary

From Grimes DE: *Infectious diseases,* St. Louis, 1991, Mosby, p. 18.

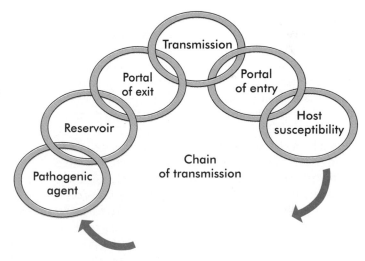

Figure 11-10 Chain of transmission for infection. The chain must be intact for an infection to be transmitted to another host. Transmission can be controlled by breaking any link in the chain. (Redrawn from Grimes DE: *Infectious diseases,* St. Louis, 1991, Mosby, p. 21.)

foodborne disease outbreak. It is advisable to have an epidemiologically trained person monitoring food preparation, storage, and serving at such occasions.

Herd Immunity

When one is dealing with infectious diseases and establishing a control plan, the concept of herd immunity is also important to consider. *Herd immunity* is the immunity level of a specific group. Immunity is "that resistance usually associated with possession of antibodies that have an inhibitory effect on a specific microorganism, or its toxin, that causes a particular infectious disease" (CDC, 1987, Principles of epidemiology: agent, p. 42). Characteristics of the different types of immunity are presented in Table 11-6.

If 100% of a given group had received measles vaccine, the herd immunity would be 100%. If 80% had received measles vaccine, the herd immunity would be at least 80%. Some people in the group have natural immunity, raising the percentage higher.

Herd immunity does not have to be 100% to prevent an epidemic or to control a disease, but it is not known just what percentage is safe. Communities usually strive to achieve at least a 90% to 95% herd immunity level. A national goal is to increase basic immunization levels among children under age 2 to at least 90% and among children in child care facilities and kindergarten through post-secondary education institutions to at least 95% (USDHHS, 1991, *Healthy People 2000,* p. 521).

It is important to realize that as herd immunity decreases, the chances for epidemics rise. In the United States a major concern is that many school-age children are not receiving immunizations for communicable disease. This greatly decreases the level of herd immunity and is a major barrier to maintaining community health.

Community health nurses are instrumental in helping the public to see the need for effective control of disease by active immunization. This will continue to be a major function of the community health nurse, because immunizing populations at risk is the most effective way to control many childhood communicable diseases (refer to Chapter 14 for immunization schedules).

Casefinding

Casefinding is a major function of epidemiologists and community health nurses. This process focuses on early diagnosis and treatment by discovery of new cases of a disease or condition. It may evolve through clinical observation or laboratory tests and may involve mass or individual testing. Opportunities for casefinding are limitless and come through home visits, clinic nursing, school visits, and prenatal classes, to name only a few. Community health nurses in these settings can pick up casefinding clues such as a tired young mother who seems unable to handle her three preschool children, possible scoliosis in a preadolescent girl, or a developmental delay in a toddler. By being alert to such clues many situations will be identified in which to use nursing skills to prevent disease and promote health. In some instances of casefinding, such as child abuse, a perceptive nurse may observe tendencies of abusive behavior in a parent and be able to assist the parent in working through these tendencies. This could prevent the abuse.

Step V: Implement Control Plan

An active effort should be made to elicit and coordinate the cooperation of the lay public, as well as private and official agencies, when putting control measures into operation. A control program that takes into consideration the beliefs, attitudes, and customs of the community is more likely to be accepted by the public than one that ignores community norms. Health education programs can help to "sell" a control program in the community, especially if they deal with current community attitudes and beliefs.

To evaluate the effectiveness of a control program, broad goals and specific objectives for the program must be identified before the program begins. Defining broad goals and specific outcome objectives such as the ones below makes it easier to determine if control efforts are successful.

Broad Goal: To increase the herd immunity level for DTP to 95% in Centerville.

Objectives: To increase the herd immunity level for DTP in census tracts 4 and 5 by 25% in 4 months by immunizing kindergarten and first-, fifth-, and tenth-grade students.

To increase the herd immunity level for DTP in census tracts 8 and 9 by 17% in 4 months by immunizing kindergarten and first-, fifth-, and tenth-grade students.

Control measures involve primary, secondary, and/or tertiary preventive activities. They include things such as disease reporting, quarantine, environmental control, human carrier control, health education, activities to decrease host susceptibility (e.g., immunizations), and technological advances.

Barriers to Control Programs

There are many barriers to the successful implementation of a control program for both infectious disease and noncommunicable conditions. Barriers to control involve factors such as unknown etiology, no known treatment, unavailable community resources, multifactorial etiology, long latency periods, and lack of reporting.

Low levels of immunity in an exposed population group increase the likelihood of disease occurrence. Mass and individual immunization programs are effective in raising immunity levels for some diseases. For many diseases, however, there are no specific prophylactic immunizations. Examples of such diseases are impetigo and STDs.

Individuals without overt disease symptoms but who harbor the disease organism can be a major vehicle in disease transmission. These individuals are known as *carriers.* Typhoid and salmonellosis are examples of diseases that are often transmitted by carriers.

With any disease and for a variety of reasons, some individuals will delay or not seek treatment. Whatever the reason, a delay in confirmation and treatment of the disease can enhance its spread and continuation and impede control plan implementation.

Individuals for whom the diagnosis is not suspected or confirmed are also barriers to the control of disease. Disease may not be confirmed for several reasons. Some people will evidence atypical symptoms of the disease in question. If clinical symptoms do not fit a disease model the disease may be missed completely or misdiagnosed. Other individuals are seen too early or too late in the course of the disease process to either suspect or confirm the disease. In these situations laboratory tests may be falsely negative or they may not be done at all because the clinical symptoms do not reflect a need. There are other times when a diagnosis cannot be confirmed because specimens (stools, emesis, or sputum) have inadvertently been destroyed or handled improperly. When working in the home or in other health care settings it is vitally important to recognize that laboratory tests are needed to confirm most infectious disease diagnoses.

Lack of reporting, often reflecting nonacceptance of a diagnosis, is one of the key barriers in a control program. This can result from clerical error, indifference, fear, shame, or any of a number of variables. In some instances professionals may not want to get involved or do not feel it appropriate to become involved. This is especially true when a social problem such as gonorrhea or child abuse is the disease or condition in question.

Community health nurses need to be acutely aware of these barriers because they are frequently in a position to help individuals, families, or health care professionals overcome them. Through the use of the referral process, knowledge of community resources, interviewing skills, and the ability to understand both health and disease processes, the community health nurse is uniquely able to assist in resolving these barriers.

Step VI: Evaluate Control Plan

An important part of the epidemiological process is evaluation. This ensures that a process can be improved the next time it is repeated. It also ensures, through the problem-solving approach, that all elements of a problem have been reviewed. The first step in evaluation is to determine how well the objectives of the process were met. This implies that before carrying out the process, objectives were clearly and

behaviorally written. The next question to be answered is how the current situation compares to the situation prior to the investigation. Finally, the practicality of the control measures should be determined. Feasibility and cost in terms of money, time, staff, facilities, and community support should be analyzed.

Step VII: Make Appropriate Report

Prompt, accurate, and concise epidemiological reporting will provide a basis for future investigations and control measures. Appropriate reporting demonstrates to the community the health professionals' accountability and clarifies the epidemiological situation. Reporting should include what was involved in the epidemiological process: diagnosis, factors leading to the epidemic, control measures, process evaluation, and recommendations for preventing similar situations.

Underreporting of many epidemiological investigations occurs. This happens for many reasons. Completion of necessary forms can be tedious and time-consuming and, therefore, neglected. Frequently there is no one person assigned the responsibility for seeing that reports are completed, so the responsibility is overlooked. Usually more effective reporting occurs when one person is designated to coordinate the reporting activities of others.

Societal and individual values and attitudes also contribute to underreporting. At times, conditions such as STDs, alcoholism, or mental illness are not discussed or reported because health care professionals are afraid to disturb the status quo in the community.

Accurate reporting is essential for the identification of major community health problems and preventive health action that would correct these problems. Treating only individuals with overt symptoms, rather than collecting and reporting data on populations at risk, does very little to prevent future health problems.

Step VIII: Conduct Research

If health services to populations are to be improved, epidemiological research is essential. Health professionals must be prepared to collect and analyze data systematically so that the gaps in knowledge relative to disease causation, prevention, and control are eliminated. The ultimate goal of epidemiology—

the prevention and control of infectious diseases, chronic conditions, and other health-related phenomena in populations—is far from being realized. Infectious diseases such as gonorrhea, syphilis, hepatitis, enteric disorders, and tuberculosis are still major health problems. In spite of scientific advances in the development of immunizations that prevent communicable diseases, epidemic outbreaks of childhood conditions, especially measles and diphtheria, continue to occur. Noninfectious conditions such as accidents and substance abuse and chronic diseases including cancer and heart conditions are fast-growing problems. Because of their complex nature, very little is known regarding their etiology or ways to prevent and control them. It is unfortunate that research in the practice setting is often lacking. Research can be exciting and challenging, especially when one discovers significant data that will aid a community to better its health status.

EPIDEMIOLOGICAL CHALLENGES OF THE FUTURE

Many contemporary challenges for epidemiologists exist. These challenges include the control of communicable and chronic diseases as well as selected psychosocial health phenomena. A major challenge on the epidemiological frontier is the control of acquired immunodeficiency syndrome (AIDS), which is at epidemic proportions in the United States today.

Communicable Disease: A Neglected Public Health Mandate

According to the Institute of Medicine's Committee for the Study of the Future of Public Health (1988), communicable disease has become a neglected mandate in the U.S. public health system. On a national level, the U.S. Public Health Service Centers for Disease Control and Prevention (CDC) in Atlanta, Georgia, is the major agency responsible for communicable disease control in this country (refer to Chapter 5). It maintains a national morbidity reporting system that collects, compiles, and publishes demographic, clinical, and laboratory data on many communicable and chronic diseases and conditions from each state. A department of each state has designated responsibility for control of communicable disease. This department

maintains a morbidity reporting system based on regulations adopted by the state board of health, which derives its authority to issue regulations from acts of the state legislature. These regulations usually specify which diseases or conditions are reportable; who is responsible for reporting; what information is required for each case reported; what manner of reporting is needed; and to whom the information is reported. State regulations also commonly require reporting of any outbreak of unusually high prevalence of any disease and the occurrence of any unusual disease. Diseases which become important from a public health standpoint (e.g., AIDS) are usually promptly added to the list of reportable diseases (CDC, 1987, Principles of epidemiology: disease, pp. 2-3).

Diseases reported by the states to the CDC are determined by the Association of State and Territorial Health Officers. The CDC compiles state data and distributes a summary of this information to the states through its publication *Morbidity and Mortality Weekly Report* (MMWR). The MMWR provides current statistics on communicable diseases and information on public health issues and conditions. The CDC provides an annual summary of disease reports from the states to the World Health Organization (WHO). However, CDC notifies WHO promptly of any reported cases of the internationally quarantinable diseases—smallpox, plague, cholera, and yellow fever—and influenza virus isolates (CDC, 1987, Principles of epidemiology: disease, p. 6).

Unfortunately, the past strides made in communicable disease control and eradication in the United States have come to be taken for granted. We have become increasingly lax in many of our communicable disease practices. Although state health authorities document investigations of disease epidemics and outbreaks, there is *no* national system for surveillance of epidemics (CDC, 1989, Surveillance, p. 694). Many children and adults in the United States are not completely immunized, and there has been an increase in the incidence of immunizable diseases such as measles and rubella (CDC, 1989, Mumps, p. 392). Measles eradication in the United States had been targeted for 1977, but that goal has not been met. Tuberculosis is on the rise in the United States (CDC, 1989, A strategic plan, p. 2), as are syphilis and hepatitis A (CDC, Mumps, p. 392). Many new sexually transmitted diseases are emerging; we have still not controlled or eradicated the old ones, and some are increasing in incidence. Appendix 11-1 provides information on some of the common communicable diseases that the community health nurse may have contact with in clinical practice. Information about commonly acquired sexually transmitted disease is given in Appendix 11-2. AIDS is discussed extensively in Chapters 14 and 16. Appendix 11-3 identifies the communicable diseases that need to be reported to the health department.

The American public needs to recognize communicable disease as a contemporary public health concern. The challenge to public health is to control the communicable diseases that already exist while meeting the demands of new communicable diseases—such as AIDS—as they develop. National goals are focusing on reducing vaccine-preventable diseases such as measles and diphtheria, epidemic-related pneumonia and influenza deaths, viral hepatitis, tuberculosis, and AIDS and HIV infection in addition to other infectious diseases including infectious diarrhea and nosocomial infections (USDHHS, 1991, *Healthy People 2000*).

Epidemiological Precautions to Prevent AIDS Transmission

AIDS is a contemporary public health challenge. Although it is discussed in greater depth in Chapters 14 and 16, the epidemiologically based precautions for minimizing transmission of the human immunodeficiency virus (HIV) are presented here.

In 1987 the CDC recommended that blood and body fluid precautions be consistently used for *all* patients to minimize transmission of the HIV and hepatitis B virus (HBV). This extension of blood and body fluid precautions to all patients is called "Universal Blood and Body Fluid Precautions" or "Universal Precautions" (CDC, 1988, p. 377). The universal precautions and other pertinent information can be found in *Mortality and Morbidity Weekly Reports* (MMWR) (CDC, 1987, HIV; 1988; 1989, Guidelines; 1989, Publications). All clinical sites should have these guidelines readily available to health care personnel.

Under universal precautions blood and certain body fluids are considered potentially infectious for human immunodeficiency virus (HIV) and hepatitis B virus (HBV). The body fluids to which universal precautions apply are listed in the box on this page. It is significant for health care professionals to remember that universal precautions are designed to protect health care providers as well as clients. Occupationally acquired AIDS/HIV infection has been

◀ **Body Fluids to Which Universal Precautions Apply and Do Not Apply** ▶

Apply	Do Not Apply*
Blood	Feces
Semen	Nasal secretions
Vaginal secretions	Sputum/saliva
Cerebrospinal fluid (CSF)	Sweat
Synovial fluid	Tears
Pleural fluid	Urine
Peritoneal fluid	Vomitus
Pericardial fluid	Breast milk
Amniotic fluid	

*Universal precautions would apply to the above body fluids if they contained visible blood. The presence of human immunodeficiency virus and hepatitis B virus has been demonstrated in some of these fluids, but the risk of transmission is extremely low or nonexistent. Epidemiological studies have not implicated these fluids in the transmission of HIV and HBV infections.

From Centers for Disease Control (CDC): Update: universal precautions for prevention of transmission of human immunodeficiency virus, hepatitis B virus, and other bloodborne pathogens in health-care settings, *MMWR* 37:377-387, June 24, 1988; and CDC: Recommendations for prevention of HIV transmission in health-care settings, *MMWR* 36(Suppl S2), August 21, 1987.

documented (refer to Table 11-7) and can be acquired in a variety of health care settings, including the client's home.

Figure 11-11 identifies important CDC HIV/AIDS prevention milestones. CDC publishes its guidelines in the *Morbidity and Mortality Weekly Report* (MMWR), which the reader is encouraged to review on a regular basis. CDC has developed health education materials on HIV/AIDS for the lay public, as well as for health care providers.

Implementation of universal precautions does not eliminate the need for other category or disease-specific isolation precautions such as those for infectious diarrhea or pulmonary tuberculosis. Special precautions are strongly recommended for oral examinations and treatments in the dental setting and during phlebotomy. In addition to universal precautions, detailed precautions have been developed for procedures and/or settings in which prolonged or intensive exposures to blood occur, such as invasive procedures, dentistry, autopsies or morticians' services, dialysis, and the clinical laboratory.

TABLE 11-7 Health-Care Workers with Occupationally Acquired AIDS/HIV Infection*

Occupation	Occupational transmission	
	Documented	Possible
Dental worker, including dentist	—	6
Embalmer/morgue technician	—	3
Emergency medical technician/ paramedic	—	7
Health aide/attendant	1	5
Housekeeper/ maintenance worker	1	5
Laboratory technician, clinical	12	12
Laboratory technician, nonclinical	1	1
Nurse	12	14
Physician, nonsurgical	4	7
Physician, surgical	—	2
Respiratory therapist	1	1
Surgical technician	1	1
Other technician/ therapist	—	3
Other health-care occupations	—	2
Total	33	69

*Reported through December 1992.
From Centers for Disease Control and Prevention: *CDC HIV/AIDS prevention: fact book, 1993,* Atlanta, Ga., 1993, The Centers, p. 20.

Tuberculosis: A Reemerging Killer

Tuberculosis (TB) has been a major killer throughout recorded history. Worldwide it continues to rank among the leading causes of mortality and morbidity. Despite unparalleled biomedical achievement of effective prophylaxis and chemotherapy, it is estimated that the annual incidence of new cases of tuberculosis is about 8 million and that this disease causes almost 3 million deaths annually worldwide (Kochi, 1991; Rubel and Garro, 1992). Until about 10 years ago tuberculosis was rapidly disappearing from the United

States. Since 1988 there has been a dramatic reversal of this trend (Multidrug-resistant tuberculosis, 1992). "In 1990, the number of reported tuberculosis cases increased 9.4% compared with 1987 and 15.5% compared with 1984" (CDC, 1992, Prevention and control of tuberculosis in U.S., p. 1). Between 1985 and 1991 there were approximately 39,000 more cases reported than would have been expected had the previous downward trend continued (CDC, 1992, National Action Plan, p. 6).

"At no time in recent history has tuberculosis been as great a concern as it is today" (CDC, 1992, National Action Plan, p. 5). In addition to the increase of reported cases, recent outbreaks of multidrug-resistant tuberculosis (MDR-TB) have posed a threat to the public's health. Factors contributing to the recent epidemic of tuberculosis in the United States include, but are not limited to, the recent AIDS epidemic, social circumstances such as homelessness and poverty, the migration of refugees and immigrants to this country, and the deteriorating public health infrastructure with a resulting lack of funding for tuberculosis surveillance and control activities. Figure 11-12 depicts the amplifying effect of HIV infection on tuberculosis morbidity and transmission.

Select epidemiological characteristics of tuberculosis are included in Appendix 11-2. Aggregates at high risk for developing the disease are presented in Table 11-8. Reducing tuberculosis to an incidence of no more than 3.5 cases per 100,000 people (baseline: 9.1 per 100,000 in 1988) is a national health objective (USDHHS, 1991, *Healthy People 2000,* p. 516). Preventive therapy for the control of tuberculous infection among high-risk populations is essential. The key strategies of the national action plan for eliminating tuberculosis focus on (1) identification and treatment of infectious cases so that they do not continue to transmit infection and (2) identification and treatment of infected people before they develop the infectious form of the disease (USDHHS, *Healthy People 2000,* p. 517). The major components in the United States' action plan to combat multidrug-resistant tuberculosis are presented in the box on p. 410.

Tuberculosis is now "the other epidemic" (Allen and Ownby, 1991) that needs to be addressed by all health care professionals across the nation. Large-scale, epidemic transmission of tuberculosis is a major threat to all health care providers and patients (Iseman, 1992). Community health nurses have and will continue to play a role in the prevention and treatment of

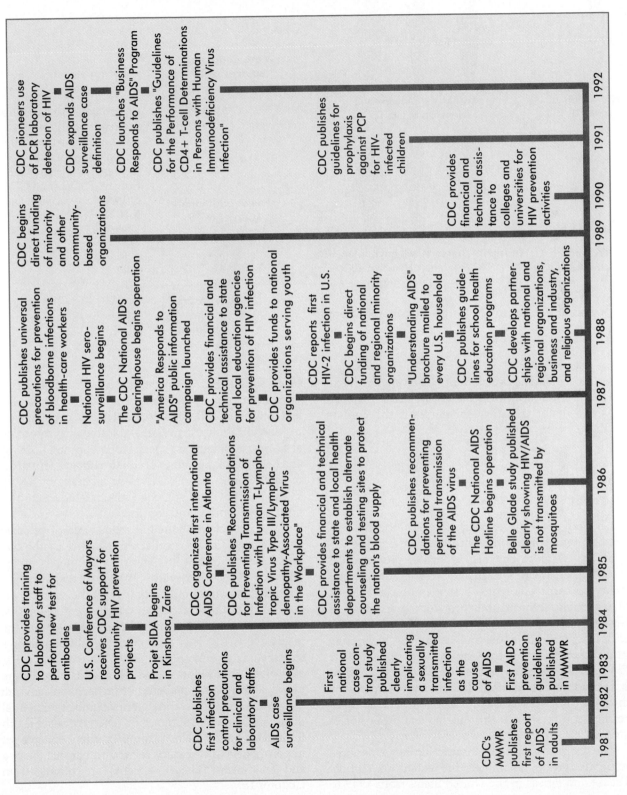

Figure 11-11 Centers for Disease Control and Prevention: HIV/AIDS prevention milestones. (From Centers for Disease Control and Prevention: *CDC HIV/AIDS prevention: fact book, 1993,* Atlanta, Ga., 1993, The Centers, p. 36.)

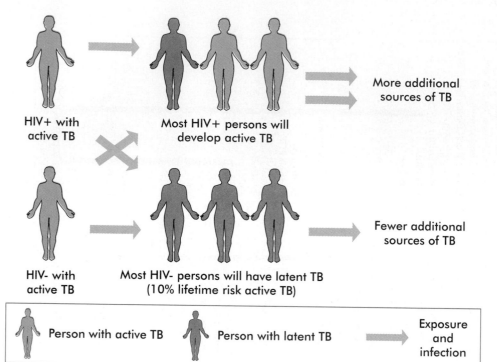

HIV+ with active TB

Most HIV+ persons will develop active TB

More additional sources of TB

HIV- with active TB

Most HIV- persons will have latent TB (10% lifetime risk active TB)

Fewer additional sources of TB

Person with active TB   Person with latent TB   Exposure and infection

Figure 11-12 The amplifying effect of HIV infection on TB morbidity and transmission. (From Centers for Disease Control and Prevention: *CDC HIV/AIDS prevention: fact book, 1993*, Atlanta, Ga., 1993, The Centers, p. 18.)

tuberculosis. Taking precautions to prevent the transmission of multidrug-resistant tuberculosis in all settings is a major challenge for nurses in the coming decade.

Chronic Disease and Conditions: An Increasing Challenge

Chapter 18 deals extensively with chronic and handicapping conditions. Chronic disease and conditions are of great concern to health professionals because they are long-term and often limit a person's ability to carry out major activities of daily living. Major activity refers to ability to work, keep house, or engage in school or preschool activities (Collins, 1986, p. 55). Chronic diseases and conditions have been studied extensively in the United States since the late 1940s. The prevalence of the diseases and conditions is increasing worldwide. Individuals experiencing chronic health problems require ongoing and comprehensive community health nursing and other health services.

The Commission on Chronic Illness, a national voluntary group, examined the extent of chronic disease and illness in the United States from 1949 to 1956. This commission defined chronic diseases as impairments or deviations from normal that have at least one of the following characteristics: permanency, residual disability, irreversible pathological causation and alteration, need for special rehabilitation training, and need for a long period of supervision, observation, or care (Commission on Chronic Illness, 1957, p. 4). These concepts still guide practice related to chronic disease prevention and control.

Currently, data about the prevalence of selected chronic conditions are collected regularly by the National Center for Health Statistics by means of the National Health Interview Survey. In this survey a condition is considered chronic if (1) the condition is described by the respondent as having been first noticed more than 3 months before the week of the interview, or (2) it is one of the conditions always classified as chronic regardless of time of onset. Examples of conditions always viewed as chronic are ulcers, emphysema, diabetes, arthritis, neoplasms, all congenital anomalies, and psychoses and other mental disorders (Collins, 1986, p. 54). The National Health Interview Survey also examines the concepts of impairment and disability related to chronic disease and conditions. These concepts are discussed in Chapter 18.

TABLE 11-8 Tuberculosis: At-Risk Aggregates

Aggregate	Select risk data
Medically underserved low-income populations, including racial/ethnic minorities and homeless	In 1990 almost 70% of all TB cases and 86% of those among children age <15 years occurred among racial/ethnic minorities. In 1990 the risk of TB (compared with the case rate of 4.2/100,000 population among non-Hispanic whites) was 9.9 times higher for Asians/Pacific islanders, 7.9 times higher for non-Hispanic blacks, 5.1 times higher for Hispanics, and 4.5 times higher for American Indians/Alaskan Natives.
Foreign-born persons entering the United States	In 1989 the overall tuberculosis rate was 9.5 per 100,000 population; for foreign-born persons arriving in the United States, the estimated case rate was 124/100,000.
HIV-infected persons	The incidence of tuberculosis in HIV-infected persons is not well established but appears to be substantially in excess of what would be expected in non–HIV-infected persons. For HIV-infected persons who have latent tuberculosis infection, the risk of developing active TB was shown in some outbreaks to be 7% to 10% per year.
Residents in institutions (e.g., nursing homes, prisons, long-term care facilities)	Nursing home residents have an incidence of tuberculosis from two to seven times higher than demographically similar persons living in other settings. Institutional settings are high-risk environments because persons with infectious tuberculosis are likely to live in these settings, the environmental characteristics are conducive to transmission, and large numbers of susceptible persons may be located in these settings. The incidence of TB among inmates of correctional institutions is more than three times higher than that for nonincarcerated adults aged 15-64 years.
Persons with medical risk factors that increase risk of diseases	Medical risk factors that substantially increase the risk of tuberculosis are: silicosis; gastrectomy; jejunoileal bypass; weight of 10% or more below ideal body weight; chronic renal failure; diabetes mellitus; conditions requiring prolonged high-dose corticosteroid therapy and other immunosuppressive therapy; some hematological disorders such as leukemia; and other malignancies.
Contacts of infectious cases	Are at extremely high risk for developing infection and disease. Most cases of tuberculosis occur in people who are already infected with tubercle bacilli. Individuals in this population who are at highest risk of developing disease are those who have been recently infected and those who are exposed to a variety of stressors.

Data from Centers for Disease Control (CDC): Prevention and control of tuberculosis in correctional institutions: recommendations of the advisory committee for the elimination of tuberculosis, *MMWR*, 38:313-320, 1989; CDC: Screening for tuberculosis and tuberculous infection in high-risk populations, *MMWR* (No. RR-8)39:1-7, 1990; CDC: Tuberculosis among foreign-born persons entering the United States: recommendations of the Advisory Committee for Elimination of Tuberculosis, *MMWR* (No. RR-18) 39:1-21, 1990; CDC: Prevention and control of tuberculosis in U.S. communities with at-risk minority populations, *MMWR* (No. RR-5) 41:1-11, 1992; CDC: Prevention and control of tuberculosis among homeless persons, *MMWR* (No. RR-5) 41:13-21, 1992.

People of any age can evidence chronic conditions; these conditions are not synonymous with old age. It should be remembered that aging is the normal process of biological, psychological, and sociological change over time. However, because aging involves a gradual lessening in levels of efficiency and functioning in the various body systems, elderly people are more likely than young people to have chronic conditions. They also are likely to have more of them.

◄ **U.S. National Action Plan to Combat Multidrug-Resistant Tuberculosis (MDR-TB)** ►

Surveillance and epidemiology: determine the magnitude and nature of the problem

Laboratory diagnosis: improve the rapidity, sensitivity, and reliability of diagnostic methods for MDR-TB

Patient management: effectively managing patients who have MDR-TB and preventing patients with drug-susceptible TB from developing drug-resistant disease

Screening and preventive therapy: identifying persons who are infected with or at risk of developing MDR-TB and preventing them from developing clinically active TB

Infection control: minimizing the risk of transmission of MDR-TB to patients, workers, and others in institutional settings

Outbreak control: facilitate collaboration of various officials and organizations in controlling MDR-TB outbreaks

Program evaluation: ensuring that TB programs are effective in managing patients and preventing MDR-TB

Information dissemination/training and education: develop a cadre of health-care professionals with expertise in the management of TB, including MDR-TB

Research: identify better methods for combating MDR-TB

From Centers for Disease Control and Prevention: National action plan to combat multidrug-resistant tuberculosis, *MMWR* 41(No. RR-11):5-48, 1992, p. 5.

The Scope of Chronic Disease

Figure 11-13 illustrates that chronic conditions are evidenced across the age spectrum. People of all ages are affected by chronic disease. Note, however, the predominance of many chronic conditions in the later years (from age 45 and on).

Differences by gender and age for select chronic conditions with the highest prevalence are shown in Figure 11-14. Females account for almost three of every five chronic sinusitis conditions and almost three of every five arthritis conditions. Women have much higher arthritis prevalence rates because they account for a greater percentage of the 56+ population for whom arthritis prevalence rates are very high (Collins, 1993, p. 11).

Chronic illness is a significant health problem in the United States. Roughly 33 million Americans have some degree of chronic activity limitation, of which 9 million have functional limitation so severe that they cannot work, attend school, or maintain a household (National Center for Health Statistics, 1989, current estimates). Chronic conditions also influence health services use and have an impact on disability days. For example, it has been found that each year heart conditions cause an average of 143.8 million bed disability days, arthritis causes 126.7 million bed disability days, and deformities or orthopedic impairments cause 120.1 million bed disability days (Collins, 1993, p. 19). A bed disability day is a day in which an individual stays in bed more than half the day because of illness or injury (Benson and Marano, 1994, p.141).

The 10 leading causes of chronic health conditions for the U.S. population as a whole are presented in Figure 11-15. Some other major causes of chronic health problems are dermatitis, migraine, visual impairments, diseases of the urinary tract, diabetes, and tinnitus. As can be seen in Figure 11-13, there are tremendous age-related variations relative to these chronic conditions.

Chapters 14 through 19 identify age-related health risks across the lifespan. When examining data about age-related risks, it is important to remember, however, that many chronic conditions found in later life have their roots in childhood or young adulthood and continue throughout the lifespan.

Why so much chronic disease? Strauss states that without question a major reason for the high rate of chronic disease in the United States is the elimination or control of infectious and parasitic diseases (Strauss, 1975, p. 3). The industrialized nations of the world are no longer greatly affected by preventable and controllable conditions. Instead, persons in these countries die from cancer, heart disease, stroke, and other long-term conditions such as diabetes.

The relatively low social value given to older people by our culture, as well as the acute care and cure orientation of health personnel, helps to explain why so little attention has been given to the care of persons with chronic conditions. This is unfortunate since there are many physical, social, and psychological components of long-term disease that require organized health care services. Long-term conditions will

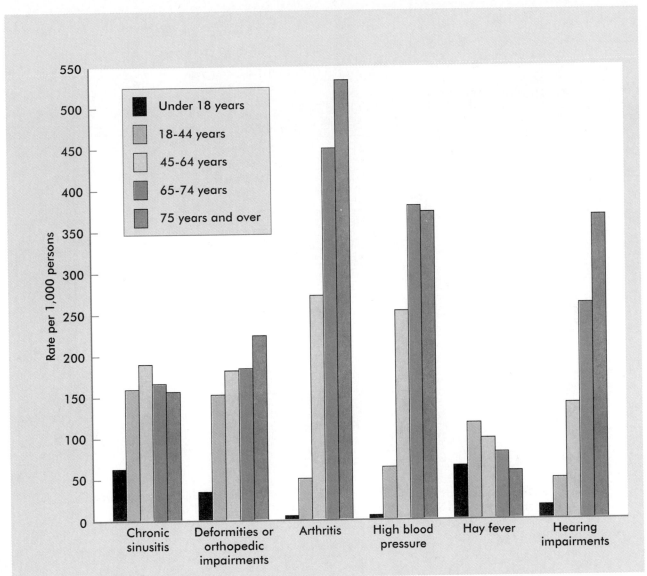

Figure 11-13   Rate per 1000 persons per year for selected reported chronic conditions with highest prevalence, by age: United States, 1986-88. (From Collins JG: *Prevalence of selected chronic conditions: United States, 1986-88,* National Center for Health Statistics, Vital Health Stat 10(182), 1993, p. 13.)

undoubtedly play a major role in U.S. health care for years to come.

Levels of Prevention for Chronic Disease

The first of a four-volume series based on the work of the Commission on Chronic Illness was appropriately titled *Prevention of Chronic Illness.* Prevention must be the underlying approach to chronic conditions or

these problems will only increase with time. Prevention on all three levels—primary, secondary, and tertiary—is essential for effective management and control of chronic conditions.

Primary prevention of many serious chronic illnesses is frequently impossible because health professionals are unable to determine the exact point in time when a condition begins. When, for example, does

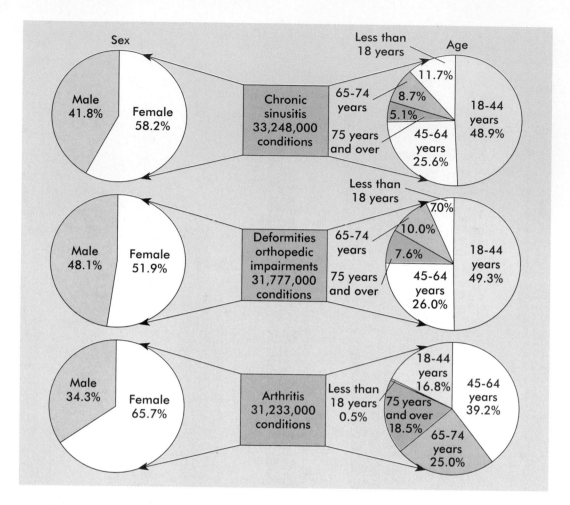

Figure 11-14   Percent distribution of selected chronic conditions with highest prevalence by sex and age: United States, 1986-88. (From Collins JG: *Prevalence of selected chronic conditions: United States, 1986-88,* National Center for Health Statistics, Vital Health Stat 10(182), 1993, p. 12.)

schizophrenia or asbestosis begin? Each of these diseases goes through a long latent period before symptoms are seen. They may stem from such variables as hereditary characteristics, occupational conditions, environmental stresses, or nutritional factors. Some chronic conditions can be prevented. Primary preventive efforts that control communicable disease, reduce accidents, emphasize adequate care during pregnancy, and suggest ways to cope with emotional stress all contribute to the prevention of certain chronic conditions. Primary prevention is an important task of the community health nurse.

Detection and treatment of chronic conditions (secondary prevention) are often possible. For many con-

ditions such as diabetes, hypertension, breast cancer, and glaucoma, large-scale national programs for early detection represent a profitable and economical approach to secondary prevention. Early diagnosis plays a significant role in the control of chronic disease and conditions.

A major secondary prevention effort relative to chronic illness occurred in the United States when the National Health Survey was authorized and conducted in 1956 to secure information about health conditions in the general population. This survey was enacted under the National Health Survey Act, which was proposed in 1955 by the U.S. Department of Health, Education, and Welfare (USDHEW). Under

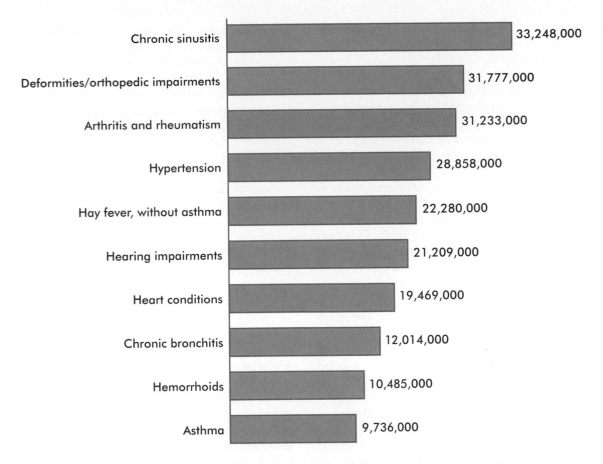

Figure 11-15 Ten major causes of chronic health conditions in the United States by number of persons, in rank order: 1986-88. (From Collins JG: *Prevalence of selected chronic conditions: United States, 1986-88,* National Center for Health Statistics, Vital Health Stat 10(182), 1993, p. 8.)

this act the Surgeon General of the Public Health Service was authorized to conduct a survey in order to produce uniform national statistics on disease, injury, impairment, disability, and related topics.

In 1972 a new survey mechanism initiated by USD-HEW, the Health and Nutrition Examination Survey (HANES), began. Persons 1 to 74 years of age were examined with emphasis on their nutritional status. Statistical data were collected on health records, fertility patterns, morbidity, and mortality. Today, HANES is the primary source of nationwide data on illnesses, disabilities, and physiological measurements.

Tertiary prevention activities, as well as primary and secondary ones, should be planned when working with people who have chronic conditions. Tertiary prevention involves rehabilitation, with the ultimate goal being cure or full restoration of the client's level of functioning. For some chronic conditions this may be impossible; hence, the ideal goal must be replaced by more limited objectives such as maximizing remaining functional potential or minimizing further deterioration. Another option would be to learn to live within the limitations that the chronic disease has imposed. A more detailed discussion of the concept of rehabilitation is presented in Chapter 18.

Approaches to the Study of Chronic Conditions

Two basic approaches to the study of chronic conditions and other diseases are retrospective and prospective studies. Retrospective and prospective studies are designed to determine if there is a relationship between a factor and a disease, as well as the intensity of that relationship. Mausner and Kramer (1985, pp. 159-174) discuss extensively the principles involved in these types of studies. Since only a brief summary of their thoughts is presented below, the reader should refer to Mausner and Kramer's text to obtain a better understanding of these approaches.

Retrospective studies look at people who are diagnosed as having a disease and compare them with those who do not have disease. The persons who do not have the disease are called *controls*. The controls come from the same general population segment as the individuals who have the condition and have the same characteristics as the study group except for the disease condition. A retrospective study examines factors in the person's past experience. One of the disadvantages of retrospective studies is that detailed information may not be available or accurate. The greatest problem, however, is finding a control group that is alike in all respects except for the condition under study. The advantages of this type of study are cost and the number of subjects needed. Retrospective studies are relatively inexpensive and require a small sampling size because cases are identified at the onset.

Prospective studies start with a group of people—a cohort—all presumed to be free from a condition but who differ in their exposure to a supposedly harmful factor. This cohort is followed over a period of time to discover differences in the rate at which disease develops in relation to exposure to the harmful factor. A major advantage of this type of study is that the cohort is chosen for study before the disease develops. The cohort is therefore not influenced by knowledge that disease exists, as in retrospective studies.

Prospective studies allow calculation of incidence rates among those exposed and those not exposed. Thus, absolute difference in incidence rates and the true relative risk can be measured. The major disadvantage is that a prospective study is a long, expensive project. A large cohort must be used, especially if the disease has low incidence. Also, the larger the number of factors to be studied, the larger the cohort must be. The loss of people from the cohort as a result of death, lack of interest, or job mobility is a major problem when a study lasts over an extended period of time. Changes in diagnostic criteria, administrative problems, loss of staff or funding, and the high cost of record keeping can all contribute to make this a study that should not be undertaken without careful planning.

Retrospective and prospective studies assist in identifying causes of disease and effective disease control mechanisms. It is not intended that this brief description of retrospective and prospective studies will prepare community health nurses to do them. The purpose is to familiarize readers with the basic concepts involved in the study of chronic conditions.

The community health nurse does, however, play an active role in the control of chronic conditions. Case finding through screening programs is a significant aspect of this part of the community health nurse's role.

Screening as a Method for Detection and Control of Chronic Conditions

Screening programs can be an efficient way to identify individuals in a community who may unknowingly have a chronic condition, as well as an infectious disease.

There are two types of screening programs whereby chronic and infectious disease is sought in apparently healthy individuals: the *single screening test,* where only one condition is being identified, such as giving a group of teachers a TB tine test, and the *multiphasic screening test,* where a battery of tests is used at one time to detect several disease conditions. Doing height and weight measurements, audiometry, and vision screening of all persons at a county fair is an example of multiphasic screening.

Screening tests do not provide a conclusive diagnosis of a disease but rather are used to identify asymptomatic individuals who may unknowingly have a problem. Anyone who evidences symptoms of a disease through a screening program should have further medical diagnostic testing. This is essential since early diagnosis and treatment are the primary goals of a screening program. Early diagnosis and treatment are particularly beneficial for conditions—such as hypertension and cancer—for which there are treatment measures available to prevent progression of the condition.

Advantages of screening programs are that often they are relatively inexpensive, take little time, need few professionals to administer them, provide opportunity for prevention, early diagnosis, and treatment, and present statistics on the prevalence of disease when there is adequate follow-up. Major disadvantages of screening programs are that people tend to substitute them for medical examination, findings of screening programs are presumptive and further testing should be done to confirm a diagnosis, screening programs often do not reach vulnerable groups of people, and conditions may be missed during screening, resulting in persons receiving a false impression of their health status.

Not all chronic conditions lend themselves to screening. Many authors have discussed criteria to consider when establishing screening programs. The following principles are seen as essential to good screening practices (Wilson and Jungner, 1968; Mausner and Kramer, 1985):

1. The condition sought should be an important health problem (affect a significant percentage of people).
2. There should be an accepted treatment for clients with recognized disease.
3. Facilities for diagnosis and treatment should be available.
4. There should be a recognizable latent or early symptomatic stage.
5. There should be a suitable test or examination (to detect the disease).
6. The test should be acceptable to the population.
7. The natural history of the condition, including development from latent to declared disease, should be adequately understood.
8. The cost of casefinding (including diagnosis and treatment) should be economically balanced in relation to possible expenditure for medical care as a whole.
9. Casefinding should be thought of as a continuing process and not a "once and for all" project.

It should be clear from reviewing these principles that although screening can be one method for early discovery of asymptomatic disease, it should be used judiciously and discriminately. Screening results need to be thoroughly evaluated and the conditions found must be treated.

Summary

The epidemiological process helps community health nurses to identify the health status of the community in which they are working and to prevent disease, chronic conditions, and other health-related phenomena such as child abuse, mental illness, and domestic violence. This process places emphasis on analyzing the needs of aggregates rather than the needs of individual clients. Like the nursing process it is a scientific, systematic problem-solving approach to the study of health needs.

There are several key concepts inherent in the understanding and utilization of the epidemiological process. These are study of aggregates at risk, natural life history of disease, levels of prevention, host-agent-environment relationships, multiple causation of disease, and person-place-time relationships. In addition to these concepts a community health nurse must understand biostatistics in order to effectively use the epidemiological process.

By applying the concepts and methods of epidemiology, community health nurses play a vital role in the prevention of disease, injuries, and social problems in a community. Through their contacts in a variety of settings they are in a key position to do casefinding, to eliminate barriers to the control of disease, and to promote health through teaching and counseling.

◄ *An Exercise in Critical Thinking* ►

Select a contemporary health problem of interest (e.g., elder abuse, teenage pregnancy, suicide, drug abuse, AIDS, tuberculosis, or homelessness) and discuss agent, host, and environmental factors that have contributed to the occurrence of this problem and have presented barriers to control. Identify primary, secondary, and tertiary preventive activities designed to reduce the condition occurrence and the role of nursing in implementing these activities.

APPENDIX 11-1

Some Common Communicable Diseases Encountered by Community Health Nurses

Disease	Etiological agent	Primary reservoir	Incubation period	Mode of transmission	Period of communicability	Symptoms	Treatment
Hepatitis A (infectious)	Virus	Humans	15-50 days (30 days average)	Person-to-person by fecal-oral route	Maximum infectivity during the incubation period and continuing for a few days after onset of jaundice; no carrier state	Abrupt and "flu-like" with loss of appetite, nausea and vomiting, abdominal discomfort, jaundice, dark brown urine, light brown stool (may be asymptomatic)	No specific treatment (bedrest, increased fluids, no alcoholic beverages, no fried or fatty foods)
Hepatitis B (serum)	Virus	Humans	2 weeks–9 months (60-90 day average)	Percutaneous or permucosal exposure to infected body fluids (blood, saliva, semen, and vaginal fluids)	Weeks before onset of symptoms and infective for entire clinical course; carrier state can exist	Onset is gradual with symptoms similar to those of hepatitis A	Same as hepatitis A
Rubella (German measles)	Virus	Humans	14-21 days	Usually person-to-person (direct contact or droplet spread)	At least 4 days before rash and at least 4 days after onset of rash; very contagious	Mild febrile illness with a macular rash (adults may experience more serious illness); rash on scalp, body, and limbs; usually lasts 1-3 days	No specific treatment (bedrest, increase fluids)
Measles	Virus	Humans	7-21 days (10 days average)	Usually person-to-person (direct contact or droplet spread)	At least 4 days before rash and at least 4 days after onset of rash; very contagious	Resembles a bad cold with eyes and nose running, red blotchy rash beginning usually on face (often behind ears) and then becoming generalized, cough, Koplik spots, more severe symptoms than in rubella; lasts about 4 days	No specific treatment (bedrest, increase fluids, place in darkened room if eyes hurt)

APPENDIX 11-1

Some Common Communicable Diseases Encountered by Community Health Nurses—cont'd

Disease	Etiological agent	Primary reservoir	Incubation period	Mode of transmission	Period of communicability	Symptoms	Treatment
Mumps	Virus	Humans	14-26 days (18 days average)	Person-to-person (direct contact with saliva or droplet spread)	At least 6 days before parotitis and up to 9 days after; very infective about 2 days before symptoms	Pain and swelling in one or both parotid glands, fever, pain on opening and shutting mouth (may need to use a straw to drink)	No specific treatment (bedrest, increase fluids)
Chicken-pox	Virus	Humans	12-21 days (14 days average)	Person-to-person (direct contact; droplet or airborne spread)	2 days before vesicles and 6 days after vesicles appear; very contagious	Sudden onset; maculopapular rash that becomes vesicular and leaves a crusty scalp; generalized rash, itchy	No specific treatment (topical applications for itching, bedrest, encourage fluids, dress in loose clothing and caution person not to become overheated)
Pink eye	Multiple agents	Humans	24-72 hours	Person-to-person by direct contact, also through contaminated clothing, fomites	Entire course of disease, until redness and discharge have disappeared	Lacrimation, eye irritation, and redness of lids; photophobia and mucopurulent discharge	Treatment dependent on causative agent
Ringworm	Fungi	Humans	4-14 days (variable)	Direct skin-to-skin or indirect contact from items such as chairs, barber clippers	As long as lesions are present	Scalp: scaly patches of temporary baldness, crusty lesions, hair may become brittle Body: flat, spreading ring-shaped lesions that are red on the periphery and vesicular or pustular in center Feet: "athlete's foot" characterized by scaling or cracking of the skin between the toes, itching	Topical fungicide: oral medication as prescribed

Data from Vaughan G: *Mummy, I don't feel well,* London, 1970, Causton and Sons, Ltd.; Tennessee Department of Health and Environment: *Protect them from harm,* Murfreesboro, Tenn., 1983, Lancer; Benenson AS: *Control of communicable diseases in man,* ed 15, Washington, D.C., 1990, American Public Health Association.

Continued

APPENDIX 11-1
Some Common Communicable Diseases Encountered by Community Health Nurses—cont'd

Disease	Etiological agent	Primary reservoir	Incubation period	Mode of transmission	Period of communicability	Symptoms	Treatment
Scabies	Mite (*Sarcoptes scabiei*)	Humans	2-6 weeks for initial infestation; 1-4 days for reinfection	Direct skin-to-skin contact; transfer may occur from clothing	As long as condition is present—until mites and eggs are destroyed by treatment	Papular or vesicular; may evidence "burrows" on skin like grayish-white threads; lesions prominent around webs of fingers, wrists, elbows, belt line; intense itching	Kwell lotion
Pediculosis	Louse	Humans	2 weeks (8-10 days average)	Direct person-to-person or indirect contact with infected personal belongings	As long as eggs or lice are alive	Scalp: itching; swollen lymph nodes; can often see nits or lice in hair. Pubic: itching; swollen glands	Kwell lotion or shampoo
Giardiasis	*Giardia lamblia*, a flagellate protozoan	Humans	5-25 days or longer (7-10 days average)	Ingestion of cysts in fecally contaminated water or food; person-to-person by hand-to-mouth transfer of cysts from feces	Entire period of infection	Chronic diarrhea, steatorrhea, abdominal cramps, bloating, frequent loose and pale greasy stools, fatigue, weight loss	Atabrine is drug of choice; metronidazole (Flagyl) is also effective; furazolidone pediatric suspension for young children and infants; enteric precautions should be used
Salmonellosis	Numerous serotypes of salmonella (bacterial); *S. typhimurium* is the most common	Humans and domestic and wild animals, including poultry, swine, cattle, rodents, and pets (e.g., dogs, cats, turtles, chickens)	6-72 hours (12-36 hours average)	Ingestion of organisms in food contaminated by feces; person-to-person by fecal-oral route	Entire period of infection, sometimes over 1 year; antibiotics can prolong this period	Acute enterocolitis, with sudden onset of headache, abdominal pain, diarrhea, nausea, and sometimes vomiting; dehydration; fever nearly always present; anorexia and loose bowels persist for days	Rehydration and electrolyte replacement with oral glucose-electrolyte solution; antibiotics (ampicillin or amoxicillin) for infants under 2 months, the elderly, and the debilitated, or patients with prolonged symptoms (antibiotics may prolong carrier state)

APPENDIX 11-1

Some Common Communicable Diseases Encountered by Community Health Nurses—cont'd

Disease	Etiological agent	Primary reservoir	Incubation period	Mode of transmission	Period of communicability	Symptoms	Treatment
Shigellosis	Shigella (Group A, *S. dysenteriae;* Group B, *S. flexneri;* Group C, *S. boydii;* Group D, *S. sonnei*); bacterial	Humans	1-7 days (1-3 days average)	Person-to-person by fecal-oral route	During acute infection and until infectious agent is no longer present (usually within 4 weeks)	Diarrhea accompanied by fever, nausea, and sometimes toxemia, vomiting, cramps, and tenesmus; blood, mucus, pus in stool	Fluid and electrolyte replacement; antimotility agents contraindicated; antibiotic therapy (e.g., ampicillin, tetracyclines), based on antibiogram of isolated strain, for patients with severe symptoms
Tuberculosis	*Mycobacterium tuberculosis* and *M. africanum* primarily from humans, and *M. bovis* primarily from cattle	Humans	From infection to demonstrable primary lesion 4-12 weeks; risk after infection may persist for a lifetime as a latent infection	Person-to-person (airborne droplet); ingestion of unpasteurized milk or dairy products	As long as sputum is positive for tubercular-bacilli; children with primary tuberculosis are generally not infectious	Imperceptible onset of cough that progressively worsens and is associated with production of mucopurulent sputum. Hemoptysis, chills, myalgia, sweating, anorexia, weight loss, or low-grade fever that persists over weeks to months may occur	Drug therapy with a combination of antimicrobial drugs (e.g., isoniazid, rifampin, and pyrazinamide) Rest/maintain adequate fluid and caloric intake
Impetigo	Bacteria (often *streptococci* or *staphylococci*)	Humans	Variable, but commonly 4-10 days	Person-to-person contact with lesions or secretions and mildly infectious through fomites	As long as purulent lesions continue	Draining, crusty skin lesions that may resemble ringworm or dry scales; often accompanied by fever, malaise, headache and loss of appetite	Antibiotics such as penicillin and erythromycin and antibiotic creams and lotions

APPENDIX 11-2

Information about Select Commonly Acquired Sexually Transmitted Diseases (STDs)

Disease	Usual symptoms	Diagnosis
Gonorrhea* (clap, dose, drip) Cause: *Neisseria gonorrhoeae* bacterium	Appear in 2-10 days or up to 30 days *Women:* 80% have no symptoms; may have puslike vaginal discharge; lower abdominal pain; painful urination *Men:* Thick, milky discharge from penis and/or painful urination; 10%-20% have no symptoms *Men and women:* Sore throat, pain and mucus when defecating; often no anal symptoms	*Women:* Culture from vagina, cervix, throat and/or rectum *Men:* Smear or culture from penis, rectum, and/or throat
Nongonococcal urethritis/ cervicitis* (NGU, NGC) Common cause: *Chlamydia trachomatis* Other causes: *Ureaplasma urealyticum; Trichomonas vaginalis; Candida albicans* and *herpes simplex virus*	Appear in 1-3 weeks *Women (NGC):* Usually have no symptoms: may have frequent uncomfortable urination: vaginal discharge *Men (NGU):* Mild to moderate discomfort on urination; thin, clear or white morning discharge from penis	*Women:* No highly definitive diagnostic tool is currently available for chlamydial infection; culture (to rule out gonorrhea) and a vaginal smear (to rule out trichomonas and yeast) *Men:* Culture (to rule out gonorrhea) and a smear
Pelvic inflammatory disease (PID)† *Affects only women* Usual causes: *Neisseria gonorrhoeae; Chlamydia trachomatis;* enteric bacteria	Onset of symptoms varies; abnormal vaginal discharge; severe pain and tenderness in lower abdominal/pelvic area; painful intercourse and/or menstruation; irregular bleeding; chills and fever; nausea, vomiting	History, culture, and examination to rule out other problems (ectopic pregnancy, appendicitis, etc.); pelvic ultrasound; laparoscopy
Human papilloma virus infection/Condylomata acuminata (HPV, genital/venereal warts) Cause: Human papilloma virus	Appear in 1-6 months; firm, flesh-colored or grayish-white warts on vulva, anus, lower vagina, penis, scrotum, mouth, throat; lesions on cervix usually not visible to the naked eye; itching	Clinical examination and Pap smear of colposcopy for lesions on cervix

Symbols indicate that a particular STD may also be contracted in the following ways:
*Infants: while in birth canal of an infected mother.
†Increased risk through use of the intrauterine device (IUD) as a method of contraception.
‡Fluid from chancre coming in contact with cuts in the skin; infants: while in infected mother's womb.
§Sharing wet towels with an infected person.
‖Change in pH balance of vagina from pregnancy, diabetes, birth control pills, antibiotics, stress, douching.
**Puncture of skin with contaminated needle; using toothbrush, razor, etc., of an infected person.
††May be spread by fingers from one hairy area to another; or by sharing linen or clothing of an infected person.
‡‡Close physical contact (sexual or nonsexual).
Data from Venereal Disease Action Coalition: *Sexually transmitted diseases: a community information and resource guide,* Detroit, 1983, United Community Services of Metropolitan Detroit, pp. 9-11; Centers for Disease Control and Prevention: 1989 sexually transmitted diseases treatment guidelines, *MMWR* 38(No. S-8):4-40, 1989; Centers for Disease Control and Prevention: 1993 sexually transmitted diseases treatment guidelines, *MMWR* 42(No. RR-14):3-59, 1993.

Possible complications	Treatment	Special considerations
Women: Pelvic inflammatory disease (10%-20% of cases) (see PID above) *Men:* Narrowing of urethra; sterility; swelling of testicles *Men and women:* Arthritis, blood infections, dermatitis, meningitis, and endocarditis *Newborns,* Eye, nose, lung, and/or rectal infections	Ceftriazone plus doxycycline or tetracycline or spectinomycin Ceftriazone	3-10 days after treatment and again in 4-6 weeks a culture test should be done (to show cure)
Women: Pelvic inflammatory disease (see PID above), cervical dysplasia (currently under study), ectopic pregnancy, and infertility *Men:* Prostatitis, epididymitis *Newborns:* Eye infections, pneumonia	Doxycycline or azithromycin (erythromycin for pregnant women)	
Sterility; chronic abdominal pain; chronic infection (of the fallopian tubes, uterus and/or ovaries); ectopic pregnancy, death	*Inpatient:* Cefoxitin IV in combination with doxycycline or clindamycin and gentamicin IV *Ambulatory:* Cefoxitin IM in combination with ceftiaxone and doxycycline or tetracycline; bedrest and no sex for at least 2 weeks	Usually the result of untreated gonorrhea or chlamydial infection Scarring of fallopian tubes may increase risk of future ectopic pregnancies IUD, if present, should be removed and replaced by another form of birth control Careful medical follow-up is essential
Blockage of vaginal, rectal, or throat openings; cervical dysplasia; cancer (currently under study)	Cryotherapy with liquid nitrogen or cryoprobe; podophyllin benzoin (contraindicated in pregnancy) or trichloroacetic acid; electrocautery	Warts and invisible lesions are highly contagious; both will continue to multiply until completely removed

Continued

Information about Select Commonly Acquired Sexually Transmitted Diseases (STDs)—cont'd

Disease	Usual symptoms	Diagnosis
Herpes, genital or oral (cold sores; fever blisters on mouth) Causes: herpes simplex virus I (HSV I; oral); herpes simplex virus II (HSV II; genital)	May occur immediately or as late as 1 year after contact or not at all; some people exhibit few or no symptoms Itching, tingling sensation followed by painful blister-like lesions that appear in clusters at the site of infection (i.e., lips, nose, inner and outer vaginal lips, clitoris, rectum, thighs, buttocks); blisters dry up and disappear generally leaving no scar tissue HSV II symptoms in women may include increased vaginal discharge, painful intercourse and urination; painless lesions on cervix may go undetected *Primary episodes:* HSV II—some experience fever, body aches, flulike symptoms, swollen lymph nodes near infected areas *Recurrent episodes:* HSV I and HSV II—generally lessen in frequency and severity over time	Culture from sore, clinical examination or Tzanck smear Definitive diagnosis only possible when lesions are present
Syphilis‡ (syph, lues, pox, bad blood) Cause: *Treponema pallidum* (spirochete bacterium)	First stage—(appears in 10-90 days, average 3 weeks): painless sores (chancres) where bacteria entered body (genitals, rectum, lips, breasts, etc.) Second stage—(1 week to 6 months after stage 1): rash; flulike symptoms; mouth sores; genital/anal sores (condylomata lata); inflamed eyes; patchy balding Latent stage—(10-20 years after stage 2): None Final stage—See possible complications	Blood test; clinical examination
Vulvovaginitis Causes: *Trichomonas vaginalis* (protozoa)§; *Candida albicans* (fungus)‖ *Gardnerella/Haemophilus vaginalis* (bacteria)**	A. *Trichomoniasis* (Trich, TV, A, B, C Vaginitis) appear in 1-6 weeks *Women:* Thin, foamy yellow-green or gray vaginal discharge with foul odor; burning, redness, itching and/or frequent urination *Men:* Usually no symptoms. May have slight, clear morning discharge from penis; itching after urination	*Women:* Vaginal smear; microscopic identification; urinalysis; culture (to rule out gonorrhea); clinical examination *Men:* Hard to diagnose

Possible complications	Treatment	Special considerations
Oral: Autoinoculation to skin or eyes *Genital:* Possible increased risk of cervical cancer; disturbance of bladder or bowel functioning (neuralgia); meningitis (nonfatal) *Newborns:* Blindness, brain damage, and/or death to baby passing through birth canal of mother with active lesions	No known cure at present The following may be helpful in reducing symptoms and/or recurrences: oral acyclovir; stress reduction techniques (yoga, meditation, etc.); keeping sores dry/clean; healthy diet and exercise; inpatient therapy in severe cases: acyclovir IV	HSV I can be found genitally and HSV II can be found orally due to oral-genital sex or autoinoculation Recurrent attacks are unpredictable but often appear at times of high stress, when fatigued, after vigorous intercourse, around menstruation, at times of other illnesses, etc. Research is inconclusive regarding whether or not herpes is occasionally contagious when there are no active lesions Many experience difficult, but not insurmountable, adjustments in self-image and sexual behavior *Women:* Should have Pap smears twice yearly and if pregnant, inform their health care provider (of their herpes); cesarean delivery is indicated if mother has active lesions at the time of delivery; *cervical lesions may go undetected because they are not painful*
Adult: Blindness, deafness (usually reversible); brain damage; paralysis, heart disease, death *Newborns:* Damage to skin, bones, eyes, teeth, and/or liver; death	Penicillin (tetracycline or doxycycline for penicillin-allergic patients; doxycycline used in nonpregnant patients only)	Many women will not notice chancre because it is painless and may be deep inside vagina Complications can be prevented if treated at 1st or 2nd stage Return for blood test 1 month after treatment and once every 3 months for 1 year
A. None	A. Metronidazole (Flagyl)	A. All partners should be treated even if they have no symptoms Cautions about Flagyl: very high doses have been shown to cause cancer in laboratory animals Should not be taken by pregnant or breastfeeding women Alcohol should be avoided when taking Flagyl as it may cause severe headaches and nausea

Continued

APPENDIX 11-2

Information about Select Commonly Acquired Sexually Transmitted Diseases (STDs)—cont'd

Disease	Usual symptoms	Diagnosis
	B. Candida infections (yeast, monilia); onset of symptoms varies	
	Women: Thick, white cottage cheese–like, foul-smelling discharge which adheres to the vaginal walls; intense itching and irritation of genitals	
	Men: usually no symptoms; dermatitis on penis	
	C. *Gardnerella infections;* onset of symptoms varies	
	Women: Thin, foul-smelling yellow-gray discharge; may have some vaginal burning	
Hepatitis B Cause: hepatitis B virus	Appear in 1-6 months, but often no clear symptoms General flulike symptoms; liver deterioration marked by darkened urine, lightened stool, yellowed eyes and skin, skin eruptions, enlarged and tender liver	Blood tests; clinical examination
Pediculosis pubis†† (crabs, cooties, lice) Cause: *Phthirus pubis* (crab louse)	Appear in 4-5 weeks Intense itching in hairy areas (usually begins in pubic hair)	Clinical examination; self-examination may reveal blood spots on underwear, eggs or nits
Scabies‡‡ (the itch) Cause: *Sarcoptes scabiei* (parasite mite)	Appear in 4-6 weeks Severe itching and raised reddish tracts; may appear anywhere on body and are caused by the mite burrowing under the skin	Clinical examination; microscopic observation

Possible complications	Treatment	Special considerations
B. *Newborns:* Mouth and throat infections	B. Miconazole nitrate, clotrimazole, butaconazole or teraconazole intravaginally	A, B, and C. Recurrent infections are common and can be prevented: tub bathing during menstruation, loose clothing and cotton panties; also avoid use of bubble bath, deodorant, tampons, scented soaps, vaginal sprays and douches (as these may irritate the vagina and/or change the pH balance)
C. None	C. Metronidazole (Flagyl) or clindamycin (effective in 50%-60% of cases)	
Chronic hepatitis; chronic acute hepatitis; cirrhosis; liver cancer; death	Bed rest; lots of fluids; a light, healthy diet and no alcohol; no specific drug therapy	Often confused with flu or a bad cold and thus not treated early Recovery usually 2-3 months Will not recur once cured Hepatitis B vaccine will provide immunity
None	Lindane (Kwell) cream, lotion, or shampoo (not recommended for pregnant or breastfeeding women); pyrethrins and piperonyl butoxide applications	Common soap will not kill crabs All clothes and linen must be washed in hot water or dry-cleaned or removed from human contact for 1-2 weeks
Secondary bacterial infection (from scratching)	Lindane (Kwell) cream, lotion, or shampoo (not recommended for pregnant or breastfeeding women) or crotamiton (Eurox) cream or lotion	Common soap will not kill the mites All clothing and linen must be washed in hot water or dry-cleaned or removed from human contact for 1-2 weeks

---

APPENDIX 11-3
Notifiable Diseases, United States

Acquired immunodeficiency syndrome (AIDS)
Amebiasis
Aseptic meningitis
Botulism, total
Brucellosis
Chancroid
Cholera
Diphtheria
Encephalitis, primary
Encephalitis, post-infectious
Gonorrhea
Granuloma inguinate
Hepatitis A
Hepatitis B
Hepatitis, non-A non-B
Hepatitis, unspecified
Legionellosis
Leprosy
Leptospirosis
Lymphogranuloma venereum
Malaria
Measles (rubeola)
Meningococcal infections
Mumps

Pertussis (whooping cough)
Plague
Poliomyelitis, paralytic
Psittacosis
Rabies, human
Rheumatic fever
Rubella (German measles)
Rubella, congenital syndrome
Salmonellosis
Shigellosis
Syphilis, total all stages
   Primary and secondary
   Congenital 1 year
Tetanus
Toxic-shock syndrome
Trichinosis
Tuberculosis
Tularemia
Typhoid fever
Typhus fever
   Flea-borne (endemic, murine)
   Tick-borne (Rocky Mountain spotted)
Varicella (chickenpox)

From Centers for Disease Control and Prevention: Summary of notifiable diseases, United States, 1992, *MMWR* 41:3, 1993.

References

Allen MA and Ownby KK: Tuberculosis: the other epidemic, *JANAC* 2:9-24, 1991.

Beach EK: *Environmental health and communicable disease module,* Ann Arbor, Mich., 1974, The University of Michigan, School of Nursing—Community Health Nursing.

Benenson AS: *Control of communicable diseases in man,* ed 15, Washington, D.C., 1990, American Public Health Association.

Benson V and Marano MA: *Current estimates from the National Health Interview Survey,* National Center for Health Statistics, Vital Health Stat 10(189), 1994.

Centers for Disease Control (CDC), Training and Laboratory Program Office: *Principles of epidemiology: agent, host, environment* (self-study course 3030-G, manual 1), Atlanta, Ga., 1987, The Centers.

CDC, Training and Laboratory Program Office: *Principles of epidemiology: disease surveillance* (self-study course 3030-G, manual 5), Atlanta, Ga., 1987, The Centers.

CDC: Recommendations for prevention of HIV transmission in health-care settings, *MMWR* 36(Suppl S2), August 21, 1987.

CDC: Update: universal precautions for prevention of transmission of human immunodeficiency virus, hepatitis B virus, and other bloodborne pathogens in health-care settings, *MMWR* 37:377-387, June 24, 1988.

CDC: Guidelines for prevention of transmission of human immunodeficiency virus and hepatitis B virus to health-care and public safety workers, *MMWR* 38(Suppl S6), June 23, 1989.

CDC: Prevention and control of tuberculosis in correctional institutions: recommendations of the advisory committee for the elimination of tuberculosis, *MMWR* 38:313-320, 1989.

CDC: Publication of MMWR recommendations and reports on HIV and hepatitis B virus in health-care and public-safety workers, *MMWR* 38:446, 1989.

CDC: Surveillance for epidemics—United States, *MMWR* 38:694-696, 1989.

CDC: A strategic plan for the elimination of tuberculosis in the United States, *MMWR* 38(Suppl S3), April 21, 1989.

CDC: ACIP: mumps prevention, *MMWR* 38:388-400, 1989.

CDC: 1989 sexually transmitted diseases treatment guidelines, *MMWR* 38(No. S-8): 4-40, 1989.

CDC: *Personal communication,* August 1990.

CDC: Screening for tuberculosis and tuberculous infection in high-risk populations, *MMWR* (No. RR-8) 39:1-7, 1990.

CDC: Tuberculosis among foreign-born persons entering the United States: recommendations of the Advisory Committee for Elimination of Tuberculosis, *MMWR* (No. RR-18) 39:1-21, 1990.

CDC: National action plan to combat multidrug-resistant tuberculosis, *MMWR* 41(No. RR-11):5-48, 1992.

CDC: Prevention and control of tuberculosis among homeless persons, *MMWR* (No. RR-5) 41:13-21, 1992.

CDC: Prevention and control of tuberculosis in U.S. communities with at-risk minority populations, recommendations of the advisory council for the elimination of tuberculosis, *MMWR* 41(No. RR-5):1-11, 1992.

CDC: Summary of notifiable diseases, United States, 1992, *MMWR* 41:3, 1993.

CDC: *CDC HIV/AIDS prevention: fact book, 1993,* Atlanta, Ga., 1993, The Centers.

CDC: 1993 sexually transmitted diseases treatment guidelines, *MMWR* 42(No. RR-14):3-59, 1993.

Collins JG: *Prevalence of selected chronic conditions, United States, 1979-81* (DHHS Pub No [PHS] 86-1583), Hyattsville, Md., 1986, National Center for Health Statistics.

Collins JG: *Prevalence of selected chronic conditions: United States, 1986-88,* National Center for Health Statistics, Vital Health Stat 10(182), 1993.

Commission on Chronic Illness: *Chronic illness in the United States, vol I: prevention of chronic illness,* Cambridge, Mass., 1957, Harvard University Press.

Communicable Disease Center: *Food-borne disease investigation: analysis of field data,* Atlanta, Ga., 1964, U.S. Public Health Service.

Doyle, Arthur Conan: *The hound of the Baskervilles,* New York, 1971, Berkley.

Duncan DF: *Epidemiology: basis for disease prevention and health promotion,* New York, 1988, Macmillan.

Friedman GE: *Primer of epidemiology,* New York, 1974, McGraw-Hill.

Grimes DE: *Infectious diseases,* St. Louis, 1991, Mosby.

Horwitz M, Pollard R, Merson M, and Martin SA: A large outbreak of foodborne salmonellosis on the Navajo Nation Indian Reservation: epidemiology and transmission, *Am J Public Health* 67:1071-1076, 1977.

Institute of Medicine—Committee for the Study of the Future of Public Health: *The future of public health,* Washington, D.C., 1988, National Academy Press.

Iseman MD: A leap of faith. What can we do to curtail intrainstitutional transmission of tuberculosis? *Annals of Internal Medicine* 117:251-253, 1992.

Kochi A: The global tuberculosis situation and the new control strategy of the World Health Organization, *Tubercle* 72:1-6, 1991.

Last JM, ed: *Maxcy-Rosenau public health and preventive medicine,* ed 12, Norwalk, Conn., 1986, Appleton-Century-Crofts.

Leavell HR and Clark EG: *Preventive medicine for the doctor in his community: an epidemiologic approach,* New York, 1965, McGraw-Hill.

MacMahon B and Pugh T: *Epidemiology principles and methods,* Boston, 1970, Little, Brown.

Mausner J and Bahn A: *Epidemiology: an introductory text,* Philadelphia, 1974, Saunders.

Mausner JS and Kramer S: *Mausner and Bahn epidemiology: an introductory text,* ed 2, Philadelphia, 1985, Saunders.

Maxcy RF and Rosenau MJ: *Preventive medicine and public health,* New York, 1965, Appleton-Century-Crofts.

Michigan Department of Public Health: *Enteric infections case history,* Lansing, Mich., undated, Division of Epidemiology.

Michigan Department of Public Health: *Infant mortality in Michigan,* Lansing, Mich., 1987, Task Force on Infant Mortality.

Michigan Department of Public Health: *Minority health in Michigan: closing the gap,* Lansing, Mich., 1988, The Department.

Multidrug-resistant tuberculosis, *Annals of Internal Medicine* 117:257-259, 1992.

National Center for Health Statistics: *Current estimates from the National Health Interview Survey, United States, 1998,* Vital and Health Statistics, series 10, No. 173, DHHS Pub. No. (PHS) 89-1501, Washington, D.C., 1989, U.S. Government Printing Office.

National Center for Health Statistics: *Health, United States, 1988,* DHHS Pub. No. (PHS)89-1232, Washington, D.C., 1989, U.S. Government Printing Office.

Prescott WH: *History of the conquest of Mexico,* New York, 1936, Random House, Inc.

Robey B: Two hundred years and counting: the 1990 census, *Pop Bull* 44(1), Washington, D.C., 1989, Population Reference Bureau.

Rubel AJ and Garro LC: Social and cultural factors in the successful control of tuberculosis, *Public Health Reports* 107:626-636, 1992.

Strauss A: *Chronic illness and the quality of life,* St. Louis, 1975, Mosby.

Strauss A, Corbin J, Fagerhaugh S, Glaser BG, Mainos D, Suezek B, and Weiner CL: *Chronic illness and the quality of life,* ed 2, St. Louis, 1984, Mosby.

Surgeon General: *Healthy people: the Surgeon General's report on health promotion and disease prevention, vol I and II,* Washington, D.C., 1979, U.S. Government Printing Office.

Tennessee Department of Health and Environment: *Protect them from harm,* Murfreesboro, Tenn., 1983, Lancer.

U.S. Bureau of the Census: *Statistical abstract of the United States,* ed 109, Washington, D.C., 1989, U.S. Department of Commerce.

U.S. Department of Health and Human Services—Public Health Service: *Health status of the disadvantaged, Chartbook 1986,* Washington, D.C., 1986, U.S. Government Printing Office.

USDHHS: *Healthy People 2000: national health promotion and disease prevention objectives, full report, with commentary,* Washington, D.C., 1991, U.S. Government Printing Office.

USDHHS: *Health status of minorities and low-income groups,* ed 3, Washington, D.C., 1991, U.S. Government Printing Office.

Vaughan G: *Mummy, I don't feel well,* London, 1970, Causton and Sons, Ltd.

Venereal Disease Action Coalition: *Sexually transmitted diseases: a community information and resource guide,* Detroit, 1983, United Community Services of Metropolitan Detroit.

Wilson JMG and Jungner F: Principles and practice of screening for disease, *Public Health Papers No 34,* Geneva, 1968, WHO.

Woodward SB: The story of smallpox in Massachusetts, *N Engl J Med* 206:1181, 1932.

Selected Bibliography

Breslow L: Risk factor intervention for health maintenance, *Science* 200:908-912, 1978.

Centers for Disease Control (CDC): Common-source outbreak of giardiasis—New Mexico, *MMWR* 38:405-406, 1989.

Christiansen EE: Family epidemiology: an approach to assessment and intervention. In Hymovich DP and Barnard MU, eds: *Family health care, vol I: general perspectives,* New York, 1979, McGraw-Hill.

Donabedian D: Computer-taught epidemiology, *Nurs Outlook* 24:749-751, 1976.

Dworkin J: AIDS education for health care professionals in an organizational or systems context, *Public Health Reports* 107:668-674, 1992.

Graham S: The sociological approach to epidemiology, *Am J Publ Health* 64:1046-1049, 1974.

Lancaster E: Tuberculosis comeback: impact on long-term care facilities, *J Gerontological Nurs* 19:6-21, 1993.

Murphy SA: Human responses to catastrophe. In Fitzpatrick JJ, Taunton RL, and Jacox AK, eds: *Annual Review of Nursing Research,* vol 9, New York, 1991, Springer.

National Institute on Disability and Rehabilitation Research: *State estimates of disability in America,* Washington, D.C., 1993, U.S. Department of Education.

Newbern VB: Dealing with infectious and contagious diseases in the South: 1900-1945, *Fam Community Health* 16:11-18, 1993.

Norr KF, McElmurry BJ, Moeti M, and Tiou SP: AIDS prevention for women: a community-based approach, *Nurs Outlook* 40:250-256, 1992.

Plani A, Schoenborn C: *Health promotion and disease prevention: United States, 1990,* National Center for Health Statistics, Vital Health Stat 10(185), 1993.

Rabinowitz S, Melamed S, Kasan R, and Ribak J: Personal determinants of health promoting behavior, *Public Health Reviews* 20:5-14, 1993.

Richards IDG and Baker MR: *The epidemiology and prevention of important diseases,* New York, 1988, Churchill Livingstone.

Tervis M: Approaches to an epidemiology of health, *Am J Publ Health* 65:1037-1045, 1975.

U.S. Department of Health and Human Services (USDHHS): *Toward equality of well-being: strategies for improving minority health,* Washington, D.C., 1993, U.S. Government Printing Office.

Valanis B: *Epidemiology in nursing and health care,* ed 2, Norwalk, Conn., 1992, Appleton & Lange.

12

Community Assessment and Diagnosis

OUTLINE

Why Assess the Community?

Diagnosing Preventive Health Needs in the Community

Methods for Assessing a Community's Health Status

Sources of Community Data

Analysis of All Available Data

Practical Tips for Implementing Community Assessment and Diagnostic Activities

---

OBJECTIVES

Upon completion of this chapter, the reader should be able to:

1. Describe the relevance of community assessment and diagnostic activities to community health nursing practice.
2. Discuss the application of the nursing process to community-oriented practice.
3. Identify parameters for assessing a community's level of functioning.
4. Summarize methods for assessing a community's health status.
5. Explain the relevance of public health statistics to community health nursing practice.
6. Summarize federal, state, and local sources for obtaining community data.
7. Formulate guidelines for implementing community assessment and diagnostic activities in the practice setting.

Chapter 2 explored the ANA's and the APHA's definitions of community health nursing practice, which state that the dominant responsibility of nurses in community health is to the community or the population as a whole (ANA, 1986 and APHA, 1981). Recently both private foundations (The Pew Charitable Trusts) and nursing organizations (ANA and NLN) confirmed the importance of focusing on the health of the community (ANA, 1991; NLN, 1993; Shugars, O'Neil, and Bader, 1991). These organizations' visions for the future emphasize a consumer-driven, community-based health care system and the need for changes in the education of health professionals to prepare them to deal with current issues in health care delivery. They advocate that health professionals be educated to address health promotion and disease prevention at aggregate and community levels, as well as the personal care level (NLN, 1993).

Health promotion and disease prevention at the community level requires the implementation of assessing, diagnosing, and organizing strategies that allow health providers to identify a unique community profile. To establish this profile, community health nurses must "see," "smell," and "hear" the community and describe its people, its environment, its health status, and its health resources. Further, they must work with community residents and systematically analyze all facets of community dynamics (described in Chapter 3) so that aggregates at risk are determined and ways to meet their needs are identified.

Community health nurses at both administrative and staff levels must become involved in community assessment, diagnostic, organizational and health planning activities in order to maintain appropriate health services for all citizens. Nursing directors and supervisors should assume leadership in establishing mechanisms for the ongoing survey of community needs and for maintaining collaborative relationships with consumers and other health care resources. They should encourage staff nurses to assess the characteristics of their work community (neighborhood, census

tract, or district), and aggregates at risk (e.g., the homeless, elderly residents in a senior citizens' high-rise building, pregnant teenagers, or Asian refugees) within these work regions. This assessment process assists staff in understanding how to effect change when resources are lacking and how to mobilize resources when they exist. Nursing administrators must provide an atmosphere within their agency that supports staff involvement in community activities; otherwise staff efforts will be focused on individual and family services.

Staff nurses must also take the initiative to expand their thinking to the community as a whole. When handling a family caseload and managing other professional responsibilities such as clinic and school activities, it is easy for community health nurses to narrow their scope of practice. The value of taking time to study the community in which the nurse practices and to implement community-focused activities is not always readily evident when work demands are heavy. Community-focused practice includes such elements as participation in health screening programs and epidemiological study, education of the community through the media, community advocacy, development of nurse-managed clinics, and outreach activities with disadvantaged populations (Anderson, 1983; Anderson and Yuhos, 1993; Boettcher, 1993; Checkoway, 1988; Storfjell and Cruise, 1984).

WHY ASSESS THE COMMUNITY?

It is essential for the community health nurse to have an understanding of community dynamics because health action occurs in the community. Every community has *patterns* of functioning or community dynamics that either contribute to or detract from its state of health. The community health nurse must recognize these patterns in order to anticipate community responses to health action and to influence the direction of health programming. Without this knowledge it is difficult to effect change.

Knowledge of community dynamics is obtained through systematic community assessment. Community assessment helps the nurse and other health care professionals to identify cultural differences in relation to consumer interests, strengths, concerns, and motivations. This assessment also assists health care professionals in analyzing processes through which community beliefs, values, and attitudes are transmit-

We are indebted to A. Josephine Brown, friend and colleague, who encouraged both faculty and students to expand their thinking beyond individual client casework to the community as a whole. Through her efforts community health nurses have learned how to use the nursing process to plan, implement, and evaluate community health programming. Content and case illustrations in this chapter reflect many of the concepts shared by her.

ted. Having this information allows health professionals to individualize health planning activities for their community.

It is important for the community health nurse to recognize that, as the traditions and health experiences in each community vary, the type of programs designed to meet consumer needs should also vary. Programs appropriate for one community or for an aggregate within a community may be ineffective in meeting the needs of other community aggregates. Calvillo (1992) substantiated this fact when she examined AIDS knowledge and attitudes among Latina women in Los Angeles compared to a national sample of Hispanic women in the United States. The Los Angeles sample had lower educational and income levels. These respondents were less knowledgeable about AIDS and held more erroneous misconceptions about the transmission of AIDS than their national counterparts. Calvillo (p. 415) also found that "women in the Los Angeles sample who were more acculturated had significantly higher knowledge scores, fewer erroneous beliefs and greater knowledge of preventive measures." These facts suggested to Calvillo that socioeconomic status, differing levels of acculturation, and ethnicity all affect educational health programming. She concluded that focused educational efforts should be established to meet the needs of Latina women in Los Angeles since it was obvious that mass media efforts were not meeting their needs.

Studies such as those conducted by Calvillo reinforce the need to study the characteristics of the community in which one is working. They demonstrate that assumptions cannot be made about community response to health promotion and disease prevention interventions, and they point out the relevance of identifying factors that facilitate or inhibit change in health beliefs. Such studies also provide data that support the need for collaborative relationships between the consumer and the health care provider to enhance the delivery of health care services.

Assessment of the community is essential if the community health nurse plans to meet the needs of all aggregates in a given community. Experiences from one community setting cannot always be generalized to another, because health needs and resources are not consistent from one community to another. Research (Burman and Steffes, 1992; Lee and Buehler, 1992) has shown, for example, that rural families who are dealing with serious illness have limited formal resources to call upon in time of need. Data about a specific community are needed if the nature and origin of health problems and the responses to health matters are to be identified.

With the curtailment of federal monies for health care programs, it is even more imperative that community needs and priorities be documented. Funds are appropriated on the basis of documented evidence that a planned health program actually reflects a need within the community. Health programs will be federally funded only when data support their need.

Purpose of Community Assessment for the Community Health Nurse

Within any community setting there will be professionals from many disciplines and concerned citizens interested in community assessment, diagnostic, organizing, and health planning activities. Since it would be impossible for any one group to handle all the health care needs of a community, efforts by many should be encouraged and supported. Equally important is the need for each discipline to define its responsibilities in relation to community-focused activities so that overlapping and uncoordinated efforts will be avoided. Unfortunately it is not uncommon to find that the linkages between various community agencies are weak and that health services are planned without taking into consideration the contributions that other health care professionals are making (refer to Chapter 5). To alter this situation, health care providers must view the community as client and understand that interdisciplinary efforts are needed to achieve wellness for the population as a whole.

Developing effective partnerships with clients and other health providers is the key to successful health planning in the future. "Public health, in a reformed health care system, will forge partnerships between communities and all levels of government. Communities and public health agencies—together—will keep the public healthy by assessing the community's health needs fully, developing the best policies to meet those needs, and assuring that all of us have access to high quality health and medical services and the highest attainable level of individual and community health" (APHA, 1993, unnumbered, forward).

In keeping with APHA's vision for the future, community health nurses must recognize that they are members of an interdisciplinary health team whose activities should not be carried out in isolation when assessing the community. Implicit in the concept of interdisciplinary functioning are several major premises which were delineated in Kane's classic writings on interprofessional teamwork. These include the following: (1) there is a common endeavor or goal that all professionals are working toward; (2) interdisciplinary teams are established to meet client needs, and therefore the client is the key member on the team; (3) professionals will share knowledge and information across disciplinary boundaries so that team goals can be reached; and (4) all disciplines will delineate and share the unique talents they have, so that the team can delegate responsibilities to appropriate team members (Kane, 1975).

The unique perspective that the community health nurse brings to an interdisciplinary community team is a holistic philosophy derived from a synthesis of nursing and public health knowledge. The community health nurse's professional experience, educational preparation, value system, and relationships with consumers provide the skills necessary to integrate biopsychosocial data into a meaningful whole. Since all parameters of human functioning and all aspects of community dynamics have an impact on the client's (community) health status, the whole must be analyzed to truly determine the needs of the consumer.

Prevention is often the one aspect of wholeness that is overlooked when community problems are analyzed and health services developed. This happens because many health care professionals have a curative rather than a preventive health philosophy. Because community health nurses, as well as other community health professionals, have educational preparation that enhances their ability to examine the preventive aspects of health behavior, they are delegated the major responsibility for monitoring preventive and health promotion practices in the community. "Only programs that systematically work to promote health and to prevent disease and injury on a community-wide basis can keep people from getting sick. It has always been the mandate of public health to prevent, rather than merely treat, our health problems" (APHA, 1993, p. 1).

The community health nurse's primary purpose in assessing the community is to identify strengths and deficiencies in relation to preventive health practices. The nurse places emphasis on examining the health care delivery system to determine if structural or process characteristics within this system impede preventive health programming. In addition, the community health nurse works with consumers and other health care professionals to improve the quality of preventive and health promotion activities when deficiencies are identified.

DIAGNOSING PREVENTIVE HEALTH NEEDS IN THE COMMUNITY

When participating in community diagnostic activities the community health nurse uses the nursing process as described in Chapter 9, but shifts emphasis from the family as client to the community as client. Data are collected from multiple sources (assessing) and analyzed in order to formulate nursing diagnoses about community health problems. Nursing diagnoses about existing health needs, community dynamics that either positively or negatively influence health action, and deficiencies in the existing health care delivery system are generated for the purpose of facilitating community organization and health planning activities. Nursing diagnoses about community strengths are also made, because it is through its strengths that a community is able to resolve its health problems. Some examples of nursing diagnoses that might be made after the community health nurse has analyzed community assessment data are listed here:

- Children in census tracts 10 and 11 are at risk for lead poisoning because most homes were built before 1950, homes are poorly repaired, and housing regulations are inadequately enforced.
- Thirty-five percent of the aging persons in the community are experiencing social isolation because recreational activities and transportation for these persons are lacking.
- Teenagers are at risk for unwanted pregnancies because health care resources in the community refuse to provide birth control information for teenagers without parental consent.
- Community health nursing services need to be increased in census tract 5, because the number of new referrals from this area exceeds the time the current nurse has available for home visiting.
- Local churches within the community readily support health education efforts.

- Service clubs within the community respond very favorably when health care professionals request financial assistance for meeting unresolved health problems.

Nursing diagnoses describe the individual's, family's, or the community's health problem/condition/(strength) and the primary etiological or related factor(s) contributing to the problem/condition that is the focus of nursing treatment (Gordon, 1993). Community-focused nursing diagnoses are derived from a synthesis of assessment data, are based on the concept of risk relative to population groups (discussed extensively in Chapter 11), and are situations primarily resolved by nursing intervention. For example, note the earlier nursing diagnosis related to teenagers in the community. Teenagers who find it difficult to obtain contraceptive services are at risk for unwanted pregnancies. A community health nurse is often in a key position to assist youth with their family planning needs through health education and program planning interventions and nursing treatment. He or she is also frequently in a position to prevent or diagnose lead poisoning among children. Since many families are unaware of the dangers of this condition and its causes (etiology), community health nurses often plan health education programs designed to inform the public about lead poisoning. They also assess the environment during home visits and travel through their districts to ascertain the extent of homes still having lead-painted surfaces (children at high risk for lead poisoning live in homes built before 1950 because lead was included in paint before this date).

Once nursing diagnoses are established, the community health nurse uses the principles of planning (refer to Chapter 13) to prioritize health needs, to determine alternative ways to resolve these needs, to develop specific objectives for health programming, and to identify ways to accomplish the stated objectives (planning). Following are a few examples of objectives that might be developed when planning a health program to meet the social needs of aging citizens in the community:

- The county commissioners will appropriate funds for a senior citizens project in census tract 2.
- St. Francis Catholic Church will donate space in their facilities once a week for recreational activities for the aging.
- Community volunteers will plan and imple-

ment recreational activities for the aging at St. Francis Church.
- The local chapter of the American Red Cross will provide transportation for aging citizens once a week, so that these persons can participate in the social activities planned at St. Francis Church.

These objectives can be met in several ways. For example, the community health nurse might make all the necessary contacts personally or delegate responsibilities to others, perhaps by obtaining volunteers. Church groups, service clubs, and social workers from community agencies, for instance, often know of individuals who are interested in volunteering their time and energies for worthy community projects. Community health nurses usually seek help from others when planning a health program because they know that active participation by consumers and other professionals promotes long-term support and involvement.

Planning must result in action (implementing), and action must be evaluated; otherwise time and effort are wasted and community needs go unresolved. When one is evaluating action, new problems often emerge. If this is the case, objectives and intervention strategies should be altered to reflect ways to resolve new and existing needs.

Diagnosing community health problems and planning action to correct these problems are often more difficult than was just indicated. The point being made above is that the community health nurse uses the nursing process—assessing, analyzing, planning, implementing, and evaluating—when intervening in affairs of the population as a whole, as well as when working with individual families. A range of community-focused nursing functions, categorized by the phases of the nursing process, is presented in the box on pp. 434-435.

How community health nurses assess the health status of populations and how they analyze community data is further elaborated on in this chapter. An overview of community organization and health planning activities is presented in Chapter 13.

METHODS FOR ASSESSING A COMMUNITY'S HEALTH STATUS

There are a variety of strategies a community health nurse can use to obtain data about community

Community-Focused Nursing Functions

Assessment

1. Identifies pertinent information about community.
2. Gathers descriptive data about the community.
3. Assesses health-related learning needs of populations.
4. Participates in identifying community health states and health behaviors, including the knowledge, attitudes, and perceptions of groups regarding health and illness.
5. Collects pertinent information about community in a systematic way.
6. Aids in community health surveys.
7. Includes members of the community as partners in the assessment process.
8. Uses basic statistics and demographic methods to collect health data.
9. Collaborates with other health care providers to assess the community.
10. Consults with community leaders to describe the community.

Analysis

11. Identifies common and recurrent health problems that have potential for illness consequences.
12. Identifies health needs of help-seeking and nonseeking populations.
13. Describes health capability of community based on assessment.
14. Applies selected epidemiologic concepts in analyzing assessment data (population-at-risk, incidence, prevalence, for instance).
15. Describes present community health problems in the perspective of time (recognizes trends).
16. Describes and analyzes resources available including patterns of utilization.
17. Analyzes data for relationships and clues to the community's health.
18. Aids/participates in analysis of community health data base.
19. Forms ideas and hypotheses concerning data gathered in community assessment to derive inferences for nursing programs.
20. Includes members of the community in analyzing assessment data.

Planning

21. Assists in developing plans to meet needs arising from gaps or deficiencies identified.
22. Develops service priorities and plans for intervention based on analysis, community expectations and accepted practice standards.
23. Participates in planning community health programs.
24. Determines priorities for community health care based on information gathered during assessment.
25. Participates with community leaders in planning to meet identified health needs.
26. Participates with others in developing health plans applicable to the community at large.
27. Develops service objectives of identified community problems.
28. Uses knowledge of change process in planning community programs.
29. Plans for community-wide or age-specific screening programs.
30. Includes members of the community as partners in planning community health programs.

Implementation

31. Mobilizes the community's collective resources to help achieve higher community health goals.
32. Functions as a health advocate for the community.
33. Serves as vital link in the communication network between all kinds of community agencies and clients.
34. Seeks opportunities to participate with other disciplines in projects to bring about changes in the availability, accessibility, and accountability of health care and related systems.
35. Sets up immunization campaigns with community leaders and public health officials.
36. Initiates and monitors disease prevention programs in the community.
37. Educates the community through media regarding health issues.
38. Organizes community groups to work on alleviating community health problems.
39. Acts as a catalyst/potentiator for community change.

From Anderson ET: Community focus in public health nursing: whose responsibility? *Nurs Outlook* 31:44-48, 1983, p. 46.

◀ *Community-Focused Nursing Functions—cont'd* ▶

40. Sets up ongoing community health education programs with community leaders and public health officials.

Evaluation

41. Monitors health services for desired quality.
42. Continually validates appropriateness of public health programs (discusses with residents, collects more data, for example).
43. Contributes information for use in evaluation of nursing programs.
44. Evaluates community response to nursing intervention.
45. Ensures necessary community health program eval-

uation data are collected accurately and systematically.
46. Analyzes results of service in relation to proportion of population served.
47. Promotes systematic evaluation of community resources.
48. Evaluates the impact of nursing activities on the health of the community as a whole.
49. Includes members of the community as partners in evaluating health programs.
50. Analyzes results of service in relation to whether community program objectives were reached.

© 1981, E. Anderson

strengths and needs. Before selecting any method for data collection, the community health nurse must first define what needs to be assessed. Establishing guidelines for assessment helps the nurse to organize the data collection process and to identify significant factors that influence a community's state of wellness.

Figure 12-1 summarizes the various parameters the community health nurse should examine when analyzing the health status of any community. It points out that the physical, social, and mental aspects of wellness are interrelated and that people and environmental and health resource characteristics make an impact on a community's state of wellness. If any one of these components changes, the balance of health is altered in the community setting. When diagnosing community needs it is important to examine all components of wellness and to identify community dynamics that detract from or enhance community growth. Chapter 3 presents the knowledge needed to analyze community dynamics.

After determining the information needed to establish appropriate nursing diagnoses about community problems, the community health nurse uses both subjective and objective data collection methods to obtain this information. These methods are discussed below. It is important to keep in mind that no one method is sufficient for obtaining a comprehensive view of how a community is functioning. In evaluating community assessment methodology, verification that adequate sampling and faithful description and

interpretation have taken place is essential (Ruffing-Rahal, 1985, p. 135).

Use an Assessment Tool

A systematic approach to data collection is needed in order to obtain a comprehensive profile of a community's level of functioning or competence. Use of a community assessment tool is one way to systematically obtain information about community dynamics and health status data. A community assessment tool helps community health nurses to identify assessment parameters, organize data in a meaningful manner, formulate diagnoses about community strengths and needs, and identify needed community intervention activities.

State and local health departments are developing community assessment tools to facilitate collection of essential community data needed for health planning. This is so because the demographics of the population are changing rapidly, significant health problems such as homelessness and AIDS are increasing, and dramatic changes are occurring in the health care delivery system. A method for systematically monitoring these changes is needed. Changes in the way funding agencies support state and local health programs have also promoted the development of community assessment tools. For example, federal health block grant monies (refer to Chapter 13 for further discussion) are allocated to the states in a lump sum. States have the

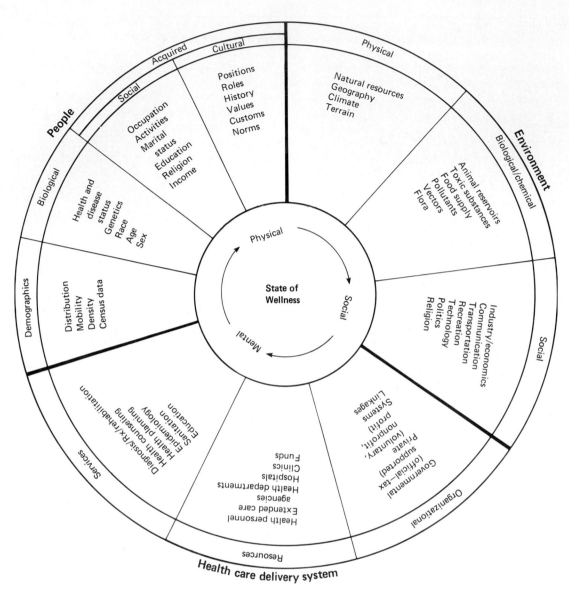

Figure 12-1   The community: its people, its environment, and its health care delivery system.

freedom to use these monies to support state and local health activities within the block grant functional areas of maternal-child health, prevention, community health services, and alcohol, drug abuse, and mental health. Local health departments and other community agencies must submit to the state a grant proposal, which includes data to support a community need, to obtain monies from the block grant allocations.

A community assessment tool to assist the beginning practitioner in obtaining community data very quickly was presented in Appendix 3-1. The assessment tool in Appendix 12-1 is systematically organized around the components of a community and community dynamics. This tool aids the practitioner in doing a comprehensive community assessment over an extended period of time.

Analyze Available Statistics

Many people immediately associate the term *statistics* with a long list of numbers, boring to read and difficult to use. If used effectively, however, statistical data can be exciting and intriguing. These data can quickly reveal facts about a community, including clues about why citizens do or do not become involved in health projects, as well as concrete information about the characteristics of the population being served. For example, one community health nurse was concerned because parents in one of the schools she serviced were not participating in health activities designed to promote child safety. When this nurse looked at census tract data, she found that 64% of the households in her district were headed by single-parent, working mothers who had marginal incomes. This information suggested to the nurse that in order to reach these women she would have to plan activities outside the traditional 8 to 5 working hours. It also pointed out to her that she was dealing with families who were at risk for financial, social, and psychological crises. These data stimulated the nurse to design health programs that were relevant to mothers' and children's needs. One program, "How to Meet Your Social Needs While Caring for Small Children," was particularly well received. This program was planned because the nurse on several home visits heard mothers complain about the lack of time for leisure activities. The expressed concerns of these mothers, coupled with knowledge obtained from census tract data, led the nurse to believe that there were other mothers in the area who had the same concern. Her nursing diagnosis was valid and resulted in a meaningful health program that was well attended. Because this one program was so well received, an ongoing activity and discussion group for these mothers was established, with equally positive results. The processes this nurse used to develop her mother's group and to maintain it are presented in Chapter 21.

Use of statistical data can be very beneficial in community health nursing practice. The nurse in the above illustration found that statistical data provided her with clues about why families were not responding to school health activities. Statistical data also helped this nurse to identify some of the possible concerns of the population she was serving; thus she was able to predict health interests and plan health programs accordingly.

Statistical data often provide the basis for decision-making in the face of uncertainty. The community health nurse frequently finds that there are several requests for nursing service and that it is necessary to plan time to benefit the greatest number of people.

Using census tract data, vital statistics, and health statistics can help community health nurses to determine where to focus their efforts. Take, for instance, the community health nurse who has several requests for the establishment of a well-baby clinic in various locations. If only one clinic can be funded, this nurse may use statistical data to document a need for a clinic in one location rather than another. The concentration of preschool children in a given area, the illness and death rates of these children, and the level of immunization protection can all be obtained from statistical data. These data provide information about where the greatest need exists and can be used to substantiate a decision a nurse might make about clinic location.

The importance of understanding and using statistical data becomes increasingly apparent to the community health nurse when decisions such as those described above must be made. Statistical data help the community health nurse to carry out many daily responsibilities more effectively. These data help the nurse to:

- Predict health needs of individuals, families, and populations
- Identify aggregates at risk
- Determine priorities when needs are greater than staff time available
- Evaluate the outcomes of nursing services
- Document accountability
- Support the need for increased funding for nursing services

Specific types of statistical data were presented in Chapter 11. It is important for health care professionals to analyze a range of available health or health-related data, such as demographic, morbidity, and mortality statistics, to assess community strengths and needs. Comparing local, state, and national statistics is equally important. Additionally, examining statistical trends over time can provide significant results. These processes help the professional to more effectively judge a community's health and needed health action. For example, if a local community's incidence rate for lung cancer is significantly higher than the incidence rate for the state and the nation over a five-year period, this community might want to initiate a prevention control program immediately. However, if this situation was noted only in a given year, the community would want to establish an effective monitoring system to determine if this was an isolated occurrence or the start of a pattern over time.

TABLE 12-1 Distribution of Reported AIDS Cases by Exposure Category and Sex in the United States, Cumulative Totals through December 1992

Horizontal Axes

	% of AIDS cases			
Exposure category (risk group)	Men (N = 221,714)	Women (N = 27,485)	Children <13 yrs (N = 4,249)	Total (N = 253,448)
Vertical Axes				
Male homosexual contact with HIV	64%			56%
IV drug users (IVDU)	20%	50%		23%
Heterosexual contact with HIV	1%	36%		7%
Male homosexual and IVDU	7%			6%
Transfusion recipient	3%	7%	7%	2%
Mother with HIV			86%	1%
Hemophiliac	1%		4%	1%
Undetermined	4%	7%	3%	4%
Total	100%	100%	100%	100%

From Centers for Disease Control and Prevention: *HIV/AIDS Surveillance Report, Year-End Edition* 9:11-12, February 1993.

Graphical Presentation of Data

Graphical presentation of data is an efficient way to show large numbers of observations at one time. Numerical figures are more easily remembered when presented graphically because data are organized and relationships are demonstrated. Tables, graphs, and charts are some of the instruments used to present statistical information symbolically. Guidelines for presenting data in this form include the following:

- Illustrate only the amount of data that is visually appealing.
- Number a table, graph, or chart if more than one is used (Table 12-1).
- Title each table, graph, or chart, including in the title information identifying *what, where,* and *when*.
- Label both the horizontal and vertical axes of the graphic presentation.
- Identify the source of the data at the bottom of the chart, including author, title of publication, publisher, date of publication, and reference page number.

When these guidelines are used, a table would look like the example presented in Table 12-1.

Graphical presentation of data has popular appeal and is frequently used to portray quickly a large number of facts. Graphs, charts, and tables can be misused or misunderstood, however, especially if one attempts to relate data that are unrelated. Also, attempting to present too many facts in one table defeats the purpose for using visual presentations of data; when this is done, it confuses rather than clarifies the events being illustrated.

Available data on a community should be used in the most effective way possible to get across the significance of a community's health problems. These data should not, however, be misrepresented on tables, graphs, and charts. If available data are not sufficient to reach decisions about a community's state of health, do not try to make them so by graphically presenting incomplete or inaccurate findings. Rather, use other methods to collect the data needed to analyze what is happening in the community.

Carry Out Surveys

Surveys are commonly conducted in community health nursing practice because existing health and health-related data are inadequate to substantiate a need for the development of a particular health program. Standard sources of data may show that suicide is one of the leading causes of death for older adolescents. This information is significant in that it focuses attention on a major health problem of this developmental age group. It is not sufficient, however, to identify health action needed in a particular community for reducing adolescent mortality as a result of suicide. Other types of information must be collected before a health project is initiated in a local community. Data about such things as the use of available mental health resources by teenagers, attitudes of professionals and consumers in relation to the needs of the adolescent, and reasons for teenage suicidal actions must be ascertained before health planning can be effective. A survey is frequently conducted to obtain this type of information.

A community survey is a systematic study designed to collect data about a community's functioning. Data about a specific segment of the population, about a particular component of the health care delivery system, or about health needs of the entire community may be collected when conducting a survey. The scope varies depending on the purpose and the financial and work force resources available. It is important to define specifically the reason for doing a survey because this process can be costly and time-consuming. On the other hand, this process can provide essential data for health programming and may save time and monies if it is planned carefully (refer to Figure 12-2).

Sometimes health care professionals become enthusiastic and attempt to speed up the survey process by decreasing planning time. This practice is not wise because planning can actually decrease the time it takes to effectively implement a survey. For example, conducting a pilot study or a small-scale survey during the planning phase can help to eliminate major problems in the survey process before an extensive study is initiated. This could significantly reduce the amount of time that is needed to obtain appropriate data.

There are a variety of ways in which a community can survey its needs. Personal interviews, telephone interviews, or written questionnaires are a few examples of the methods that can be used to collect data about community health problems and strengths. It is important to select carefully survey methods and tools because resources and needs vary from one community to another. Reviewing the literature about what other professionals are discovering in their work is useful.

Surveys should be used to obtain data that are not

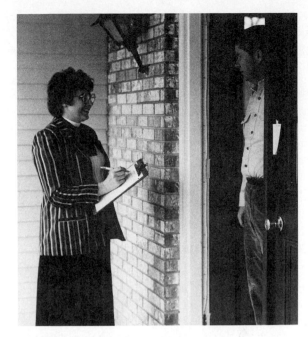

Figure 12-2 House-to-house surveys assist health care professionals in obtaining a comprehensive understanding of their local communities. A well-planned survey can provide data about such things as resource use patterns, social concerns, and specific health needs of a particular community. The public health professional pictured was a member of an epidemiological team that was conducting a city-wide family health study. Higher than average infant deaths prompted the local health department to initiate this study. The results of the survey helped the health department to focus its maternal-child health (MCH) efforts. Ten years after the survey was completed, this local community no longer qualified for special state MCH funds because of its low infant mortality rate. (Courtesy Henry Parks, photographer.)

available from other sources. Generally, accurate data can be obtained about vital events (births, deaths, or marriages), but morbidity data are often incomplete. Disease rates and data about health-related phenomena (alcoholism, mental disorders, child abuse) are usually only estimates because of the lack of adequate reporting. It is frequently unknown how many individuals are affected by these conditions or how many affected are receiving adequate care. Surveys may be able to elicit such data. In addition, a survey can help to determine comprehensive needs of a particular segment of a population. Census information provides data about a census tract in relation to income, housing, education, and transportation. It does not provide data about specific health problems, social needs, or health care resources.

Data obtained from a survey provide the foundation for more extensive investigation of health needs in a community. Research is frequently conducted after surveys are completed to explore the potential cause-and-effect relationships between differing community phenomena. Surveys do not provide sufficient evidence to substantiate cause-and-effect conclusions because generally there are very few controls built into a survey design (Polit and Hungler, 1987).

Conduct Focus Group Interviews

Conducting focus group interviews is another approach for obtaining information about health needs and strengths from a community's perspective. "The focus group interview or discussion is a qualitative approach to learning about population subgroups with respect to conscious, semi-conscious and unconscious psychological and sociocultural characteristics and processes" (Basch, 1987, p. 411). The focus group method is useful for obtaining culturally relevant and community-specific assessment data because it aids health care providers in gaining an understanding of a range of community attitudes and beliefs about a problem. It also assists the health professional in obtaining data about peoples' perceived needs and priorities and their preferences regarding health programming (Gonzalez, Gonzalez, Freeman, and Howard-Pitney, 1991, p. 19).

The standard focus group format is similar to the processes used with small groups (Basch, 1987; Gearhart-Pucci and Haglund, 1992; Krueger, 1989). The leader or moderator uses a variety of leadership interventions to establish the focus groups, to promote a supportive group atmosphere, and to accomplish specific goals. These interventions are discussed in Chapter 21 and include such things as finding an appropriate and easily accessible setting, creating a nonthreatening climate in which all members feel safe to participate, and facilitating group process by clarifying and highlighting significant issues.

Like other small groups, a focus group usually lasts no more than 1 to 3 hours. A focus group differs from many small groups in that the participants are usually homogenous with respect to characteristics such as age, sex, and social variables. Focus group interviews

are structured around a specific set of questions designed to identify community needs and strengths. This structure is established to learn about and assist the community as a whole, rather than individual group participants (Basch, 1987).

When using the focus group approach to assess community problems, several groups that represent varying aggregates at risk are identified in order to obtain a range of opinions about community problems and preferences and priorities for health programming. For example, if health care professionals want to learn about the accessibility of preventive health care services in a community, they may discuss this issue with a group of senior citizens, parents of young children, teenagers, low-income families, and individuals representing an ethnic group in the community. Only with this type of representation can the health care professional obtain data about perceived need in relation to the community as a whole. Key informants can assist health care providers in identifying appropriate focus group participants. Focus group interviews are an efficient way of gathering information about a target group's perspective on an identified concern (Gearhart-Pucci and Haglund, 1992).

Conduct Research

Research to document the effectiveness of nursing services and to identify cause-and-effect relationships is critically needed in the community health nursing setting. Funders of health care services are demanding concrete data that support the need for nursing personnel, the need for certain health programs, and the value of using one intervention strategy rather than another. If qualitative data are not available, funders evaluate effectiveness only on the basis of quantitative counts, such as the numbers of home, school, or clinic visits. When this happens the quality of nursing care can suffer.

Research can help the health care professional to document effectiveness of quality, as well as to identify community needs and to propose intervention strategies that best meet these needs. Illustrative of this is the study conducted by Street Health, a community-based nursing organization in Toronto that operates clinics for women and men who are homeless or underhoused (Crowe and Hardill, 1993, p. 21). Recognizing that they lacked quantitative data to document both the health problems of their homeless clients and barriers to services—structural and attitudinal—the Street Health nurses established a research survey project to obtain the data needed to strengthen their lobby efforts for homeless people. This survey showed that homeless women and men had health problems similar to the general population but that the prevalence of many health problems, such as emphysema, chronic bronchitis, and epilepsy, was significantly greater in the homeless population than the general public. It also showed that life circumstance had a tremendous impact on homeless persons' abilities to cope with these problems and that there were a number of barriers preventing the homeless from receiving appropriate and/or compassionate care (Crowe and Hardill, pp. 22-23). Based on these survey results, Street Health developed over 40 recommendations that target a variety of community health agencies and educational institutions. For example, Street Health has recommended that emergency room staff receive sensitivity training about the community they serve, that the Ministry of Health prohibit all publicly funded health care institutions from refusing care to individuals who do not have their health card, and that Toronto's metro police develop a standing order to address the problem of discriminatory treatment of and violence towards homeless people (Crowe and Hardill, p. 23). The Street Health nurses are currently using these research findings to advocate needed health services for their clients.

Research use is a critical component of professional nursing practice. It is imperative that the community health nurse be familiar with research in the field and integrate research findings into clinical nursing practice. Reading journals and attending professional conferences are important ways to remain current on research related to nursing practice. The *Annual Review of Nursing Research* is a unique nursing research reference that has been published every year since 1983. Each volume has chapters summarizing nursing research in selected areas by experts in the field. A number of areas that have been addressed in the *Review* would be of interest to community health nurses.

"Not all nurses need to conduct research, but all should use it to guide their practice" (Lusk, 1993, p. 153). The ANA has spelled out a research role for nurses at all levels of preparation (ANA, 1989). Research is every nurse's business! Research-based knowledge in community health nursing is rapidly evolving and nurse researchers are an integral part of the scientific community, helping to move nursing into the 21st century. Nursing and related health research is incorporated throughout this text, with referenced research studies in most chapters.

Time must be provided so that practitioners can investigate clinical practice issues and concerns. Only in this way can a profession remain viable. Collaborative relationships established between service settings and academic environments can facilitate practitioners' involvement in research. Research can be stimulating and challenging to practitioners, especially if they have support and encouragement from individuals who are involved in clinical research on a regular basis. On the national level, a major thrust in nursing research is aimed at community-based practice. The National Institute of Nursing Research's priorities are outlined in Chapter 24.

Contact Key Community Informants

Research and surveys tend to focus on the present. Since a community's current characteristics are an outgrowth of its historical development, it is beneficial to interview consumers and community leaders to identify what has gone on in the past and how the past is affecting the present. The values, attitudes, and interests of previous community leaders often subtly influence the current direction of health planning. Contact with key community persons, or *informants,* can help community health nurses to understand why there is resistance to certain health programs, how to reduce resistance to change, and with whom nurses might work to enhance their productivity in the community setting.

Directors of housing projects, clergy, professionals in other health care agencies, local politicians, owners of long-established businesses, and unofficial community spokespersons are some of the individuals a nurse might contact to obtain information about community dynamics. These individuals can help the nurse to gain knowledge about the power relationships within a local area, community values and attitudes, and environmental factors that enhance or detract from a community's state of health. Unofficial spokespersons often provide the most candid opinion of how the consumer views health and the health care delivery system. Clergy, agency clients, and cultural organizations such as International Neighbors or the Polish club, can frequently assist a community health nurse in identifying these unofficial spokespersons.

A community health nurse should use every opportunity available to relate to community people outside and within the agency. The opportunities are limitless and require only motivation on the part of the nurse and supervisory support to take advantage of them. A visit to the local library can provide very valuable information about a community's history. On the other hand, talking with people the nurse meets while carrying out regular caseload responsibilities can be just as valuable. Spontaneous interchange often provides an atmosphere for free, honest communication. This type of dialogue also helps to create a positive image in relation to what health care professionals are doing to improve the health of people. The ability to relate to others in the community, such as school principals, physicians, administrators in mental health agencies, secretaries, and clergy, is essential if one wants to diagnose community needs accurately.

Observe, Listen, and Analyze

Data about a community can be obtained daily by observing, listening, and analyzing. What the environment looks like when the nurse drives in the district, how families are dressed when they are seen in the clinic setting, and who relates to whom during community meetings all provide the community health nurse with clues about a community's state of health.

Participant observation during significant community events such as community health and political meetings, social gatherings, religious ceremonies, and special celebrations is an important process for community health nurses. This process can assist the health care provider in learning about people's behavior and practices and their differences and similarities. During this process the nurse might notice how business is conducted, how decisions are made, who attends community events, health concerns of community residents, and differences in attitudes about service usage (Gonzalez, Gonzalez, Freeman, and Howard-Pitney, 1991; Randall-David, 1989). Participant observations help the community health nurse to identify significant cultural differences in the community and health concerns that need to be addressed. They also aid the nurse in identifying key informants.

Community health nurses who are really interested in the welfare of their community will take time to analyze what has been observed and heard. They will be alert to environmental conditions that adversely affect the state of a community's health. If, when driving through the district, a nurse finds older homes in poor repair, he or she can raise questions about the potential for lead poisoning and the need for enforcement of housing legislation. An astute nurse will not ignore observations or accept them as a matter of fact without trying to effect change.

Analysis of community observations must focus on strengths in addition to needs, because it is through a community's strengths that health problems are resolved. One community health nurse, for example, was able to effect environmental changes in her district because she identified that the parents in the area were genuinely concerned about the welfare of their children. Rat-infested vacant lots in the neighborhood presented a serious threat to the children who played in them. This nurse, with the assistance of a minister, was able to mobilize parents' energies so that the garbage from these lots was removed and rats were killed. Maintaining the lots as suitable play areas became a major community project.

A community health nurse who views the community as the unit of service is more likely to meet the needs of individual families than the nurse who focuses only on family health care needs. Family problems are interrelated with community problems and often cannot be resolved until changes occur within the community system. A nurse needs to collect data on the community in order to determine the extent to which family health problems are influenced by community values, attitudes, and beliefs. Frequently, families from differing ethnic backgrounds are labeled "social" problems because they do not relate to social systems in the same way as middle-class Americans. When this is the case, change will not occur if the community health nurse works only with individual families. In these situations the community health nurse needs to help social systems adapt to different cultural values and attitudes and must help families learn how to interact with social systems unfamiliar to them.

SOURCES OF COMMUNITY DATA

There are numerous federal, state, and local agencies and individuals that a community health nurse can contact in order to obtain data about the community. Some have been mentioned previously in this chapter and are summarized here to give a composite picture of the multiple sources of data one can use when diagnosing community needs.

The only federal agency specifically established for the collection and dissemination of health data is the National Center for Health Statistics. This agency conducts the National Health Survey, which provides valuable information on the health and illness status of U.S. residents (refer to Chapter 11). In addition, this agency provides official information on vital statistics and data about the supply and use of health resources (Office of the Federal Register, 1988).

Several other federal agencies will supply health data on request. The Alcohol, Drug Abuse, and Mental Health Administration, the Health Resources and Services Administration, and the Centers for Disease Control and Prevention are a few examples of such agencies. Appendix 12-2 presents selected sources of data on the health of the U.S. population, the availability and use of health services, and health care expenditures. The *United States Government Manual,* which can be purchased from the Superintendent of Documents, U.S. Government Printing Office, Washington, D.C., is a valuable reference for identifying other government agencies that disseminate health data. This manual describes the purposes and programs of most federal agencies, and is updated regularly.

The importance of obtaining data from the Bureau of the Census on the size, distribution, structure, and change of populations in the United States cannot be overemphasized. These data demonstrate patterns over time and provide general characteristics of a community's total population. Knowing that there is a high concentration of individuals 65 years and over, or of children ages 1 through 5 in a community, assists health care professionals in predicting the types of health problems and health care services needed in a particular community. For example, a community health nurse who knows from census tract data that 30% of the people in his or her census tract are 65 years or older should become concerned if limited or no geriatric families are in the caseload and then investigate why referrals for this age group are not being received.

In addition to helping individual staff nurses, census tract data help nursing administrators to determine where nursing services are most needed. Knowledge about the concentration of people, the economic status, and housing conditions in an area assists administrators in predicting aggregates at risk in segments of their community. Often state health departments will help local health departments use census tract data to identify at-risk groups. State health departments have statistical divisions that provide consultation in relation to data collection and analysis.

State health departments are a major source of data for identifying the health status of citizens in a particular state. Vital statistics, morbidity data, health work force, and resource information are usually collected and disseminated by this agency. The department of education, the bureau of mental health, and the office of services to the aging are some other state agencies that supply health and health-related information. Obtaining a state directory of social agencies will help each reader to determine which agencies in her or his state furnish information about specific health needs in local communities. The number of state agencies that supply health and health-related data are too numerous to list here.

On the local level, some key sources for obtaining community data are the chamber of commerce, city planner's office, health department, county extension office, intermediate school districts, libraries, health and welfare professionals, hospital records, clergy, community leaders, and consumers. Again, sources are too numerous for all of them to be listed here. Most cities and counties have social services directories that provide information on the major health and welfare resources in their community. Experienced practitioners can also help new community health nurses to identify the most appropriate source for obtaining specific data about the area in which they are functioning.

Legislators and public officials on all three levels of government are usually more than willing to assist the health care professional in analyzing social and health care legislation. Laws and ordinances related to community health reflect the values and priorities of a community, the state, and the federal government. Every health care professional should be familiar with legislation that influences the health of his or her community. Specific laws and ordinances are discussed throughout this text. Here it is sufficient to emphasize the importance of studying legislative trends in order to gain an understanding of a community's priorities in relation to health care issues.

ANALYSIS OF ALL AVAILABLE DATA

Data should not be collected merely for the sake of having data. Unfortunately this is often the case. Daily activity reports, vital statistics, and census data are frequently collected, but just as frequently filed in a drawer without being used. This benefits no one. Once community data are assembled they should be

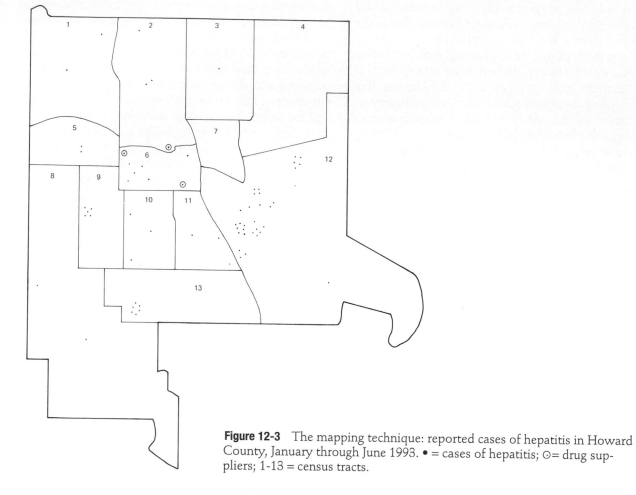

Figure 12-3 The mapping technique: reported cases of hepatitis in Howard County, January through June 1993. • = cases of hepatitis; ☉= drug suppliers; 1-13 = census tracts.

organized in a meaningful way so that patterns of functioning and trends can be ascertained. Many techniques can be used to synthesize community data. Charts, figures, and tables are often used for this purpose. Graphic presentation of population distributions, morbidity data, or vital statistics for several decades can be very effective in pinpointing significant community problems. Growth or lack of growth in a community, for instance, can be identified when population distributions are graphically visualized. Lack of growth in a community can be a very serious problem because many federal and state health funds are allocated on a per capita basis; that is, a given amount of money is allocated for each person residing in the area.

Mapping is another technique that facilitates data analysis. Dotted scatter maps can be used to deter-

mine at a glance such things as high-risk populations, poor environmental conditions, the distribution of illness, disease, and health, and the accessibility of health care services. When this technique is used, school districts or political jurisdictions are usually outlined on a county map. Point symbols or spots are then distributed within these divisions as specified events happen (disease, death, health-related phenomena, or condemned housing), at the exact locations where the events occurred. Figure 12-3, Reported Cases of Hepatitis in Howard County, illustrates the mapping technique. The clustering of hepatitis cases in census tracts 12, 13, and 9 was related to an outbreak of hepatitis that occurred in a trailer camp in census tract 12. Relatives and friends from census tracts 9 and 13 had contact with family and friends in census tract 12 while they were in a communicable state. An epidemiological investigation provided evidence showing that a major outbreak of hepatitis had occurred in a very short time period. The clustering of hepatitis cases in census tract 6 was a result of drug problems.

Dotted scatter maps can be very impressive and useful, but they can also be misleading if the population base is not analyzed. One geographical area may have far fewer cases than another because there are far fewer people in that area. Calculating rates, ratios, and percentages aids in making comparisons between census tracts. These descriptive statistics also help to compare the occurrence of significant events with other communities and with state and national rates.

Comparing community rates with state and national rates is very beneficial. It can highlight specific health problems and community strengths. It helps a community determine priorities for program planning. If a community's infant and maternal mortality rates, for instance, are much higher than state and national rates, a community would want to examine carefully its maternal-child health programming. On the other hand, a community may find, when making these comparisons, that its maternal-child health statistics are far superior to those of other areas. This in turn could demonstrate to the community the value of maintaining adequate health programs for these two age groups in the population.

Analysis of data often supports the need for further data collection. This is illustrated in the following case situation:

▶ The health department became aware of a maternal infant health problem in one census tract of a large urban area. This census tract was a residential rental area with basement efficiency apartments renting for $540.00 or higher per month. The population was 75% students and young working people, referred to as the "swinging singles." Of the remaining 25%, 20% were elderly first-generation Jewish merchants, and 5% were young black families living in the city housing project. The area had a high reported incidence of mugging, purse snatching, and apartment thefts, with rumors of drug manufacturing, pushing, and usage.

Few referrals were made to the health agencies in the area; casefinding was negligible; records of nursing services showed few home visits to individuals in this district. The explanation given for this situation was that the majority of the population in this census tract was either at school or working and, therefore, inaccessible to agency personnel during the working day. Evening office hours were scheduled by private physicians and several health clinics in the area. The health department became particularly concerned about the lack of referrals from this census tract when they analyzed the infant and maternal death rates for the entire county. It was discovered that only in this census tract did these rates significantly vary from national statistics.

Infant and maternal mortality rates for the specified census tract were:

23.4 infant deaths per 1000 live births
5.2 maternal deaths per 1000 live births

Infant and maternal mortality rates in the United States during the same time period were:

10.1 infant deaths per 1000 live births
3.1 maternal deaths per 1000 live births

It was obvious from the vital statistics that something had to be done to improve the health status of mothers and children in this area. However, more specific data were needed to determine causes of death, health status of area residents, and use of health care services, as well as related health problems, including socioeconomic difficulties, drug use, and attitudes about the "establishment." Personnel from a drug clinic and the student organization at a local college assisted the health department in collecting the data they needed. Lack of transportation, extremely limited incomes, lack of knowledge, inadequate nutrition, and resistance to normal channels of health care were some of the major problems identified. The establishment of a neighborhood health clinic, staffed mostly by college students and area residents, produced positive results. Data analysis at the end of 3 years reflected a significant decrease in both the infant and maternal mortality rates for this area.

This situation dramatically illustrates the importance of analyzing data once they are compiled. Community diagnostic activities are carried out so that appropriate decisions about health planning can be made. If data are not analyzed, health action probably will not occur.

PRACTICAL TIPS FOR IMPLEMENTING COMMUNITY ASSESSMENT AND DIAGNOSTIC ACTIVITIES

Community assessment and diagnostic activities are exciting and challenging. It should be apparent, however, that they cannot be left to chance. If these activities are to be implemented effectively, time for planning, assessing, and analyzing must be set aside and administrative support must be available. Equally important is the need to always keep the framework of the "community" in clear perspective when providing nursing care. Community dynamics that adversely affect the health status of individuals, families, and aggregates at risk should not be ignored. Nursing intervention strategies should be planned to resolve community problems and the needs of individual clients.

New practitioners often experience feelings of frustration and disillusionment when first entering the practice setting because there are tremendous gaps between reality and the ideal. Presented below are suggestions for bridging some of these gaps in relation to community activities.

Do Preliminary Community Assessment during Orientation Period

It is only natural for newly employed nurses to want immediate involvement in client casework. Reading policy and procedure manuals and attending orientation meetings can be tiring and less than rewarding. It is important, however, to remind yourself that orientation periods are designed to facilitate functioning in all aspects of one's job responsibilities. Do not overplan family visits during this time period. Rather, balance family and community activities so that time is available to learn about community dynamics and population characteristics. Allowing time in your schedule to engage in the following activities during the orientation period will help you to function more effectively in the community health setting.

- Analyze census tract and vital statistics data to learn about population characteristics in your district.
- Attend case conferences and community meetings (PTA, social service council, citizen group activities) with an experienced employee.

- Attend a board of health meeting to identify the values and attitudes of those responsible for policy-making in the health department.
- Drive through your district, observing environmental conditions, interactions between people, and the location of health care and welfare resources, recreational facilities, local churches, school systems, and shopping areas (refer to Figure 12-4).
- Shop in your district to determine cost of essentials such as food and clothing.
- Make field visits with personnel from other departments in your agency (environmental health, mental health, or nutrition).
- Observe in clinic settings (well-baby, STD, adult screening, or prenatal).
- *Ask questions.*

Most agencies allow new employees to help design their own orientation. The above activities should be planned for, even if similar experiences were available during your course of study in the academic environment. In the educational setting these types of experiences are planned so that students have the opportunity to apply theoretical concepts in the practice setting. Educational experiences cannot, however, provide the practitioner with the specific information needed to understand the unique characteristics of the population being served.

Discuss Community Problems during Supervisory Conferences

In community health nursing practice the practitioner is frequently unable to meet client needs because of deficiencies in the health and welfare systems. There may also be insufficient time to work comprehensively with all the families referred to the nurse. These difficulties should be discussed with the nursing supervisor because the supervisor is in a favorable position for initiating major change in community systems. In addition, the supervisor can provide support and assistance in relation to caseload management activities and give suggestions about innovative intervention strategies for dealing with community problems. For example, it is not uncommon for the nursing supervisor to help the staff develop a new well-baby clinic when child health services are lacking. It is also not uncommon for the nursing supervisor

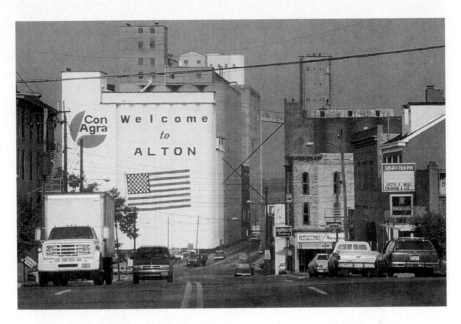

Figure 12-4 Direct observation of a community provides the nurse with valuable assessment data.

to provide support and assistance when a staff member wants to establish group activities in order to expand her or his services to a larger number of clients.

Include Community-Focused Activities in Evaluation Tools

Staff-level community-focused activities are seldom evaluated or rewarded. As a result, very little priority is placed on these types of activities and the focus of service shifts from the community as a whole to individual clients. To alter this pattern the practitioner must take time to revise evaluation tools and procedures so that community activities are assessed during the evaluation process. Only if this is done will time be allocated for community work. Listed below are a few examples of items you might want to include under a community service category on a staff evaluation tool:

- Assesses health needs and strengths of specific populations (school, clinic, industry) in assigned district
- Works with nursing supervisor to discern health action needed for at-risk aggregates in assigned district
- Works with the nursing supervisor to develop intervention strategies (group work, clinic ser-

vices) for aggregates at risk in assigned district
- Collaborates with other professionals on health-planning projects for aggregates at risk in the community

Summary

Meeting the health needs of at-risk aggregates is a major function of the community health nurse. A nurse must know the community before this responsibility can be effectively carried out. A variety of strategies must be used to assess the health status, the health capability, and the health action potential of the nurse's community. Data must be analyzed, as well as collected, so that target groups for nursing service can be identified. Use of the nursing process facilitates implementation of these activities.

There are numerous professionals and consumers who will assist the community health nurse in identifying community health problems and strengths. Interdisciplinary collaboration and consumer participation must be fostered during the community assessment and diagnostic processes because no one person alone can appropriately diagnose community needs.

Exploring the community, its organization, and its activities is extremely rewarding because it gives a clearer picture of community health action. It provides the foundation for health planning activities that are designed to improve the health status of high-risk groups. It further helps the community health nurse to assist individual families more effectively because often family health problems cannot be resolved until changes occur in the health care delivery system. It may be difficult for the community health nurse to integrate community-focused activities into an already busy schedule, but it is essential to do so in order to meet the needs of individuals, families, and aggregates at risk.

◀ *An Exercise in Critical Thinking* ▶

You are a community health nurse who works for a local health department that was directed by the city commissioners to develop short- and long-range plans to combat local community violence. The agency's violence task force, of which you are a member, recognizes that it has insufficient data to make decisions about specific community interventions. Thus, the committee's first goal is to assess community perceptions regarding this problem and to collect and analyze quantitative data relative to the nature of the problem. Taking into consideration that there are several types of violence (e.g., child and elder abuse, domestic violence, homicide, and intentional and unintentional injury) that occur in a community, identify the key informants who could assist your task force in obtaining the community's perspective about the problem. Additionally, discuss the kinds of quantitative data you would need to document the extent of the violence in your community and where and how you might obtain this data. Further, discuss how community attitudes about violence could facilitate or inhibit your data collection process.

Community Assessment Tool: Overview of Its People, Environment, and Systems

Community _____　　　　　　　　　　　　　　　　　Date _____

Check (✔) appropriate column*	Strength	Potential need	Problem	Description/comments
I. *People*				
A. Vital and demographic statistics 1. Population density				
2. Population composition a. Sex ratio				
b. Age distribution				
c. Race distribution				
d. Ethnic origin				
3. Population characteristics a. Mobility				
b. Socioeconomic status				
c. Level of unemployment				
d. Educational level				
e. Marriage rate				
f. Divorce rate				
g. Dependency ratio				
h. Fertility rate				
i. Head of household				
4. Mortality characteristics a. Crude death rate				
b. Infant mortality rate				
c. Maternal mortality rate				
d. Age-specific death rate				
e. Leading causes of death				
5. Morbidity characteristics a. Incidence rate (specific diseases)				
b. Prevalence rate (specific diseases)				
B. History of community (i.e., founding, cultural groups)				
C. Values, attitudes, and norms				
D. Individual and family living practices				

*Place check in only one column—strength, potential need, or problem.

NOTE: The material presented in Chapters 3, 4, 5, 11, 12, and 13 and the cultural assessment tool in Chapter 7 are especially helpful to the nurse when using this assessment tool. The nurse initially collects available data and then adds to this assessment on an ongoing basis.

Continued

Community Assessment Tool: Overview of Its People, Environment, and Systems—cont'd

Check (✔) appropriate column	Strength	Potential need	Problem	Description/comments
1. Types of families				
2. Number of children per family				
3. Leisure activities				
II. *Environmental* A. Physical 1. Natural resources				
2. Geography, climate, terrain			.	
3. Roads/transportation				
4. Boundaries				
5. Housing (types available by percent, condition, percent rented, percent owned)				
6. Other major structures				
B. Biological and chemical 1. Water supply				
2. Air (color, odor, particulates)				
3. Food supply (sources, preparation)				
4. Pollutants, toxic substances, animal reservoirs or vectors				
5. Flora and fauna				
6. Is this a predominantly urban, suburban, or rural community? (How is land used?)				
III. *Systems* A. Health 1. Preventive health care practices and facilities (list)				
2. Treatment health care facilities (e.g., acute care, medical, and surgical hospitals) (list)				
3. Rehabilitation health care facilities (e.g., alcoholism) (list)				
4. Long-term health care facilities (e.g., nursing homes) (list)			.	

Community Assessment Tool: Overview of Its People, Environment, and Systems—cont'd

Check (✔) appropriate column	Strength	Potential need	Problem	Description/comments
5. Respite care services for special population groups (list)				
6. Hospice care services (list)				
7. Catastrophic health care facilities and services (list)				
8. Special health services for population groups (what and how provided) a. Preschool				
b. School age				
c. Adult or young adult				
d. Occupational health				
e. Adults and children with handicapping conditions				
9. Voluntary health care resources				
10. Sanitation services				
11. Health work force (population ratios)				
12. Health education activities				
13. Methods of health care financing (approximate percent) a. Private pay				
b. Health insurance				
c. HMO				
d. Medicaid/Medicare				
e. Worker's Compensation				
14. Prevalent diseases and conditions (list)				
15. Linkages with other systems				
16. Health care resource overall availability				
17. Health care resource overall use				

Continued

Community Assessment Tool: Overview of Its People, Environment, and Systems—cont'd

Check (✔) appropriate column	Strength	Potential need	Problem	Description/comments

B. Welfare
  1. Official (public) welfare resources
    a. General (list; e.g., Department of Social Services)				

b. Safety and protection (list; e.g., fire department)				
2. Voluntary welfare resources (list)				
3. Transportation resources (public and private)				
4. Facilities to meet needs (e.g., shopping areas, public housing)				
5. Special services for population groups (list)				
6. Resource accessibility				
7. Resource use				
C. Education 1. Public educational facilities (list)				
2. Private educational facilities (list)				
3. Libraries (list)				
4. Educational services for special populations a. Pregnant teens				
b. Adults				
c. Developmentally disabled children and adults				
d. Other				
5. Resource accessibility				
6. Resource use				
D. Economic 1. Major industry and business (list)				
2. Banks, savings and loans, credit unions (list)				

Community Assessment Tool: Overview of Its People, Environment, and Systems—cont'd

Check (✔) appropriate column	Strength	Potential need	Problem	Description/comments
3. Major occupations (list)				
4. General socioeconomic status of population				
5. Median income				
6. Percent of population below poverty level				
7. Percent of population who are retired				
E. Government and leadership 1. Elected official leadership (list with title)				
2. Nonofficial leadership (list with title affiliations)				
3. City offices (location, hours, services)				
4. Accessibility to constituents				
5. Support of community resources				
F. Recreation 1. Public facilities (list)				
2. Private facilities (list)				
3. Recreational activities frequently used (list)				
4. Leisure activities frequently used (list)				
5. Coordination with educational recreation facilities and programs				
6. Programs for special population groups a. Elderly				
b. People who are handicapped				
c. Others				
7. Resource accessibility				
8. Resource use				
G. Religion 1. Facilities by denomination (list)				

Continued

Community Assessment Tool: Overview of Its People, Environment, and Systems—cont'd

Check (✔) appropriate column	Strength	Potential need	Problem	Description/comments
2. Religious leaders (list)				
3. Community programs and services				
4. Resource accessibility				
5. Resource use				
IV. *Community dynamics* (describe) A. Communication (diagram and describe)				
1. Vertical (community to larger society)				
2. Horizontal (community to itself)				
3. Specific resources (e.g., television, radio, newspapers)				
V. *Major sources of community data* A. Government (list, e.g., local health department, city planning office)				
B. Private (list, e.g., chamber of commerce)				

Questions for the Community Health Nurse

1. In general, are resources readily available and accessible?
2. What does the community see as its major strengths and needs?
3. How self-sufficient is the community in meeting its perceived needs?
4. What does the community health nurse see as the community's major strengths and needs?

5. Health care
   a. How does the community view and use the health care system? (Specify cultural barriers.)
   b. What does the community see as its health care needs?
   c. What are the goals and major activities of the health system?
   d. How self-sufficient is the community in meeting its health needs?

Community Assessment Tool: Overview of Its People, Environment, and Systems—cont'd

Community Health Care Goals and Activities to Implement Them

Date	Goals	Activities to Implement

Assessor _____ Date_____

Assessor _____ Date_____

Assessor _____ Date_____

APPENDIX 12-2

Selected Sources of Data on the Health of the United States Population, the Availability and Use of Health Sources, and Health Care Expenditures

Source of data	Type of data
Department of Health and Human Services	
National Center for Health Statistics (NCHS)	Only federal agency specifically established for the collection and dissemination of health data.
National Vital Statistics System	Collects and publishes data on births, deaths, marriages, and divorces in the United States: The recording of births and deaths has been complete since 1933.
National Survey of Family Growth	Conducted by NCHS periodically since 1963; latest survey was 1988. This survey is designed to provide national data on the demographic and social factors associated with childbearing, adoption, and maternal and child health. Factors examined include sexual activity, marriage, unmarried, cohabitation, divorce and remarriage, contraception and sterilization, infertility, breastfeeding, pregnancy loss, low-birth weight, and use of medical care for family planning, infertility, and prenatal care. Interview data are obtained from a sample of women ages 15-44 years.
National Health Interview Survey (NHIS)	A nationwide, continuing, sample survey; data are collected through personal household interviews on personal and demographic characteristics, illnesses, injuries, impairments, chronic conditions, utilization of health resources, and other health topics.
National Health Examination Survey (NHES)	A nationwide, continuing sample survey, established in 1960-1962. Data were collected through direct standardized physical examinations, clinical and laboratory tests, and measurements on the total prevalence of certain chronic diseases and the distributions of various physical and physiological measures including blood pressure and serum cholesterol levels. In 1971, the survey name was changed to the *National Health and Nutrition Examination Survey.*
National Health and Nutrition Examination Survey (NHANES)	A nationwide, continuing, sample survey where health-related data are obtained by direct physical examinations, clinical and laboratory tests, and related measurement procedures. A major purpose of this survey is to measure and monitor indicators of the nutritional status of the American people. The first NHANES was conducted from 1971 through 1974 and obtained detailed examination data on cardiovascular, respiratory, arthritic, and hearing conditions. The second NHANES was conducted from 1976 through 1980, and obtained detailed data on diabetes, kidney and liver functions, allergy and speech pathology, as well as the nutritional status of U.S. residents. Periodic follow-up of the total cohort strengthens this data base.
National Master Facility Inventory (NMFI)	NMFI is a comprehensive file of inpatient health facilities (hospitals, nursing and related care homes, and other custodial or remedial care facilities) in the United States.
National Hospital Discharge Survey (NHDS)	A continuing, nationwide sample survey which collects data about discharges from short stay hospitals.
National Nursing Home Survey (NNHS)	Two sample surveys (August 1973 through April 1974 and May through December 1977) done to obtain data about nursing homes, their expenditures, residents, staff, and discharged patients (1977 survey only).
National Ambulatory Medical Care Survey (NAMCS)	NAMCS is a continuing national probability sample of ambulatory medical encounters in the offices of nonfederally employed physicians.
National Medical Care Utilization and Expenditure Survey (NMCUES)	NMCUES is a national sample survey which examined health expenditures for and use of personal health services and individual and family insurance coverage during 1980. It also checked, through an administrative records survey, the eligibility status of the household survey respondents for the Medicare and Medicaid programs.

From *National Center for Health Statistics: Health, United States, 1991,* Hyattsville, Md., 1992, Public Health Service, pp. 305-321.

APPENDIX 12-2

Selected Sources of Data on the Health of the United States Population, the Availability and Use of Health Sources, and Health Care Expenditures—cont'd

Source of data	Type of data
Health Resources and Services Administration	
Bureau of Health Professions	This bureau evaluates both the current and future supply of health manpower in the various occupations. It also designates Health Manpower Shortage Areas for three federal programs: the National Health Service Corps and the Loan Repayment and Scholarship programs. These shortage area designations are also used to determine funding priorities for other programs.
Centers for Disease Control and Prevention (CDC)	
Center for Infectious Diseases	This center maintains a national morbidity reporting system, which collects demographic, clinical, and laboratory data on conditions such as rabies, aseptic meningitis, diphtheria, tetanus, encephalitis, foodborne outbreaks, and others. One of its primary purposes is to maintain national surveillance of infectious diseases. Currently, a major surveillance system has been established by this center to deter epidemiological trends relative to AIDS. The *AIDS Surveillance* is conducted by health departments in each state, territory, and the District of Columbia. Using a standard confidential case report form, the health departments collect information on each identified AIDS case. The pamphlet, *Morbidity and Mortality Weekly Report (MMWR)*, published by CDC provides extremely valuable, up-to-date information on a broad base of public health concerns and issues, as well as current statistics on infectious diseases.
Epidemiology Program Office (EPO)	EPO, in partnership with the Council of State and Territorial Epidemiologists (CSTE), operates the *National Notifiable Diseases Surveillance System.* The purpose of this system is primarily to provide weekly provisional information on the occurrence of diseases defined as notifiable by CSTE.
Center for Chronic Disease Prevention and Health Promotion	This center maintains an *Abortion Surveillance* system which provides epidemiological data on abortions in all states in the United States.
Center for Prevention Services	This center conducts a U.S. Immunization Survey which is used to estimate the immunization level of the nation's child population against the vaccine preventable diseases. Periodically, immunization level data are also collected on the adult population.
Alcohol, Drug Abuse, and Mental Health Administration	
National Institute on Alcohol Abuse and Alcoholism	Funds national surveys of drinking habits, which provide data on trends in alcohol consumption.
National Institute on Drug Abuse	This institute conducts *National Household Surveys on Drug Abuse* to obtain data on trends in use of marijuana, cigarette, and alcohol among youths 12-17 years of age and young adults 18-25 years of age
National Institute of Mental Health	The Institute conducts surveys of inpatient and outpatient psychiatric facilities and studies to determine characteristics of patients served by these facilities.
Health Care Financing Administration	
Bureau of Data Management and Strategy	This bureau compiles annual estimates of public and private expenditures for health by type of expenditure and source of funds. It also maintains a Medicare statistical program which tracks the eligibility of employees and the benefits they use, the certification status of institutional providers, and the payments made for covered services.

Continued

APPENDIX 12-2

Selected Sources of Data on the Health of the United States Population, the Availability and Use of Health Sources, and Health Care Expenditures—cont'd

Source of data	Type of data
Department of Commerce	
Bureau of the Census	This bureau has taken a census of the United States population every ten years since 1790. It also conducts a monthly Current Population Survey (CPS) to provide estimates of employment, unemployment, and other characteristics of the general labor force, the population as a whole, and various subgroups of the population.
Department of Labor	
Bureau of Labor Statistics	This bureau prepares monthly the *Consumer Price Index* (CPI) which is a measure of the changes in average prices of the goods and services purchased by urban wage earners and by clerical workers and their families. The CPI shows trends in medical care prices based on specific indicators of hospital, medical, dental, and drug prices. This bureau also publishes data on employment and earnings.
Environmental Protection Agency	This agency collects data on the five pollutants for which National Ambient Air Quality Standards have been set (refer to Chapter 17) and maintains a National Aerometric Data Bank (NADB).
National Institutes of Health (NIH)	NIH through its National Cancer Institute maintains 11 population-based cancer registries known as the Surveillance, Epidemiology and End Results (SEER) Program. This program provides data on all residents diagnosed with cancer during the year and follow-up information on previously diagnosed patients.
National Institute for Occupational Safety and Health (NIOSH)	NIOSH conducted the *National Occupational Hazard Survey* (NOHS) between February 1972 through June 1974 to obtain data on employee exposure to particular chemicals and physical agents in various industries. Beginning in 1981, NIOSH began a second national survey of worksites patterned after NOHS, known as the *National Occupational Exposure Survey (NOES)*.
United Nations	The statistical office of this organization prepares the *Demographic Yearbook,* which is a comprehensive collection of international demographic statistics.
Alan Guttmacher Institute	This institute is the research and development division of the Planned Parenthood Federation of America, Inc. It conducts, on an annual basis, a survey of abortion providers. This institute also prepares educational documents related to other fertility issues such as teenage pregnancy.
American Hospital Association (AHA)	AHA annually surveys hospitals in the United States to obtain data about characteristics of clients served by the hospital, services provided, demographic and geographic characteristics (e.g., bed size and location), length of hospital stays, and the like.
American Medical Association (AMA)	AMA has maintained a master file of physicians since 1906. From 1920 to 1957 AMA also conducted annual censuses of all hospitals registered by the Association.
Public Health Foundation	The Association of State and Territorial Health Officials (ASTHO) Reporting System, operated by the Public Health Foundation, is a statistical system that provides comprehensive information about the public health programs of state and local health departments. This system was established in 1970.

References

American Nurses Association, Community Health Nursing Division: *Standards of community health nursing practices* (Pub No CH-10), Kansas City, Mo., 1986, The Association.

American Nurses Association (ANA): *Education for participation in nursing research,* Kansas City, Mo., 1989, The Association.

American Nurses Association: *Nursing's agenda for health care reform,* Kansas City, Mo., 1991, The Association.

American Public Health Association, Public Health Nursing Section: *The definition and role of public health nursing in the delivery of health care,* Washington, D.C., 1981, The Association.

American Public Health Association (APHA): *Public health in a reformed health care system: a vision for the future,* Washington, D.C., 1993, The Association.

Anderson ET: Community focus in public health nursing: whose responsibility? *Nurs Outlook* 31:44-48, 1983.

Anderson J and Yuhos R: Health promotion in rural settings: a nursing challenge, *Nurs Clinics of North America* 28:145-157, 1993.

Basch C: Focus group interview: an underutilized research technique for improving theory and practice in health education, *Health Education Quarterly* 14:411-448, 1987, Winter.

Belville R, Indyk D, Shapiro U, Dewart T, Moss JZ, Gordon G, and Lachapelle S: The community as a strategic site for refining high perinatal risk assessments and interventions, *Social Work in Health Care* 16:5-19, 1991.

Boettcher JH: Promoting maternal infant health in rural communities: the Rural Health Outreach Program, *Nurs Clinics of North America* 28:199-210, 1993.

Burman M and Steffes M: Home health care and hospice services in rural areas. In Western Institute of Nursing: *Communicating nursing research, silver threads: 25 years of nursing excellence, Vol. 25,* Boulder, Colorado, 1992, The Institute, p. 426.

Calvillo ER: AIDS knowledge and attitudes among Latinas. In Western Institute of Nursing: *Communicating nursing research, silver threads: 25 years of nursing excellence, Vol 25,* Boulder, Colorado, 1992, The Institute, p. 415.

Centers for Disease Control and Prevention: *HIV/AIDS Surveillance Report, Year-End Edition,* February 1993:1-23.

Checkoway B: Community-based initiatives to improve health of the elderly, *Danish Medical Bulletin,* Special Supplement, Series No. 6, 1988, pp. 30-36.

Community Health Nursing Faculty: *Public health statistics notes,* East Lansing, Mich., 1968, Michigan State University.

Crowe C and Hardill K: Nursing research and political change: the Street Health Report, *The Canadian Nurse* 88:21-24, 1993.

Duncan DF: *Epidemiology: basis for disease prevention and health promotion,* New York, 1988, Macmillan.

Gearhart-Pucci L and Haglund BJA: Focus groups: a tool for developing better health education materials and approaches for smoking intervention, *Health Promotion International* 7:11-15, 1992.

Gonzalez U, Gonzalez J, Freeman U, and Howard-Pitney B: *Health promotion in diverse cultural communities,* Palo Alto, Calif., 1991, Health Promotion Resource Center, Stanford Center for Research in Disease Prevention.

Gordon M: *Manual of nursing diagnosis, 1993-1994,* St. Louis, 1993, Mosby.

Kane RA: *Interprofessional teamwork,* Syracuse, N.Y., 1975, Syracuse University School of Social Work.

Krueger, RA: *Focus groups—a practical guide for applied research,* London, 1989, Sage Publications.

Lee H and Buehler J: Exploration of perceived needs and adequacy of resources for rural families with cancer. In Western Institute of Nursing: *Communicating nursing research, silver threads: 25 years of nursing excellence,* vol 25, Boulder, Colorado, 1992, The Institute, p. 424.

Lusk SL: Linking practice and research, *American Association of Occupational Health Nurses Journal* 41:153-157, 1993.

Maternal and Infant Task Force on AIDS: *Perinatal AIDS in Michigan,* Lansing, Mich., 1988, Michigan Department of Public Health.

Mausner JS and Kramer S: *Mausner and Bahn Epidemiology—an introductory text,* ed 2, Philadelphia, 1985, Saunders.

National Center for Health Statistics: *Health, United States, 1988,* DHHS Pub No (PHS)89-1232, Washington, D.C., 1989, US Government Printing Office.

National Center for Health Statistics: *Health, United States, 1991,* Hyattsville, Md., 1992, Public Health Service.

National League for Nursing: *A vision for nursing education,* New York, 1993, The League.

Office of the Federal Register: *United States government manual, 1988/89,* Washington, D.C., 1988, The Office.

Polit DF and Hungler BP: *Nursing research: principles and methods,* ed 3, Philadelphia, 1987, Lippincott.

Randall-David E: *Strategies for working with culturally diverse communities and clients,* Bethesda, Md., 1989, The Association for the Care of Children's Health.

Ruffing-Rahal MA: Qualitative methods in community analysis, *Public Health Nurs* 2:130-137, 1985.

Shugars DA, O'Neil EH, and Bader JD, eds: *Healthy America: practitioners for 2005, an agenda for action for U.S. health professional schools,* Durham, N.C., 1991, The Pew Health Professions Commission.

Storfjell JL and Cruise PA: A model of community-focused nursing, *Public Health Nurs* 1:85-96, 1984.

United States Department of Health and Human Services (USDHHS): *Health status of the disadvantaged chartbook, 1986,* Washington, D.C., 1986, U.S. Government Printing Office.

Selected Bibliography

Bracht N, ed: *Health promotion at the community level,* London, 1990, Sage Publications.

Finnegan L and Ervin NE: An epidemiological approach to community assessment, *Public Health Nurs* 6:147-151, 1989.

Flynn BC: Developing community leadership in healthy cities: the Indiana Model, *Nurs Outlook* 40(3):121-126, 1992.

Goeppinger J: Health promotion for rural populations: partnership interventions, *Family and Community Health* 16:1-10, 1993.

Hamilton P: Community nursing diagnosis, *Adv Nurs Sci* 5(3):21-36, 1983.

Hanchett E: *Community health assessment: a conceptual tool kit,* New York, 1979, Wiley.

Muecke MA: Community health diagnosis in nursing, *Public Health Nurs* 1:23-35, 1984.

Schultz PR: When client means more than one: extending the foundational concept of person, *Adv Nurs Sci* 10:71-86, 1987.

Schwab M, Neuhauser L, Morgen S, Syme SL, Ogar D, Roppel C, and Elite A: The Wellness Guide: towards a new model for community participation in health promotion, *Health Promotion International* 7:27-36, 1992.

Smith MC and Barton JA: Technologic enrichment of a community needs assessment, *Nurs Outlook* 40(1):33-37, 1992.

13

Community Organization
and Health Planning
for Aggregates at Risk

OBJECTIVES

Upon completion of this chapter, the reader should be able to:

1. Describe the concepts of community organization and health planning.
2. Compare the nursing, epidemiological, and health care planning processes.
3. Analyze the steps of the health care planning process.
4. Use concepts from epidemiology to carry out health planning.
5. Use community assessment data and diagnoses in health planning activities.
6. Describe how to work with communities as partners to solve contemporary health problems.

7. Describe seven epidemiological trends that influence health care planning.
8. Describe five demographic trends that make an impact on planning for future health care needs.
9. Identify significant legislation that has influenced health planning activities.
10. Describe barriers to health planning.
11. Discuss the use of health planning concepts in community health nursing practice.
12. Summarize key principles involved in health planning.

Chapter 2 describes how aggregates at risk and the community are the client for the community health nurse. A distinguishing feature of this specialty area is a focus on interventions that protect and promote the health of communities; this chapter describes how nurses put that concept into practice. Problems that contemporary community health nurses frequently encounter include crack-addicted neonates, family violence, child abuse, and drug and alcohol abuse. Further, declining family incomes, lack of access to health care, and growing hunger and homelessness face too many people. These are awesome problems that require interventions different from those developed by nurses working with individual clients and family members. Community health nurses use community-based health promotion efforts that stimulate community organization. They are involved in policy decisions that address the environmental, social, and behavioral variables making an impact on the health of families.

Lillian Wald, the founder of modern community health nursing, was a role model for this behavior. She described how nurses helped to make the community a positive environment that facilitates the self-actualization of individuals through the life span. In describing how nurses from Henry Street Settlement House functioned, she wrote that the nurses are "enlisted in the crusade against disease and for the promotion of right living, beginning even before life itself is brought forth, through infancy, into school life, on through adolescence. . . . The nurse is being socialized, made part of a community plan for the communal health. Her contribution to human welfare, unified and harmonized with those powers which aim at care and prevention, rather than at police power and punishment, forms part of the great policy of bringing human beings to a higher level" (Wald, 1915, p. 60). Wald noted early in her career that working with political leaders to change the social and physical environment was as important as helping individuals modify their health behaviors. This activist changed child labor laws, helped build playgrounds, and established school nursing, all examples of how political and social structures influence the health of communities, aggregates, families, and individuals.

We are indebted to Assistant Professor Nancy Watson, who helped faculty and students at the University of Rochester to understand basic concepts of population-based health planning. Content and illustrations in this chapter reflect many of her ideas.

Community organizations using health care planning processes facilitate work with communities as partners, assisting and motivating aggregates to bring about changes; these changes are designed to solve health problems and to create environments that prevent health problems from developing. Using this approach to deal with health concerns means that community health nurses shift from a one-to-one reactive model of care to a multidisciplinary, proactive, community-based model that involves the community in problem identification and resolution.

Major recent public health documents reflect the emphasis on working with communities to solve current health problems. *Healthy Communities 2000: Model Standards* was published in 1991 and put into practice the objectives of *Healthy People 2000* (USDHHS, 1991). This latter document was discussed in Chapter 5; it serves as a statement of the nation's health objectives for the year 2000. *Healthy Communities 2000* (APHA, 1991) provides a tool for community use in working toward these objectives. Documents from the American Nurses Association (1980, 1986) and the American Public Health Association (1981) support the role of the nurse in health planning. These organizations believe that the dominant responsibility of nurses in community health is to the community or the population as a whole and that the nurse must acknowledge the need for comprehensive health planning to implement this responsibility. Nursing's *Agenda for Health Care Reform: An Agenda for Action* (ANA, 1991) addresses the need to work with communities for equitable distribution of health care in the United States. This document emphasizes primary care, cost controls, and health care benefits for all. Currently most major nursing and public health organizations have documents discussing health care reform, using multidisciplinary efforts and client coalitions to promote health and welfare changes.

DEFINING HEALTH PLANNING

Health planning is an ongoing process whereby information about a community is systematically collected and used to structure a usable community health plan that empowers communities to choose strategies for health.

This scientific problem-solving approach helps a community to evaluate and bring about specific changes in its health care delivery system. The health planning process for aggregates at risk involves the

13-1 Comparison of the Nursing, Epidemiological, and Health Care Planning Processes

Nursing process	Epidemiological process	Health planning process

Assessing
    Data collection to determine nature
      of client problems
	I. Determine the nature, extent, and scope
	    of the problem
	    A. Natural life history of condition
	    B. Determinants influencing condition
	      1. Primary data (essential agent)
	        a. Parasite, bacterium, or virus
	        b. Nutrition
	        c. Psychosocial factors
	      2. Contributory data
	        a. Agent
	        b. Host
	        c. Environment
	    C. Distribution patterns
	      1. Person
	      2. Place
	      3. Time
	    D. Condition frequencies
	      1. Prevalence
	      2. Incidence
	      3. Other biostatistical
	        measurements
		Preplanning
		Assessment

Analyzing
    Formulation of nursing diagnoses
      or hypotheses
	II. Formulate tentative hypothesis(es)
	III. Collect and analyze further data to test
	     hypothesis(es)
		Policy development

Planning	IV. Plan for control	
Implementing	V. Implement control plan	Implementation
Evaluating	VI. Evaluate control plan	Evaluation
Revising or terminating	VII. Make appropriate report VIII. Conduct research	

same steps used in the individual and family-centered nursing process: assessing, analyzing, planning, implementing, and evaluating. Basic concepts of epidemiology and biostatistics (Chapter 11), and management (Chapter 22) are used to refine decision-making and diagnostic skills and to expand intervention options during the health planning process.

Table 13-1 illustrates how the steps in the problem-solving approach can be used in various situations. This chapter discusses in detail each step of the aggregate- and community-focused health planning process, using the scientific problem-solving approach. It emphasizes the importance of generating citizen participation during this process.

The emphasis in health planning is on the health of aggregates at risk within the community, and problems, solutions, and actions are defined on this level. By comparison, in clinical nursing the emphasis is on the individual as the unit of service (Williams, 1977, p. 251). In community health nursing the family is the unit of service and the client is the community.

Another distinguishing feature of aggregate-based health planning is its focus on the prevention of existing health problems in the population being served, as well as on the promotion of health and well-being. Chapters 14 through 20 will focus on aggregates, using a developmental framework. For each age group, existing health problems are pre-

Trends Affecting Health Care Planning

Epidemiological Trends

1. Diseases of the aging including cardiovascular, cancer, diabetes, osteoarthritis, cognitive impairment, and advancing age, place crucial demands on the health care system. With the number of people growing older, these demands will increase.
2. Diseases of life-style and behavior, including obesity, trauma, substance abuse, sexually transmitted diseases, teenage pregnancy, occupational and environmental hazards, and the homeless and disabled, mean that social policies have to change and that health education should take place in non-traditional forms.
3. Diseases and technology have brought about a marked reduction in premature mortality and an overall reduction in morbidity. These changes have also produced social, legal, and ethical dilemmas.
4. The AIDS epidemic has produced immeasurable human suffering and costs of 2.3 billion dollars annually. In the absence of a cure or vaccine this epidemic will spread.
5. Infant mortality rates place the United States at twenty-second in the world; there are large discrepancies in deaths of infants between whites and African-Americans.
6. Enhanced understanding of diseases is helping researchers to understand that people do not progress from health to disease but that genetic predisposition interacts with exposure to various physical, chemical, and biological factors. Preventing disease is much more complex than once thought.

7. Environmental factors that pre-dispose and or cause disease are present. Our industrial age has created conveniences but at a price. The world will need to choose between convenience and environmental destruction in some cases.

Demographic Trends

1. The aging population is increasing with those 65+ increasing to four million by 1995. The population over age 85 will grow steadily to 15.5 percent by 2010.
2. The baby boom generation, those born between 1946 and 1964 reversed a downward trend and added 1.5 million persons each year of the boom. This group is one of the best educated generation and will place demands on the health care sector over the next 50 years.
3. A declining younger population will produce smaller numbers for schools and colleges.
4. Racial and ethnic diversity, including growth in the African-American and Hispanic-American populations will make an impact on all aspects of the health care system since both groups are currently underserved and underrepresented in health care.
5. Changes in the family unit mean that a mother, father, and two children are no longer the norm. Locations and hours of delivery of health care will need to change as will the traditional set of medical problems focusing on emotional health and well-being.

From Shugars DA, O'Neil EH, and Bader JD, eds.: *Healthy America: practitioners for 2005, an agenda for action for U.S. health professional schools,* Durham, N.C., 1991, The Pew Health Professions Commission, pp. 31-32, 39-40.

sented, at-risk aggregates identified, and preventive intervention strategies discussed.

Trends Affecting Health Care Planning

To assist community residents in planning programs that meet health care needs requires an understanding of the demographic and epidemiological trends in the United States. Prevailing attitudes, as well as these trends, influence both the services needed and the organization of these services. The box above presents a summary of trends; an examination of them makes it clear that the health care delivery system will

be dealing with unprecedented demands that will require creative planning and programming.

The Community Health Nurse and Health Planning

The community health nurse is particularly well qualified to work with a community's citizens in carrying out population-based health planning. Each day the nurse sees the needs of aggregates at risk within the community through home visits, clinics, classes, schools, and other nursing activities. She or he is able to obtain a composite picture of the health

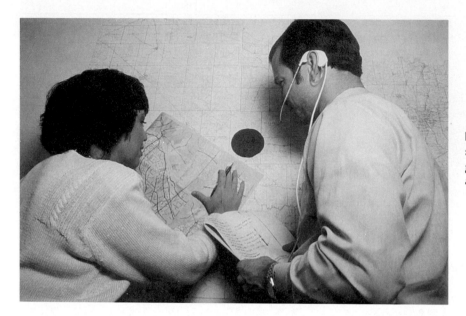

Figure 13-1 Health planners study aggregates within specific geographical and political boundaries using maps and other tools.

needs of an aggregate such as lack of prenatal care, family planning services, or public transportation. The nurse's continual, comprehensive contact with the community makes her or him knowledgeable about available resources and gaps in service provision. The staff nurse should share these assessed health needs with supervisory personnel, and together they can discuss the alternatives to the situation. The agency's philosophy of service, policies, priorities, and staff variables will affect the alternatives offered. By sharing assessed needs with people in an agency who are in a position to assist in implementing change, the nurse is taking a beginning step in health planning for the needs of the community.

Nurses usually see only the "tip of the iceberg" when diagnosing problems common to families in their caseloads. What has been assessed, however, can become the basis for an epidemiological investigation of community needs, because the family is the smallest epidemiological group (Taylor and Knowelden, 1964, p. 303). Epidemiological studies examine groups of families in an agency's geographical area. They frequently involve investigation of needs in census tracts or specific political boundaries such as cities, towns, or counties (refer to Figure 13-1).

Health needs of aggregates can also be dealt with by building on research studies and known problems and solutions. How this is done is illustrated by graduate students in community health nursing at the University of Texas who assessed an aggregate at risk, nearby immigrant and refugee Hispanic persons. Evidence showed that this community of approximately 100,000 Central American immigrants fared poorly in terms of both potential and realized access to medical care. The purpose of the assessment was to gather information to document systematically whether expanded public health services were needed in the area, and, if so, what types of services were needed (Rojas-Urruita and Aday, 1991). Bilingual interviewers spoke with 242 people; questions adapted from a 1976 interview on access to medical care were part of the interview schedule. The results indicated that 67% of this group sought health care compared to 87% of the general population for comparable illnesses. One in ten persons in the study population had been denied access to medical care for some reason. Study findings were given to both local and county health authorities and other area agencies. "The result was a series of meetings with agency personnel and community representatives that resulted in proposals from the city health department, for, in the short run, establishing a storefront public health clinic in the area, and for the long term, developing a multiservice center to provide preventive and treatment-related care . . . " (Rojas-Urruita and Aday, 1991, p. 25). The project demonstrated that research can both identify problems and promote the implementations of solutions to reduce community problems.

The primary goal of health planning activities such as those just described is to develop comprehensive health care options for all citizens in the community. Working with one community aggregate helps health planners in developing comprehensive services for all.

THE HEALTH CARE PLANNING PROCESS*

As illustrated in Table 13-1, the phases of the health care planning process have different labels but, in essence, they are the same problem-solving phases used in both the epidemiological process and the nursing process. Professionals from all disciplines use the health planning process. Thus, learning the terminology related to their problem-solving approaches is important because it unites scientific thinking across disciplines. Since health planning most often requires interdisciplinary team effort, it is crucial that team members have a common framework from which to work. The health planning process provides this framework.

The health care planning process is orderly and logical; it is a tool that helps those using it to organize large amounts of community data that describe community problems and strengths, as well as health planning solutions. For purposes of discussion, the health care planning process is divided into five phases: preplanning, assessment, policy development, implementation, and evaluation. Each of these phases is separately described, but in reality they are overlapping and inseparable.

The Preplanning Phase

Into this phase is built the foundation for the rest of the process. Before developing policies for health planning, it is crucial that planners test their ideas and validate that what they perceive as a problem is also seen by others as a problem severe enough to warrant changes. The planning organization and environment needs to be "tested" to ascertain whether there are sufficient resources and commitment to devote to the work required to bring about the change. Preliminary expectations and skeleton organizational plans need to be outlined. These sound like simple commonsense

---

*Christine DeGregorio, Ph.D., while a University of Rochester doctoral student in political science, first wrote the phases and steps of the community planning process as outlined here. Much of the content and many of the illustrations in this section reflect her thinking and creativity. It is used with her permission.

comments; in reality these very basic parts to the process are often skipped and positive results are then difficult to achieve.

The preplanning phase has six steps: (1) obtaining community and consumer support and participation, (2) development of a broadly defined problem statement, (3) statement of a goal, (4) delineation of a timetable that accounts for the remaining four phases of the process, (5) assessment of resources for the task that needs to be accomplished, and (6) planning for data collection strategies to be used. Each of these steps helps to build a framework needed for future planning activities.

Obtaining Community and Consumer Support and Participation

Encouraging people to be involved in making decisions and addressing policy issues that make an impact on their quality of health helps to ensure that programs will progress beyond the ideas of the planners. Changes in individual behavior and community relationships, as well as in the social environment, are necessary to reduce the morbidity and mortality associated with problems encountered by community health nurses. For example, teenagers can be taught the importance of wearing seat belts, driving the posted speed limits, and not drinking while driving. However, this behavior is enhanced with roads that have adequate shoulders and no hidden curves and by stiff penalties for breaking the traffic laws. Since many traditional health promotion approaches that focused on changing individual behavior have failed, a variety of new models to promote consumer participation have been tested. Phrases including community participation, community organization, community empowerment, and empowerment education reflect the movement to have people "buy into" the changes needed for healthy living. Community organization activities are designed to stimulate conditions for change and to mobilize citizens and communities for health action. A major goal during this process is to empower the community to use its resources to accomplish significant community goals, decided primarily by community representatives and consistent with local values (Bracht and Kingsbury, 1990, pp. 66-67). Community empowerment is the process of increasing a group's control over consequences that are important to their members and to others in the broader community (Braithwaite and Lythcott, 1989, p. 283).

The process of empowering communities can be facilitated in various ways. Schlaff (1991), in a prize-winning idea for the 1990 Secretary's Award for Innovation in Health Promotion and Disease Prevention, described an ideal scenario in one city: a health center worked with the Neighborhood Council to deal with health problems; the council was an elected body of residents and activists representing the community. The health center director reported directly to the council and working with them were Community Health Workers who reflected the ethnic and cultural diversity of the community. Community Health Workers carried out health education in homes; people indigenous to the population of concern also assisted planners in accurately defining problems that needed correction. The program combined the use of community organization, efforts to form organizational structures involving members of the community, and the use of lay health workers who lived in the community where they worked.

Another illustration of empowering a community to change both the health behavior of individuals and their collective health is the Abbotsford Community Nursing Center in Philadelphia. The Center is located in a tenant-managed public housing development and delivers primary health services ranging from prenatal to geriatric care. Need for the services offered were in part based on a resident-administered survey that defined the major health issues in the community. Residents have control of the 12-member board that makes final decisions about program design, hiring of personnel, and policy. Residents of the project are hired to be the outreach workers, drivers, security personnel, and receptionists. Using these indigenous resources puts money directly back into the community being served and also brings information about the community to the Center. The outreach workers visit households in the development on a regular basis, provide information on health education and prevention issues, and follow up on missed appointments and concerns such as prenatal and postnatal difficulties. The Center is *community driven,* which means that the residents have control both over the resources and ownership in the results of the program (Resources for Human Development, Inc., and the Abbottsford Homes Tenant Management Corporation, Program Abstract). This behavior illustrates well the first step of program planning: obtaining community and consumer support and participation.

Development of a Broadly Defined Problem Statement

A problem is a condition that is sufficiently distressing that change to bring relief is desired or sought. An example of a broadly defined problem statement from which policy development could begin might be the following: "Deaths from motor vehicle accidents for people 15 to 24 years of age in Jones County have substantially increased over the past year." This statement has a broad, yet clear, focus. All involved in the planning process would know that the concern is increased motor vehicle accidents for a certain age group in a specific area in a given year.

Statement of a Goal

A goal is a general statement of intent or purpose that provides guidance for the activities that are to take place. A goal emanating from the above problem statement might be, "The Jones County Health Department will work toward reducing the rate of fatalities from motor vehicle accidents among people 15 to 24 years of age by 10% in 3 years."

Delineation of a Timetable That Accounts for the Remaining Four Phases of the Process

In order to develop a realistic timetable planners must have a general idea of what they plan to accomplish in the months ahead. After a specific goal is delineated, health planners have a preliminary discussion about what needs to be done to achieve the stated goal. This discussion focuses on examining the nature of the tasks to be accomplished and what is feasible for the agency or community to do, considering other priorities.

Table 13-2 presents a sample health planning timetable. As discussed earlier, this table illustrates how the phases overlap and build on one another.

Assessment of Resources for the Task That Needs to Be Accomplished

Resources can be positive or negative, and they can be both internal (part of the organization) and external to an organization. Positive resources include money, enthusiasm for the goal, space in which to work, time, technical expertise (such as ability to work on a computer or knowledge of the planning process), and experienced workers who have popularity, esteem and charisma, and commitment to the goal. Negative resources can include a deficit of any of the above.

TABLE 13-2	Timetable for Jones County Health Department's Motor Vehicle Accident Project

Phases	Time in months											
	Dec	Jan	Feb	Mar	April	May	June	July	Aug	Sept	Oct	Nov
Preplanning	―――											
Assessment		――――――――										
Policy development				―――――――――――――								
Implementation							――――――――――――					
Evaluation									―――――――――			

Resources may be found within the organization or elsewhere. Space and money, for example, may need to be obtained from voluntary community agencies and technical expertise requested from a university. Knowing the community in which one works helps the community health nurse to quickly identify valuable resources during the planning process (refer to Chapter 12).

One of the most valuable health planning resources is a committee that works toward the goal and that has power and authority to make decisions. To be viable the committee must have tasks assigned to it that are crucial to the goal; the committee must also have an audience that expects results. Health planning committee members should be chosen on the basis of their interpersonal skills, their knowledge of the planning process, their commitment to the goals, and their power and authority within the agency. Not every committee member will likely have all of these ingredients for successful planning; however, these ingredients must be present in some degree if successful planning is to take place. Inexperienced planners should be part of the group so that learning can take place for future planning activities. The planning committee may need to be trained in the planning process if this is an entirely new activity for committee members. Help with the process may be obtained from a variety of community resources such as the United Way, the county health planning council, and local university faculty members.

An example of how community leaders are organized and trained to deal with health problems is the collaborative effort between the Indiana University School of Nursing Institute of Action Research for Community Health, the Indiana Public Health Association, and six Indiana cities (Flynn, Rider, and Bailey, 1992). Healthy Cities Indiana is a community development approach to health promotion and involves a public-private partnership in developing healthier cities. Citizens participate in examining problems and solutions to promote healthy cities; community leadership development that supports health promotion is fundamental. Central to the process is the local health city committee that represents the community. Its members come from various sectors of the city including arts and culture, business, dentistry, education, employment, environment, finance, health and medical care, local government, media, parks, and other areas such as religion and transportation. The Healthy Cities Indiana program emphasizes experiential learning with these leaders, teaching what people want and need rather than setting goals for them. Emphasis is on the committee's ability to deal with the community's problems and the development of its own capabilities and resources. When needed, external resources are used. Chapter 3 discusses this committee in more detail.

Planning That Delineates the Data Collection Strategies to Be Used

A plan needs to be developed to assess the problem of concern. When developing this plan the planning group focuses on *what* data are needed, from *whom* they need input, *how* they should obtain data, *who* will be responsible for collecting the data, and *when* the data collection process will be completed. For example, the Jones County Health Department planning group would want active participation from parents,

13-3 Jones County Health Department Motor Vehicle Accident Project: Worksheet for Planning Data Collection Strategies

Goal: Reduce the rate of motor vehicle accidents among 15- to 24-year-old youth in Jones County.
Rationale for Goal: The rate of fatal motor vehicle accidents (MVA) among 15- to 24-year-old youth has increased 5% in the past year.

Type of data	Data source	Collection method	Time for completion	Responsibility of
Data Collection Plan for Organizational Assessment:				
Characteristics of accident victims	Clients	Personal interview	April 30, 1993	Staff CHN
Epidemiological data	Accident reports and interview data	Review of reports	April 30, 1993	Planning committee
___	___	___	___	___
___	___	___	___	___
Data Collection Plan for Community Assessment:				
Causes of accidents	Law enforcement officers	Mail survey	April 30, 1993	Planning committee
Content covered in driver education courses	Driver education staff	Telephone interview	April 30, 1993	Planning committee
___	___	___	___	___
___	___	___	___	___

teachers, legislators, and police officers when they examine vehicle fatalities.

The plan for data collection should be written in sufficient detail, so that all involved parties are clear about what needs to be accomplished. A worksheet such as the one presented in Table 13-3 facilitates the planning process.

At the conclusion of these five steps, the planning group should have a good grasp of the problem, should be aware of the power and authority they have from the involved community, should know their strengths and weaknesses, and should have delineated the time frame for the process. The group is then ready to move to the next phase of the planning process: *assessment.*

The Assessment Phase

In population-based planning,

A specific population is analyzed to determine its health problems. The health system is then studied to determine how it must function if those problems are to be addressed. Population-based planning can be contrasted with demand or resource-based planning, which begins by examining the capabilities and/or utilization of the health population (USDHEW, 1979, Guidelines, p. 5).

In population-based planning, three steps in the assessment phase of the health care planning process are completed. These are (1) conducting a needs assessment, (2) setting priorities upon which the planning committee can focus, and (3) specifying objectives to which organizational and community resources can be applied. Each of these steps assists planners to become more specific as they progress through the planning process.

Conducting a Needs Assessment

A needs assessment is a systematic method of gathering information about populations. This assessment helps to detect and measure problems and determine the relevance, adequacy, and appropriateness of services designed to combat them. It analyzes the need for human services through multiple measurement approaches. It also delineates population strengths, such as concerned citizen groups, that can be tapped when developing policies and implementation strategies.

Defining the parameters of the population to be studied is an area of concern to the planning committee. Will it be the county? Will it be a school district? Will it be a town or a city or a metropolitan area? Chapter 12, in the section entitled "Methods for Assessing a Community's Status," presents guidelines for defining these parameters.

Assessing a population's needs is a complex matter that goes beyond defining who the population actually is. Needs are relative, and they are based on values, culture, history, and the experiences of the individual, the family, and the community. Human needs are not easily identified, but are diffuse and related. For example, motor vehicle deaths may be related to poor roads that are the result of a low-level tax base for road construction, due to high unemployment. Human needs often change, because communities which influence human need are dynamic and their needs are in a constant state of flux; a need today may not be a need next year. Most importantly, translating assessed needs into community programs is greatly influenced by the availability of human and financial resources in addition to the availability of technology. Thus, a needs assessment must analyze community resources in addition to the characteristics of the population and the nature of the problem being encountered by the population.

Community resources should be identified when the nature of the problem is examined. When examining the nature and extent of the problem, planners discern trends over a certain period of years and cite the problem's significance, implications, and comparisons with norms or other standards. The following

assessment tool, designed to collect data about motor vehicle accidents in Jones County, can be used as a guide when collecting data about other health problems in a community:

1. Community assessment of the problem of fatalities from motor vehicle accidents
   a. Mortality data
   b. Morbidity data (incidence and prevalence) trends in recent years
   c. Demographic characteristics associated with mortality and morbidity (at-risk aggregates) in the defined community
   d. Local factors, such as road conditions, thought to influence trends
   e. Lifestyle of population groups
      (1) Environmental characteristics promoting health or illness
      (2) Economic base of population, income, and occupation
      (3) Health behaviors, such as drinking patterns, that influence health states
   f. Local perception of needs, problems, or priorities
2. Community resources
   a. Health services, strengths, and limitations
   b. Usage rates for health services
   c. Population coverage
3. Extent of knowledge related to the problem under consideration
   a. Magnitude of the problem in other populations: national and state data
   b. Etiological factors (*results* of case-control and cohort studies or theories)
   c. Physiological, sociological, and psychological processes related to pathology
   d. Inferences for *primary* prevention and early detection of problems
   e. Treatment potential
      (1) Inferences for therapeutic strategies at the individual, family, or aggregate level
      (2) Inferences for *secondary* and *tertiary* prevention (both of above are based on *results* of clinical trials and other types of evaluative studies or theories)

How and where health planners obtain this data is presented in the section "Sources of Community Data" in Chapter 12.

A community will be readier to act if it believes that a given issue is important and if the issue affects a number of people. People in a community will also be readier to act if they have had previous success with community action and if there is a network of organizations to facilitate change (Brown, 1991, p. 442). Chapter 3 discusses types of communities; those classified as anomic, transitory, stepping-stone, or diffuse will likely have more difficulty with community organization and change than will parochial or integral communities (refer to p. 87 for a description of these types of communities).

Setting Priorities

The next step in the assessment phase of the planning process is to set priorities in relation to the problems. There are three approaches to setting priorities in the planning process (MacStravic, 1978). The first and most common is to set priorities based on the *severity of the problem* or the desirability of some objective. Using the mortality problem in Jones County as an example, the first priority might be to reduce the fatalities for the group under study to at least the rate of 2 years past, since it increased by 5% in the past year. Another method of setting priorities is to focus on a measure of the *problem's susceptibility to solution.* In order to use this kind of approach, planners need to know the kinds of solutions that are available. The assumption is that, besides knowing the severity of the problem, planners must also know if anything can be done about it and then give highest priority to problems for which the solutions are known. The continuing example of motor vehicle accidents in Jones County provides another priority based on solution-oriented methods: prevent alcohol intake among teenagers, since assessment has demonstrated a causal relationship between teenage drinking and car accidents. The final method of setting priorities is to use outcome-oriented methods that focus primarily on the *cost benefit of specific interventions.* The logic of this method is that planners should give highest priority to the action that will yield the best return. Given the information that the planning committee likely has about the problem of fatalities among teenagers in Jones County, its priority when using the outcome-oriented method might be to raise the drinking age in Jones County to 21.

Whatever method is used by the planning committee to set priorities, the priority chosen will affect the timing and the amount of resources allocated to that priority.

Specify Objectives

The last step in this assessment phase is to specify objectives to which organizational and community resources can be applied over a specified period of time. Objectives are specific, concrete, measurable statements of outcomes that need to be accomplished in order to eventually reach a broad goal. They are intended to guide the operations of the agency to reach the goal.

Objectives focus on the what and when. They specify *results,* not strategies for getting results. For example, two objectives that help to reach the goal of reducing the rate of fatalities from motor vehicle accidents might be (1) define who is at risk for motor vehicle accidents among people aged 15 to 24 years in Jones County by March 1995 and (2) lower the fatality rate for people aged 15 to 24 years in Jones County by 5% in the next year.

Spiegel and Hyman (1978, pp. 16-18) designed criteria for testing the feasibility of objectives. As planners write their objectives, they need to keep these criteria in mind:

- The organization should have the authority to undertake the objectives.
- Objectives should be within the capabilities of the agency in terms of organization, personnel, equipment, facilities, and techniques.
- Objectives should fall within budget restrictions.
- Objectives should fit into the available timetable.
- Objectives should be legal and consistent with the ethical and moral values of the community affected.
- Objectives should be practical and must be implementable.
- Objectives must be acceptable to those who are responsible for carrying them out.
- Minimum negative side effects should result from the achievement of the objectives.
- Objectives should be measurable in concrete terms.

At the conclusion of the three steps of the assessment phase, planners will know the details of the problem under consideration. They will also know the resources available both within and outside the organization and the community that can help deal with the problem. When this information is known, health planners concentrate on the third step in the planning process, *policy development.*

The Policy Development Phase

Policy development involves the determination of strategies to achieve the objectives that emerge as the result of the assessment done in phase two of the planning process. These strategies include methods for allocating resources such as money, personnel, and equipment. The strategies also clarify relationships that affect rights, status, and resources. In this phase planners pay attention to social and political parameters: where are the greatest resources? Where is there resistance to the objectives? What methods or strategies could best achieve the objectives? Will one of the strategies be a modification of what already exists or will it be even better communication than what exists? Will the strategies to meet the objectives involve contracts with other organizations and/or support for these organizations so that they can better meet the objective? Answers to these questions will result in an allocation of resources, the identification of responsibilities, and, finally, the establishment of an action plan that has tasks, responsibilities, and a time frame clearly delineated.

Sound social policy and value considerations provide the guidelines for the allocation of community resources, program development, and coordination. Policy development is frequently a process of negotiation among the different groups involved in the planning process: consumers, service providers, decision makers, and resource persons. Further, during the policy development phase planners must anticipate expected changes in services, legislation, and general trends, and then must foresee what impact these changes will have on the local community. A balance must be achieved that will most effectively use community resources to meet the needs perceived by ordinary citizens, as well as needs perceived by professionals with expertise.

The need for sound public policies cannot be overemphasized. A renowned community health nurse has described how the health of people in the United States is the result of the environments in which they live and the patterns which they follow (Milio, 1981). She further writes about how these patterns and environments are shaped by public policy that is, in turn, shaped by available information. For example,

Milio (1988) suggests that the United States adopt public policy measures already used in other countries such as Norway, where a comprehensive farm, food, and nutrition policy has the goal of improving national dietary policies, improving poor rural areas, and offering support to farm families. A 10-member steering committee is multidisciplinary and includes government officials and food cooperatives, retailers, educators, and researchers. Although change is not occurring rapidly, it is taking place.

Health care planners should develop this kind of mind-set as they think about solutions to problems; policy decisions are constantly being made that affect the health of Americans—through management of the ecology, the economy, and farm and factory production, distribution, and consumption.

It is easier to discuss the policy development phase of the planning process by dividing it into four steps: (1) assess various strategies to achieve objectives, (2) match tasks with resources, (3) negotiate new organizational liaisons as needed, and, finally, (4) establish contracts as needed. The result will be an action plan.

Assess Various Strategies to Achieve Objectives

Generating alternatives to meet the objectives written in phase two is one of the most exhilarating steps in the process. It is a time to be creative and innovative, to exercise a flair for originality.

Certain methods for generating various strategies have proved to be the most efficient and effective way to meet the objectives. Simple idea generation, or writing down ideas in a group is one. Another well-known one is *brainstorming*—throwing caution to the wind and citing any idea that comes to mind. *Think tanks* (getting together to talk over the problem with people who are involved in it) and *forced association* (exploring relationships between words) are two more methods of generating strategies. Spiegel and Hyman (1978) describe in detail how to generate various alternatives. The strategies chosen to reach the objectives will be based on their cost. They are also affected by accountability (whom does the public associate with the outcomes of the strategy), as well as whether the decisions about the strategy are attributed to the decision-maker.

Match Tasks with Resources

After several strategies have been chosen for each objective, resources need to be assigned to make

13-4   Jones County Health Department: One Action Plan for the Motor Vehicle Accident Project

Objective: To raise the drinking age to 21 in Kentucky by 1995.

Action steps	Date	Person responsible
Get support of the 15 Jones County PTAs	March 15, 1994	Eigsti
Get support of all district legislators	March 15, 1994	Clemen and Jones
Put one article each month of the year in the "Democrat and Chronicle"	Monthly	Alexander
Get support of grocery association	August 1, 1994	McGuire

certain that the task or strategy is accomplished. This results in an action plan specifying the work activities needed to achieve the objective. It includes what is to be done, who is responsible, and by what date each step should be completed. It should be possible to accomplish action steps in 1 to 12 months; each objective may have many action steps. For example, if one objective is "To raise the drinking age to 21 in Kentucky by 1995," the action plan that matches strategies with resources to achieve that objective might look like the one presented in Table 13-4.

Step two of the policy development phase results in an action plan that delineates specific action steps with responsible individuals, along with a realistic time frame. This type of plan facilitates the completion of necessary health planning activities.

Negotiate New Organizational Liaisons and Establish Contracts As Needed

These steps help planners to complete action steps. For example, if Ms. Alexander is responsible for a monthly newspaper article regarding the need to raise the drinking age to 21, she will need to have a firm commitment from the editor that the paper will print it. This may involve a visit by administrative personnel in the health department to the editorial director of the newspaper and a written or verbal agreement that such a plan is feasible. This may also be the situation if support from legislators is desired; liaison activities with community organizations interested in causes of motor vehicle accidents among youth and the health department who then, together, ask for political support is likely to be necessary. These two steps may be the most difficult, and yet the most important aspects

needed to achieve positive outcomes from program planning activities.

Table 13-5, showing the planning sequence, summarizes the differences between goals, plans, objectives, and action steps, as well as the following parameters of each of these: functions, leadership, data base, time span, and accountability. Having an awareness of these differences is important, because each level of planning must be completed to ensure effective and efficient community health planning.

The Implementation Phase

The fourth phase of the health care planning process is implementation. All the work of the other phases finally leads to achievement of concrete outcomes in the real world. Implementation is, to a great extent, a political process that requires that those seeking to bring about change be very aware of the various forces present in the community. Will these forces help the changes to take place or can they be mobilized to provide support for the changes? Implementation involves incentives for people to change, public hearings, and advocacy for change. This phase calls for trust, rapport, and patience to work out new and difficult relationships and to respond to the unanticipated ramifications of the change.

In short, implementation is carrying out the plan. It involves organizing, delegating, and managing work so that the action steps prepared in the last phase are completed and objectives are accomplished within the specified time. These are the questions that planners need to answer in the implementation phase: What is to be done? How will it be done? Who will do it? What

TABLE 13-5 The Planning Sequence

Planning level	Function	Primary leadership	Data base	Time-span	Accountability
Goals	To provide broad purpose and general direction for the organization	Board	Ideology, values, role, mission	Infinite	Everyone
Plans	To provide definitive direction and a plan for the organization	Chief executive Planning chairman Planning committee Adopted by board	Operational Societal (issues & trends) Opinions of community leaders, key internal lay & staff leaders	2-5 years	President, planning chairman, executive director
Objectives	To provide measurable specification of attainable outcomes within operational goals	Unit executives Unit boards and committees	Operational Clients Community Opinions of key internal lay and staff leaders of operating units	1 year	Executive director, specific staff
Action steps	To provide specification of steps to be taken and activities to be conducted to achieve objectives; persons responsible; completion dates	Unit Executives Staff	Operational Available resources	1-12 months	Individual staff

Developed by Christine DeGregorio, Ph.D., while a doctoral student in political science, University of Rochester, Rochester, N.Y.

are the deadlines for each step? Who will monitor progress? How and when will the solution be evaluated?

A flowchart of activity that anticipates management problems is used throughout this phase. Two common methods of plotting this activity are program evaluation and review technique (PERT) charts and Gantt or Milestone charts.

A PERT chart (Figure 13-2) is designed to show the varied components that make up a planning system and the sequence and relationships among these components. It helps to evaluate progress toward planning objectives, aids in finding potential and actual problems, and predicts the likelihood of reaching objectives.

The first step in developing a PERT network is to specify the program objective(s) clearly and to visualize all the individual tasks needed to complete the program in a clear manner. In the following diagram, *event* (shown within the circles) represents the start or completion of a specified step in the program. Since it is an event, it does not consume time. An *activity* takes time and resources to progress from one event to the next; therefore the activity is represented by lines connecting circles or the events. An activity needed to accomplish event 1 on Figure 13-2, "Planning Task Legitimized," might be to meet with the executive director of the agency to gain the director's support for the program.

Events are typically represented by numbers that

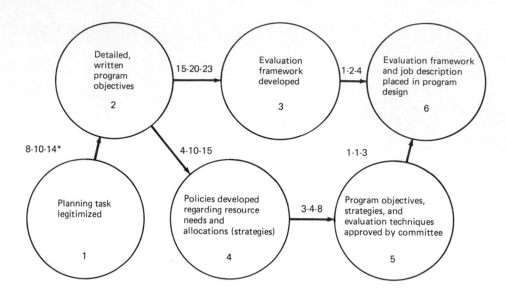

Figure 13-2 PERT chart sample sheet. (Developed by Christine De Gregorio, Ph.D., while a graduate student in Political Science, University of Rochester.)

are not necessarily in sequential order. Numbering makes the identification and location of events and activities possible, since each event becomes known by its number and each activity by the numbers of the events at its start and completion. Since PERT is primarily concerned with control over time, three estimates for time are assigned to each activity. These help to measure the uncertainty and are estimated by people most familiar with the activity involved. The type of time estimates used in a PERT chart are:

1. *Optimistic time.* An estimate of the minimum time an activity will take, based on "everything going right the first time"
2. *Most likely time.* An estimate of the normal time an activity will take if you were to repeat the activity over and over
3. *Pessimistic time.* An estimate of the maximum time an activity will take should a string of bad luck occur. (If one goes beyond this length of time, the program will not be completed.)

The three time estimates are usually written over the arrows that represent the activities in the PERT with "optimistic time" first, "pessimistic time" last, and "most likely time" in the middle. For example, in Figure 13-2 event 1, "Planning Task Legitimized," could optimistically be completed in 8 weeks. However, it is most likely that this event will be done in 10 weeks or even in 14 weeks maximum. Thus, the time estimates would be written like this: 8-10-14.

Gantt is the name of the person who first promoted the second type of program time line. In a simple Gantt Timeline (Figure 13-3) the project is indicated by major events rather than a breakdown of the elements of that event. For example, "train staff" may be noted on the chart. The event may have several major elements that will not be indicated on a simple Gantt. These might include needs assessment of staff, internal training resources, needed external resources, development of training materials, actual training, and evaluation of future training. On the chart this process would be indicated by a line or arrow. If planners wanted to explain what occurred in that time frame they would have to provide an additional explanation narrative to accompany the Gantt Timeline.

In a Gantt Milestone grid one might use a small triangle to indicate the actual event. In combining these two types of charting, the process and the actual event on the chart, planners might use a dotted line to indicate a preplanning or postplanning evaluation process and a triangle to indicate the event.

The Gantt Milestone is a good tool to use when there are many complex areas of program development that would require a very complex PERT chart. Planners use the Gantt Milestone approach to program development as a backup to needs assessment, program planning, and budget development. When one of these techniques is used, it is best to list what must be done, who will do it, and when it must be done. With such planning charts many program or project directors have been able to avoid planning too many tasks

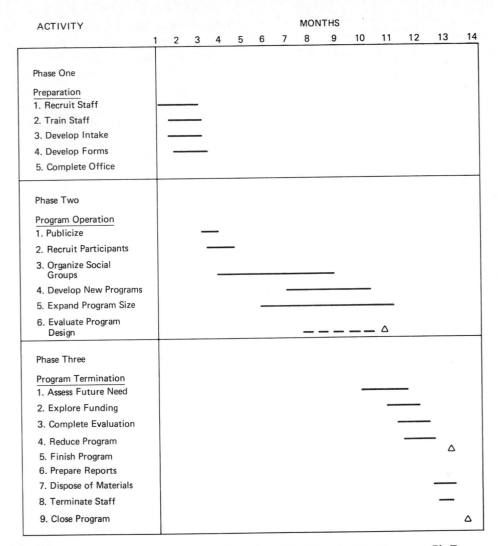

Figure 13-3   Gantt or milestone chart. (Developed by Christine De Gregorio, Ph.D., while a graduate student in Political Science, University of Rochester.)

for the same time period or tackling less urgent tasks until all essential tasks have been completed.

It is important to monitor the implementation plan to make certain that the correct sequence of activities needed to reach the program objectives is being carried out. This monitoring also enables the organization to identify successful and unsuccessful strategies and helps to monitor the progress being made in the achievement of objectives. While monitoring the implementation phase, the emphasis among planners is on the next phase of the health planning process—evaluation.

The Evaluation Phase

The fifth phase of the health care planning process, evaluation, is best seen as a continuous feedback process; it looks back upon actions to determine their effectiveness in order to make decisions regarding future actions. Figure 13-4 illustrates the feedback nature of the evaluation process.

There are three steps in the evaluation phase: documenting progress, comparing achievements against a performance standard, and preparing for needed modifications. If any one of these steps is ignored, the evaluation process will be incomplete.

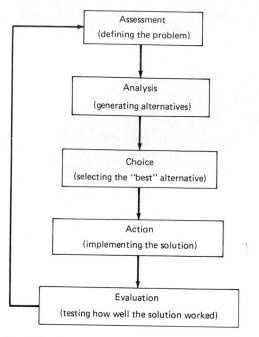

Figure 13-4 Summary of the planning process. (Developed by Christine De Gregorio, Ph.D., while a graduate student in Political Science, University of Rochester.)

Document Progress

Keeping accurate and complete records of successes and problems in the process is a key activity to a productive evaluation. The following critique can be made of the planning document:

1. Are problems clearly defined?
2. Are the problems documented?
3. Are the solutions appropriate?
4. Do the solutions have many associated risks?
5. Is the envisioned scope of change satisfactory?
6. What impact will the change have on rights, resources, and structures?
7. Are the risks worth the gains?
8. Are the objectives feasible?
9. Is the evaluation plan appropriate?

With the information obtained by asking these questions, planners can move to the next step in the evaluation phase.

Compare Achievements Against a Performance Standard

Performance standards are based on the objectives which were written in the assessment phase of the process. For each action step written to reach each objective, criteria or standards should be established before implementation. For example, if the objective is "to raise the drinking age to 21 years of age by 1995," and one of the action steps is to get support of the 15 Jones County Parent Teacher Associations, standards to evaluate this action step might be:

1. High achievement—support of all 15 PTAs
2. Adequate achievement—support of 10 PTAs
3. Inadequate progress—less than 10 PTAs support

Standards for evaluation should be established before implementing of action steps. In addition, ways to determine if the standards were met should be developed. The method to obtain data about PTA support might involve a verbal report from the coordination PTA group. This method would be delineated on an action plan (refer to Table 13-4) as follows:

1. Source of data: verbal report from coordination PTA group
2. Time: March 1994
3. Responsibility: Mary Cox, CHN

This kind of information should be collected for each action step so that there are objective data about the manner in which each objective is accomplished. Collecting objective data helps planners to more effectively evaluate progress. Objective data are usually more accurate than are subjective data. For example, "knowing you have support" of the PTA groups is far more significant than "thinking you have support." In addition, funders of health programs respond more favorably to objective data than they do to subjective information.

Prepare for Needed Modifications

The information obtained in the final step of the evaluation phase is used by planners to make decisions about the changes that need to be made in the objectives and associated action plans. The following questions need to be asked about the planning process:

1. Have any key informants been left out of the community planning process—citizens, professionals, leaders?
2. Was an adequate decision-making process used?
3. Have responsibilities and tasks been allocated appropriately?
4. Has there been negative feedback or a destructive impact (lost trust or commitment or heightened resistance) thus far?
5. What positive community responses (improved cooperation, trust, problem solving, heightened commitment, or greater resources) have occurred thus far?

As Figure 13-4 demonstrates, evaluation is a cycling process. "Although evaluation looks to past performance as planning looks to future performance, both are dependent upon skilled use of information in making decisions . . . to build in evaluation means to build into our thinking an analytic approach to what we are doing . . . it means continually asking the simple but pertinent question about every program action: Why should this be done?" (Arnold, Blankenship, and Hess, 1971, p. 282).

All five phases of the planning process—preplanning, assessment, policy, development, implementation, and evaluation—are interrelated and are, in reality, not carried out separately in the manner that they have been presented. When the basic elements included in each phase are followed, planners have a much greater likelihood of success than when they are passed over. The health care planning process is a valuable tool for planners who wish to bring about change to solve a difficult problem.

Planners need to consider a number of other broad principles when planning for population groups. These broad principles assist planners to make knowledgeable decisions when progressing through all phases of the planning process.

KEY PRINCIPLES INVOLVED IN HEALTH PLANNING

When studying the subject of comprehensive health planning for aggregates at risk, a number of principles emerge.

Community Diagnosis

Understanding the concepts presented in Chapter 12 relative to community diagnosis, along with the epidemiological variables of person, place, and time, is essential to answer the key questions that health planners must ask as they assess health planning needs. *Person* involves the "who" of community diagnosis. The cultural, ethnic, psychosocial, spiritual, and biological characteristics of the person variable must be considered when planning health services. These characteristics influence how persons define health and illness. Since these terms do not have a common meaning to all people, it is crucial to identify how the population being served views these concepts. If, for instance, a population narrowly defines health as the absence of disease, this population would probably respond more favorably to the provision of curative care than to the provision of preventive care.

Place describes the setting where services are planned. It may be rural or urban, the inner city or suburbia. When examining the characteristics of place the availability, accessibility, and cost of present services should be analyzed. Size is also a factor to consider when looking at place. A community with 1000 residents will have different needs than a community that has a population of 1 million. The cost to deliver health services, the kinds of personnel and financial resources that are available, and the complexity involved in planning and implementing services are some factors that vary among populations of different sizes.

The basic unit of service in health planning is the population to be served and its distribution. Any planning should take into consideration population size and distribution and needs as reflected by health statistics. Population size and mortality and morbidity rates for the future should be estimated. Future demands on the health care delivery system are determined in this way.

Time, in relation to urgency, needs to be considered when doing health planning. If the problem under consideration, for example, is an emergency such as influenza among aging citizens, immediate action must be taken. Other health problems such as accident prevention may not require immediate action but can necessitate action over time.

Long-term action makes more complex demands on the health planner. When long-term intervention is needed, mechanisms must be established to ensure that evaluation occurs periodically during the intervention phase, that coordination of all persons involved in the process is supported, and that public awareness of the problem and the health program is maintained.

It is extremely important to determine the appropriate time to initiate the health program under consideration. Analyzing community values and attitudes, availability of resources, and cost-benefit factors helps the health planner to determine the appropriate time to begin health-planning intervention.

Examining a community's developmental history is another significant factor to consider when looking at the time variable. An older, inner-city ethnic community would probably have more set values and attitudes about health and illness than would a newer community such as a prospering subdivision. Analyzing how values and attitudes have evolved over time in an older community assists the health planner in identifying key community leaders who can influence value and attitude changes and acceptance of intervention strategies that have facilitated health behavior change in the past.

Planning for Comprehensive Care

A comprehensive health care system plans for preventive, episodic, and catastrophic health care services for the entire population. Preventive services focus on the prevention of condition occurrence. Episodic services are diagnostic, curative, and restorative. Catastrophic services are designed to handle emergency and disaster situations and to help families who incur health situations beyond the scope of their financial resources.

Within the health care system are various patterns for providing comprehensive services to populations. Generalized and specialized school health services, as well as generalized and specialized medical care offices, are examples of the types of patterns used to deliver health care. However, within each of these patterns, comprehensive care needs to be built into the program. How the nurse in the school setting plans for the delivery of comprehensive services to the school-age population is discussed in depth in Chapter 15. Planning preventive focused immunization programs against measles, rubella, and diphtheria, developing protocols for the handling of episodic health care needs such as outbreaks of "nuisance" diseases, and establishing guidelines for handling emergency or catastrophic incidents are examples of some of the activities a nurse in the school setting would carry out to ensure that comprehensive care is available for the entire schoolage population.

Total Health Programs

The concept of a total health program is basic to comprehensive health care. Rather than thinking of a nursing program offering health services, planners should identify the role of nursing in a health care program in addition to the role of other disciplines, such as physicians, occupational therapists, nutritionists, and social workers. Ministers, priests, rabbis, pharmacists, health educators, school personnel, architects, physicians, psychiatrists, social workers, and environmentalists bring skills that aid clients with specific problems: the rabbi deals with spiritual affairs, the pharmacist deals with medicine regimens, and the nutritionist deals with nutritional concerns. The nurse's unique role is to be able to collate all of the information gathered by other professionals and to synthesize it when analyzing health care situations. In addition, the nurse is in a key position to collect data that provide a foundation for understanding the health care needs of aggregates. For example, as the nurse visits homes he or she learns where and how families obtain food, prepare it, and eat it. The nurse may also learn where and how people buy medications, how well they follow prescribed therapy, and where health care services are or are not available.

The community health nurse is skilled in forming health care plans based on clients' lifestyles and the cultural and socioeconomic factors of the community. This knowledge, as well as data collected during home visiting, should be transmitted to other members of the health team when health planning for groups within the community takes place.

Operating Within an Interdependent System

Numerous voluntary and official agencies at the local, state, and federal level have detailed programs that contribute to successful methods for preventing disease and promoting the health of both aggregates at risk and the community. Much of this text has presented facets of these contributions, beginning with the multiple voluntary organizations such as the American Heart Association and the United Way and the work of health departments at the local, state, and federal levels. Although the most effective point for health promotion and disease prevention is the community (Kreuter, 1992, p. 136), the responsibilities and contributions of all of these organizations to the health of the local community is critical.

Thus, health care professionals planning health intervention programs need to develop techniques of working within an interdependent system that connects local, state, and federal planning efforts.

One technique, developed in 1983 at the Centers for Disease Control, is PATCH: Planned Approach to Community Health. PATCH is designed to "strengthen state and local health departments' capacities to plan, implement, and evaluate community-based health promotion activities targeted toward priority health problems" (Krueter, 1992, p. 135). PATCH uses the existing system of official public health agencies, but it nutures leadership to develop intervention programs wherever it can be found. *Horizontal* and *vertical* networks are key to PATCH; at each level—local, state, and federal—coalitions, collaboration, and partnerships are required. Further, from the top federal level down to the local health department, leaders are expected to work together to strengthen each other. PATCH builds strongly on the concept of community empowerment discussed earlier in this chapter, but in the process it provides practical skills-based programs of technical assistance where health education leaders in state health agencies can work with people at the local level to establish needed programs; the health care planning process as presented in this chapter is the methodology used to develop programs. Community health professionals can expect to see an increased emphasis on working interdependently to achieve health for all of the citizens of the world. An entire volume of *The Journal of Health Education* (1992, 23:3) explicates the PATCH concept in greater detail.

SIGNIFICANT HEALTH LEGISLATION

Health planning began with the establishment of area-wide councils in the 1930s, which were formed to raise and allocate money for hospital construction and modernization. The members on these hospital councils were laypersons involved in philanthropic and civic affairs and professionals such as hospital administrators (National Academy of Sciences, 1980, p. 13). For a long time health planning was primarily reactive. Only after a health problem affected a large number of people was there an attempt to solve it. Beginning with some of President Johnson's Great Society programs in the 1960s, however, health planning was emphasized at the federal level. Described in Chapter 5, the Heart Disease, Cancer, and Stroke Amendment (Public Law 89-239), known as the Regional Medical Program, involved professionals in health planning. In 1966 the Comprehensive Health Planning and Public Health Service Amendment (Public Law 89-749) was passed. This was a significant document written to enable states and communities to plan for better use of health resources. There were many problems with this law, one being that no new plans could interfere with existing patterns of private practice of medicine and dentistry. The law was also inadequately funded. Because of these problems, other legislative action was taken in the mid-1970s.

The National Health Planning and Resources Development Act of 1974 (Public Law 93-641) was signed by President Gerald Ford on January 4, 1975. Its purpose was to provide funding for program development activities and services that would improve the delivery of health care in local communities. It was hoped that this legislation would improve accessibility of health care services, curtail rising costs, and monitor the quality of care being provided.

The goals of the National Health Planning and Resources Development Act were clearly delineated in the preamble. The preamble stated that this law was passed "to facilitate the development of recommendations for a national health planning policy, to augment area wide and state planning for health services, manpower and facilities, and to authorize financial assistance for the development of resources to further that policy" (Rubel, 1976, p. 3).

The terms of Public Law 93-641 ended the existing Hill-Burton Act (1947-1974), Regional Medical Programs (1966-1974), and the Comprehensive Health Planning Programs (1966-1974). All of these programs were designed to correct health care delivery problems but none of them had the power to be comprehensive.

There were two new titles in Public Law 93-641: title XV and title XVI. Title XVI provided federal financial assistance for construction and modernization of health care facilities. Title XV created a national network of local health systems agencies (HSAs), state health planning and development agencies (SHPDAs), and statewide health coordinating councils (SHCCs). These agencies were regulatory and were responsible for health planning and the development of resources under the law. The HSAs were very important elements of Public Law 93-641. They were geographically located in designated regions where effective planning and development of resources could be implemented at the community level. Their purpose was to improve the health of residents in the area by increasing the availability, continuity, and quality of health services while simultaneously limiting the costs of health care. Decreasing duplication of services was also a major goal of these HSAs.

Public Law 93-641 also created a new National Council for Health Policy (NCHP). This council was located within the Department of Health and Human Services, and made recommendations to the secretary of the Department on national health policy planning.

There were several major elements in the law that represented a new approach to planning for health services (Rubel, 1976, p. 4). First, there was an emphasis on strong local planning and local control over the development of services. All segments of the health care system, including providers of care, consumers, and third-party payers, must be part of health-planning boards. Second, the *certificate of need* (CON) program was to ensure that states did not develop health services that were not needed. Last, there were incentives to states to hold the cost of health care down.

The Demise of Public Law 93-641

The system of federally mandated health planning continued for 7 years. During this time HSAs were taken seriously as planning agencies, as evidenced by the fact that there was extensive investment of time and energy by volunteers in the activities of HSAs; newspapers regularly carried stories of their work; and the field of health law developed as hospitals and consumers hired attorneys to aid them in deliberations with the HSAs.

However, there were also problems. Political conservatives did not like government regulation of health care and many resented what they perceived to be the interference of the federal government in local government. Some critics felt that the program did not save enough money, and others felt that there was not sufficient concern for quality care.

By 1981 the Reagan administration proposed eliminating federal health planning requirements by 1982. Its arguments for this goal were that Public Law 93-641 had not controlled costs and that states should be making their own planning decisions. Further, regulation of supply was counter to free market competition.

The Omnibus Budget Reconciliation Act passed in 1981 (discussed in Chapter 20) ended the federal mandate for planning under Public Law 93-641. Under the Reconciliation Act, states could request that all funding for HSAs be eliminated. Further, this act stipulated that HSAs were no longer required to collect data or review existing facilities and proposed federal grants. Appropriations for funding HSAs were reduced from their high of $167 million in 1980 to $64 million for 1981. The result was that there was not enough money to support HSAs at the staffing levels required by law. Finally, in 1987, HSA legislation was repealed.

The Development of Health Block Grants

Another piece of legislation passed during the Reagan administration that had a tremendous impact upon health care planning in the 1980s was the development of health block grants (refer to Chapter 4). Block grants were part of the Federal Omnibus Budget Reconciliation Act (Public Law 97-35), which reorganized the amount and type of federal health care expenditures. The act had two effects: traditional federal categorical grant programs and the funding for these programs were reduced by 25%. This legislation affected four areas of health care: maternal and child health; prevention; community health services (primary care); and alcohol, drug abuse, and mental health.

A *block grant* is a funding mechanism through which the federal government supports a state or local health program. Normally a block grant is a lump sum given by the federal government to a state unit such as a health department; the state unit has the freedom (under some broad restrictions) to finance various activities within the block grant functional area. Categorical grants also make federal money available to state and local units for health care programs. However, categorical grants can be used only for specifically designated programs and are usually limited to activities narrowly defined by federal laws. Thus, categorical grants allow much less flexibility in the use of funds than do block grants.

Health block grants affect four vital areas of concern to professionals who care about the health and well-being of population groups. In particular, mothers and children are one of the most vulnerable populations affected by this new legislation. Since funding for these programs was reduced under the block grant funding mechanism, the challenge for the future will be to provide cost-effective care for vulnerable aggregates. History shows that needs are not being met.

Future Legislation

The decade of the 1990s will most certainly produce dramatic changes in health care legislation because millions of Americans have no health care coverage and costs are out of control. For the federal government medical costs have become "the fastest growing major item, increasing at more than 8% annually at a time when inflation is only about 5%" (Time, November 25, 1992, p. 35). President Bill Clinton was elected in 1992 with a mandate by the American people for health care reform. At the state level health care reform has already altered the system: in 1992 Vermont and Minnesota created a health care authority with the goal of developing a single-payor insurance plan like Canada's. Nurses in both of these states played major roles in bringing about change.

The Health Insurance Association of America, reflecting the change in public thinking, proposed a plan that would require insurance coverage for all Americans. The proposed plan reflects the realization that comprehensive health legislation is "almost certain to come, with or without insurer's participation, in the Clinton Administration" (Eliason, 1992, p. 1).

Changes in federal regulations and health care guidelines in 1992 posed challenges and advances for nurses. A new federal agency, the Agency for Health Care Policy and Research, issued guidelines for treating Medicare patients with postoperative pain, decubiti, and urinary incontinence. The guidelines set standards for these nursing problems for institutions receiving Medicare reimbursement for clients. Further, the Health Care Financing Administration granted "deemed status" to the Community Health Accreditation Program and the Joint Commission for the Accreditation of Health Care Organizations, meaning that accredited home care agencies will not have to undergo annual Medicare or Medicaid surveys to qualify for reimbursement. This action was an acknowledgement of the professional accountability of nurses for providing care with excellence.

Another milestone for nursing in 1992 was the election of the first nurse in history to Congress. Bernice Johnson, a black woman from Texas, was one of nine nurses who ran for this office and the only one who won. She stressed pay equity for women, preschool education, on-site child care, parental leave, reproductive choice, subsidized housing, and better health care (News, 1992, p. 71). Making changes in the health of individuals and communities means that public policy must change. Nurses increasingly have role models working in the public arena to produce change.

COLLABORATION FOR INTERDISCIPLINARY FUNCTIONING

Although community health nursing is exciting and challenging, nurses in this specialty area encounter problems that can be overwhelming: pregnant women addicted to crack, aging people living alone with no caretakers, child and spouse abuse, and clients having difficulties obtaining access to care, all accompanied by the terrible conditions of poverty. Nurses cannot solve these crises alone; we need to work competently with other disciplines and professions to begin to solve them. Interdisciplinary functioning and collaboration is a learned skill: individuals working in one group do not automatically come together as a united team. Understanding the definitions of interdisciplinary functioning and collaboration and the factors that facilitate team work help the nurse to participate in a setting that includes other professions.

Collaboration is the process of working jointly with others. An interdisciplinary team is a group of people "who have a unified direction, who are committed to achieving common objectives, and who are focused on an integrated outcome . . . " (Mariano, 1989, p. 286). Mariano discusses three factors that make an impact upon collaboration: goal and role conflict, decision-making skills, and communication skills. Goals need to be clear to all team members and the role or the skills that each professional contributes toward that goal must be made clear. Competent professionals know their own strengths, limitations, and contributions, and are capable of communicating these to others. The process used in decision-making by the team is influenced by these factors and is successful when there is respect for the contributions of everyone (refer to Tables 15-5 and 20-3 for the role contributions of various disciplines on the health care team). Data available for making the decisions need to be adequate as well. Synthesizing information from multiple sources such as clients, families, and health records for the purpose of obtaining a comprehensive picture of client situations is another crucial aspect of collaboration. Communication skills, enhanced by respect and knowledge of the goals and roles of team members, succeeds with a climate of openness and the guarantee that people can express thoughts freely.

BARRIERS TO HEALTH PLANNING

Each step in the process of health planning goes down neatly on paper. Carrying out the process in "real life" is a different and challenging activity. There are several barriers to health planning that need to be acknowledged. Some of these, such as unavailability and inaccessibility of resources, inadequate knowledge, and lack of commitment to health planning, were addressed previously. Others are presented in the following section.

A major barrier to effective health planning is a lack of understanding of the term *health*. Health is an elusive state that is difficult to define. What causes health is not easy to enumerate. It is possible to list healthy behaviors, but no one can guarantee health because both health and disease are affected by multiple interrelated variables (multiple causation principle). Epidemiological research has not yet been sufficient to document what these multiple causes are for many conditions or what health actions most effectively promote health and prevent disease. Thus, it is difficult for health planners to develop health action strategies for many situations. As more epidemiological research is conducted this barrier should become less acute.

The disease-oriented focus in our present health care delivery system presents another key barrier to health planning. Health promotion and prevention concepts are very often not accepted by laypersons and professionals alike in this system. Skyrocketing health costs have severely disrupted the country's health care system and thus community health prevention programs have been badly neglected. Basically what has happened is that persons spend so much money curing illness that there is little money left for preventive health care.

Lack of sufficient money and personnel is a constant barrier. Health may not be a priority for communities so that energy and money are spent in other directions. Health planning is often a political rather than a technical or analytical exercise, and it is possible to see an ongoing contest between local, state, and federal governments for control of planning agencies and money.

Noncompliance with health-planning activities is also a barrier. In the United States freedom of choice is a highly prized right. Safety belts save lives, but one chooses whether or not to use them, even when existing laws mandate their use. Healthy behaviors can be presented as options but that is all. Differing values promote different priorities. If an individual is not motivated to seek preventive care, preventive health-planning action will be ineffective.

The health care system in the United States is an enormous industry that has unbelievable growth each year. Health care is a basic part of the American economy; it is inevitable that it does not function perfectly. Efforts are being made, however, to improve the quality of health care in our country.

Health care providers are being confronted with awesome tasks when facing issues such as AIDS and lack of insurance coverage for many Americans. Clearly, health care reform with changes in the health care delivery system is demanding restructuring of the organizational culture. We will continue to see "changes in leadership orientations, and increasing flexibility to accommodate flattening of organizational authority systems. Incorporated in these changes are needs for the implementation of a more collaborative model of team building for the delivery of public health nursing services. Collaborative models should include the consumers of our services to whom we must listen" (Graham, 1992, p. 73).

The nursing profession's reason for being is caring for others, a revolutionary concept in health policy. "The challenge to nurses and other health and social activists is one of leadership, of rebuilding communities, of reclaiming spaces and places for humane and caring interactions, and of articulating a compelling vision of another way for society and its people to be. The challenge is ultimately one of transforming such a vision into a reality of rebuilt and reclaimed communities. . . . nursing needs to consider its role in creating new realities that ensure that caring is a core value in both health and social policies" (Moccia, 1990, p. 76).

Summary

Health planning for aggregates at risk is a major function of the community health nurse. In any community setting there are aggregates at risk for specific health problems. The developmental framework helps the community health nurse to identify these groups across the life span.

Empowering a community to choose strategies for health based on appropriate information, resources, and support enables that community to self-determine its health (McMurray, 1991). This is the highest goal a community health nurse can help an aggregate to achieve.

Community health nurses provide unique contributions during the health planning process. Educational experiences prepare nurses to comprehensively analyze needs of families and populations. Clinical practice brings them in touch daily with consumer concerns and helps to identify gaps or duplication in the health care delivery system.

Currently there are obvious deficiencies in the health care delivery system, which warrant health planning action. Health care services are frequently fragmented, extremely costly, and often lacking for specific segments of the population. However, there has been a positive trend evolving that places emphasis on developing new ways to meet the health care needs of all citizens.

Involvement in health planning activities can be exciting and rewarding. Nurses are increasingly recognizing the importance of actively participating on health planning teams and engaging in political activities aimed at changing health policy.

◀ *An Exercise in Critical Thinking* ▶

The article in Appendix 13-1 (Mahon J, McFarlane J, and Golden K: De Madres a Madres: a community partnership for health, *Pub Health Nurs* 8(1):15-19, 1991) describes how community health nurses used the health care planning process to begin solving the problem of lack of prenatal care in an aggregate at risk. Analyze how the concepts of community empowerment and education were used in the program. What changes would you make to increase community involvement in the program?

APPENDIX 13-1

De Madres a Madres: A Community Partnership for Health

Joan Mahon, M.S., R.N., Judith McFarlane, R.N., Dr.P.H., and Katherine Golden, B.S.N., R.N.

Abstract To increase the number of Hispanic women who begin early prenatal care, a community partnership for health was initiated among the general public, businesses, 14 volunteer mothers, and one community health nurse. Volunteer mothers living in the targeted community were taught how to identify Hispanic women at risk for not starting early prenatal care, and how to provide social support and community resource information within a culturally acceptable milieu. At the end of the first year of the partnership, over 2000 women at risk for not starting early prenatal care had been contacted by the volunteer mothers.

Address correspondence to Judith McFarlane, R.N., Professor and Director, de Madres a Madres: A Community Partnership for Health, Texas Woman's University, College of Nursing, 1130 M.C. Anderson Boulevard, Houston, TX 77030.
Joan Mahon is the clinical nurse associate with de Madres a Madres and Katherine Golden is research associate. Both are at Texas Woman's University.

This program was aided by grant CHE-255 from the Texas Gulf Coast Chapter, March of Dimes Birth Defects Foundation.

As a single teenage mother, I felt alone and frightened when I was pregnant. I asked myself what I was going to do, how I would manage, where I could go for help, and who would help me. Women in my community need information and support during pregnancy.
—19-year-old single parent and volunteer mother in de Madres a Madres

A NATIONAL DISGRACE

Almost 40,000 infants die each year before their first birthday due to low birth weight. The cost of intensive care, special education, and social services for these infants and their families can average $400,000 over the children's life. In comparison, the cost of routine prenatal care is $400 (American Public Health Association, 1989a). The Surgeon General's goal for the nation was that by 1990, 90% of all pregnant women would begin prenatal care within the first three months of pregnancy (USDHHS, 1980). Based on the 1978–1986 rate of progress, however, the nation will not meet this goal until the year 2094, 100 years after the target date (Children's Defense Fund, 1989). As reported by the American Public Health Association (1989b), maternal and infant health has clearly suffered and markedly declined in recent years, as chronicled by 12 key indicators, including prenatal care, rates of low birth weight, and infant mortality.

A WIDENING MINORITY GAP

Compounding the problem are major disparities between the maternal and infant health of white and minority Americans (USDHHS, 1989). Between 1984 and 1985 there was no improvement in the proportion of infants with low birth weight. Among black and nonwhite infants, the frequency of low birth weight increased (Children's Defense Fund, 1989).

Low birth weight, infant mortality, and pregnancy complications are clearly associated with inadequate prenatal care. To improve access to prenatal care, the National Institute of Medicine (1988) set forth a seminal document detailing demographic risk factors associated with insufficient prenatal care, barriers to the use of prenatal care, and recommendations to improve the use of prenatal care. The report profiled Hispanic women as substantially less likely than non-Hispanic white mothers to begin prenatal care early, and 3 times as likely to obtain late or no care. Moreover, Hispanic mothers as a group are more likely than non-Hispanic black mothers to begin prenatal care late or not at all. Clearly, when compared to non-Hispanic white and black women, Hispanic women are at far greater risk to not receiving early prenatal care; many receive no prenatal care. In addition to minority status, age is a major indicator, with teenagers and mothers over age 40 years being at highest risk of receiving late or no prenatal care. Women with less than a high school education are also at increased risk. Finally, poverty was cited as one of the most important correlates of insufficient prenatal care.

In Houston, the fourth largest city in the nation, the minority health gap is widening. According to the latest figures from the City of Houston Health Department (1988), 68.6% of pregnant women initiate prenatal care during the first trimester; for Hispanic women the figure falls to 60.4%. Stated another way, 40% of the Hispanic women in Houston do not receive early prenatal care. The 1989–1990 Texas State Health Plan designated access to prenatal and maternity care for low-income pregnant women in Texas as the top priority issue. Texas accounts for 8% of all births nationally. Nearly 1 in every 12 infants in this country who died in 1985 was a Texas resident (Texas Department of Health, 1988). Improving birth outcomes in the state would have a major impact on meeting the Surgeon General's goals for the nation.

CULTURALLY RELEVANT SOCIAL SUPPORT AND INFORMATION TO FACILITATE EARLY PRENATAL CARE

With the Hispanic woman at high risk for not receiving early prenatal care, innovative approaches to provide access to care are essential. Barriers were well defined and verified by the National Institute of Medicine (1988) as sociodemographic (age, education, parity), system access (transportation, clinic availability, insurance), and cultural-personal (fear, stress, depression, denial). To mitigate barriers to prenatal care, de Madres a Madres: A Community Partnership for Health was initiated in a Hispanic community. (De Madres a Madres means "from mothers to mothers.")

The program is a collaborative effort among the general public, businesses, and volunteer mothers to identify Hispanic women at risk for not starting early prenatal care. Other objectives are to provide social support and information on community resources within a culturally acceptable framework. The value of social support in promoting a healthy pregnancy is well supported in the literature (Nuckolls, Cassel, & Kaplan, 1972; Norbeck & Tilden, 1983; Omer et al., 1987; Gray, 1987; American Nurses Association, 1987). The use of lay volunteers and paraprofessionals to offer education and support services in the home setting to pregnant women is also widely reported in the literature (National Institute of Medicine, 1988; Heins, Nance, & Ferguson, 1987; Olds et al., 1986). The conceptual basis for the program was drawn directly from a community as client model (Anderson and McFarlane, 1988). An analysis of each community system was completed to yield community strengths and portals for intervention as well as identify community leaders and levers for change. Community as client information was used to strategize planning, implementation, and evaluation of the de Madres a Madres program.

The pregnant women in all cited studies received intensive social support by volunteers or lay professionals after they initiated prenatal care in a clinic setting, which for most was in the second or third trimester. No program has been reported to date that offers targeted support and information to high-risk women before they enter the health care system. De Madres a Madres proposed culturally relevant social support and community resource information to identified at-risk women before they entered the system. The premise was that culturally relevant social support coupled with community resource information would enable pregnant women to transcend barriers to early prenatal care.

The program will be evaluated by the number of women who begin early prenatal care before as compared to after implementation of the program. The percentage of pregnant women who obtain early prenatal care at the neighborhood health clinic, located within the target community and the only provider of public prenatal care, will be evaluated for the two years of the program and compared to a two-year period before the program was initiated. Additional variables include the number of at-risk women visited by the volunteer mothers, and the number of health and social service referrals completed by the volunteer mothers. Finally, structured interviews of at-risk women who are assisted by the volunteer mothers will be used to evaluate the program. Requirements for the volunteer mothers include residence in the community, at least 18 years of age, and completion of an eight-hour training program offered by the community health nurse. Community awareness, involvement, commitment, and ownership are the essential program elements.

Community Awareness and Recruitment of Volunteer Mothers

Begun in 1989 and funded by a two-year community service grant from the local chapter of the March of Dimes, de Madres a Madres employed one master's-prepared community health nurse (CHN). Based on the fact that Houston's Hispanic women are the least likely to obtain early prenatal care, an inner-city Hispanic community was selected by the March of Dimes for program implementation. This community has a population of 13,555, of which 34% are women of childbearing age. Median family income is $12,782, and 19% of the households receive public assistance. The CHN completed a community assessment that identified 31 key community leaders.

The 31 community leaders, many of whom were Hispanic, included school principals, the clergy, civic leaders, attorneys, social service administrators, a state representative, health care providers, elected city council representatives, school board members, and law enforcement officers. Most were visited individually several times. The objectives and purpose of the program were explained during each visit. Each community leader was asked for names of potential volunteer mothers. (Since most community leaders were men, sharing the names of women yielded an endorsement for the program from the male hierarchy.)

Simultaneously, the CHN made formal presentations about the program at scheduled community functions, including school meetings, civic association gatherings, church functions, and crime-prevention meetings. At least 100 people attended most formal meetings and learned about de Madres a Madres. In addition, informal presentations were made by the community health nurse at community health fairs, school-sponsored fiestas, and church-supported bazaars and social events.

The CHN assimilated herself into community activities, and on a typical day might begin by visiting with a cluster of women at the local bakery to learn of their concerns during pregnancy and perceived barriers to care. The next stop might be a discussion with the school nurse regarding how the de Madres a Madres program could be integrated into the nurse's regularly scheduled group meeting with pregnant teens. Then on to churches in the area to meet with lay groups of volunteer women interested in outreach and community service. The evening might consist of making a formal presentation on the program at a neighborhood meeting to prevent crime, followed by informal chats with women interested in becoming volunteer mothers.

The community assessment and establishment of trust between the CHN and residents was the lengthiest phase of the program. It was quickly learned that, although most of the 13,000 residents were considered of Hispanic ethnicity, the residents segregated themselves by nation of birth. For example, second-generation Mexican-Americans would not associate with newly immigrated Mexicans, and neither group would mingle with Guatemalans, El Salvadorans, or Nicaraguans. Values, beliefs, and health practices were nationality specific. It was necessary to recruit volunteer mothers from each group. In addition to nation of origin, immigration status differed widely and was a definite barrier to prenatal care. Women in the amnesty program were at highest risk of not receiving prenatal care and, like teen mothers, required special efforts on the part of the volunteer mothers and CHN.

Community Commitment and Involvement

At the end of nine months, 14 volunteer mothers had completed the eight-hour training session with the CHN. They ranged in age from 19 to 65 years, had experienced roles from teenage mother to grandmother, and, because of their positions in the community, came into daily contact with women at risk for not starting early prenatal care. The women met in small groups for two hours and were guided through information on the importance of early prenatal care, how to identify women at risk for not starting early care, resources for pregnant women, and effective supportive communication skills. The mothers learned and shared their perceptions of the many barriers to obtaining care during pregnancy. Information was provided on how effective listening and social support can decrease isolation and enable pregnant women to obtain resources and early prenatal care. The volunteer mothers learned how to be advocates for healthy pregnancies. The following is an outline of the curriculum.

A. Role as advocate
1. Overview of de Madres a Madres: A Community Partnership for Health
2. Importance of volunteer neighborhood mothers
3. Volunteer role in the home and the community
B. Resources in the community
1. Health, food, job training, education, financial aid, transportation, housing
C. Communication/support techniques
1. Development of trust; use of empathy; verbal skills relating to trust and empathy
2. Nonverbal skills relating to trust and empathy; use of touch
D. Effective supportive communication skills
1. Techniques for effective communication; barriers to communication; ways of facilitating communication
E. Aspects of quality prenatal care
1. Places to receive prenatal care; probable cost; what the visit will entail; outcome of good prenatal care; maternal complications from lack of prenatal care; ambivalence about pregnancy and fears of prenatal care
F. Health resources (detailed description)
1. Agencies offering prenatal care; eligibility requirements; how agencies coordinate care

G. Low-birth-weight infants, known causes
   1. Prenatal care
   2. Nutrition
   3. Substance abuse
   4. Stress (battering)
H. Family dynamics, interpersonal relationships
   1. Supportive family relationships
   2. Spousal abuse
I. Importance of social support, Effects of stress on pregnancy
   1. Methods to decrease stress and increase problem solving skills
   2. Effective listening; decreasing isolation; guiding to proper resources; role modeling
   3. Increasing mother's self-worth

Strategies for presenting the curriculum varied. Some of the content was taught during a visit to the local hospital's intensive care unit for low-birth-weight infants. Other sessions focused on role playing and group sharing of experiences. Guest speakers discussed how to obtain health and social services programs for pregnant women. Volunteers who completed the training program were given a tote bag with the program name and logo. They proudly carried the bag daily and turned queries about the logo into discussion session about the program with colleagues at work as well as the general public.

A great deal of camaraderie developed among the volunteer mothers, who established a strong social support network for each other. Such group support was essential for the successful coping of these volunteers as they assisted women in dire circumstances. The mothers met regularly with the CHN to discuss their experiences and plans for community events, and receive additional and updated information. They also met informally as a group and began to establish an organizational infrastructure with leadership positions.

Because these mothers were of the same culture and spoke the same language as women in their community, information was offered in a culturally acceptable milieu. Methods of providing the information varied. One mother invited women into her home to discuss concerns and community resources for a healthy pregnancy. Others visited women in their homes. Several of them were present at the food pantry in the community where they offered social support and community resource information with 75 to 100 women weekly. Many of the women who frequented the pantry were undocumented residents and unaware of how to obtain care for their pregnancy without fear of reprisal.

Although the fact of pregnancy is frequently obvious, exact status was not solicited. The basic premise of de Madres a Madres is primary prevention. If at-risk women are offered culturally relevant information, they will be able to use it when a pregnancy is confirmed. It also was assumed that mothers would share the information with family and friends, creating a ripple effect of information throughout the community. The volunteer mothers were taught that information is empowering and contact is success. The at-risk women would choose when and how to use the information.

The volunteer mothers planned and implemented several communitywide events to share information, including a de Madres a Madres party for all women in the community and an information booth at community functions. A brochure that included community resources and a video about the program were developed for use by the volunteers. A small purse mirror with community resource numbers was given to all mothers visited by the volunteers.

A COMMUNITY PARTNERSHIP FOR HEALTH

Community ownership follows community awareness, involvement, and commitment. To facilitate community ownership, the second year of the de Madres a Madres program will focus on strengthening involvement of the business community, including financial support for the program. The CHN will assist the community in exploring sources for continuation funding, including the United Way and Hispanic Chamber of Commerce. A community advisory board will be formed, with representatives from business, community leaders, and volunteer mothers. A task of the board will be to assume future direction and support mechanisms for the program.

After the first year of the program, more than 2000 at-risk women had received information from a volunteer mother. The type of woman seen daily is exemplified by Olivia.

Olivia, age 21, was five months pregnant and a recent immigrant to Houston. She did not speak English and had not begun prenatal care. After seeing a notice about a de Madres a Madres event, she walked the one mile to the neighborhood elementary school where the program was being held. At the event, Olivia learned about community resources including the location of the prenatal clinic and health and social service agencies. A volunteer mother arranged to visit her the next day. During the home visit, Olivia stated that she was in need of basic food staples for her family, and that her husband was physically abusive. The volunteer mother offered information about the shelter for battered women, location of neighborhood food pantries, and eligibility requirements for specific health and social services. After contact with the volunteer mother, Olivia initiated prenatal care, enrolled in the Women, Infants, and Children (WIC) program, and received weekly food staples from the neighborhood pantry.

Maternal and child health is essential for a healthy and prosperous community. De Madres a Madres developed a community support network to form a partnership of the general public, businesses, and volunteer mothers to protect and promote the health of pregnant women. When a volunteer mother with two children who works full time was asked why she donated her time, her reply was quick and sure, "Why would I not help these women? This community is my home. I care about these women."

Article References

American Nurses' Association. (1987). *Access to prenatal care: Key to preventing low birthweight.* Kansas City, MO: Author.

American Public Health Association. (1989a). The nation's health [editorial] Washington, DC: Author.

American Public Health Association. (1989b). *Monitoring children's health: Key indicators.* Washington, DC: Author.

Anderson, E., & McFarlane, J. (1988). *Community as client. Application of the nursing process.* Philadelphia: J.B. Lippincott.

Children's Defense Fund. (1989). *The health of American's children. Maternal and child health data book.* New York: Author.

City of Houston Health Department. (1988). *The health of Houston 1984–1986.* Houston: Author.

Gray, L. (1987). A descriptive study on perceived social support among clients assessed by public health nurses. Unpublished thesis, Texas Woman's University, Houston, Texas.

Heins, H. C., Nance, N. W., & Ferguson, J. E. (1987). Social support in improving perinatal outcome: The resource mothers program. *Obstetrics and Gynecology, 70,* 263–266.

National Institute of Medicine. (1988). *Prenatal Care: Reaching Mothers, Reaching Infants.* Washington, DC: National Academy Press.

Norbeck, J. S., & Tilden, V. P. (1983). Life stress, social support, and emotional disequilibrium in complications of pregnancy: A prospective multivariate study. *Journal of Health and Social Behavior, 24,* 30–46.

Nuckolls, K. B., Cassel, J., & Kaplan, B. H. (1972). Psychosocial asserts, life crises and the prognosis of pregnancy. *American Journal of Epidemiology, 95,* 431–441.

Olds, D. L., Henderson, C. R., Tatelbaum, R., & Chamberlin, R. (1986). Improving the delivery of prenatal care and outcomes of pregnancy: A randomized trial of nurse home visitation. *Pediatrics, 77,* 16–28.

Omer, H., Elizur, V., Barnea, T., Friedlander, D., & Palti, Z. (1987). Psychological variables and premature labour: A possible solution for some methodological problems. *Journal of Psychosomatic Research, 30,* 559–565.

Texas Department of Health. (1988). *1989–90 Texas state health plan.* Texas Statewide Health Coordinating Council. Austin: Author.

U.S. Department of Health and Human Services. (1980). *Promoting health/preventing disease: Objectives for the nation.* Washington, DC: Government Printing Office.

U.S. Department of Health and Human Services. (1989). *Health, United States, 1988.* Washington, DC: Government Printing Office.

References

American Nurses Association: *A conceptual model of community health nursing* (Pub No Ch-10 2M), Kansas City, Mo., 1980, The Association.

American Nurses Association: *Standards of community health nursing practice* (Pub No CH-10), Kansas City, Mo., 1986, The Association.

American Nurses Association: Nursing proposes health care reform, *American Nurse* 23(2):1, 1991.

American Public Health Association, Public Health Nursing Section: *The definition and role of public health nursing in the delivery of health care,* Washington, D.C., 1981, The Association.

American Public Health Association: *Healthy communities 2000: model standards—guidelines for community attainment of the year 2000 national health objective,* ed 3, Washington, D.C., 1991, The Association.

Arnold M, Blankenship L, and Hess J: *Administering health systems, issues and perspectives,* Chicago, 1971, Aldine & Atherton.

Bracht N and Kingsbury L: Community organization principles in health promotion: a five-stage model. In Bracht N, ed.,: Health promotion at the community level, Newbury Park, Calif., 1990, Sage, pp. 66-88.

Braithwaite RL and Lythcott N: Community empowerment as a strategy for health promotion for black and other minority populations, *JAMA* 261(2):282-283, January 13, 1989.

Brown ER: Community action for health promotion: a strategy to empower individuals and communities, *International J of Health Services* 21(3):441-456, 1991.

Eliason F: Insurers change their minds on universal health coverage, *New York Times Business Diary,* Section 3, December 6, 1992, p. 1.

Flynn BC, Rider MS, and Bailey WW: Developing community leadership in healthy cities: the Indiana model, *Nurs Outlook* 40(3):121-126, 1992.

Graham KY: Health care reform and public health nursing, *Public Health Nurs* 9:6, 73, 1992.

Kreuter MW: PATCH: its origin, basic concepts and links to contemporary public health policy, *J Health Education* 23(3):135-139, 1992.

MacStravic R: Setting priorities in health planning: what does it all mean? *Inquiry* 15:20-24, 1978.

McMurray A: Advocacy for community self-empowerment, *International Nursing Review* 38:19-21, 1991.

Mahon J, McFarlane J, & Golden K: De madres a madres: a community partnership for health, *Public Health Nurs* 8(1):15-19, 1991.

Mariano C: The call for interdisciplinary collaboration, *Nurs Outlook* 37(6):285-288, 1989.

Milio N: *Promoting health through public policy,* Philadelphia, 1981, FA Davis.

Milio N: Public policy as the cornerstone for a new public health: local and global beginnings, *Fam Community Health* 10(2):57-64, 1988.

Moccia P: Reclaiming our communities, *Nurs Outlook* 38(2):73-76, 1990.

National Academy of Sciences, Institute of Medicine: *Health planning in the United States: issues in guidelines development,* Washington, D.C., 1980, The National Academy.

News: In a first, Texas elects a nurse legislator to Congress, *Am J Nurs* 92(12):71, 80, 1992.

Resources for Human Development, Inc. and Abottsford Homes Tenant Management Corporation: *Project abstract,* Philadelphia, Pa., undated.

Rojas-Urruita X and Aday LS: A framework for community assessment: designing and conducting a survey in a Hispanic immigrant and refugee community, *Public Health Nurs* 8(1):20-25, 1991.

Rubel EJ: Implementing the National Health Planning and Resources Development Act of 1974, *Public Health Rep* 91:3-8, 1976.

Schlaff AL: Boston's Codman Square community partnership for health promotion, *Public Health Reports* 106(2):186-191, 1991.

Shugars DA, O'Neil EH, and Bader JD, eds.: *Healthy America: practitioners for 2005, an agenda for action for U.S. health professional schools,* Durham, N.C., 1991, The Pew Health Professions Commission.

Sofarer S: Community health planning in the United States: a postmortem, *Fam Community Health* 10(4):1-12, 1988.

Spiegel AD and Hyman HH: *Basic health planning methods,* Germantown, Md., 1978, Aspen Systems.

Taylor I and Knowelden J: *Principles of epidemiology,* ed 2, Boston, 1964, Little, Brown.

Time: *Cover story: condition: critical,* November 25, 1992, 34-42.

U.S. Department of Health, Education, and Welfare (USDHEW): *Guidelines for the development of health systems plans and annual implementation plans,* Hyattsville, Md., 1979, Bureau of Health Planning.

U.S. Department of Health and Human Services: *Prevention '82* (DHHS Pub No PHS 82-50157), Washington, D.C., 1982, U.S. Government Printing Office.

U.S. Department of Health and Human Services: *Healthy People 2000: national health promotion and disease prevention objectives, full report, with commentary,* Washington, D.C., 1991, Public Health Services.

Wald L: *House on Henry street,* New York, 1915, Henry Holt.

Williams CA: Community health nursing—what is it? *Nurs Outlook* 25:250-254, 1977.

Selected Bibliography

American Nurses Association: *Community-based nursing services: innovative models,* Kansas City, Mo., 1986, The Association.

Anderson ET and McFarland J: *Community as client,* Philadelphia, 1988, Lippincott.

Bagwell M and Clements S: *A political handbook for health professionals,* Boston, 1985, Little, Brown.

Battista RN and Lawrence RS, eds: *Implementing preventive services,* New York, 1988, Oxford University Press.

Bremer A: Revitalizing the district model for the delivery of prevention-focused community health nursing services, *Fam and Community Health* 10(2):1-10, 1987.

Clabots RB and Dolphin D: The multilingual videotape project: community involvement in a unique health education program, *Public Health Rep* 107(1):75-80, 1992.

DeBella S, Martin L and Siddall F: *Nurses' role in health care planning,* New York, 1986, Appleton-Century-Crofts.

Ducanis AJ and Golin AK: *The interdisciplinary health care team: a handbook,* Germantown, Md., 1979, Aspen Publishers.

Editors of Nursing 91: The nurse-doctor game, *Nurs 91* 21(6):60-64, 1991.

Emery KR: Developing a new or modified service: analysis for decision making, *Health Care Super* 4(2):30-38, 1986.

Fagin CM: Collaboration between nurses and physicians: no longer a choice, *Nurs and Health Care* 13(7):354-363, 1992.

Gottschalk J and Teymour L: Envisioning the future: challenges in community health nursing, *J of Nurs Admin* 22(6):11-12, 1992.

Leipert B: Notes from the field. Shifting gears—changing paradigms: a vision for community health nursing, *Public Health Nurs* 9(2):138-139, 1992.

Navarro U: Why some countries have national health insurance, others have national health services, and the United States has neither, *Int J Health Services* 19:384-404, 1989.

Oda DS: The imperative of a national health strategy for children: is there a political will? *Nurs Outlook* 37:206-208, 1989.

Rosenbaum S and Johnson KA: Providing health care for low-income children: reconciling child health, goals with child health financing realities, *Milbank Q* 64:442-478, 1986.

Salem DA and Levine IS: Enhancing mental health services for homeless persons: state proposals under the MHSH block grant program, *Public Health Rep* 104:241-248, 1989.

Shamansky SL and Graham KY: Pushing out the boundaries, *Public Health Nurs* 6(1):113, 1989.

Stein LI, Watts DT, and Howell T: The doctor-nurse game revisited, *New Engl J of Med* 322:546-594, 1990.

Spotts H and Schewe C: Communicating with the elderly consumer: the growing health care challenge, *J Health Care Market* 9(3):36-44, 1989.

Wheelan TL and Hunger JD: *Strategic management and business policy,* ed 3, Reading, Mass., 1989, Addison-Wesley.

Winkelstein W: Determinants of worldwide health, *Am J Publ Health* 82(7):931-932, 1992.

Zerwekh JV: At the expense of their souls, *Nurs Outlook* 39(2):58-61, 1991.

Unit Five

Meeting the Needs of Aggregates At Risk Across the Life Span

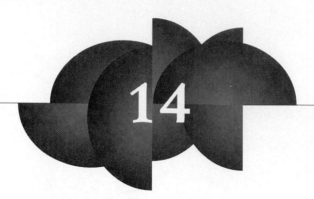

14

Needs and Services of Children from Birth to 5 Years

OBJECTIVES

Upon completion of this chapter, the reader should be able to:

1. Describe U.S. trends in infant and maternal mortality and why health care professionals are concerned about these trends.
2. Discuss the 1990 Federal Program Objectives for Pregnancy and Infant Health.
3. Discuss the leading causes of mortality among infants and children 1 to 5 years of age.
4. Analyze factors associated with high-risk pregnancies and births.
5. Discuss common health problems for infants and children 1 to 5 years of age.

6. Analyze health promotion needs of families with children in the newborn to 5-year-old age group and community health nursing interventions to address these needs.
7. Discuss significant legislation that has influenced maternal and child health care delivery.
8. Describe barriers to the delivery of services to the newborn to 5-year-old population and their parents.
9. Identify the roles assumed by the community health nurse to promote maternal, infant, and child health.

The vast majority of children in the United States are healthy, and efforts at preventing disease and reducing injuries among this population mean that there will be further improvements in their health. The U.S. infant mortality rate declined from 14.1 per 1000 live births in 1977 to 9.2 in 1990; the mortality rate of children between the ages of 1 and 9 years also substantially declined during this time period (Congress of the United States, OTA, 1987, 1; USDHHS, 1993, Child Health '92, pp. 16, 22).

However, when the infant mortality rate for the United States is compared with the same rate in other developed countries, there is a striking reason for the concern of those who care about the public's health: this nation ranks lower than 23 other industrialized countries. Since 1980 Japan has had the lowest infant mortality rate in the world. In 1987 the risk of a child dying in infancy in Japan was less than half that of a child in the United States (refer to Figure 14-1). About 1 percent of all babies born in the United States die in the first year of life, and two thirds of these deaths occur in the first 28 days of life (Congress of the United States, OTA, 1987, p. 2)

The infant mortality rate and the maternal mortality rate have been used as indicators of a nation's health since the turn of the century for several reasons: they are basic vital statistics collected in most countries and they are closely related to adequate nutrition, housing, sanitation and other environmental conditions (refer to Chapter 6). In 1900 deaths of mothers and children were major contributors to mortality figures: approximately 60 mothers died for every 10,000 pregnancies that produced live-born infants; of every 1000 live births, 100 infants did not survive the first year of life (Pickett and Hanlon, 1990, p. 400).

Statistics such as these motivated concerned individuals to develop community maternal-child health programs; nursing assumed a major leadership role in this effort (refer to Figure 14-2). Lillian Wald, the pioneer community health nurse and feminist, helped establish milk stations in 1903 at the Henry Street Settlement House in New York City to ensure the safety of milk for babies. Diarrhea caused by contaminated milk in the summer months was the cause of many deaths. The City of New York followed this example and in 1911 authorized the establishment of 15 milk stations:

A nurse is attached to each station to follow into the homes and there lay the foundation, through education, for hy-

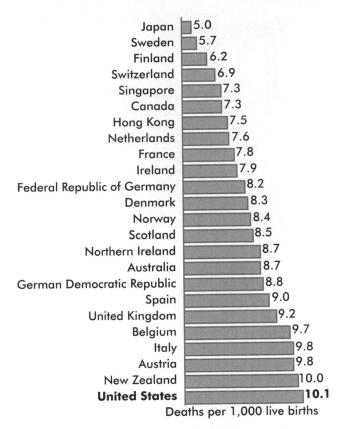

Figure 14-1 Comparison of national infant mortality rates: 1987. (From USDHHS, Public Health Service: *Child health USA '91,* DHHS Pub No. HRS-M-CH91-1, Washington, D.C., 1991, U.S. Government Printing Office, p. 17.)

gienic living. A marked reduction in infant mortality has been brought about and moreover, a realization, on the part of the city, of the immeasurable social and economic value of keeping the babies alive. (Wald, 1915, p. 57)

Traditionally, childbearing women, infants, and children are considered to be the most dependent and vulnerable members in a society. As the society develops there is a trend toward greater concern for this segment of the population. The health of a society's children ensures that society's future, so this concern for infants and children is justified on economic, as well as other, grounds.

The high U.S. infant mortality rate is the result of the extraordinary number of low-birth-weight babies born in this country. "Low birthweight so overwhelms other health problems of early childhood that it cannot

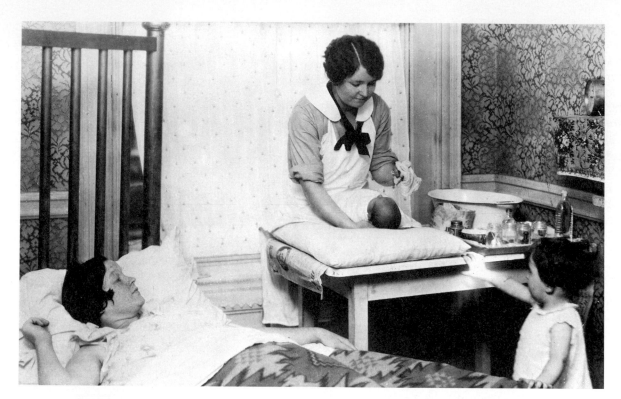

Figure 14-2   A community health nurse from the Visiting Nurse Service of New York City visits a mother with a new baby at home in the early 1930s. (Courtesy Visiting Nurse Service of New York City.)

be ignored" (Congress of the United States, OTA, 1987, p. 2). Though there has been remarkable progress in reducing infant mortality, as was noted above, the decline in mortality has slowed and continues to lag. This slowdown seems to be the result of an increase in the number of live births in the lowest birth weight category, an outcome of rapid advances in the technology of neonatal intensive care units and the concentration of high-risk births in sophisticated perinatal centers. "The number of reported live births under 500 grams in this country increased more rapidly in the 1980s than did live births at all other birthweights. The vast majority of newborns under 500 grams die in infancy; thus an increase in the reported number of live births in this category would have the effect of pushing up the U.S. infant mortality rate" (Congress of the United States, OTA, p. 5).

These facts about infant mortality are important to the community's health because babies and children are our nation's most important resource. A nation's infant mortality rate is a measure of its success in combating poverty, ignorance, and disease (Mason, 1991, p. 475).

Tragically, poverty among the children of the United States is pervasive: one in five children is poor, and children are twice as likely to be poor as any other group of Americans, including the elderly.

"In 1989, when the poverty rate was 11.4 percent for the elderly, 10.2 percent for nonelderly adults, and 18.1 percent for children ages six through 17, the poverty rate for children younger than six was 22.5 percent. Nearly one-quarter of America's infants and preschoolers were in families that did not have enough income to meet their most basic needs. The normal development of these infants and preschoolers is being jeopardized by the nation's tolerance of these abnormally high poverty rates" (Johnson, Miranda, Sherman, and Weill, 1991, p. 7).

Poverty rates have always been higher for black children than for white children; however, white child poverty grew faster than black child poverty, and rates for Latino children grew the fastest of all three groups.

Healthy People 2000: National Health Promotion and Disease Prevention Objectives (USDHHS, 1991, p. 29-30), provided the following statement about poverty and children's health:

Health disparities between poor people and those with higher incomes are almost universal for all dimensions of health. Those disparities may be summarized by the findings that people with low income have death rates that are twice the rates for people with incomes above the poverty level.

No single indicator of health status makes the connection between poverty and poor health more clearly than does infant mortality. Poor pregnancy outcomes including prematurity, low birth weight, birth defects, and infant death are linked to low income, low educational level, low occupational status, and other indicators of social and economic advantage.

The National Health Promotion and Disease Prevention Objectives (USDHHS, 1991, Healthy People) for Infant and Maternal Health are listed in the box on p. 494. The objectives emphasize the major health concerns of infants including low birth weight, congenital anomalies, sudden infant death syndrome, and respiratory distress syndrome. They include maternal factors associated with these concerns and prenatal care. Special population groups including low-income, black, American Indian/Alaska natives, and Hispanic women, and black and American Indian/Alaska native infants are targeted.

Figure 14-3, which presents infant mortality rates for the United States from 1950 to 1986 by specified race, graphically illustrates that the color of an infant's skin is a measure of the chances of that infant's survival. Infant mortality rates for all races declined substantially from 1950 to 1986, with the greatest decline for Native Americans. However, the rate for blacks is still substantially higher than that for all other races (USDHHS, Public Health Service, 1990, Health Status of the Disadvantaged, p. 33)

The National Commission to Prevent Infant Mortality was created by Congress (Public Law 99-660) in 1986 to establish a national strategic plan for the United States, designed to reduce infant mortality and morbidity (National Commission to Prevent Infant Mortality, 1989, Home visiting). The Commission's plan for action was presented to Congress in August, 1988, in its report entitled "Death Before Life: The Tragedy of Infant Mortality." The commission focused on practical solutions for improving maternal

and child health and identified two major goals: 1) that every pregnant woman and infant receive adequate care, the woman as soon as she knows she is pregnant and the infant from the moment of birth; and 2) that maternal and child health and well-being become a national priority (National Commission to Prevent Infant Mortality, 1988, August).

Infant mortality is a critical problem; each year about 40,000 babies die before their first birthday (National Commission to Prevent Infant Mortality, 1988, Infant Mortality and the Media). All sectors of society—government, communities, healthprofessionals , business, and industry—must focus attention on this problem. Infant mortality is very costly to society in both human and economic terms (National Commission to Prevent Infant Mortality, 1988, 1985 Indirect Costs).

Both public and private efforts were initiated in the 1980s to combat infant and maternal mortality. The Healthy Mothers, Healthy Babies Coalition was started in December 1980 by six national organizations, one of which was the American Nurses Association, following the Surgeon General's Workshop on Maternal and Infant Health. This coalition is now a cooperative venture of 80 national voluntary, health professional, and government organizations. It is focusing on high-level prenatal, obstetric, and neonatal care; preventive services during the first year of life; education of health professionals; and broad public information activities aimed at pregnant women and their families (Arkin, 1986).

COMMON HEALTH RISKS

This chapter discusses the health concerns common to the newborn to 5-year-old age group and presents how poverty and race/ethnic origin affect these concerns. Interventions using a population-based approach are advanced. Though the problems are extraordinary, there are encouraging solutions occuring at the national level. Successful intervention programs dealing with the disadvantaged are also discussed in this chapter.

Morbidity and mortality among the newborn to 5-year-old population present a major public health concern. In the process of growing up, children encounter injuries and illnesses that interfere with normal functioning. Jack and Jill's broken crown and Humpty Dumpty's fall off the wall are common experiences known to every child.

◀   *Healthy People 2000: Maternal and Infant Health Objectives*   ▶

Health Status Objectives

- Reduce the infant mortality rate to no more than 7 per 1,000 live births. (Baseline: 10.1 per 1,000 live births in 1987)
- Reduce the fetal death rate (20 or more weeks of gestation) to no more than 5 per 1,000 live births plus fetal deaths. (Baseline: 7.6 per 1,000 live births plus fetal deaths in 1987)
- Reduce the maternal mortality rate to no more than 3.3 per 100,000 live births. (Baseline: 6.6 per 100,000 in 1987)
- Reduce the incidence of fetal alcohol syndrome to no more than 0.12 per 1,000 live births. (Baseline: 0.22 per 1,000 live births in 1987)
- Reduce low birth weight to an incidence of no more than 5 percent of live births and very low birth weight to no more than 1 percent of live births. (Baseline: 6.9 and 1.2 percent, respectively, in 1987)
- Increase to at least 85 percent the proportion of mothers who achieve the minimum recommended weight gain during their pregnancies. (Baseline: 67 percent of married women in 1980)
- Reduce severe complications of pregnancy to no more than 15 per 100 deliveries. (Baseline: 22 hospitalizations prior to delivery per 100 deliveries in 1987)
- Reduce the cesarean delivery rate to no more than 15 per 100 deliveries. (Baseline: 24.4 per 100 deliveries in 1987)
- Increase to at least 75 percent the proportion of mothers who breastfeed their babies in the early postpartum period and to at least 50 percent the proportion who continue breastfeeding until their babies are 5 to 6 months old. (Baseline: 54 percent at discharge from birth site and 21 percent at 5 to 6 months in 1988)

- Increase abstinence from tobacco use by pregnant women to at least 90 percent and increase abstinence from alcohol, cocaine, and marijuana by pregnant women by at least 20 percent. (Baseline: 75 percent of pregnant women abstained from tobacco use in 1985)
- Increase to at least 90 percent the proportion of all pregnant women who receive prenatal care in the first trimester of pregnancy. (Baseline: 76 percent of live births in 1987)
- Increase to at least 60 percent the proportion of primary care providers who provide age-appropriate preconception care and counseling. (Baseline data available in 1992)
- Increase to at least 90 percent the proportion of women enrolled in prenatal care who are offered screening and counseling on prenatal detection of fetal abnormalities. (Baseline data available in 1991)
- Increase to at least 90 percent the proportion of pregnant women and infants who receive risk-appropriate care. (Baseline data available in 1991)
- Increase to at least 95 percent the proportion of newborns screened by State-sponsored programs for genetic disorders and other disabling conditions and to 90 percent the proportion of newborns testing positive for disease who receive appropriate treatment. (Baseline: For sickle cell anemia, with 20 States reporting, approximately 33 percent of live births screened [57 percent of black infants]; for galactosemia, with 38 States reporting, approximately 70 percent of live births screened)
- Increase to at least 90 percent the proportion of babies aged 18 months and younger who receive recommended primary care services at the appropriate intervals. (Baseline data available in 1992)

From USDHHS, Public Health Service: *Healthy people 2000: national health promotion and disease prevention objectives,* full report, with commentary, Washington, D.C., 1991, U.S. Government Printing Office, pp. 110-111.

There are health problems common to the newborn to 5-year-old age group that can be prevented, as well as problems that necessitate secondary and tertiary prevention. In order to plan health services for this group, the community health nurse should be familiar with factors that increase children's risk for morbidity and mortality. Having this knowledge facilitates application of the three levels of prevention and casefinding.

Figures 14-4 and 14-5 show the leading causes of death for children under 1 year and children 1 to 9

years. About two thirds of all infant deaths occur in the neonatal period—the first 28 days of life (U.S. Congress, OTA, 1988, p. 4). Infants most at risk during this period are low-birth-weight babies or those weighing less than 5½ pounds. These babies are 40 times more likely than normal-weight infants to die during the neonatal period (Institute of Medicine, 1985). Congenital anomalies cause a significant number of infant deaths during both the neonatal and postneonatal (28 days to 1 year) periods. The most important cause of death during the postneonatal period is

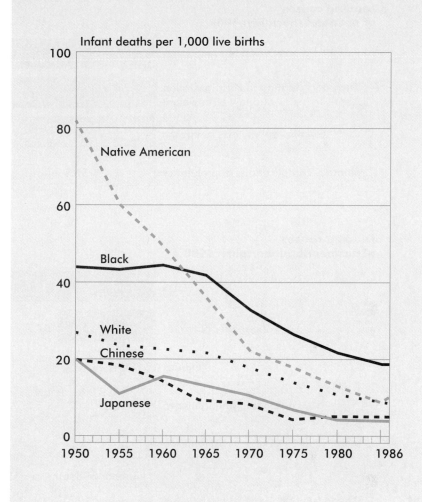

Figure 14-3 Infant mortality rates by specified race: United States, selected years, 1950 to 1986. (From USDHHS, Public Health Service: *Health status of the disadvantaged. Chartbook 1990, DHHS Pub No. (HRSA) HRS-P-DV 90-1,* Washington, D.C., 1990, U.S. Government Printing Office, p. 33.)

sudden infant death syndrome (SIDS). SIDS accounts for more than one third of all postneonatal deaths. Economic and educational deprivation, the continuing high rate of teenage pregnancy, and barriers impeding access to prenatal, perinatal, and infant care, particularly for disadvantaged groups, are other factors known to have a negative impact on infant survival (Task Force on Infant Mortality, 1987; USDHHS, Office of Disease Prevention and Health Promotion, 1986). As children become mobile, accidental injuries become the major cause of death.

Risks before Birth

Factors associated with high-risk pregnancies (refer to the box on p. 498) have been known for a considerable length of time and have not changed signifi-

cantly in recent years. These factors are important because they provide the basis for the high mortality and morbidity rates during the first year of life and contribute to the high maternal mortality rates. They are danger signs signaling threat to the newborn and the mother. Those caring for the pregnant mother can effectively use these high risk indicators to identify mothers and infants who have special care needs and can benefit from preventive interventions.

Many of the same elements that influence infant mortality have an effect on maternal mortality. Among the most important of these are the continuing high rate of teenage pregnancy; late entry into prenatal care; barriers impeding access to maternity care; inadequate "systems" of care for high-risk women; and the continuing high rate of unintended births (USDHHS, Office of Disease Prevention and Health Promotion,

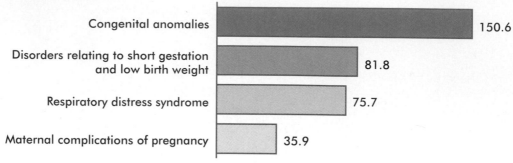

**Leading causes
of neonatal mortality: 1988**

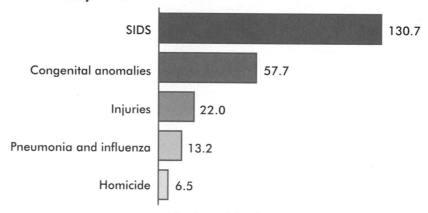

**Leading causes
of postneonatal mortality: 1988**

Number of deaths per 100,000 live births

Figure 14-4   Neonatal and postneonatal mortality, 1988. (From USDHHS, Public Health Service: *Child health USA '91,* DHHS Pub No HRS-M-CH-91-1, Washington, D.C., 1991, U.S. Government Printing Office, p. 19.)

1986, pp. 41-42). As is demonstrated in the box on p. 498, socially and economically deprived persons are more likely than others to have high-risk pregnancies. This is at least partially explained by the lack of adequate prenatal care, which is unavailable to many population groups, including the inner city and rural poor, teenage mothers, and disadvantaged ethnic groups (e.g., black, Hispanic, and Native American women).

Early, regular prenatal care results in improved pregnancy outcomes: numerous studies have demonstrated that prematurity and infant mortality rates are lowest when prenatal care begins before the fourth month of pregnancy and continues with at least eight prenatal visits (Rosenbaum, Layton, and Liu, 1991). However, in spite of the effectiveness of timely prenatal care, almost one fourth of all pregnant women

receive late or no care (National Center for Health Statistics, 1988). Trends in the use of prenatal care are disturbing. Since 1980 the percentage of all births in women who have had late or no prenatal care has risen among all races, with this trend most pronounced among black women (Brown, 1989).

Numerous personal and system barriers limit participation in prenatal care (refer to box on p. 499). Economic status and health insurance coverage play large roles in determining whether or not a woman obtains prenatal care (Brown, 1989). Nevertheless, the number of women of childbearing age without insurance is increasing, while at the same time the cost of maternity care is rising: some 15 million women have no insurance to cover maternity care; 10 million of these women have no insurance of any sort (Alan Guttmacher Institute, 1987).

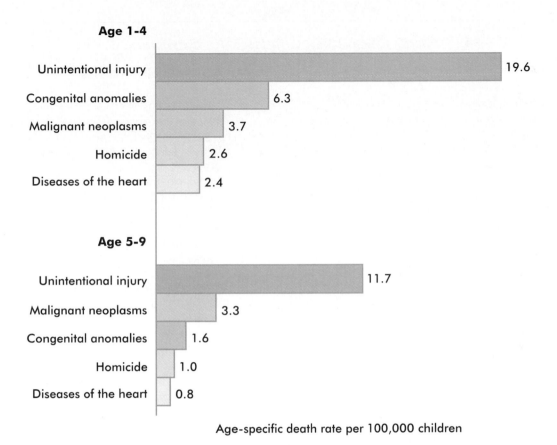

Age 1-4

Unintentional injury 19.6
Congenital anomalies 6.3
Malignant neoplasms 3.7
Homicide 2.6
Diseases of the heart 2.4

Age 5-9

Unintentional injury 11.7
Malignant neoplasms 3.3
Congenital anomalies 1.6
Homicide 1.0
Diseases of the heart 0.8

Age-specific death rate per 100,000 children

Figure 14-5 Leading causes of death in children ages 1-9: 1988. (From USDHHS, Public Health Service: *Child health USA '91,* DHHS, Pub No HRS-M-CH-91-1, Washington, D.C., 1991, U.S. Government Printing Office, p. 24.)

There is a substantial racial disparity in the timely receipt of prenatal care. In 1988 79% of white mothers, compared to 61% of black mothers, received early prenatal care. Women younger than 20 years are less likely than older women to receive early prenatal care (USDHHS, 1991, Child Health USA '91, p. 48). Further, 6% of infants born in 1988 were born to women who received no care or received care only during the third trimester of pregnancy (refer to Figure 14-6).

Although financial factors significantly affect a woman's decision to obtain prenatal care, other socio-demographic, system-related, and attitudinal barriers must be addressed by health care professions (refer to box on p. 499). Women who have insurance also delay or receive no prenatal care. Reasons for lack of participation in prenatal care vary among high-risk groups. For example, adolescents frequently cite fear as a reason for not seeking health care services. Women who are experiencing stressful life situations, charac-

terized by daily problems and struggles, often attach a low value to prenatal care. More recently, it is believed that drug abuse could be a prominent reason for insufficient use of prenatal services (Brown, 1989).

Community-wide, well-coordinated initiatives are needed to address problems related to pregnancy and insufficient prenatal care. Since needs vary among different segments of the population, a comprehensive array of programs must be developed (Alan Guttmacher Institute, 1989; Chamberlin, 1988; National Commission to Prevent Infant Mortality, 1989, Home visiting). As previously discussed, coalition- or constituency-building among all sectors of society is a must to enhance service delivery to mothers and children. There is renewed interest in the importance of home visiting to reach geographically isolated and/or other disadvantaged groups (Chamberlin; National Commission to Prevent Infant Mortality). Home visiting activities can improve many health

◀ *Factors Associated with High-Risk Pregnancy* ▶

1. Demographic Factors

  a. Lower socioeconomic status
  b. Disadvantaged ethnic groups
  c. Marital status: unwed mothers
  d. Maternal age
   (1) Gravida less than 16 years of age
   (2) Primigravida 35 years of age or older
   (3) Gravida 40 years of age or older
  e. Maternal weight: nonpregnant weight less than 100 lb or more than 200 lb
  f. Stature: height less than 62 in (1.57 m)
  g. Malnutrition
  h. Poor physical fitness

2. Past Pregnancy History

  a. Grand multiparity: six previous pregnancies terminating beyond 20 weeks' gestation
  b. Antepartum bleeding after 12 weeks of gestation
  c. Premature rupture of membranes, premature onset of labor, premature delivery
  d. Previous cesarean section or mid- or high-forceps delivery
  e. Prolonged labor
  f. Infant with cerebral palsy, mental retardation, birth trauma, central nervous system disorder, or congenital anomaly
  g. Reproductive failure: infertility, repetitive abortion, fetal loss, stillbirth, or neonatal death
  h. Delivery of preterm (less than 37 weeks) or postterm (more than 42 weeks) infant

3. Past or Present Medical History

  a. Hypertension or renal disease or both
  b. Diabetes mellitus (overt or gestational)
  c. Cardiovascular disease (rheumatic, congenital, or peripheral vascular)
  d. Pulmonary disease producing hypoxemia and hypercapnia
  e. Thyroid, parathyroid, and endocrine disorders
  f. Idiopathic thrombocytopenic purpura
  g. Neoplastic disease
  h. Hereditary disorders
  i. Collagen diseases
  j. Epilepsy

4. Additional Obstetric and Medical Conditions

  a. Toxemia
  b. Asymptomatic bacteriuria
  c. Anemia or hemoglobinopathy
  d. Rh sensitization
  e. Habitual smoking
  f. Drug addiction or habituation
  g. Chronic exposure to any pharmacological or chemical agent
  h. Multiple pregnancy
  i. Rubella or other viral infection
  j. Intercurrent surgery and anesthesia
  k. Placental abnormalities and uterine bleeding
  l. Abnormal fetal lie or presentation, fetal anomalies, oligohydramnios, polyhydramnios
  m. Abnormalities of fetal or uterine growth or both
  n. Maternal trauma during pregnancy
  o. Maternal emotional crisis during pregnancy

Modified from Vaughn VC, McKay RJ, and Behrman RE, eds, and Nelson WE, senior ed: *Textbook of pediatrics,* ed 11, Philadelphia, 1979, Saunders.

outcomes, including increasing attendance in cost-effective prenatal care, encouraging healthy behaviors, and discouraging harmful activities during pregnancy such as smoking and drug use (National Commission to Prevent Infant Mortality, 1989, Home visiting).

Risks after Birth

Once a baby is born, gestational age, birth weight, and environment are significant factors in the chances for survival. The newborn period (birth to 1 month) is particularly important since the majority of all infant deaths occur within the first 28 days of life (USDHHS, 1985, Prevention 84/85, p. 53).

As stated earlier, infant mortality rates remain high in this country compared to other industrialized countries. Most U.S. infant deaths occur among low-birth-weight infants (those under 2500 grams). Though we have achieved dramatic declines in infant mortality over the years, we have done this with the use of technology to save increasingly smaller babies. Thus the rates of low birth weights have not changed; however, the number of small babies who survive

Barriers to Use of Prenatal Care

I. Sociodemographic

Poverty
Residence: inner-city or rural
Minority status
Age: <18 or >39
High parity
Non–English-speaking
Unmarried
Less than high school education

II. System-Related

Inadequacies in private insurance policies (waiting periods, coverage limitations, coinsurance and deductibles, requirements for up-front payments)
Absence of either Medicaid or private insurance coverage of maternity services
Inadequate or no maternity care providers for Medicaid-enrolled, uninsured, and other low-income women (long wait to get appointment)
Complicated, time-consuming process to enroll in Medicaid
Availability of Medicaid poorly advertised
Inadequate transportation services, long travel time to service sites, or both
Difficulty obtaining child care
Weak links between prenatal services and pregnancy testing
Inadequate coordination among such services as WIC and prenatal care

Inconvenient clinic hours, especially for working women
Long waits to see physician
Language and cultural incompatibility between providers and clients
Poor communication between clients and providers exacerbated by short interactions with providers
Negative attributes of clinics, including rude personnel, uncomfortable surroundings, and complicated registration procedures
Limited information on exactly where to get care (phone numbers and addresses)

III. Attitudinal

Pregnancy unplanned, viewed negatively, or both
Ambivalence
Signs of pregnancy not known or recognized
Prenatal care not valued or understood
Fear of doctors, hospitals, procedures
Fear of parental discovery
Fear of deportation or problems with the Immigration and Naturalization Service
Fear that certain health habits will be discovered and criticized (smoking, eating disorders, drug or alcohol abuse)
Selected lifestyles (drug abuse, homelessness)
Inadequate social supports and personal resources
Excessive stress
Denial or apathy
Concealment

From Brown S: Drawing women into prenatal care, *Family planning perspectives* 21(2):75, March/April 1989. © The Alan Guttmacher Institute.

with handicaps is substantial and presents important fiscal and health problems for the nation.

"The most striking factor in the U.S. experience remains the racial disparity in rates of low birthweight (LBW). The LBW rate for black Americans is twice that of whites and other racial/ethnic groups, and is well above the objectives (for the nation) set for 1990. This higher rate of LBW is paralleled by higher infant mortality rates, although unlike LBW, the mortality rates are declining. What accounts for this difference?" (Berendes, Kessel, and Yaffe, 1991, p. 6). Research suggests that genetic or inherited differences in addition to structural racism may account for some of the differences. For example, as a group, black college-educated couples in this country have infant mortality rates that are 90% higher than for white college-educated parents. The mortality is primarily related to a much higher rate of death associated with premature delivery (Hogue and Hargraves, 1993, p. 10). Table 14-1 depicts the factors that have an impact on intrauterine growth and gestational duration and thus the weight of the infant. Many of these factors can be modified to prevent prematurity. The intervention programs listed in this chapter address these factors at either the primary or secondary level of prevention.

The costs of low-birth-weight infants are high in both human and economic terms: a low-birth-weight infant costs more than twice as much as a normal-birth-weight infant. Birth defects, chronic illnesses, institutional or foster care, and special education

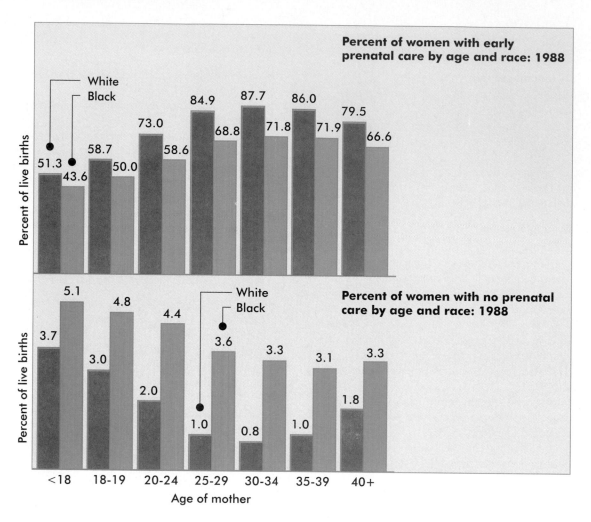

Figure 14-6   Percentage of women receiving early or no prenatal care by age and race: 1988. (From USDHHS, Public Health Service: *Child health USA '91,* DHHS, Pub No HRS-M-CH-91-1, Washington, D.C., 1991, U.S. Government Printing Office, p. 48.)

needs all contribute to this cost (Robert Wood Johnson Foundation, 1991, p. 36). From a human perspective, families experience considerable stress when dealing with the needs of a low-birth-weight infant.

Problems developing before the infant reaches 1 month of age are usually related to gestational age and birth weight and in utero problems. Problems after 1 month are more often related to environmental factors. Here the community health nurse plays a significant role in prevention, especially in relation to morbidity.

Parent-Child Bonding

Parent-child bonding can be adversely affected when an infant is separated from its primary caregiver

for a period of time. This separation can occur when an infant is premature or otherwise at risk and must have long-term health care away from parents. Even with normal hospital deliveries, mothers may not see their infants for 12 to 24 hours following delivery. Studies have shown that this period is crucial for the formation of attachment bonds between mothers and their babies and is important for establishing mothering behavior (Klaus and Kennell, 1976). Klaus and Kennell (p. 124) hypothesize that all disorders of mothering, ranging from a persisting concern about a minor abnormality to abuse and neglect of children, are in part the end result of separation in the early newborn period.

Another problem associated with high-risk in-

TABLE 14-1   Factors Assessed for Independent Causal Impact on Intrauterine Growth and Gestational Duration

	Genetic and constitutional	Demographic and psychosocial	Obstetric	Nutritional	Maternal morbidity during pregnancy
Factors assessed	Infant sex[1] Racial/ethnic origin[1] Maternal height[1] Maternal prepregnancy weights[3]	Maternal age[2,4] Socioeconomic status[2,4] Marital status Maternal psychologic factors	Parity[1] Birth or pregnancy interval Sexual activity Intrauterine growth and gestational duration in prior pregnancies In utero exposure to diethylstilbestrol[3] Prior induced abortion Prior stillbirth or neonatal death Prior infertility Prior spontaneous abortion[3]	Gestational weight gain[1] Vitamin B_6 Caloric intake[1] Energy expenditure, work, and physical activity Protein intake/status Iron and anemia Folic acid and vitamin B_{12} Calcium, phosphorus, and vitamin D Other vitamins and trace elements Zinc and copper	General morbidity and episodic illness[1] Malaria[1] Urinary tract infection Genital tract infection

[1]Established direct determinants of intrauterine growth include infant sex, racial/ethnic origin, prepregnancy weight, paternal height and weight, maternal height and weight, parity, prior LBW, gestational weight gain, caloric intake, general morbidity, malaria, cigarette smoking, alcohol consumption, and tobacco chewing.
[2]Established indirect determinants of intrauterine growth include maternal age and socioeconomic status.
[3]Factors with well-established direct causal impact on gestational duration include prepregnancy weight, prior prematurity, prior spontaneous abortion, in utero diethylstilbestrol exposure, and cigarette smoking.
[4]Factors with well-established indirect causal impact on gestational duration include maternal age and socioeconomic status.
From Kramer MS: *The etiology and prevention of low birthweight: current knowledge and priorities for future research.* In Berendes H, Kessel S, and Yaffe S, eds: *Advances in the prevention of low birthweight: an international symposium,* Washington, D.C., 1991, National Center for Education in Maternal and Child Health, p. 35.

fants—those who are small or have other physical, familial, and psychological problems—can be their failure to thrive. A child who fails to thrive is one whose weight and sometimes height fall below the fifth percentile for the child's age (Whaley and Wong, 1991, p. 616). Three general categories of failure to thrive have been defined (Whaley and Wong, p. 617):

- **Organic failure to thrive (OFTT),** which is the result of a physical cause, such as congenital heart defects, neurologic lesions, microcephaly, chronic urinary tract infection, gastroesophageal reflux, renal insufficiency,

malabsorption syndrome, endocrine dysfunction, or cystic fibrosis. This category accounts for less than half of all FTT.

- **Nonorganic failure to thrive (NFTT),** which has a definable cause that is unrelated to disease. NFTT is most often the result of psychosocial factors, such as inadequate nutritional information by the parent; deficiency in maternal care or a disturbance in maternal-child attachment; or a disturbance in the child's ability to separate from the parent, leading to food refusal to maintain attention (Chatoor and others, 1985). NFTT has been described under a variety of less acceptable names, including maternal deprivation, environmental deprivation, and deprivation dwarfism.

- **Idiopathic failure to thrive,** which is unexplained by the usual organic and environmental etiologies but may also be classified as NFTT. Both categories of NFTT account for the majority of cases of FTT.

Causes of failure to thrive include poverty, inadequate nutritional knowledge, health beliefs such as fad diets, family stress, feeding resistance, and insufficient breast milk (Whaley and Wong, 1991, p. 617). Whaley and Wong have suggested that nursing care for families who have children that fail to thrive must include support that encourages adaptive mothering behaviors and promotes mother-child attachment. The nursing care should also include teaching specific nurturing techniques, including adequate feeding and interaction with the environment. Assistance to the family in resolving problems that interfere with their ability to provide a nurturing environment is another important element of nursing care. Dealing with families who have a parent-child disturbance is difficult; Whaley and Wong (p. 618) discuss this care in depth.

Child Maltreatment

Child maltreatment involves direct harm or intent to injure, including intentionality without physical injury. Different types of child maltreatment occur, including physical and/or psychological abuse and neglect and sexual abuse. In general, *abuse* refers to acts of commission such as beating or excessive chastisement. *Neglect* refers to acts of omission such as failure to provide adequate food, clothing, or emotional care. However, the line separating the two is a very thin one (U.S. Congress, OTA, 1988, p. 167).

The problem of child maltreatment is growing. There were almost 2.7 million reports of suspected abused or neglected children nationwide in 1991, meaning that 42 of every 1000 children may have been reported. Estimates indicate that between 35% to 50% of cases reported are substantiated upon investigation. This number of reports represents an increase of 40% since 1985; an estimated 1383 children died from abuse or neglect in 1991 (USDHHS, 1993, Child Health USA '92, 1993, p. 29).

Child abuse or neglect is a cumulative problem since the scars that result from such behavior have long-term effects. The most damaging aspect of child abuse and neglect is on the developmental process and emotional growth of the child. Abused children do not feel safe and are unable to trust others—Erikson's first stage in development.

"The most important parental risk factors for child maltreatment are those related to poverty and unemployment and a history of abuse as a child" (U.S. Congress, OTA, 1988, p. 176). Parents may follow *their* parents' method of child rearing: if it was characterized by abuse and neglect, their child-rearing style may duplicate their own experience. At the same time, it is possible that intergenerational violence could be related in part to the perpetuation of poverty from one generation to the next (U.S. Congress, OTA, p. 175).

Parents of abused children often do not understand normal growth and development patterns and expect too much of their children. As a result, the child is criticized and physically and emotionally punished. A sense of failure and lack of confidence and faith in one's own abilities often results in abused and neglected children who in turn may abuse and neglect others.

Family functioning patterns in households experiencing parent-child violence reflect a disturbance in parental nurturing skills as a result of many factors (Garbarino, 1977). These include blocks to the role transition of parent because of inability to develop the role of caregiver. The parents may also have had inadequate role models. Such parents lack knowledge about what is involved in parenting, both physically and emotionally, and thus do not know what to expect realistically of themselves or their children. Abusing parents often consider their own needs more important than their children's needs: they have an inappropriate concept of the legitimacy and value of their own needs when ranked with their children's needs. Expecting children to fulfill parents' needs is another problem. Abusing parents feel that they are unable to have any effect and control over events inside and outside the family. Unfortunately, these same families are often characterized by great demands for adjustment to stresses such as moves, job changes, and illnesses. Difficulties may also arise when children begin demanding independence, pushing away from families, or when they are negativistic.

Garbarino also suggests that abusing families are socially isolated from support systems. This isolation may be a result of mobility patterns, characteristics that alienate others, social stresses that cut families off from potential and actual supports, and social service agencies that are unable to identify and care for high-risk families.

Community health nurses need to be alert to situations where abuse and neglect might occur and intervene before they happen. Marital strain, poverty, isolation, and overwhelmed parents are signals to be heeded. Premature births or having children with developmental disabilities are stressful situations that need to be noted. Parents who expect infants to be responsible for their acts and who respond with physical punishment also bear watching.

Mental retardation, emotional disorders, and learning disorders can be other evidences of a less-than-positive nurturing environment for infants. Organic pathological factors are contributors to these disorders, but psychosocial and other factors also influence the development of these disorders. A summary of physical and behavioral indicators that can assist nurses in identifying child abuse and neglect can be found in Chapter 15.

Presently there are no states with enough resources and personnel to deal adequately with the increasing number of reported cases of abuse and neglect, not to mention working with families who have already been identified as needing care.

Sudden Infant Death Syndrome

Another sequel to high-risk pregnancy may be the sudden infant death syndrome (SIDS). In the United States, 2 of every 1000 live-born infants die annually from SIDS. It is the number one cause of death in infants between the ages of 1 month and 1 year. Although SIDS was identified as early as in the writings of the New Testament, no single cause for this condition has been discovered. It is suspected that SIDS is caused by a combination of events and some type of biochemical, anatomical, or developmental defect or deficiency (National SIDS Clearinghouse, 1989). Helping parents handle grief and guilt feelings is the major role of the community health nurse in these situations. The impact of death on siblings is another area where the nurse must intervene.

Increasingly, communities are setting up crisis teams to assist families who have experienced a child's death from SIDS. One health department in a northern city employs a pediatric nurse practitioner who works full-time with such families. She facilitates family adjustment as they work through the grief process after death has come to a seemingly healthy infant.

Helping families to deal with their feelings about future parenting is very important (Chan, 1987).

Public health professionals may have a significant preventive intervention role as well as a therapeutic role when dealing with SIDS. A 7-year study of unexpected infant deaths in England suggested that home visiting by health visitors was directly related to a reduction in mortality of infants scored to be at risk for unexpected infant death (Carpenter, 1983, p. 724). The scoring system for ascertaining who was at risk included factors such as the mother's age, her previous pregnancies, duration of the second stage of labor, mother's blood group, birth weight, single or multiple birth, if the infant was breastfed or bottle-fed, and presence of urinary infection of mother during pregnancy.

Home visits by health visitors were made for SIDS preventive follow-up every 2 weeks for 3 months and every month for up to 6 months to those infants scoring at high risk. "The reduction in mortality attributed directly to the effect of increased visiting of high-risk infants is numerically similar to the number of lives saved by treating cancers in children. This suggests that home visiting by health visitors is highly cost-effective" (Carpenter, 1983, p. 723).

Acute Illnesses

Respiratory diseases and other conditions such as diarrhea result in short-term disability and account for many doctor visits for infants. These diseases caused much death in the past. Today there is less mortality from these conditions, but a tremendous amount of professional time is spent in controlling acute illnesses. The nurse in the pediatric clinic or the nurse who makes home visits will see these kinds of problems and will need the expertise to explain their origin and treatment to parents.

Problems of Children Ages 1 to 5

Children do change in their capacities. As developmental growth occurs, infants and children's needs and problems become different.

Accidental Injuries

In 1988 about 38% of all deaths among children ages 1 through 4 were caused by injuries (National Safety Council, 1991, p. 6). Figure 14-7 depicts deaths in 1988 due to injuries in this age group as compared to deaths from cancer and congenital anomalies. As

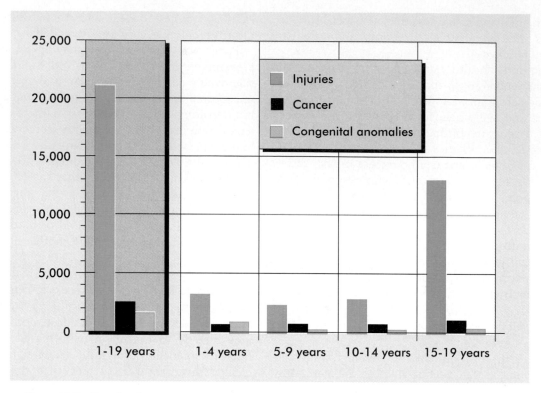

Figure 14-7 Deaths due to injuries vs. deaths from cancer and congenital anomalies, 1988. (From Children's Safety Network: *A data book of child and adolescent injury,* Washington, D.C., 1991, National Center for Education in Maternal and Child Health, p. 2.)

former Surgeon General C. Everett Koop said, "If a disease were killing our children in the proportions that injuries are, people would be outraged and demand that this killer be stopped" (Children's Safety Network, 1991, p. 2).

Figure 14-8 shows that fires and burns caused the greatest number of injury deaths among toddlers and preschoolers, with drownings, pedestrian injuries, and motor vehicle occupant injuries also causing a significant number of deaths. Primary prevention of many of these deaths is possible.

Accidental injuries disproportionately strike the young, which is costly to society from many perspectives. Accidental injuries can cause tremendous social and emotional stress, significant activity limitation, and financial burdens. "More than half of the impairments caused by injuries result in activity limitations: seventy percent of impairments due to injuries are deformities or orthopedic impairments" (National Institute on Disability and Rehabilitation Research,

1989, p. 26). It is not difficult to see that accidents are a major health problem and that present education and legislation are not as effective as they should be in combating a problem that is preventable.

Respiratory and Gastrointestinal Problems

Upper respiratory infections become a common cause of illness in the 1- to 5-year-old age group, especially when these children begin to play in groups. Upper respiratory infections can be minor and cause only minimal interference to living. Others can be life-threatening, especially when no treatment is obtained. Lower respiratory tract infections result generally from infections of the upper respiratory tract.

Minor gastrointestinal problems are almost as common as respiratory infections. The use of epidemiology in examining the numbers of cases in a family and a community helps to determine whether the causative agent is communicable. Epidemiological investigation also helps to identify significant environmen-

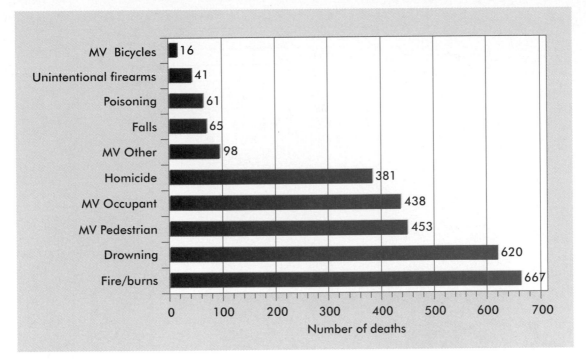

MV = Motor vehicle.

Figure 14-8 Number of deaths by cause for toddlers and preschoolers ages 1-4, 1988. (From Children's Safety Network: *A data book of child and adolescent injury,* Washington, D.C., 1991, National Center for Education in Maternal and Child Health, p. 8.)

tal conditions that need changing, especially when a child has repeated infections. In one day-care center, for example, repeated episodes of diarrhea among a number of the children led the supervisor to look for a cause. It was discovered that feeding bottles were left in tote bags until the noon feedings and that spoiled milk was the result. After its epidemiological investigation the day-care center began to refrigerate bottles immediately upon the arrival of infants and parents.

Prompt treatment of acute conditions, ongoing medical care, educating parents about good health care practices, and early detection of illness can help to prevent or curtail respiratory and gastrointestinal problems.

Chronic Conditions

Chronic conditions are important because of their long-term effects. They can significantly limit a child's normal activities and increase health care usage. In 1990 over 3.5 million, or 5.2%, of children ages 1 through 19 were limited in their activities due to

chronic illnesses and impairments (USDHHS, 1991, Child Health USA, '91, p. 28). Children with activity limitations have 2½ times as many physician contacts and spend over 11 times as many days in the hospital as do other children: they account for 40% of all hospital days among children ages 1 through 19 (USDHHS, Office of Maternal and Child Health, 1989, pp. 45-46).

Cancer is the third leading cause of mortality in children 1 through 4 years of age (National Safety Council, 1991). The types of cancers seen in children differ from those seen in adults. Those affecting children are the leukemias, embryonal tumors, and sarcomas. Regular medical follow-up can aid in early diagnosis of such conditions.

Under the category of chronic problems come children with developmental disabilities such as phenylketonuria, Down syndrome, cerebral palsy, blindness, mental retardation, or deafness. Also included are children with physical health problems such as diabetes, rheumatoid arthritis, and kidney disease.

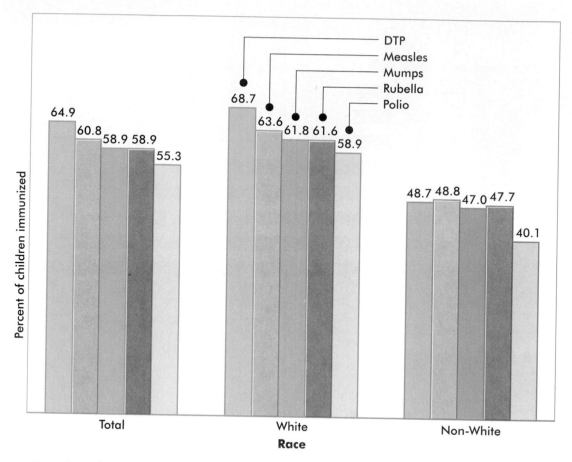

Figure 14-9   Immunization rates for children ages 1 to 4 by race and vaccine, 1985. (From USDHHS, Public Health Service: *Child health USA '91,* DHHS Pub No HRS-M-CH-91-1, Washington, D.C., 1991, U.S. Government Printing Office, p. 49.)

These children present problems to their families that demand special attention, study, and creative problem-solving.

Between 100,000 and 200,000 babies born each year in the United States are mentally retarded. The causes of the retardation can be identified in only one fourth of the cases. In the other three fourths, inadequacies in prenatal and perinatal care, nutrition, child rearing, and social and environmental opportunities are suspected as causes (USDHHS, 1985, Prevention '84/'85). Many of these suspected causes can be dealt with in some manner by the community health nurse.

Communicable and Preventable Diseases

Preventable communicable diseases are still a major community health problem. The seven major child-hood diseases—poliomyelitis, mumps, tetanus, diphtheria, rubella, pertussis, and measles—can cause permanent disability and death. In spite of the fact that effective immunizations have been available for several decades to protect children from these diseases, a significant number of preschool children are not adequately immunized.

Figure 14-9 depicts the immunization rates for children ages 1 through 4 by race and vaccine. More than one third of white children and over one half of non-white children in this age group have not been properly immunized against five common childhood diseases. Recent reports of measles outbreaks indicate that there are some geographical areas and demographic groups with "dangerously low immunization levels" (USDHHS, 1991, Child Health USA '91, p. 49). In 1990 a measles epidemic caused 89 deaths, the

TABLE 14-2 Some Complications from Selected Childhood Diseases for which Immunizations are Available

Complications	Mumps	Measles (rubeola)	Rubella	Rubella (in utero)	Polio	Tetanus	Pertussis	Diphtheria
Mental retardation		X	X	X			X	
Brain damage		X	X	X			X	
Meningoencephalitis	X	X	X	X				
Paralysis					X			X
Blindness		X	X	X				
Deafness	X	X	X	X				X
Pancreatitis	X							
Juvenile-type diabetes	X							
Orchitis (postpubertal)	X							
Oophoritis (postpubertal)	X							
Sterility (males)	X							
Pneumonia	X	X				X	X	X
Heart damage, pericarditis	X							X
Polyarthritis			X					
Hepatitis	X							
Nephritis	X							X
Cerebral hemorrhage							X	
Muscle spasm						X		
Death	X	X	X	X	X	X	X	X

Modified from Garner MK: Our values are showing: inadequate childhood immunization, *Health Values: Achieving High Level Wellness* 2:130, 1978; Hoekelman RA, Blatman S, Brunell PA, Friedman SB, and Seidel HM: *Principles of pediatrics health care of the young*, New York, 1978, McGraw-Hill; Scipien GM, Barnard MU, Chard MA, Howe J, and Phillips PJ: *Comprehensive pediatric nursing*, ed 3, New York, 1986, McGraw-Hill.

largest number of reported deaths from measles in two decades. This epidemic is predictive of other immunization problems in the health care delivery system (Interagency Committee to Improve Access to Immunization Services, 1992, p. 244).

Table 14-2, relating complications from childhood diseases, summarizes the problems that can result from the preventable childhood diseases. The contributing factors that allow children, especially preschoolers, to remain unimmunized include the lack of consumer awareness, understanding, and responsibility; the complicated vaccine schedule, which easily can be misunderstood; the increased mobility of families, which can lead to fragmented health care; inadequate funding for immunization research at the federal level; resistance by public school systems to comply with state immunization requirements; and apathy because the evidences of childhood disease are no longer obvious.

Many reasons for inadequate immunization protection can also be found within the health care system. For example, providers frequently fail to take advantage of opportunities to provide vaccines to at-risk persons, particularly children, during regular visits to health care facilities. Clinic hours and locations may not be "user friendly."

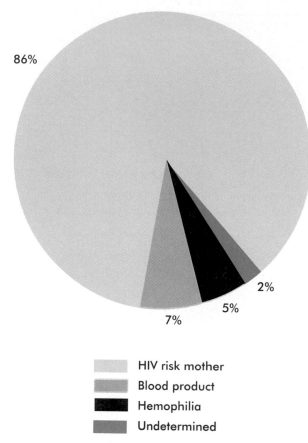

86%

7%

5%

2%

◼ HIV risk mother

◼ Blood product

◼ Hemophilia

◼ Undetermined

Figure 14-10 Cumulative total pediatric AIDS by exposure category through December 1992, United States. (From Centers for Disease Control and Prevention: *HIV/AIDS Surveillance report,* February 1993, p. 9.)

Pediatric AIDS

Pediatric acquired immunodeficiency syndrome (AIDS) is a major public health problem in the United States. As of June 1993 there were 4710 cases of AIDS among children under 13 years of age, and these numbers continue to grow daily. The majority of pediatric AIDS cases are the result of transmission from infected mothers, with a disproportionate number of cases occurring in black and Hispanic children (USDHHS, 1991, Child Health USA '91, p. 32). In 1992 86% of the pediatric HIV infection cases to date were acquired from HIV-risk mothers (mothers with/at risk for HIV infection), 7% were associated with transmission of blood and blood products, and 5% were of children who had hemophilia or other coagulation disorders (refer to Figure 14-10) (CDC, 1993, February).

The epidemiological characteristics of AIDS victims are discussed in Chapter 16. Children with AIDS have characteristics similar to those of heterosexual adults with AIDS, particularly women: the majority of perinatally acquired pediatric AIDS cases are related to intravenous (IV) drug abuse or sexual contact with IV drug abusers; the geographical areas most heavily affected by perinatal transmission of AIDS are the New York City metropolitan area, northern New Jersey, and southern Florida; and the majority of children with perinatally acquired HIV infection are black or Hispanic and are inner-city residents of low socioeconomic status (Rogers, 1987, p. 17). Perinatally acquired AIDS is usually seen in children under the age of 2 (Berry, 1988, p. 341).

Professionals working with families who have children with AIDS must address an array of complex medical, social, and emotional problems. The children must be kept comfortable and well nourished, protected from opportunistic infections, and must receive nurturing parenting (Berry, 1988). Families need supportive assistance to help them to handle the physical care needs of their children, obtain adequate financial and health care resources, and cope with the stresses related to the progression of the disease. These families frequently need an advocate in the health care delivery system and the community and help in coordinating health care services. "Emotional support is an absolute necessity for these families because each family member is experiencing stress" (Berry, p. 344). Family members can experience social isolation, fear, guilt, financial burdens, grief, and physical stress. The community health nurse assumes a major role in helping families to deal with these emotions and experiences. The community health nurse also plays a significant role in educating families, professionals, and communities about AIDS prevention. Pediatric AIDS must be prevented! It cannot be cured!

Lead Poisoning

At present, lead poisoning is one of the most common preventable *environmental* diseases of childhood in the United States. Mental retardation, learning disabilities, and other neurological handicaps are the needless results of this condition. Infants and young children are at highest risk for complications of lead toxicity (Coppens, Hunter, Bain, Gatewood, Gordon, and Mailloux, 1990).

In 1990 an estimated 3 million children under 6 years of age had blood lead levels (BLLs) of more than 10 µ/dl. Regardless of race, children in poverty are more vulnerable to lead exposure than children not living in poverty (USDHHS, 1993, Child Health USA '92, p. 27).

There are two principal routes of exposure to lead:

TABLE

14-3   Environmental Sources of Lead Potentially Harmful to Children

Source	Method of ingestion
Lead-based paint chips or flakes*	Many small children habitually eat chips or flakes of peeling paint
Dust from lead-based wall and ceiling paints	Inhaled by persons in the rooms
Airborne lead (about 1 kg per person per year)	About 5 percent from industrial sources and 90 percent** from burning leaded gasoline
Cigarette smoke	Nonsmokers, too, ingest lead when inhaling cigarette smoke
Drinking water	Especially in cities where water pipes are old or known to contain lead, or both
Vegetables cooked in lead-containing water	Vegetables can concentrate lead from cooking water by a factor of five or more
Food	Especially vegetables grown in urban plots, where both soil and air are often heavily contaminated
Ethnic remedies	Traditional remedies from Mexico (azarcon or greta), Southeast Asia (paylooah), India (surma), and Tibet (unknown ayurvedic) have been associated with high blood lead levels.
Snow and ice contaminated by automotive exhaust fumes, especially in urban areas	Children who eat snow and lick icicles ingest significant amounts of lead
Paper coated with pigments containing lead	Children may chew or swallow pieces of such papers; the papers may be burned in fireplaces or incinerators, releasing lead into the air; lead in the pigments may leach into groundwater from dumps or landfills

*The leading cause of high-dose lead exposure among children in the United States is lead-based paint.

**In the United States this is changing because most cars now use unleaded gasoline.

Modified from Drummond AH: Lead poisoning in children, *J School Health* 51:44, 1981. Copyright 1981, American School Health Association, Kent, Ohio; CDC: lead poisoning associated with use of traditional ethnic remedies—California, 1991-1992, *MMWR* 42:521-524, 1993; CDC: *Preventing lead poisoning in young children: a statement by the Centers for Disease Control,* Atlanta, Ga., October 1991, USDHHS, Public Health Service.

ingestion and inhalation (Chadzynski, 1986). Some important sources of lead are described in Table 14-3. Lead-containing paint is the major source for children in the United States; approximately 12 million children are exposed to leaded paint in older homes. However, a significant number of children are also exposed to lead from contaminated drinking water (10.4 million children), gasoline (5.6 million children), dust/soil (5.9-11 million children), and food (1 million children) (CDC, 1988, Childhood lead poisoning).

Lead poisoning is not confined to poor children in deteriorated neighborhoods; no economic or racial subgrouping of children is exempt from the risk of adverse health effects from lead toxicity (CDC, 1988, Childhood lead poisoning). Children from some ethnic groups (e.g., Hmong, Chinese, and Hispanic) are exposed to lead through folk remedies used to treat minor ailments. Chinese herbal medicines, Pay-loo-ah, an Asian folk medicine used for treating fever in children, and Azarcon, a Mexican folk remedy for

"empacho" or chronic indigestion, have been identified as sources of lead poisoning among children (Chadzynski, 1986).

Because of the seriousness of this problem, the Centers for Disease Control and Prevention in 1991 revised its childhood lead poisoning prevention policy statement to recommend lowering the BLL of concern from 25 µg/dl to 10 µg/dl (CDC, 1993, State activities, p. 165). In addition, the CDC introduced a multitiered approach for dealing with the problem including environmental management, medical follow-up based on elevated BLL, universal screening of all young children, and primary prevention such as identification and remediation of sites of poisoning.

Although knowledge about its etiology, pathophysiology, and epidemiology has increased significantly in the past two decades, childhood lead poisoning continues to remain a major public health problem. Each year this condition causes death, mental retardation, and other problems in thousands of children. The long-term effects of lead poisoning can be subtle; the neurological defects may not be discovered until a child enters school and the teacher notes a slight deficiency in the child's performance. The increasing number of children being observed with long-term effects of lead toxicity, with blood levels much lower than previously believed harmful, is an area of major concern. It is estimated that several million children are exposed to low-dose levels of lead (CDC, 1988, Childhood lead poisoning).

Eliminating pediatric lead poisoning will require substantial effort and expense. This condition will not be eradicated until lead hazards are identified and removed from the environment. The likelihood of this occurring in the near future is doubtful because of the extensive prevalence of lead in the environment; it is estimated that lead paint remains on 30 to 40 million dwellings in the United States (Chadzynski, 1986).

A comprehensive, community-wide approach is essential in order to control lead poisoning among children. To be successful, a lead toxicity prevention program must include environmental management in addition to screening and diagnostic and treatment approaches. These approaches should focus on controlling lead exposure in high-risk areas, epidemiological investigation of environmental hazards, casefinding, early diagnosis and treatment, dissemination of educational materials to professionals and the public, and the passage of effective legal regulations. Community health nurses assume responsibility for many of these activities.

Several problems need to be addressed to achieve successful control of lead poisoning. Physicians and other health professionals, as well as the public, are often not aware of the magnitude of this problem. As a result there is a high rate of recurrence of lead toxicity among children because of the lack of epidemiological follow-up of reported cases. Children are treated and then sent back into the same environment that produced the poisoning; the cycle then repeats itself.

Some other problems that need to be addressed are weak and ineffective housing laws, lack of enforcement of existing laws, the cost of eliminating lead from the environment, limited housing for low-income families, inability to reach many high-risk children, and access to care issues for disadvantaged populations. To resolve many of these problems, priority must be placed on public education about environmental hazard identification and elimination.

Nutritional Inadequacies

Another condition seen by the community health nurse when working with children aged 1 to 5 is nutritional inadequacy and anemia. Inadequate diets can cause growth retardation. "Although growth retardation is not a problem for the vast majority of young children in the United States, among some age and ethnic subgroups of low-income children up to 16 percent of individuals aged 5 and younger are below the fifth percentile. The prevalence of growth retardation is especially high for Asian and Pacific Islander children aged 12 through 59 months, Hispanic children up to age 24 months, and black infants in the first year of life. The Asian and Pacific Islander children who show the greatest prevalence of low height for age include those of Southeast Asian refugee families" (USDHHS, 1991, Healthy people 2000, Full report, pp. 116-117). The goal for the nation is to reduce growth retardation among low-income children ages 5 and younger to less than 10% by the year 2000.

Two feeding problems commonly seen by the nurse are overfeeding of infants and young children and too early an introduction of foods other than milk or formula. Feeding solid foods at an early age is viewed by parents as a developmental milestone and thus they push the infant before he or she is ready. There appears to be little evidence to support giving solids before the age of 3 to 4 months, because the result of this practice is the replacement by solids of the milk the infant needs for growth. Another result is that the child may be overfed if the amount of milk given is not decreased when solids are given. Solids are not digested well by young children because of their immature gastrointestinal systems. Spoon feeding begun too early can result in frustration for both parent and child.

The most prevalent form of anemia in the United States is dietary iron deficiency (CDC, 1992, Pediatric Nutrition Surveillance). Although the prevalence of anemia in U.S. children has declined substantially since 1980, children screened through the Pediatric Nutrition Surveillance System (PedNSS) in 1991 still had a significantly higher prevalence of anemia than other children. The PedNSS uses data from selected public health and nutrition programs such as WIC, Healthy Start, EPSDT, well-child clinics, and other programs funded from maternal and child health block grants. Of the 6,339,720 screened in 1991, the overall prevalence of anemia was 20% to 30% for the PedNSS population, much higher than the 5% national prevalence for young children (CDC, Pediatric Nutrition Surveillance, p. 21). Infants and children particularly at risk are those who are born prematurely, have perinatal blood loss, have congenital heart disease, are irritable and anorexic, have pica or disturbed sleep patterns, and are fed homogenized cow's milk before the age of 9 months. Cow's milk induces enteric blood loss and significantly influences the occurrence of iron-deficiency anemia. Breastfeeding is being advocated to reduce the prevalence of nutritional deficiencies among infants. However, current trends are not encouraging. Since 1982 there has been a slight but continuing decline in breastfeeding. Women least likely to breastfeed are those who are low-income, black, under 20 years of age, and/or living in the southeastern region (USDHHS, Office of Maternal and Child Health, 1989, p. 19). The year 2000 Objective for the Nation is to "increase to at least 75 percent the proportion of mothers who breastfeed their babies in the early post partum period and to at least 50 percent the proportion who continue breastfeeding until their babies are 5 to 6 months old" (USDHHS, 1991, *Healthy People 2000*, p. 123). The 1991 PedNSS data indicate that only 36% of this population were breastfed at the time of hospital discharge, and by 6 months of age only 15% were still being breastfed (CDC, 1992, Pediatric nutrition surveillance, p. 21).

Another problem, overnutrition, results from the popular notion that to be healthy is to be fat and the equating of rewards for good behavior with food. Obesity is not condoned for adults, but fat children are often considered cute. Unfortunately, childhood fat may not disappear in adulthood. Plotting body weight in comparison with body height helps parents and nurses to determine whether obesity is a problem.

Compared with children in many other countries, children in the United States have higher blood cholesterol levels and higher intakes of saturated fatty acids and cholesterol. Adults in this country have higher blood cholesterol levels and higher rates of cardiac heart disease (CHD) morbidity and mortality than do adults in many other countries. High blood cholesterol is seen in families as a result of both environmental and genetic factors. Further, children with high cholesterol levels are more than likely to have high levels as adults. Thus one way to prevent CHD in adults is to lower the average levels of blood cholesterol in children (USDHHS, NIH, 1991, p. 21).

The National Cholesterol Education Program has described a strategy to accomplish this task by combining a population approach with an individualized approach (USDHHS, NIH, p. 3). The population approach focuses on school meals, the nutrition teaching of health professionals, the way government agencies provide education and labeling, the food industry's preparation and distribution of food, and the work of the mass media in programming. The individual approach focuses on meticulous screening of those at risk and drug and diet therapy. Lowering cholesterol levels in children is one example of primary prevention of CHD in adults.

Community health nurses play a significant role in preventing nutritional deficiencies. Many children experience inadequate diets related to knowledge deficits of parents, cultural food patterns, and financial difficulties. Community health nurses are often in a unique position to identify these problems, to instruct regarding needed alterations in eating habits, to provide information about food preparation on a low-income budget, and to make appropriate referrals to community resources that deal with nutritional problems.

Dental Problems

Poor dental hygiene is another significant problem that begins in the preschool years. Although the prevalence of dental caries increases with age, children 5 through 9 years of age in 1987 had an average of four baby teeth affected by decay (USDHHS, Office of Maternal and Child Health, 1989, p. 26). It is estimated that 5% of children aged 2 through 4 years have "bottle-mouth caries," a condition caused by sucking at bedtime on a bottle containing milk or juice. Prevalence of baby bottle tooth decay increases dramatically among low-income children; 53% of children from low-income families and Native American children have this condition (USDHHS, 1991, Child Health USA '91, p. 30). Other causes of dental caries among preschool children include, but are not limited to, eating foods high in sugars, eating frequent between-meal snacks without brushing teeth, and the cariogenicity of some liquid medications such as Pen-Vee-K and phenytoin (Dilantin).

Unfortunately, it is often only after children reach school age that parents become concerned with dental hygiene, and by then much damage may have been done to the teeth. The appearance of their mouths contributes to the way people feel physically and emotionally, and the financial cost of dental repair can be very high.

Behavioral Problems

Disturbance of sleep patterns, toilet training, eating, and relationships with strangers and continual whining and crying are some behavioral problems often seen by the nurse who works with children. Parents will often have questions about problems in these areas that seem minor but can cause daily discomfort to a family and develop into more major problems.

HEALTH PROMOTION NEEDS

Identifying areas where families and larger groups can increase the state of their health, where they are working toward maximizing their potential, is one of the most exciting and challenging aspects of family and community health nursing.

Health promotion in the newborn to 5-year-old age group is particularly important because this period provides the foundation for the physical, intellectual, and emotional health for the rest of the child's life.

The nurse needs to remember that behavior changes with age in a patterned, predictable manner. Behavior has form and shape just as physical patterns do. All growth, whether physical or emotional, implies organization.

Norms for various ages can be dangerous if they are used as absolute standards because each child develops with a different rhythm. Making diagnoses from the behavior a child exhibits takes knowledge, skill, and experience. However, norms for various ages can be guides for planning health promotion programs. The Denver Developmental Screening Test and the Washington Guide, which are discussed later, provide normal growth and development ranges.

Health professionals across the nation recognize the value of health promotion services for the newborn to 5-year-old age population group. They also recognize that there is still much to be accomplished in order to protect our nation's most precious resources—our children.

Health Promotion before Birth

Good health begins before a child is conceived. Children need to be wanted and planned, and people need to learn how to be parents. Becoming pregnant does not confer readiness for children because an individual does not automatically put aside all personal needs to prepare for a child's world, which is in itself not a rational world. Thus parent education needs to start early. It needs to become a part of school curricula, community organizations, and church groups. Parenting programs need to include information regarding the physical aspects of child care; nutrition for the mother and the child; the physical, intellectual, and emotional development of children; and the stresses of role changes for parents. Some schools use the team approach, with the teacher, the school nurse, the social worker, and the nutritionist all working together to promote nurturing parenting skills.

The nurse in the school setting can help teachers and administrators plan parenting classes at the junior- and senior-high level. Accompanying information on parenting must include courses on responsible sexuality, the physiology of sexual development, the part optional parenthood and contraception play in teenagers' sexuality, and the consequences of poor health practices during adolescent years.

State teenage pregnancy initiatives to reduce unintended pregnancy among adolescents have increased significantly since 1985 and include actions such as programs to enhance life options, school-based clinics that provide contraceptives and a broad range of physical and mental health services and family life education (Alan Guttmacher Institute, 1989).

The nutrition of the female throughout her life plays a role in the health of the children she delivers. As girls become responsible for their own nutrition and can make choices about what they eat, they need to know what proper nutrition is. They also need to be aware that their choices are affecting the health of their future children. The school setting is an appropriate place to teach this kind of information. Health professionals must include adolescents' preferences for fast foods (those prepared with minimum time in franchise restaurants) when planning lunch meals and doing nutritional counseling. Fast foods are eaten as meals and as snacks and, for many people, they provide a significant proportion of their daily caloric intake. Nutritionists have developed "nutrient profiles" of fast foods, some of which contain significant quantities of nutrients. The community health nurse can use these profiles to make eating of fast foods more positive.

Fathers-to-be are often neglected in family life and parenting programs. Males can play a major role in preventing unintentional pregnancies and sexually transmitted diseases, both of which cause significant problems related to conception and pregnancy. However, males need appropriate information to develop responsible decision-making about sexuality. They also need an opportunity to obtain information necessary to develop nurturing parenting skills.

Health Promotion during Pregnancy

Pregnancy is a developmental task for both parents. Parents need support throughout pregnancy because this is a time of change and of strong emotions, some positive, some negative, and most ambivalent. How people feel about pregnancy varies widely and depends on whether or not the parents are married, whether they have other children, whether the mother is working, whether memories of their childhood are positive or negative, and how they feel about their own parents. Lack of support can cause the parents to feel stress, can delay preparation for the infant, and can retard bond formation. Supportive intervention efforts during pregnancy and the few months following the birth can improve maternal and child health outcomes (National Commission to Prevent Infant Mortality, 1989).

Currently many health departments, neighborhood centers, and hospital outpatient clinics have established maternal support services (MSS) to ensure healthy pregnancies for at-risk mothers. These programs provide funding for prenatal care and home visits by a multidisciplinary team, and include social services, health care, and outreach services. With the emphasis on early discharge after birth and an increased interest in home deliveries, the need for community health nursing services for this aggregate is increasing.

Prenatal classes, groups such as LaLeche League, and visits by the community health nurse can help with this kind of support. The nuclear family system of the United States and the mobility of many Americans often means that the parents do not have other family members, family physicians, close friends, or neighbors who can be helpful in this period.

Concerns that parents have during the time of pregnancy, which should be addressed during prenatal classes, involve preparing for labor and delivery, how to physically prepare the home environment for the new baby, whether or not to breastfeed, whether or not the new mother should work outside the home, and how to prepare other siblings for the additional family member. Moreover, the mother needs to know

that alcohol, smoking, and other drugs can adversely affect the fetus; she should, of course, begin seeing her obstetrician or family doctor as soon as she suspects she is pregnant.

Parents should know that their genetic backgrounds can play a crucial role in their child's health. Ideally this concern would occur before marriage, but often it does not. Down syndrome, Tay-Sachs disease, sickle-cell anemia, cystic fibrosis, hemophilia, and Huntington's disease are some diseases that have a genetic origin. When parents know that these diseases are in their family constellations, they have several choices. They can have genetic testing before conception, they can adopt, or they can choose not to bear a child. They can also choose to conceive and then have genetic testing to ascertain whether or not the fetus carries the disease. Another alternative is to conceive and deliver without having genetic tests. If couples know about genetic problems before they marry, they may also make the decision not to marry. The community health nurse needs to be able to help people look at alternatives and provide sources of genetic counseling. There are an increasing number of genetic counseling centers throughout the country.

Expectant parents need more than knowledge to make the transition to parenthood successfully. They need the chance to review the various situations that arise in parenting, compare different ways of dealing with them, and develop their own style of parenting. Nurses have used prenatal class settings to provide clarification about the role of the parent, to do actual role modeling by actively discussing problems and exploring alternatives, and to provide opportunities for role rehearsal. Role rehearsal can be done by using case studies and situations with the opportunity for parents to react and respond. Case studies and sharing of personal experiences to stimulate problem-solving can be used with parents throughout any of the developmental and maturational crisis periods they may experience with their children.

Home births have had a mild resurgence of popularity. The cries for home births are a "healthy adaptation to the public's depersonalization of medical practice" (Editorial, 1983, p. 637). Hospitals have created birth centers that involve the family in the birth process and facilitate early discharge to home. This discharge can take place as early as 4 hours postdelivery in some cases. The importance of this resurgence in home births for community health nurses is that they need to be skilled in handling nursing care needs of mothers and babies during the

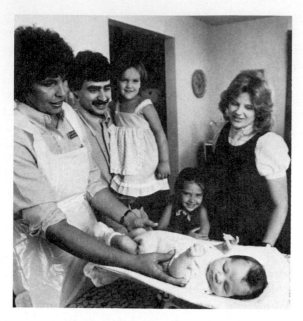

Figure 14-11 A community health nurse whose services are financed under the auspices of the Genessee Region Home Care Association visits an infant only 24 hours old. (From Genessee Region Home Care Association, Rochester, New York.)

immediate postdelivery period. The nurse shown in Figure 14-11 is visiting a family with an infant only 24 hours old. Insurance benefits for this family include coverage for nursing visits, laboratory tests, and homemaking services.

Health Promotion after Birth

The community health nurse should be aware that sometimes health services are not offered to new parents between the postpartum hospital discharge and the sixth-week checkup. The mother is often not in optimum physical condition after experiencing a loss in blood volume, rapid weight loss, and displacement of internal organs during the birth process. Yet she needs to meet the needs of a dependent infant whose respirations are not well established, who is undergoing massive blood changes, and who may be weak, dehydrated, and irritable. In addition, when the mother goes from the protected hospital environment to the home setting, she needs to adjust to role changes and the responsibility of infant care. Nurses in the hospital who work with parents postpartum should make selective referrals of those families needing the services that a community health nurse can offer. The nurse, with observation, is able to "pick up" stresses and provide needed help.

The community health nurse has an important role in the referral process from hospital to home with families who have newborns. The community health nurse can discuss with the hospital nurse the types of families who need referrals. The hospital nurse should assess the entire family situation, assess the parent-child bonding, and make appropriate referrals based upon this information. The referral process is based upon the hospital nurse's assessment, and it is vital that she or he understand what an appropriate referral is and what the community health nurse can do with families who have newborns.

Table 14-4 is a compilation of concerns with which new parents may desire help during the puerperium. The puerperium is a short period of time, but it can be a highly troubled one if needed help is not present. These concerns should be taken into consideration when a nurse is identifying parents for referral or when a community health nurse is making a home visit.

SUPPORTING FAMILIES

The goal of supporting families is to strengthen them, ensuring the well-being and healthy development of their children. Families are supported by helping parents to cope with the stresses of daily life; giving parents new information about child development and rearing so that parents in turn can better support their own children; reducing the isolation that parents feel, bringing them into contact with other parents; and referring parents to needed services and agencies, ideally before there is a crisis (Allen, Brown, and Finlay, 1992, p. 6). In today's complex world no family has all of the knowledge and resources needed to meet their needs. With more births to teens, with declining family incomes, with growing hunger and homelessness and with increasing lack of access to health care, parenting requires the help of the community. "Parents in different circumstances need different kinds of help and different levels of support, but all parents need some kind of help at one time or another" (Allen, Brown, and Finlay, p. 13). Lillian Wald recognized the need to support families when she created the Henry Street Settlement House in New York City in the early part of this century. Her "home" offered health care and helped people with housing and employment and other social service needs.

The most contemporary impetus to the family support movement has been Head Start, the comprehensive preschool program for disadvantaged chil-

14-4 Percentages of Mothers Noting Specific Concerns During the Puerperium

Area of concern	Percent of mothers concerned			Area of concern	Percent of mothers concerned		
	Minor concern	Major concern	Total		Minor concern	Major concern	Total
Return of figure to normal	30	65	95	Discomfort of stitches	33	20	53
Regulating demands of husband, housework, children	42	48	90	Breast care	40	10	50
				Constipation	35	15	50
				Setting limits for visitors	27	23	50
Emotional tension	48	40	88	Interpreting infant's behavior	27	23	50
Fatigue	28	55	83				
Infant behavior	47	33	80	Breast soreness	35	13	48
Finding time for self	45	33	78	Hemorrhoids	25	23	48
Sexual relations	53	20	73	Labor and delivery experience	28	20	48
Diet	33	40	73				
Feelings of isolation, being tied down	42	28	70	Father's role with baby	22	23	45
				Lochia	35	5	40
Infant's growth and development	45	25	70	Other children jealous of baby	27	13	40
Family planning	25	43	68	Other children's behavior	25	15	40
Exercise	23	45	68				
Infant feeding	43	25	68	Infant's appearance	18	20	38
Changes in relationship with husband	35	25	60	Traveling with baby	27	8	35
				Clothing for baby	20	10	30
Physical care of infant	45	13	58	Feeling comfortable handling baby	15	8	23
Infant safety	33	25	58				

From Gruis M: Beyond maternity: postpartum concerns of mothers, *Am J Maternal Child Health* 2:185, 1977.

dren. The creators of this program of the 1960s recognized the interrelatedness of health, nutrition, parent involvement, and children's learning. Each parent with a child in Head Start is asked to volunteer time as a classroom aide and to attend parent education meetings with the goal of helping the parents to become better teachers of their own children. Each Head Start program also has a parent council with policy-making responsibilities. "Today more than one-third of the Head Start's paid employees nationwide are former Head Start parents who were inspired to continue their education as a result of their participation in Head Start activities" (Allen, Brown, and Finlay, 1992, p. 14).

The fundamental principles of family support were presented in Chapter 8. What is advocated is a holistic approach that emphasizes the importance of the family unit, comprehensively addressing the needs of all family members. Families can have interrelated needs that require coordination of service when numerous resources are used. Community health nurses intervene in this situation and prevent crises by connecting families to support services in the community.

Single Parents

Adolescent single parents and their infants are at high risk both emotionally and physically. Help with parenting skills for this age group is a high priority for the community health nurse. Adolescents usually have not completed their own physical, mental, and emotional growth, and becoming responsible for another human being presents both a maturational and a situational crisis for them. Prenatal and postnatal clinics set up for intensive and personal care for this group, as well as alternative education classes within the school system, have been ways in which this has been accomplished. Chapter 15 discusses adolescent parenthood further.

Divorced, single, or separated parents often find themselves fulfilling the roles of individual, father, mother, breadwinner, homemaker, and citizen. This can be an overwhelming situation unless appropriate resources are available and utilized. The community health nurse is able to help single parents look at the reality of their situation and at the options and resources available to them. Community groups, such as Parents Without Partners and local family counseling centers, may be helpful. Many times these parents are functioning quite well in relation to the responsibilities they encounter. The positive aspects and actions evidenced should be reinforced.

The single father can be at a greater disadvantage for receiving societal supports than the single mother. Many programs have been designed and implemented for maternal-child health, since this is considered the natural occurrence. The father, whose involvement with his children has only recently received societal sanction, often finds himself less prepared and with fewer supports in his dual-parent role.

Another dilemma of the single parent is that of the "weekend parent." Many divorced parents are put in the role of seeing their children on a limited basis. They are unsure of their role with their children and have many concerns about how to facilitate their children's developmental growth. Again, the nurse, with counseling and referral to appropriate resources, can be helpful and can facilitate adjustment to the weekend parent role.

Preventive Health Care

Newborn Assessment

Assessment of the newborn is viewed as a decisive foundation for early casefinding and preventive care. The kinds of observations that are made help to determine the nursing and medical care that the infant will receive, as well as the kind of parenting that is given.

During the assessment the nurse should get baseline data about the infant's surface features, move-

ment patterns, and general health for comparisons with future examinations. Since health promotion is the concern, systematic periodic assessment over a period of time is important. The developmental approach, rather than the traditional disease-oriented model, should be the focus. Parental involvement in the assessment process helps the nurse to see how the family interacts. It also provides the opportunity to begin anticipatory guidance and problem-solving.

The Neonatal Behavioral Assessment Scale developed by T. Berry Brazelton (Brazelton, 1973) is a valid and useful method for observing, making judgments, and scoring selected reflexes, motor responses, and interactive behavioral responses of newborns. The main focus of the scale is on the observation and rating of the infant's interactive behavior. It measures a total of 27 behavioral responses of the infant organized into the following six categories:

1. Habituation—how soon the infant diminishes responses to specific stimuli
2. Orientation—when and how often the infant attends to auditory and visual stimuli
3. Motor maturity—how well the infant coordinates and controls motor activities
4. Variation—how often the infant coordinates and controls motor activities
5. Self-quieting abilities—how often, how soon, and how effectively the infant uses personal resources to console himself or herself
6. Social behaviors—smiling and cuddling behaviors

Using the Brazelton scale points out vividly that newborns are able to control their responses to external stimuli. Generally, the abilities of newborns have been underestimated by both parents and health professionals.

Anticipatory Guidance

Anticipatory guidance in helping parents to know what to expect of their children at different stages is one of the *most basic and significant* health promotion needs of parents. Through anticipatory guidance parents can gain knowledge about average development, and thus they will not expect too much or too little from their children. They can also learn that, although there are patterns, each child is unique within a pattern. Parents readily acquire literature on growth and development from the hospital or pediatrician. The community health nurse should be familiar with this material and explain to parents that it is to be used a guide.

Parents are able to assess quite accurately their children's problems when they are given adequate information. This is logical because their proximity makes them frequent observers. Parents' assessment is important because how they define health or behavior as a problem influences interaction in the home and the child's further development.

Since an infant's growth and development is so rapid during the first 2 years, it is imperative that periodic and systematic screening be done. An illustration of this is the infant's reflexes, which are present during the first weeks and then develop into purposeful movements as the central nervous system develops. Periodic comprehensive assessment and use of the developmental model facilitates the study of an infant's growth, early behavior patterns, and general development. If, for example, the infant's reflexes are questionable in symmetry, equality, or movement, this might be a sign of immaturity or a lack of integration in the central nervous system. These might also be signals of serious impairment of the central nervous system. Periodic screening and evaluation helps parents and professionals to evaluate more carefully the questionable status of the reflexes and to plan stimulation that enhances sensory development.

Baseline information compiled through periodic assessment is the key to planning early intervention. It allows for objectivity in conclusions that can be made about an infant's early development and can aid in planning interventions. The baseline data also serve as a basis for self-comparison of an infant or child over a period of time. It is imperative that the nurse know "normal" expectations for development so that what is unusual, abnormal, or delayed can be quickly recognized.

There are numerous schedules available for preventive child health care. Appendix 14-1 presents a summary of the health care that should be provided at specified intervals. Table 14-5 presents the recommended immunization schedule for infants and children. Children whose immunization program has been delayed will have a different schedule (refer to Tables 14-6 and 14-7). Providing parents a written immunization schedule can help to prevent confusion. Effective anticipatory guidance helps parents to determine when children should have immunizations and the value of them.

The resurgence of measles in the United States during the period 1989-1991, due to the failure to vaccinate children at the recommended age of 12 to 15 months, provided an impetus for the National Vaccine Advisory Committee (NVAC) to establish standards for pediatric immunization practices (see the box on p. 521). These standards have been approved by the U.S. Public Health Service and endorsed by the American Academy of Pediatrics (CDC, 1993, Standards for Pediatric Immunization Practice, p. 1).

"The measles epidemic signaled that the immunization delivery system must be changed immediately if the nation's children are to be fully protected" (CDC, 1993, Standards for Pediatric Immunization Practice, p. 2). Health care professionals need to take advantage of all health care visits as opportunities to provide vaccinations, advocate for third-party reimbursement for vaccinations, and eliminate barriers that impede efficient vaccine delivery. Long waiting periods, appointment-only services, prevaccination physical examinations that impede the timely receipt of immunizations, inadequate supply of vaccines, and needless deferment of indicated immunizations are examples of system barriers (CDC, Standards for Pediatric Immunization Practices). Appendix 14-2 presents the true contraindications and precautions to vaccinations and describes when needless deferment of immunizations occur.

Hepatitis B (HBV) infection has become a major public health problem. The reported incidence of acute hepatitis B increased by 37% from 1979 to 1989 and an estimated 1 million persons with chronic HBV infection are potentially infectious to others. Long-term sequelae such as chronic liver disease are problems of people chronically infected (USDHHS, PHS, 1991, Recommendations of The Immunization Practices Advisory Committee, p. 1).

In the United States children become infected with HBV through a variety of means, including perinatal transmission and after birth contact with a household chronic carrier. A comprehensive strategy to prevent HBV must eliminate transmission during infancy and childhood; thus infants and children should receive hepatitis B vaccine during routine health visits. Universal infant vaccination will reduce acute hepatitis B and hepatitis B–associated chronic liver disease over the long term—a cost-effective measure. Table 14-8 provides the guides to postexposure immunoprophylaxis for exposure to hepatitis B virus.

Immunizations are a crucial component of preventive health care. Further components in the preventive child health care schedule are the history to be obtained from parents and physical measurements to be done. The Denver Developmental Screening Test (Erickson, 1976, pp. 173-192) and the Washington

TABLE 14-5   Recommended Schedule for Routine Active Vaccination of Infants and Children*

Vaccine	At birth (before hospital discharge)	Months							4–6 years (before school entry)
		1–2	2†	4	6	6–18	12–15	15	
Diphtheria-tetanus-pertussis§			DTP	DTP	DTP		DTaP/DTP¶		DTaP/DTP
Polio, live oral			OPV	OPV	OPV**				OPV
Measles-mumps-rubella							MMR		MMR††
Haemophilus influenzae type b conjugate									
HbOC/PRP-T§,§§			Hib	Hib	Hib		Hib¶¶		
PRP-OMP§§			Hib	Hib			Hib¶¶		
Hepatitis B***									
Option 1	HepB	HepB†††				HepB†††			
Option 2		HepB†††		HepB†††		HepB†††			

*See Table 14-6 for the recommended immunization schedule for infants and children up to their seventh birthday who do not begin the vaccination series at the recommended times or who are >1 month behind in the immunization schedule.

†Can be administered as early as 6 weeks of age.

§Two DTP and Hib combination vaccines are available (DTP/HbOC [TETRAMUNE™]; and PRP-T [ActHIB™, OmniHIB™] which can be reconstituted with DTP vaccine produced by Connaught).

¶This dose of DTP can be administered as early as 12 months of age provided that the interval since the previous dose of DTP is at least 6 months. *Diphtheria and Tetanus toxoids and acellular pertussis vaccine (DTaP) is currently recommended only for use as the fourth and/or fifth doses of the DTP series among children aged 15 months through 6 years (before the seventh birthday).* Some experts prefer to administer these vaccines at 18 months of age.

**The American Academy of Pediatrics (AAP)recommends this dose of vaccine at 6–18 months of age.

††The AAP recommends that two doses of MMR should be administered by 12 years of age with the second dose being administered preferentially at entry to middle school or junior high school.

§§HbOC: [HibTITER®] (Lederle Praxis). PRP-T: [ActHIB™, OmniHIB™] (Pasteur Merieux). PRP-OMP: [PedvaxHIB®] (Merck, Sharp, and Dohme). A DTP/Hib combination vaccine can be used in place of HbOC/PRP-T.

¶¶After the primary infant Hib conjugate vaccine series is completed, any of the licensed Hib conjugate vaccines may be used as a booster dose at age 12–15 months.

***For use among infants born to HBsAg-negative mothers. The first dose should be administered during the newborn period, preferably before hospital discharge, but no later than age 2 months. Premature infants of HBsAg-negative mothers should receive the first dose of the hepatitis B vaccine series at the time of hospital discharge or when the other routine childhood vaccines are initiated. (All infants born to HBsAg-positive mothers should receive immunoprophylaxis for hepatitis B as soon as possible after birth.)

†††Hepatitis B vaccine can be administered simultaneously at the same visit with DTP (or DTaP), OPV, Hib, and/or MMR.

Modified from CDC: General recommendations on immunization: recommendations of the Immunization Practices Advisory Committee, *MMWR* 43(no. RR-1), January 28, 1994, p. 9.

Guide (Barnard and Erickson, 1976, pp. 75-95) are valuable tools that assist the nurse in checking for developmental landmarks, giving norms for their attainment. Areas of concern to parents about infants include nutrition, frequency and amounts of feedings, weaning, sleeping patterns, teething, handling of the genitals, and dealing with common illnesses. After the first year of life, the child matures and new behavior patterns develop. Parents thus have additional areas of concern after a child is a year old, such as how to provide adequate nutrition when appetite decreases. This is normal because the child is also having a decrease in growth. Other concerns during this period include sleep disturbances and nightmares, nocturnal enuresis, bowel and bladder training, thumbsucking, temper tantrums, masturbation, stuttering, negativism, and the increased need for independence and exploration. A thoughtful hearing of questions in relation to these concerns gives the nurse an idea of how the parents perceive the problem. Answers based

14-6 Recommended Accelerated Immunization Schedule for Infants and Children <7 Years of Age Who Start the Series Late* or Who Are >1 Month Behind in the Immunization Schedule† (i.e., Children for Whom Compliance with Scheduled Return Visits Cannot Be Assured)

Timing	Vaccine(s)	Comments
First visit (≥4 mos of age)	DTP§, OPV, Hib¶,§, Hepatitis B, MMR (should be given as soon as child is age 12-15 mos)	All vaccines should be administered simultaneously at the appropriate visit.
Second visit (1 mo after first visit)	DTP§, Hib¶,§, Hepatitis B	
Third visit (1 mo after second visit)	DTP§, OPV, Hib¶,§	
Fourth visit (6 wks after third visit)	OPV	
Fifth visit (≥6 mos after third visit)	DTaP§ or DTP, Hib¶,§, Hepatitis B	
Additional visits (Age 4–6 yrs)	DTaP§ or DTP, OPV, MMR	Preferably at or before school entry.
(Age 14-16 yrs)	Td	Repeat every 10 yrs through-out life.

DTP, Diphtheria-tetanus-pertussis; *DTaP,* Diphtheria-tetanus-acellular pertussis; *Hib, Haemophilus influenzae* type b conjugate; *MMR,* Measles-mumps-rubella; *OPV,* Poliovirus vaccine, live oral, trivalent; *Td,* Tetanus and diphtheria toxoids (for use among persons ≥7 years of age)

*If initiated in the first year of life, administer DTP doses 1, 2, and 3 and OPV doses 1, 2, and 3 according to this schedule; administer MMR when the child reaches 12–15 months of age.

†See individual ACIP recommendations for detailed information on specific vaccines.

§Two DTP and Hib combination vaccines are available (DTP/HbOC [TETRAMUNE™]; and PRP-T [ActHIB™, OmniHIB™] which can be reconstituted with DTP vaccine produced by Connaught). DTaP preparations are currently recommended only for use as the fourth and/or fifth doses of the DTP series among children 15 months through 6 years of age (before the seventh birthday). DTP and DTaP should not be used on or after the seventh birthday.

¶The recommended schedule varies by vaccine manufacturer. For information specific to the vaccine being used, consult the package insert and ACIP recommendations. Children beginning the Hib vaccine series at age 2–6 months should receive a primary series of three doses of HbOC [HibTITER®] (Lederle-Praxis), PRP-T [ActHIB™, OmniHIB™] (Pasteur Merieux; SmithKline Beecham; Connaught), or a licensed DTP-Hib combination vaccine; or two doses of PRP-OMP [PedvaxHIB®] (Merck, Sharp, and Dohme). An additional booster dose of any licensed Hib conjugate vaccine should be administered at 12–15 months of age and at least 2 months after the previous dose. Children beginning the Hib vaccine series at 7–11 months of age should receive a primary series of two doses of an HbOC, PRP-T, or PRP-OMP-containing vaccine. An additional booster dose of any licensed Hib conjugate vaccine should be administered at 12–18 months of age and at least 2 months after the previous dose. Children beginning the Hib vaccine series at ages 12–14 months should receive a primary series of one dose of an HbOC, PRP-T, or PRP-OMP-containing vaccine. An additional booster dose of any licensed Hib conjugate vaccine should be administered 2 months after the previous dose. Children beginning the Hib vaccine series at ages 15–59 months should receive one dose of any licensed Hib vaccine. Hib vaccine should not be administered after the fifth birthday except for special circumstances and noted in the specific ACIP recommendations for the use of Hib vaccine.

Modified from CDC: General recommendation on immunization: recommendations of the Immunization Practices Advisory Committee, *MMWR* 43(No. RR-1), January 28, 1994, p.10.

on the child's development are supportive and help to eliminate some major concerns and problems.

Helping parents to know when a child is ill enough to call a doctor is important. This action can help to prevent minor upper respiratory infections (URIs) and gastrointestinal (GI) upsets from becoming major problems. Fever of 101° F for over 24 hours is a signal to parents to call the health care provider.

The possibilities for preventive health care are varied and almost endless when helping parents to

14-7 Recommended Immunization Schedule for Persons ≥ 7 Years of Age Not Vaccinated at the Recommended Time in Early Infancy*

Timing	Vaccine(s)	Comments
First visit	Td†, OPV§, MMR¶, and Hepatitis B**	Primary poliovirus vaccination is not routinely recommended for persons ≥ 18 years of age.
Second visit (6–8 weeks after first visit)	Td, OPV, MMR††,¶, Hepatitis B**	
Third visit (6 months after second visit)	Td, OPV, Hepatitis B**	
Additional visits	Td	Repeat every 10 years throughout life.

MMR, Measles-mumps-rubella; *OPV,* Poliovirus vaccine, live oral, trivalent; *Td,* Tetanus and diphtheria toxoids (for use among persons ≥7 years of age)

*See individual ACIP recommendations for details.

†The DTP and DTaP doses administered to children <7 years of age who remain incompletely vaccinated at age ≥7 years should be counted as prior exposure to tetanus and diphtheria toxoids (e.g., a child who previously received two doses of DTP needs only one dose of Td to complete a primary series for tetanus and diphtheria).

§When polio vaccine is administered to previously unvaccinated persons ≥18 years of age, inactivated poliovirus vaccine (IPV) is preferred. For the immunization schedule for IPV, see specific ACIP statement on the use of polio vaccine.

¶Persons born before 1957 can generally be considered immune to measles and mumps and need not be vaccinated. Rubella (or MMR) vaccine can be administered to persons of any age, particularly to nonpregnant women of childbearing age.

**Hepatitis B vaccine, recombinant. Selected high-risk groups for whom vaccination is recommended include persons with occupational risk, such as health-care and public-safety workers who have occupational exposure to blood, clients and staff of institutions for the developmentally disabled, hemodialysis patients, recipients of certain blood products (e.g., clotting factor concentrates), household contacts and sex partners of hepatitis B virus carriers, injecting drug users, sexually active homosexual and bisexual men, certain sexually active heterosexual men and women, inmates of long-term correctional facilities, certain international travelers, and families of HBsAg-positive adoptees from countries where HBV infection is endemic. Because risk factors are often not identified directly among adolescents, universal hepatitis B vaccination of teenagers should be implemented in communities where injecting drug use, pregnancy among teenagers, and/or sexually transmitted diseases are common.

††The ACIP recommends a second dose of measles-containing vaccine (preferably MMR to assure immunity to mumps and rubella) for certain groups. Children with no documentation of live measles vaccination after the first birthday should receive two doses of live measles-containing vaccine not less than 1 month apart. In addition, the following persons born in 1957 or later should have documentation of measles immunity (i.e., two doses of measles-containing vaccine [at least one of which being MMR], physician-diagnosed measles, or laboratory evidence of measles immunity): a) those entering post-high school educational settings; b) those beginning employment in health-care settings who will have direct patient contact; and c) travelers to areas with endemic measles.

Modified from CDC: General recommendations on immunization: recommendations of the Immunization Practices Advisory Committee, *MMWR* 43(No. RR-1), January 28, 1994, p.11.

learn to handle childhood illness. Questions such as the following help a community health nurse to determine what information parents need in order to prevent serious illness: Do the parents have a thermometer and do they know how to use it? Do they understand the meaning of dehydration? Do they know basic first aid and when to call a physician?

Accident Prevention

Since accidents are the major cause of death after the age of 1 year, prevention of them is critical. Appendix 14-3 summarizes typical actions that cause

accidents and lists precautions to take at varying age levels to avoid accidents.

It has long been recognized that a child's environment significantly influences his or her state of health. The most common site of accidental injuries to children under the age of 15 is the home (USDHHS, 1989, Office of Maternal and Child Health, p. 27). Human, as well as physical, factors in the home can lead to accidents. For example, parents' lack of knowledge about childhood growth and development can contribute to accidents. Parents who lack this understanding often neglect to "safety-proof" the child's environment. Infants and toddlers need to be protected from

◀ *Standards for Pediatric Immunization Practices* ▶

1. Immunization services are readily available.
2. There are no barriers or unnecessary prerequisites to the receipt of vaccines.
3. Immunization services are available free or for a minimal fee.
4. Providers utilize all clinical encounters to screen and, when indicated, vaccinate children.
5. Providers educate parents and guardians about immunization in general terms.
6. Providers question parents or guardians about contraindications and, before vaccinating a child, inform them in specific terms about the risks and benefits of the vaccinations their child is to receive.
7. Providers follow only true contraindications.
8. Providers administer simultaneously all vaccine doses for which a child is eligible at the time of each visit.
9. Providers use accurate and complete recording procedures.
10. Providers co-schedule immunization appointments in conjunction with appointments for other child health services.
11. Providers report adverse events following vaccination promptly, accurately, and completely.
12. Providers operate a tracking system.
13. Providers adhere to appropriate procedures for vaccine management.
14. Providers conduct semi-annual audits to assess immunization coverage levels and to review immunization records in the patient populations they serve.
15. Providers maintain up-to-date, easily retrievable medical protocols at all locations where vaccines are administered.
16. Providers practice patient-oriented and community-based approaches.
17. Vaccines are administered by properly trained persons.
18. Providers receive ongoing education and training regarding current immunization recommendations.

From CDC: Standards for pediatric immunization practices, *MMWR* 42 (No RR-5):3, 1993.

hazards in the environment. They lack the cognitive development needed to understand what things or activities could lead to injury. Developmental characteristics that place young children at risk for specific types of accidents are identified in Appendix 14-3. Providing parents with this type of information can help them to identify potential hazards in a child's environment.

Parents cannot remove all environmental hazards and they *cannot* and *should not* control their children 24 hours a day. However, with a combination of child supervision, education of parents, and legislative and environmental changes to get rid of hazards, accidents can be reduced. Families need an understanding of the philosophy of accident prevention. As specified by the National Safety Council, it is not a barrage of do's and dont's but rather it is doing things the right way in the interest of the welfare of others.

One method the nurse can use to improve the family approach to accident prevention is accident analysis after an accident occurs. What, how, to whom, where, when, and why did the accident happen? Families must understand that the purpose of this is not to fix blame but rather to prevent a recurrence. Often, teaching the parent who is the primary care provider for the child will have an impact on accident

| TABLE **14-8** | Guide to Postexposure Immunoprophylaxis for Exposure to Hepatitis B Virus |

Type of exposure	Immunoprophylaxis
Perinatal	Vaccination + HBIG*
Sexual—acute infection	HBIG = Vaccination
Sexual—chronic carrier	Vaccination
Household contact—chronic carrier	Vaccination
Household contact—acute case	None unless known exposure
Household contact—acute case, known exposure	HBIG = vaccination
Infant (<12 months)—acute case in primary care-giver	HBIG + vaccination
Inadvertent—percutaneous/permucosal	Vaccination = HBIG

*HBIG = Hepatitis B immune globulin.
From USDHHS, Public Health Service: *Recommendations of the Immunization Practices Advisory Committee. Hepatitis B. virus: a comprehensive strategy for eliminating transmission in the United States through universal childhood vaccination,* Atlanta, Ga., 1991, CDC, p. 6.

◀ *Effective Interventions to Prevent Child and Adolescent Injury* ▶

Planning and Prioritizing

- A broad-based coalition representing the community of interest;
- surveillance tools and methods to lidentify and monitor the number of injuries;
- the use of E codes to aid in the ascertainment of injury causes; and
- selection of priority areas for injury control.

Comprehensive Multifaceted Approach

- Evaluation of prevention strategies to determine effectiveness;
- dissemination and universal implementation of effective strategies;
- targeting of high-risk groups, such as low income; and
- incorporation of prevention messages and efforts into service systems for children and adolescents.

Institutionalization and Acceptance

- Coordination of local, State and Federal efforts;
- institutionalization of injury prevention programming;
- enforcement of existing legislation protecting children; and
- development of a societal norm of a 'safe childhood and adolescence.'

From Children's Safety Network, *A data book of child and adolescent injury,* Washington, D.C., 1991, National Center for Education in Maternal and Child Health, p. 61.

prevention. The nurse can help this parent to be alert to hazards in the environment when home visits are made.

The Safe Kids Coalition is a nationwide effort to prevent childhood injury. It is a growing network of 121 state and local coalitions in 41 states, created by the Children's National Medical Center in Washington, D.C. (phone 202-745-5000) with major funding from Johnson and Johnson. The injury intervention strategies used by the coalition are those described by White in Chapter 2 and include enforcement, engineering, education, and evaluation. An underlying belief of coalition members is that solutions to the injuries sustained by children in accidents will not come from Washington or the media but rather when everyone in a community is involved. For example, in Allentown, Pennsylvania, the local group has sponsored a bike rodeo to teach children and parents about safety in this area. They also sponsored a safety carnival and in-service programs for elementary school teachers. The Safe Kids Coalition is a place for professionals concerned about the prevention of major problems in the newborn to 5 years age group to place their efforts.

The box above summarizes interventions for preventing child and adolescent injury from preventable accidents as described by the Children's Safety Network, Maternal and Child Health Bureau (1991). These interventions are part of the efforts of the Safe Kids Coalition as well.

Prevention of Child Maltreatment

As previously mentioned in this chapter, abuse and neglect are symptoms of stress in a family. The conditions of poverty, undernutrition, unemployment, overcrowding, restricted physical surroundings, and inadequate education support this problem. Knowledge currently available tells us that antenatal poverty and nutritional deficits produce a high-risk infant; at the same time, high-quality medical care is least available to the very people who are at highest risk. The high-risk infant and ill-prepared parents have the fewest resources for achieving the best health possible. Communities can deal with these poverty problems at a local level. However, the nation needs to deal with them at a federal level to make the most impact.

To save a child from the serious effects of abuse and neglect, nurses need to be alert when they notice that families are having children very quickly with no relief between pregnancies. The danger signs of marital stress, isolation, and overwhelmed parents need to be seen also. Premature births, where questionable bonding has taken place, indicate a need for priority service, as do families where there are children with developmental disabilities and chronic disease.

Every parent needs to know how children grow and develop; the concept that babies are responsible for their acts and can think and reason like an adult is all too commonly believed and must be corrected.

Education of personnel, including judges, attor-

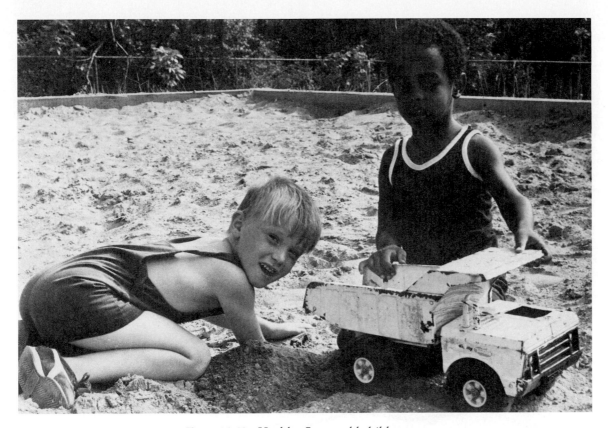

Figure 14-12   Healthy 5-year-old children.

neys, social workers, and doctors, is necessary so that abused children are found, identified as such, and then given treatment. Parents must not be treated as criminals but rather given help so that their stress is alleviated. Equally important are the rights of children.

Social institutions such as churches and schools need to be used to help support families. In our mobile society where people move frequently, families can feel isolated and alone and uncared for. Homemaker services, big brothers and sisters, and parent aides, as well as community volunteers, could fill some of the gaps experienced by families who are isolated.

Preschool Assessments

Kindergarten and preschool health assessments are excellent developmental points at which to look at the physical, intellectual, and emotional growth of children. At this time parents are increasingly aware of and concerned about the learning and thought competency of their children. They want to know that their children are ready to begin school. A child's

ability to learn, see, perform appropriate gross and fine motor tasks, follow instruction, speak, communicate, and relate socially with others are all indicators of readiness for school (refer to Figure 14-12). The Denver Developmental Screening Test is one method used by community health nurses to look at these areas.

Preschool assessments also provide an excellent opportunity to enforce state immunization laws so that all children receive immunizations before they are in school. Evidence suggests that a sizable number of preschoolers are not fully immunized. Recent surveys examining immunization status of children starting school in nine cities documented that only 52% to 71% of these children had been vaccinated against measles by their second birthday and only 10% to 42% had completed their immunization series (CDC, Retrospective Assessment, 1992).

Day Care For Children

In 1990 more than 50% of the preschool children in the United States had mothers in the workforce, a twofold increase since 1970. Figure 14-13 depicts this

**Children with mothers in
the work force: 1970-1990**

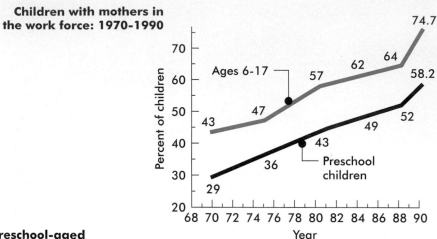

**Place of care for preschool-aged
children: 1977-1987**

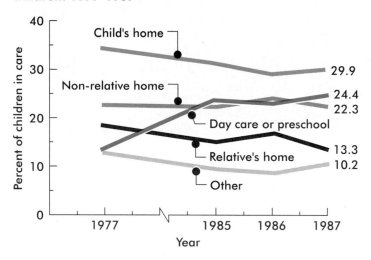

Figure 14-13 Children with mothers in the work force, 1970-1990, and place of care for preschool-aged children, 1977-1987. (From USDHHS, Public Health Service: *Child health USA '91,* DHHS Pub No. HRS-M-CH-91-1, Washington, D.C., 1991, U.S. Government Printing Office, p. 14.)

dramatic increase. One fourth of these children spent the time their mothers were working in non-residential day care centers. Women who work full time tend to use day care centers while women who work part time tend to use in-home care. Figure 14-13 also depicts the shift in child care arrangements in the past ten years from in-home care to day care or nursery school settings. The importance of this information for community health nurses is threefold: as parents, nurses may need assistance with finding safe and affordable child care, and further, nurses may be able to assist their clients with this important activity. Additionally, community health nurses can assist day care providers in facilitating a safe and healthy environment for the children they serve. Each year an estimated 7% of all children in day care required medical treatment for injuries (Selecting a safe day

care center, 1992, p. 32). The Safe Kids Coalition suggests that parents visit centers, ask questions about services offered, and observe. Look at precautions taken for the prevention of falls from stairs and windows, storage of cleaning supplies, types of toys and their cleanliness—the kinds of concerns that parents have for the safety of children at home. Space for play and the ratio of staff to children are other concerns. The National Association for the Education of Young Children in Washington, D.C., has lists of accredited day care centers across the country.

GENERAL CONCEPTS OF HEALTH PROMOTION

Health promotion needs are based on the developmental tasks and common health problems of the specific population group. For the newborn to 5-year-old and parenting population, the following factors should be considered when developing a health promotion program:

1. A monitoring system to identify high-risk infants and parents
2. An organized community program to combat problems such as accidents and child abuse
3. An organized system for provision of preventive health services, such as physical examinations and immunizations
4. Health education program to meet anticipatory guidance needs of parents and children
5. A well-established procedure for follow-up care of clients with identified health care needs
6. Passage and revision of significant legislation, such as the enforcement of immunization laws

AGGREGATES AT PARTICULAR RISK AMONG THOSE UNDER 5 YEARS OF AGE

Infants and children cannot speak or act on their own behalf; they are dependent on the adults around them to do for them what must be done to ensure a healthy happy life. The fact that very young children are twice as likely to live in poverty than any other age group, accompanied by the fact that the number of children in poverty increased by more than 2.2 million in only a decade, should strike fear into the thoughts of professionals who care about the health of the children of the United States (Johnson, Miranda, Sherman, and Weill, 1991, p. 5). Adults who live around children have not adequately spoken or acted on their behalf. This section discusses three aggregates at particular risk: the homeless, those with fetal alcohol syndrome, and children who are technology-dependent.

The Homeless

Families, mainly mothers with small children, were the fastest-growing group of homeless people in the 1980s. It is difficult to comprehend that there are thousands of families in this country, headed by women, who have no permanent home (Francis, 1991, p. 90). Having no home hurts children and their families in many ways, but what it obviously does is compromise access to the formal health care system, prenatal care, insurance coverage, sanitary environments, and immunizations. Children in homeless shelters have diarrhea, elevated blood lead levels, and asthma at higher rates than other children. Nutrition and emotional stability are other factors compromised by homelessness; the job of simply being a child must be out of the question in a shelter with dozens of other people and no privacy and certainty about life.

A subgroup at high risk among the homeless are runaway girls. Recent indications are that this population includes increasing numbers of women who are pregnant: one study of homeless girls in 19 cities found that 30% of the girls 16-19 years of age were pregnant (Athey, 1989, p. 5). Rarely do these adolescents receive prenatal care and they are subjected to both physical and sexual abuse. Further, they are vulnerable to drug and alcohol abuse.

The key causes of homelessness are poverty, the shortage of low-income housing, and lack of the support needed by families with special needs or in times of particular stress. Addressing these factors takes initiatives from all levels of government, from corporate and business communities, and from community groups and religious congregations (Mihaly, 1991, p. 220). The American Nurses Association has included homelessness among the issues it advocates for in Washington, D.C., as have many other state associations. Nurses can contact the legislative committee of their state nurses' association for information about what their associations are doing to support this issue. Athey's report (1989) includes descriptions of six programs serving pregnant and homeless adolescents.

Fetal Alcohol Syndrome

Fetal alcohol syndrome (FAS) has been called the most common, best known, most preventable cause of mental retardation in the western world. This syndrome is caused by a pregnant woman's heavy use of alcohol, and diagnosis is based on the following symptoms in the infant: retarded growth, a pattern of facial abnormalities, and abnormalities of the central nervous system that can include mental retardation (Masis and May, 1991, p. 484). Fetal alcohol effect and alcohol-related birth defect are manifestations of lower amounts of alcohol ingested during pregnancy. Because there is no cure for this syndrome, primary prevention is of utmost importance. Studies indicate that the incidence of FAS is about 1.3 to 2.2 per 1000 live births (Masis and May).

Female alcoholics are frequently ostracised in our society and thus have been left to produce a number of

TABLE 14-9   Summary of OTA Estimates of the Size of the Technology-Dependent Child Population, 1987

Defined population	Estimated number of children
Group I:	
Requiring ventilator assistance…	680 to 2,000
Group II:	
Requiring parenteral nutrition….	350 to 700
Requiring prolonged intravenous drugs……………	270 to 8,275
Group III:	
Requiring other device-based respiratory or nutritional support…………………	1,000 to 6,000
Rounded subtotal (I + II + III)……………	**2,300 to 17,000**
Group IV:	
Requiring apnea monitoring……	6,800 to 45,000
Requiring renal dialysis…………	1,000 to 6,000
Requiring other device-associated nursing……………	Unknown, perhaps 30,000 or more

From U.S. Congress, Office of Technology Assessment: *Technology dependent children: hospital v. home care—a technical memorandum,* OTA-TM-H-38, Washington, D.C., May 1987, U.S. Government Printing Office, p. 4.

children with FAS before they themselves die prematurely. Masis and May (1991) describe a hospital-based, comprehensive approach to the prevention of FAS that combines clinical assessment, community outreach, and epidemiological knowledge to attack the resulting birth defects. One of the striking results of this program was its acceptance by the women referred to it: of 48 who were referred, only 3 refused outright. The outstanding success of this program could be a model for others.

Children Who Are Technology-Dependent

Over the past two decades it has become increasingly possible to save smaller and sicker newborns. Twenty years ago, nine of every 10 babies born weighing less than 1000 grams (2.2 lb) died. Today, with the median birth weight at 7 lb 8 oz, up to 75% of the babies who weigh between 1.7 and 2.2 lb survive.

It is the rare low-birth-weight infant, however, who does not suffer serious complications such as brain or pulmonary hemorrhages, heart failure, or infections—among other problems. Further, the number of babies born each year with multiple defects totals about 30,000.

An increasing number of these babies receive sophisticated treatment at birth and grow into young children whose lives are regulated by technology. One such group of children are infants who are ventilator-dependent.

Increasing numbers of parents are opting to care at home for their children whose lives are regulated by technology. "Technology-dependent" is a term used to describe a small subset of the disabled child population who rely on life-sustaining medical technology and who typically require complex, hospital-level nursing care. Table 14-9 is a summary of the estimates of the size of this population in 1987. Both the numbers in this aggregate and the group types are increasing and the children in groups I, II, and III in Table 14-9 may double in the next few years (U.S. Congress, OTA, 1987, p. 4).

Many health care professionals consider the home setting better than the hospital when all the needs of children are considered. This can happen only when parents want their children home, when families can cope with living with the child amid the intrusion of health care providers in the home, and when the effectiveness of home care services including equipment, respite care, social and psychological supports, and professional caregivers are adequate. The financing of home health care for this aggregate is problematic because many of the families frequently lack private insurance. Further, "virtually all very-long-term technology-dependent children requiring a high level of nursing assistance will exceed the limits of their families' private insurance policies, will be uninsurable in the self-purchase insurance market because they are poor risks, and will end up on Medicaid" (U.S. Congress, OTA, 1987, p. 7). As alternatives to hospital care become more widely available, the incentive will be present to discharge these children quicker and sicker into the community, even before adequate preparations have been made. (U.S. Congress OTA, p. 8). Community health nurses involved in planning for their discharges will need to watch for this scenario. Further, nurses in the community will need high-level technical skills.

Appendix 10-1 reveals one mother's graphic story of her struggles to keep her ventilator-dependent child at home and the strengths and weaknesses of the health care team who aided the family in its struggle. Families who have children with special needs, such as ventilator-dependent children, need coordinated, comprehensive health care services that ensure continuity of care. They also need to have a clear understanding of the referral process and community resources that can promote family stability and concrete assistance during times of stress. Chapters 8, 10, and 18 are helpful to review when visiting families in the community who have "special" children.

SIGNIFICANT HEALTH LEGISLATION

During the past 70 years there has been much federal legislation and many demonstration projects concerned with the health of infants and mothers in America. The Children's Bureau was established in 1912. White House Conferences on Children and Youth have been held every 10 years since 1910. The Shepherd-Towner Act of 1921 created maternal and child health services at the state level, supported by the federal government. Title V of the Social Security Act of 1935 provided for grants to states for maternal and child health services and services to crippled children. The Emergency Maternity and Infant Care Program existed during the 1930s. The need for community mental health programs was recognized in the 1960s. The Eighty-ninth Congress, during President Johnson's time in office (1963-1968), brought huge changes in child health legislation with the establishment of the Office of Economic Opportunity and its Headstart Program, Medicaid, and the National Institutes of Child Health and Human Development. Some of the significant current legislation follows.

There are seven major public programs designed to meet the needs of women and children in this country. These programs are the preventive health and health services block grant; maternal and child health block grant; Early and Periodic Screening, Diagnosis, and Treatment portion of Medicaid; childhood immunization program; childhood lead poisoning prevention; community health centers; and migrant health centers (General Accounting Office, 1992, p. 1). Table 14-10 provides significant data related to each of these programs. A broad range of health, welfare, and environmental services are provided by them. An-

other significant program that provides needed maternal and child health services is the Women, Infants, and Children Program (WIC). As presented in Chapter 4, WIC is a federal nutrition and health program administered by the U.S. Department of Agriculture that makes food available to at-risk pregnant and lactating women, and infants and children up to the age of 5 years.

Though they fill tremendous needs for many women and children, it is problematic that objectives overlap, that coordination between programs is lacking, and that requirements for the programs are not well-defined. Further, resource limitations may result in fewer services than those authorized to be made available. When services are listed as optional they may not be made available because grantees may only choose to provide the required services paid for by these funds. Thus services provided by one state or grantee may not be provided by another (GAO, 1992, p. 17).

Fragmentation, categorization, and lack of coordinated services was addressed in the 1990s by private foundations and the federal government. The concept of "One-Stop Shopping" was used to describe a client-centered system that facilitates access to care by enhancing coordination and integration of the many programs available to women (Macro Systems, Inc., 1990, p. iv). Major issues related to the delivery of maternal and child health services are currently being discussed under Clinton's Health Care Reform mandate. These discussions could significantly alter present maternal and child health programs.

Child Maltreatment

The Child Abuse Prevention and Treatment Act (Public Law 93-247) was signed into law in 1974 in response to the need for a nationwide effort to solve this complex problem. This act created the National Center on Child Abuse and Neglect as the primary place where the federal government can focus its efforts on identifying, treating, and preventing child abuse and neglect (Combating child abuse, 1988, p. 369). To carry out the mandates of the act, the National Center has begun programs in four areas: demonstration and research, information gathering and dissemination, training and technical assistance, and assistance to states. In 1962 the Children's Bureau developed and promoted a model state child abuse mandatory reporting law that, in effect, states that professionals or child care workers must report sus-

TABLE 14-10 Programs Serving Low-Income Mothers and Children in the United States: Program Objectives and Target Population*

Program and authority	Program objectives and target population
Community Health Centers Grant (CHC) (Section 330, Public Health Service [PHS] Act)	This program provides preventive and primary health care services and case management of other services to medically underserved populations;[a] each CHC must demonstrate the capability to serve all age groups, and should be able to identify populations in its service area with special health care needs.
Migrant Health Centers Grant (MHC) (Section 329, PHS Act)	This program provides preventive and management of other services to migrant and seasonal farmworkers and their families; in defining its appropriate role, each center assesses the needs of its target population.
Maternal and Child Health Block Grant (M&CH) (Title V, Social Security Act [SSA])	This block grant program seeks to improve the health of mothers and children who do not have access to adequate health care,[b] particularly those from low-income families: direct services include preventive and primary care for children, prenatal care and delivery services, and postpartum care, but this funding also helps to support the state service delivery infrastructure; other services must also be provided for children with special health care needs (rehabilitative services for certain categories of children under 16 who are disabled).
Childhood Lead Poisoning Prevention Program (CLPPP) (Lead Contamination Control Act, 1988)	This program provides states with resources to establish and expand programs to prevent childhood lead poisoning; program activities may include screening for lead poisoning, referral for medical treatment and environmental intervention, follow-up, and education about lead poisoning. It targets high-risk children under 6 years of age.
Childhood Immunization Program (CIP) (Section 317, PHS Act)	This program provides states with resources to establish and maintain programs to immunize children against vaccine-preventable diseases; CIP funds may be used for the planning and implementation of immunization programs, for vaccine purchase, and for assessment of immunization status.
Preventive Health and Health Services Block Grant (PHHS) (Title XIX, part A of PHS Act)	This block grant program provides states with resources for comprehensive preventive health services. Each state determines the target population to be served.
Medicaid/Early and Periodic Screening, Diagnosis, and Treatment (EPSDT) (Title XIX, SSA)	This program seeks to diagnose physical and mental problems in low-income children under 21 and to provide treatment to correct any conditions found.

*All seven programs are authorized to address the health care needs of women, children, or both, but each targets a slightly different population, and the type of services available under each program varies.
[a]Medically underserved populations are designated by the Department of Health and Human Services (HHS) according to the percentage of population with income below the poverty level, percentage of population 65 years of age and over, infant mortality rate, and physicians per 1,000 population.
[b]The Maternal and Child Health Block Grant provides both grants to states and funding for set-aside programs. In this fact sheet, we are reporting only on the grants to states.
From General Accounting Office: *Federally funded health services: information on seven programs serving low-income women and children,* GAO/HRD-92-73FS, Gaithersburg, Md., May 1992, The GAO, pp. 10-11.

pected child abuse to the appropriate officials. Public Law 93-247 reinforced this mandate.

The Child Abuse Prevention and Treatment Act of 1974 has been amended several times in the past decade and a half. In 1988 Congress passed legislation to reauthorize three programs designed to prevent and treat child abuse and domestic violence and to encourage the adoption of hard-to-place children. This legislative act was entitled "The Child Abuse Prevention, Adoption, and Family Services Act of 1988" (Public Law 100-294). It consolidated into one act the Child Abuse Prevention and Treatment Act of 1974, the Child Abuse Prevention and Treatment and Adoption Reform Act of 1978, and the Family Violence Prevention and Services Act of 1984.

Public Law 100-294 mandates funding to support state and local efforts designed to prevent abuse and family violence and to identify and treat the victims. It also ensures funding of the National Center on Child Abuse and Neglect, a national commission on child and youth deaths, a project to study the nationwide incidence of family violence, and initiatives to eliminate barriers to the adoption of older children, minority children, and children with physical and mental handicaps. Additionally, it mandates support of professional training and research activities (USDHHS, Administration for Children, Youth, and Families, 1988).

The states have acted on Public Law 100-294 in various ways and community health nurses must know the laws that are in effect in the states in which they are working. Health care professionals are directly affected by this law and by state child protection laws that require the reporting of child abuse and neglect.

Fertility-Related State Laws

In recent years several states have enacted fertility-related laws: in 1982 alone, 45 such laws were passed. These new laws cover such issues as sterilization, abortion, insurance benefits for pregnancy-related health care, family planning services and information, and maternal and infant health. Much of the legislation reflected a growing concern about the health problems of low-income women, infants, and children.

In 1991 a decision by the Supreme Court, Rust v. Sullivan, upheld legislation specifying that no federal funds could be used in programs where abortion is a method of family planning. Thus nurses working in clinics using federal monies could not inform their clients that abortion was an alternative. The decision was a disturbing one because people's access and equity in health care information was at stake: women who could afford to pay private providers could be informed that abortion was a legal option, but poor women did not have that option (Murphy, 1991, p. 238). The day after his inauguration, January 22, 1993, President Bill Clinton used the power of an executive order to reverse the Supreme Court decision in the Rust v. Sullivan case. That day was also the 20th anniversary of Roe v. Wade, the decision that established the constitutional right to abortion.

Developmental Disabilities

Scientific advances in recent decades have made it possible to save infants who previously would have died at birth. However, this phenomenon has created special challenges for health care professionals. The number of infants and children with developmental disabilities is increasing significantly. These children need assistance to help them to achieve their maximum potential. Because this assistance was often very costly and not available for many children with developmental disabilities, the Congress has passed, in the past decade and a half, two significant pieces of legislation that were designed to promote early intervention with handicapped and at-risk young children.

The Education for All Handicapped Children Act (Public Law 94-142) was enacted in November 1975. This act entitles all handicapped children between the ages of 6 and 18 to a free and appropriate education regardless of the type of handicap or the degree of impairment. It also allows incentive monies for providing services to children beginning at age 3 and for young adults between 18 and 21. This act is discussed more extensively in Chapter 15.

The Education of the Handicapped Act Amendments of 1986 (Public Law 99-457) significantly expanded services to preschool children 3 to 5 years old and at-risk infants and toddlers up to age 3 years. This law created two new federal programs—the preschool grant program and the handicapped infants and toddlers program. By 1990-1991 state educational agencies had to provide a free and appropriate education for all handicapped children beginning at the age of 3. Significant federal funding was allocated to support the preschool grant program. The handicapped infants and toddlers program was established to reduce the potential for developmental delays, help families to meet the special needs of their handicapped children and toddlers, minimize institutionalization of handicapped individuals, and reduce educational costs to society. Incentive funding for this program has helped states to develop and implement quality early intervention programs and to coordinate early intervention services. Community health nurses are active participants on the multidisciplinary teams that are providing services to infants and toddlers under this program.

On July 26, 1990, President George Bush signed into law the Americans with Disabilities Act, which prohibits discrimination on the basis of disability in employment. For the first time, employers in both the private and public sector cannot discriminate because an individual is disabled (Smith, 1992). Chapter 18 discusses the implications of this act in depth.

BARRIERS TO HEALTH CARE

Major barriers to the delivery of services to the newborn to 5-year-old population and their parents have been discussed earlier in this chapter and in Chapter 13. The following case situations illustrate some specific problems parents have in obtaining care for themselves and their children under 5 years of age.

▶ **Sue was 17 years old when she became pregnant. Her husband, Tom, age 18, worked as a gas station attendant. His income provided only the basic necessities of food and rent but was too high to allow them any public assistance. Sue decided to "save" money by waiting for antepartum care until near her EDC. Upon her first antepartum visit to the doctor 1 month before delivery, she was found to be severely hypertensive and diabetic. Her infant weighed 10 lb at birth and required 1 month's hospitalization. Sue and Tom felt that they were severely criticized by the health personnel for not receiving adequate antepartum care.**

▶ **Diane and Jim Jones have four children under 5 years of age. Jim has a job-related back injury and is unemployed. The Joneses have a Medicaid card and they use the outpatient department of a large teaching hospital in their city for medical care. They go there only when they absolutely must. The family has no car and uses the city bus line, which involves three transfers for the 4-mile trip. With**

four children, Mrs. Jones finds this most difficult, especially in cold weather. When she does arrive at the hospital, she must wait several hours and then sees a different physician each time so that she must repeatedly give her family's health histories. Mrs. Jones feels that "the people in that hospital don't care about or understand me and my kids."

As part of the *Healthy Mothers, Healthy Babies* campaign initiated by the U.S. Department of Health and Human Services to help achieve the maternal and infant health objectives for the nation (Bratic, 1982), a study was carried out to document the perceived barriers to seeking health care and information among women of a lower socioeconomic status. Three major barriers were identified ("Healthy Mothers" Market Research: How to Reach Black and Mexican American Women, 1982): (1) *low priority of preventive health care,* because it takes considerable energy for many of these mothers to meet basic needs and because government funding sources do not adequately finance preventive health services, (2) *difficulties encountered within the health care system,* including communication barriers, perceived negative attitudes of staff, and the unavailability or inappropriateness of educational materials, and (3) *low motivation to adopt good health practices,* because many clients generally have a day-to-day orientation, multiple life problems, and a support group that does not understand or support certain health habits or practices.

THE ROLES OF THE COMMUNITY HEALTH NURSE

The community health nurse plays a number of roles in providing service to the newborn to 5-year-old age group. The following paragraphs describe some of these roles.

Advocate-Planner

Since the children in the newborn to 5-year-old age group cannot speak for themselves, the nurse becomes an advocate. This can involve pointing out to caregivers the safety hazards in the environment and urging necessary changes. On a broader level, the nurse is an advocate for the development of day care centers in a community and publicizes the inadequacy of health and medical care for economically disadvantaged families. This role of advocate means that the nurse must be involved in the political process to correct issues such as unemployment, lack of adequate income, overcrowding, and the cycle of poverty, which can ultimately be solved only with legislative changes. Attitudes of assertiveness, a knowledge of the political process, and a willingness to take risks are necessary tools for this role.

Teacher

The community health nurse needs to be a teacher. This role includes demonstrating information about child care to families and involving parents in the learning process. Helping parents to understand good nutrition for this age group, or why safety seats and belts are necessary in cars, means involvement of all concerned in the process of teaching and learning and changing values and attitudes. The community health nurse is well versed in the developmental tasks of this age group. Teaching parents about these tasks is a form of anticipatory guidance and assists in task accomplishment.

Group Worker

In order to meet the needs of the newborn to 5-year-old population, the community health nurse needs to be attuned to opportunities for group teaching and counseling. Working with the LaLeche League or Parents Anonymous, a crisis intervention program set up to help prevent damaging relationships between parents and their children, are options. Other possibilities are numerous. One community health nurse, for example, had in his caseload area a large mobile park. Within the park he found five families who had children in special school classes because of developmental disabilities, each of whom expressed a need for help with their child. This staff nurse helped the parents form a weekly discussion group and the results were that isolated families received mutual supportive help in the form of babysitting, shared meals, and problem-solving about how to deal with difficult situations.

Coordinator

Coordinating community resources is another significant role of the community health nurse. Numerous services are available to families, and this is positive. However, families can feel uncared for and torn apart when the department of social services, Med-

icaid screening clinic, the community health nurse, the school nurse, and the child guidance center all request the same information in detail, or when these same health professionals do not communicate with each other and therefore plan different goals. Professionals need to be careful to ask the permission of a family before they share information regarding that family with another professional or agency. They should seek this permission as soon as they realize that families are working with multiple agencies.

Closely tied to this role is the facilitating role of the nurse. Helping families and the larger community to understand their rights as people and to understand services offered in the community all facilitate the better utilization of these services. The nurse helps families work toward desired change. Every community has persons with ideas and skills; all that needs to be done is to give them direction and reinforcement. Milio's *9226 Kercheval: The Storefront That Did Not Burn* is the classic story of how one community health nurse helped an inner-city area establish its own day care center (Milio, 1970). This nurse found that people saw a great problem with children who were not cared for while mothers worked. She acted as a catalyst to assist in solving the problem and was a facilitator and enabler as well.

Casefinder

Because of the nurse's proximity to infants and children, casefinding has been a strategic role for many years. At-risk children are identified and followed periodically as they develop. Disabilities are lessened when treatment is begun early, and some can be prevented by primary intervention. A system needs to be established in each community to periodically screen all children for problems. The Early Periodic Screening, Diagnosis, and Treatment Program (EPSDT) of Medicaid is one schedule that can be followed.

The North American Nursing Diagnosis Association accepted "altered parenting," "high risk for altered parenting," and "weak mother-infant or parent-infant attachment" as appropriate diagnostic terms in nursing and acceptable nursing diagnoses for clinical testing (Gordon, 1993). These diagnoses are presented in Tables 14-11, 14-12, and 14-13. The defining characteristics developed by the Association provide practitioners with useful parameters for casefinding when working with families with children.

14-11   The North American Nursing Diagnosis Association: Nursing Diagnosis for
Altered Parenting

Nursing diagnosis: altered parenting

Definition: Inability of nurturing figure(s) to create an environment which promotes optimum growth and
development of another human being. (Adjustment to parenting, in general, is a normal maturation process
following birth of a child.)

Etiological or related factors	Defining characteristics
Knowledge or skill deficit (specify: parenting skills, developmental guidelines, etc.)	Inattentive to infant/child needs*
Fear (specify focus)	Inappropriate caretaking behaviors, (toilet training, feeding, sleep/rest, etc.)*
Social isolation	History of child abuse or abandonment by primary caretaker*
Physical impairment (blindness, etc.)	Actual alteration:
Mental or physical illness	Verbalization cannot control child
Support system deficit (between/from significant other[s])	Abandonment of infant/child
Interrupted parent-infant bonding (e.g., illness of newborn)	Runaway
	Incidence of physical and psychological trauma
Family or personal stress (financial, legal, recent crisis, cultural change, multiple pregnancies)	Lack of parental attachment behaviors
Unmet social, emotional, or developmental needs (of parenting figures)	Inappropriate visual, tactile, auditory stimulation
	Negative identification of infant's/child's characteristics
Interruption in bonding process (i.e., maternal, paternal, other)	Negative attachment of meanings to infant's/child's characteristics; verbalization of resentment toward infant/child
Unrealistic expectations (self, infant, partner)	Verbalization cannot control child
Perceived threat to own survival (physical and emotional)	Evidence of physical and psychological trauma to infant/child
Lack of role identity	Constant verbalization of disappointment in gender or physical characteristics of the infant/child
Lack of, or inappropriate, response of child	Verbalization of role inadequacy
Physical or psychosocial abuse (of nurturing figure)	Verbal disgust at body functions of infant/child
Limited cognitive functioning	Noncompliance with health appointments for infant/child or self
	Inappropriate or inconsistent discipline practices
	Frequent accidents (infant/child); frequent illness (infant/child)
	Growth and development lag of infant/child
	Verbalizes desire to have child call parent by first name versus traditional, cultural tendencies
	Child receives care from multiple caretakers without consideration for the needs of the infant/child
	Compulsively seeks role approval from others

*Denotes critical, or major, defining characteristics.
From Gordon M: *Manual of nursing diagnosis* 1993-1994, St. Louis, 1993, Mosby, pp. 313, 315.

Epidemiologist

Collecting data on health problems and care is an important epidemiological role. Nurses are concerned about why parents do not use available health services and what motivates those who do. A community health nurse carried out a study to determine answers to these concerns and found that users of child health services had access to free medical care, were younger, and had more children than nonusers (Selwyn, 1978, p. 231). Reasons why people do and do not use health care are important elements in planning health services.

When the community health nurse visits parents after accidental poisoning incidents, the nurse can add to the epidemiological understanding of the predisposing and immediate causes of the accident and make recommendations to prevent them from occurring again. If it were the case that 75% of the families who have poisoning accidents have other health problems, there is evidence that this kind of stress leads to poisoning accidents.

A good record system in the health agency will help nurses to collect data on health problems, to plan interventions, and to evaluate care given. These data can provide information on changing health needs and necessary health services.

A good record system will collect data on the newborn to 5-year-old child that provide the basis for a health history on which later events in the family system can be compared and built.

Clinic Nurse

Community health nurses have long worked in well-baby clinics where, at regular intervals, the health of children up to the age of 5 is assessed, immunizations are given, and parents have the opportunity to discuss concerns of growth and development. This role has been expanded to an assessment and treatment role. Nurses deal with problem behavior such as delayed play, immature social behavior, and temper tantrums. With the nurse's knowledge of child development, behavior modification, and management techniques, the roles of observer, consultant, and counselor to parents, preschool teachers, and day care workers are valuable in dealing with minor problems that can develop into major ones.

Home Visitor

A well-known role of the nurse caring for the needs of the newborn to 5-year-old age group is that of the

---

TABLE 14-12 **The North American Nursing Diagnosis Association: Nursing Diagnosis for High Risk for Altered Parenting**

Nursing diagnosis: high risk for altered parenting

Definition: Presence of risk factors during prenatal or childbearing period that may interfere with process of adjustment to parenting.

Defining characteristics (risk factors)

Unavailable or ineffective role model
History of physical and psychosocial abuse (of nurturing figure)
Support system deficit (between/from significant others)
Unmet social, emotional, developmental needs (of parenting figures)
Interruption in bonding process (maternal, paternal, other)
Unrealistic expectation (self, infant, partner)
Perceived threat to own survival (physical, emotional)
Physical impairment (blindness, etc.)
Physical or mental illness
Presence of stress (financial, legal, recent personal crisis, cultural change, multiple pregnancies)
Knowledge or skill deficit (specify: parenting skills, developmental progression, etc.)
Limited cognitive functioning
Lack of role identity
Lack of, or inappropriate, response of child to relationship
Social isolation
Fear (specify focus)

From Gordon M: *Manual of nursing diagnosis 1993-1994,* St. Louis, 1993, Mosby, p. 311.

---

community health nurse who visits parents and babies in their homes. Each health department sets its own priorities and standards for the care of parents and children. This ranges from the prenatal and postnatal referral of each pregnancy to the referral of only those mothers and infants at high risk. The broad background of community health nurses equips them with skills to help establish the standards as to which newborns and parents will be visited. In particular, families that are poor, uneducated, or headed by

TABLE 14-13 The North American Nursing Diagnosis Association: Nursing Diagnosis for Weak Mother-Infant Attachment or Parent-Infant Attachment

Nursing diagnosis: weak mother-infant attachment or parent-infant attachment

Definition: Pattern of unreciprocal bonding relationship between parent and infant or primary caretaker and infant

Etiological or related factors	Defining characteristics
Parental anxiety	Minimal smiling, close contact, enfolding, talking to baby
Fear (specify)	Does not assume "en face" position, eye-to-eye contact
Parent-infant separation	Minimal touching, stroking, patting, rocking, holding, kissing of infant
Perceived low parenting competency (infant care)	except when necessary to feed or change diapers
Low (infant) social responsiveness	Does not attempt comforting responses to crying or continues unsuccessful methods
Support system deficit	Low reciprocal interaction pattern (e.g., minimal smiling, babbling response to touching, kissing, etc.)
Family stress	Irritable infant or low responsiveness to parent
	Few positive comments about infant; expressions of disappointment
	Bottle propped or tense posture during breastfeeding
	Infrequent visitation of hospitalized infant (e.g., less than twice a week)
	Prenatal history of ambivalence, negative feelings regarding pregnancy
	High-risk adolescent parent, physically or mentally ill parent

From Gordon M: *Manual of nursing diagnosis 1993-1994,* St. Louis, 1993, Mosby, pp. 321, 323.

teenage parents often face barriers to getting the health care or social support services they need. Many experts believe that providing services in the home reduces these barriers. They also believe that home visiting for prenatal counseling or parenting education for this population group can address problems before they become irreversible or extremely costly (General Accounting Office, July 1990, pp. 2-3).

The nurse who visits in the home, especially when both parents are present, is in a privileged position to closely and periodically assess the baby's, the parents', and the family's development. The nurse can also identify stress, help parents deal with problems of poor bonding, provide role modeling for bonding and parenting, give anticipatory guidance, and help reinforce positive behavior. The nurse aids families in using community resources as necessary. For example, when parents and a new baby with a diagnosis of spina bifida, Down syndrome, or cleft palate come home from the hospital, it is most often the community health nurse who introduces the family to the resources of the special health care services, known as crippled children services in some states, for financial aid, to the physical therapy offered by the intermedi-

ate school program, or to the interdisciplinary diagnostic services of university-affiliated centers. This same nurse will likely be one of the persons to help parents as they go through the grief process related to having a baby who is less than "perfect." The nurse can also be alert to signs of stress within the family in this situation; living 24 hours a day with a helpless infant who has additional problems can be an overwhelming problem for some families. Homemakers, parent's aides, and parent-support groups are useful when families are in such a situational crisis.

One of the major characteristics of handicapped children, and particularly the mentally retarded, is some delay in reaching developmental milestones in self-help skills. It is sometimes assumed that these skills will develop without intervention as a result of physical growth and maturation. Often this is not the case and the child is unable to function independently. This leads to institutionalization, enormous financial and personal expenditures, and waste of human potential. With the use of behavior modification technology, most self-help skills can be attained by handicapped persons, including those who are profoundly retarded. The community health nurse is in a unique position to help families with these skills. Beginning immediately after birth with early infant stimulation is essential. The goal is that each person attain his or her own potential. The nurse can aid the family in recognizing this potential and give guidance in the process of reaching it. Time needed to exercise and teach the young child with developmental disabilities can lead to the neglect of other children. Parents and nurse must be cognizant of this situation.

Summary

The years from birth to age 5 provide the foundation for a child's lifelong physical, mental, and social development. The child's health and that of the parents is inextricably interwoven, and both have health care needs that the community health nurse can help to fill.

Utilization of the developmental health promotion model to assess the needs of young children provides a positive way to prevent many of the major health problems of those newborn to 5 years of age, or at least weaken their impact. This is the challenge for community health nurses!

Children are our nation's greatest resource. Decreasing infant and maternal mortality rates reflect this value, as does legislation such as Medicaid, which provides health care for at least a segment of the newborn to 5-year-old population.

◀ *An Exercise in Critical Thinking* ▶

The following case study, "Lilly's Anger" (Dangelmaier, 1992, p. 41), describes a public health nurse whose caseload was at-risk pregnant women and infants. Describe the skills the nurse used as she cared for Lilly and her baby.

———————————— LILLY'S ANGER ————————————

I am a public health nurse providing home visits to "at risk" pregnant women and infants. The women and infants I see generally live in rural settings.

Perhaps the most challenging aspect of my work is trying to engage the client who, for a combination of reasons, is not initially receptive to help from someone perceived as an "outsider." The following situation provides insight to the challenges and complexities routinely encountered by public health nurses such as myself.

I first encountered Lilly approximately ten months ago. She was eight months pregnant and was found to have some abnormalities in her blood work at the last checkup. She needed to have an ultrasound immediately to determine if the baby was okay. The clinic was unable to reach Lilly by phone and asked me to stop by her home and urge her to get into the clinic as soon as possible for further assessment.

Lilly's need for help on the one hand, and resistance to any kind of intervention on the other hand, quickly surfaced in my initial contact. To begin with, she was very angry. Angry about being awakened from her sleep—I learned she worked nights in a laundry. Angry about having relinquished her first child and the pressure her parents were putting on her to do it again. Angry about her negative experiences with the Department of Social and Health Services. Angry at the prospect of the second ultrasound. "Didn't I just have one a month ago? Can things change all that much in four weeks?"

Speaking in a loud voice and in a forceful manner, Lilly had no difficulty letting me know her thoughts about her pregnancy and her generally less than desirable circumstances. Her anger and frustration were intensified by her imposing figure. Lilly is about six feet tall, large framed, has bright red hair, and is developmentally delayed. I found her presentation rather intimidating, especially in view of the dark and dreary house into which I had been invited to state my business. However, the fact that I allowed Lilly to vent seemed to be having a quieting effect. I tried as much as possible to validate her concerns, and as a result, she gradually became more open to having the second ultrasound. In fact, I actually dialed the number so she could set up the appointment. By the time I left Lilly's home, she was also indicating that she "might" be receptive to another visit. "But don't call until the late afternoon."

Driving away from Lilly's home, I reflected on what had transpired and wondered if I would ever see her

From Dangelmaier A: Lilly's anger. In Zewekh J, Primomo J, and Deal L, eds: *Opening doors: stories of public health nursing,* Olympia, Wa., 1992, Washington State Department of Health, Parent-Child Health Services, pp. 41-45.

again. Given the number of problems in this case, on-going help was certainly needed, but would Lilly be open to it?

Attempts to make contact by phone got nowhere, so I decided to "drop-in" about four weeks after my first visit. My hope was that it was late enough in the day so Lilly would be up from her sleep and receptive to my visit. Apparently, my willingness to listen to her during my first visit rather than retreat during her burst of anger and frustration, earned a certain measure of respect and acceptance. Lilly invited me in and we began to explore in greater detail the concerns and issues touched on during my first contact. This conversation opened the way for me to introduce some thoughts on how she might deal with the problems at hand.

Lilly had followed through with the second ultrasound which didn't reveal any abnormalities. However, because her blood pressure was up, she was advised to terminate her work and go on bed rest for the balance of her pregnancy—a matter of a week or so. Lilly said she had also decided to keep the baby in spite of the pressure from her parents. With her boyfriend gone, her parents antagonistic, and no apparent circle of friends, it was evident that Lilly had no adequate "support system." Lilly had none of the items she needed for the baby, such as layette and car seat and she was undecided whether to breastfeed or bottle feed. I was relieved and encouraged to hear that Lilly would be receptive to my help in acquiring the necessary items and in obtaining information on how to deal with her bed rest. She also had concerns about how to provide appropriate care for her newborn. Her anxiety was prompted by her complete lack of experience. Having relinquished her first child, the opportunity to learn these skills had been forfeited.

To help expand Lilly's support base, I asked if she might also be willing to see our social worker, who could provide some guidance. She said she was. In fact, at this point in our relationship, she seemed open to exploring whatever ideas and resources I felt might be helpful. The visit ended with the understanding I would return in three days, hopefully with additional information and some of the baby items she needed.

As I left Lilly's, I reflected again on all that had occurred. It was clear we had progressed in our relationship. Lilly was now actively participating in identifying her concerns and exploring resources that could meet her needs. I also thought about one of my primary objectives in this relationship: when possible, to assist Lilly in accomplishing tasks on her own rather than doing them for her. My purpose was to help Lilly gain some much needed confidence and increase her skill level. Hopefully, her trust in me and the strength of our relationship had evolved to the point where she would be comfortable rather than resistant to help. My goals were twofold: assist Lilly to feel competent in meeting the challenges of being a new mother, and help her gain the strengths, confidence and knowledge to seek appropriate help when necessary.

I was able to visit Lilly one more time before the baby was due. I provided her with some information she was interested in and was able to locate both a layette and car seat for the baby. Equally important, the visit provided the opportunity to obtain Lilly's consent for on-going visits in the months following delivery.

Some eight months have passed since Lilly delivered a normal infant girl. The baby is happy and thriving. Monthly visits have allowed me to provide support and the chance to teach Lilly additional skills in caring for her baby. It has been interesting to observe Lilly's increasing ability to cope with problems that have arisen.

In the last few months Lilly has had to deal with being evicted from her rental home, seeing her boyfriend leave again, and continuing criticism from her parents. In spite of this, she interacts positively with the baby and provides good infant care. Lilly has also taken the initiative to find a full-time sitter so that she can work rather than be on welfare. She is comfortable in seeking out resources when needed, as evidenced by her participation in the WIC program, social service counseling, and the low-cost housing authority. She has demonstrated considerable growth in self-confidence and her capacity to function in general. She openly discusses the value of my visits and laughingly reflects back on our shaky beginning. We both agree that our relationship has grown. No longer is getting in touch with Lilly a problem. In fact, she seems quite comfortable in calling me, sharing her concerns, and inviting me to "come and see baby Sarah." I will probably continue regular visits until the baby is a year old. I know that when I no longer provide visits to this family, Lilly and I will both miss the positive working relationship we have come to enjoy. It has been a growing experience for both of us.

I could have given up on Lilly after my first stressful contact. I'm glad I didn't!

Suggested Schedule for Preventive Child Health Care

Age	History*	Measure-ment†	Physical examination	Develop-mental landmarks*‡	Discussion and guidance*	Procedures†,§	Attending
1 month	Initial Eating Sleeping Elimination Crying At every visit mother should be asked for questions	Height Weight Head circum-ference Temper-ature Evalua-tion of hearing	Complete¶	Eyes follow to mid-line Baby re-gards face *While prone, lifts head off table*	Vitamins Sneezing Hiccoughs Straining, with bowel movements Irregular respiration Startle reflex Ease and force of urination Night bottle Colic "Spoiling" Accidents	PKU Urinalysis Hep B-2 (Option 1)*** Hep B-2 (Option 2)	MD and assistant
2 months	Health Sensory-motor develop-ment Eating Sleeping Elimination Happiness	Height Weight Head circum-ference Temper-ature	Complete or obser-vation**	*Vocalizes Smiles re-sponsively*	Solid foods Immuni-zations Thumb-sucking	DTP-1 tOPV-1 Hib-1 HbOC/ PRP-T Hib-1 PRP-OMP Urine screening	MD and/or assistant
3 months	Health Eating Sleeping Elimination Crying Other behavior	Height Weight	Complete or obser-vation**	Holds head and chest up to make 90 degree angle with table Laughs	Feeding Accidents Sleeping without rocking Coping with frus-trations		

*May be accomplished in part by assistant if physician desires. Much of this may be accomplished in part by appropriate pamphlets or leaflets where deemed desirable.

†Usually accomplished by assistant.

‡Age given for landmarks indicates approximate age at which 90 percent of children have accomplished test. Adapted from Denver Developmental Screening Test.

§Immunization schedules updated from CDC: General recommendations on immunization: recommendations of the Immunization Practices Advisory Committee, MMWR 43 (No. RR-1), January 28, 1994, p. 9.

¶By physician. observation of child, completely undressed, by assistant trained to observe respiration, skin, musculature, motor activities, and so forth.

**Obvious deviations from normal must be checked by physician.

***For use among infants born to HBs Ag-negative mothers. The first dose should be administered during the newborn period, preferably before hospital discharge, but no later than age 2 months (refer to Table 14-5).

NOTE: Italicized items indicate report of parent and may be accepted as proof of accomplishment. May be obtained by assistant.

Reprinted with permission from Committee on Standards of Child Health Care, Council on Pediatric Practice, American Academy of Pediatrics, 1972. Copyright American Academy of Pediatrics 1972 and 1977.

Continued

APPENDIX 14-1

Suggested Schedule for Preventive Child Health Care—cont'd

Age	History*	Measurement†	Physical examination	Developmental landmarks*‡	Discussion and guidance*	Procedures†,§	Attending
4 months	Health Eating Sleeping Elimination Other behavior Sensory-motor development Current living situation Parent-child interaction	Height Weight Head circumference Temperature	Complete§	Holds head erect and steady when held in sitting position *Squeals* Grasps rattle Eyes follow object for 180 degrees	Feeding Schedule to fit in with family Attitude of father Respiratory infections	DTP-2 tOPV-2 Hib-2 HbOC/ PRP-T Hib-2 PRP-OMP Hep B-3	MD and/or assistant
5 months	Health Eating Sleeping Elimination Sensory-motor development	Height Weight Temperature	Complete or observation¶	*Smiles spontaneously* *Rolls from back to stomach or vice versa* Reaches for object on table	Feeding Vitamins (if not previously mentioned)		MD and/or assistant
6 months	Health Eating Sleeping Elimination Other behavior Sensory-motor development	Height Weight Head circumference Temperature Evaluation of hearing	Complete or observation¶	No head lag if baby is pulled to sitting position by hands	Feeding Accidents Night crying Fear of strangers Separation anxiety Description of normal micturition	DTP-3 OPV-3 Hib-3 HbOC/ PRP-T Hep B-4 (Option 1)—between 6-18 months Hep B-4 (Option 2)—between 6-18 months	MD and/or assistant
8-9 months	Health Eating Sleeping Elimination Sensory-motor development	Height Weight Temperature	Complete or screening¶	Sits alone for seconds after support is released	Use of cup Eating with fingers Fear of strangers Accidents		MD and/or assistant

APPENDIX 14-1

Suggested Schedule for Preventive Child Health Care—cont'd

Age	History*	Measurement†	Physical examination	Developmental landmarks*‡	Discussion and guidance*	Procedures†,§	Attending
8-9 months	Behavior			Bears weight momentarily if held with feet on table Looks after fallen object Transfers block from one hand to the other Feeds self cracker	Need for affection Normal unpleasant behavior Discipline		
10 months if last exam at 8 months	Health Eating Sleeping Elimination Behavior Sensory-motor development Speech development Current living situation Parent-child interaction	Height Weight Temperature	Complete or observation**	*Pulls self to standing position* *Stands holding on to solid object (not human)* Pincer grasp; picks up small object using any part of thumb and fingers in opposition *Says Da-da or Ma-ma* Resists toy being pulled away *Plays peek-a-boo* Makes attempt to get toy just out of reach	Toilet training: when to start Normal drop in appetite Independence vs. dependency Discipline Instructions for use of syrup of ipecac	Hemoglin or hematocrit	MD and/or assistant

Continued

APPENDIX 14-1
Suggested Schedule for Preventive Child Health Care—cont'd

Age	History*	Measure-ment†	Physical examination	Develop-mental landmarks*‡	Discussion and guidance*	Procedures†,§	Attending
10 months if last exam at 8 months				*Initial anxiety toward strangers*			
12 months	As for 10 months	Height Weight Head circum-ference Temper-ature	Complete¶	*Cruises: walks around holding onto fur-niture* *Stands alone 2-3 sec-onds if outside support is removed* *Bangs together two blocks held one in each hand* *Imitates vocalization heard within preceding minute* Plays pat-a-cake	Negativism Likelihood of respiratory infections "Getting into things" Weaning from bottle Proper dose of vitamins Control of drugs and poisons	Tuberculin test (intra-dermal preferred) Between 12-15 months MMR-1 Hib-booster HbOC/ PRP-T Hib-booster PRP-OMP Urinalysis	MD and assistant
15 months	As for 10 months	Height Weight Temper-ature	Complete or obser-vation**	*Walks well* Stoops to recover toys on floor Uses Da-da and Ma-ma specifically for correct parent Rolls or tosses ball back to examiner *Indicates wants by pulling, pointing, or appropriate verbalization (not crying)*	Temper tantrums Obedience	DTaP/DTP	MD and/or assistant

APPENDIX 14-1
Suggested Schedule for Preventive Child Health Care—cont'd

Age	History*	Measurement†	Physical examination	Developmental landmarks*‡	Discussion and guidance*	Procedures†,§	Attending
15 months				*Drinks from cup without spilling much*			
18 months	As for 10 months	Height Weight Temperature	Complete¶	Puts one block on another without its falling off *Mimics household chores like dusting or sweeping*	Reaction toward and of siblings Toilet training Speech development	Hib	MD and assistant
21 months	As for 10 months Peer reaction	Height Weight Temperature	Complete or observation**	Walks backward and upstairs Feeds self with spoon *Removes article of clothing other than hat* *Says three specific words besides Da-da and Ma-ma*	Manners "Poor appetite"		MD and/or assistant
2 years	Health Eating Sleeping Elimination Toilet training Sensory-motor development Speech Current living situation Peer and social adjustment	Height Weight Temperature Hearing	Complete¶	Kicks a ball in front of him with foot without support *Scribbles spontaneously— purposeful marking of more than one stroke on paper*	Need for peer companionship Immaturity: inability to share or take turns Care of teeth	Hemoglobin and/or hematocrit Urinalysis	MD and assistant

Continued

APPENDIX 14-1
Suggested Schedule for Preventive Child Health Care—cont'd

Age	History*	Measure-ment†	Physical examination	Developmental landmarks*‡	Discussion and guidance*	Procedures†,§	Attending
2 years				Balances four blocks on top of one another *Points correctly to one body part* Dumps small objects out of bottle after demonstration *Does simple tasks in house*	From this point on, guidance may be indicated by the mother's answers to a questionnaire about behavior and emotional problems		
2½ years	As for 2 years	Height Weight Temperature	Complete¶	*Throws overhand after demonstration* Names correctly one picture in book, e.g., cat or apple Combines two words meaningfully	*Guidance from questionnaire answers* Dental referral Perversity and decisiveness		MD and/or assistant
3 years	As for 2 years	As for 2 years Blood pressure	Complete¶	Jumps in place *Pedals tricycle* Dumps small article out of bottle without demonstration *Uses plurals*	*Guidance from questionnaire answers* Sex education Nursery schools: qualifications of a good one	As for 2 years	MD and assistant

APPENDIX 14-1

Suggested Schedule for Preventive Child Health Care—cont'd

Age	History*	Measure-ment†	Physical examination	Develop-mental landmarks*‡	Discussion and guidance*	Procedures†,§	Attending
3 years				*Washes and dries hands*	Obedience and dis-cipline		
4 years	As for 2 years	As for 2 years Vision ("E" chart) Blood pressure	Complete¶ Fundus exami-nation	Builds bridge of three blocks after demon-stration Copies circle and cross *Identifies longer of two lines* Knows first and last names Understands what to do when "tired" *Plays with other children so they interact—tag* *Dresses with supervision*	*Guidance from question-naire answers* Kindergarten Use of money Dental care	As for 2 years Between 4-6 years (before school entry) DTaP/DTP OPV-4 MMR-2	MD and assistant
5 years	As for 2 years (omit toilet training) Kinder-garten	As for 2 years Vision ("E" chart) Color blindness Audiometer Blood pressure	Complete¶	Hops two or more times Catches ball thrown 3 feet Dresses without supervision *Can tolerate separation from mother for a few minutes without anxiety*	*Guidance from question-naire answers* Readiness for school Span of attention: how to increase it	As for 2 years	MD and assistant

---

APPENDIX 14-2

Guide to Contraindications and Precautions to Vaccinations*

True contraindications and precautions	Not true (vaccines may be administered)
General for all vaccines (DTP/DTaP, OPV, IPV, MMR, Hib, HBV)	

Contraindications	Mild to moderate local reaction (soreness, redness, swelling) following a dose of an injectable antigen
Anaphylactic reaction to a vaccine contraindicates further doses of that vaccine	Mild acute illness with or without low-grade fever
Anaphylactic reaction to a vaccine constituent contraindicates the use of vaccines containing that substance	Current antimicrobial therapy
	Convalescent phase of illnesses
Moderate or severe illnesses with or without a fever	Prematurity (same dosage and indications as for normal, full-term infants)
	Recent exposure to an infectious disease
	History of penicillin or other nonspecific allergies or family history of such allergies

DTP/DTaP	

Contraindications	Temperature of <40.5 C (105 F) following a previous dose of DTP
Encephalopathy within 7 days of administration of previous dose of DTP	Family history of convulsions§
	Family history of sudden infant death syndrome
Precautions†	Family history of an adverse event following DTP administration
Fever of ≥40.5°C (105°F) within 48 hrs after vaccination with a prior dose of DTP	
Collapse or shocklike state (hypotonic-hyporesponsive episode) within 48 hrs of receiving a prior dose of DTP	
Seizures within 3 days of receiving a prior dose of DTP§	
Persistent, inconsolable crying lasting ≥3 hrs within 48 hours of receiving a prior dose of DTP	

DTP = Diphtheria-tetanus toxoid and pertussis vaccine	IPV = Inactivated poliovirus vaccine
DTaP = Diphtheria and tetanus toxoids and acellular pertussis vaccine	MMR = Measles-mumps-rubella vaccine
	Hib = *Haemophilus influenzae* type b vaccine
OPV = Oral poliovirus vaccine	HBV = Hepatitis B vaccine

*This information is based on the recommendations of the Advisory Committee on Immunization Practices (ACIP) and those of the Committee on Infectious Diseases (Red Book Committee) of the American Academy of Pediatrics (AAP) as of October 1992. Sometimes these recommendations vary from those contained in the manufacturer's package inserts. For more detailed information, providers should consult the published recommendations of the ACIP, AAP, American Association of Family Practice Physicians, and the manufacturer's package inserts.

†The events or conditions listed as precautions, although not contraindications, should be carefully reviewed. The benefits and risks of administering a specific vaccine to an individual under the circumstances should be considered. If the risks are believed to outweigh the benefits, the vaccination should be withheld; if the benefits are believed to outweigh the risks (for example, during an outbreak or for-eign travel), the vaccination should be administered. Whether and when to administer DTP to children with proven or suspected under-lying neurologic disorders should be decided on an individual basis. It is prudent on theoretical grounds to avoid vaccinating pregnant women. However, if immediate protection against poliomyelitis is needed, OPV, not IPV, is recommended.

§For children with a personal or family (siblings or parents) history of convulsions, acetaminophen should be considered before DTP is administered and thereafter every 4 hours for 24 hours.

¶There is a theoretical risk that the administration of multiple live-virus vaccines (OPV and MMR) within 30 days of one another if not administered on the same day will result in a suboptimal immune response. There are no data to substantiate this lack of response.

**Persons with a history of anaphylactic reactions following egg ingestion should be vaccinated only with extreme caution. Protocols that have been developed for vaccinating such persons should be consulted (*J Pediatr* 1983; 102:196–9, *J Pediatr* 1988;113:504–6).

††Measles vaccination may temporarily suppress tuberculin reactivity. If testing cannot be done the day of MMR vaccination, the test should be postponed for 4–6 weeks.

From CDC: Standards for pediatric immunization practice, *MMWR* 42(No RR-5):12-13, 1993.

Guide to Contraindications and Precautions to Vaccinations—cont'd

True contraindications and precautions	Not true (vaccines may be administered)
OPV¶	
Contraindications Infection with HIV or a household contact with HIV Known altered immunodeficiency (hematologic and solid tumors; congenital immunodeficiency; and long-term immunosuppressive therapy) Immunodeficient household contact **Precaution†** Pregnancy	Breast-feeding Current antimicrobial therapy Diarrhea
IPV	
Contraindication Anaphylactic reaction to neomycin or streptomycin **Precaution†** Pregnancy	
MMR¶	
Contraindication Anaphylactic reactions to egg ingestion and to neomycin** Pregnancy Known altered immunodeficiency (hematologic and solid tumors; congenital immunodeficiency; and long-term immunosuppressive therapy) **Precaution†** Recent (within 3 months) immune globulin administration	Tuberculosis or positive skin test Simultaneous TB skin testing†† Breast-feeding Pregnancy of mother of recipient Immunodeficient family member or household contact Infection with HIV Nonanaphylactic reactions to eggs or neomycin
Hib	
None identified	
HBV	
None identified	Pregnancy

APPENDIX 14-3
Accident Prevention at Various Age Levels

Typical accidents	Normal behavior characteristics	Precautions
First Year		
Falls	After several months of age can squirm and roll, and later creeps and pulls self erect	Do not leave alone on tables, etc., from where falls can occur
Inhalation of foreign objects	Places anything and everything in mouth	Keep crib sides up
Poisoning	Helpless in water	Keep small objects and harmful substances out of reach
Burns		Use infant car seat
Drowning		Have syrup of ipecac at home
Second Year		
Falls	Able to roam about in erect posture	Keep screens in windows
Drowning	Goes up and down stairs	Place gate at top of stairs
Motor vehicles	Has great curiosity	Cover unused electrical outlets; keep electric cords out of easy reach
Ingestion of poisonous substances	Puts almost everything in mouth	Keep in enclosed space when outdoors; not in company of an adult
Burns	Helpless in water	Keep medicines, household poisons, and small sharp objects out of sight
		Keep handles of pots and pans on stove out of reach and containers of hot food from edge of table
		Protect from water in tub and in pools
		Use safety belts and car seats
2-4 Years		
Falls	Able to open doors	Keep doors locked when there is danger of falls
Drowning	Runs and climbs	Place screen or guards in windows
Motor vehicles	Can ride tricycle	Teach about watching for automobiles in driveways and in streets
Ingestion of poisonous substances	Investigates closets and drawers	Keep firearms locked up
Burns	Plays with mechanical gadgets	Keep knives, electrical equipment out of reach
	Can throw ball and other objects	Teach about risks of throwing sharp objects and about danger of following balls into street
		Use safety belts and car seats
5-9 Years		
Motor vehicles	Daring and adventurous	Use seat belts
Bicycle accidents	Control over large muscles more advanced than control over small muscles	Teach techniques and traffic rules for cycling
Drowning		Encourage skills in swimming
Burns	Has increasing interest in group play; loyalty to group makes him willing to follow suggestions of leaders	Keep firearms locked up except when you can supervise their use
Firearms		

Modified from Vaughn VC, McKay RJ, Behrman RE, eds, and Nelson WE, senior ed: *Textbook of pediatrics,* ed 11, Philadelphia, 1979, Saunders, p. 264. Adapted from Shaffer TC: *Pediatr Clin North Am* 1:426-427, May 1954.

References

Alan Guttmacher Institute: *Blessed events and the bottom line: the financing of maternity care in the United States,* New York, 1987, The Institute.

Alan Guttmacher Institute: *Teenage pregnancy in the United States: the scope of the problem and state responses,* New York, 1989, The Institute.

Allen M, Brown P, and Finlay B: *Helping children by strengthening families: a look at family support programs,* Washington, D.C., 1992, Children's Defense Fund.

American Academy of Pediatrics, Committee on Infectious Diseases: Measles, reassessment of the current immunization policy, *Pediatrics* 84(6):110-113, 1984.

American Nurse: *Nursing represented on Clinton transition team,* 25:1, Washington, D.C., January 1993, American Nurses Association.

Arkin EB: The Healthy Mothers, Healthy Babies Coalition: four years of progress, *Public Health Rep* 101:147-156, 1986.

Athey J: *Pregnancy and childbearing among homeless adolescents: report of a workshop,* University of Pittsburgh, October 16-17, 1989, Public Health Social Work Training Program, Division of Public and Community Health Service.

Barnard KE and Erickson ML: *Teaching children with developmental problems,* St. Louis, 1976, Mosby.

Berendes H, Kessel S, and Yaffe S, eds: *Advances in the prevention of low birthweight: an international symposium,* Washington, D.C., 1991, National Center for Education in Maternal and Child Health.

Berry RK: Home care of the child with AIDS, *Pediatr Nurs* 14:341-344, 1988.

Bowling JM and Riley P: *Access to prenatal care in North Carolina,* Raleigh, N.C., 1987, North Carolina State Center for Health Statistics.

Bratic E: Healthy Mothers, Healthy Babies Coalition—a joint private-public initiative, *Public Health Rep* 97:503-509, 1982.

Brazelton TB: *The neonatal behavioral assessment scale,* Philadelphia, 1973, Lippincott.

Brown S: Drawing women into prenatal care, *Family Planning Perspect* 21(2):73-80, 88, 1989.

Bureau of the Census: Fertility of American women: June 1988, *Current Population Reports, Series P-20, No 436,* Washington, D.C., 1989, U.S. Government Printing Office.

Carpenter RG: Prevention of unexpected infant death, *Lancet* i:723-727, 1983.

Centers for Disease Control and Prevention (CDC): Childhood lead poisoning—United States: report to the Congress by the Agency for Toxic Substances and Disease Registry, *MMWR* 37(32):481-485, August 19, 1988.

CDC: *HIV/AIDS surveillance report,* January, 1990.

CDC: *HIV/AIDS surveillance report,* February 1993.

CDC: Lead poisoning associated with use of traditional ethnic remedies—California, 1991-1992, *MMWR* 42:521-524, 1993.

CDC: Pediatric Nutrition Surveillance System—United States, 1980-1991. In CDC surveillance summaries, *MMWR* 41(No. SS-7):1-24, 1992.

CDC: General recommendations on immunization: recommendations of the Immunization Practices Advisory Committee, *MMWR* 43(No. RR-1), January 28, 1994, entire issue.

CDC: Retrospective assessment of vaccination coverage among school-aged children—selected U.S. cities, 1991, *MMWR* 41:103-107, 1992.

CDC: *Preventing lead poisoning in young children: a statement by the Centers for Disease Control,* Atlanta, Ga., October 1991, USDHHS Public Health Service.

CDC: Progress toward achieving the national 1990 objectives for immunization, *MMWR* 37:613-617, October 1988.

CDC: State activities for prevention of lead poisoning among children—U.S., 1992, *MMWR* 42:165-172, 1993.

CDC: Standards for pediatric immunization practices, *MMWR* 42:(No. RR-5) 1-13, 1993.

CDC: Supplementary statement of contraindications to receipt of pertussis vaccine, *MMWR* 33:169-171, 1984.

Chadzynski L: *Manual for the identification and abatement of environment lead hazards,* Washington, D.C., 1986, Division of Maternal and Child Health.

Chamberlin RW, ed: *Beyond individual risk assessment: community wide approaches to promoting the health and development of families and children,* Washington, D.C., 1988, The National Center for Education in Maternal and Child Health.

Chan MM: Sudden infant death syndrome and families at risk, *Pediatr Nurs* 13(3):166-168, 1987.

Chatoor I, Dickson L, Schaefer S, and James E: A developmental classification of feeding disorders associated with failure to thrive: diagnosis and treatment. In Drotar D, ed: *New directions in failure to thrive,* New York, 1985, Plenum Press.

Child Nutrition Amendments of 1986, National Defense Authorization Act, Public Law 99-661.

Children's Safety Network: *A data book of child and adolescent injury,* Washington, D.C., 1991, National Center for Education in Maternal and Child Health.

Combating child abuse, *Congressional Q Almanac* 44:369, 1988.

Committee on Labor and Public Welfare, Subcommittee on Health, United States Congress (hearing): *School-age mothers and child health act,* 1975, Washington, D.C., November 4, 1975, U.S. Government Printing Office.

Congress of the United States, Office of Technology Assessment: *Healthy children: investing in the future. Summary,* Washington, D.C., 1987, U.S. Government Printing Office.

Coppens NM, Hunter PN, Bain JA, Gatewood AK, Gordon DA, and Mailloux MS: The relationship between elevated lead levels and enrollment in special education, *Family Commun Health* 12(4):39-46, 1990.

Dangelmaier A: Lilly's anger. In Zewekh J, Primomo J, and Deal L, eds: *Opening doors: stories of public health nursing,* Olympia, Wash., 1992, Washington State Department of Health, Parent-Child Health Services, pp. 41-45.

Drummond AH: Lead poisoning in children, *J School Health* 51:43-47, 1981.

Editorial: The valley of the shadow of birth, *Am J Public Health* 73(6):635-637, 1983.

Erickson ML: *Assessment and management of developmental changes in children,* St. Louis, 1976, Mosby.

Francis MB: Homeless families: rebuilding connections, *Publ Health Nurs* 8(2):90-96, 1991.

Garbarino J: The human ecology method of child maltreatment: a conceptual model for research, *J Marriage family* 39:721-735, 1977.

Garner MK: Our values are showing: inadequate childhood immunization, *Health values: achieving high level wellness* 2:129-133, 1978.

General Accounting Office: *Federally funded health services: information on seven programs serving low-income women and children,* GAO/HRD-92-73FS, Gaithersburg, Md., May 1992, The office.

General Accounting Office: *Home visiting: a promising early intervention strategy for at-risk families,* GAO/HRD-90-83, Gaithersburg, Md., July 1990, Author.

Gordon M: *Manual of nursing diagnosis 1993-1994,* St. Louis, 1993, Mosby.

Gruis M: Beyond maternity: postpartum concerns of mothers, *Am J Maternal Child Health* 2:182-188, 1977.

Health Care Financing Administration (HCFA): *State Medicaid manual, part 5: early and periodic screening, diagnosis, and treatment (EPSDT),* HCFA Pub No 45-4, Baltimore, Md., 1988, Printing and Publications Branch, Office of Management and Budget.

"Healthy mothers" market research: how to reach black and Mexican American women, Contract No 232-81-0082. Submitted to USDHHS, PHS, September 14, 1982 by Juarez and Associates, Inc., 12139 National Blvd, Los Angeles, Calif.

Hoekelman RA, Blatman S, Brunell PA, Friedman SB, and Seidel HM: *Principles of pediatrics: health care of the young,* New York, 1978, McGraw-Hill.

Hogue CR and Hargraves MA: Class, race, and infant mortality in the United States, *Am J Public Health* 83(1):9-11, 1993.

Hopp JW and Rogers EA: *AIDS and the allied health professions,* Philadelphia, 1989, FA Davis.

Interagency Committee to Improve Access to Immunization Services: The Public Health Service action plan to improve access to immunization services, *Public Health Reports* 107(3):243-251, May-June 1992.

Institute of Medicine: *Preventing low birthweight,* Washington, D.C., 1985, National Academy Press.

Johnson CM, Miranda L, Sherman A, and Weill JD: *Child poverty in America,* Washington, D.C., 1991, Children's Defense Fund.

Kennell J, Voos D, and Klaus M: Parent infant bonding. In Helfer RE and Kempe CH, eds: *Child abuse and neglect: the family and the community,* Cambridge, Mass., 1976, Ballinger.

Klaus MH and Kennell JH: *Maternal-infant bond,* St. Louis, 1976, Mosby.

Kleinman J: *Perinatal and infant mortality, recent trends in the United States, proceedings of the international collaborative effort perinatal and infant mortality, vol 1,* DHHS Pub No. (PHS) 85-1252, Hyattsville, Md., 1985, National Center for Health Statistics.

Koop CE: Excerpt from keynote address. In Silverman BK, ed: *Report of the Surgeon General's workshop on children with HIV infection and their families,* DHHS Pub No HRS-D-MO 87-1, 1987, pp. 3-5.

Kramer MS: The etiology and prevention of low birthweight: current knowledge and priorities for future research. In Berendes H, Kessel S, and Yaffe S, eds: *Advances in the prevention of low birthweight: an international symposium,* Washington, D.C., 1990, National Center for Education in Maternal and Child Health.

Macro Systems, Inc.: *One stop shopping for perinatal services: identification and assessment of implementation methodologies,* Washington, D.C., 1990, National Center for Education in Maternal and Child Health.

Masis KB and May PM: A comprehensive local program for the prevention of fetal alcohol syndrome, *Public Health Reports* 106(5):484-494, 1991.

Mason JO: Today's challenges to the Public Health Service and to the nation, *Public Health Reports* 106(5):473-477, 1991.

Mihaly LK: *Homeless families: failed policies and young victims,* Wash-ington, D.C., January 1991, Children's Defense Fund Child, Youth and Family Futures Clearinghouse.

Milio N: *9226 Kercheval: the storefront that did not burn,* Ann Arbor, 1970, University of Michigan Press.

Miller CA, Fine A, Adams-Taylor S, and Schorr LB: *Monitoring children's health: key indicators,* Washington, D.C., 1986, American Public Health Association.

Murphy E: Celebrating the Bill of Rights in the year of Rust vs. Sullivan, *Nurs Outlook* 39(5):238-239, 1991.

National Center for Health Statistics: Advance report of final natality statistics, 1986, *Monthly Vital Stat Rep* 37(3), Hyattsville, Md., 1988, The Center.

National Commission to Prevent Infant Mortality: *Home visiting: opening doors for America's pregnant women and children,* Washington, D.C., 1989, The Commission.

National Commission to Prevent Infant Mortality: *Infant mortality and the media,* Washington, D.C., May 1988, The Commission.

National Commission to Prevent Infant Mortality: *1985 indirect costs of infant mortality and low birthweight,* Washington, D.C., May 1988, The Commission.

National Commission to Prevent Infant Mortality: *Death before life: the tragedy of infant mortality,* Washington, D.C., August 1988, The Commission.

National Institute on Disability and Rehabilitation Research: *Chartbook on disability in the United States, an Info Use report,* Washington, D.C., 1989, The Institute.

National Safety Council: *Accident facts, 1991 edition,* Chicago, 1991, The Council.

National SIDS Clearinghouse: *Fact sheet: what is SIDS?* McLean, Va., 1989, The Clearinghouse.

Oliva G, Fahrner R, Sokal K, and Weeams R: *Women and infants at risk for HIV infection: guidelines and protocols for prevention and care,* San Francisco, 1989, Department of Public Health, Family Health Bureau, Perinatal AIDS Project.

Pickett G and Hanlon JJ: *Public health administration and practice,* St. Louis, 1990, Mosby.

Prevention Briefs: Lead poisoning threat to 1 in 25 preschoolers, *Public Health Rep* 98(1):51, 1983.

Robert Wood Johnson Foundation: *Challenges in health care: a chartbook perspective 1991,* Princeton, N.J., 1991, The Foundation.

Rogers MF: Transmission of human immunodeficiency virus infection in the United States. In Silverman BK, ed: *Report of the Surgeon General's workshop on children with HIV infection and their families,* DHHS Pub No HRS-D-MC 87-1, Rockville, Md., 1987, USDHHS, Division of Maternal and Child Health, pp. 17-19.

Rosenbaum S, Layton C, and Liu J: *The health of America's children,* 1991, Children's Defense Fund.

Schneider J, Aurori B, Armenti L, and Soltanoff D: Impact of community screening on diagnosis, treatment and medical findings of lead poisoning in children, *Public Health Rep* 96:143-149, March-April 1981.

Scipien GM, Barnard MU, Chard MA, Howe J, and Phillips PJ: *Comprehensive pediatric nursing,* ed 3, New York, 1986, McGraw-Hill.

Selecting a safe day care center. Solving the day care puzzle: how to choose the safest center for your child, *Pennsylvania Nurse* 47(10):32, Harrisburg, Penn., October 1992, Pennsylvania Nurses Association.

Selwyn BJ: An epidemiological approach to the study of users and nonusers of child health services, *Am J Public Health* 68:231-235, 1978.

Shaheen E, Alexander D, and Barbero GJ: Failure to thrive: a retrospective profile. In Schwartz JL and Schwartz LH, eds: *Vulnerable infants: a psychosocial dilemma,* New York, 1977, McGraw-Hill.

Smith LL: Coping with disability. Nurse administrators' obligations under the Americans with Disabilities Act, *J Nursing Admin* 22(3):29-31, 1992.

Task Force on Infant Mortality: *Infant mortality in Michigan,* Lansing, Mich., 1987, Michigan Department of Public Health.

U.S. Congress, Office of Technology Assessment: *Technology dependent children: hospital v. home care—a technical memorandum,* OTA-TM-H-38, Washington, D.C., May 1987, U.S. Government Printing Office.

U.S. Congress, Office of Technology Assessment: *Healthy children: investing in the future,* OTA-H-345, Washington, D.C., 1988, U.S. Government Printing Office.

U.S. Department of Health Education and Welfare (USDHEW): *Healthy people, the Surgeon General's report on health promotion and disease prevention,* DHEW Pub No PHS 79-55071, Washington, D.C., 1979, U.S. Government Printing Office.

US Department of Health and Human Services (USDHHS), Administration for Children and Families: *Child abuse and neglect: a shared community concern,* DHHS Pub No (ACF)92-30531, Washington, D.C., March 1992, U.S. Government Printing Office.

USDHHS, Children's Bureau: *National Center on child abuse and neglect: research symposium on child neglect, February 23-25, 1988,* Washington, D.C., 1988, U.S. Government Printing Office.

USDHHS, Public Health Service: *Child health USA '91,* DHHS Pub No HRS-M-CH-91-1, Washington, D.C., 1991, U.S. Government Printing Office.

USDHHS, Public Health Service: *Child health USA '92,* DHHS Pub No. HRS-M-CH-92-6, Washington, D.C., March 1993, U.S. Government Printing Office.

USDHHS, Public Health Service: *Health of the disadvantaged chart book-II,* DHHS Pub No (HRA) 80-633, Washington, D.C., 1980, Health Resources and Services Administration.

USDHHS, National Institutes of Health: *National cholesterol education program: report of the expert panel on blood cholesterol levels in children and adolescents,* NIH Pub. No. 91-277732, Washington, D.C., September 1991, U.S. Government Printing Office.

USDHHS, Public Health Service: *Health status of the disadvantaged. Chartbook 1990,* DHHS Pub No (HRSA) HRS-P-DV 90-1, Washington, D.C., 1990, U.S. Government Printing Office.

USDHHS, Public Health Service: *Healthy people 2000: national health promotion and disease prevention objectives, full report, with commentary,* Washington, D.C., 1991, U.S. Government Printing Office.

USDHHS: *Promoting health, preventing disease: objectives for the nation,* Washington, D.C., 1980, U.S. Government Printing Office.

USDHHS, Public Health Service: *Prevention '84/'85,* Washington, D.C., 1985, U.S. Government Printing Office.

USDHHS, Public Health Service: *Recommendations of the Immunization Practices Advisory Committee: general recommendations on immunization,* Atlanta, Ga., 1989, CDC.

USDHHS, Public Health Service: *Recommendations of the Immunization Practices Advisory Committee: Hepatitis B. virus—a comprehensive strategy for eliminating transmission in the United States through universal childhood vaccination,* Atlanta, Ga., 1991, CDC.

USDHHS, Office of Disease Prevention and Health Promotion: *The 1990 health objectives for the nation: a midcourse review,* Washington, D.C., 1986, U.S. Government Printing Office.

USDHHS: *Health status of minorities and low income groups,* DHHS Pub No (HRSA) HRS-P-DV 85-1, Washington, D.C., 1986, Health Resources and Services Administration.

USDHHS: *Prevention '86/'87: federal programs and progress,* Washington, D.C., 1987, U.S. Government Printing Office.

USDHHS, Administration for Children, Youth and Families: *Child Abuse, Prevention, Adoption and Services Act of 1988,* Washington, D.C., 1988, U.S. Government Printing Office.

USDHHS, Public Health Service: *The Surgeon General's report on nutrition and health,* DHHS (PHS) Pub No 88-5021, Washington, D.C., 1988, U.S. Government Printing Office.

USDHHS, Public Health Service: *Parents' guide to childhood immunization,* Atlanta, Ga., 1988, CDC.

USDHHS, Public Health Service: *Promoting health/preventing disease: year 2000 objectives for the nation (draft for public review and comment),* Washington, D.C., 1989, U.S. Government Printing Office.

USDHHS, Office of Maternal and Child Health: *Child health USA '89,* Washington, D.C., 1989, U.S. Government Printing Office.

Vaughn VC, McKay RJ, and Behrman RE, eds, and Nelson WE, senior ed: *Textbook of pediatrics,* ed 11, Philadelphia, 1979, Saunders.

Wald L: *The house on Henry Street,* New York, 1915, Holt.

Whaley LF and Wong DL: *Nursing care of infants and children,* ed 4, St. Louis, 1991, Mosby.

World Health Organization (WHO): *Air quality guidelines for Europe, Copenhagen,* 1987, WHO Regional Office for Europe, pp. 242-261.

Selected Bibliography

Ahmann E: *Home care for the high risk infant: a holistic guide to using technology,* Rockville, Md., 1986, Aspen.

Bomar PJ: Perspectives on family health promotion, *Family Commun Health* 12(4):1-11, 1990.

Children's Defense Fund: *The nation's investment in children: an analysis of the president's FY 1990 budget proposals,* Washington, D.C., 1989, The Fund.

Flage L: Changing household structure, child-care availability, and employment among mothers of preschool children, *J Marriage Family* 51:51-63, 1989.

Kamerman SB: Toward a child policy decade. *Child Welfare* 68:371-390, 1989.

Kodadek S: When a child is handicapped: parents' perspectives on the experience. In *Family Nursing Continuing Education Project, Nursing of families' acute or chronic illness,* Portland, Ore., 1988, Oregon Health Sciences University.

Kryder-Coe JH, Solomon LM, and Molnar J, eds: *Homeless children and youth: a new American dilemma,* New Brunswick, N.J., 1991, Transaction Publishers.

Mason JO: Reducing infant mortality in the United States through "Healthy Start", *Public Health Reports* 106(5):479-483, 1991.

Notkin S, Rosenthal B, and Hopper K: *Families on the move: breaking the cycle of homelessness,* New York, 1990, Edna McConnell Clark Foundation.

Radecki SE: A racial and ethnic comparison of family formation and contraceptive practices among low income women, *Public Health Reports* 106(5):494-501, 1991.

Planning Health Services for the School-Age Child

OBJECTIVES

Upon completion of this chapter, the reader should be able to:

1. Identify the rights of children as delineated in the Children's Charter.
2. Explain how fluctuations in the birth rates since World War II have affected health planning for the school-age population.
3. Describe the major childhood mortality and morbidity risks and the community health nurse's role in decreasing these risks.
4. Discuss the role of the community health nurse when working with families who have children with chronic handicapping conditions.
5. Analyze select psychosocial problems of childhood and adolescence and discuss community health nursing interventions for addressing these problems.

6. Discuss the components of a comprehensive school health program.
7. Describe the role of the community health nurse in the school setting.
8. Summarize how health and educational legislation affect the delivery of health care services to the school-age population.
9. Compare and contrast role responsibilities of select disciplines on the school health team.
10. Formulate guidelines for implementing community health nursing role responsibilities in the school setting.

Children are one-third of our population and all of our future.

SELECT PANEL FOR THE PROMOTION OF
CHILD HEALTH (1981)

During the twentieth century a concerted effort has been made to improve the health status of all children. However, the goals of the 1930 Children's Charter (refer to the box on p. 552-553)—which emphasized that children, regardless of their race, color, or creed (Figure 15-1) should have an environment and life experiences allowing them to develop to their fullest potential—are still far from realized.

Since the turn of the century there have been major achievements in relation to the health status of school-age children and the services provided for them. In the early 1960s Wallace noted three particularly noteworthy advances: (1) a decrease in mortality in this age category; (2) the expansion of organized school health services; and (3) the recognition that adolescents have special problems and needs (Wallace, 1962, p. 25). Despite these accomplishments, there remains a sizable number of children who will never reach their fullest potential. Although health care in the United States is considered a right rather than a privilege, there is still failure to meet the health needs of specific segments of the population. Children of racial minorities, children from poor, central-city, and rural families, and children with handicapping conditions continue to have a high incidence of mortality and morbidity. They also use health care services less frequently than the population as a whole (Director's Task Force on Minority Health, 1988; U.S. Congress, OTA, 1988; USDHHS, Office of Disease Prevention and Health Promotion, 1986; USDHHS, Office of Maternal and Child Health, 1989). Evidence indicates that children are increasingly being underserved by the U.S. health care system (Alan Guttmacher Institute, 1987; National Commission to Prevent Infant Mortality, 1989; U.S. Congress, OTA). Improving children's access to health care will be a major challenge for health professionals throughout the next decade.

Providing effective and efficient health and welfare services for all segments of the school-age population is no easy task. Demographic, vital, and morbidity statistics reveal that professionals need to deal with an array of health risks when planning health and welfare services for this population group. The following review of these risks clearly illustrates the complex nature of the difficulties encountered when health care professionals work with school-age children.

Historically, community health nurses have assumed a major role in developing child health services. Lillian Wald initiated a special project in New York City schools in 1902 to demonstrate to city officials the value of preventive health counseling in relation to the needs of school-age children (Kalisch and Kalisch, 1986). Since that time, nursing services to meet the needs of our youth have grown steadily. Community health nurses are now working with children in a variety of settings, including their homes, schools, clinics, and residential settings for special aggregates at risk. In order to plan nursing services for children in a variety of settings, the community health nurse must have knowledge about their needs and an understanding of the range of services required to meet these needs.

DEMOGRAPHIC, VITAL, AND MORBIDITY STATISTICS

Knowledge and use of statistical data about this age group are essential for the nurse to carry out effective health planning and implementation activities. Statistical data help the community health nurse to identify how many people need nursing services and what type of services can best help the population to resolve its health problems (refer to Chapter 11). Since health needs and services differ with age, it is important to analyze the composition of the population and the mortality and morbidity statistics specific to the particular age group under consideration.

Composition of the Population

One of the most significant characteristics of a country's population composition is age structure. It is important to examine this variable because health risks are frequently age-related, and the absolute number of people in a particular age category influences the amount of resources needed to provide adequate health care services.

The age structure of the population in the United States has been changing. Fluctuations in the birth rates since World War II and dramatic changes in life

◀ *The Children's Charter* ▶

President Hoover's White House Conference on Child Health and Protection, recognizing the rights of the child as the first rights of citizenship, pledges itself to these aims for the children of America.

I For every child spiritual and moral training to help him to stand firm under the pressure of life

II For every child understanding and the guarding of his personality as his most precious right

III For every child a home and that love and security which a home provides; and for that child who must receive foster care, the nearest substitute for his own home

IV For every child full preparation for his birth, his mother receiving prenatal, natal, and postnatal care; and the establishment of such protective measures as will make childbearing safer

V For every child health protection from birth through adolescence, including: periodical health examinations and, where needed, care of specialists and hospital treatment; regular dental examinations and care of the teeth; protective and preventive measures against communicable diseases; the insuring of pure food, pure milk, and pure water

VI For every child from birth through adolescence, promotion of health, including health instruction and a health program, wholesome physical and mental recreation, with teachers and leaders adequately trained

VII For every child a dwelling-place safe, sanitary, and wholesome, with reasonable provisions for privacy; free from conditions which tend to thwart his development; and a home environment harmonious and enriching

VIII For every child a school which is safe from hazards, sanitary, properly equipped, lighted, and ventilated. For younger children nursery schools and kindergartens to supplement home care

IX For every child a community which recognizes and plans for his needs, protects him against physical dangers, moral hazards, and disease; provides him with safe and wholesome places for play and recreation; and makes provision for his cultural and social needs

X For every child an education which, through the discovery and development of his individual abilities, prepares him for life; and through

training and vocational guidance prepares him for living which will yield him the maximum of satisfaction

XI For every child such teaching and training as will prepare him for successful parenthood, home-making, and the rights of citizenship; and, for parents, supplementary training to fit them to deal wisely with the problems of parenthood

XII For every child education for safety and protection against accidents to which modern conditions subject him—those to which he is directly exposed and those which, through loss or maiming of his parents, affect him indirectly

XIII For every child who is blind, deaf, crippled, or otherwise physically handicapped, and for the child who is mentally handicapped, such measures as will early discover and diagnose his handicap, provide care and treatment, and so train him that he may become an asset to society rather than a liability. Expenses of these services should be borne publicly where they cannot be privately met

XIV For every child who is in conflict with society the right to be dealt with intelligently as society's charge, not society's outcast; with the home, the school, the church, the court and the institution when needed, shaped to return him whenever possible to the normal stream of life

XV For every child the right to grow up in a family with an adequate standard of living and the security of a stable income as the surest safeguard against social handicaps

XVI For every child protection against labor that stunts growth, either physical or mental, that limits education, that deprives children of the right of comradeship, of play, and of joy

XVII For every rural child as satisfactory schooling and health services as for the city child, and an extension to rural families of social, recreational, and cultural facilities

XVIII To supplement the home and the school in the training of youth, and to return to them those interests of which modern life tends to cheat children, every stimulation and encouragement should be given to the extension and development of the voluntary youth organizations

Continued

XIX To make everywhere available these minimum protections of the health and welfare of children, there should be a district, county, or community organization for health, education, and welfare, with full-time officials, coordinating with a statewide program which will be responsive to a nationwide service of general information, statistics, and scientific research. This should include:

(a) Trained, full-time public health officials, with public health nurses, sanitary inspection, and laboratory workers

(b) Available hospital beds

(c) Full-time public welfare service for the relief, aid, and guidance of children in special need due to poverty, misfortune, or behavior difficulties, and for the protection of children from abuse, neglect, exploitation, or moral hazard

For every child these rights, regardless of race, or color, or situation, wherever he may live under the protection of the American Flag.

expectancy have significantly altered the age distribution in the nation over the past three decades. Table 15-1 illustrates the changes that have occurred since 1960. Overall, aging of the population is evident. In 1991 the median age reached a high of 34.3 years. The increasing median age is driven by the aging of the population born during the "baby boom" (1946 to 1964) after World War II (U.S. Bureau of the Census, 1993, Population Profile).

Changing birth rates have greatly influenced the distribution of the school-age population in the past 30 years. The decrease in the number of preschool children, from 11.2 percent in 1960 to 7.4 percent in 1975, and the increase in the 18-to-65-year-old population during the same period are the direct result of these changes. The baby boom immediately following World War II expanded the preschool population in the 1960s and the 18-and-above population group in the 1970s. The declining birth rate of the 1970s is reflected in the decline of the 1975 preschool percent distribution. The decline in the overall U.S. birth rate has, however, leveled off since the mid-1970s. "The annual *number* of births during 1989-1991 was the highest experienced in the United States since the peak Baby Boom years of 1954 to 1964" (U.S. Bureau of the Census, 1993, Population Profile, pp. 2-3). Births increased during this time period due to increased rates of childbearing—not because of increases in the number of women of childbearing age (U.S. Bureau of the Census, Population Profile).

Shifts in the age distribution of a population in such a short time present special difficulties for health professionals. This is especially true when they are attempting to predict what health services are needed

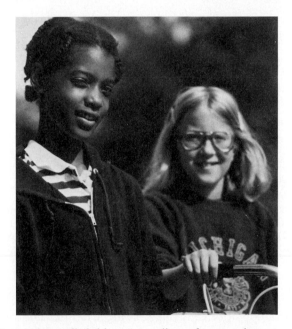

Figure 15-1 All children, regardless of race, color, or creed, need positive life experiences in order to develop to their fullest potential.

for a specific age group in the future. When birth rates fluctuate it is easy to have either an overabundance or an underabundance of health personnel and services. Health professionals in the 1950s and 1960s, for example, were underequipped to handle the number of school-age children resulting from the postwar baby boom.

What the future holds is unknown. The fluctuations in birth rates and fertility in the United States over the last four decades illustrate that family-size preference has varied in response to financial and

15-1 Number of Resident Population by Age, Sex, and Race, United States, 1960, 1970, 1975, 1980, 1985, 1991*

Sex, age, and race	Unit	Year					
		1960	1970	1975	1980	1985	1991
Total							
Both sexes, all ages	Million	180.7	203.3	215.5	226.5	241.1	252.6
Age Distribution							
Under 5 years old	Million	20.3	17.2	16.1	16.3	18.0	19.2
5-17 years old	Million	44.2	52.5	51.0	47.4	45.0	45.9
18 years old and over	Million	116.1	133.5	148.3	162.8	175.7	187.5
25-34 years old	Million	22.9	24.9	31.3	37.1	42.0	43.1
35-44 years old	Million	24.2	23.1	22.8	25.6	31.8	39.4
45-64 years old	Million	36.2	41.8	43.8	44.5	44.9	46.8
65 years old and over	Million	16.6	20.0	22.7	25.5	28.5	31.8
Median age	Year	29.4	28.0	28.7	30.0	31.5	34.4
Racial Distribution							
White	Million	160.0	178.1	187.2	194.8	202.8	NA
Black	Million	19.0	22.6	24.7	26.6	28.9	NA
Percent of resident population	Percent black	11.0	11.1	11.5	11.8	12.2	12.4
Persons of Spanish origin	Million	NA†	9.1	NA	14.6	16.9	NA

Resident population as of July 1.
†NA, not available.
1960 Data from U.S. Bureau of the Census: *U.S.A. statistics in brief, 1978: a statistical abstract supplement,* Washington, D.C., 1978, U.S. Department of Commerce, unnumbered pages; 1970 through 1987 data from U.S. Bureau of the Census: *U.S.A. statistics in brief, 1988: a statistical abstract supplement,* Washington, D.C., 1988, U.S. Department of Commerce, unnumbered pages; 1991 data are from U.S. Bureau of the Census: *Statistical abstract of the United States: 1992,* ed 112, Washington, D.C., 1992, U.S. Government Printing Office; and U.S. Bureau of the Census: *Population profile of the United States: 1993,* Current Population Reports, Series P23-185, Washington, D.C., 1993, U.S. Government Printing Office.

social conditions and can do so in the future. "The total fertility rate is the number of births 1,000 women would have if they were to experience the fertility rates at each age prevailing in a particular year" (U.S. Bureau of the Census, 1993, Population profile, p. 3.) The total fertility rates for 1990-1991 were higher than any seen in the United States since the early 1970s (U.S. Bureau of the Census, Population profile). A difference of only one additional child per family can have a tremendous impact on the range of services needed for the school-age population in the future.

Figure 15-2 displays the U.S. population by age group in 1991. Although the 21-years-and-under age group is declining relative to other age groups in the population, the absolute number of children in this age range is increasing. "Between 1980 and 1991, there

was a 14.4% increase in the number of children under 5 years of age" (USDHHS, 1993, Child Health USA '92, p. 9). There were about 25 million more children younger than 22 in 1991 than in 1950 (USDHHS, Child Health USA '92, p. 9).

A younger school population is evolving. The increasing demand for preprimary school enrollment presented real challenges for the health and educational systems in the 1980s and is projected to do so in the future. The number of children 3 or 4 years old enrolled in nursery school increased from 1.0 to 2.6 million between 1970 and 1991; the proportion increased from 14.1% in 1970 to 34.1% in 1991 (U.S. Bureau of the Census, 1993, Population Profile, p. 12).

In 1991 there were 63.9 million students enrolled in school, including 14.1 million college students. The

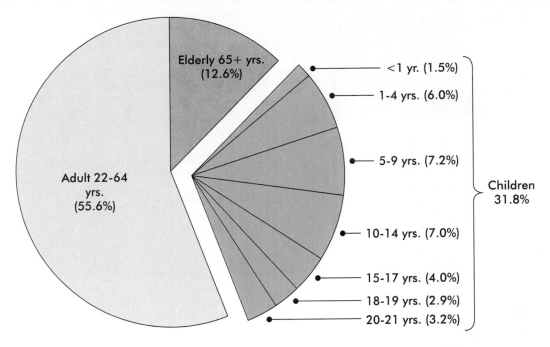

Figure 15-2 U.S. population by age group: 1991. (From USDHHS: *Child health USA '92,* Washington, D.C., 1993, U.S. Government Printing Office, p. 9.)

box at right displays the number of students at each level. These numbers are certainly not small and support the need to plan *organized* health services that address the primary health care needs of students at various development stages. When planning for these health services it is imperative to analyze local and national statistics, since there are striking differences in the birth and fertility rates in different segments of the population. Between 1990 and 1991, for example, the nation's under-5 population grew by 2.5%, but in some states (District of Columbia, Nevada, and California) the rate of increase was over 5% (U.S. Bureau of the Census, 1993, Population profile, p. 7).

Community health nurses who work with the school-age population encounter a variety of physical, psychosocial, cultural, environmental, and developmental health problems and concerns. Because this chapter emphasizes planning health services, only general morbidity and mortality statistics and growth and development data will be presented here. The reader can obtain a comprehensive understanding of childhood problems and specific growth and development characteristics by referring to *Nursing Care of Infants and Children* (Whaley and Wong, 1991).

Total School Enrollment in 1991 (in Millions)

All ages	**63.9**
Nursery school	2.9
Kindergarten	4.2
Elementary (1-8)	29.6
High school (9-12)	13.1
College	14.1

From U.S. Bureau of the Census: *Population profile of the United States: 1993,* Current population reports, Series P23-185, Washington, D.C., 1993, U.S. Government Printing Office, p. 12.

Childhood Mortality Risks

The leading causes of deaths by specific childhood age groups are presented in Figure 15-3. Injuries, cancer, congenital anomalies, homicide, and diseases of the heart are the leading causes of death for children ages 1 to 9 years old. For children ages 10 to 19, suicide replaces heart disease as a major killer. Although childhood mortality rates have substantially declined in the past several decades, death rates attributed to

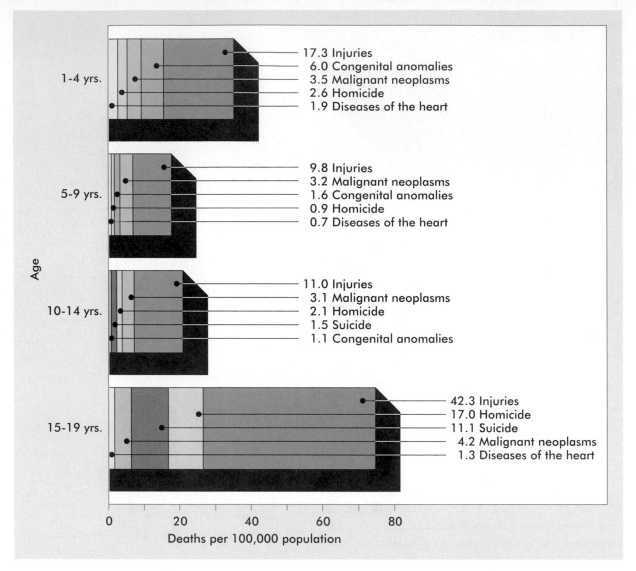

Figure 15-3   Leading causes of childhood deaths by age groups: 1990. (Modified from USDHHS: *Child health USA '92,* Washington, D.C., 1993, U.S. Government Printing Office, pp. 22, 31.)

suicide and homicides have increased significantly since 1960.

When reviewing statistical data such as those presented in Figure 15-3, keep in mind that these rates vary significantly within segments of the population. For example, the homicide rate for black adolescents ages 15 to 19 is over eight times the rate for their white counterparts. Conversely, the rate of suicide in 15 to 19-year-olds is almost twice as high for white adolescents as for black teens (USDHHS, 1993, Child Health USA '92, p. 31).

It is striking to note (refer to Figure 15-3) that the majority of childhood deaths could be prevented. It

has long been recognized that environmental, social, and behavioral factors greatly influence the occurrence of mortality across the life span. It was noted in our first national health plan that approximately "50 percent of our United States' deaths are due to unhealthy behavior or lifestyle; 20 percent to environmental factors; 20 percent to human biological factors; and only 10 percent to inadequacies in health care" (USDHEW, 1979, p. 9).

Injuries

Although deaths from unintentional injury have declined significantly since 1950, injuries remain the leading cause of death for children of all ages. Motor vehicle accidents are the single largest contributing cause of injury deaths for children of any age (USDHHS, 1993, Child Health USA '92, p. 22). Adolescents are particularly at risk for motor vehicle–related injuries; for adolescents ages 15 to 19 years, the death rate for this cause is at least five times the rate for any other childhood age category of unintentional injury deaths. The rate of motor vehicle deaths for white adolescents ages 15 to 19 is almost twice that of blacks (USDHHS, Child Health USA '92, p. 32).

Following motor vehicle accidents, fires and related burns and drowning are also leading causes of childhood unintentional injury deaths. Children ages 1 to 4 have the highest death rates from these causes, with rates approximately three times the rate for children ages 5 to 9 (USDHHS, 1993, Child Health USA '92, p. 23). Among children under 5, drownings occur most frequently in swimming pools and home spas. Household fires are a particular risk to children, with children under 5 who live in substandard housing at special risk (USDHHS, 1991, Healthy People 2000, p. 13).

A significant challenge for community health professionals in the next decade is to find ways to reduce fatalities from injuries. An important role of the community health nurse is to promote driving safety among adolescents and young adults, including identifying at-risk individuals. Driving without wearing a seat belt or while under the influence of alcohol or other drugs increases an individual's risk for becoming a motor vehicle fatality. Data reflect that a significant number of adolescents engage in risk-taking behaviors. Less than one fourth (24.3%) of all students in grades 9-12 who participated in the national school-based Youth Risk Behavior Survey (YRBS) in 1990 "always" used safety belts when riding in a motor vehicle driven by someone else (CDC, 1992, Safety-Belt, p. 111). Although the estimated number of alcohol-involved drivers in fatal crashes has decreased significantly since 1982, the year alcohol-related traffic crash data first became available, alcohol use among youth is still a major concern. National survey results on drug use for 1992 reflect that seven of eight students (88%) have tried alcohol by twelfth grade and more than half of all seniors (51%) have used it in just the past month. Thirty percent of twelfth graders in this study reported being drunk in the past 30 days (Johnston, O'Malley, and Bachman, 1993, National Survey, p. 45).

The community health nurse can also assume a major role in preventing accidents and injuries in younger school-age children through health education activities designed to prevent poisonings, fires, falls, and other causes of accidents. The Consumer Product Safety Commission (1-800-638-CPSC) provides material on consumer product safety including product hazards, product defects, and injuries sustained in using products. This information can help the nurse to plan sound educational programs. The National Child Safety Council Childwatch (1-800-222-1464) answers questions and distributes literature on safety and sponsors the Missing Kids program (publicized through milk cartons).

Homicide

In 1974, for the first time in our country's history, homicide became a major killer of children and young adults. Since 1960 the rate of homicide has nearly tripled and has become the fourth leading cause of death of children ages 1-9; for adolescents 10-14 it ranks third, and for youth 15-19 it is the second leading cause of death. As previously mentioned, black adolescents ages 15-19 have a significantly higher homicide death rate than whites (USDHHS, 1993, Child Health USA '92, p. 31). The homicide rate for Hispanic and American Indians/Alaska Natives in reservation states is also much higher than the rate for the general population (USDHHS, 1991, Healthy People 2000, p. 228). Children at special risk among all ethnic and minority groups are presented in the box on p. 558.

Certainly no one factor accounts for the increase in homicide among children. Poverty has been identified as a critical variable because of the high incidence of homicide among impoverished ethnic and minority groups. The use, manufacture, and distribution of drugs is another important factor associated with homicide (USDHHS, 1991, Healthy People 2000, p. 239). Family breakup, the availability of handguns, characteristics of adolescence that make a teenager prone to violence, and societal attitudes that portray violence as an acceptable conflict resolution strategy are some other factors that should be considered when planning strategies to reduce childhood mortality resulting from violence (USDHHS, Office of Disease Prevention and Health Promotion, 1986; USDHHS, Office of Maternal and Child Health, 1986; National Committee for Injury Prevention and Control and Education Development Center, 1989).

Community health nurses must work closely with all agencies in the community to *prevent* homicide in

◀ *Children At Risk for Homicide* ▶

Youth with high-risk behaviors
- Juvenile offenders
- Youth with histories of fighting or victimization
- Drug/alcohol abusers
- Drug dealers
- Weapon carriers
- Gang members
- School dropouts
- Unemployed youth
- Homeless youth
- Relocated and immigrant youth
- Youth living in poverty

Young children (10 years or less)
- Abused or neglected children
- Children who have witnessed violence
- Children with behavioral problems
- Children living in poverty

From USDHHS: *Healthy People 2000: national health promotion and disease prevention objectives, full report, with commentary,* Washington, D.C., 1991, U.S. Government Printing Office, p. 228-229; National Center for Injury Prevention and Control: *The prevention of youth violence: a framework for community action,* Atlanta, GA, 1993, Centers for Disease Control and Prevention, p. 6.

the school-age population. Comprehensive programs to prevent childhood homicide must involve many sectors of the community and multiple approaches to the problem. Activities for preventing youth violence usually employ one of three general prevention strategies: education, legal and regulatory change, and environmental modification (National Center for Injury Prevention and Control, 1993, p. 11). The box below displays examples of interventions used under each strategy category. Community health nurses assume a significant role in planning and implementing violence control interventions.

Suicide

Since 1960 the incidence of suicide among youth has been steadily increasing; it was the third leading cause of death for persons ages 15 to 19 in 1990, and the fourth leading cause of death for children 10 to 14 years of age (USDHHS, 1993, Child Health USA '92, p. 31). Suicide is a large contributor to death in adolescents; the suicide rate has more than tripled among youth in the past 30 years (CDC, 1992, Youth suicide prevention, p. 2).

Health professionals view suicide as a problem of extreme importance in the adolescent population be-

◀ *Activities to Prevent Youth Violence* ▶

Education

Adult mentoring
Conflict resolution
Training in social skills
Firearm safety
Parenting centers
Peer education
Public information and education campaigns

Legal/Regulatory Change

Regulate the use of and access to weapons
- Weaponless schools
- Control of concealed weapons
- Restrictive licensing
- Appropriate sale of guns

Regulate the use of and access to alcohol
- Appropriate sale of alcohol
- Prohibition or control of alcohol sales at events
- Training of servers

Other types of regulations
- Appropriate punishment in schools
- Dress codes

Environmental Modification

Modify the social environment
- Home visitation
- Preschool programs such as Head Start
- Therapeutic activities
- Recreational activities
- Work/academic experiences

Modify the physical environment
- Make risk areas visible
- Increase use of an area
- Limit building entrances and exits
- Create sense of ownership

From National Center for Injury Prevention and Control: *The prevention of youth violence: a framework for community action,* Atlanta, Ga., 1993, Centers for Disease Control and Prevention, p. 11.

cause it is an indicator that social, emotional, and physical stress is great. Rapidly changing societal values, population mobility, and economic pressures have presented adolescents with decision-making conflicts that result in uncertainty and stress (refer to Figure 15-4).

The extent of the suicide problem is much greater than the recorded figures indicate. Because suicide is viewed by our culture as a cowardly and disgraceful act, it is often concealed by families and medical personnel. Many suicides are not recorded as such on the death certificate, and it can be difficult to differentiate between suicide and death resulting from an accident. The result is that the recorded incidence reflects only a portion of the deaths caused by suicide. In addition, when one looks at the rate of attempted suicide, the problem becomes even more significant because suicide attempts far exceed actual suicides. Of the 12,272 students in grades 9-12 who participated in CDC's Youth Risk Behavior Survey in 1991, 29% had thought seriously about attempting suicide, 19% had made a specific plan to attempt suicide, 7% actually attempted suicide, and 2% made a suicide attempt that resulted in an injury or poisoning that had to be treated by a doctor or nurse (Centers for Disease Control and Prevention, 1992, Behaviors Related to, p. 771).

"Suicide clusters" and the possible "contagion" effect of adolescent suicide is a growing public concern. A suicide cluster is the occurrence of suicides or attempted suicides closer together in space and time than is considered usual for a given community. It is estimated that suicide clusters account for approximately 1% to 5% of all suicides among adolescents and young adults. In a cluster, suicides occurring later in the cluster often appear to have been influenced by earlier suicides. Thus a community-wide intervention approach is needed to address this problem. Persons at risk need to be identified and interviewed, personal counseling services should be provided for close friends/relatives of the victims and potentially suicidal adolescents, and the community needs to be supported in a way that minimizes sensationalism (Centers for Disease Control and Prevention, 1988, CDC recommendations).

As with homicide, a comprehensive community-focused approach that emphasizes prevention and is linked as closely as possible with professional mental health resources is needed to combat youth suicide (Centers for Disease Control and Prevention, 1992,

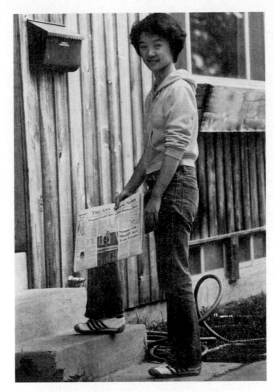

Figure 15-4 Accelerated societal changes have exposed American youth to increased opportunities and increased stresses. American youth are exposed much earlier than their previous counterparts to such things as human sexuality concerns, pressures from peers to use alcohol and drugs, and varying lifestyles. Community health nurses are often in a favorable position to detect youth who are having difficulty coping with the demands of life.

Youth Suicide). Currently a broad spectrum of youth suicide prevention programs in the United States use a variety of prevention strategies. The eight strategies outlined in the box on p. 560 focus on enhancing recognition of suicide, referral, and promoting activities designed to address known or suspected risk factors. Most youth suicide prevention programs target adolescents despite the fact that the suicide rate among young adults 20-24 years of age is generally twice as high as the rate among adolescents 15-19 years of age. Greater prevention efforts need to be targeted toward young adults (CDC, Youth Suicide, pp. x-xi).

Community health nurses, especially those functioning in the school setting, are in a key position to detect troubled youth and to work with the

◀ *Youth Suicide Prevention Strategies* ▶

- **School Gatekeeper Training**
  Directed at school staff to help them identify students at risk of suicide, refer such students for help, and respond in cases of a tragic death or other crisis in school.
- **Community Gatekeeper Training**
  Provides training for community members such as clergy, police and recreation staff to aid them in identifying youths at risk of suicide, and referring these youth for help.
- **General Suicide Education**
  Provides students with facts about suicide, alert them to suicide warning signs, and provide them with information about how to seek help for themselves or for others.
- **Screening Program**
  Involves administration of a standardized instrument to identify high-risk youth in order to provide more thorough assessment and treatment for a smaller, targeted population.
- **Peer Support Programs**
  Designed to foster peer relationships, competency development and social skills as a method to prevent suicide among high-risk youth.
- **Crisis Centers and Hotlines**
  Provide emergency counseling for suicidal people.
- **Means Restriction**
  Designed to restrict access to firearms, drugs, and other common means of committing suicide.
- **Intervention After a Suicide**
  Designed in part to help prevent or contain suicide clusters and to help youth effectively cope with feelings of loss that come with the sudden death or suicide of a peer.

From Centers for Disease Control and Prevention: *Youth suicide prevention programs: a resource guide,* Atlanta, Ga., 1992, The Centers, pp. ix-x.

community in planning a comprehensive suicide prevention program. It is important to move beyond an individual-focused approach. A community-oriented approach that uses a variety of intervention strategies is needed to address the nation's suicide problem.

Congenital Anomalies

Each year approximately 100,000 infants are born in the United States with serious congenital anomalies, and the proportion of these infants who survive into childhood is increasing yearly (USDHHS, 1993, Child Health USA '92, p. 20). Many factors increase the risk for congenital anomalies. "One-fourth of all congenital anomalies are caused by genetic factors, suggesting a need for preconception counseling for both men and women" (USDHHS, 1991, Healthy People 2000, p. 10). Poverty, poor housing, malnutrition, pregnancy at a young age, use of alcohol and cigarettes, and inadequate medical care also increase the likelihood that illness, disability, or death will occur. It has been shown that mothers in all age categories who are disadvantaged are at risk for producing an unhealthy child (Binsacca, Ellis, Martin, and Petitti, 1987; National Center for Health Statistics, 1989; Stockwell, Swanson, and Wicks, 1988; Task Force on Infant Mortality, 1987). The risk of having an abnormal birth increases as a mother's consumption of alcohol and smoking increase (USDHHS, Healthy People 2000). Young mothers and mothers who have inadequate health care are more likely to have low-birth-weight babies than other mothers. Low-birth-weight infants have a high incidence of congenital malformations. It is obvious from these facts that a preventive health program designed to reduce childhood mortality related to congenital malformations must include ways to eliminate poor environmental and social conditions, to expand the use of prenatal services by young and disadvantaged mothers, and to alter unhealthy behaviors (alcohol consumption and smoking) that increase the risk for abnormal births.

Malignant Neoplasms

Cancer is a significant contributor to the causes of death in children 1 through 14 years of age. It is the leading cause of death *by disease* in children in the 1-to 14-year-old age group. Leukemia is the most frequent cancer in children 9 years of age and under: lymphomas are the most common form of cancer in children 10 to 14 years of age. Leukemia accounts for almost one third of the deaths from cancer in childhood (American Cancer Society, 1994). It is estimated that 8200 new cases of cancer will be diagnosed in the United States among children aged 1 to 14 years in 1994 (American Cancer Society, 1994).

Cancer places a tremendous burden on families and society. The severe nature of this condition and the prolonged treatment needed cause pain and anguish for both the child and the family. Cancer in childhood also causes financial hardship for many families because funding for catastrophic illness is frequently not available. Health planning efforts for cancer should focus on providing early detection, treatment, and supportive services, funding for research, and monies to eliminate individual financial hardships. Community health nurses can significantly assist families in coping with childhood cancer by providing hospice care services and by helping them to obtain needed resources from community agencies (Martinson, Armstrong, Geis, Anglim, Gronseth, Macinnis, Kersey, and Nesbit, 1978). The American Cancer Society, for instance, supplies dressings and equipment free of charge. Other community agencies such as departments of social services and Crippled Children's Association provide funds for medical treatment. Helping parents to establish and maintain support networks is an important role for nurses working with families who are coping with childhood cancer (Lynam, 1987).

Childhood Morbidity Risks—Acute Conditions

The incidence of acute conditions in childhood is difficult to ascertain because (1) many acute conditions are not reportable; (2) reportable acute conditions are often not reported; and (3) acute illness is frequently treated at home and as a result is not brought to the attention of health professionals. Data from the National Health Surveys since 1956 do give estimated patterns of incidence over time. According to this survey, acute conditions are illnesses and injuries that were first noticed less then 3 months before the reference date of the interview, and were serious enough to have had an impact on behavior (Adams and Benson, 1991, p. 3).

The major types of acute illness for children ages 6 through 16 fall into five major categories. In order of frequency, these are respiratory conditions, infective and parasitic diseases, injuries, digestive system conditions, and all other conditions. School-age children miss approximately 3.8 days of school per year due to these conditions. The number of school-loss days per year per 100 children has not changed significantly over the past two decades (U.S. Bureau of the Census, 1992, Statistical abstract).

Respiratory conditions account for over 50% of the reported acute illnesses among school-age children.

These conditions are frequently ignored because "everyone gets a cold or an earache"; colds and earaches are "a normal part of life." However, these seemingly minor illnesses must not be disregarded. It has long been recognized that they do interfere with activities of daily living and may often lead to serious, chronic disabilities. In a study by Heazlett and Whaley (1976, p. 146), it was noted that the common cold—the respiratory condition with the highest incidence rate—affected adversely to a significant degree the perceptual and learning performance of junior high students. Otitis media, the third leading reason for pediatrician contact, can, if untreated, result in permanent hearing loss and/or chronic ear infection. In 1988 about 25% of the children who responded to the National Health Interview Survey on Child Health reported they had had repeated ear infections during their lifetime (Hendershot, 1989). Diseases of the respiratory system were the major cause of hospitalization of children 1 through 9 years of age in 1990 (USDHHS, 1993; Child Health USA '92, p. 24).

Infective and parasitic diseases are of concern to all health personnel because of their contagious nature. Many of them, such as scabies, impetigo, ringworm, and head lice, are still considered "diseases of the poor and unclean" even though this myth has been disproved. Children who have experienced these conditions are often socially isolated from their peers and labeled "dirty kids" even after treatment ceases. The reader will find the American Public Health Association Handbook, *Control of Communicable Diseases in Man* (Benenson, 1990), an extremely useful resource when identifying and recommending follow-up for any of these communicable conditions. It must be remembered, however, that physical care and treatment is not sufficient. The social stigma associated with these diseases is often more devastating than the disease itself. Epidemiological investigation (refer to Chapter 11) to determine the source of infection is essential in order to prevent further disease incidence and the social stigma associated with infective and parasitic diseases.

Injuries disproportionately strike the young. Injuries are the leading cause of death and a major cause of morbidity and disability among children and youth (USDHHS, 1991, Healthy People 2000). The most common single site of injuries to children under age 15 is the home. "Injuries occurring at school account for about 21 percent of all injuries among children aged 10 through 14 years" (USDHHS, Office of Maternal and Child Health, 1989, pp. 23, 27). Injuries present a significant burden on society. "One in every nine children is hospitalized for accidental or other injuries before age 15; 10 million emergency room visits per year are made for accidents or other injuries" (U.S. Congress, OTA, 1988, p. 5). Data from U.S. Consumer Product Safety Commission's National Electronic Injury Surveillance System (NEISS) reveal that sports and recreation are responsible for more treatments in hospital emergency rooms than any other category of injuries (Verhalen, 1987, pp. 673-674). Sports are the most frequent cause of injury for both male and female adolescents (Ostrum, 1993, p. 335).

Males have a significantly higher rate of nonfatal injuries than females because of differences in activities and behavior such as participation in contact sports. Better-planned sports programs might substantially reduce the number of sports-related injuries. Monitoring environmental conditions in homes and schools and promoting highway safety and regulations, such as child safety seat laws, could also significantly decrease childhood injuries.

Diseases of the digestive system, such as stomach ache, vomiting, diarrhea, Hirschsprung disease, celiac disease, appendicitis, and colitis, were the third leading cause of hospitalization of children aged 1 through 14 years in 1990 (USDHHS, 1993, Child Health USA '92, p. 24). Some of these diseases have a psychosocial etiology or are aggravated by psychosocial stresses. An astute community health nurse will assess for stressors in addition to physical causes when working with children who have digestive tract problems. This is especially important when a child has recurrent unexplained abdominal pains. Some key variables to consider when physical causes for digestive conditions have been ruled out are inadequate nutrition; family conflict; separation due to death, divorce, and illness; child abuse; tense classroom atmosphere; unfavorable teacher-student relationships; poor academic achievement; unrealistic expectations for performance; and lack of peer support.

Childhood Morbidity Risks— Chronic Conditions

Childhood chronic conditions are of special concern to health professionals for several reasons. First, these conditions may inhibit normal developmental processes and cause disability in later life. Second, the

stress of chronic illness frequently affects significant others in addition to the child who has the chronic condition. Last, prevention, treatment, and management services for chronic conditions are costly because of the long-term nature of these conditions and the number of persons affected by them.

The nation's wars dramatically illustrated the need to focus attention on preventing chronic health problems in our youth. During both World War I and World War II, a significant number of men were rejected for military service because of existing chronic conditions such as dental problems, psychiatric difficulties, and orthopedic abnormalities. In spite of recognition since the early 1920s that the health status of our nation's youth was far from ideal, 15% of the 18-year-olds were rejected for military service in 1965 because they had chronic handicapping conditions. Two thirds of these conditions could have been prevented if they had been detected before age 15 (Travis, 1976, p. 4).

It is estimated that approximately 10% to 15% of all children have some form of chronic health condition, many of which are mild. However, more than 4.1 million (6%) children aged 1-19 years were limited in their usual activities because of chronic illnesses and impairments in 1991 (USDHHS, 1993, Child Health USA '92, p. 26). The percentage of children with limitation of activity has doubled since 1960. As can be seen in Figure 15-5, disadvantaged children are more likely to be limited in activity because of chronic conditions than their wealthier counterparts (USDHHS, Child Health USA '92, p. 26).

Table 15-2 presents the types of chronic handicapping conditions of childhood. Among persons under 18 years of age the leading causes of chronic conditions, in rank order, are hay fever or allergic rhinitis without asthma, chronic sinusitis, chronic bronchitis, asthma, dermatitis, and deformities or orthopedic impairments (Collins, 1993).

Asthma tends to limit a child's activity more than other respiratory conditions and is a main cause of days lost from school in this age group. In 1988, 6% of the sample children in the National Health Interview Survey on Child Health had had asthma, about 7% had had hay fever, and about 8% had had eczema or skin allergies (Hendershot, 1989).

Community health nurses provide supportive assistance in a variety of ways to families whose children have chronic conditions. They assist these families in obtaining adequate health care, in making necessary adjustments in family lifestyle, and in ob-

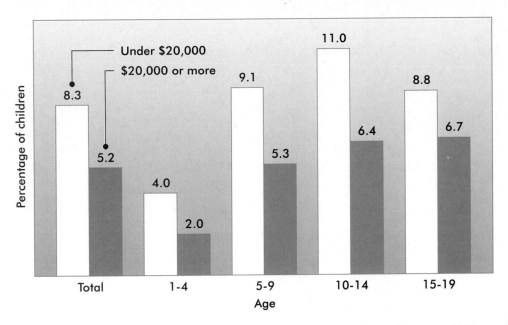

Figure 15-5   Limitation of activity due to chronic conditions by age and income: 1991. (From USDHHS: *Child Health USA '92,* Washington, D.C., 1993, U.S. Government Printing Office, p. 26.)

taining community resources that will help them to promote their child's growth and development. *Compuplay* is one such resource. Compuplay Resource Centers serve families with children 2 to 14 years of age with physical, mental, sensory, or behavioral disabilities. These centers provide computer play classes, software lending libraries, and local in-service training for professionals. Families interested in this resource can obtain further information by writing to the INNOTEK Director, National Lekotek Center, 2100 Ridge Avenue, Evanston, Ill., 60204 or by calling 708-328-0001 (Compuplay Centers, 1988, p. 5). Other resources that may be helpful to families dealing with a chronic illness are identified in Chapter 18. Families appreciate learning about these resources.

Community health nurses also assume a significant role in assisting school-age children to accept peers who have a chronic condition. A program to help children adjust to other children with chronic disabling conditions is *Kids on the Block.* This program is a puppet presentation showing puppets in wheelchairs, with assistive devices, and with various physical and mental conditions. This program stimulates discussion of childrens' feelings about peers who are different. Educational and health professionals can obtain more information about *Kids on the Block* by contacting 1-800-368-KIDS.

In addition to chronic diseases, school-age children may experience many chronic social problems that present serious difficulties for both themselves and their families. Homelessness, for example, is becoming increasingly prevalent among families with children. This problem is discussed extensively in Chapters 14 and 16. Four other social problems of particular concern to community health nurses who are working with school-age children are child maltreatment, teenage parenthood, sexually transmitted diseases (STDs), and drug abuse. None of these difficulties is unique to the school-age population. However, because a sizable proportion of our youth is experiencing these problems, a discussion of them is warranted.

Child Maltreatment

As a result of increased reporting requirements in recent years, it is now known that child maltreatment is reaching epidemic proportions among the school-age and the preschool population. Child maltreatment can involve physical and/or psychological abuse and neglect and/or sexual abuse.

In 1991 there were almost 2.7 million reports of suspected abused or neglected children nationwide. This represented an increase of 40% since 1985. In 1991 53% of the substantiated child maltreatment cases involved neglect, 21% involved physical abuse,

TABLE 15-2 Types of Chronic Childhood Handicapping Conditions

Categories of conditions	Types of conditions
A. Disorders of the central nervous system (CNS)	1. Poliomyelitis 2. Cerebral palsy 3. Epilepsy and other seizure disorders 4. Spina bifida 5. Spinal cord and cranial injury
B. Sensory disorders	1. Speech disorders: cleft lip, palate, articulation defects, stuttering, mutism 2. Hearing impairment, including deafness 3. Vision impairments
C. Cosmetic disorders	1. Facial deformities: severe acne, severe scarring 2. Burns 3. Scoliosis 4. Dwarfism 5. Cleft lip, palate 6. Many CNS disorders
D. Mobility disorders (muscular and skeletal systems)	1. Various orthopedic disorders 2. Thalidomide deformities 3. Osteogenesis imperfecta 4. Amputations 5. Muscular dystrophy 6. All the CNS disorders
E. Systemic disorders	1. Diabetes 2. Hemophilia, sickle cell anemia, and other blood dyscrasias 3. Cystic fibrosis 4. Asthma 5. Arthritis 6. Heart disease 7. Kidney disease
F. Malignancies	1. Leukemia 2. Other cancers
G. Mental retardation	1. Borderline 2. Severe 3. Many CNS disorders
H. Psychiatric disorders	1. Schizophrenia and psychosis 2. Severe affective disturbances 3. Personality disorders 4. Long-term behavior disorders
I. Severe developmental disorders	1. Failure-to-thrive syndrome 2. Autism
J. Persistent learning disability	

From Select Panel for the Promotion of Child Health: *Better health for our children: a national strategy,* vol IV, DHHS Pub No (PHS) 79-55071, Washington, D.C., 1981, U.S. Government Printing Office, p. 324.

and 13% involved sexual abuse (USDHHS, 1993, Child Health USA '92, p. 29). "Many experts believe that sexual abuse is the most underreported form of children maltreatment, because of the 'conspiracy of silence' which often characterizes these cases" (DePanfilis and Salus, 1992, p. 8). Data dealing with reported child neglect reflect that the average age for all maltreated children is 7.3 years. Children who experienced serious physical injuries are young, with an average age of 5.3 years. Emotionally maltreated children are on the average 8.1 years old (AAPC, 1986). An estimated 1383 children died from abuse or neglect in 1991 (USDHHS, Child Health USA '92, p. 29).

Several groups of children at risk for child maltreatment have been identified. Substantial physical force is most likely to be used against children under 5 or against 15- to 17-year-old youths (AAPC, 1986, p. 173). The risk of being sexually abused for girls between 10 and 12 years of age is more than double the average rate for all girls between 1 and 18 years. Girls are more likely to be sexually victimized than boys (Finkelhor and Araji, 1986). Statistics also reveal that disabled children and youths, as well as those who are relatively unresponsive socially, have an increased risk of being abused. Children from families with four or more children also show higher rates of abuse and neglect (Clearinghouse on Child Abuse and Neglect Information, 1992).

The average age of the abuser is 31 years, reflecting that maltreating parents range from young to old (AAPC, 1986; U.S. Congress, OTA, 1988). As was previously discussed in Chapter 14, "the most important parental risk factors for maltreatment of children are poverty, unemployment, and a history of abuse as a child" (U.S. Congress, OTA, p. 176). A relatively high number of parents who were abused as children abuse their children. Although abuse occurs in families of all socioeconomic levels, parents in poor families or those who are experiencing unemployment are most likely to maltreat their children. Children from families whose annual income is less than $15,000 experience maltreatment almost seven times more frequently than children from higher income families (Clearinghouse on Child Abuse and Neglect Information, 1992, p. 6). However, it is significant that in the majority of poor families children are not abused (U.S. Congress, OTA).

Although reporting of child maltreatment has improved in the last decade, this problem continues to be underreported and is often not identified. All health care professionals, including the community health nurse, must expand their efforts to identify undetected abuse and neglect in school-age children. Presented in Table 15-3 is a summary of physical and behavioral indicators that can assist nurses in identifying child abuse and neglect. Using data such as those previously discussed relative to risk factors can help professionals to identify potential abusers and victims of maltreatment. Strategies aimed at preventing initial maltreatment or a recurrence should be focused on changing risk factors that have been demonstrated to have a major influence on child maltreatment. For example, strategies designed to reduce poverty-related stresses, such as referring families to community agencies for financial aid, are appropriately aimed at eliminating a significant risk factor of child maltreatment (U.S. Congress, OTA, 1988).

The problems of child abuse and neglect are compounded for professionals who work with the school-age population because often they must deal with the lasting effects of conditions which existed during infancy and the preschool years. Longitudinal studies are beginning to report findings which indicate that there are long-term detrimental consequences of child abuse. Children who are abused during early childhood tend to have difficulty establishing trust, have more aggressive and behavioral problems than children who have not been abused, and frequently manifest a general air of depression, unhappiness, and sadness. Children who are sexually abused initially exhibit anger, hostility, and sexual problems, but long-term more serious problems such as diminished self-esteem, fear, and depression emerge (Dubowitz, 1986). In addition, data suggest that long-term effects of child maltreatment may include other problems such as juvenile delinquency, attempted suicide, substance abuse, truancy, and runaway behavior (Lindberg and Distad, 1985; McCord, 1983). There are an estimated 1 million runaways in the United States (National Center on Child Abuse and Neglect, 1986).

The effects of maltreatment can be devastating and the costs to society extremely high. Professionals and community citizens must join together to deal with this critical problem. To ensure that all children reach their optimal level of functioning, mechanisms must be established for early identification, reporting of actual or suspected abusing situations, and early and adequate intervention. "The impact of abuse can be minimized by early recognition and timely response

15-3 Physical and Behavioral Indicators of Child Abuse and Neglect

Type of CA/N*	Physical indicators	Behavior indicators
Physical abuse	Unexplained bruises and welts: 　On face, lips, mouth 　On torso, back, buttocks, thighs 　In various stages of healing 　Clustered, forming regular patterns 　Reflecting shape of article used to 　　inflict (electric cord, belt buckle) 　On several different surface areas 　Regularly appear after absence, 　　weekend, or vacation Unexplained burns: 　Cigar, cigarette burns, especially on 　　soles, palms, back, or buttocks 　Immersion burns (socklike, glovelike, 　　doughnut-shaped on buttocks or 　　genitalia) 　Patterned like electric burner, iron, 　　etc. 　Rope burns on arms, legs, neck, or 　　torso 　Infected burns, indicating delay in 　　seeking treatment Unexplained fractures or dislocations: 　To skull, nose, facial structure 　In various stages of healing 　Multiple or spiral fractures Unexplained lacerations or abrasions: 　To mouth, lips, gums, eyes 　To external genitalia 　In various stages of healing Bald patches on the scalp	Feels deserving of punishment Wary of adult contacts Apprehensive when other children cry Behavioral extremes 　Aggressiveness 　Withdrawal Frightened of parents Afraid to go home Reports injury by parents Vacant or frozen stare Lies very still while surveying 　surroundings Will not cry when approached by 　examiner Responds to questions in monosyllables Inappropriate or precocious maturity Manipulative behavior to get attention Capable of only superficial relationships Indiscriminately seeks affection Poor self-concept
Physical neglect	Underweight, poor growth pattern, 　failure to thrive Consistent hunger, poor hygiene, 　inappropriate dress Consistent lack of supervision, 　especially in dangerous activities or 　long periods Wasting of subcutaneous tissue Unattended physical problems or 　medical needs Abandonment Abdominal distention Bald patches on the scalp	Begging, stealing food Extended stays at school (early arrival 　and late departure) Rare attendance at school Constant fatigue, listlessness, or falling 　asleep in class Inappropriate seeking of affection Assuming adult responsibilities and 　concerns Alcohol or drug abuse Delinquency (e.g., thefts) States there is no caretaker

*CA/N = child abuse and neglect.

TABLE 15-3 Physical and Behavioral Indicators of Child Abuse and Neglect—cont'd

Type of CA/N	Physical indicators	Behavior indicators
Sexual abuse	Difficulty in walking or sitting Torn, stained, or bloody underclothing Pain, swelling, or itching in genital area Pain on urination Bruises, bleeding, or lacerations in external genitalia, vaginal, or anal areas Vaginal or penile discharge Venereal disease, especially in preteens Poor sphincter tone Pregnancy	Unwilling to change for gym or participate in physical education class Withdrawal, fantasy, or infantile behavior Bizarre, sophisticated, or unusual sexual behavior or knowledge Poor peer relationships Delinquent or runaway Reports sexual assault by caretaker Change in performance in school

Emotional maltreatment	Speech disorders
	Lags in physical development
	Failure to thrive
	Hyperactive or disruptive behavior
		Habit disorders (sucking, biting, rocking, etc.)
		Conduct and learning disorders (antisocial, destructive, etc.)
		Neurotic traits (sleep disorders, inhibition of play, unusual fearfulness)
		Psychoneurotic reactions (hysteria, obsession, compulsion, phobias, hypochrondria)
		Behavior extremes:
		  Compliant, passive
		  Aggressive, demanding
		Overly adaptive behavior:
		  Inappropriately adult
		  Inappropriately infant
		Developmental lags (mental, emotional)
		Attempted suicide

From Heindl C, Krall CA, Salus M, and Broadhurst DD: *The nurse's role in the prevention and treatment of child abuse and neglect,* Washington, D.C., 1979, National Center on Child Abuse and Neglect, Children's Bureau, Administration for Children, Youth and Families, Office of Human Development Services, p. 10.

to the child. Access to good health, education, and social services foster resilience in children regardless of the specific nature of the stressor" (Humphreys and Ramsey, 1993, pp. 53-54).

Both health professionals and the public need educational opportunities that will increase their knowledge about child abuse and neglect and help them to intervene effectively with abusive families. The *Clearinghouse on Child Abuse and Neglect* (P.O. Box 1182, Washington, D.C., 20013, 703-385-7565 or 1-800-394-3366) was established in 1975 by the federal govern-

ment to assist communities with their educational needs relative to child maltreatment. This clearinghouse disseminates information and resource materials on all types of child maltreatment, responds to public inquiries, and has a computerized data base that maintains updated statistics. Hotline services are also readily available to help communities and troubled families. The *National Child Abuse Hotline* (1-800-422-4453) provides information, professional counseling, and referrals for treatment. The *Parents Anonymous Hotline* (1-800-421-0353; 1-800-352-0386 in California) provides information on self-help groups for parents involved in child maltreatment.

Teenage Parenthood

While the birth rate for adolescents aged 15 to 19 years declined between 1970 and 1986, the birth rate for young adolescents (under 15 years of age) remained essentially unchanged during this time period. There was also a substantial increase in births to younger adolescents, and the incidence of induced abortions increased steadily among this age group. Black adolescents are almost twice as likely to be single parents as white teens. However, the proportion of births increased significantly more for single white teenagers aged 15 to 19 years (181% increase) than for single black teens (43%) between 1970 and 1986 (National Center for Health Statistics, 1988).

Each year in the United States one adolescent in 11, aged 15 through 19, becomes pregnant. This figure is significantly higher than that of Canada, England, or France, where fewer than one teen in 20 becomes pregnant (USDHHS, 1993, Child Health USA '92, p. 33). The problem of teenage pregnancy has become extensive enough that the federal government has established the Office of Adolescent Pregnancy Programs in the Department of Health and Human Services (200 Independence Avenue, SW., Room 736E, 202-245-7473). The primary mission of the office is to prevent adolescent pregnancy and improve the quality of care for pregnant adolescents.

Over 1 million U.S. teenagers became pregnant in 1988, of which 28,000 were under 15 years of age. Almost one half (48%) of all pregnancies to teenagers ended in a live birth: 39% ended in an induced abortion; and a spontaneous abortion occurred in 14%. Nearly one half of all pregnancies to adolescents under 15 years of age were reported to end in abortion (USDHHS, 1993, Child Health USA '92, p. 33).

Data suggest that the United States has a higher rate of teenage pregnancy than any other industrialized country because these teenagers are less likely to practice contraception. When they do, they are likely to practice it less effectively than do teenagers in European countries (Jones, Forrest, Goldman, Henshaw, Lincoln, Rosoff, Westoff, and Wulf, 1985; Irwin, Brindis, Brodt, Bennett, and Rodriguez, 1991). Teenagers account for about one third of all the unintended pregnancies in the United States; three quarters of these pregnancies occur among adolescents who are not using any method of contraception (Westoff,

1988). Mosher and Horn (1988, p. 33) found that only 17% of young women aged 15 to 24 make their first family planning visit before they begin having intercourse, and 73% wait an average of 23 months after first intercourse to begin using services. "The percentage of female adolescents who were sexually experienced increased from 47% in 1982 to 55% in 1990" (USDHHS, 1993, Child Health USA '92, p. 33).

Several factors influence nonuse or inconsistent use of birth control among teenagers (Orr, 1984; Irwin, Brindis, Brodt, Bennett, and Rodriguez, 1991). Many are poorly informed about their sexual development, believing that they are too young to get pregnant or not knowing how women conceive. Others find it difficult to obtain contraceptive services, feel it is morally wrong to use birth control measures, or believe that contraceptive use interferes with the pleasures of sex and can be dangerous to one's health. Some want to become pregnant to fulfill needs of love, attention, and belonging. Black and Hispanic adolescent girls are particularly at risk for unintended pregnancies (USDHHS, 1991, Healthy People 2000). Levy, Perhats, and Johnson (1992) found that adolescents with developmental disabilities are also at risk for unintended pregnancies.

Van Dover (1985) has demonstrated that contracting (refer to Chapter 9) can positively influence both family planning knowledge and behavior with young, sexually active women. She found "that clients with whom she contracted achieved significantly higher knowledge scores and showed significant increases in contraceptive consistency than did the routine clinic-care control group" (pp. 53-54).

The multiplicity and complexity of needs manifested during teenage parenthood mandate close coordination among professionals from all disciplines. Pregnancy can pose serious physical and psychosocial health problems and concerns for the teenage parents, their families, and the community at large. The involved teenagers are dealing with two developmental crises, adolescence and parenthood, which may result in adverse, long-lasting psychosocial consequences if effective intervention is not available.

Medically, both the teenage mother and her baby are at high risk. Children born to teenage parents have a much higher neonatal, postnatal, and infant mortality rate. These babies have a higher incidence of prematurity, low birth weight, and respiratory distress. The mothers tend to have more physical problems throughout their pregnancy. Considering that adolescence is a period when marked physical changes and rapid growth occurs, it is understandable that the additional stress of pregnancy increases a teenage mother's susceptibility to health difficulties. Toxemia, hypertension, nutritional deficiencies, prolonged labor, pelvic disproportion, and cesarean sections are a few complications of pregnancy common to the teenage mother (Osofsky, 1985; U.S. Congress, OTA, 1988; USDHHS, 1991, Healthy People 2000).

Parenthood in adolescence can present a number of special problems. Adolescent mothers face increased risks of single parenthood, incomplete education, poverty, unemployment, and welfare dependency (Hoffman, Foster, and Furstenberg, 1993). Financially, teenagers are often not able to provide for such basic needs as food, clothing, and shelter. Frequently they need assistance from social service agencies to adequately care for themselves and their children. Because they are not prepared for a career, it is difficult for them to obtain productive employment. Often a pregnant teenager drops out of school, which increases the likelihood that future employment opportunities will be limited and that social isolation from peers will occur. In addition to peer isolation, teenage parents frequently feel rejected by their families. Dependence on welfare systems, school disruption, unstable home situations, and limited peer support often result in further pregnancies outside of marriage. Every effort should be made to ensure that teenage parents, both mother and father, are able to achieve the developmental tasks of adolescence. They need counseling that will help them to deal with the role of adolescence, as well as the role of parenthood. Their families need assistance with resolving their negative feelings so that they can help their children to handle successfully their new roles.

The Adolescent Family Life Bill of 1981 and the Adolescent Family Life Demonstration Projects Amendments of 1983 have assisted professionals in providing both physical and psychosocial services to teenage parents and their families. The goals of these legislative acts are as follows:

(1) find effective means, within the context of the family, of reaching adolescents before they become sexually active; (2) to promote adoption as an alternative for adolescent parents; (3) to establish innovative, comprehensive, and integrated approaches to the delivery of care services for pregnant adolescents; (4) to encourage and support research projects and demonstration projects concerning the societal causes and consequences of adolescent premarital sexual relations, contraceptive use, pregnancy, and child rearing; (5) to support evaluative research to identify services which alleviate, eliminate, or resolve any negative consequences of adolescent premarital sexual relations and adolescent childbearing for the parents, the child, and their families; and (6) to encourage and provide for the dissemination of results, findings, and information from programs and research projects relating to adolescent premarital sexual relations, pregnancy, and parenthood (Perovich and Tipon, 1984, p. 186).

The Adolescent Family Life (AFL) program was incorporated into the Omnibus Budget Reconciliation Act of 1981 (Public Law 97-35, which is presented in Chapter 4). In 1988 12 research projects and 88 care and prevention demonstration projects were funded under this program. The prevention projects target teens not yet sexually active and promote adolescent abstinence. The care projects provide comprehensive, integrated services to improve the immediate health outcomes for mother and child and their prospects for a productive future. The AFL program supports research that examines adolescent sexuality and pregnancy (USDHHS, Public Health Service, 1988).

A major assessment of adolescent health and health services completed by the U.S. Congress' Office of Technology Assessment (OTA) in April 1991 highlighted a need to consider adolescent health as a national priority (OTA, 1991, Vols. I, II, III). OTA found that adolescents often face formidable barriers in trying to obtain basic health care and that "the conventional wisdom that American adolescents as a group are so healthy that they do not require health and related services is not justified" (OTA, 1991, Vol. I, p. 6). OTA suggested that Congress may want to (1) improve U.S. adolescents' access to health services; (2) restructure and invigorate federal efforts to improve adolescent health; and (3) improve adolescents' environments (OTA, 1991, Vol. I, p. 1). This report could have a significant influence on the type of services available to adolescents in this decade.

Individual counseling with teenage parents is necessary but not sufficient to prevent unintended adolescent pregnancies. The Panel on Adolescent Pregnancy and Childbearing (1987) believed that "the responsibility for addressing adolescent pregnancy should be shared among individuals, families, voluntary organizations, communities, and governments, and that public policies should affirm the role and responsibility of families to teach human values"

(p. 120). This panel further recommended that prevention of adolescent pregnancy had the highest priority and that needs of young adolescents and disadvantaged youth be given priority if resources are inadequate to address all the needs. Making contraceptive methods available and accessible to sexually active teens, addressing adolescent sexuality from the perspective of both sexes, and promoting strategies that help adolescents to develop the necessary capabilities to make and carry out responsible decisions about sexual and fertility behavior were also recommended by the Panel on Adolescent Pregnancy and Childbearing.

Sexually Transmissible Diseases (STDs)

One alarming consequence of the increased sexual experimentation among youths is the dramatic rise in the incidence of sexually transmissible diseases in this age category. As with most social problems, hard data reflect only the tip of the iceberg. Professionals frequently do not accurately report the occurrence of sexually transmissible diseases, and many nonapparent subclinical infections go untreated. From estimated reports over time, however, it is apparent that sexually transmissible diseases, especially gonorrhea, chlamydial infections, syphilis, and herpes have reached epidemic proportions in recent years (USDHHS, 1991, Healthy People 2000; CDC, 1992, Division of STD/HIV Prevention).

Sexually transmitted diseases (STDs) are among the most common infectious diseases in the United States today (National Institute for Allergy and Infectious Diseases, 1987, An introduction). During the 1980s public and professional interest in the STD problem escalated because this problem expanded at an alarming rate, both in its scope and in its complexity. There is now a greater understanding of both the range of agents transmitted through sexual contact and the relationship of STD to reproductive and other health problems. Acquired immunodeficiency syndrome (AIDS) emerged as a major threat during the 1980s.

The most common STDs are AIDS, chlamydial infections, genital herpes, genital warts, gonorrhea, and syphilis. Appendix 11-2 presents information about these and some of the other commonly acquired sexually transmitted diseases that affect adolescents and adults. STDs affect both sexes from all backgrounds and economic levels. However, they are most prevalent among teenagers and young adults.

Almost 12 million cases of sexually transmitted diseases occur annually, 86% of them in people aged 15 through 29 years (Centers for Disease Control and Prevention, 1990, Division of STD/HIV). Of grave concern is the growing segment of children affected with pediatric AIDS (refer to Chapter 14). "If the incidence of AIDS in children continues to increase, within the next 10 years, AIDS may become the fifth leading cause of death among children of all ages in this country" (USDHHS, National Institute of Child Health and Human Development, 1993, p. 1). It is estimated that for every child with AIDS reported to the CDC, anywhere from 2 to 3 children may be HIV-infected (USDHHS, National Institute of Child Health and Human Development). We are currently dealing with only the "tip of the pediatric AIDS iceberg." However, as was discussed in Chapter 11, the portion of the iceberg that is submerged is the most insidious and potentially dangerous portion of the clinical spectrum of disease (Figure 15-6). Among our nation's youth many STDs are submerged.

STD Action Coalitions and local health departments are valuable resources for the nurse working with adolescents who suspect they may have a STD. Immediate treatment is essential. When diagnosed and treated early, almost all STDs can be treated effectively (USDHHS 1991, Healthy People 2000). However, many young people suffer serious permanent complications from these infections. For example, every year an estimated 1 million women have an episode of pelvic inflammatory diseases (PID), the most serious and common complication of STDs among women. About one fifth of these PIDs are experienced by teenagers. PID can lead to infertility, tubal pregnancy, chronic pelvic pain, and other serious consequences. Over 100,000 women become infertile as a result of PID each year (USDHHS, Healthy People 2000).

Any community health nurse working with the school-age population must realize that the occurrence of sexually transmitted diseases is a *major* health problem in this age category. Programs that provide preventive, curative, and educative services for all children in the population served by the nurse must be planned. Use of the epidemiological process (Chapter 11) and the principles of health planning (Chapter 13) will facilitate the accomplishment of such a task. For readily accessible STD information, the nurse or client may want to utilize the VD Hotline at 1-800-227-8922. This hotline provides information on all types of STDs

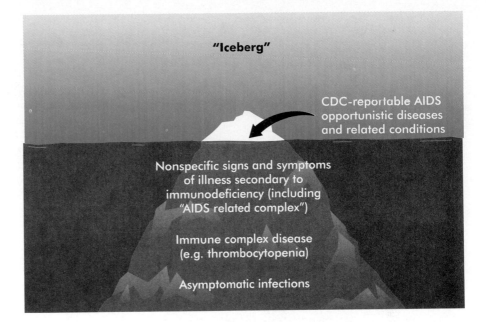

Figure 15-6 The clinical spectrum of HIV infection. (From USDHHS, National Center for Nursing Research: *HIV infection: prevention and care, a report of the NCNR priority expert panel on HIV infection,* NIH Pub No. 90-2417, Bethesda, Md., 1990, The Center, p. 25.)

and confidential referrals for diagnosis and treatment. The American School Health Association and United Way sponsor this service.

Drug Abuse

Illegal use of drugs, like sexual experimentation and STDs, is a serious national health problem among youth. Since 1975 the Monitoring the Future Project at the University of Michigan's Institute for Social Research has conducted a yearly survey to collect data on the range of substance use among American youth. Figure 15-7 presents data obtained by this project. It illustrates the prevalence and recency of use of 11 types of drugs among American high school seniors in 1992. Smokeless tobacco, marijuana, cigarettes, and alcohol are the most common substances used by American adolescents (Johnston, O'Malley, and Bachman, 1993, National survey results).

Data from the Monitoring the Future Project reveal that there was a marked increase in drug use by high school seniors from 1975 to 1978, but during the 1980s and early 1990s this trend slowed down. However, the 1992 survey findings of nearly 50,000 8th-, 10th-, and 12th-grade students across the country point to some troublesome warning signals. "While the long-term decline in the use of a number of drugs among the 12th-graders continued in 1992, some of their key beliefs and attitudes began to move in the wrong direction, perhaps presaging a reversal of the previous

declines in drug use among seniors, as well" (Johnston, O'Malley, and Bachman, 1993, News Release, p. 2). In 1992, for the first time in recent years, there was a statistically significant decline among 12th-graders in the perceived risk of LSD, heroin, and amphetamines; declines for marijuana, cocaine, and barbiturates were also evident but statistically nonsignificant. Additionally, Johnston, O'Malley, and Bachman (News Release, p. 1) noted modest but statistically significant increases in the use of select drugs among 8th-graders. Increases were noted in the use of marijuana, cocaine, crack, LSD, other hallucinogens, stimulants, and inhalants. "In 1992, eighth-graders were significantly less likely to see cocaine or crack as dangerous and (nonsignificantly) less likely to see marijuana use as dangerous than eighth-graders in 1991" (Johnston, O'Malley, and Bachman, News Release, p. 2). It has been found that changes in the perceived dangers of drugs can play a major role in reducing the use of some drugs.

The 1992 findings from the Monitoring the Future Project suggest that our nation cannot afford to be lax in the attention given to the control of drug abuse among youth. Overall, drug use among high school students and young adults remain wide-spread. Although there are regional and population differences in the use of illicit drugs among young people, no community is free of illegal drug use by this group (Johnston, O'Malley, and Bachman, 1993, National survey results).

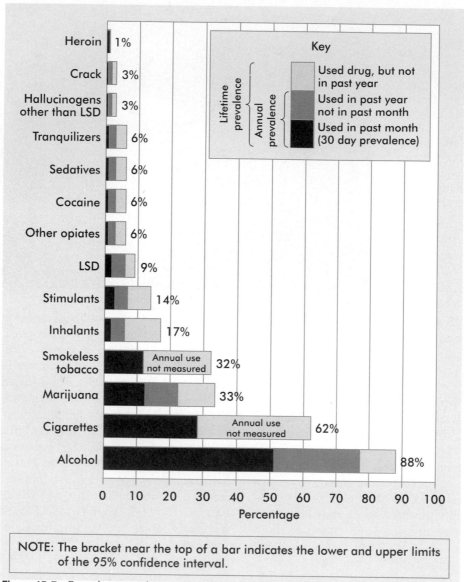

Figure 15-7 Prevalence and recency of use of various types of drugs: class of 1992. (From Johnston LD, O'Malley PM, and Bachman JG: *National survey results on drug use from monitoring the future study, 1975-1992,* vol I, NIH Pub. No 93-3597, Washington, D.C., 1993, U.S. Government Printing Office, p. 37.)

Multiple factors contribute to illegal drug use among our youth. One key variable is availability. The more widely used drugs are those reported to be most available. Other significant variables are peer influence, community norms, personality factors such as low self-esteem, family dysfunction, lack of supervision, and child maltreatment (Goodstadt, 1989; Johnston, O'Malley, and Bachman, 1993, Na-

tional survey results; U.S. Congress, OTA, 1988; Young, Werch, and Bakema, 1989). Children may resort to taking drugs to escape poor home environments and unhappy social situations and to mask such feelings as sadness, boredom, hopelessness, fear, and anger. Children from homes where there is a lack of affection and discipline need extra attention and support from adults so that their psychosocial developmental needs will be met through supportive relationships rather than through drug use.

Data suggest an urgent need for health care professionals to focus attention on the drug problem among youth. Multiple health interventions are essential to successfully prevent and resolve drug abuse. Drug abuse prevention programs have traditionally employed one or both of two strategies: educational or social control through policy, and regulation or legislation (Goodstadt, 1989, p. 247). Goodstadt, after reviewing the research and theory related to these strategies, promotes the joint development and implementation of educational and policy strategies to combat drug abuse in school settings. To be effective, a drug prevention program must have support from the school, family, peers, and community.

In order to provide the type of support needed by youth who use illegal drugs, community health nurses must have an understanding of the dynamics associated with drug use and knowledge about the developmental characteristics of this age group. Having knowledge about effective drug prevention strategies is also essential. Professionals who specialize in working with clients who are drug abusers are valuable resource persons and should be consulted when the nurse is having difficulty handling drug problems.

For the youth, parent, or professional interested in obtaining drug abuse information, several national hotlines are available. The National Cocaine Hotline (1-800-COCAINE) answers questions on the health risks of cocaine and provides referral services. The National Federation of Parents for Drug-Free Youth (1-800-554-KIDS) provides referrals for parents of children with drug and alcohol problems. The National Parents' Resource Institute for Drug Education (PRIDE: 1-800-241-7946) provides a broad range of educational and professional materials on drug-related issues and will refer families to appropriate organizations. The National Institute on Drug Abuse (NIDA) hotline (1-800-662-HELP) provides general information on drug abuse and AIDS (as it relates to intravenous drug users) and offers referrals to drug rehabilitation centers. The Target Resource Center (1-800-366-6667) is a service of the National Federation of State High School Associations, and provides information on school programs, publications, videotapes, and other drug education materials. It also makes referrals to organizations for alcohol and drug abuse information.

DEVELOPMENTAL TASKS OF SCHOOL-AGE CHILDREN

Stuffed rabbit
Seven years my nocturnal security
Now neglected worn and eyeless
Lying in the memory-choked attic
Stabbed by blunt dusty shafts of sunlight
Recalling to me
Evenings of forbidden play beneath giggle-muffling blankets
Recalling to me the day that I grew
Too big
Too old
To sleep with innocence while hugging security.
I'll leave you here stuffed rabbit,
You're dead
But God, what a long slow funeral we're having!
Gregory Smith, written at age 18

All school-age children must accomplish certain developmental tasks to achieve happiness and self-fulfillment. The author of "Stuffed Rabbit," above, was describing the overall task of adolescence: "relinquishing a child's life-style and attaining an adult life-style" (Nicholson, 1980, p. 11). He was giving up secure patterns of behavior to achieve emotional independence.

Social scientists such as Erikson, Havighurst, Freud, Piaget, and Sullivan have provided professionals with a variety of ways in which to explain human development. The manner and sequence of growth and development are universal and predictable features of childhood. However, children's behavioral responses do vary and are influenced by the culture and environment in which they live (Whaley and Wong, 1991).

To work effectively with all age groups, community health nurses must have knowledge of normal growth and development processes. They must also understand how these processes are influenced by psychosocial factors and how they affect families as well as individuals. As children, for example, become increasingly independent of parents and seek support and advice from others (peers, teachers, significant adults outside the home), parents can experience a great deal of anxiety. During these times they may need reassurance that they are not "losing" their children and an opportunity to express feelings of frustration and fear of failing as a parent. Supportive intervention can help parents to cope successfully with stresses associated with normal growth and development.

When working with children it is critical for all health care professionals to observe for lags in normal growth and development. Early casefinding and intervention can prevent permanent disability. A comprehensive biopsychosocial and cultural assessment should be done with every child and family when the child is not performing at the appropriate developmental age level. Chapters 7 and 14 present tools for facilitating this assessment. Intervention should be started immediately if a developmental disability is confirmed (refer to Figure 15-12).

Developmental Disabilities

Developmental disabilities are increasingly identified among school-age children and present significant stresses to those affected. Although estimates of the number of children handicapped by developmental disabilities vary significantly, it is known that several million children and their families are dealing with this problem. A diagnosis of a handicapping condition constitutes a crisis for a family and may require multiple adjustments in their lifestyle. Community health nurses frequently assume a significant role in promoting physical and psychosocial well-being among families by addressing the issues related to developmental disabilities.

As of 1978, the definition of developmental disabilities is found in Public Law 95-602 (Comprehensive Rehabilitation Service Amendments of 1978) and reads as follows:

"Developmental disability" means a severe, chronic disability of a person which—
a) Is attributable to a mental or physical impairment or a combination of mental and physical impairments;
b) Is manifested before the person attains age 22;
c) Is likely to continue indefinitely;
d) Results in substantial functional limitations in three or more of the following areas of major life activity;
   i. Self-care
   ii. Receptive and expressive language
   iii. Learning
   iv. Mobility
   v. Self-direction
   vi. Capacity for independent living, and
   vii. Economic sufficiency; and
e) Reflects the person's need for a combination and sequence of special, interdisciplinary, or generic care, treatment, or other services which are of lifelong or extended duration and are individually planned and coordinated.

The major life activity for preschool children is play, and for school-age children is learning or school.

More than 4.1 million (6%) children aged 1-19 were limited in their usual activities because of chronic illnesses and impairments in 1991 (USDHHS, 1993, Child Health USA '92, p. 26). Mental retardation is the chronic condition most likely to cause limitation of activity, with 83.6% of persons affected having limitation of major or outside activities (Collins, 1993, Prevalence of Selected Chronic Conditions, p. 2). Problems such as mental retardation, "learning disabilities," cerebral palsy, epilepsy, blindness, autism and other emotional difficulties, speech and hearing impairments, and orthopedic difficulties can affect learning abilities. Environmental factors can also influence a child's progress along the growth and development continuum.

As with average children, the degree to which children with developmental disabilities adjust successfully as healthy individuals varies. The nature and quality of their previous and current life experiences and their physical, emotional, and cognitive status greatly influence how well children with developmental disabilities progress. Typically these children have different life experiences from average children, and these differences are weighted in a negative direction. Clinical experience reveals that often children with developmental disabilities have deficient socializing experiences, both in quantity and quality, during childhood (Clemen and Pattullo, 1980, p. 197).

Numerous variables affect the socioadaptive capacity of children with developmental disabilities. The interdependence of these variables is graphically shown in Figure 15-8. An overwhelming number of the factors are influenced by environmental conditions. Few of them are inherent in the child, immutable to change (Clemen and Pattullo, 1980, p. 226).

In spite of the passage on November 29, 1975, of Public Law 94-142, Education for All Handicapped Children Act, there are still many children who are not receiving the services they need to develop to their fullest potential. It is extremely important for health professionals to focus attention on casefinding when working with school-age children so that developmental disabilities are identified early. It is also important for health professionals to assume an advocacy role when they identify that children with handicapping conditions are not receiving the health services they need. Parents should be assisted in obtaining necessary resources and should be informed of their rights, including the mandates of Public Law 94-142. The National Information System for Health Related

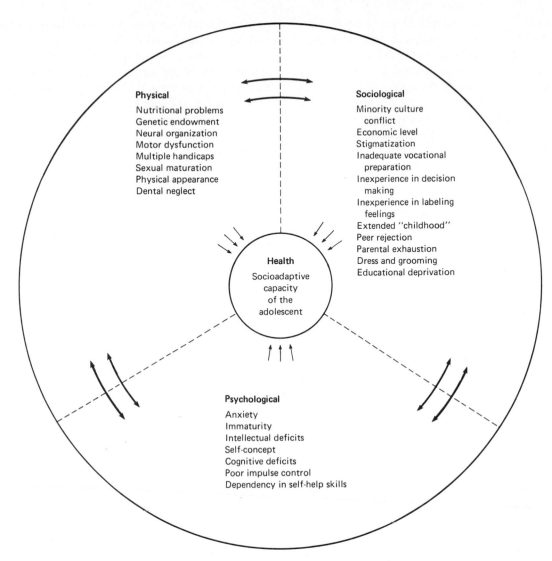

Figure 15-8 Factors influencing the health and socioadaptive capacity of the adolescent with mental retardation. (Modified from Figure 12, Concept of multiple causation in mental retardation, in Garrard SD: Mental retardation in adolescence, *Pediatric Clinics of North America* 7(1):150, 1960; and Clemen S and Pattullo A: The adolescent with mental retardation. In Howe J, ed: *Nursing care of the adolescent,* New York, 1980, McGraw-Hill, p. 226.)

Services (NIS) helps families who have developmentally disabled and chronically ill children up to age 12 to obtain needed services. This organization makes referrals to support groups and sources of financial, medical, and legal assistance and can be reached at 1-800-922-9234 or 1-800-922-1107 (South Carolina).

Public Law 94-142 mandates that every school system receiving special federal educational funds must provide a "free, appropriate education for all handicapped children between the ages of six and eighteen, regardless of the type of handicap or the degree of impairment." It also provides incentive monies to extend services to children beginning at age 3 and for young adults between 18 through 21. Public Law 99-457, passed in September, 1986 made some significant changes to Public Law 94-142. This law created a new Preschool Grant Program that mandates that children beginning at the age of 3 have the "right to education." It also created a new Handicapped Infants and Toddlers Program that dispenses incentive monies to provide educational services for handicapped and at-risk infants and toddlers. Public Law 99-457 is discussed more extensively in Chapter 14.

Under Public Law 94-142 school systems that do not have appropriate diagnostic and therapeutic facilities and personnel are legally bound to purchase whatever is required. In addition to full educational opportunities, the other rights covered by this law are as follows:

1. Due process safeguards that assist parents in challenging decisions regarding their children
2. Education in the mainstream to the fullest extent possible
3. Assurance that tests and other evaluation materials do not reflect cultural or racial bias
4. A "child-find" plan to identify all children within the state who have special needs

Many states have been more progressive than the federal government in planning services for handicapped children and have mandated services for a wider age range (e.g., birth to 25 years). The Developmental Disabilities Assistance and Bill of Rights Act (Public Law 95-602) and subsequent amendments to this act have assisted states in expanding services to persons with developmental disabilities in the 1980s. This act ensures availability of funds to help states provide comprehensive services to persons whose needs cannot be met under the Education for All Handicapped Children Act, the Rehabilitation Act of 1973, or other health, education, or welfare programs (Michigan State Planning Council for Developmental Disabilities, 1983). A more extensive discussion of this legislative act and other acts that provide services for individuals with a handicapping condition can be found in Chapter 18.

Children with developmental disabilities, like all school-age children, need organized, comprehensive community health services designed to foster optimal growth. The coordination of services between professional disciplines cannot be overemphasized. No one community system can provide the entire spectrum of services needed by the school-age population. Lack of coordination results in duplication of efforts, inefficient use of time and energies, inconsistent messages, and deficiencies in services. One community health nurse, for example, visited a family who had a newborn infant with Down syndrome. The nurse referred the family to the intermediate school district for diagnostic and follow-up services. The physical therapist, the occupational therapist, and the psychologist from this special service division of the educational system visited the family to assess their needs. Although each of these disciplines provided a valuable service, it was difficult for the family to work with all of them. Alert intervention on the part of the community health nurse kept the family from rejecting the offered services.

Since most children attend school, the school is a logical environment in which to promote the health of all children. The components of an effective school health program will be elaborated on in the next section. The reader should remember, however, that health services rendered in the school environment must be viewed within the context of the broader community. School health cannot be separated from the ecological and social conditions of the home and the community.

SCHOOL HEALTH PROGRAM

As early as 1850, the importance of health promotion activities in the school environment was stressed. At that time Lemuel Shattuck (1850, pp. 178-179) wrote the following:

Every child should be taught, early in life, that, to preserve his own life and his own health and the lives and health of others, is one of his most important and constantly abiding duties. Some measure is needed which shall compel children to make a sanitary examination of themselves and their associates, and thus elicit a practical application of the lessons of sanitary science in the everyday duties of life. The recommendation now under consideration is designed to furnish this measure. It is to be carried into operation in the use of a blank schedule, which is to be printed on a letter sheet, in the form prescribed in the appendix, and furnished to the teacher of each school. He is to appoint a sanitary committee of the scholars, at the commencement of school, and, on the first day of each month, to fill it out under his superintendence. . . . Such a measure is simple, would take a few minutes each day, and cannot operate otherwise than usefully upon the children, in forming habits of exact observation, and in making a personal application of the laws of health and life to themselves. This is education of an eminently practical character, and of the highest importance.

There are several key concepts delineated in Shattuck's writings that have relevancy for current school health practices. Specifically, the following ideas extracted from Shattuck's comments are important to consider when establishing a school health program:

1. All citizens have the responsibility to preserve life and promote health in the community. In order to assume this responsibility, lay persons and health professionals need *knowledge* (sanitary sciences) and an opportunity to *apply* health principles in daily living situations. It is both logical and useful to help children in the school setting to learn healthy habits of functioning, because children spend a considerable amount of time in this environment.

2. "Sanitary examination" can prevent spread of communicable disease. Even though there has been a drastic reduction in the incidence of communicable conditions, school-age children are still very susceptible to these conditions because they are constantly exposed to them and are in environmental situations that support the spread of agents (refer to Chapter 11). Whenever a large number of individuals is confined in a limited space, such as a school environment, the likelihood of transmission of disease from one individual to another increases. The significance of sanitary examinations in the school setting should not be underestimated. It is also important to recognize that laypersons (children, parents, and school personnel) can learn how to observe for signs and symptoms of illness. Health care professionals do not have to routinely conduct sanitary examinations. Their time can be better spent in helping others to care for themselves.

3. Health education is an appropriate function for the school system because it provides children with skills that assist them to function effectively in society and to meet their individual health care needs. Educational curricula should be designed so that learners obtain the knowledge and skills necessary to cope adequately with the demands and stresses of situations they will be encountering after leaving the educational environment. Individuals must handle health matters constantly throughout life.

4. A "sanitary committee" or health council should be used to monitor the effectiveness of the school health program. Without such a committee, it is often found that the health component of school services is neglected.

Today comprehensive school health programs incorporate Shattuck's ideas and several other activities aimed at promoting healthful living. Modern school health activities are divided into three basic interrelated categories: (1) health services, (2) health education, and (3) healthy school environment. The latest national survey conducted by the American School Health Association to determine the status of school health in America reflects that in 43 states (86%) a legal basis for health education has been established through educational codes or other state legislation. Almost two thirds of the states have a legal basis for health service programming and almost four fifths have a legal basis for healthful school environment (Lavato, Allensworth, and Chen, 1989).

In order to provide all of the services discussed under these three categories, a school system must develop mechanisms that will facilitate interdisciplinary teamwork. Interdisciplinary coordination and collaboration is the key to successful implementation of a comprehensive school health program.

Health Services

School health services are designed to protect and promote the health of all students and all school personnel. Health service programming includes such things as periodic screenings for hearing and vision disorders and scoliosis, provision of emergency care, development of a care management plan for children with handicaps, and the provision of nutritionally adequate meals.

The type of health services needed in a school setting will vary from community to community, depending on the availability of other community resources and the characteristics of the population being served. Before developing a school health program, health professionals, school personnel, and community citizens should jointly study the needs of their community in order to identify what specific health services must be provided in the school environment. School health services should not duplicate community services already available. Rather, they should augment community services so that the comprehensive health care needs of the school-age population are met. For example, if a community lacks accessible health services for children and youth, the school may provide comprehensive health services in the school setting. Currently approximately 300 school-based clinics operate in elementary, middle, and high schools in the United States (Passarelli, 1994, p. 144). There are also school-linked clinics and other health service models for children in many states

(Center for the Future of Children, 1992; Passarelli). These types of clinics are located in most major cities and many rural areas to improve children's access to health care. However, in some school settings very few health services are provided because the community has an adequate number of health personnel, accessible clinic services for disadvantaged populations, and families in the school district who are financially stable.

Regardless of the resources available in the community, certain basic health services should be provided in all school systems. Procedures should be established to achieve the following objectives:

1. To appraise the health status of students and school personnel on a continual basis
2. To counsel students, parents, teachers, and others regarding appraisal findings
3. To encourage health care to correct remedial defects
4. To provide emergency care for injury or sudden illness
5. To prevent and control infectious diseases
6. To identify children with handicapping conditions and to arrange for educational programs that will enhance the maximum potential of these children
7. To maintain a record-keeping system that complies with state laws (immunization) and that documents the health needs of special children

To accomplish these objectives health education, health promotion, and environmental inspection activities must be integrated. Having one person in the school system responsible for coordinating this integration is essential.

Health Education

Health education is a process that helps people to make sound decisions about personal health practices and about individual, family, and community well-being. Knowledge alone does not necessarily foster appropriate health habits. In order to facilitate effective decision-making in health matters, the school system should provide every child with the opportunity to acquire *knowledge* essential for understanding healthy functioning, develop *attitudes* and *habits* that foster preventive health behaviors, and practice health *skills* conducive to effective living (Stone, Perry, and Luepker, 1989). To achieve these goals, the child, the

family, and the community must be involved in the educational process. This is essential because the development of sound health habits is influenced by a variety of forces including such things as societal norms, beliefs and attitudes of significant others, and the internal motivations and beliefs of the individual.

Eberst (1984, p. 102) has developed a model (Figure 15-9) depicting the multiple factors that exert an influence on health habits. He views health as a quality of life which encompasses at least six overlapping dimensions (mental, physical, vocational, emotional, social, and spiritual) that synergistically interact. He believes that the multiple factors identified in Figure 15-9 exert an influence on each dimension of health and that school health education can exert a greater influence on some of these factors than others. The Eberst model supports Stone, Perry, and Luepker's (1989) contention that emphasis needs to be placed on more creative and effective home-based and family-based health promotion programs to complement and reinforce school health programs. Schools can not be successful in isolation of the family.

A *planned* series of *integrated* health educational activities based on input received from students, parents, community citizens, health care professionals, and educators is needed to ensure that health education will become an integral component of a school's curriculum. Informal health counseling with individual students and special health projects such as "know your heart" and "maturational processes" are valuable but can never adequately prepare children to make sound decisions about all the personal, family, and community health needs they will encounter. Special health projects usually have a narrow focus. When only this instructional modality is used to disseminate information about health and health-related phenomena, students become very knowledgeable about certain health needs, such as dental hygiene and nutritional requirements, but learn very little about other relevant health issues.

Unfortunately, too many school districts rely on uncoordinated, incidental methods when planning ways to handle health education in their curricula. Teachers are often requested to cover specific health topics throughout the year, but frequently they are unaware of the health content that has been presented to their students in previous years. When this happens, some concepts are repeated from one year to another and others are not covered at all. Respondents to the 1987 National Adolescent Student Survey re-

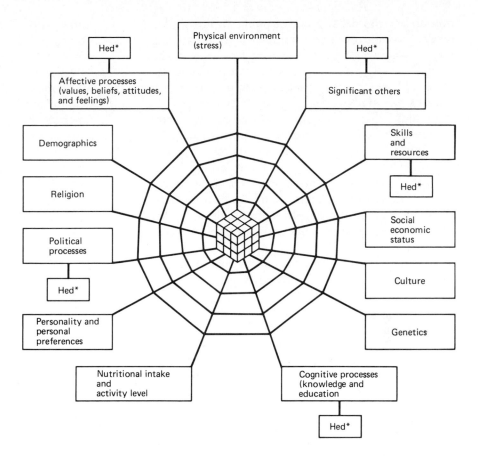

Figure 15-9 The "spider web" of factors exerting influence on health. (From Eberst RM: Defining health: a multidimensional model, *J School Health* 54:102, 1984. Copyright, 1984, American School Health Association, Kent, Ohio 44240.)

ported on the health instruction they received since the beginning of the seventh grade. While most had received instruction on the effects of drugs and alcohol (84%), nutrition and choosing healthy foods (74%), and how to prevent unintentional injuries (65%), fewer students received instruction on ways to avoid fighting and violence (43%); on AIDS (35%); on STDs (32%); on suicide prevention (28%); and on selecting health products and services (27%) (Centers for Disease Control and Prevention, 1989, p. 148).

The School Health Education Evaluation (SHEE), conducted from 1982 through 1984, provides evidence that exposure to a school health education curriculum can result in substantial changes in health-related knowledge, practices, and attitudes, and that such changes increase with the amount of instruction. SHEE estimates that the potential impact of these changes is large and could greatly affect the nation's health. Data from the SHEE program suggest that school health education is an effective strategy for improving the health behaviors of youth (Centers for Disease Control and Prevention, 1986, pp. 593, 595).

Curriculum planning for health instruction is the responsibility of all professionals in the school system. The school nurse is often asked to assume a major role in organizing health education activities. A school nurse's educational preparation and clinical experience and contact with the community puts her or him in a favorable position for understanding the essential concepts of health and illness and for coordinating activities between the school and the community. It is crucial to remember, however, that a school nurse alone cannot implement a sound health education program. Without administrative support and active involvement of all teachers, it would be impossible to achieve appropriate selection and sequencing of health content throughout the grade levels or to obtain sufficient time for health educational activities.

When planning a health education curriculum it is beneficial to have a conceptual framework for organizing the selection and sequencing of all health education activities. Many states have developed models of comprehensive school health education that can be obtained from the department of education and/or the department of public health. These models provide a valuable framework for organizing curriculum-development activities. However, to be used effectively, teachers and health care professionals must understand the concepts being presented and must be prepared to adequately address them.

In addition to curriculum models there are many excellent educational materials and audiovisual aids available to school nurses who are designing health programs for their specific school populations. Some companies, such as Lever Brothers, produce educational materials that address childhood health needs. Local and state health departments and departments of education often maintain information about where to obtain these materials.

Health educational activities in the school system should be aimed at promoting both physiological and psychosocial functioning. Students must be helped to analyze how normal growth and development progresses and to discuss their needs in relation to the maturational process. They should also be assisted in seeing how ineffective health practices can be altered and how they can prevent physical and psychosocial distress. In addition, it is important for children to learn how environmental forces affect the health status of all community citizens and to identify ways to promote healthy community functioning.

Healthy School Environment

Environmental factors that affect the health and well-being of children in the school setting are numerous. Psychosocial and physical aspects of the environment need to be monitored to ensure an optimal setting for student learning. A healthy school environment is one that promotes optimum psychosocial and physical growth and development among school-age children and school personnel. It provides an atmosphere that fosters sound mental health and favorable social conditions. It is organized in a way that reduces unhealthy stress and eliminates safety hazards for all students and school personnel.

A healthful school environment has the following features:

1. An architectural design that takes into consideration the developmental characteristics of the population being served, the needs of disabled students and staff, and the needs of the instructional program
2. A comfortable environment that has adequate seating, lighting, heating, ventilation, toilet fa-

cilities, and drinking fountains
3. An organized safety program, including provisions for emergency care and adequate transportation
4. An established mechanism to ensure safe, sanitary conditions
5. A recreational program that allows all students to participate
6. A planned schedule of school activities that takes into account the physical and psychosocial needs of children at varying grade levels
7. An organized school lunch program that provides nutritious foods, adequate time for good personal hygiene, and sufficient facilities for comfortable eating
8. An established program that provides psychosocial counseling and consultation services for staff and students

No one professional discipline can plan and implement all the services described in these three components—health services, health education, healthy school environment—of a total school health program. The role of nursing in the school setting is described in the following section. The reader should keep in mind, however, that effective teamwork is essential for successful school health programming.

THE ROLE OF THE COMMUNITY HEALTH NURSE IN THE SCHOOL HEALTH PROGRAM

Since the turn of the century when Lillian Wald placed Lina Rogers, the first school nurse, in the New York City schools, the role of nursing in the school health program has been evolving. Control of communicable disease is no longer the primary focus of nursing service. It is now recognized that the school nurse has a significant contribution to make in all aspects of the total school health program as illustrated in "A Day in the Life of a School Nurse" (Burton, 1992). The American Nurses Association's Standards of School Health also illustrate the complexity of school nursing. In 1966 the ANA identified 20 functions and 83 related activities for staff-level school nurses (ANA, 1966, pp. 4-14). These functions and activities were designed to enhance the educability of all school-age children and to improve the health of all citizens in the United States. They were developed to ensure that the ANA's philosophy of school nursing, discussed later in this chapter, would be implemented in the school setting.

A DAY IN THE LIFE OF A SCHOOL NURSE

If you had told me 10 years ago that I would be working for a public school system, I would have said you were crazy! But here I am, in 1992, working in a field that I believe is truly on the "cutting edge" of health care—school nursing.

When I took this job, I really had no idea what I was getting into. In fact, my husband encouraged me to take this position because he thought that it would be a "fluff" position supervising nurses as they handed out band-aids, and that the vacation time looked good.

For the past five years, I have held the position of nursing supervisor for the Lawrence Public Schools in Lawrence, Mass.

Lawrence is a poor city of 63,000 people, known for its negative health status indicators and largely minority population. The public school population of 11,000 students is 77 percent minority, mostly Hispanic newcomers. Lawrence has the highest teen pregnancy rate and one of the worst drug abuse problems in Massachusetts. Those problems, combined with a 44 percent high school drop-out rate and the lowest basic skills scores in the state, make our youth some of the neediest in the country.

A solid grasp of the nursing process has been the cornerstone of my practice. In the first months of employment as the nursing supervisor for the school district, I undertook a complete needs assessment that included interviews with principals, nursing staff and the community as a whole. I then invited these people to work with me on the Lawrence School Health Advisory Council. When the assessment was completed, I developed a plan for comprehensive health education and school health services, including school-based health centers at the high school, and at the elementary/middle level, developed and implemented a comprehensive health education program in grades K-12, integrated AIDS education into the health education program, and developed a comprehensive substance abuse program. I am proud to say that even with severe budget cuts, five years later, we are right on target.

What I have discovered is that school nursing is truly an opportunity to practice primary prevention at its best. It is exciting, challenging and fun! Every day is different, so it is difficult to choose one day to describe my life.

This day begins at 7:30 AM. I need to deliver syringes and sharps containers to a middle school and make sure everything is in order for the school nurse to immunize 6th grade students with the second dose of MMR vaccine. I have arranged for two other school nurses to help. There are about 100 students who need to be immunized today.

The next stop is an 8 AM meeting with my boss, the assistant superintendent of schools. I am meeting with him to bring him up to date on the Drug Free Schools Project. We have been fortunate this year to have received over $1 million in grants to develop and implement a comprehensive substance abuse prevention program in the schools. The project includes curriculum development, setting up student assistance teams, peer leadership, children of alcoholics support groups, parent education groups, teacher and administrator training and policy development. Since I am the "health person" in the school district, anything to do with health, AIDS, drugs, sex, teen pregnancy or violence gets directed to me. This is primary prevention!

It is now 9 AM. On the way to my office I stop at the community health center to meet with staff who serve the teen health center at the high school. I need to bring them up to date on Medicaid billing issues and new forms that were presented at a meeting with the state health department last week.

I arrive at my office that is located in a K-8 elementary school around 10 AM. There is a stack of messages waiting for me that need to be returned. I answer these calls. One of the calls is to a parent who needs bus transportation for her child who just had surgery. I need to approve all medical transportation. Another call is from the superintendent's office. "Send over copies of our AIDS curriculum . . . another school district is interested in what we are doing." They need the information yesterday! Another call is from a principal—she needs a nurse in the building every day for a child with a G-tube. Still another call is from one of the school nurses—there are 15 cases of chicken pox in her school today!

It is now 10:30 AM, and I need to prepare for a School Health Advisory Council meeting scheduled for this afternoon.

At noon, I attend a meeting of the Lawrence Violence Prevention Coalition. This community coalition was formed to develop a community response to increasing violence in the city. The question here, as in most community groups, is "What are the schools doing, and why are they not doing more?"

At 2 PM, the School Health Advisory Council meets. This council is made up of students, parents, teachers, school administrators, school nurses, as well as health and human services professionals from the community. This group of people provide me with the guidance and support I need to do my job. Because several parents on the council are more comfortable speaking Spanish, I meet with them 30 minutes before the meeting to provide them with an orientation to the agenda so that they will feel more comfortable and be able to provide input during the meeting.

At this council meeting, I present our health services budget as well as a review of the health services staffing pattern and health status of our kids. Today, I do not have good news to report. I have been instructed to present a level-funded budget to the school committee, but this actually means a budget cut. A nurse who left the system five months ago will probably not be replaced.

We have 1,218 children with some type of health problem, an increase of more than 200 since last year. This includes 428 children with asthma, an increase of 125 students since last year. We also have a significant increase in the number of students with active seizure disorders, kidney disease, heart disease and leukemia. The need for direct nursing services has increased with twice the number of children requiring medication in school this year. Also with the mandates of Special Education, more children with complex needs are being brought into the system. The needs of these children range from intermittent catheterization and G-tube feedings to case management and clinical services. The council discusses my report in detail. They are concerned about decreases in staff with the increased need for services. Council members, including parents, offer to speak at upcoming school committee meetings in support of the health program.

It has been a busy day, but a good one. I believe that, at least for this day, I have shown how effective school nurses can be, and what a vital role nurses play in bridging the gap between the health care and education communities. With the severe fiscal constraints faced by school districts, difficult decisions are made everyday. The purpose of the school system is to educate children. However, the basic health and safety needs of children must be met in order for them to learn. Because attitudes and health behaviors that school-age children develop will be carried into adulthood, the schools need to accept responsibility for educating the whole child.

School nurses play a vital role in helping the school meet this responsibility. They are truly on the cutting edge of health promotion and health services. They practice primary prevention at its best!

As a final note, I add that my husband now says I am the only person he knows who can take a perfectly simple job and make it complicated.

Peg Trainor Burton is the nursing supervisor for the Lawrence Public Schools in Lawrence, Mass. A diploma graduate of St. Mary's School of Nursing in Clarksburg, W.Va., Burton earned a BSN at Duquesne University, Pittsburgh, Pa., and a master's degree at Boston University School of Nursing, where she specialized in community health nursing. She holds current certification as a family nurse practitioner. Burton is a member of ANA, the National Association of School Nurses, the American School Health Association and the American Public Health Association.

From Burton PT: A day in the life of a nurse: school nursing on cutting edge of prevention, *The American Nurse* 24:23, 1992, September. Reprinted by permission of the American Nurses Association.

Philosophy of School Nursing

School nursing is a highly specialized service contributing to the process of education. That it is a socially commendable, economically practical, and scientifically sound service can be well demonstrated. It must be diligently pursued through health and educational avenues to the end that positive health among all the citizenry of this country will be a reality.

The professional nurse, with her experience and knowledge of the changing growth and behavioral patterns of children, is in a unique position in the school setting to assist the children in acquiring health knowledge, in developing attitudes conducive to healthful living, and in meeting their needs resulting from disease, accidents, congenital defects, or psychosocial maladjustments.

Nursing provided as part of a school program for children is a direct, constructive, and effective approach to the building of a healthful and dynamic society. (ANA, 1966, p. 1.)

The ANA's most current standards for school nursing are displayed in the box on p. 583. Extensive structure, process, and outcome criteria for measuring the achievement of these standards can be found in the document *Standards for School Nursing Practice* (ANA, 1983). In this document, "the purpose of school nursing is to enhance the educational process by the modification or removal of health-related barriers to learning and by promotion of an optimal level of wellness (ANA, 1983, p. 1). The latest standards for school nursing developed by the National Association of School Nurses confirm this purpose and identify standards of practice similar to those written by the ANA (Proctor, Lordi, and Zaiger, 1993).

School nursing is an exciting, rewarding field of nursing practice that provides numerous opportunities for creative, independent functioning. Needs of

◀ ***Standards of School Nursing Practice*** ▶

Standard I. Theory

The school nurse applies appropriate theory as basis for decision making in nursing practice.

Standard II. Program Management

The school nurse establishes and maintains a comprehensive school health program.

Standard III. Nursing Process

The nursing process includes individualized health plans which are developed by the school nurse.

Standard IV. Interdisciplinary Collaboration

The school nurse collaborates with other professionals in assessing, planning, implementing, and evaluating programs and other school health activities.

Standard V. Health Education

The nurse assists students, families, and groups to achieve optimal levels of wellness through health education.

Standard VI. Professional Development

The school nurse participates in peer review and other means of evaluation to assure quality of nursing care provided for students. The nurse assumes responsibility for continuing education and professional development and contributes to the professional growth of others.

Standard VII. Community Health Systems

The school nurse participates with other key members of the community responsible for assessing, planning, implementing, and evaluating school health services and community services that include the broad continuum of promotion of primary, secondary, and tertiary prevention.

Standard VIII. Research

The school nurse contributes to nursing and school health through innovations in theory and practice and participation in research.

Reprinted with permission from *Standards of School Nursing Practice* © 1983, American Nurses Association, Washington, D.C., pp. 3-15.

the population being served, community resources, patterns for delivery of service, and federal, state, and local funding and regulations influence how each of these nurses functions.

Patterns for Providing School Nursing Services

Two administrative patterns are being used to provide nursing services in the school setting: specialized and generalized. Specialized services are provided by school nurses who are employed by the board of education. These nurses are accountable to school administrators and work only with the school-age population. Some health departments are developing special school-health units within the health department. These specialized school nurses are accountable to the community health nursing director. Generalized services are provided by community health nurses hired by health departments or visiting nurse associations. These nurses function part time in the school setting as part of a generalized community health nursing program. They work with all at-risk populations in their assigned area.

There is a great deal of controversy about which pattern for delivering school nursing services is most appropriate. Clinical experience has shown that both patterns can be effective. Mechanisms must be established, however, to ensure that:

- The school nurse is a sanctioned member of the school health team
- Health care for the school-age child is provided within the context of the family and the community
- The nurse serving the school-age population has an understanding of the health needs and the growth and development characteristics of the school-age child
- School health services are adequately financed by the community
- The school nurse has professional *nursing* supervision

The activities of generalized and specialized school nurses vary among school systems. Unfortunately, there are many educational systems that use the nurse only to provide first aid and emergency care. Others, however, use the nurse in a comprehensive manner such as Burton described on p. 581 and 582.

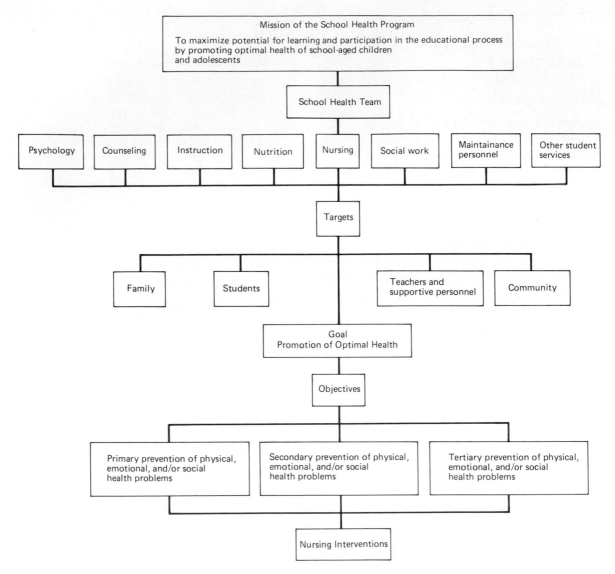

Figure 15-10 Rustia's school health promotion model. (From Rustia J: Rustia school health promotion model, *J School Health* 52(2):109, 1982. Copyright 1982, American School Health Association, Kent, Ohio 44240.)

A school nurse who is able to clearly articulate her or his role and functions and who demonstrates clinical expertise to all members of the school health team is more likely to be used appropriately than one who has trouble defining what it is a school nurse has to offer.

Functions of the Nurse on the School Health Team

School nurses frequently have difficulty defining what it is they have to contribute to the school health team and thus they are often used in a very narrow context. Traditionally nurses are seen as the profes-

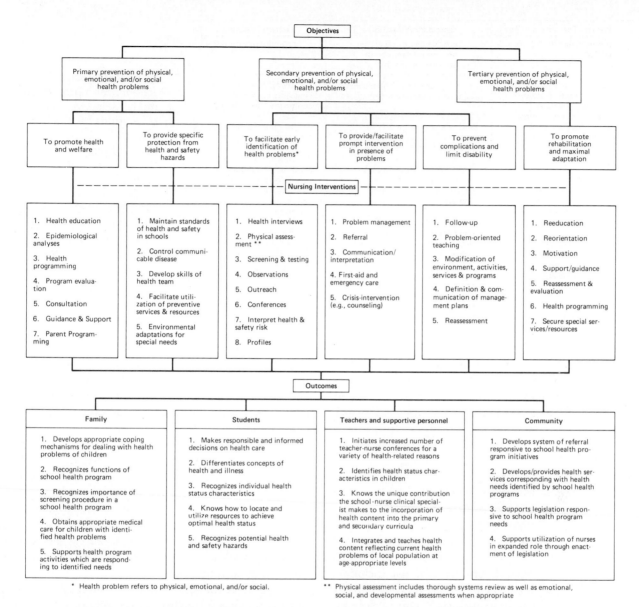

Figure 15-11 Rustia's school health promotion model: delineation of nursing interventions and client outcomes. (From Rustia J: Rustia school health promotion model, *J School Health* 52(2):109, 1982. Copyright 1982, American School Health Association, Kent, Ohio 44240.)

sionals who provide first aid, give injections, inspect for communicable disease, or counsel dirty children. In any school system the nurse must sell what she or he has to offer by demonstrating that these traditional views of nursing are very limited and not an effective way to use a nurse's talents.

Rustia's school health promotion model (Figures 15-10, 15-11, and 15-12) clearly illustrates that nurses have multiple functions in the school setting and that these functions involve nursing interventions beyond traditional physical health care activities. Clinical experience has shown that professionals from other

Primary Prevention — To promote health and welfare	Secondary Prevention — To provide and/or facilitate prompt intervention in presence of health problem	Tertiary Prevention — To promote rehabilitation
1. Teacher conferences to determine special needs of teachers in working with handicapped/terminal children; provide support and guidance. Be involved in IEP development.*	1. Document student problems by direct observation techniques.	1. Identify inconsistent behaviors in teachers/staff and counsel accordingly.
2. Frequent parent/teacher/ nurse conferences to assure consistency between home/ school in management of behavior and learning, goal setting.	2. Consult with physician and render appropriate primary care, e.g., postural drainage programs.	2. Interpret physician and special therapy instructions.
3. Assess and record developmental progress and revise individual education plan accordingly.	3. Refer to school or other resources for additional psychoeducational testing and evaluation.	3. Coordinate services to assist families in their psychological adjustment to a chronically ill child and assess family coping periodically.
	4. Counsel directly with child and family about problems, feelings, behavior, etc.	4. Plan classroom and building adaptations to maximize ability to function.
	5. Participate on committees for admission, review, or dismissal of handicapped students in Special Education.	5. Assess home environment, identify needs, and suggest modifications.

Figure 15-12 Rustia's school health promotion model: selected nursing interventions for children and adolescents with handicapping conditions. (From Rustia J: Rustia school health promotion model, *J School Health* 52(2):109, 1982. Copyright, 1982, American School Health Association, Kent, Ohio 44240.)

disciplines have a greater respect for school nurses who assume functions beyond the traditionally defined ones than for school nurses who limit their functioning to the provision of routine physical health care. Described below are the various functions a nurse should implement in the school setting.

Advocacy

There still are too many school-age children who are not receiving the health care they deserve. Outreach to assist families to more effectively enter the health care system and a reevaluation of the methods for delivering services to children are needed if this trend is to be changed. Every professional, including the school nurse, must speak out for our children.

The nurse in the school setting is in a prime position to identify children who have health needs and who need more effective health care services. The school nurse must take the initiative to help the families of these children to obtain medical, socioeconomic, and emotional counseling on a continuing basis. If services are lacking, the school nurse should become actively involved in influencing funders to allocate monies for such services. It is known, for instance, that developmentally the adolescent has different needs than younger school-age children. Often, however, community services that specifically address the needs of the adolescent are lacking or inadequate (National Commission on the Role of the School and the Community in Improving Adolescent Health, 1990). A concerned school nurse will have knowledge about the factors that affect an adolescent's use of health care and will take action to promote the development of programs designed to meet the unique needs of this developmental age group.

The school nurse should be an advocate for needed health services within the school system, as well as within the community. It is not uncommon for the school nurse to identify environmental conditions that are unsafe, or gaps in health education programs, or deficiencies in the delivery of personal health services. These situations must not be ignored by the school nurse because they may prevent children from reaching their maximum potential.

In order for the school nurse to successfully carry out the advocacy function in the school setting, the legal issues involved in delivering care to children must be understood. The nurse must also be knowledgeable about legislative programs that finance health care services for our youth.

Since laws and health services vary from one state to another, every nurse functioning in the school setting should become familiar with those that exist in his or her state (Knecht, 1981, p. 606). There are, however, some basic issues with which all nurses must deal when working with school-age children. Specifically, issues related to parental consent for the health care of minors, confidentiality in relation to the health record, laws requiring the reporting of child abuse and neglect, and legislation mandating that children with special needs have equal educational opportunities should be examined carefully.

School-age children are minors. Parental consent is generally necessary for minors to receive health care treatment for such things as immunizations, medical treatment by a physician, and special psychological testing for learning difficulties. Children may be treated by a physician in any emergency situation without parental consent. Since, however, it is very difficult to establish what constitutes an emergency, every school should develop policies that deal with emergency situations. An emergency consent form which includes the following information should be on file for each child:

- Child's full name, address, and telephone number
- Where to reach the parents during school hours
- Whom to call if the parents cannot be reached
- The name, address, and telephone number of the child's family physician
- The family's preference for hospital care
- Insurance or Medicaid numbers
- Any known allergies or chronic health problems of the child
- Parent's consent for ambulance transportation

In addition to the emergency form, every school should have a teacher who is designated as the school's primary first-aid person. This is crucial because the school nurse is often responsible for serving many school buildings and thus is frequently not available when emergencies occur. The permanent staff member assigned the responsibility for handling emergency first aid should take refresher first-aid courses as needed.

The parental consent regulations were designed to protect the rights of minors. It is increasingly recognized that children, especially adolescents, have not had access to certain health care services because they could not or would not obtain parental consent (OTA, 1991, Adolescent Health, vol. III). Thus many states have changed their laws so that minors who are emancipated or sufficiently mature to understand the consequences of their decision can obtain certain types of health care treatment without parental consent. Age stipulations for when minors can seek help on their own vary from state to state.

Laws that allow minors to seek medical treatment without parental consent usually deal with human sexuality problems, drug abuse, and mental health services. In almost all states minors can receive medical treatment for STDs on their own. In some states phy-

sicians can diagnose pregnancy and provide prenatal care, contraceptive services, and drug abuse and other mental health assistance without parental consent (OTA, 1991, Adolescent Health, vol. III, pp. 127-130).

Health laws and educational laws are not necessarily the same. Youth, for instance, may receive health education relative to contraceptive practices in a medical clinic but may not be allowed to receive this same information in the educational setting. Professionals providing health care services must learn how both health and educational laws influence their practice in a particular state. Health care professionals should be advocates for change if these laws do not agree with their philosophy of professional practice.

Confidentiality regarding a client's health record is a legal issue that concerns every health care provider in the school system. Indiscriminate sharing of school records resulted in the passage of the Family Privacy and Education Act of 1974. This act mandates that "parents of students under 18 years of age, attending educational institutions receiving federal funds, may view their child's educational records on request and may seek expungement or correction of false or inaccurate entries. No information can be released outside of the school setting without proper parental authorization. This right devolves on students themselves once they become 18" (Hofmann, 1978, p. 531). Generalized school nurses are technically not official members of the school system, which could present a problem when they need to use the school records. Some school systems have coped with this dilemma by adopting a policy which makes the generalized school nurse an official member of the school staff.

Besides the Family Privacy and Education Act of 1974, several other pieces of federal legislation influence the delivery of health care services to the school-age population. Most of these have already been described in Chapters 4 and 14 or other sections of this chapter: Medicaid, EPSDT, maternal child health, family planning, dental health, crippled children and child support laws, and the McKinney Homeless Assistance Act all ensure funding for essential child health or health-related services. The 1993 Family and Medical Leave Act (refer to Chapter 4) could assist families in dealing more effectively with situations involving ill children. Under this act, employees working for private employers who have fifty or more employees are entitled to up to 12 weeks unpaid leave in a year's period to care for sick family members, including children.

Legislation related to child nutrition programs (National School Lunch Programs, School Breakfast Program, Child Care Food Program, Summer Food Service Program, Special Milk Program, Supplemental Food Program for Women, Infants, and Children, and Commodity Supplemental Food Programs) currently provides funds for child health services, as it has historically. The National School Lunch Program is the oldest and largest of the child nutrition programs. It was started in the 1930s to safeguard the health and well-being of American children and to encourage the consumption of nutritious foods. Most of the other child nutrition programs were initiated in the 1960s after passage of the Child Nutrition Act of 1966. The Omnibus Budget Reconciliation Act (OBRA) of 1980, Public Law 96-499, included many changes in the child nutrition programs. These changes and the legislative history of child nutrition programs are summarized in the document *Child Nutrition Programs: Description, History, Issues, and Options* prepared by the Committee on Agriculture, Nutrition, and Forestry (1983). Frequently youth who should be benefiting from child nutrition programs are not. A concerned school nurse should work to alter this situation if it exists in the school system. A nurse can accomplish this by helping others to see the correlation between poor nutrition and illness, which may influence people in power to support a process that facilitates rather than hinders use of federal school-lunch monies. The nurse can also achieve changes by regularly monitoring legislative regulations. OBRA legislation throughout the 1980s and early 1990s has expanded services to low-income children, including nutritional services.

The Child Abuse Prevention, Adoption and Family Service Act, the Education for All Handicapped Children Act, the School Age Mother and Child Acts, and the Adolescent Family Life Bill, all of which were previously discussed, were passed to protect the rights of high-risk children. School personnel must report suspected abuse or neglect to the legal authorities. They must also provide educational services for all handicapped children and pregnant mothers if they desire to remain in school.

The Adoption Assistance and Child Welfare Act of 1980 (Public Law 96-272) was also passed to protect the rights of high-risk children. This piece of legislation is considered to be one of the most significant welfare bills of the past two decades. It was designed to encourage permanent placement of children, either with their natural families or through adoption, and to discourage foster care arrangements. It is hoped that, through this legislation, children will no longer be allowed to drift in the legal system, being shifted from one foster home or institution to another. Public Law 96-272 is particularly significant for hard-to-place children. In the past, too many of these children never experienced a stable family life because some families who were interested in adopting them could not afford to do so. Many hard-to-place children have special needs requiring financial expenditures that a normal family budget cannot handle. Now families can adopt special children and obtain federal assistance to help them pay for these expenses. In addition, services are available for children, especially adolescents, who cannot remain in their homes or live in a foster care setting (Calhoun, 1980, p. 2). Children who are hard to place are more likely to be found because Public Law 96-272 requires states to conduct an inventory on such children.

State and federal legislation is written to promote and protect the health of school-age children. Compulsory school attendance acts, required immunization before school entry, legislation on health education in the school system, and laws that exclude ill children are some examples of state legislation that assist children to reach their optimal health status. One national health action, the enactment of the National Childhood Immunization Initiative of 1977, is assisting states to better enforce their immunization requirements. The National Childhood Vaccine Injury Act of 1988 promotes permanent access to immunization records and prevention of complications from certain vaccines and toxoids. This act requires that health care providers permanently record vaccinations and mandates the reporting of selected events after vaccination related to side effects from specific vaccines and toxoids (Centers for Disease Control and Prevention, 1988, National Childhood Vaccine).

A knowledge of federal and state laws helps school nurses to speak out on behalf of children when services are not being provided. Laws also provide legal backing for encouraging parents to assume responsibility for acting in the best interest of their children. In addition, laws require health professionals to carry out an advocacy function when they identify that the rights of children are being abused.

Casefinding

"Every child has a right to have an education which will meet his individualized needs and to have care and treatment for handicapping conditions so that he can learn more effectively" (1930 Children's Charter). Casefinding is essential if these goals are to be accomplished. All personnel in the school system have a responsibility to identify as early as possible children at risk for physical, behavioral, social, or academic disabilities.

The school nurse uses a variety of methods for identifying at-risk children. Observing their appearance and behavior during their daily school activities is one way to quickly discern which students need more extensive follow-up. Many orthopedic problems, for example, have been picked up by an alert school nurse who has watched children in the school setting walk down the hall during recess. Eating lunch in the school cafeteria has helped other school nurses to identify children with poor dietary habits. Walking out on the playground during recess frequently assists school nurses in determining which children are having difficulty relating with their peers.

Incidental observations like those mentioned above are extremely valuable, but they do not replace the need for periodic, systematic health observations. The school nurse should meet with every teacher in the school system to encourage them to observe on a regular basis the health status of all students in the classroom. Teachers are the key persons in a health appraisal program. Their position in the classroom setting provides them with frequent opportunities to make significant observations of each child's health status. The school nurse can help to enhance a teacher's observational skills by discussing signs and symptoms of illness, by developing teacher health observational forms, and by responding to teachers' concerns about a particular child's health. In-service programs for all teachers in the school system can also sharpen teachers' observational skills. One school nurse, for instance, noted a significant increase in the number of student referrals from teachers after she showed the film *Looking at Children* to the faculty in one of her elementary schools. This film was developed by Metropolitan Life Insurance Company for the purpose of promoting improved observations of children by teachers. Many local and state health departments have these educational materials available for loan to local school districts.

Teachers' concerns should be taken seriously, because they observe children daily and they are likely to identify abnormal behaviors more quickly than any other member of the school health team. Our clinical experiences have dramatically supported this statement. One of us, for example, received a referral from a kindergarten teacher because a pupil in her classroom looked pale and tired. The teacher was also concerned because it took this child longer than most children to get up after a fall on the playground. The child was seen by his family physician and found to have a congenital heart defect, a condition that had never been diagnosed before even though the child had been seen regularly by medical personnel.

Planned comprehensive screening sessions are another way to systematically observe a child's health status. School nurses should see that such programs are developed, but they do not necessarily need to conduct all screening tests themselves. Hearing and vision technicians, school aides, teachers, social workers, nutritionists, and all other members of the health team can play a vital role in a screening program. Height and weight measurements, hearing and vision tests, dental examinations, and immunization checks have traditionally been conducted in the school settings. In many school settings a more comprehensive screening is being done to identify children at risk. In addition to the traditional procedures, screening for scoliosis, urinary tract infections, anemia, and psychosocial difficulties is being done. Identifying the characteristics of the population being served will help the community health nurse to determine what type of screening program to initiate in the school setting in which she or he is working. Remember that children from all socioeconomic backgrounds have health problems that may not be obvious to them or their families. One middle-class mother was very appreciative of the school's vision screening program after her 6-year-old daughter was found to have serious visual difficulties. The mother reported to the school nurse that, after her daughter obtained glasses, for the first time her daughter was able to see leaves on the trees. Without glasses, this 6-year-old child could see only large masses in her environment. Her mother felt distraught that her daughter's eye problem had not been detected sooner.

Screening programs have identified many students in the school setting who have health problems. It is a waste of time and money to screen for defects, however, if follow-up health activities are neglected. Follow-up is a school nurse's most important function in a screening program. The school nurse can direct families to appropriate agencies for diagnostic, treatment, and rehabilitation services and can find funds for these services if necessary. The Lions' Club, for instance, frequently provides funds for glasses when the client is of school age.

Contact with students in the health clinic and review of school records are other methods school nurses use to identify high-risk children. The school nurse should be alert to problems other than the stated concern when a child visits the health clinic. Orthopedic, visual, dental, and relationship difficulties are often identified while the nurse is putting on an adhesive bandage or comforting a crying child. Earlier in this chapter the problems of teenage parents were discussed. Too often the needs of the father are neglected. When a pregnant, unwed teenage mother visits the health clinic, the school nurse should not forget that there is another person involved in this girl's situation: single teenage fathers do need help. The school nurse can frequently help a teenage father by discussing with the mother the feelings that he might be experiencing and the services available to him for verbalizing his concerns. The nurse can also meet with the father in the clinic or home setting to identify what assistance he needs or can provide. The Teen Father Collaboration project (Sander and Rosen, 1987) has demonstrated that some teenage fathers are interested in contributing to the well-being of their children and take advantage of social services available to them.

Reviews of school records help the school nurse to discern those children who should be contacted in the school setting or families that should be visited in the home. Frequently school nurses identify significant health problems that should be discussed with both school personnel and families when they examine school entry physicals. One school nurse, for example, noted that a kindergarten child's blood pressure was extremely high. Follow-up revealed several interesting facts: (1) the physician thought that this child's blood pressure was elevated because he was anxious about seeing a physician; (2) the child's father had hypertension; and (3) the teacher had noted that the child's ears turned bright red with physical exertion. This child was indeed hypertensive and was placed under the care of a cardiac specialist because the school nurse took the time to review health records and did not ignore health problems identified during this review.

Review of absenteeism records, along with health records, is another way of identifying high-risk children. Studies have shown that students who are frequently absent from school have a high prevalence of health problems and are at risk for future illnesses and absenteeism. Preventive intervention services may help families and children when a nurse intervenes with children at risk for high absenteeism. Helping families is probably the best way to help their children. Referring them to community resources, for instance, may help these families to meet their basic human needs for clothing, shelter, and food, and could reduce the number of illnesses experienced by their children.

High-risk children are present in any school system. When school nurses discover that they are spending all of their time providing first-aid services, they should carefully evaluate their nursing practice. School nurses must regularly determine if steps have been taken to identify children in need. Sitting in the health clinic is not an effective way of delivering nursing services in the school setting.

Community Liaison Activities

Some of the most important factors that the school nurse must consider when working with school-age children are the beliefs, values, and resources of the community where these children reside. The health status of individuals is greatly affected by the beliefs and values that exist in the home and the community and by health resources available to meet their needs. The interrelationship among all of these variables cannot be ignored when health programs are being planned to resolve problems encountered by the school-age population. The problems of STDs and teenage pregnancies, for example, can be dealt with in the school setting only when the values and beliefs present in the home and the community allow this to happen.

School nurses have more opportunities than other school personnel to unite all of these variables. They have the freedom and flexibility to visit families in their homes and to coordinate services between the home, the school, and other community agencies. Viewing the health status of children at school often provides school nurses with data necessary for identifying health priorities and needs in the community. Health needs of school-age children tend to reflect needs of the community in general. When children lack dental care, for instance, this is frequently so because limited community services exist to meet their dental needs.

School nurses must engage in community liaison activities in order to meet the needs of all school-age children. No school system has adequate resources to handle all the health problems experienced by the children it serves. Cooperative planning and collaboration between the educational system and other community agencies who are assisting children can serve only to enhance the effectiveness of the school's health program.

Community involvement should be sought by the school nurse during all stages of the health-planning process. Health programs conducted at school that fulfill health needs as identified by the community are far more successful than programs that ignore community priorities. Perceptions of health problems differ from community to community. Thus it is important for community health nurses working in the school setting to ascertain from their consumers what constitutes the communities' most pressing health problems.

Community liaison activities can be challenging and rewarding for several reasons. Working with others in parent-teacher organizations or community agencies can strengthen the school health program. This, in turn, can increase a nurse's satisfaction because children who need help are receiving it. Community liaison activities also expose school nurses to different viewpoints, which help nurses to expand their range of alternative solutions for health problems. In addition, these activities enhance creative thinking through stimulation by others, facilitate continuity of care, and increase community participation in health programming. Community interest groups are more motivated to implement a health program if they have participated in designing that health program. School nurses, through their involvement with groups, can gain a greater appreciation of community issues, demands, and needs.

Consultation

Nurses bring to the school setting a unique set of skills which allow them to become valuable, contributing members of the school health team. Specifically, there are three major areas where nursing differs from other disciplines in the school setting. First, nurses have been prepared to assess comprehensively all the variables that have an influence on a child's health status. Nurses' understanding of normal growth and development, as well as disease processes, provides them with the knowledge needed for identifying both physical and psychosocial health problems and for determining how to handle health concerns. Teachers frequently ask school nurses questions about disease conditions such as diabetes, epilepsy, hepatitis, or

scabies. They may question if a child is ill, when to send a child home when he or she is not feeling well, or whether a child with a chronic condition should be allowed to participate in recreational activities. Children with heart problems or other chronic conditions are frequently overprotected by school personnel until medical recommendations are interpreted by the nurse. It is also not uncommon for the school nurse to encounter fear when infectious diseases are present in the school system and school personnel do not understand the etiology of communicable diseases or how to prevent the spread of these diseases. One teacher, for example, became so upset after she heard that one of her students had hepatitis that she moved the child's desk into the hall and immediately called the school nurse. She wanted the nurse to talk with her class about "what to do when they got hepatitis." The teacher was sure that everyone in the classroom would become ill, because all she knew about this condition was that it was contagious. Her anxiety was reduced once the nurse explained the etiology and the mode of transmission of this disease process and the treatment needs of the ill child. Appendix 11-1 summarizes some of the common communicable diseases encountered by community health nurses in the school settings.

The nurse's preparation for dealing with the family as the unit of service is a second major area of uniqueness. Family problems may affect a child's functioning in the school setting and often problems of all family members need to be addressed before a child's functioning in school changes. Problem behavior such as poor school attendance, aggressive behavior, use of drugs, or withdrawal from school activities often signals that a child's family is having difficulty. The adolescent depicted in the following case situation had a high absenteeism record until the school nurse helped her mother to obtain medical care for herself.

▶ **Pattie Lynne Babcock was a 14-year-old junior high school student who was missing an average of 2 days of school per week when the school social worker referred her to the generalized school nurse. Even though Pattie only had a functional heart murmur, her mother would relate any illness she had to her "bad heart." The school social worker felt that Pattie Lynne's mother needed help with understanding how her fears were affecting Pattie Lynne's perceptions of her health. Mrs. Babcock was very receptive to the nurse's visit. She had** been widowed recently and "wasn't sure how to care for Pattie Lynne properly." During the nurse's first home visit, Mrs. Babcock related that she hadn't been feeling well lately. Her heart pounded so fast at times that she feared she might have a heart attack. She had trouble with her vision but felt it was because she was getting old. Mrs. Babcock had a history of hypertension but had stopped taking her blood pressure medication "because it made her feel worse." The nurse found her blood pressure to be 210/116 and stressed the need for immediate medical follow-up. Mrs. Babcock reluctantly made an appointment with her family physician while the nurse was in the home. She felt she had too many other things to take care of to worry about herself. Using crisis intervention principles, the school nurse in this situation helped Mrs. Babcock to identify what it was she had to handle and then encouraged her to work on one thing at a time. The nurse's promise to return motivated Mrs. Babcock to seek medical care. During the nurse's second visit the following week, Mrs. Babcock reported that she was feeling better physically and was also able to verbalize that she thought she was going to die. She could identify that when she was afraid, "it was nice to have Pattie Lynne home with me." She also saw how her fear of having a heart attack altered her perceptions of Pattie Lynne's heart murmur. The school nurse continued to make home visits until Mrs. Babcock developed mechanisms to cope with the changes in her life. Like all school-age children, Pattie Lynne continued to miss a day of school periodically. Her attendance record improved dramatically, however, once the nurse assisted Mrs. Babcock in dealing with her problems.

Extensive knowledge of community resources and the referral process is the third unique skill the school nurse has to contribute in the school setting. There are many families within school systems who do not have a regular source of medical supervision. Other families have their own physician and dentist but cannot afford to use these services. One student community health nurse came back to the health department disturbed following her second visit to an inner-city junior high school. She was appalled at the number of children who had obvious dental caries and questioned why their parents did not care enough about them to obtain dental care. A staff nurse suggested to her that limited financial resources might be prevent-

ing many of these families from obtaining the dental supervision they needed. When the student contacted the parents of these children, she found that in fact this was the case. After she discussed the services available at the health department dental clinic, two families requested that all of their children be referred to this resource. School personnel were appreciative of these referrals and identified several other children who needed dental assistance.

Parents and school personnel do *care*. If school nurses demonstrate that they are willing to use the unique skills they have, both families and other members of the school health team will confer with them regularly. The opportunities are endless. School nurses who reflect a genuine interest in the welfare of children and their families, a nonthreatening, accepting attitude toward other professionals seeking advice, and competency in decision-making based on sound scientific principles are more likely to be used effectively than school nurses who do not demonstrate these characteristics.

Epidemiological Investigation

Health services in a school setting should be designed to meet the needs of the total school population. Health counseling and instruction with individual students reaches only the tip of the iceberg in a given population. Nurses must use the epidemiological process to identify *aggregates at risk* and to plan and implement scientific health programming.

Effective school nurses organize the data they have to identify factors that influence the health status of school-age populations. The characteristics of populations are studied in order to determine the most appropriate intervention strategies to meet their needs. One school nurse used health records, data obtained during home visits, contact with students in the health clinic, and census tract information to substantiate the need for a breakfast program in the school system. These data revealed several significant facts. Children frequently came into the health clinic complaining of a stomach ache because they had not eaten breakfast. Fifty-five percent of the children came from one-parent homes where the income was minimal. Of the 167 children enrolled in this elementary school, 110 qualified for a free lunch program. During home visits, the school nurse made numerous community referrals because families did not have adequate financial resources to meet their basic needs. In addition, several children from this school district, who were screened through the Medicaid EPDST program at the health department, had been diagnosed as having nutritional anemia. All of these data were organized and shared with the school principal. Seeing the hard facts, he agreed with the nurse that federal funds should be sought to support a breakfast program in order to improve the nutritional status of students in the school district.

An epidemiological approach to school health is a prevention-oriented approach. In the situation just mentioned, the nurse worked to prevent nutritional problems such as anemia and to prevent learning difficulties in the future; children who are ill often do not learn well. Prevention is far less costly than treatment.

There are numerous situations in the school setting that require primary preventive intervention. Accidents, for example, are the leading cause of death in the school-age population. Astute school nurses may be able to identify factors that cause accidents in the school setting by analyzing their health records and by observing their school environments. Identifying commonalities among children who receive care for accidents can result in eliminating environmental factors that increase the potential for hazardous accidents. Debris in the playground, unsupervised play, and playground equipment inappropriate to the developmental age level of children are some factors that may need to be changed in the school setting to reduce frequent accidents.

Accurate and complete record-keeping is essential if epidemiological studies are to be effective. Too often nursing services are not well documented and it is impossible to retrieve data about what was done by the school nurse to solve a health problem. A record system must be designed to allow for complete and efficient recording of data. A cumulative record of each child's health status should be maintained and records of children with special health problems tagged. A tagging system allows for quick analysis of the needs of the population as a whole. If 50 children in a school system, for example, have problems with obesity, group counseling sessions and changes in curriculum planning may be warranted.

It is imperative for community health nurses in the school setting to evaluate the results of their interventions. When nurses work with aggregates, the epidemiological process is the tool that most appropriately helps them to examine the results of their group intervention strategies (refer to Chapter 11). *Until*

nurses begin to document what they have accomplished, they will not be used to their fullest potential.

Health Counseling

Children and youth are currently facing difficult and complex health problems and concerns. They are exposed much earlier than their previous counterparts to issues such as sexuality concerns, varying lifestyles, pressures from peers to use alcohol and drugs, knowledge about health problems, decisions regarding future career planning, and family disruption and disorganization. Often they have knowledge about these issues but they do not understand how to deal with them. They have a need to discuss their feelings and emotions with a nonthreatening adult. Because the school nurse does not evaluate a student's academic performance, which helps students to view her or him as nonthreatening, and because students may have physical health complaints when experiencing emotional stress, the school nurse is frequently the first member of the school health team to identify a student's need for counseling. The school nurse should take advantage of these opportunities and assist these students in obtaining the help they need.

As in other settings, the nurse in the school uses the family-centered nursing process to determine appropriate management goals and intervention strategies. Too often in the school setting, however, data are hurriedly collected because other children are waiting to see the nurse. Problems are missed when this is done and intervention strategies are inappropriate to the child's needs. The case situation that follows illustrates the need to collect sufficient data to diagnose a child's actual health problems and to plan a variety of intervention strategies to resolve these problems.

▶ **Lindsey Elizabeth, a first-grader, was lying on the cot in the health clinic when the community health nurse arrived for her weekly visit. The school secretary reported to the nurse that Lindsey had just come into her office crying because she had a stomach ache. When asked by the school nurse how she was feeling, Lindsey sobbed and stated, "My stomach hurts." A physical examination revealed that no one area hurt more than another and that with a little attention Lindsey stopped crying. When she was asked if her parents knew she did not feel well this morning, her answer was, "My mother doesn't love me anymore. She went away."**

The nurse helped Lindsey to verbalize her feelings of rejection and let her know that she understood how much it hurts to lose someone you love. A hug by the nurse assisted Lindsey in recognizing that others did care about her and so she was ready to go back to class that day. The nurse realized, however, that Lindsey had received only temporary relief from her distress. She had a conference with her teacher and ways to give Lindsey special attention were discussed. In addition, the nurse contacted Lindsey's father. He was very angry that his wife had left and found it extremely difficult to talk to his children about what was happening. Fortunately he was concerned about how his separation was affecting Lindsey and agreed to seek family counseling at a local mental health clinic. Lindsey's mother never did return home. Her father, however, learned how to deal with his anger and gradually was able to allow his children to talk about their mother. This, coupled with support from an empathic teacher, helped Lindsey to function more effectively in the school setting.

Elementary school children often verbalize their feelings more readily than do older school-age children. Since one of the developmental tasks of adolescence is to achieve emotional independence from parents and other adults, students at the junior or senior high level may test the school nurse before they share their real concerns. One such case is described here:

▶ Noel, a 14-year-old junior high student, wandered into the health clinic during class breaks 3 weeks in a row with minor physical complaints. Finally he asked the nurse if he could talk with her alone. He wanted to know "how a person could tell if he had VD." Further discussion revealed that Noel was having nocturnal emissions and thought he had gonorrhea because he had learned in a health class that a purulent discharge occurred with this disease. Noel had never heard about nocturnal emissions and was fearful that his wet discharges at night were due to gonorrhea. He was greatly relieved when he found out that he was normal. The nurse encouraged him to return to the clinic if he had other questions and suggested that his father might be able to talk with him about other developmental changes that occur during adolescence. The need to discuss normal developmental changes as well as to review how STDs are trans-

mitted was also shared with the teacher responsible for the eighth-grade health class.

Health counseling opportunities such as the ones described above are numerous and present in all school settings. Nurses who are attuned to the developmental needs and the social characteristics of the population they are serving will not be "Band-Aid" pushers. Rather, they will take time to find out from other school personnel which students have health problems and will be alert for students who need to talk.

Health Education

The ultimate goal of nursing intervention is to help the client to help himself or herself. Through health education activities in the school setting, school nurses are preparing children and their families, school personnel, and the community to make sound health decisions. They recognize that the population they serve needs adequate knowledge and the opportunity to explore values and attitudes about health matters before they can assume responsibility for maintaining their personal health status.

The following examples demonstrate that the nurse in the school setting has both direct and indirect responsibilities in relation to health education. Nurses use the principles of teaching and learning to carry out effectively their health education responsibilities:

1. *Incidental health education with students.* A second-grader was advised to keep his hands clean to avoid infection after his nail was pulled away from the skin of the right forefinger during gym class. A 14-year-old junior high girl was helped to understand body changes during adolescence after frequent visits to the health clinic with menstrual cramps. Dental hygiene was discussed with a 10-year-old boy who had several dental caries. A tenth-grader was helped to see the relationship between her frequent headaches and her refusal to wear her glasses.
2. *Incidental health education with school personnel.* A seventh-grade teacher was advised to see his family physician after several spontaneous nose bleeds. The etiology and prevention of ringworm were discussed with a first-grade teacher when she informed the school nurse that three children were absent from school because of this condition.

3. *Incidental health education with parents.* A young mother of three children, ages 5 years, 3 years, and 1 month, was given a pamphlet on breast-feeding during a nurse-parent conference. She was breast-feeding for the first time and was late for the conference because of breast discomfort. A father of a second-grader was taught to watch for signs and symptoms of brain concussion after his son was hit on the head by a swing in the playground.

4. *Planned direct health teaching.* Child care, including such things as feeding, bathing, and dressing, was demonstrated to a group of school-age parents. Physical and emotional maturational changes were reviewed with a sixth-grade class the first time a new teacher was covering this topic with the students. What a school nurse does was discussed with first-graders. Opportunities in nursing were shared with senior high students during a career day.

5. *In-service health education.* Teachers in an elementary school were shown the film *Looking at Children* to help them identify common childhood health problems. Parents were shown the maturational films their fifth-graders were to see so that they could respond to their children's questions. A drug education workshop was conducted for junior high teachers after a sharp increase in the incidence of drug usage was noted in their school system.

6. *Curriculum planning.* Diet planning was integrated into the health class after the school nurse noted on student records that a sizable number of students had anemia or were obese. The school nurse was asked to serve on the school health committee after sharing with the school administrators several health concerns of parents she encountered while making home visits.

7. *Health instruction planning with teachers.* A resource file designed to help teachers understand common health problems was established after one school nurse received numerous requests for such information. A second-grade teacher was provided with information about dental health, was given dental models to demonstrate effective dental care, and was helped to obtain pamphlets on dental hygiene when she requested that the school nurse conduct a unit on dental care for her class. The nurse felt that the teacher knew her students better than she did and could more effectively develop teaching strategies appropriate to their needs.

The nurses in these situations all believed in the value of health education as an appropriate strategy to help clients help themselves. They involved all members of the school health team, including parents and students, so that health education would be an ongoing process, even when the nurse was not available. Health education is an essential component of any school health program. School nurses can play a very significant role in ensuring that this component is not neglected. They must, however, be careful not to assume the responsibilities of others when functioning in the school setting: health education should be *integrated* into the overall curriculum. This will never occur if the school nurse continually teaches sporadic health classes. Helping teachers to assume responsibility for health education activities is a much more beneficial approach. There may be times when a teacher is very uncomfortable with a particular topic. Demonstrating that sensitive issues can be handled effectively in the classroom setting often reduces a teacher's fears about covering this topic in the future. If, however, teachers continually ask to have the nurse present certain health topics, the need for in-service education with the teachers should be considered. It is impossible for nurses to carry out their other functions in the school setting if all their time is spent teaching in the classroom.

Home Visiting

Parents are vital members of the school health team. They are ultimately responsible for the health care of their children and they greatly influence their children's health practices. Contact with parents in the home environment is a most effective way of increasing their understanding and involvement with their child's health problems. Home visits also demonstrate that the school nurse cares about parents as individuals and respects their parental rights.

At times home visiting is the only way to obtain a comprehensive picture of a child's health status. Family dynamics do have an impact on a child's functioning. Assessment of parent-child relationships is best obtained in the client's natural setting. Observations of how the child is physically handled, of environmental conditions, and of interactions between a child, the parents, and siblings is more easily assessed in the home environment. These observations provide a different type of data than a conference with a parent in the health clinic. Parents may not be aware of how they interact with their children so that what they verbalize may not always be what is actually occurring.

Most parents do care about their children, and they desire to do the very best they can to help them develop normally. Sometimes they do not take action when their child has a health problem because they do not understand why it is necessary to do so or know what they should do to resolve the problem. At other times health care is not obtained because the family has multiple pressures they must deal with first. Fear, guilt, and not knowing that a problem exists are some other reasons why health action is not taken. A home visit by a concerned nurse can serve as a catalyst for motivating parents to seek help for their child's health needs.

The school nurse cannot possibly visit at home every child served in the school system. Children who manifest needs or difficulties such as the following should receive priority for home visits:

1. History of many absences due to illness
2. Behavioral problems that interfere with academic functioning or that adversely affect social relationships with peers
3. Adjustment difficulties related to a chronic condition such as diabetes, epilepsy, heart defects, or obesity
4. Suspected child abuse or neglect
5. Special programming needs in relation to a developmental disability
6. Lack of medical follow-up on an identified health problem
7. Pregnancy
8. Frequent exposure to infectious diseases

Home visiting can be rewarding and extremely beneficial. It frequently is the key which opens the door to a happier life for many children. The following case situation describes how a home visit helped one 8-year-old child to positively increase her interactions with her peers:

▶ **Tammie Baxter was referred to the school nurse because she had a pronounced body odor. Her peers shunned her, and she appeared to be a lonely child. Tammie's teacher had many questions about her home environment and the health status of her parents. She had heard that Tammie's father was ill as a result of complications of diabetes. A very receptive mother answered the door when the school nurse made her first home visit. The nurse discovered that a family of seven was living in a five-room home that was composed of a living room, a kitchen, two bedrooms, and a bath. All five Baxter children, ages 8, 6, 4, 2, and 1, were sleeping on mattresses on the floor in one bedroom. Tammie smelled like urine, not because she was ill, but because three of her siblings had enuresis. She had limited clothes because the family was having severe financial problems. Tammie's difficulties with personal hygiene were resolved quickly once her mother discovered how the other children were treating her. A referral was made to a community clothes closet so that Tammie could be dressed like her peers. Tammie's teacher was amazed at how quickly her personal hygiene changed after this referral. A little extra attention from the teacher also helped to alter Tammie's relationships with her classmates.**

A long-term helping relationship between the Baxter family and the school nurse evolved from this one simple teacher referral. Tammie was not, however, the focus of the conversation on subsequent visits. Her father was indeed in need of medical care. Mr. Baxter was laid off from work at an industrial plant because he was showing sugar in his urine; a telephone call between the community health nurse working in the school and the industrial nurse clarified that Mr. Baxter could return to work as soon as his diabetes was under control. Several community referrals helped this family to obtain medical care.

Team Participation

No one discipline can meet the needs of all the school-age children. Team cooperation and collaboration are essential if children are to receive the health services they deserve. The school nurse who has a "me" philosophy rather than a "we" philosophy will quickly become frustrated and will soon recognize that it is impossible to achieve goals without the help of others.

In order for school health nurses to carry out their functions effectively and efficiently, they must provide nursing services within the framework of the total health program, working cooperatively with other school personnel. Understanding the roles of each member of the school team (Table 15-4) can facilitate planning and implementation of nursing services. The role definitions presented in Table 15-4 are only guidelines. When entering a new school system, every nurse should spend time with all of these individuals to determine how they function in that given system.

Interdisciplinary functioning can be stimulating and rewarding. For this to happen, all team members must define how they can integrate their specific skills into an effective group effort that emphasizes a common endeavor. A philosophy of care must also be delineated and goals established which are acceptable to all.

No team effort with school-age children will be successful unless the central figures on the team are the child and involved family. Planning *for* others does not work. Rather, they must be *involved* in decision making before they can internalize health beliefs and attitudes and change health behavior.

Practical Tips for Role Implementation

Implementing multiple and varied functions is a formidable task. This is especially true for the nurse in the school setting because the school's primary goal is to educate students, not to provide health care services. School nurses must demonstrate that what they have to offer will enhance a child's learning. In addition, school nurses must often deal with diverse role expectations. School administrators, teachers, parents, and students frequently define the nurse's role differently from how the nurse defines it because they have had various encounters with nurses in the past. It is important for school nurses to avoid panic or withdrawal when they do not initially accomplish what they have hoped to or when they experience role conflicts. It takes time to develop a meaningful role in any setting. Provided below are some suggestions for facilitating the role implementation process in the school setting.

Define Your Philosophy of Nursing Practice

If school nurses cannot articulate the role of the nurse in the school health program, they cannot expect other members of the health care team to use them as they would like to be used. Reviewing the literature devoted to school nursing and the school health policies developed by your agency will provide you with information needed to formulate a philosophy of practice with which you can feel comfortable.

Study Your Community

Understanding the needs of the population you are serving is essential. Children, families, and school personnel will respond more quickly to your suggestions if you demonstrate a sensitivity to their concerns and if you support your comments with data. Review the students' health records to identify their pressing health problems. Analyze census tract data to determine the characteristics of the families in the school district. Talk with students and teachers as you walk around the school building. Avoid sitting in the health clinic. Leave the school setting and drive through the area in which your school is located. Do a community analysis (refer to Chapters 3 and 12).

Contact Key People

A school nurse who takes the initiative to contact school personnel and community groups responsible for the implementation of the school health program is more likely to become quickly involved than one who functions in isolation. Meet with the school principal before school starts. Explain your role and determine a time when you can orient teachers to the nursing services you have to offer. Find out the name of the president of the PTA and the student health council. A telephone call to these individuals may open the doors to the community and the student body.

Demonstrate Your Skills

The best way to help others to understand what it is you do is to show them what you can do. Follow up quickly on the referrals sent to you by other school personnel. Share with them the results of your interventions. A nurse who too quickly states that an activity is not the nurse's responsibility is apt to make other members of the team hesitant to use her or him. Often the nurse is requested to provide first aid or to inspect for communicable disease because individuals making these requests are afraid to handle these situations. Respond to their concerns by first caring for the children and then providing school personnel with information so that they can handle these situations in the future.

15-4 Role Descriptions for Selected Members of the School Health Team

Discipline	Role description
Principals	School administrators who are responsible for planning and providing direction for all activities carried out to meet the goals of the school, including nursing services.
Teachers	Staff members who are responsible for the educational aspects of the school program. Teachers enhance the total school health program by conducting health education activities in the classroom and by identifying children who have physical and emotional health problems that impede learning.
Teacher consultants	Pupil personnel specialists* who have advanced training for handling educational programming for children with special learning needs such as reading problems, mental retardation, and emotional disturbances.
Teachers, homebound	Pupil personnel teachers, specially trained to deal with physical handicaps and the educational implications of these conditions. These persons work in the home with children who have been certified by a physician as being unable to physically attend school due to a noninfectious physical disability. These individuals provide both educational instruction and counseling services for homebound students.
School social workers	Pupil personnel specialists who provide direct counseling services for a child and family, if the child is demonstrating adjustment difficulties in the school setting. School social workers apply the principles and methods of social casework to help students to enhance their social and emotional adjustment and to adapt to change. The primary purpose of their intervention is to reduce impediments to learning. These individuals are often used as resource persons by all other members of the school health team.
Screening technicians	Pupil personnel staff trained to identify particular health problems, usually vision and hearing difficulties, through the use of screening tests.
Volunteers	Lay staff who receive in-service education to carry out defined tasks for other staff members. Responsibilities should relate to the in-service training they have received. Careful selection, training, and supervision by professional staff is a must if these individuals are to be utilized successfully in the school setting.
Therapists, physical	Pupil personnel specialists who treat muscular disabilities of children on a prescriptive order from the child's physician. Their services are designed to enable students to improve their physical health status so that their physical health problems do not impede learning.
Therapists, speech	Pupil personnel specalists who work with children who have difficulty producing and combining certain sounds in words, who are unable to speak with reasonable fluency, who speak with an abnormally pitched voice, or who have physical anomalies such as cerebral palsy. Speech therapists help children to develop normal speech patterns which help them to more effectively develop social relationships and to advance academically.
School psychologists	Pupil personnel specialists whose major responsibility is to determine the reasons for a child's inability to learn. These specialists are often known as the school diagnosticians because the primary purpose of their service is to identify or diagnose causes of learning problems. These individuals use psychological tests, such as IQ and personality tests, during the psychological assessment. Parental permission must be obtained before a child can be tested by these specialists. The amount of direct counseling a psychologist does with a child varies from one school to another. Usually, however, this person functions as a consultant to other school personnel. Psychologists in other settings are often more involved in direct counseling services.

*Pupil personnel division—a special service division of a local board of education. Pupil personnel specialists in this division are accountable to the superintendent of schools.
Modified from Jackson County Intermediate School District: *Special education services available to Jackson County,* Jackson, Mich., undated.

Communicate with All Members of the School Health Team

Do not wait for others to come to you. Relate with teachers in their lounge and in their classroom. Ask questions about the students that will help you to determine where your services are most needed. Share in writing or in person when you have followed up on a referral. Use the bulletin board to provide health information to students. *Talk with the school secretary.* She or he probably knows the students and their families as well as any other person in the building.

Organize Your Activities

A school nurse who just lets things happen frequently does not accomplish goals. Establish a calendar of activities for the year. Be specific about the goals you want to accomplish. Know when you will orient the teachers to your services, when you will provide in-service education, when you will review student records, and when you will follow up on student health problems. A tickler system (refer to Chapter 21) can help you to monitor student follow-up needs. *A calendar is a must.* If you do not plan your time, others will plan it for you.

Set Priorities

A nurse cannot be all things to all people. Identify what needs to be done and then determine what you can handle, considering the time you have available. Request consultation from the school health team to establish priorities significant to the needs of the population being served.

Document Your Activities

People respond favorably to concrete data. Keep a daily record of your activities. Use these records with others to substantiate what you have done, to support the need to set priorities, and to document the need for a new health program or changes in the existing health program. *Remember, changes generally do not occur when concrete data are lacking.*

Summary

Traditionally, community health nurses have assumed a major role in planning health services for school-age children. Currently they work with this population group in a variety of settings such as the home, the school, clinics, and residential settings for children with special needs. A family-centered, prevention-oriented, interdisciplinary approach is the most effective way to meet the needs of school-age children, regardless of the setting in which the nurse is functioning.

In 1991 in the United States there were approximately 63.9 million persons enrolled in school who needed health services. Community health nurses who work with these children encounter an array of physical, psychosocial, cultural, environmental, and developmental health problems and concerns. A well-organized, comprehensive health care system that takes into consideration the developmental characteristics of children and adolescents is essential if youth are to reach their maximum potential.

Since most children attend school, the school is a logical environment in which to promote the health of all children. The role of the community health nurse in the school health program has been evolving since the turn of the century. Initially a school nurse was seen as the professional who provided first aid, gave injections, inspected for communicable diseases, or counseled "dirty" children. Now, she or he is an advocate, a health counselor, a health educator, an epidemiologist, a consultant, a community health planner, and a coordinator. Teamwork is essential for successful implementation of these roles. The central figures on the team *must* be the school-age child and his or her family.

Working with school-age children and their families can be challenging and rewarding. A philosophy of nursing practice that stresses the need to help others help themselves and focuses on the client's strengths reaps the nurse the most benefits.

◀ *An Exercise in Critical Thinking* ▶

Considering the characteristics of the students in the high school you attended and the school environment, discuss the health needs of this group of adolescents and strategies you would use to address these needs. Additionally, identify factors in that environment that would facilitate or hinder the implementation of health education efforts, health services programming, and environmental engineering strategies.

References

Adams PF and Benson V: *Current estimates from the National Health Interview Survey,* National Center for Health Statistics, Vital Health Stat: 10(181), 1991.

Alan Guttmacher Institute: *Blessed events and the bottom line: financing maternity care in the United States,* New York, 1987, The Institute.

American Association for Protecting Children. *Highlights of official child neglect and abuse reporting—1984,* Denver, Co., 1986, American Humane Association.

American Cancer Society: *Cancer facts and figures—1994,* Atlanta, Ga., 1994, The Society.

American Nurses Association: *Functions and qualifications for school nurses,* New York, 1966, The Association.

American Nurses Association: *Standards of school nursing practice,* Kansas City, Mo., 1983, The Association.

Benenson A, ed: *Control of communicable diseases in man,* ed 15, Washington, D.C., 1990, American Public Health Association.

Binsacca DB, Ellis J, Martin DG, and Petitti DB: Factors associated with low birthweight in an inner-city population: the role of financial problems. *Am J Public Health* 77:505-506, 1987.

Burton PT: A day in the life of a nurse: school nursing on cutting edge of prevention, *The American Nurse* 24:23, 1992, September.

Calhoun JA: The 1980 Child Welfare Act: a turning point for children and troubled families, *Children Today* 9:2-4, 1980.

Center for the Future of Children: School linked services, *The Future of Children* 2(1)6-144, 1992.

Centers for Disease Control and Prevention (CDC): The effectiveness of school health education, *MMWR* 35(38):593-595, 1986.

CDC: National Childhood Vaccine Injury Act: requirements for permanent vaccination records and for reporting of selected events after vaccination, *MMWR* 37:197-220, 1988.

CDC: CDC recommendations for a community plan for the prevention and containment of suicide clusters, *MMWR* 37(S-6):1-12, 1988.

CDC: Results from the National Adolescent Student Health Survey, *MMWR* 38(9):147-150, 1989.

CDC: *Division of STD/HIV Prevention Annual Report, 1989,* Atlanta, Ga., 1990, USDHHS.

CDC, Division of STD/HIV Prevention: *Sexually transmitted disease surveillance, 1991,* Atlanta, Ga., 1992, The Centers.

CDC: Behaviors related to unintentional and intentional injuries among high school students—United States, 1991, *MMWR* 41:771-772, 1992.

CDC: Safety-belt and helmet use among high school students—United States, 1990, *MMWR* 41:111-114, 1992.

CDC: Unintended childbearing: pregnancy risk assessment monitoring system—Oklahoma, 1988-1991, *MMWR* 41:933-936, 1992.

CDC: *Youth suicide prevention programs: a resource guide,* Atlanta, Ga., 1992, The Centers.

Clearinghouse on Child Abuse and Neglect Information: *Child abuse and neglect: a shared community concern,* Washington, D.C., 1992, U.S. Government Printing Office.

Clemen S and Pattullo A: The adolescent with mental retardation. In Howe J, ed: *Nursing care of the adolescent,* New York, 1980, McGraw-Hill.

Collins JG: *Prevalence of selected chronic conditions, United States, 1986-88,* National Center for Health Statistics, Vital Health Stat 10(182), Washington, D.C., 1993, U.S. Government Printing Office.

Committee on Agriculture, Nutrition, and Forestry, United States Senate: Child nutrition programs: description, history, issues, and options, *Legislative hearings of the 98th Congress, 1st Session,* Washington, D.C., 1983, U.S. Government Printing Office.

Compuplay Centers provide computer resources, *NARICQ* 1(3):5, 1988.

DePanfilis D and Salus MK: *A coordinated response to child abuse and neglect: a basic manual,* Washington, D.C., 1992, U.S. Government Printing Office.

Director's Task Force on Minority Health: *Minority health in Michigan, closing the gap,* Lansing, Mich., 1988, Michigan Department of Public Health.

Dubowitz H: *Child maltreatment in the United Stats: etiology, impact and prevention,* Washington, D.C., 1986, U.S. Congress, Office of Technology Assessment.

Eberst RM: Defining health: a multidimensional model, *J School Health* 54:99-103, 1984. Copyright 1984, American School Health Association, Kent, Ohio, 44240.

Enos WF, Conrath TV, and Byer JC: Forensic evaluation of the sexually abused child, *Pediatrics* 78:385-398, 1986.

Fergusson J, Ruccione K, Waskerwitz M, Perin G, Diserens D, Phil M, Nesbit M, and Hammond GD: Time required to assess children for the late effects of treatment, *Cancer Nurs* 10:300-310, 1987.

Finkelhor D and Araji S: *A source book on child sexual abuse,* Beverly Hills, Calif., 1986, Sage.

Garrard SD: Mental retardation in adolescence, *Pediatr Clin N Am* 7:147-164, 1960.

Goodstadt MS: Substance abuse curricula vs. school drug policies, *J School Health* 59:246-250, 1989.

Heazlett M and Whaley R: The common cold: its effects on perceptual ability and reading comprehension among pupils of seventh-grade class, *J School Health* 96:145-146, 1976.

Hein H, Burmeister L, and Papke K: The relationship of the unwed status to infant mortality, *Obstetrics and Gynecology* 76:763-768, 1990.

Heindl C, Krall CA, Salus M, and Broadhurst DD: *The nurse's role in the prevention and treatment of child abuse and neglect,* Washington, D.C., 1979, National Center on Child Abuse and Neglect, Children's Bureau, Administration for Children, Youth and Families, Office of Human Development Services.

Hendershot GE: *The 1988 National Health Interview Survey on Child Health: new opportunities for research,* Atlanta, Ga., 1989, National Center for Health Statistics.

Hoekelman RA, Blatman S, Brunell PA, Friedman SB, and Seidel HM, eds: *Principles of pediatrics: health care of the young,* New York, 1978, McGraw-Hill.

Hofmann AD: Legal issues of child health care. In Hoekelman R, Blatman S, Brunell P, Friedman S, and Seidel H: *Principles of pediatrics: health care of the young,* New York, 1978, McGraw-Hill.

Hoffman SD, Foster EM, and Furstenberg FF: Reevaluating the costs of teenage childbearing, *Demography* 30:1-13, 1993.

Humphreys J and Ramsey AM: Child abuse. In Campbell J and Humphreys J: *Nursing care of survivors of family violence,* St. Louis, 1993, Mosby, pp. 36-67.

Hutchins U, Kessel S, and Placek P: Trends in maternal and infant health factors associated with low infant birth weight, United States, 1972 and 1980, *Public Health Rep* 99:162-172, 1984.

Hyche-Williams J and Waszak C: *School-based clinics: 1990,* Washington, D.C., 1990, Center for Population Options.

Irwin CE, Brindis CD, Brodt SE, Bennett TA, and Rodriguez RQ: *The health of America's youth: current trends in health status and utilization of health services,* San Francisco, Calif., 1991, University of California at San Francisco.

Jackson County Intermediate School District: *Special education services available to Jackson County,* Jackson, Mich., undated.

Johnston LD, O'Malley PM, and Bachman JG: *National survey results on drug use from Monitoring the Future Study, 1975-1992,* vol. I, NIH Pub. No 93597, Washington, D.C., 1993, U.S. Government Printing Office.

Johnston LD, O'Malley PM, and Bachman JG: *News release, national survey results on drug use from the Monitoring the Future Study 1975-1992,* vol I, Ann Arbor, Mich., 1993, The University of Michigan.

Jones EF, Forrest JD, Goldman N, Henshaw SK, Lincoln R, Rosoff JI, Westoff CF, and Wulf D: Teenage pregnancy in developed countries: determinants and policy implications, *Family Plan Perspect* 17(2):53-63, 1985.

Kalisch PA and Kalisch BJ: *The advance of American nursing,* ed 2, Boston, 1986, Little, Brown.

Knecht LD: Consent and confidentiality: legal issues in adolescent health care for the school nurse, *J School Health* 51:606-609, 1981.

Lavato C, Allensworth D, and Chen F: *School health in America: an assessment of state policies to protect and improve the health of students,* ed 5, Kent, Ohio, 1989, American School Health Association.

Levy SR, Perhats C, and Johnson MN: Risk for unintended pregnancy and childbearing among educable mentally handicapped adolescents, *School Health* 62:151-153, 1992.

Lindberg FH and Distad LJ: Survival response to incest: adolescents in crisis. *Child Abuse Neglect* 9:521-526, 1985.

Lynam MJ: The parent network in pediatric oncology, supportive or not? *Cancer Nurs* 10:207-216, 1987.

Martinson I, Armstrong G, Geis D, Anglim M, Gronseth E, Macinnis H, Kersey J, and Nesbit M: Home care for children dying of cancer, *Pediatrics* 62:106-113, 1978.

McCord J: A forty-year perspective of the effects of child abuse and neglect, *Child Abuse and Neglect* 1:265, 1983.

Metropolitan Life: *Looking for health,* New York, 1969, Metropolitan Life.

Michigan State Planning Council for Developmental Disabilities: *Developmental disabilities three year state plan: Fy 1984-86,* State of Michigan, Lansing, Mich., 1983, Michigan Department of Mental Health.

Mosher WD and Horn MC: First family planning visits by young women, *Family Plan Perspect* 20:33-40, 1988.

National Center on Child Abuse and Neglect: *A report to the Congress: joining together to fight child abuse,* Washington, D.C., 1986, U.S. Government Printing Office.

National Center for Health Statistics (NCHS): Advance report of final natality statistics, 1986, *Monthly Vital Statistics Report,* vol 37, no. 3, suppl DHHS Pub No (PHS) 88-1120, Hyattsville, Md., 1988, U.S. Public Health Service.

NCHS: *Health, United States 1988,* DHHS Pub No (PHS) 89-1232 Public Health Service, Washington, D.C., 1989, U.S. Government Printing Office.

National Center for Injury Prevention and Control: *The prevention of youth violence: a framework for community action,* Atlanta, Ga., 1993, Centers for Disease Control and Prevention.

National Commission to Prevent Infant Mortality: *Home visiting: opening doors for America's pregnant women and children,* Washington, D.C., 1989, The Commission.

National Commission on the Role of the School and the Community in Improving Adolescent Health: *Code blue: uniting for healthier youth,* Alexandria, Va., 1990, National Association of State Board of Education, pp. 1-52.

National Committee for Injury Prevention and Control and Education Development Center, Inc.: *Injury prevention: meeting the challenge,* Newton, Mass., 1989, Education Development Center, Inc.

National Institute for Allergy and Infectious Diseases: *An introduction to sexually transmitted diseases,* Bethesda, Md., 1987, The Institute.

National Institute for Allergy and Infectious Diseases: *Pelvic inflammatory disease,* Bethesda, Md., 1987, The Institute.

National Research Council, Institute of Medicine, Committee on Trauma Research: *Injury in America,* Washington, D.C., 1985, National Academy Press.

National Safety Council: *Accident facts, 1988 edition,* Chicago, Ill., 1988, The Council.

Nicholson SW: Growth and development. In Howe J, ed: *Nursing care of adolescents,* New York, 1980, McGraw-Hill.

Number of U.S. births climbed again in 1990, matching 1962 level, *Family Planning Perspectives* 25:236-237, 1993.

O'Day B: *Preventing sexual abuse of persons with disabilities: a curriculum for hearing impaired, physically disabled, blind and mentally retarded students,* Santa Cruz, Calif., 1983, Network Publications.

Office of Technology Assessment (OTA): *Adolescent health, vol I: summary and policy options,* Washington, D.C., 1991, U.S. Government Printing Office.

Office of Technology Assessment: *Adolescent health, vol II: background and the effectiveness of selected prevention and treatment services,* Washington, D.C., 1991, U.S. Government Printing Office.

Office of Technology Assessment: *Adolescent health, vol. III: crosscutting issues in the delivery of health and related services,* Washington, D.C., 1991, U.S. Government Printing Office.

Olds DL, Henderson CR, Tatelbaum R, and Chamberlain, R: Improving the delivery of prenatal care and outcomes of pregnancy: a randomized trial of nurse home visitation, *Pediatrics* 77:16-28, 1986.

Orr MJ: Private physicians and the provision of contraceptive services to adolescents, *Family Plan Perspect* 16:83, 1984.

Osofsky HJ: Mitigating the adverse effects of early parenthood, *Contemp Ob-Gyn* 25(1):57-59, 65, 68, 1985.

Ostrum GA: Sports-related injuries in youths: prevention is the key—and nurses can help, *Pediatric Nursing* 19:333-342, 1993.

Panel on Adolescent Pregnancy and Childbearing, National Research Council: *Risking the future: adolescent sexuality, pregnancy, and childbearing,* Washington, D.C., 1987, National Academy Press.

Passarelli C: School nursing: trends for the future, *J School Health* 64:141-146, 1994.

Perovich JD and Tipon ES, eds: *United States code service: lawyers edition,* 42USCS The Public Health and Welfare §§295f-300z-10, Rochester, N.Y., 1984, Lawyers Co-operative Publishing.

Prevalence of disability in childhood, *Disability Stat Bull* 1:2, Spring, 1988.

Proctor S, Lordi S, and Zaiger D: *School nursing practice—roles and standards,* Scarborough, Me., 1993, National Association of School Nurses.

Rustia J: Rustia school health promotion model, *J School Health* 52(2):108-115, 1982. Copyright, 1982, American School Health Association, Kent, Ohio 44240.

Sander JH and Rosen JL: Teenage fathers: working with the neglected partner in adolescent child bearing, *Family Plan Perspect* 19:107-110, 1987.

Select Panel for the Promotion of Child Health: *Better health for our children: a national strategy,* vol IV, DHHS Pub No (PHS) 79-55071, Washington, D.C., 1981, U.S. Government Printing Office.

Shattuck L: *Report of the Sanitary Commission of Massachusetts,* Boston, 1850, Dutton and Wentworth.

Spencer MJ and Dunklee P: Sexual abuse of boys, *Pediatrics* 78:83, 1986.

Stockwell EG, Swanson DA, and Wicks JW: Economic status differences in infant mortality by cause of death, *Public Health Rep* 103:135-142, 1988.

Stone DB and Rubinson LG: Suicide among teenagers reflects troubled society, *American Medical Association* 230:1246, December 2, 1979.

Stone EJ, Perry CL, and Luepker RV: Synthesis of cardiovascular behavioral research for youth health promotion, *Health Educ Q.* 16:155-169, 1989.

Task Force on Infant Mortality: *Infant mortality in Michigan,* East Lansing, Mich., 1987, Michigan Department of Public Health.

Travis G: *Chronic illness in children: its impact on child and family,* Stanford, Calif., 1976, Stanford University Press.

U.S. Bureau of the Census: *U.S.A. statistics in brief, 1978: a statistical abstract supplement,* Washington, D.C., 1978, U.S. Department of Commerce.

U.S. Bureau of the Census: *U.S.A. statistics in brief, 1988: a statistical abstract supplement,* Washington, D.C., 1988, U.S. Department of Commerce.

U.S. Bureau of the Census: *Statistical Abstract of the United States: 1992,* ed 112, Washington, D.C., 1992, U.S. Government Printing Office.

U.S. Bureau of the Census: *Population profile of the United States: 1993,* Current Population Reports, Series P23-185, Washington D.C., 1993, U.S. Government Printing Office.

U.S. Congress, Office of Technology Assessment: *Healthy children: investing in the future,* OTA-H-345, Washington, D.C., 1988, US Government Printing Office.

U.S. Department of Health, Education and Welfare (USDHEW): *Healthy people: the Surgeon General's report on health promotion and disease prevention,* DHEW Pub No PHS 79-55071, Washington, D.C., 1979, U.S. Government Printing Office.

USDHHS, Office of Disease Prevention and Health Promotion: *The 1990 health objectives for the nation: a midcourse review,* Washington, D.C., 1986, U.S. Government Printing Office.

USDHHS, Office of Maternal and Child Health: *Surgeon General's workshop on violence and public health report,* DHHS Pub No HRS-D-MC 86-1, Rockville, Md., 1986, The Office.

USDHHS: *Prevention '86/'87: federal programs and progress,* Washington, D.C., 1987, U.S. Government Printing Office.

USDHHS, Public Health Service: *Adolescent family life program: fact sheet,* Washington, D.C., 1988, The Service.

USDHHS, Office of Maternal and Child Health: *Child health USA '89,* HRS-M-CH 8915, Washington, D.C., 1989, Bureau of Maternal and Child Health Recourses Development.

USDHHS, National Center for Nursing Research: *HIV infection: prevention and care, a report of the NCNR priority expert panel on HIV infection,* NIH Pub No. 90-2417, Bethesda, Md., 1990, The Center.

USDHHS: *Healthy people 2000: national health promotion and disease prevention objectives, full report, with commentary,* Washington, D.C., 1991, U.S. Government Printing Office.

USDHHS: *Child health USA '92,* Washington, D.C., 1993, U.S. Government Printing Office.

USDHHS: National Institute of Child Health and Human Development: *The new face of AIDS: a maternal and pediatric epidemic,* Washington, D.C., 1993, The Institute.

Van Dover LJW: *Influence of nurse-client contracting on family planning knowledge and behaviors in a university student population,* unpublished doctoral dissertation, Ann Arbor, 1985, University of Michigan School of Nursing.

Verhalen RD: Other unintentional injuries, *Public Health Rep* 102:673-675, 1987.

Wallace H: *Health services for mothers and children,* Philadelphia, 1962, Saunders.

Westoff CF: Contraceptive paths toward the reduction of unintended pregnancy and abortion, *Family Plan Perspect* 20(1):4-13, 1988.

Whaley LF and Wong DL: *Nursing care of infants and children,* ed 4, St. Louis, 1991, Mosby.

Young M, Werch CE, and Bakema D: Area specific self-esteem scales and substance use among elementary and middle school children, *J School Health* 59:251-254, 1989.

Selected Bibliography

Atwood JD and Donnelly JW: Adolescent pregnancy: combating the problem from a multi-systemic health perspective, *Health Ed* 40(4):219-227, 1993.

Center for the Future of Children: School linked services, *The Future of Children* 2(1), 6-144, 1992.

Center for the Future of Children: U.S. health care for children, *The Future of Children* 2(2):4-212, 1992.

Children's Defense Fund: *The state of America's children 1992,* Washington, D.C., 1992, The fund.

Errecart MT, Walberg HJ, Ross JG, Gold RS, Fiedler JL, and Kolbe LJ: Effectiveness of teenage health teaching models, J School Health 61:26-30, 1991.

Glynn TJ: Essential elements of school-based smoking prevention programs, *J School health* 59:181-188, 1989.

Henshaw SK, Kenney AM, Somberg D, and Van Vort J: *Teenage pregnancy in the United States: the scope of the problem and state responses,* Washington, D.C., 1989, The Alan Guttmacher Institute.

Jackson MM: Tuberculosis in infants, children, and adolescents: new dilemmas with an old disease, *Pediatric Nursing* 19:437-442, 1993.

Johnson CM, Miranda L, Sherman A, and Weill JD: *Child poverty in America,* Washington, D.C., 1991, Children's Defense Fund.

Katz M, Gunn WJ, and Inverson DC: Design of the school health education evaluation, *J School Health* 55:301-304, 1985.

Kirby D, Waszak C, and Ziegler J: Six school-based clinics: their reproductive health services and impact on sexual behavior, *Family Planning Perspectives* 23:6-16, 1991.

McGovern JP and DuPont RL: Student assistance programs: an important approach to drug abuse prevention, *J School Health* 61:260-264, 1991.

Natapoff JN and Essoka G: Handicapped and able-bodied children's ideas of health, *J School Health* 59:436-440, 1989.

Rosenbaum S, Layton C, and Liu J: *The health of America's children,* Washington, D.C., 1991, Children's Defense Fund.

16

Health Promotion Concerns of Adult Men and Women

OBJECTIVES

Upon completion of this chapter, the reader should be able to:

1. Discuss the developmental stages and tasks of adulthood and how achievement of developmental milestones can enhance growth.
2. Discuss the roles of adults in relation to nursing interventions for wellness.
3. Summarize the national priorities for adult health promotion and protection and preventive health activities.
4. Rank and discuss the major causes of mortality and morbidity for the adult male and female population.

5. Understand gender influences on health needs and behaviors.
6. Discuss factors that increase adults' risk for mortality and morbidity.
7. Discuss the community health nurse's role in maintaining the health of adult men and women.
8. Describe common situational crises experienced during adulthood and nursing interventions that assist adults in coping with these crises.
9. Describe aggregates of risk in the adult male and female populations.

Adults are the caretakers of the young and the old. Men and women are the leaders, the employers, the employees, the college students, the college teachers, the childbearers, the parents of developing families, the breadwinners of the nation, the grandparents of grandchildren, and the caregivers of their aging parents. They advocate for the vulnerable and lead community groups. Simultaneously adults are developing as individuals and need to be concerned with their own health. This chapter discusses health concerns for adult men and women in contemporary society based on major developmental influences. Health risks for this population group and health promotion interventions dealing with these risks are included as well. Finally, aggregates at risk in the adult population are presented. Note that the adult with a handicapping condition is discussed in Chapter 16; occupational health issues for men and women are presented in Chapter 17. The needs of mothers and fathers of the newborn, infant, and young child are discussed in Chapter 14. The caregiving responsibilities for aging family members of men and women, but especially women, are identified in Chapter 20.

Through the 1980s the total population grew about 1% each year, with the largest annual increase among those 35 to 44—the people born at the beginning of the baby boom. The next largest increase was among those 85 and older. These facts lead to predictions that by 2030, 22% of Americans will be more than 65 years of age. Today that rate is 12% (Robert Wood Johnson Foundation, 1991, p. 2). Figure 16-1 depicts the population of the United States by age and race, 1950 and 1989. The black and Hispanic populations are growing faster than the white population and, while the middle years bulge is obvious among these groups, they have a higher proportion of children and a smaller proportion of older adults than the white population (Robert Wood Johnson Foundation, p. 2).

Among both blacks and whites the life expectancy for females exceeds that for males; however, the discrepancy between the sexes is greater for blacks than for whites. In 1987 female life expectancy exceeded male life expectancy by 8.4 years among blacks but only by 6.7 years among whites (USDHHS, 1991, Health status of minorities, p. 16). These statistics influence mortality and morbidity sex differences in the adult population: though they live longer, females experience more chronic diseases than males.

DEVELOPMENTAL TASKS OF ADULTHOOD

Significant personality growth and development occurs during adulthood (Erikson, 1963, 1982; Havighurst, 1972; Stevenson, 1977). Human beings change and learn and pass through developmental stages that require achievment of predictable tasks. Accomplishment of these tasks provides a foundation for growth; if they are not accomplished, future development can be jeopardized or altered. As with all ages there are individual differences in how adults achieve developmental tasks.

The development of adults is complex because they concurrently have individual, family, and community responsibilities. Development is also influenced by numerous variables including interpersonal relationships, established patterns for coping, available support systems, community relationships, and societal mandates, norms, roles, and expectations. Table 16-1 illustrates the complexity of the developmental stages and tasks of adulthood.

Erikson's Intimacy, Generativity, and Ego Integrity

Erik Erikson's (1963) classic work on developmental theory stressed the importance of psychosocial components in development. Erikson wrote that development was a continuous process and that delays or crisis at one developmental stage could diminish successful achievement of other stages. His psychosocial theories address stages of development, developmental goals and tasks, psychosocial crises, and coping processes (Newman and Newman, 1975; Taylor, Lillis, and LeMone, 1989, p. 155). Erikson described eight developmental stages from birth to death, three of which apply to the 18- to 65-year-old population. According to Erikson (1963, 1982) these stages are *intimacy* (young adult), *generativity* (middle adult), and *ego integrity* (older adult). A brief summarization of these developmental stages follows.

Young adults are involved in an intense search of self. At the same time they are at the developmental stage of *intimacy* and need to begin to relate to others and become partners in friendships and in sexual, work, and community relationships. It is a time for development of close personal relationships based on commitment to others. In addition, they must develop the ethical strength to abide by these commitments,

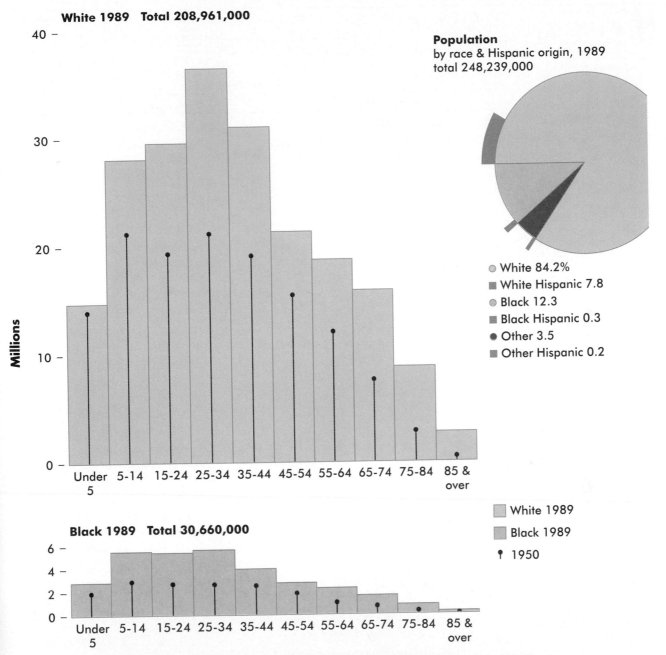

Figure 16-1 Population of the United States by age and race, 1950 and 1989. (From Robert Wood Johnson Foundation: *Challenges in health care: a chartbook perspective 1991,* Princeton, N.J., 1991, The Foundation, p. 3.)

even when this may call for significant sacrifices and compromises. Young adults may experience conflicting values and ideas as they try to sort out what life means to them and what types of commitments they want to make. The young adult who is successful in achieving intimacy will develop the ability to love; unsuccessful resolution can result in isolation and self-absorption.

As life continues into middlescence, it is expected that the adult will guide and care for the younger

TABLE 16-1 Developmental Tasks of the Adult (Ages 18-65): Major Goals—
to Develop Intimacy, Generativity, and Ego Integrity

| Young adult | Middlescent | |
	Middlescence I	Middlescence II
Age: 18-29 years	**Age: 30-50 years**	**Age: 51-65 years***
1. Establishing autonomy from parents or parent surrogates	1. Developing socioeconomic consolidation	1. Maintaining flexible views in occupational, civic, political, religious, and social positions
2. Choosing and preparing for an occupation	2. Evaluating one's occupation or career in light of a personal value system	2. Keeping current on relevant scientific, political, and cultural changes
3. Developing a marital relationship or other form of companionship	3. Helping younger persons to become integrated human beings	3. Developing mutually supportive (interdependent) relationships with grown offspring and other members of the younger generation
4. Developing and initiating parenting behaviors for use with own, and other's, offspring	4. Enhancing or redeveloping intimacy with spouse or most significant other	4. Reevaluating and enhancing the relationship with spouse or most significant other or adjusting to his or her loss
5. Developing a personal lifestyle and philosophy of life	5. Developing a few deep friendships	5. Helping aged parents or other relatives progress through the last stage of life
6. Accepting one's role as a citizen and developing participatory citizen behaviors	6. Helping aging persons progress through the later years of life	6. Deriving satisfaction from increased availability of leisure time
	7. Assuming responsible positions in occupational, social, and civic activities, organizations, and communities	7. Preparing for retirement and planning another career when feasible
	8. Maintaining and improving the home and other forms of property	8. Adapting self and behavior to signals of the accelerated aging process
	9. Using leisure time in satisfying and creative ways	
	10. Adjusting to biological or personal system changes that occur	

*In her text, Stevenson assigns the age range for Middlescence II to be 50-70 years.
Material on middlescence from Stevenson JS: *Issues and crises during middlescence,* New York, 1977, Appleton-Century-Crofts, pp. 18, 25.

generation and assist the older one. This involves an ability to care and do for others, and when these attributes exist the adult becomes *generative* in nature. Generativity is viewed in terms of procreativity, productivity, and creativity, and is cyclical in nature.

Caring or generative adults help to promote these same qualities in children. Economic and social conditions are making it more difficult to achieve this developmental task. For example, with an increasing number of women working, there is less time for generativity and the responsibilities it entails.

If generativity is not reached, stagnation can occur. Stagnated adults do not demonstrate the need or inclination to care for others. Instead they are egocentric and self-absorbed.

Toward mid-to-late middlescence the adult establishes *ego integrity,* which involves reassessment of self. This is a contemplative process that involves looking at where one has been and where one is going, and examining personal values, decisions, and lifestyles. One also strives to accomplish major educational, career, family, personal, and civic aspirations during this stage of life, and to become self-fulfilled. If life aspirations are not fulfilled, adulthood can be a time of disillusionment, disenchantment, and despair. However, the person who has achieved ego integrity knows and likes himself or herself and is able to accept individual strengths and weaknesses. The person is able to distinguish between the things over which she or he does and does not have control and can accept those things that cannot be changed. Despair is likely to occur if ego integrity is not reached.

In order to promote wellness and to enhance an adult's self-care capabilities, the community health nurse needs to have an understanding of the processes involved in developing intimacy, generativity, and ego integrity. Adults should be moving toward accomplishment of these developmental tasks, if health is to be maintained. The community health nurse can facilitate accomplishment of adult developmental tasks through anticipatory guidance, stress and crisis intervention, health risk appraisal, teaching, referral to appropriate community resources, and health promotion activities.

The Roles of the Adult and Nursing Intervention

When examining the developmental tasks of adulthood and the roles assumed by the adult in achieving these tasks, it can be seen that life for an adult is complex and changing. Major roles assumed by the adult are varied and include parent, grandparent, individual, spouse or companion, son or daughter, citizen, friend, leisure-time user, and worker. A role assumed in one setting will often influence a role assumed in another. A person may not be developmentally ready to assume another role when chronological age requirements dictate change, or unexpected situations make the role assumption mandatory. Examples of role changes that people often are not prepared to make are mandatory retirement at age 65 years and parenthood when a pregnancy was unplanned.

Individual

The adult's role as an individual is an extremely important one. The adult is his or her own person with individual experiences, thoughts, and feelings; when working with adults, nurses should obtain information about their individual needs. Labeling and stereotyping must be avoided, and plans of care should be developed to meet the needs of the individual.

The community health nurse should always remember that all adults need to define what is personally important to them and set personal life goals. This concept can create conflict for the nurse, especially when the goals of clients differ from those of the nurse. The nurse who recognizes that accepting the client's right of self-determination generates trust, cooperation, and self-esteem finds it easier to handle this conflict.

An example of when a client's and nurse's values may differ can be seen in the contemporary issue of women's striving for equality. Today, for example, many women have a career outside the home. This can create feelings of anxiety and insecurity in some women who do not have outside work interests. These women may enjoy staying at home but also question if something is wrong with them because they do not have interests similar to "all" other women. A community health nurse working with such women should keep in mind that the goal is to help clients to learn what is self-fulfilling for them. Work outside the home is not the only way to achieve happiness and satisfaction. The nurse should assist women who are having these conflicts to determine why they are having them; is it because they want to change their style of living or because they feel society expects them to do so? The nurse can also help these women to explore the alternatives they have for achieving self-fulfillment. The nurse should guard against stressing career alternatives over others. At times, options which have been rewarding to the nurse are emphasized; *remember that various lifestyles are healthy, not abnormal.*

The individual needs to be prepared physically, mentally, and socially to take on the future in a manner that will promote personal growth and development. The changes that the adult experiences can produce frustration, confusion, and lack of direction. The nurse is able to help adults cope with these changes by providing supportive guidance. Familiarizing adults with the developmental tasks that they are facing, helping adults to explore how these tasks might be achieved, and emphasizing that stress is normal when one encounters new and different situations are a few examples of supportive activities that may enhance adaptation or promote growth when adults are experiencing stress.

Parent/Grandparent

The generative aspect of middlescence is explicit when the roles of parent and grandparent are discussed. One extends oneself to one's children and grandchildren. In the role of parent the adult is expected to maintain the family physically and emotionally, take part in the allocation of family resources and the division of labor, and assist in the socialization process. In addition, the generative person also extends herself or himself to others outside the family. One does not have to be a biological parent to be generative.

Parenting in the young adult years has been discussed in depth in Chapter 14. Parenting issues in the middle years often involve dealing with the developmental concerns of their adolescent children. This situation can be particularly stressful for middlescent adults because they must adapt to stresses associated with two developmental stages: adolescence and middlescence. It is helpful for the nurse to discuss the developmental tasks of adolescence with parents, which can help them to understand that some of what they thought was rebellious and abnormal is a part of normal adolescent development. Although this may not make living through the series of events easier, it helps to reassure and give hope. It also helps parents to see where normal growth and development may have gone astray and where professional help may be needed. Parents who have accomplished the developmental tasks of middlescence are more likely to foster independence in their children and relinquish control than those who have not. Middlescent parents who have not faced the developmental issues of their life period find it difficult to "let go." The community health nurse can assist parents in achieving this generational balance; helping each person progress along his or her developmental continuum should be the major goal.

A primary task of the parent in the middle years is launching children from the parental home. Launching is a time when the young adult becomes independent and autonomous, and the family maintains a state in which other members can successfully function. Launching can be a prolonged period. Many more different roles, responsibilities, and relationships occur in the early stages of launching than in the later stages. The permanence of the launching situation has much to do with the adjustment to it. Also, it is not just the launching activity but the surrounding psychosocial variables that will have a great effect on its success. The nurse can help parents through this process by discussing with them the tasks involved in launching along with ways to accomplish them. Assisting parents in identifying ways, other than child rearing, to achieve satisfaction is one of the most significant activities a community health nurse performs when working with launching families. Adolescents and young adults have a greater chance of achieving healthy independence when their parents support their efforts.

Sons are often allowed more emancipation during the launching process than daughters. Knafl and Grace (1978, p. 514) note that parents provide sons with earlier and more frequent opportunities for independent action, give them more privacy in personal affairs, and hold them to less exacting filial and kinship obligations than daughters. This pattern of functioning can cause family conflict and stress, especially if daughters are about the same age as sons. Helping parents to identify the differences in their behavior when dealing with similar issues may help them to evaluate and change their behavior.

The community health nurse can help parents to be aware of how their involvement with their children should change during launching. Parents must become less directive and recognize that young adults need time to sort out what they want from life. Launching is often a time when parents reflect on how they have raised their children. They frequently evaluate their parenting on the basis of how their children have progressed toward financial independence and whether or not they have established a stable, happy home. Many parents do not consider a child fully launched until these two tasks have been achieved (Knafl and Grace, 1978, p. 311).

Duvall and Miller (1985, p. 276) have discussed the family developmental tasks involved in launching as follows:

1. Adapting physical facilities and resources for releasing young adults
2. Meeting launching-center families' costs

3. Reallocating responsibilities among grown and growing offspring and their parents
4. Developing increasingly mature roles within the family
5. Interacting, communicating, and appropriately expressing affection, aggression, disappointment, success, and sexuality
6. Releasing and incorporating family members satisfactorily
7. Establishing patterns for relating to in-laws, relatives, guests, friends, community pressures, and impinging world pressures
8. Setting attainable goals, rewarding achievement, and encouraging family loyalties within a context of personal freedom

It is important that children recognize the stresses their parents may be experiencing during the launching period. Too often the focus of nursing intervention is only on the parent. Parents are frequently made to think that what they are doing is "all wrong." Adolescents and young adults need to understand that they are not the only ones experiencing stress and that they need to take responsibility for their own actions. The rights of the parents, as well as those of the children, should be protected. This is illustrated in the following case situation:

▶ **John Michael, age 22, decided to live with his parents because he wanted to save money to buy a condominium. He expected to live free of charge, to have no household responsibilities in his parents' home, and to come and go as he pleased. Conflicts arose when John's parents did not agree with his plans. His parents were experiencing financial stress. They had two other children in college and had just finished spending a considerable amount of money for John's education. John was making an adequate salary and they expected him to contribute financially toward family expenses, at least by paying for his groceries. They also felt that he should assume responsibility for some of the household chores, just as he would do if he were living independently. John became angry. He wanted the freedom of adulthood without having to assume the responsibilities that went along with this freedom.**

The community health nurse was involved with John's family because Mrs. Michael was a newly diagnosed diabetic. It was during her third home visit that the nurse identified the stress between John and his parents. During the visit, John's mother was tense, almost to the point of being in tears. Observing her distressed state, the nurse encouraged her to verbalize her feelings and afterward made arrangements to meet jointly with John and his parents. During this conference, the nurse requested that each family member share his or her perceptions of what was happening. Emphasis was also placed on identifying alternative ways to resolve the family conflict and on assisting each family member to see his or her needs and responsibilities.

One issue that became apparent during this conference was that John realized his parents also had needs and were experiencing stress. Just as parents must examine the developmental needs of their children, adult children also must be capable of looking at the developmental needs of their parents. Children often fail to do this, especially when they are working toward establishing self-identity. The child at launching age is able to relate at least partially to the needs of his or her parents, but may need some help in recognizing this fact.

In addition to launching, grandparenting is also encountered in the middle years. Some middlescents experience significant anxiety when their first grandchild arrives because they perceive this event as a sign that they are getting "old." Other middlescents are delighted and eagerly wait for grandchildren. Often grandparents find that they have more time to spend with their grandchildren than they did with their own children. A grandparent can greatly enhance the growth of younger generations. Duvall (1962, p. 409) states:

Children need grandparents who have come to terms with life and accept it philosophically as parents have not yet learned or have not had the time to do. When those who are at the beginning of the journey hold hands with those who have travelled a long way and know all the turns in the road, each gains the strength needed by both.

Adults who have achieved generativity, intimacy, and ego integrity are more likely to hold hands with their grandchildren than those who have not achieved these strengths. The birth of a grandchild to them is not viewed as a negative sign of aging, but rather it is seen as a process that extends and expands their lives.

Spouse or Companion

Adulthood is a time spent in developing and re-developing relationships with a spouse or significant others. A significant other can be anyone with whom the adult has a close, meaningful relationship. With today's many lifestyles it is completely possible that there will be a significant other who is not a spouse. This significant other may be part of a heterosexual or homosexual relationship. Being nonjudgmental about various lifestyles is essential if the community health nurse is to help the adult achieve self-fulfillment.

Adulthood is a time to enjoy joint activities and to spend time in a companion relationship. Once the problems associated with the raising of a family have been significantly resolved, as in later middlescence, the adult can look in new directions for ways to use physical, mental, and social energies. It is important for the couple to maintain separate interests and activities while developing, maintaining, or redeveloping complementary relationships.

Establishing satisfying sexual relationships is a major task of adulthood. However, it is an area often overlooked during the nursing assessment and nurse-client interactions. Clients frequently do not raise sexuality concerns unless encouraged by the health care professional to do so. Specific issues that might need to be addressed during a health interview with an adult include family planning concerns, sexual experimentation before marriage, incompatibility problems, prevention of sexually transmitted diseases, and cultural norms that inhibit the development of meaningful sexual interactions.

The human sexual and emotional responses to menopause and the climacteric can adversely affect spouse or companion relationships. The nurse can help partners to be aware of the changes that each is experiencing and encourage an emotionally supportive relationship. Adults experiencing these changes should be assisted in seeing that they are normal and do not necessarily have to interfere with sexual activities.

Son or Daughter

Adults are striving for independence from their parents and at the same time are trying to maintain or establish meaningful relationships with them. During this time adults can experience role reversal with their parents. As parents age, some become less able to carry out activities of daily living for themselves. Adult children may then be placed in the position of helping

aging parents progress through these later years. Adults need to assist these aging persons without dominating their lives and without taking over decision-making for them. They must achieve a balance without feeling guilty for doing too little or too much and must realize that it is only possible to do one's best with the resources that are available.

The community health nurse should encourage the adult who is caring for aging parents to verbalize feelings. This is especially important to do when the question of whether to place the parent in a nursing home or other extended-care facility arises. It is essential at this time to identify the needs of both the adult and the adult's parents and how the needs of each can be met.

During the middlescent period it is also important to deal with the eventual death of aging parents and relatives. Burial arrangements and the handling of personal affairs should be discussed, and plans should be made. In a society that does not often deal openly with death, this is not an easy task. Health care professionals need to be comfortable talking about dying, death, and grief. Situations involving death and dying are inevitable, yet the American public has little involvement or teaching in death education. For many Americans, death education comes late in life, if it comes at all, and they are often not equipped to deal with death in relation to themselves or others.

Certain life skills can enhance the individual's ability to cope with death and dying situations. These skills include decision-making ability, successful coping behaviors, information sharing and processing ability, and values clarification. Knowledge of the grief process, coupled with these life skills, should assist the adult in resolving grief associated with death. A great number of middlescents experience death for the first time with the loss of a parent. The death of the remaining parent is a major crisis point in the adult's life. Death becomes more of a reality as one approaches middlescence, and there is often the urge to make more of one's life before it is too late. Death education and helping a family work through the grieving process are important community health nursing activities.

It is also crucial for adults to realize that when aging parents talk about death they are not emotionally disturbed. This is a normal developmental occurrence that should not be denied simply because it arouses difficult feelings. Assisting aging parents to resolve their feelings about death can help adults in accepting their own eventual death and other grief, dying, death, and loss situations.

Citizen

During the early adult years persons are usually involved in civic memberships and responsibilities. These involvements often directly affect their families, such as membership in a parent-teacher organization, block clubs to improve their environment, and political elections when school millage is an issue. During middlescence the individual tends to become engaged to a greater degree in civic activities because family responsibilities lessen and there is stability in occupational endeavors.

People in middlescence are accorded the highest positions in American society, including the presidency, company top executive jobs, and high military and civil positions. They are often also expected to take an active role in civic activities. Middlescents have much influence in the community and may run for federal, state, and local offices. They are sought as community leaders and often serve as community volunteers. Adults are valuable resources as volunteer staff and supporters for health projects in the community. However, the middlescent who does not experience a lessening in home and work responsibilities will have less time for such activities unless other adjustments are made. This is increasingly becoming a problem, because two-career families are frequently postponing the onset of parenthood.

The existence of people available to carry out civic activities is critical to the survival of the nation. Not having persons in leadership and volunteer positions would be a great loss for this country. Community health nurses can help make adults aware of their importance to the community and assist them in understanding the need for balancing citizen commitments with family and individual responsibilities.

Friend

Adulthood is a time of life when developing and maintaining a few deep friendships is beneficial and rewarding. It is also a time when one has decreased contact with members of the immediate family, because of mobility, death, or launching of children. Having friends that one can count on and enjoy being with helps to provide support and pleasure when family contacts are limited. Middlescent adults often find it satisfying to have friends with whom they can share their activities.

The community health nurse frequently encour-

TABLE 16-2   Comparison of Work and Leisure

Dimension	Work	Leisure
Decision-making control	Relatively more external	Relatively more internal
Spatial parameter	Continuity of space	Freedom of space
Time parameter	Structured time	Nonstructured time
Social structure	Permanence of structure	Transiency of structure
Activity	Defined activity	Emerged activity

From Stevenson JS: *Issues and crises during middlescence,* New York, 1977, Appleton-Century-Crofts, p. 72.

ages the adult to mobilize additional friendship support in times of stress. Sharing ways to meet other adults with similar interests is helpful. Volunteer work with health or other community agencies, social clubs in the community, church activities, or adult discussion groups are some of the options that the nurse could explore with the adult who has limited friendships. Some adults will prefer not to develop or maintain these friendships.

Leisure-Time User

Leisure is not an easy word to define; it means many things to many people. Leisure is antithetical to work as an economic pursuit. It is a planned activity that promotes growth and is pleasurable. Table 16-2 differentiates between work and leisure activities. *Internal motivation* is the key factor to consider when working with clients who do not plan leisure activities.

In our society many adults do not seriously engage in leisure-time activity. We are work-oriented, and leisure activity is given a lower priority than other activities. When leisure activity does occur, it is largely in the environments of home and community. Some adults limit their leisure activities mainly to the home setting because they have a number of responsibilities that closely tie them to this environment. However, for the person with many responsibilities at home, leisure time may be more relaxing and fulfilling outside that setting.

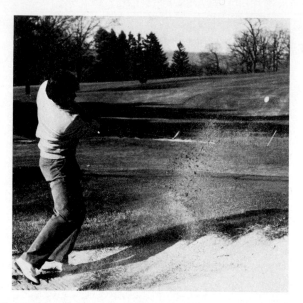

Figure 16-2   Using leisure time in satisfying and creative ways is a significant developmental task of middles-cents, but one that is frequently neglected by career-oriented individuals. Effective use of leisure time can reduce stress, promote sound mental health, and provide satisfying outlets and relationships. This busi-nessman finds that golfing on a regular basis helps him to better deal with the pressures of a busy work en-vironment. While he enjoys his career activities very much, he also recognizes that work cannot fulfill all his needs. (Courtesy Henry Parks.)

Using leisure time in satisfying and creative ways is a developmental task for adulthood (Stevenson, 1977). The community health nurse should encourage the adult to make a conscious effort to devote time to these activities. Otherwise, an important developmental area is being overlooked (refer to Figure 16-2). People need time in which to enjoy themselves and relax. The great amount of free time that often accompanies later life will be better spent if individuals have developed leisure-time activities that are satisfying to them.

Frequently the adult needs help in examining why he or she does not engage in leisure activities. Often it will be found that many adults do not know how to use the free time they have and thus they devote all their time to work or other responsibilities. The nurse can assist these individuals by helping them to identify interests they have had in the past or would like to develop now, as well as to explore ways in which they can meet their current interests. Take for example, the case of Sara Washington:

▶ Sara Washington was a 40-year-old divorced woman with no children. She was referred to the community health nurse for health supervision visits by her family physician following hospitaliza-tion for severe hypertension. After her divorce Sara devoted herself to work. She was an interior de-signer who was well respected in her field; promo-tion came very rapidly. Most of her social involve-ments were work-related.

Sara's recent hospitalization scared her. When the community health nurse took a social history on her first home visit, she replied, "I know I can't keep working like I have been, but I get bored when I don't have something to do. There is very little social life for a woman my age in this town. My peers are all married or divorced themselves. Those who are divorced are like me, they work all the time."

Community health nursing intervention helped Sara to discover how much she missed contact with people on a personal level, the types of social activi-ties she might explore, her fears about getting in-volved, and the middlescent's need for leisure-time activities to achieve normal growth and develop-ment. Sara had enjoyed cooking, entertaining friends, art, and drama before her divorce. Support-ive encouragement by the community health nurse facilitated her involvement once again in these ac-tivities. She especially enjoyed dance lessons and found that they provided several opportunities for socializing. "You know, when one takes the time, it really isn't that difficult to find something fun to do," stated Sara during one of the nurse's home visits.

Adults who have experienced a stressful life event such as divorce may use work to reduce their tension and anxiety. Unfortunately, this develops into a regu-lar pattern of functioning whereby work becomes the central focus of life and leisure activity is eliminated. An astute community health nurse might prevent this from happening by providing anticipatory guidance and supportive encouragement when encountering adults during times of heightened stress.

Worker

The health of the worker and the role of the occupational health nurse are discussed in Chapter 17. Work as a major adult role is discussed here. Working is generally essential to one's economic stability and has psychological implications for the individual as well.

The young adult is in a stage of training for, and deciding upon, a career. The middlescent may be at a career peak and derives much satisfaction from her or his job; this is usually the time of maximum power and influence. Americans in executive positions are often 40 to 65 years old and earn a large part of the nation's income.

By the time a person reaches middlescence, career patterns are usually well established. It will be found, however, that some adults are in the process of changing careers or are dissatisfied with their present ones. The community health nurse must realize that both of these situations can be difficult for the adult and may require crisis intervention services. Through the use of the nursing process, the community health nurse can help these adults to identify why they are dissatisfied with their career choice, what options or alternatives are open, and the career planning resources available in the community, including agencies like career counseling centers, state employment security commissions, and departments of vocational rehabilitation.

Job dissatisfaction is often related to other personal difficulties; stresses at work can be compounded when an adult has home pressures to handle. This was the case with Ed Sorka.

▶ **Ed Sorka was a 29-year-old husband and father of two daughters, ages 3 and 5. He became disillusioned with his job because "his boss demanded too much and gave too few rewards." Ed's wife had multiple sclerosis that was getting progressively worse. She required help with activities of daily living and found it hard to participate in social events. Ed was a devoted husband and father. All his spare time was spent with his family. He found it difficult to talk about his wife's condition or his need for leisure activities; verbalizing stress encountered at work was much easier for him to handle. When the community health nurse helped him to examine both work and home stresses, Ed discovered that he really did not want to change jobs but that he did need time for himself. Arrangements were made for homemaker services to reduce the demands on Ed's time.**

Some adults change jobs or careers out of necessity and not by choice, because of changes in the job market or personal health problems. These individuals and their families can experience intense stress, especially if the adult who is changing careers derived great satisfaction from the previous work. The McSweeney

family, for instance, had an increased incidence of health problems when Mr. McSweeney returned to college to prepare for another career.

▶ **George McSweeney was a 38-year-old engineer, husband, and father of three school-age children. As a result of industrial noise he lost 50% of his hearing. Unable to continue functioning at his job, he returned to college to prepare for another career. Financially his family had few difficulties because Mr. McSweeney received workers' compensation and federal scholarship monies. The community health nurse encountered the McSweeney family after they had repeatedly taken Lisa, their 10-year-old daughter, into the emergency room for treatment of an asthmatic condition. The nurse was well received by the family because both parents were unsure of when to seek medical care for their daughter. The nurse discovered that Lisa's condition had been under good control until the family moved and she had to change schools. In addition, she found that Mr. McSweeney was having tension headaches regularly; a medical evaluation ruled out organic problems. Lisa had fewer asthma attacks and Mr. McSweeney had fewer headaches as the family began to verbalize the frustrations associated with the multiple changes they had recently experienced.**

Stress on the family system can also occur when a wife returns to work during the middlescent years. Many wives stay home during the young adult years to raise a family and to tend the home. As home responsibilities decrease, there are an increasing number of women in middle years who seek employment. Both spouses' working generates a number of considerations. Dual career family situations greatly affect the amount of time that either spouse has available for civic, leisure, or other activities outside the home and work. With the combined incomes, however, dual careers can give increased financial flexibility and allow families to purchase services, such as housekeeping and lawn maintenance, that they do not have time to do. This situation gives the family more choices in relation to recreational activities and plans for the future. A wife who works outside the home can also create changes in roles and role expectations that result in stress. The husband may now be expected to assume more responsibility for household chores, meal patterns may change, and the wife may develop interests that do not include her husband. Families who have a flexible division of labor are more likely to adjust to these changes than families whose roles are rigidly allocated (refer to Chapter 7).

As the adult approaches middlescence, retirement is another area for which planning is needed. Many people look forward to retirement and see it as an opportunity for doing things that they were previously unable to do. Others dread it because they either do not want to cease working or realize that they are not financially stable enough to enjoy it. Success in retirement depends on planning for it during this period of life. Chapter 19 discusses ways in which families can plan for aging and deal with issues associated with retirement.

The variety and diversity of the roles adults assume are only part of the complicated experience of being an adult. Being an adult is not an easy task, and, thus, individual health concerns are put aside for family or civic issues. Often, health care professionals do not focus on the health care needs of the well adult: Screening programs are overlooked, primary prevention activities are neglected, and mental health needs may be left unseen. It must not be forgotten that the well adult also has health needs.

The Human Body in Adulthood

Achieving health for the adult involves maintaining physical, mental, and social well-being. Most adults are considered healthy, but the well adult has many health care needs. These needs may be overlooked due to the self-sufficient nature of the adult and the caretaker role accorded to her or him by society. A combination of the two may put an adult in the position of being "too busy" or "too involved" to look after personal health. It can be difficult to persuade the well adult to obtain health care and to practice preventive health habits. The human body during adulthood is briefly discussed to help illustrate some of the physical and mental changes that the adult experiences.

The human body is constantly undergoing physical and mental changes. During adulthood the person begins to develop an acute awareness of growing older and is faced with adjusting to a changing body image as physical alterations occur. This adjustment is often difficult in American society, as the beauty and stamina of youth are prized. The incidence of chronic and handicapping conditions increases with age and these conditions can also affect how one views oneself.

Several physical changes occur in the human body during adulthood. The senses of taste and smell begin to diminish. Vision is usually well maintained in early adulthood, but presbyopia (farsightedness) is extremely common by middlescence. Presbyopia is caused by a decreased lens elasticity that reduces the power of accommodation. It hinders the ability of the individual to view objects at close range, and glasses may be necessary for reading or close work. After age 30 the cornea begins to lose transparency and the pupil decreases in size. These changes allow less light to be admitted to the eye and result in poor illumination.

Permanent sensorineural hearing loss as a result of aging (presbycusis) accelerates during middlescence. The person experiencing presbycusis has decreased auditory acruity for higher tones and may have difficulty engaging in normal conversation, including talking over the telephone. The duration and type of noise exposure that a person encounters during earlier life influences how soon presbycusis begins. For example, the person exposed to industrial noise and the avid hunter may experience presbycusis earlier than their counterparts because of more extensive sensorineural hearing damage during youth.

Metabolic function—the combining of food with oxygen to create energy—decreases during adulthood. This, coupled with the fact that the person is often becoming more sedentary, can mean increased weight. The basal metabolism rate gradually decreases by middle age with a resultant need for reduction in caloric intake of approximately 7.5% (Murray and Zentner, 1989, p. 471).

Decreasing elasticity of the blood vessels, especially the coronary arteries, predisposes the middlescent to cardiovascular disease. Many middlescents evidence the symptomatology of cardiac conditions, such as shortness of breath, chest pains, and dyspnea on exertion. Incidence of death from cardiovascular disease is on the rise in adulthood.

In middlescence the female's ovarian estrogen production and menstruation cease. This event is called *menopause* and usually occurs between the ages of 45 and 55 years. The symptoms that a woman experiences during menopause are an interplay of physiological, sociological, and psychological changes. The physiological changes are largely a result of decreased ovarian activity and the resultant estrogen deficiency. Menopause does not have to affect one's sexual enjoyment or pleasure. However, the capability to have children ceases. The point of cessation of childbearing ability is still somewhat in question. To be safe, it has been recommended that a woman continue to use a reliable method of birth control for at least 1 year after she has gone 12 consecutive months without a menstrual period (Caldwell, 1982).

Once the female passes through menopause her childbearing capabilities cease. This often has greater psychological meaning than physical significance. Some of the physical symptomatology that may be evidenced during menopause are hot flashes, sweating, chills, dizziness, headaches, palpitations, and atrophic vaginitis. Psychological symptomatology includes depression, change in sexual drive, insomnia, fatigue, headache, irritability, and backache.

In middlescence the male passes through a period called the *climacteric* when the testes decrease, but do not cease, testosterone production. During this time the testes atrophy slightly, sperm production decreases, and, in about 20% of men, hypertrophy of the prostate begins (Murray and Zentner, 1989, p. 468). The male usually goes through this period between ages 50 and 60. He may or may not experience any physical symptoms. Psychological symptoms such as irritability, easy frustration, depression, and change in sexual drive are sometimes evidenced. Many people are not aware that this period exists for men and are often bewildered by male behavior during the climacteric.

Decalcification of the bones, a condition called *osteoporosis,* begins in middlescence. When this happens, the bones become fragile and are easily broken. Vertebral compression can occur and results in backache, headache, and other problems.

As a person ages, the amount of skeletal muscle decreases and muscle cells are replaced by adipose and connective tissue. As a result of these changes, adults have decreased muscle tone, a flabbier appearance, and decreased muscle strength. Exercise will help to maintain muscle tone and strength. The adult can engage in a variety of activities and sports, but it is advised that individuals check with a physician before beginning any vigorous exercise routine. The adult should exercise consistently, gradually increasing the amount to avoid overexertion.

An example of how an adult undergoing the physical changes of middlescence can be affected by these changes is seen in the following case situation.

▶ **Marge, a 50-year-old widow and mother of three daughters, ages 24, 27, and 30, is a typical example of how many people react to body changes during middlescence. She sought help at a local adult screening clinic because she perceived that the physical changes she was undergoing were making her look older than her chronological age. She wanted to maintain a youthful look and stated, "I am having a hard time getting old. I fear the physical changes and the dependency associated with aging." These thoughts were triggered when Marge's oldest daughter celebrated her thirtieth birthday.**

By the standards of her culture Marge was doing well. She had an established career and had just recently developed an intimate relationship with a man that could lead to marriage. She was loved and respected by her children and had frequent contact with them without interfering in their lives. Friends enjoyed being with her and described her as intellectually stimulating and fun. Marge, however, could focus only on her physical changes and was experiencing anxiety in relation to them. She was questioning whether she should terminate her relationship with her male companion so that she would not be hurt in the future. "Men only marry beautiful women."

The community health nurse who saw Marge at the adult screening clinic made arrangements to visit her at home. This nurse used the principles of crisis intervention to help her sort out reality. Marge was helped to identify her strengths and to look more realistically at the changes in her physical appearance. She was assisted in seeing that she had several alternatives open to her regarding her life and that withdrawing from personal relationships could increase her social aging process. Marge gradually began to realize that if she focused on her physical appearance alone, she could lose the joys of life she had already achieved.

Marge is not atypical of the many adults with whom the community health nurse will work. The physical changes of the aging process can be difficult to handle. The development of generativity, intimacy, and ego integrity helps an individual to adapt to physical changes associated with the aging process, because these life goals give meaning and direction to one's future.

Even though physical functioning changes or decreases, mental function can be maintained or increased during adulthood. Cerebral capacity begins to weaken relatively slowly, unless other factors such as cerebrovascular occlusion or depression occur. At age 70 the person can be as intellectually capable as at age 30 and has a greater experiential base than in youth to draw from when making decisions (Division of Gerontology, 1957, p. 58). General intelligence of the middlescent is greater than at any other time of life.

HEALTHY PEOPLE 2000: NATIONAL HEALTH PROMOTION AND DISEASE PREVENTION OBJECTIVES

"*Healthy People 2000* offers a vision for the new century, characterized by significant reductions in preventable death and disability, enhanced quality of life, and greatly reduced disparities in the health status of populations within our society" (USDHHS, 1991, Healty people, p. 1). The concepts of *Healthy People 2000* built upon the work of *Healthy People: The Surgeon General's Report on Health Promotion and Disease Prevention* (USDHEW, 1979) and *Promoting Health/Preventing Disease: Objectives for the Nation* (USDHEW, 1980). These publications were based upon the concepts that responsible and enlightened behavior is the key to good health, that the correlation between poor health and lower socioeconomic status is well-documented, and that health promotion and disease prevention are opportunities to reduce the tremendous expenditures of this country on health care.

Twenty-two priority areas for *Healthy People 2000* were presented in Chapter 4. It is an important observation for this chapter that all of these priority areas are influenced by the adult, including those focused on children and adolescents (since adults are their parents) and those focused on older adults (since their adult children are often their caretakers and advocates). Further, as a result of their energy and independence, adults can assume personal responsibility for their health with less difficulty than younger or older people. The priority areas specific to adults focus on physical activity and fitness, nutrition, tobacco, alcohol and other drugs, family planning, mental health and mental disorders, violent and abusive behavior, unintentional injuries, diabetes, heart disease and stroke, cancer, sexually transmitted diseases, and HIV infection.

Minority Health in the United States

People in the United States are healthier now than ever before. In spite of this fact there continues to be a high number of deaths and illnesses experienced by U.S. racial and ethnic populations. In 1984 the Department of Health and Human Services organized the Secretary's Task Force on Black and Minority Health to analyze this disparity. The Task Force found that the gap between minority and majority health was most dramatic when measured in "excess deaths." Excess deaths are defined as deaths that would not have occurred if minorities had the same age and sex-specific death rate as the majority population. Approximately 40% of all minority deaths fall into this category (Office of Minority Health—Resource Center, 1989, Cancer hits, p. 1). Over 80% of minority excess deaths fell into the six categories of heart disease/stroke, homicide/accidents, cancer, infant deaths, chemical dependency, and diabetes. The Task Force generated extensive recommendations meant to improve the health of minority populations.

As a result of Task Force efforts and findings the Office of Minority Health (OMH) was established to develop, coordinate, and monitor a national strategy to promote minority health, and implement Task Force recommendations. The OMH-Resource Center (OMH-RC) was established in 1987. This resource center maintains information on federal, state, and local minority health-related resources, serves as a minority health information center, stimulates the development of minority health resources, and publishes fact sheets on minority health. The OMH-RC can be contacted by calling 1-800-444-MHRC.

Figure 16-3, Death Rates by Age and Race: United States, 1986, displays the disparity in deaths among the races. Deaths among minorities exceeded those among whites in all age groups except those 15 to 19 and those 85 and over. A compelling difference among minorities as compared to whites is *socioeconomic status*. Poverty and near-poverty are the basis of many health problems experienced by blacks, Hispanics, Asian and Pacific Islanders, and American Indians and Alaskan Natives. However, even if "the socioeconomic effects are set aside, disparities experienced by these population groups will be observed. Simply put, some differences in survival and health are not solely explained by poverty or other environmental factors" (USDHHS, 1991, Health status of minorities, p. 32).

Efforts are being made to try to reduce the gap in the minority health status. Community health nurses can be instrumental in getting health education materials and programs to minority groups, ensuring that these materials are culturally sensitive, improving accessibility to services and serving as advocates for minority health and research. Empowering communities to

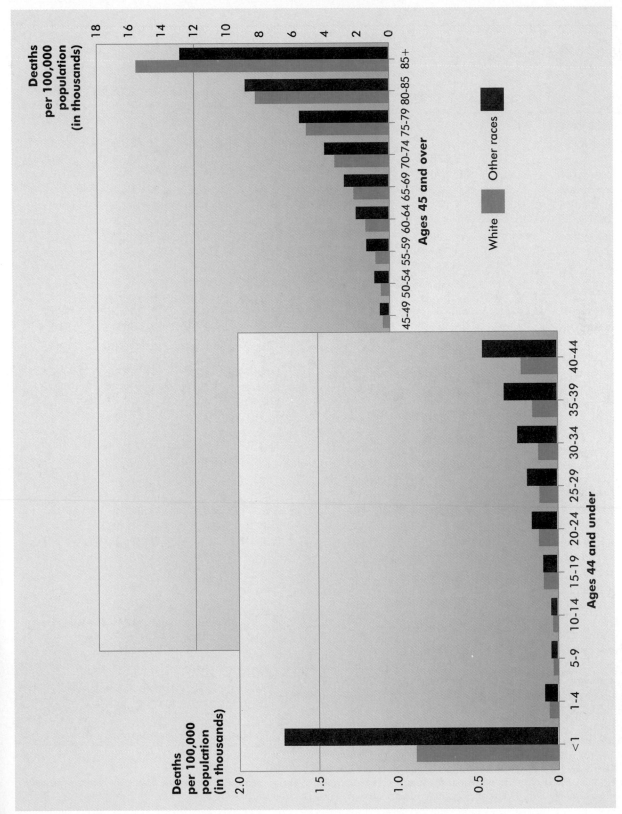

Figure 16-3 Death rates by age and race: United States, 1986. (From USDHHS: *Health status of the disadvantaged: chartbook 1990,* DHHS Pub No. (HRSA) HRS-P-DV 90-1, Washington, D.C., 1991, U.S. Government Printing Office, p. 27.)

TABLE 16-3 Deaths and Death Rates by Adult Age and Sex, 1991

Cause	Number of deaths			Death rates*		
	Total	Male	Female	Total	Male	Female
15 to 24 years						
All Causes	**36,452**	**27,549**	**8,903**	**100.1**	**148.0**	**50.0**
Accidents	**15,278**	**11,534**	**3,744**	**42.0**	**62.0**	**21.0**
Motor vehicle	11,664	8,468	3,196	32.0	45.5	18.0
Drowning	907	823	84	2.5	4.4	0.5
Firearms	542	507	35	1.5	2.7	0.2
Poison (solid, liquid)	414	334	80	1.1	1.8	0.4
Fires, burns	256	172	84	0.7	0.9	0.5
Homicide	8,159	6,923	1,236	22.4	37.2	6.9
Suicide	4,751	4,073	678	13.1	21.9	3.8
25 to 44 years						
All Causes	**147,750**	**104,261**	**43,489**	**179.9**	**255.2**	**105.3**
Accidents	**26,526**	**20,561**	**5,965**	**32.3**	**50.3**	**14.4**
Motor vehicle	15,082	11,142	3,940	18.4	27.3	9.5
Poison (solid, liquid)	3,694	2,914	780	4.5	7.1	1.9
Drowning	1,475	1,332	143	1.8	3.3	0.3
Falls	1,093	926	167	1.3	2.3	0.4
Fires, burns	884	599	285	1.1	1.5	0.7
Cancer	22,228	10,164	12,064	27.1	24.9	29.2
Human immunodeficiency virus infection	21,747	19,263	2,484	26.5	47.1	6.0
Heart disease	15,822	11,497	4,325	19.3	28.1	10.5
45 to 64 years						
All Causes	**368,754**	**227,464**	**141,290**	**788.9**	**1,011.2**	**582.6**
Cancer	134,117	72,193	61,924	286.9	320.9	255.4
Heart Disease	105,359	74,258	31,101	225.4	330.1	128.3
Stroke (cerebrovascular disease)	14,464	7,791	6,673	30.9	34.6	27.5
Accidents	**13,693**	**9,750**	**3,943**	**29.3**	**43.3**	**16.3**
Motor vehicle	6,616	4,458	2,158	14.2	19.8	8.9
Falls	1,355	1,038	317	2.9	4.6	1.3
Poison (solid, liquid)	872	553	319	1.9	2.5	1.3
Fires, burns	636	438	198	1.4	1.9	0.8
Drowning	611	518	93	1.3	2.3	0.4
Chronic obstructive pulmonary disease	12,769	6,874	5,895	27.3	30.6	24.3
Chronic liver disease cirrhosis	10,497	7,301	3,196	22.5	32.5	13.2

*Deaths per 100,000 population in each age group.
Source: Deaths are latest figures from National Center for Health Statistics.
Rates are National Safety Council calculations. The all causes and accident totals for each age group include deaths not shown separately.
From National Safety Council: *Accident Facts,* 1994 edition, Chicago, 1994, The Council, p. 7.

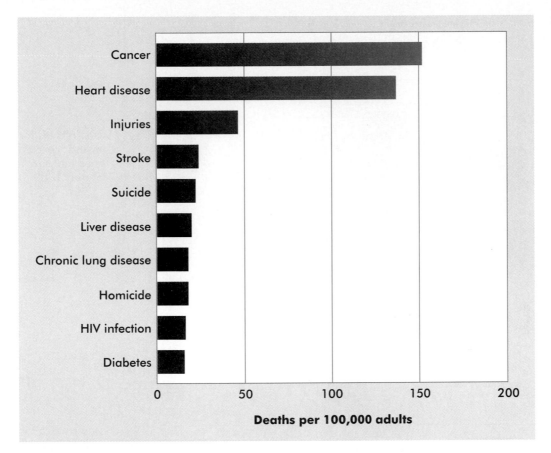

Figure 16-4   Leading causes of death of adults aged 25 through 64, 1987. (From USDHHS: *Healthy people 2000: national health promotion and disease prevention objectives, full report, with commentary,* Washington, D.C., 1991, U.S. Government Printing Office, p. 19.)

make decisions about their own health care needs and solutions as discussed in Chapter 13 is one intervention that can help to reduce the disparity in health status between whites and minorities in this country.

GENDER INFLUENCES ON HEALTH NEEDS AND BEHAVIORS

As discussed in Chapter 11, personal factors including gender, age, race, socioeconomic status, stress, and lifestyle and behavior influence the epidemiology of disease occurrence and resolution. Of these factors, gender has frequently been neglected in health care practice and research. There is, however, a growing recognition that women and men have unique health risks and needs which often require special health planning and programming. The Women's Health Initiative Project, started in 1991 by the National Institutes of Health, could provide significant data to facilitate health planning for women. Much of the research in the past has used male subjects.

In surveys that examine people's perception of their own health, only 6% of those 15 to 44 report their health as fair or poor. By comparison, among those 65 and older, 29% rate their health as poor (Robert Wood Johnson Foundation, 1991, p. 100). However, illness and deaths that are wholly or in part preventable with changes in lifestyle do occur in the age group of 25 to 65 (USDHHS, 1991, Healthy people, p. 19). Table 16-3 depicts deaths and death rates by age and sex in 1991. Figure 16-4 portrays pictorially the leading causes of death of adults aged 25 through 64 for 1987. Figure 16-5 breaks down the two leading causes of death, cancer and heart disease, by race and sex, using data from 1989. Note that black males have the highest rates of death for both of these disease; white females have the lowest rates for both diseases.

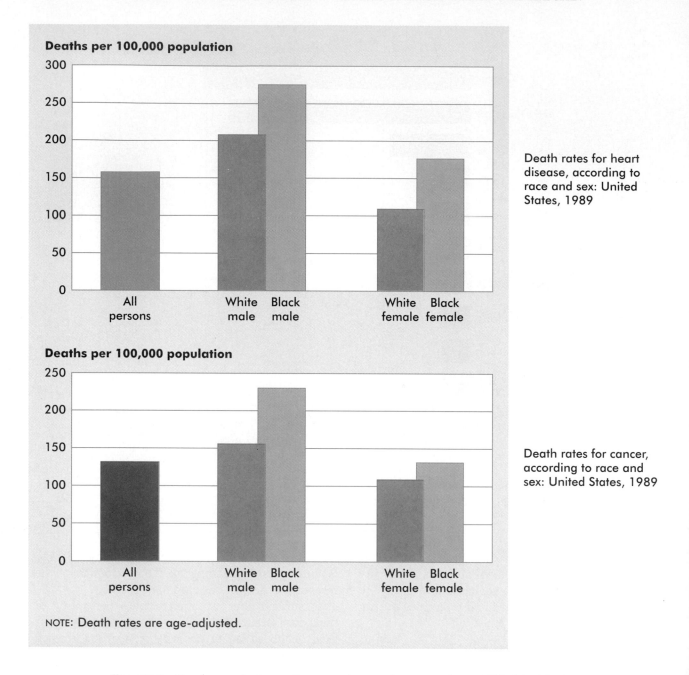

Deaths per 100,000 population

Death rates for heart disease, according to race and sex: United States, 1989

Deaths per 100,000 population

Death rates for cancer, according to race and sex: United States, 1989

NOTE: Death rates are age-adjusted.

Figure 16-5 Death rates for heart disease and cancer by race and sex, 1989. (Modified from the U.S. National Center for Health Statistics: *Health, United States, 1991,* Hyattsville, Md., 1992, Public Health Service, pp. 28-29.

Several major health risk factors are associated with the five leading causes of death in the United States: cancer, heart disease, stroke, injury, and chronic lung disease. Consumption of fat, obesity, exercise, cigarette smoking, alcohol intake, drug abuse, and seatbelt use are all related to these causes of death; all have implications for people's behavior (USDHHS, Healthy people, p. 20).

Health status statistics demonstrate that mortality and morbidity risks of females and males differ. In America women live longer than men (refer to Figure 16-6). "White women have the longest life expectancy

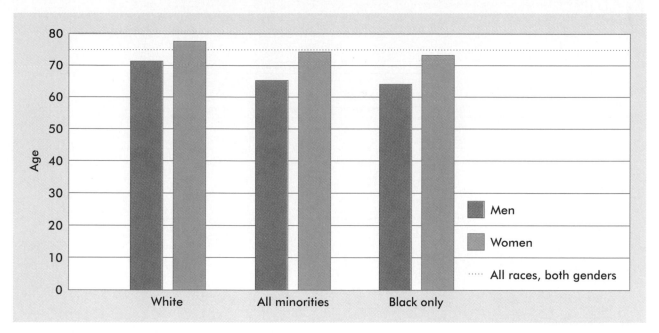

Figure 16-6   Life expectancy at birth by race and gender, 1988. (From the Robert Wood Johnson Foundation: *Challenges in health care: a chartbook perspective 1991,* Princeton, N.J., 1991, The Foundation, p. 5.)

(78.9 years) and black men have the shortest (64.9 years). Black women fare much better than black men and slightly better than white men" (Robert Wood Johnson Foundation, 1991, p. 4) but they still fare significantly worse than white women with a life expectancy of 73.4 years. Socioeconomic status (SES) and lifestyle patterns have a greater influence on overall life expectancy of males and females than do genetic and biologic factors. Genetic and biological forces have a significant impact on select disease-specific mortality rates by gender and race (e.g. cancer of prostate, uterine cancer, and sickle cell anemia).

Although the majority of adult men and women in the United States rate their health as excellent, very good, or good (refer to Table 16-4), women have a higher prevalence of chronic conditions (refer to Figure 16-7). For example, women are affected two to three times more often than men by rheumatoid arthritis (Lawrence, Hocberg, Kelsey, McDuffie, Medsger, and Felts, 1989). Gender differences related to selected other chronic conditions are discussed throughout this chapter. One reason that women have a higher prevalence of chronic conditions than men is that many of these disorders are associated with aging and women generally live longer than men (Robert Wood Johnson Foundation, 1991; Horton, 1992).

In general women report more acute illness episodes and higher rates of restricted-activity days and bed-disability days than do men (Adams and Benson, 1990). Although women use medical and preventive services more frequently than do men, and are more often in contact with physicians, studies have shown that females receive fewer therapeutic and diagnostic interventions than their male counterparts. Further research is needed to identify the reasons for females' lack of access to selected health care interventions (Horton, 1992).

Both men and women have health service use and access issues that need to be addressed by health care professionals from different perspectives. The women's movement that began in the 1960s helped many women to the realization that they controlled their own bodies and their own health. This social and political movement challenged the traditionally male-dominated health care system and has helped to make it less hierarchical with more power for clients in decision-making and with more of an emphasis on prevention (Allen and Whatley, 1986). Childbirth and menstruation, previously seen as "diseases," are now viewed as part of the normal female physiological processess. The pain of labor and nausea in pregnancy are no longer dismissed as psychogenic. One result of

16-4 Number of Persons and Percent Distribution by Respondent-Assessed Health Status, According to Select Age, Race and Gender: United States, 1990*

		Respondent-assessed health status					
Characteristic	All persons[1]	All health statuses[2]	Excellent	Very Good	Good	Fair	Poor
	Number in thousands	Percent distribution					
All persons[3]................	246,098	100.0	39.5	28.6	22.5	6.9	2.6
Sex and Age							
Male							
All ages......................	119,364	100.0	42.2	28.4	20.9	6.0	2.5
Under 5 years...........	9,768	100.0	52.4	28.0	16.5	2.7	0.4
5-17 years...............	23,319	100.0	52.5	28.2	17.1	2.0	0.2
18-24 years..............	12,242	100.0	49.9	28.7	18.1	2.8	0.4
25-44 years..............	39,299	100.0	44.9	31.0	18.9	4.1	1.2
45-64 years..............	22,324	100.0	31.7	27.4	25.5	10.3	5.2
65 years and over......	12,414	100.0	18.4	22.3	32.0	18.1	9.3
Female							
All ages......................	126,734	100.0	36.8	28.8	24.0	7.7	2.7
Under 5 years...........	9,317	100.0	54.0	28.3	15.0	2.4	0.2
5-17 years...............	22,248	100.0	52.2	27.8	17.6	2.1	0.3
18-24 years..............	12,781	100.0	39.5	33.3	22.4	4.1	0.7
25-44 years..............	40,760	100.0	38.5	31.5	23.0	5.8	1.3
45-64 years..............	24,261	100.0	26.9	26.9	29.7	11.5	5.0
65 years and over......	17,367	100.0	16.3	23.3	32.6	19.2	8.7
Race and Age							
White							
All ages......................	207,125	100.0	40.6	29.0	21.6	6.4	2.4
Under 5 years...........	15,387	100.0	54.5	28.9	14.2	2.1	0.3
5-17 years...............	36,674	100.0	54.9	28.0	15.3	1.6	0.2
18-24 years..............	20,362	100.0	45.7	31.8	18.8	3.2	0.5
25-44 years..............	67,571	100.0	43.2	31.7	19.7	4.3	1.1
45-64 years..............	40,339	100.0	30.6	27.7	27.1	10.0	4.6
65 years and over......	26,791	100.0	17.4	23.2	32.8	18.2	8.3
Black							
All ages......................	30,371	100.0	32.1	25.7	28.4	10.1	3.8
Under 5 years...........	2,986	100.0	46.8	24.8	23.0	5.1	0.3
5-17 years...............	7,137	100.0	39.8	27.8	27.5	4.4	0.5
18-24 years..............	3,535	100.0	38.2	26.3	29.2	5.6	0.8
25-44 years..............	9,422	100.0	31.6	27.8	28.8	9.5	2.2
45-64 years..............	4,786	100.0	18.0	21.9	31.8	18.8	9.5
65 years and over......	2,505	100.0	13.0	18.6	28.3	24.0	16.1

*Data are based on household interviews of the civilian noninstitutionalized population.
[1]Includes unknown health status.
[2]Excludes unknown health status.
[3]Includes other races and unknown family income.
From Adams PF and Benson V: *Current estimates from the National Health Interview Survey 1984,* 10(181), Hyattsville, Md., 1991, National Center for Health Statistics, Vital Health Stat., pp. 112-113.

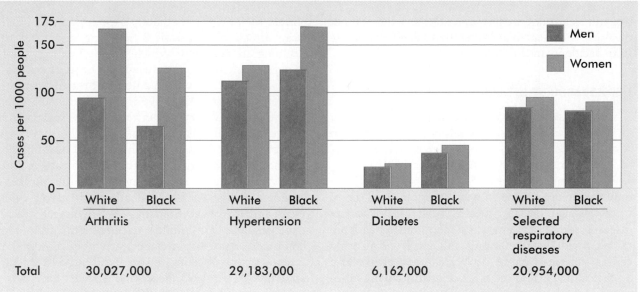

NOTE: Data are not age-adjusted.

Figure 16-7 Prevalence of selected chronic conditions by race and gender, 1988. (From the Robert Wood Johnson Foundation: *Challenges in health care: a chartbook perspective 1991,* Princeton, N.J., 1991, The Foundation, p. 71.)

the women's movement is a system that is increasingly kinder for all consumers. Men, however, also have issues that arise from their gender and their roles in society. A vivid example is the death rates among men from accidents, homicides, and suicides; as Table 16-3 demonstrates, the rates for men 15 to 24 is much higher than those of females. Further, men in our culture are frequently taught that intimacy is not a trait that is acceptable for males. There are men seeking to change these issues so that they are not held captive by sterotypes of gender. Nurses need to remain sensitive to issues of gender in our society and the attitudes held by many people, and work to change those that are damaging.

HEALTH RISKS FOR ADULT MEN AND WOMEN: SELECTED CAUSES OF MORBIDITY AND MORTALITY

As was illustrated in the previous sections, adult men and women have several health risks that are amenable to community health nursing intervention. The three major causes of death among adults will be discussed to demonstrate the role the nurse can play in promoting the health of men and women.

Accidents

Accidents are the leading cause of death among all persons ages 1-37. Among persons of all ages, accidents are the fifth leading cause of death. For those ages 15-24, accidents kill more people than homicides, the next leading cause of death (National Safety Council, 1994, p. 7). Table 16-3 details the kinds of accidents that kill people ages 15 to 64 years of age. This table also graphically depicts that males have much higher rates of deaths from accidents in all categories at all ages. This is related to numerous factors from the occupations in which men engage to attitudes about "what it means to be a man" in our society.

Accidental death rates continued a downward trend in the 1990s (National Safety Council, 1994). Lower rates of alcohol use, increased seatbelt use, and changes in speed limits contributed to this reduction (USDHHS, 1991, Healthy people, p. 19).

The community health nurse can play a major role through health education and health promotion activities to prevent premature deaths in the adult population. Health education activities geared to fire safety, home safety, water safety, seat belt use, general motor vehicle safety, CPR training, health risk information awareness, stress reduction, and poison control and treatment are just some of the activities that the nurse can use to help lower the adult mortality rate from accidents in this country.

Cardiovascular Disease

Cardiovascular diseases are the number one killer in America. These diseases kill almost one million Americans each year—close to one person every 33 seconds (American Heart Association [AHA], 1992, 1993 Heart and Stroke Fact Statistics, p. 1). If statistics hold true, close to one in two Americans will die of cardiovascular disease. Deaths from cardiovascular diseases add up to almost as many deaths as from cancer, accidents, pneumonia, influenza, and all other causes combined (AHA, 1993 Heart and Stroke Fact Statistics, p. 1). The majority of deaths from cardiovascular diseases are from heart attacks, stroke, hypertensive disease, rheumatic heart disease, and congenital heart defects. Cardiovascular disease is responsible for more days of hospitalization than any other single disorder. Cardiovascular disease can be disabling. It is the greatest cause of permanent disability claims among workers under age 65 years in the United States, and is responsible for more days of hospitalization than any other single disorder (USDHEW, 1979, p. 56).

Heart attacks are the number one cause of death in America. Although the death rate from heart attacks has dropped significantly in the last decade, more than 500,000 Americans die from heart attacks each year (AHA, 1992, 1993 Heart and Stroke Fact Statistics, p. 8). Over 1,500,000 Americans suffer heart attacks each year. The nurse can be instrumental in reducing morbidity and mortality from heart attacks. He or she can educate clients about risk factors such as dietary habits, smoking, alcohol use, stress, and family history. The nurse can also encourage families to learn cardiopulmonary resuscitation, be aware of the warning signals of a heart attack, and be acquainted with emergency community resources and telephone numbers. The American Heart Association (Fact Sheet, 1992, p. 1) lists the warning signals of heart attack as 1) uncomfortable pressure, fullness, squeezing, or pain in the center of the chest lasting 2 minutes or longer, 2) severe pain spreading to the shoulders, neck, or arms, and 3) severe pain, lightheadedness, fainting, sweating, nausea, or shortness of breath. The Association notes that not all these warning signs occur in every heart attack, and if any of these begin, the person

should seek help immediately. About one half of all heart attack victims wait 2 hours or longer before deciding to get help, which greatly reduces their likelihood of survival because most heart attack victims who die do so within 2 hours of the first awareness of symptoms (AHA, 1992, 1993 Heart and Stroke Fact Statistics). The nurse can help families understand the need for immediate action.

Strokes rank third among all causes of death in the United States, behind heart attacks and cancer. Annually more than 500,000 Americans suffer strokes, resulting in close to 150,000 deaths (AHA, 1992, 1993 Heart and Stroke Fact Statistics). When direct medical expenses and community resource utilization are combined with lost income and productivity, the cost of stroke is estimated to be about $18 billion annually (AHA, 1993 Heart and Stroke Fact Statistics). No one can calculate the cost of stroke in terms of human suffering, lost income, and years of potential life lost.

Stroke is a major cause of long-term disability. Approximately 2 million people in the United States have been disabled by strokes. Many victims are disabled by paralysis and suffer resultant speech/language and memory deficits. Again, the nurse can do much to decrease morbidity and mortality through health education activities such as risk factor education. The long-term rehabilitation needs of persons with stroke can cause great emotional and psychological distress for both client and family. The nurse can be instrumental in helping the family work through the adaptation and rehabilitation process, and assist in resource coordination and utilization.

More than 63 million Americans have hypertension linked to the incidence of heart attack and stroke. At least 32,000 Americans die from hypertension annually (AHA, 1992, 1993 Heart and Stroke Fact Statistics). Black Americans are at much higher risk for developing hypertension than white Americans. Controlling high blood pressure has been shown to be one of the most effective means available for reducing mortality in the adult population (U.S. Preventive Services Task Force, 1989).

The box on p. 625 lists the risk factors associated with heart disease and stroke. Americans are becoming increasingly aware of these risk factors. Major risk factors that cannot be changed include heredity, age, and sex (presently American men are at greater risk of experiencing a heart attack than women). Risk factors that can be alleviated include cigarette smoking, high blood pressure, elevated blood cholesterol, nutrition, stress, and level of physical activity.

The death rate as a result of heart attack is nearly twice as high among cigarette smokers (almost 47 million Americans) as among nonsmokers; heart attacks are approximately twice as frequent among diabetics as among nondiabetics; and diabetic women have five times the risk of arteriosclerotic heart disease as other women (USDHEW, 1979, pp. 57-59). Coronary heart disease and heart attacks are twice as frequent in inactive Americans as in active Americans (Monmaney, 1988, p. 60). It has been known for more than 20 years that elevated serum cholesterol levels put one at risk for developing cardiovascular disease. It is estimated that about 60 million Americans over the age of 20 years are candidates for medical advice and intervention for high blood levels of cholesterol (Sempos, Fulwood, Haines, Carroll, Anda, Williamson, Remington, and Cleeman, 1989, p. 45).

An organization actively involved in cardiovascular education, treatment, and research is the American Heart Association. The association was founded in 1924 to promote the exchange of information about heart disease. It has more than 1850 affiliates in all 50 states; a main commitment is to research. This commitment involved an investment of almost $69,000,000 in 1989, and since 1949 the association has invested more than $820 million in cardiovascular research (AHA, 1989, 1990 Research; AHA, 1989, Research). The lifesaving efforts of this organization are to be applauded. The nurse should make the client aware of this excellent community resource.

As has been mentioned, the community health nurse should focus on primary prevention activities in relation to cardiovascular disease. The nurse can help to make clients aware of cardiovascular risk factors and what can be done to decrease them, encourage clients to have regular medical supervision, and make them aware of available community resources. The health education activities of the nurse in this area cannot be overestimated. Americans have remarkable knowledge gaps about how to protect themselves against the disease that is most likely to kill them (Monmaney, Springen, Hager, and Shapiro, 1988, p. 57).

Cancer

Cancer, the leading cause of death in men and women ages 25 through 64, is actually many diseases

◄ ***Risk Factors Associated with Heart Disease and Stroke*** ►

1. Smoking
2. Consistent hypertension
3. Elevated cholesterol
4. Diabetes
5. Overweight
6. Inactivity
7. Genetic predisposition
8. Sex (male)
9. Age

From American Heart Association: *Fact sheet on heart attack, stroke, and risk factors,* Dallas, Tx., 1992, The Association, p. 3.

and is associated with a variety of risk factors. Though cancer mortality rates have not changed significantly over time, there have been changes in mortality for some age groups and for some cancers. Estimates are that 30% of cancer deaths are linked to smoking and that another 35% may be linked to diet (USDHHS, 1991, Healthy people, p. 19). Table 16-5 presents the risk factors associated with cancer at the primary and secondary levels of prevention. Table 16-3, presented earlier in this chapter, depicts cancer deaths in each age group, as well as the number of male and female deaths in each age group. Note that men and women ages 15 to 24 die from more violent causes but, as they age, death rates from cancer increase. Figure 16-4 showed pictorially the importance of cancer to the deaths of men and women ages 25 to 64.

The box on p. 627 presents the five leading cancers of concern to consumers and providers. Note the importance of gender and race to each of these groups of cancer. For example, breast cancer is the second most common cause of cancer deaths for women; lung cancer has increased 15% for black men, 12% for white men, 12% for black women, and 8% for white women.

A study by the National Center for Health Statistics (NCHS) puts yearly medical costs for cancer at $104 billion (ACS, 1993, p. 4). It accounts for 10% of the total cost of disease in the United States. The immense toll that cancer takes in human pain, suffering, and death cannot be measured in dollars.

The National Cancer Institute is the chief source of cancer information, education, and research. The Institute publishes pamphlets on different types of

TABLE

16-5 Cancer Prevention: Factors Associated with Cancer

Risk factor	Data about risk
Alcohol	Oral cancer and cancers of the larynx, throat, esophagus, and liver occur more frequently among heavy drinkers of alcohol especially when accompanied by smoking cigarettes or chewing tobacco.
Smokeless tobacco	Use of chewing tobacco or snuff increases risk of cancer of the mouth, larynx, throat, and esophagus and is a highly addictive habit.
Estrogen	Estrogen treatment to control menopausal symptoms can increase risk of endometrial cancer. However, including progesterone in estrogen replacement therapy helps to minimize this risk. Consultation with a physician will help each woman to assess personal risks and benefits. Continued research is needed in the area of estrogen use and breast cancer.
Occupational hazards	Exposure to several different industrial agents (nickel, chromate, asbestos, vinyl chloride, etc.) increases risk of various cancers. Risk of lung cancer from asbestos is greatly increased when combined with cigarette smoking.
Smoking	Cigarette smoking is responsible for 90% of lung cancer cases among men and 79% among women—about 87% overall. Smoking accounts for about 30% of all cancer deaths. Those who smoke two or more packs of cigarettes a day have lung cancer mortality rates 15 to 25 times greater than nonsmokers.
Sunlight	Almost all of the more than 700,000 cases of basal and squamous cell skin cancer diagnosed each year in the U.S. are sun-related (ultraviolet radiation). Epidemiological evidence shows that sun exposure is a major factor in the development of melanoma and that incidence increases for those living near the equator.
Ionizing radiation	Excessive exposure to ionizing radiation can increase cancer risk. Most medical and dental x-rays are adjusted to deliver the lowest dose possible without sacrificing image quality. Excessive radon exposure in homes may increase risk of lung cancer, especially in cigarette smokers. If levels are found to be too high, remedial actions should be taken.
Nutrition and diet	Research is showing the important role nutrition plays in preventing cancer. Evidence indicates that people may reduce their cancer risk by observing these nutrition guidelines:
	1. **Maintain desirable weight.** Individuals 40% or more overweight increase their risk of colon, breast, prostate, gallbladder, ovary, and uterus cancers. Physicians can recommend a suitable diet and exercise regimen to help maintain appropriate weight and body fitness.
	2. **Eat a varied diet.** A varied diet eaten in moderation offers the best hope for lowering the risk of cancer.
	3. **Include a variety of vegetables and fruits in the daily diet.** Studies have shown that daily consumption of vegetables and fresh fruits is associated with a decreased risk of lung, prostate, bladder, esophagus, colorectal, and stomach cancers.
	4. **Eat more high-fiber foods such as whole grain cereals, breads, and pasta, vegetables, and fruits.** High-fiber diets are a healthy substitute for fatty foods and may reduce the risk of colon cancer.
	5. **Cut down on total fat intake.** A diet high in fat may be a factor in the development of certain cancers, particularly breast, colon, and prostate.
	6. **Limit consumption of alcohol, if you drink at all.** The heavy use of alcohol, especially when accompanied by cigarette smoking or smokeless tobacco use, increases risk of cancers of the mouth, larynx, throat, esophagus, and liver.
	7. **Limit consumption of salt-cured, smoked, and nitrite-cured foods.** In areas of the world where salt-cured and smoked foods are eaten frequently, there is higher incidence of cancer of the esophagus and stomach. Modern methods of food processing and preserving appear to avoid the cancer-causing by-products associated with older methods of food treatment.

Modified from American Cancer Society: *Cancer facts and figures—1993,* Atlanta, Ga., 1993, The Society, pp. 19-20.

Five Leading Cancers of Concern for Adult Men and Women

Lung cancer is the most common—and most preventable-cancer in the United States for both men and women, and is increasing as large numbers of smokers grow older. Smoking is responsible for more than 85 percent of all lung cancer deaths. Since 1975, lung cancer incidence has risen more than 15 percent for black men, about 12 percent for black women, 12 percent for white men, and 8 percent for white women.

- **Colorectal cancer** is the second leading cause of death due to cancer. Some studies have suggested that high fat and/or low fiber diets increase the risk of colorectal cancer. Since 1969, death rates from these cancers have fallen among white men and women, remained about the same for black women, and increased markedly for black men. Although there is no general agreement that screening for colon cancer definitely reduces mortality among those not at high risk, consensus recommendations have suggested screening by digital rectal exams, fecal occult blood testing, and sigmoidoscopy for those over age 50.

- **Breast cancer** has become the second most common cause of cancer deaths among women, having been surpassed by lung cancer in the past decade. However, the incidence of breast cancer is more than twice that of lung cancer in women. Early diagnosis of breast cancer improves the chance of survival significantly, with 90 percent of those diagnosed when the cancer was localized reaching the 5-year survival mark. Breast cancer death rates could be reduced 30 percent with regular screening. Some evidence suggests that high-fat diets may increase the risk of breast cancer.

- **Cervical cancer** can be cured if detected early. Increased use of the Pap test has contributed to a 50-percent drop in cervical cancer deaths among both black and white women since 1969. However, black women continue to have 3 times the cervical cancer death rate of white women. Although the death rates have been decreasing, the *in situ* rates have risen in younger women aged 15 through 19.

- **Oropharyngeal cancer**-cancer of the mouth and throat-accounts for 13.2 per 100,000 in 1987. Increased risk has been linked both to use of tobacco products and to heavy alcohol use.

From USDHHS, *Healthy people 2000: national health promotion and disease prevention objectives, full report, with commentary,* Washington, D.C., 1991, U.S. Government Printing Office, pp. 19-20.

cancer that give a description of the cancer, its incidence, causes and prevention, detection and diagnosis, stages, treatment, and advances. The institute publishes *Taking Time: Support for People with Cancer and the People Who Care about Them,* an excellent resource the nurse can share with families. *Taking Time* covers such topics as sharing the diagnosis, sharing feelings, coping within the family, assistance, self-image, the world outside, living each day, and resources.

By dialing 1-800-4-CANCER (1-800-638-6070 in Alaska) one can access the Cancer Information Service of the National Cancer Institute (U.S. Department of Health and Human Services). This service provides information on community agencies and services, answers questions, and mails publications and a publication list. It also provides information about active treatment centers for specific types of cancer.

The National Cancer Institute has developed the PDQ (Physician Data Query), a computerized data base designed to give doctors quick and easy access to the latest treatment information for most types of cancer, descriptions of clinical trials that are open for patient entry, and the names of organizations and physicians involved in cancer care (National Cancer Institute, 1989, p. 11). To gain access to PDQ a doctor can use an office computer with a telephone hookup and a PDQ access code or the services of a medical library with online searching capability. Patients can call 1-800-4-CANCER to get PDQ information.

The American Cancer Society is at the forefront of private sector cancer education and research in the United States. It traces its origins to 1913 when the American Society for the Control of Cancer was founded to disseminate knowledge concerning the symptoms, treatment, and prevention of cancer; to investigate conditions under which cancer occurs; and to compile statistics on cancer. It is one of the oldest and largest voluntary health agencies in the United States today, with more than 3200 chapters. American Cancer Society public education programs reached more than 70 million Americans in 1992 (ACS, 1993, p. 27). The society is involved in professional education, publishes *Cancer Nursing News* (sent to about 90,000 nurses around the country), supports professorships in

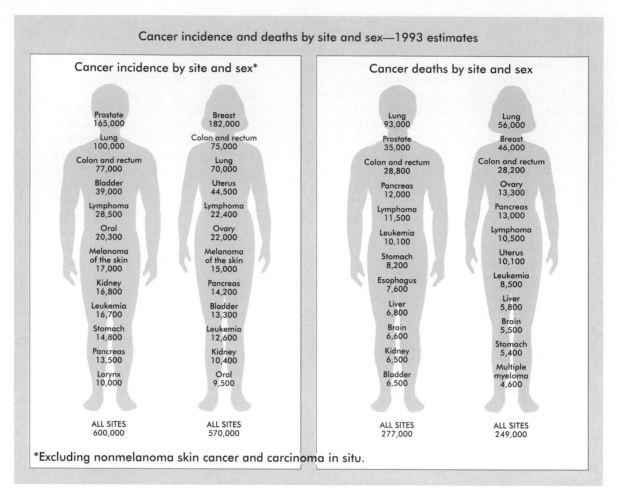

Figure 16-8 Cancer incidence and deaths by site and sex—1993 estimates. (From American Cancer Society: *Cancer Facts and Figures—1993*, Atlanta, Ga., 1993, The Society, p. 12.)

clinical oncology, and offers clinical oncology awards. Society service and rehabilitation activities include the following resource and information services: *CanSurmount*—a short-term home visitor program for patients and families of patients; *Reach to Recovery*—a patient visitor program that addresses the needs of women who have had breast cancer; laryngectomy rehabilitation volunteers in coordination with the International Association of Laryngectomees (IAL); and ostomy rehabilitation volunteers in coordination with the United Ostomy Association.

The nurse plays a central role in health education and in assisting families to locate available resources. The nurse can help the family with a member who has cancer to adjust to and cope with the situation, using the principles of crisis intervention and grieving as discussed in Chapter 8. Hospice care is discussed in Chapter 20.

Figure 16-8 presents the cancer incidence and death rates by site and sex. Table 16-6 portrays the trends in survival by site. It is encouraging to note that the survival rates for many cancers, with the exception of lung cancer, are increasing. Although skin cancer has the highest incidence it is amenable to treatment and does not carry a high mortality rate. Lung cancer and colon/rectum cancer carry relatively high mortality rates. Lung cancer now rivals breast cancer as the leading cause of cancer death in American women (ACS, 1993). Unfortunately, diagnostic procedures such as chest x-ray films and sputum examinations usually do not reveal lung cancer until it has already spread. In adult men, 90% of all lung cancer deaths

16-6 Trends in Cancer Survival, by Race: Cases Diagnosed in 1960-63, 1970-73, 1974-76, 1977-79, 1983-88

	White					Black				
	Relative 5-year survival					Relative 5-year survival				
Site	1960-63[1]	1970-73[1]	1974-76[2]	1977-79[2]	1983-88[2]	1960-63[1]	1970-73[1]	1974-76[2]	1977-79[2]	1983-88[2]
All sites	39	43	50	51	54*	27	31	39	39	38
Oral cavity & pharynx	45	43	55	54	54	—	—	36	36	32
Esophagus	4	4	5	6	9*	1	4	4	3	6*
Stomach	11	13	14	16	16*	8	13	16	15	17
Colon	43	49	50	53	59*	34	37	46	48	48*
Rectum	38	45	49	50	57*	27	30	42	38	46
Liver	2	3	4	3	6*	—	—	1	6	5
Pancreas	1	2	3	2	3*	1	2	2	4	5*
Larynx	53	62	66	68	67	—	—	59	55	53
Lung & bronchus	8	10	12	14	13*	5	7	11	11	11
Melanoma of skin	60	68	80	82	83*	—	—	69†	52‡	68†
Female breast	63	68	75	75	79*	46	51	63	63	62
Cervix uteri	58	64	69	69	68	47	61	63	62	55*
Corpus uteri	73	81	89	86	84*	31	44	60	58	54
Ovary	32	36	36	38	39*	32	32	41	40	37
Prostate	50	63	68	72	78*	35	55	58	62	63*
Testis	63	72	79	88	93*	—	—	76†	—	84†
Urinary bladder	53	61	74	76	79*	24	36	48	55	59*
Kidney & renal pelvis	37	46	52	51	55*	38	44	49	52	53
Brain & nervous system	18	20	22	24	25*	19	19	27	28	32
Thyroid gland	83	86	92	92	94*	—	—	87	92	93
Hodgkin's disease	40	67	72	73	78*	—	—	69	73	74
Non-Hodgkin's lymphoma	31	41	48	48	52*	—	—	48	50	43
Multiple myeloma	12	19	24	25	26*	—	—	27	34	29
Leukemia	14	22	35	37	38*	—	—	31	30	29

Source: Cancer Statistics Branch, National Cancer Institute.
[1]Rates are based on End Results Group data from a series of hospital registries and one population-based registry.
[2]Rates are from the SEER Program. They are based on data from poulation-based registries in Connecticut, New Mexico, Utah, Iowa, Hawaii, Atlanta, Detroit, Seattle-Puget Sound and San Francisco-Oakland. Rates are based on follow-up of patients through 1989.
*The difference in rates between 1974-76 and 1983-88 is statistically significant ($p < 0.05$).
†The standard error of the survival rate is between 5 and 10 percentage points.
‡The standard error of the survival rate is greater than 10 percentage points. —Valid survival rate could not be calculated.
From American Cancer Society: *Cancer facts and figures—1993,* Atlanta, Ga., 1993, The Society, p. 17.

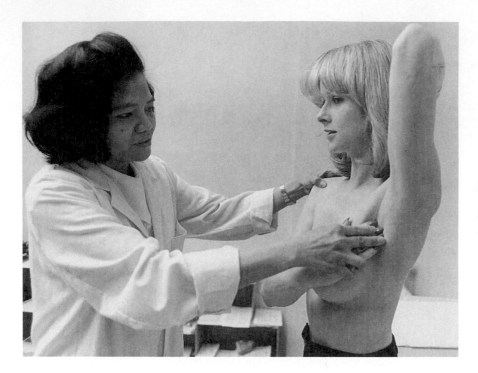

Figure 16-9 Breast self-examination being taught by a health care worker. (Courtesy American Cancer Society.)

have a direct relationship to smoking (USDHHS, 1989). Fortunately several effective screening procedures are now available to detect breast cancer and cancers of the colon or rectum. Women can do regular self-examination of the breasts (refer to Figure 16-9), and can have a physical examination and mammography.

Cancer in Minorities

The health status of Americans as a whole has improved over the past generation. However, studies by the Secretary's Task Force on Black and Minority Health (U.S. Department of Health and Human Services, Public Health Service) reflect that there continues to be a disparity in deaths and illnesses experienced by racial and ethnic groups (OMH-RC, 1989, Cancer and Minorities, p. 1). A study by the Centers for Disease Control and Prevention showed that the death rate for blacks is 2.5 times higher than for whites and that in 31% of the cases the difference cannot be explained on the basis of health risk factors and family income (Friend, 1990, p. 1D).

Cancer disproportionately strikes minority groups; a recent report by the Secretary's Task Force on Black and Minority Health found wide gaps in cancer death rates between minorities and whites (OMH-RC, 1989, Cancer hits, p. 1). Data from the Task Force, compar-

ing mortality of minorities and whites, reveal the following: Japanese living in the United States have a higher incidence of stomach cancer; Chinese living in the United States have a higher incidence of cervical and stomach cancers; Hawaiians have a higher incidence of lung and stomach cancers and the highest rate of breast cancer; Native Americans have higher rates of gallbladder, stomach, cervical, and lung cancers; and blacks have a higher rate of lung cancer.

Table 16-7 shows cancer rates in 1986 by sex and race for selected cancer sites, and the percent excess of black rates over white for these sites. Considering first all cancer sites among males, cancer incidence rates among blacks exceed the comparable white rates by 19%, while among females black incidence is lower than white by 2% (USDHHS, 1991, Health status of minorities, p. 135).

Smoking and Health

It has been 30 years since the publication of *Smoking and Health: Report of the Advisory Committee to the Surgeon General of the Public Health Service* (USDHEW, 1964). This report, prepared by an independent body of scientists that had been approved by the Tobacco Institute and eight health organizations, reviewed more than 7000 studies (Warner, 1989, p. 141; USDHHS,

TABLE 16-7 Age-Adjusted Cancer Incidence Rates* by Sex and Race, and Percent Excess of Black Rates over White for Selected Cancer Sites: United States 1986

Sex and site	White	Black	Percent excess, black rates over white
Male			
All sites	423.4	502.0	18.6
Oral cavity and pharynx	15.9	23.7	49.1
Esophagus	5.1	20.9	309.8
Stomach	10.7	17.9	67.3
Colorectal	61.4	55.8	−9.1
Colon	42.3	41.2	−2.6
Rectum	19.1	14.6	−23.6
Pancreas	10.7	15.1	41.1
Lung and bronchus	80.3	128.1	59.5
Prostate	87.7	123.4	40.7
Urinary and bladder	31.5	16.2	−48.6
Non-Hodgkin's lymphoma	16.1	10.9	−32.3
Leukemia	12.9	9.6	−25.6
All sites shown (number)	332.3	421.6	
All sites shown (percent)	78.5	84.0	
Female			
All sites	332.3	325.5	−2.0
Colorectal	42.4	46.9	10.6
Colon	31.6	36.3	14.9
Rectum	10.8	10.5	−2.8
Pancreas	7.8	13.2	69.2
Lung and bronchus	37.0	43.0	16.2
Breast	107.3	93.3	−13.0
Cervix uteri	7.8	15.5	98.7
Corpus uteri	22.3	13.8	−38.1
Ovary	13.2	8.8	−33.3
Non-Hodgkin's lymphoma	10.8	6.2	−42.6
All sites shown (number)	248.6	240.7	
All sites shown (percent)	74.8	73.9	

*Rates are per 100,000, age-adjusted by the direct method to the 1970 U.S. population.
NOTE: Data based on National Cancer Institute's Surveillance, Epidemiology, and End Results Program's population-based registries in Atlanta, Detroit, Seattle-Puget Sound, San Francisco-Oakland, Connecticut, Iowa, New Mexico, Utah, and Hawaii.
Source: National Center for Health Statistics, Health, United States, 1988, Department of Health and Human Services Pub. No. (PHS) 89–1232, Washington, D.C., U.S. Government Printing Office, 1989, Table 46, p. 91.
From USDHHS: *Health status of minorities and low-income groups,* ed 3, Washington, D.C., 1991, U.S. Government Printing Office, p. 145.

1989, p. viii). The document, often referred to as the first Surgeon General's Report on Smoking and Health, stated that there was a causal relationship between cigarette smoking, lung cancer, and other serious diseases, and that remedial action was necessary. It stirred a wave of controversy, unrest, opposition, and legislation on the issue of smoking and health.

As a result, Congress passed the Federal Cigarette Labeling and Advertising Act of 1965 and the Public Health Cigarette Smoking Act of 1969. These laws required that health warnings be printed on cigarette packages, banned cigarette advertising in the broadcast media, and increased public awareness of the hazards of smoking. In 1964 the U.S. Public Health

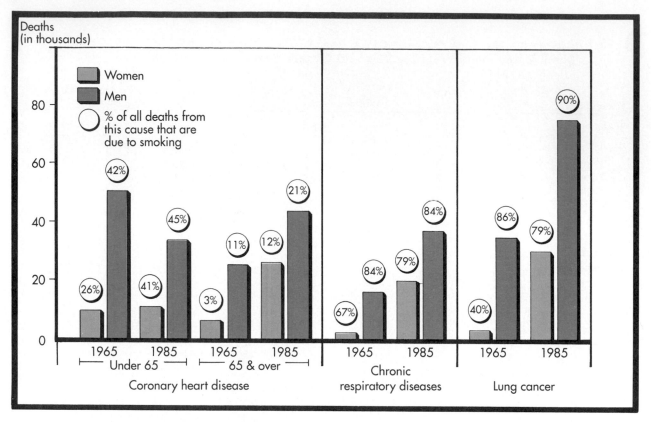

Figure 16-10 Deaths related to cigarette smoking for selected causes by gender, 1965 and 1985. (Data from U.S. Centers for Disease Control and Prevention: *Reducing the health consequences of smoking: 25 years of progress: a report of the Surgeon General,* Rockville, Md., DHHS Pub. No. (CEC)89-8411, 1989, pp. 154-158. (From the Robert Wood Johnson Foundation: *Challenges in health care: a chartbook perspective, 1991,* Princeton, N.J., 1991, The Foundation, p. 61.)

Service established the National Clearinghouse for Smoking and Health that is now the Office on Smoking and Health. This office has published more than 20 reports on the health consequences of smoking. Since the 1964 report *every* Surgeon General of the United States has reinforced that smoking is one of the most significant causes of disease and death. Figure 16-10 illustrates deaths related to cigarette smoking for selected causes by gender.

Cigarette smoking is the largest single preventable cause of illness and premature death in the United States, amounting to 390,000 deaths each year in the United States. Cigarette smoking is a major risk factor for lung cancer and other cancers, including laryngeal, esophageal, and urinary bladder cancer, for coronary artery disease, chronic obstructive lung disease, some forms of cerebrovascular disease, spontaneous abortion, retarded fetal growth and fetal or neonatal death (Rice, 1991, p. 296).

In 1987 about 32% of men and about 27% of women were cigarette smokers. While black men were more likely to be smokers than their white counterparts, the percent of women interviewed who said they were currently smoking was relatively equal by race in 1987 (USDHHS, 1991, Health status of the disadvantaged, p. 54). Table 16-8 depicts the number of cigarettes smoked per day by people 20 years of age and over by sex and race during the years 1965 to 1985. White men and women who smoked were more likely to be heavy smokers (25 or more cigarettes daily) than their black counterparts.

Cigarettes remain one of the most heavily advertised products in the United States. Cigarette advertising campaigns are increasingly aimed at women, youth, minorities, and blue-collar workers (Cigarette advertising, 1990, p. 261).

Radio and television advertisements for cigarettes

TABLE 16-8	Cigarettes Smoked per Day by Persons 20 Years of Age[1] and Over, by Sex and Race: United States Selected Years, 1965-1985.

(Percent of current smokers[3])

	Less than 15				25 or more			
Sex and Race	1965	1976	1980[2]	1985	1965	1976	1980[2]	1985
White males	27.7	22.3	20.0	21.7	26.0	33.3	37.3	36.6
Black males	49.8	43.7	48.4	52.9	8.6	10.8	13.8	10.7
White females	43.7	34.3	30.7	32.8	13.3	20.9	25.2	22.7
Black females	70.3	64.5	61.1	61.2	4.6	5.6	8.6	6.6

[1]Age adjusted.
[2]Based on data for the last 6 months of 1980.
[3]A current smoker is a person who has smoked at least 100 cigarettes and who now smokes; includes occasional smokers.
NOTE: Excludes unknown amount smoked.
Source: *Health, United States,* 1987, National Center for Health Statistics, DHHS Pub. No. (PHS) 88-1232.
From USDHHS: *Health status of the disadvantaged. Chartbook 1990,* DHHS Pub No (HRSA) HRS-P-DV 90-1), Washington, D.C., 1991, U.S. Government Printing Office, p. 55.

are no longer allowed; programs and literature aimed at helping the smoker to stop smoking have been published; the rights of nonsmokers are being stressed; nonsmoking areas have been designated in many public places and on public transportation; and higher cigarette taxes have been levied. As of 1988 more than 320 communities had adopted laws or regulations restricting smoking in public places (USDHHS, 1989, p. 9). Many workplaces have banned smoking, limited it to specific areas, or are phasing it out, and some department stores are banning cigarette sales in vending machines. Smoking is now banned on air flights of 6 hours or less in the United States, accounting for 99.8% of daily domestic flights.

Smoking and Pregnancy

Smoking during pregnancy increases the risk of stillbirth, miscarriage, premature birth, and low-birth-weight infants (USDHHS, 1989, p. 19). There is evidence that heavy smoking (two or more packs per day) by pregnant women can cause birth defects such as mental retardation, facial anomalies, and heart defects (New pattern, 1985, A3). A study conducted by the University of Maryland School of Medicine showed that pregnant women who participated in antismoking intervention programs cut their smoking in half, and on an average gave birth to infants who were heavier and larger than those who did not stop or cut back (APHA, 1984, Anti-smoking, p. 11). A self-help

cessation program for pregnant women showed that this low-cost prenatal intervention can significantly affect smoking behavior (Ershoff, Mullen, and Quinn, 1989, p. 182). Unfortunately, many women are not aware of the risk factors smoking poses for pregnancy (USDHHS, p. 19).

Passive Smoking and Smokleless Tobacco

Passive inhalation of smoke (passive smoking) and smokeless tobacco are public health issues related to smoking that have received increased attention in recent years. Studies have shown that nonsmokers are at increased health risks from passive inhalation and that smokeless tobacco use is related to certain cancers and conditions.

Each year 53,000 nonsmokers die from exposure to cigarette smoke (ACS, 1993, p. 22), and an unknown number of people develop illnesses from such exposure. Many deaths from passive smoking involve exposure at the home and workplace. The Environmental Protection Agency has stated that nonsmokers in public buildings cannot avoid exposure to the ill effects of tobacco smoke unless smokers are quarantined and are provided with separate ventilation systems. Smoke persists in buildings long after smoking stops, and the most practical way to eliminate the exposure is to remove the source.

Research studies have shown increased lung cancer risk among passive smokers and several studies have pointed to increased heart disease risk in passive smokers. There is some evidence that risk from passive inhalation of smoke increases with age. The health of children is adversely affected when parents smoke; they experience more episodes of bronchitis and pneumonia during the first years of life, (ACS, 1993, p. 22). Children in households that include adult smokers have more restricted-activity and bed-disability days than children living with nonsmokers (Byrd, Shapiro, and Schiedermayer, 1989, p. 968).

Smokeless tobaccos, such as snuff and chewing tobacco, are emerging as a health concern. It has been estimated that 12 million Americans, including 3 million under the age of 21, use snuff and chewing tobacco (National campaign, 1990, A10). Unfortunately, many states have not passed laws that prohibit the sale of smokeless tobacco to children.

This threat to health was vividly described in *Sean Marsee's Smokeless Death* (Fincer, 1985), an article about a teenage athlete who died of oral cancer related to his use of smokeless tobacco. Annually there are 29,000 new cases of oral cancer and 9000 deaths from this cause, with 70% related to tobacco use. Research has linked snuff and oral cancer and former Surgeon General C. Everett Koop has declared that smokeless tobacco does pose a cancer threat.

In response to the threat, the Comprehensive Smokeless Tobacco Education Act of 1986 (Public Law 99-252) was passed, which established a program of public education to inform people of the health dangers of smokeless tobacco products. It supports educational programs and public service announcements, and research on the effects of smokeless tobacco on human health. It also regulates the labeling of smokeless tobacco products and advertising of them—provisions similar to those of the Cigarette Smoking Act of 1969.

SOME CRISES OF ADULTHOOD AND NURSING INTERVENTION

Life comprises a series of *life change events* (refer to Table 7-4). The number, duration, and type of these events will vary with individuals. A life event that is major for one person may not be considered major for another.

Unlike young children, who have parents or others to support and guide them through the experience of life change events, the adult often does not have adequate support available during times of heightened stress or may not use the help that is available because dependency is feared. Our society emphasizes self-sufficiency during adulthood, and even a mature adult may experience feelings of insecurity when seeking assistance from others. Many adults must learn that *interdependency* is a mature state.

Examples of some life change events include the following: leaving the parental home, obtaining job education and training, pursuing a career, marriage, childbearing, child rearing, child launching, providing for an aging parent, pursuing leisure-time activities, and experiencing the death of a parent. Life change events that are more or less expected usually evoke what could be termed *normative stress*. However, other life change events induce stress that goes beyond what could be considered normative, and may necessitate developing new interpersonal relationships, coping mechanisms, and resources. Examples of some of these life change events are divorce or separation, loss of a child, loss of a job, development of a chronic health condition, and career changes. If these events occur in rapid succession, the adult may have difficulty adapting and may experience crisis.

An example of what can happen when major life events occur in rapid succession is seen in the Stephen Johns case situation:

▶ **In a period of less than 14 years, Mr. Johns, 32 years old, left home to enter college, completed a college education, entered a career, married, bought a house, had a child, changed jobs, moved to a new residence, became divorced, moved to another residence, changed jobs again, and experienced the death of a parent. These were all significant life events for Mr. Johns, and the rapid succession of their development left him in a confused and disorganized state. He was overwhelmed with his life and began to question whether it had meaning. Thus he sought counseling at a local mental health clinic. Through work with a psychiatric nurse therapist, Mr. Johns was able to establish life goals and take action to achieve these goals. This made him comfortable about himself as a person and gave direction and meaning to his life. He began to recognize his own strengths and to work within and accept his limitations. He began to reach out to others and saw that interdependency can be therapeutic.**

Although major life events may not always be

experienced this rapidly, or in this magnitude, significant stresses do occur during adulthood. While experiencing these stresses adults are also trying to achieve a balance between their responsibilities to family and society, to develop as individuals, and to maintain health. These tasks in themselves produce stress. Thus when sudden or unexpected situational difficulties arise, such as divorce, death, or changes in job and residence, the individual is at risk for crisis.

Helping Clients In Crisis

The crisis state may be experienced at any time throughout adult life. When mobilizing coping mechanisms during times of stress, the adult has many life experiences from which to draw. These experiences, however, do not necessarily prepare one to handle all the events that occur throughout adulthood. At each developmental stage there are new or different events requiring adaptation. The following quote from Knafl and Grace (1978, p. 265) vividly portrays the pressures one deals with during middlescence:

He (the middlescent) realizes that the choices of the past have limited his choices in the present. He can no longer dream of infinite possibilities. He is forced to acknowledge that he has worked up to or short of his capabilities. Goals may or may not have been reached; aspirations may have to be modified. The possibility for advancement becomes more remote. He will have to go on with ever-brighter, ever-younger men and women crowding into competitive economic, political and social arenas. In the United States success is highly valued, and is measured by prestige, wealth or power. To be without these by middle age causes stress, and the likelihood of achieving them diminishes with age.

When adults are in crisis, they should be helped to look at the circumstances that precipitated the crisis and modify them to reduce future occurrences. The nurse is supportive of the client without leveling judgment and helps the client and family to assess the resources and support systems they have available and to make plans for the immediate future. As discussed in Chapter 8, the mastery of a crisis provides opportunities for personal growth and development.

A major goal of community health nursing practice in relation to crisis is prevention. To achieve this goal, the community health nurse recognizes early signs and symptoms of heightened stress (refer to Chapter 8) and helps individuals who are experiencing these symptoms to mobilize appropriate coping mechanisms.

The supports people use during crisis and time of need will vary. Emotional support, encouragement, assistance with problem-solving, companionship, and tangible aid have been shown to be helpful to people who are dealing with a crisis. Individuals experiencing a crisis will look for caregivers who provide these interventions (Figley and McCubbin, 1983, p. 11).

AGGREGATES AT RISK IN THE ADULT MALE AND FEMALE POPULATION

As with any age group, there are persons at special risk in the adult population who require concentrated community health nursing intervention. Similar problems that affect large numbers of people deserve attention with programming that addresses primary, secondary, and tertiary prevention efforts. In addition to crises that stem from normative stress and the accomplishments of developmental tasks, adults in contemporary society face overwhelming issues such as depression, homelessness, unemployment, substance abuse, violence, poverty, and HIV infection. Other aggregates with special concerns, because they are not an accepted part of society, include gays and lesbians and men and women who are incarcerated.

Depression in Adult Men and Women

Depression is the most common, most treatable, and possibly the most painful of mental illnesses in the United States (Thompson, McFarland, Hirsch, and Tucker, 1993, p. 1321). Depression in women is common between the ages of 25 and 44 and between 55 and 70 (National Mental Health Association [NMHA], 1988). Twenty-five percent of all women and 11.5% of all men will experience a depressive episode but only one third will seek treatment (NMHA). Research shows that depression is often recurrent. Major depression is the most common serious mental disorder in women: about 7 million women in our nation have a diagnosis of major depression (USDHHS, 1985; McGrath, Keita, Strickland, and Russso, 1990).

Freud viewed depression as aggression turned inward. Depression has been described as chronic frustration stemming from environmental stresses in family, social, or work environments beyond the coping ability and resources of the client. Depression can result when stress is intensified. All persons experience times when they feel low or discouraged, but the depressed feelings are usually acute and self-limiting. Depression becomes a serious problem when it is chronic and affects the ability to cope with the events, roles, and responsibilities of daily living. Depression is often precipitated by a loss of some kind: death, separation, or loss of job, status, or health.

Some symptoms of depression include general sadness and despair, difficulty in making decisions, difficulty in carrying on a conversation, trouble concentrating, trouble sleeping, tiredness, listlessness, loss of appetite, eating binges, social regression, loss of or decreased libido, and decreased self-esteem. People who are depressed may be overly sensitive to what other people say or do, may be angry with others and not trust them, and may withdraw from others due to a fear of being among people.

Persons who are depressed are often not aware that they are suffering from this condition. They know that they do not feel well and thus may seek medical help for minor physical problems. That is why it is so important for the community health nurse to systematically collect a complete health history (refer to Chapter 9) when working with adult clients. If data are collected only on the client's complaint about physical health, depression can be overlooked.

Maintaining two-way communication between the client and nurse is essential. People who are depressed generally like feedback on what is going on, to know that someone has listened to them, and that someone is available for support and assistance. Unfortunately, all too often the depressed client is excluded from social contacts; family, friends, and even professionals may isolate depressed clients in an attempt to protect the client from further hurt or stress. This social isolation serves to reinforce the client's feelings that no one cares.

Depressed individuals who are assessed to be potentially suicidal should be referred for psychotherapy. Some nurses are afraid to assess for suicide potential because they fear their questioning may precipitate a suicide attempt. However, suicide is not prevented by avoiding conversation about it. It is prevented by helping clients get the assistance they need to deal with stresses in their daily lives.

Encountering clients who are depressed is common in community health nursing practice. At times the client is able to resolve the depressed state by using the supportive assistance of the community health nurse and significant others, such as family, friends, relatives, and lovers. At other times additional mental health counseling is necessary. However, depression will continue to exist until the individual is able to successfully mobilize coping mechanisms that enhance growth. Most chronic depressions are related to unresolved psychosocial difficulties. Crisis and normative stress are self-limiting; chronic depression is not.

The nurse can assist the client in community resource use such as community mental health centers and self-help groups. Other sources of information and referral for the client and family are groups such as the Foundation for Depressive Illness (1-800-248-4344), and the National Mental Health Association (703-684-7722). On the federal level, the National Institute of Mental Health is charged with improving the understanding, treatment, and rehabilitation of the mentally ill; preventing mental illness; and fostering the mental health of the people. NIMH is involved in prevention activities. It sponsors Project D/ART (Depression/Awareness, Recognition and Treatment). Project D/ART is concerned with ameliorating the public health problem of depression and aims to improve the identification, assessment, treatment, and clinical management of depressive disorders through an educational program focused on the general public, primary care providers, and mental health specialists. Project D/ART is involved with many voluntary and professional organizations and provides information and materials for the general public as well as professional audiences. NIMH can be contacted at 301-443-4515.

Those Who Abuse Alcohol and Other Drugs

Alcoholism is the largest drug problem in the United States today; some 10% of the adult population has a chronic, heavy intake of alcoholic beverages (Williams, Stinson, Parker, Harford, and Noble, 1987, p. 81). Nearly 10.5 million adults show symptoms of alcoholism and 7.2 million are alcohol abusers. Seventy percent of 12- to 17-year-old youths have used alcohol (USDHHS, 1987, Prevention '86/'87, p. 40), and an estimated 4.6 million teenagers have serious alcohol problems (USDHHS, Prevention '86/'87, p. 61). The per capita consumption is above 2.65 gallons of alcohol for every resident above the age of 14 years—up from 2.25 gallons in 1945 (USDHHS, Prevention '86/'87, p. 41). Cirrhosis is the ninth leading cause of death among adults, and as many as 90% of cases are associated with excessive use of alcohol (USDHHS, Prevention '86/'87, p. 40). Nearly one half of all traffic deaths are alcohol related, fetal exposure to alcohol is the leading cause of mental retardation, and alcohol abuse and dependency cost the United States more than $136 billion in 1989 (Sperling, 1990, p. D1). Although more men than women abuse alcohol and drugs, the problem for women is substantial. Life expectancy for women alcholics is decreased by 15 years (Leslie and Swider, 1986, p. 114).

Besides contributing to cirrhosis of the liver, alcoholism contributes to such health problems as nutritional deficiencies, pancreatitis, and cancer. It is a factor in other leading causes of adult deaths including accidents, suicides, and homicides. Studies show that careless handling of smoking materials by intoxicated persons is dangerous and contributes to substantial numbers of burn injuries, death, and property damage.

The psychosocial consequences of alcoholism are immense. Such consequences include disruption of family life, loss of on-the-job productivity, and lowered self-esteem. The families of alcoholics are victims of alcoholism themselves.

The adverse effects of alcohol on fetal development has been a health concern for more than 250 years. The infants of mothers who consume large amounts of alcohol suffer from low birth weight, birth defects, and/or mental retardation (USDHHS, 1983, Health, p. 19). The terms *fetal alcohol syndrome* and *alcohol-related birth defects* are often seen in the literature. However, public awareness of these conditions is still limited. Women of childbearing years, especially pregnant women, need to know the effects of drinking on their fetuses. The nurse's health history should include questions about drinking habits. However, adequate answers are not always provided when this question is asked. Thus the nurse observes for signs and symptoms of increased alcohol consumption during pregnancy. This, coupled with information on alcohol and pregnancy that should be shared with every expectant mother, may help to cut down on alcohol abuse during pregnancy. Alcohol abuse includes both chronic drinking and binge drinking: studies have shown that binge drinking can have disastrous effects.

Passive intervention measures such as the use of flame retardant fabrics and smoke detectors, identification and reduction of stairway hazards, sanctions against the sale and use of alcohol, sanctions against drunk drivers, and greater alcohol intoxication screening in health care settings and at work can all help.

Former Surgeon General C. Everett Koop recommended the following measures: a massive increase of alcohol-related public service ads to match the number of beer, wine, and spirit ads; an increase in the federal excise tax on liquor and a state tax to be used for education programs; elimination of "happy hours" and drink discounts; an end to alcohol ads that use celebrities and ads that appear on college campuses; a halt to liquor makers sponsoring sports events, rock concerts, and other programs where the majority of the audience is under age 21; an immediate reduction in the legal blood-alcohol level for motorists to 0.08% and a further reduction to 0.04% by the year 2000 (Cox, 1989). Although these measures would help to curb alcoholism in the United States, they are passive and do not involve the person who has an alcohol-related problem. They also have not been acted upon to any degree. Such measures, coupled with those in which the person is actively involved in treatment, are necessary.

Self-help groups such as Alcoholics Anonymous, Children of Alcoholics, and counseling services are available for alcoholics and their families. The National Council on Alcoholism (1-800-NCA-CALL) is a voluntary organization that offers information and referral services. Many places of work have alcoholism programs or work closely with community programs. The community health nurse can carry out health education activities, offer support, remain nonjudgmental, and encourage the client to use available resources.

The National Institute on Alcohol Abuse and Alcoholism (NIAAA) provides a national focus to increase knowledge and promote effective strategies to deal with the health and psychosocial problems associated with alcoholism. It sponsors research programs, much of which is targeted at prevention, and programs including youth awareness, fetal alcohol awareness, and national drunk driving awareness, among others. The National Clearinghouse on Alcohol and Drug Abuse (301-468-2600) offers information, educational materials, and referral sources.

Other drug use is also a dominant concern among adult men and women. Surveys in 1988 found that 21 million Americans had used cocaine at least once, and 21 million also had used marijuana in the last year. Among high school seniors in 1992, 40.7% have tried an illicit drug (Johnston, O'Malley, and Bachman, 1993). As with alcohol, drug use is linked to other concerns such as violent crime, transmission of HIV, and developmental problems in infants.

Drug use was a direct or contributing factor in 6,756 deaths in major U.S. cities in 1988. Accidental overdose was the most common cause of these deaths, and over 70% of them were among men. Alcohol and cocaine, in combination with heroin/morphine, codeine, Valium, and methadone, are the top six drugs causing deaths (Robert Wood Johnson Foundation, 1991, p. 58). Figure 16-11 shows that more than half of all drug-related deaths occur among people 30-49. When such deaths occur in people over 60 the majority are considered suicides (Robert Wood Johnson Foundation, p. 58). There is also a disproportionate number of drug deaths among minorities, also depicted in Figure 16-11.

Other drug-related deaths are those from violent crimes linked to drug use and the drug trade. According to a 1986 survey of state prisons, 28% of inmates who had been convicted of murder and 32% of inmates who had been convicted of rape were under the influence of drugs and or alcohol at the time the crime was committed (Robert Wood Johnson Foundation, 1991, p. 58)

Illicit drug use is related to the HIV epidemic, which is growing the fastest among intravenous drugs users. It also contributes to low-birth-weight and premature infants; in some communities one of every 10 infants is born to a mother who used illicit drugs during her pregnancy. The devastating effects of illegal drugs hit hardest among some of the most vulnerable population groups in our country: the poor, women and children, minorities, and those infected with HIV. They also kill a population of young adult males who will never have the opportunity to contribute their skills to society.

Treatment for drug and alcohol abuse takes place in detoxification units, residential centers, methadone clinics, outpatient programs, hospitals, or other facilities (Bennett and Woolf, 1991, p. 228). Only 12% of people receive this kind of formal treatment; many more seek informal settings such as Alcoholics Anonymous. Most people seek treatment after intense pressure from family and friends, employers, or legal authorities (Robert Wood Johnson Foundation, 1991, p. 62). There are, however, about 67,000 people on the average waiting for services from publically funded drug treatment programs; the number of days between a request for treatment and admission in 1989 was 45 for residential treatment and 22 days for outpatient programs. Funding sources for alcohol and

drug treatment comes from several places: fee-for-service provided under 60% of the funding for treatment; grants from local, state and the federal government provide about 30%. Costs of treatment mandate research to identify what kind of treatment is most effective for different types of clients. Figure 16-12 presents federal expenditures for drug control by type of activity: about 71% of the total federal expenditures for drug control are used for law enforcement activities. By contrast, only 25% of federal drug control funds are used for treatment and prevention and 4% for research and development.

The community health nurse's role with clients who are substance abusers is to begin with an assessment. Essential data from which to base an evaluation for treatment includes four categories (Bennett and Woolf, 1991, p. 229): alcohol and drug history, physical assessment, psychological assessment that includes the motivation for treatment, and social assessment that includes family supports. Assessment guides (Estes, Smith-DiJulio, and Heinemann, 1980; Smith, Wesson, and Linda, 1980) are available to the practitioner to facilitate data collection. The nurse is also knowledgeable about referring sources and payment systems for the client and family and uses the referral process (refer to chapter 10) for those who want these services. Further roles include that of researcher regarding the most effective treatment modalities and who becomes addicted. Working at local, state, and federal levels to develop policies for the primary, secondary, and tertiary treatment of this problem are also avenues of nursing activities.

Men and Women Changing Jobs or Careers

The case situations on the worker role presented earlier in the chapter illustrate that deciding to alter one's work role can result in crisis and indecision. During this time a major reorganization is required in one's life, and the stresses encountered should not be underestimated. This is particularly true if changing a job or a career was not a voluntary decision, such as when a person is fired or laid off from a job. However, even if the decision was a voluntary one, it still may not have consensus within the family.

The adult's and his or her family's perceptions of the situation should be ascertained. Does the individual see it as a new and challenging adventure or as a threat to personal and economic security? The community health nurse should be especially sensi-

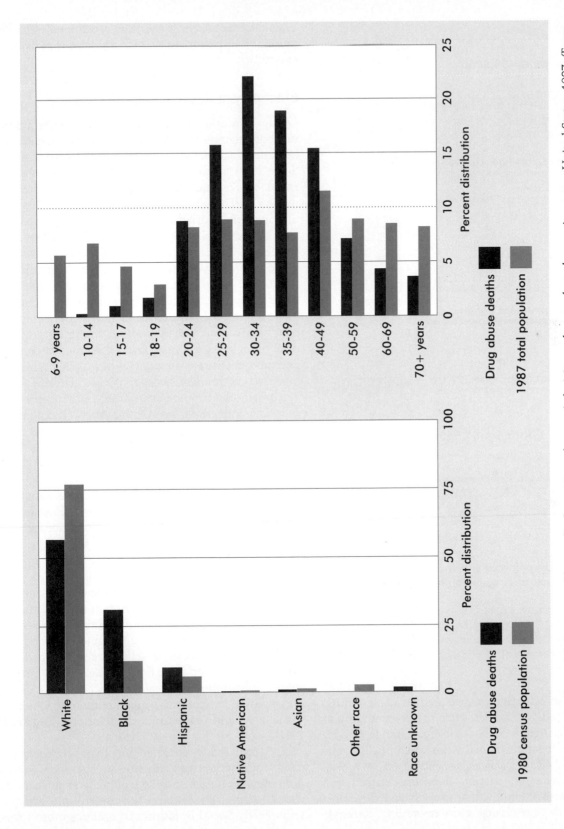

Figure 16-11 Drug abuse deaths reported by medical examiners by race/ethnicity and age, selected reporting areas: United States, 1987. (From USDHHS: *Health status of the disadvantaged: chartbook 1990*, DHHS Pub. No. (HSRA) HRS-P-DV 90-1, Washington, D.C., 1991, U.S. Government Printing Office, p. 93.)

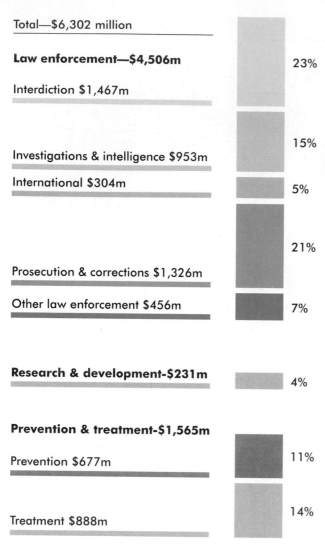

Total—$6,302 million

Law enforcement—$4,506m   23%

Interdiction $1,467m

                                     15%
Investigations & intelligence $953m

International $304m   5%

                                     21%

Prosecution & corrections $1,326m

Other law enforcement $456m   7%

Research & development-$231m   4%

Prevention & treatment-$1,565m

Prevention $677m   11%

                                     14%
Treatment $888m

NOTE: "Other law enforcement" includes state and local assistance, and regulation and compliance.

Figure 16-12 Federal expenditures on drug control by type of activity, 1989. (From the Robert Wood Johnson Foundation: *Challenges in health care: a chartbook perspective 1991,* Princeton, N.J., 1991, The Foundation, p. 67.)

tive to the distresses that can occur when an individual is changing jobs or careers, since this is becoming a frequent occurrence in our society. Change is not always easy. It can result in a more satisfying life or it can result in dissatisfaction, depending on how the client views what is happening. Support or encouragement can facilitate individual growth and development and make the change more rewarding. Referral

to outside counseling agencies, vocational rehabilitation, or employment service agencies may be necessary.

Unemployed Adult Men and Women

Layoffs among white and blue collar workers in the most prestigious companies in the United States have become an agonizing, almost daily theme in the news. Since 1980 "some 4.3 million jobs have been eliminated by Fortune 500 companies, and another 1.4 million defense industry jobs are in the process of disappearing. Individuals 55 and over are particularly at risk for unemployment: between October 1991, and October 1992, the rate of unemployment for people 35 and over was several times that of people 16 through 54" (Stern, 1993, p. 25). No one is exempt from this situation which can create devastation for a family; however, some groups are more at risk for unemployment than others. The unemployment rate has significant differences by race and ethnicity; the lowest unemployment rate was for whites, at 5.3% and the highest was for blacks at 13.0% (USDHHS, 1991, Health status of minorities). Rural residents are also especially vulnerable to unemployment. Rural unemployment rates rose more rapidly than urban rates throughout the 1980s. By 1986 this rate was 26% higher than that for urban residents (O'Hare, 1988; U.S. Bureau of Labor Statistics, 1987).

Health care professionals are concerned about unemployment because there are strong relationships between health status and level of education, as well as between health status and level of income. In 1986 13.5% of the total population, more than 32 million Americans, lived below the poverty level.

Families experiencing unemployment may at first draw closer to work on common goals, but tension usually mounts as work responsibilities are redistributed, roles are altered, and family goals are modified (Kaforey, 1984). Role reversal between husband and wife may occur, and there is an increased frequency of marital disruption and role conflict (Moen, 1983). Unemployment can cause increased family violence, instability, and economic deprivation (Voyanoff, 1983).

Social stigma is attached to unemployment, because society does not sanction it. The unemployed family may become socially isolated and suffer from shock, shame, and altered self-esteem and lifestyle (Hill, 1978). Social isolation can produce more stress for the family and should be minimized.

The unemployed person and family are psychologically vulnerable. The unemployed worker may evidence lowered self-esteem, anxiety, apathy, decreased appetite, inertia, feelings of helplessness, and suffer from a variety of psychosomatic conditions (Swineburne, 1981; Krystal, Moran-Sackett, and Cantoni, 1983). Madonia (1983) found that approximately 80% of unemployed respondents were more frustrated than when they were employed, and 70% stated that they were frequently agitated and experienced tension. Moreover, the children of the unemployed have shown symptoms of increased stress. Such families need help working through these feelings. They have suffered a loss; they need to be able to recognize the validity of their loss and be able to grieve for it.

Unemployment generates stress that can cause health problems. People who are unemployed often do not feel well physically (Madonia, 1983), and they may have physical symptoms such as chest pains, shortness of breath, dizziness, dry mouth, eczema, weakness, and inability to sleep (Krystal, Moran-Sackett, and Cantoni, 1983). Children of the unemployed experience a higher rate of illness than other children (Margolis and Farran, 1981). People who are unemployed are often unable to afford health care services because they lose health care benefits. During an average month in 1990, about 35 million Americans were uninsured. This represented 13.9% of the population and was an increase of 1.3 million from the previous year. Over the past decade the number of uninsured has increased by 11 million (Himmelstein and Woolhandler, 1992, p. 3). Figure 16-13 presents this data graphically. In 1991 more people were uninsured than at any time since the passage of Medicare and Medicaid in the 1960s.

Unemployment is a major crisis physically, socially, emotionally, and financially. Nurses can help families understand what is happening and encourage them to use appropriate community resources. Although unemployment necessitates family adjustment, change, and adaptation, the stress experienced can be minimized, and positive growth can occur.

The Homeless

Homelessness is a growing problem in the United States resulting from three factors: the deinstitutionalization of psychiatric patients, the economic reces-

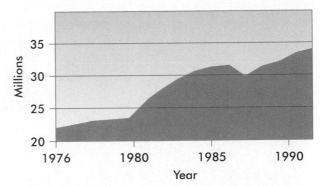

Figure 16-13 Number of uninsured Americans, 1976-1991. (From Himmelstein DU and Woolhandler S: *The national health program chartbook*, Cambridge, Mass., 1992, Center for National Health Program Studies, p. 4.)

sion, and the reduction of funding for social programs (Kinzel, 1991, p. 181) (refer to Figure 16-14). It is estimated that there are as many as 2 to 3 million homeless people in the United States (Lindsey, 1989, p. 78; Bowdler, 1989). Demographics on the homeless show that their average age is 35 to 40 years; at least one half are nonwhite; approximately one fourth are female; and approximately one third have a high school education (Bowdler and Barrell, 1987, p. 135). The homeless population is becoming ever younger, with more and more children being included in this group. It is estimated that 100,000 or more American children go to sleep homeless every night (Mihaly, 1991).

Young families are the fastest-growing group of homeless people in the United States. Most at risk are young and one-parent families, whose poverty rates have increased dramatically in recent years. One-parent families, usually headed by women, represent three fourths of all homeless families nationwide (Mihaly, 1991, p. 3). Some authorities suggest that one half of the homeless population may have severe and chronic mental disorders, 10% to 15% may seriously abuse drugs, and 40% to 50% abuse alcohol (Ryan, 1989, p. 14). However, "the fundamental cause of homelessness among children today is the rapidly growing gap between the incomes of poor, minority, and young families and the cost of available housing" (Mihaly, p. 10).

New York City alone houses almost 10,000 homeless individuals and 5000 families each night, with an annual budget of over $312 million (Lindsey, 1989, p. 78). Most homeless individuals have no regular source

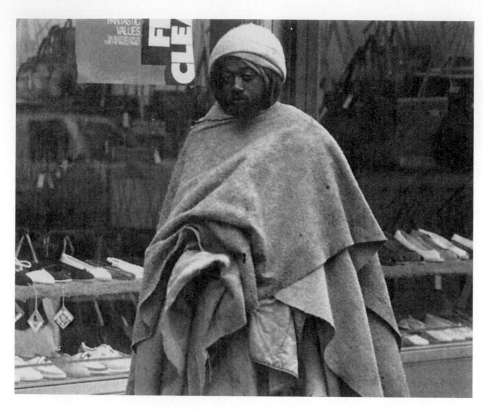

Figure 16-14 Homelessness is often the cause and effect of multiple social and chronic health problems. (Courtesy Brian Lafferty.)

of health care and the majority are without health insurance (Robertson and Cousineau, 1986, p. 561). There is a great need to enhance the mental health resources available to the homeless.

People who are homeless have a high prevalence of physical problems, mental disorders, substance abuse, and infectious/parasitic diseases (Bowdler and Barrell, 1987, p. 135). They are nearly constantly exposed to the elements; experience overcrowding and unsanitary conditions; have high rates of alcoholism, hypertension, drug abuse, trauma, and mental illness; are more susceptible to communicable diseases and conditions such as tuberculosis, influenza, scabies, lice, and pneumonia; and suffer from a variety of nutritional deficiencies (With neither, 1989, pp. 21, 31). "Many communities report that substance abuse and emotional distress are results, not causes, of homelessness" (Mihaly, 1991). Homeless children may not receive necessary immunizations, putting them at increased risk of serious communicable disease. In New York City is was found that homeless children were three times more likely than their housed poor counterparts to be behind in their immunizations (Mihaly, 1991).

Another study revealed that 50% of homeless children had immunization delays and 16% had various chronic physical disorders including asthma, anemia, and malnutrition. Skin ailments, ear infections, eye disorders, dental problems, upper respiratory infections, and gastrointestinal problems were common (Berne, Dato, Mason, and Rafferty, 1990, p. 8). The mental health of these children was profoundly affected as well: developmental delays, depression, anxiety, suicide ideation, sleep problems, shyness, withdrawal, and aggression were in evidence.

Peripheral vascular disease is common among homeless people who have been on the streets for long periods of time because they stand for extended periods. This causes gravitational and mechanical obstruction to the deep venous system and increases venous pressure (With neither, 1989, p. 31).

Homeless people are often isolated from the mainstream of society. Children do not have regular schooling or friends. Families find themselves without the necessary support or resources to cope with even minor problems and difficulties. One study carried out by nurse researchers discovered that a recurring theme from homeless people whom they studied was the need for interaction with a caring person. "The feeling that no one cares, a lack of self-worth, and a sense of limited control over their lives may lead to depression, hopelessness, and finally illness. The extent and effectiveness of health-seeking behaviors among this group are limited because of decreased trust, decreased motivation for self-care, and isolation from social and health care systems" (Kinzel, 1991, p. 189).

On a national level, the Stewart B. McKinney Homeless Assistance Act (Public Law 100-77) was enacted to help meet the needs of the homeless population. The act provides assistance to protect and improve the lives and safety of the homeless, with special emphasis on elderly, handicapped persons and families with children. It established the Interagency Council on the Homeless and numerous grant programs. The Act authorized emergency food and shelter, supportive housing, programs for primary health care, substance abuse services, community mental health care, adult education, education for children and youth, job training, and studies of homelessness.

Community health centers, federally supported by Section 330 of the Public Health Service Act, are emerging to assist disadvantaged populations. The purpose of these centers is to provide high-quality, *managed* care for those people who are most likely to lack access to health services because of geographical isolation or financial barriers (National Association of Community Health Centers, 1986, p. 1). More than 600 such centers are active. They serve over 5 million people, of whom 60% are female, 64% are members of a minority group, 45% are children, and 60% have incomes under the poverty level (National Association of Community Health Centers, p. 1). Despite the expansion of these types of health centers, the need for these services far exceeds current capacity (Mihaly, 1991).

Nurses have demonstrated innovative approaches to caring for the homeless (Park, 1989; Woolley, 1985). Three traditional approaches that have been used to provide health care to the homeless are outpatient departments of hospitals or clinics, on-site services, and comprehensive outreach. Berne and her colleagues (1990) have described a model program that has the resources to meet at least some of the needs of this population group: comprehensive pediatric mobile units travel to children living in shelters and hotels in New York City. Public health nurses and social workers who are on-site at the homeless centers identify clients and do initial assessments, and nurse

practitioners and physicians from the units diagnose and treat problems. Routine health maintenance is addressed and community resources such as WIC are used. Trevor's Place in Philadelphia and Lillian Wald's Henry Street Settlement House in New York provide supportive 24-hour care to families and are other models to follow.

Chronic Illness Among Adults

Chronic illness is a major health problem in the American population (refer to Chapters 11 and 18). Illness for the individual or family is a normal part of the life cycle. We all expect at some point in time to have a case of the flu, a cold, or even minor surgery. Acute, nondisabling illness can often be handled by normal resources and copying mechanisms. It does not involve major lifestyle adaptation. If the illness becomes chronic, disabling, or terminal, however, the family situation can become quite stressful.

When the adult is afflicted with a chronic health condition, major life changes and hardships can occur. These hardships can include strained family relationships, modifications in family activities and goals, increased health care tasks and time constraints, increased financial stress, need for housing adaptation, social isolation, medical concerns, and grieving (Figley and McCubbin, 1983, pp. 25-26.) The individual and family may also demonstrate changes in work, school, and community experiences as a result of the illness.

The extent to which lifestyle changes occur during chronic illness varies, depending on the degree of disability encountered and the adult's perception of the event. Role reversal, changes in sexual behavior, and alterations in self-image are a few examples of the problems experienced by clients who have developed debilitating chronic illness during adulthood. The adult who is not progressing well along the developmental continuum may regress, become depressed, or become dependent when chronically ill. He or she may resist treatment and techniques to make recovery faster, or become self-absorbed, not relate to others well, and use the illness as an escape from responsibility.

Northouse (1984) has described three phases of the impact of cancer on a family's life: initial, adaptation, and terminal. Northouse examined adaptation and found that copying with the demands of this phase draws some families together and pulls others apart. Researchers built on his findings and examined this phase by looking at a small group of families where the mother had a chronic illness (Hough, Lewis, and Woods, 1991). Among these families, poorly adjusted ones had a higher number of stressors with which they were dealing, and expressed low marital satisfaction and depression. In the well-adjusted families the illness was viewed in a positive light—that is, a greater appreciation of life for the present was developed. Further, the families viewed themselves as competent and effective even after the illness. Finally, well-adjusted families stated that they were more sensitive and empathic about the needs of others. These findings can aid the nurse in assessing which families might have more trouble dealing with this crisis. The nurse can help the well-adjusted adult to resume as normal a level of independence and functioning as possible and provide the support and encouragement needed for the individual to do so. The nurse can assist the client and family by making them aware of the medical course of the client's condition, giving anticipatory guidance, and encouraging them to take an active role in health care decision-making.

Nurses can help the chronically ill adult accept the interdependency needed to deal successfully with his or her condition. They should not make unrealistic promises of recovery or an optimistic prognosis if this is not the case. There may be no guarantee that treatment will improve the level of disability, and false hopes prevent the client from confronting and working through the crisis.

Use of both the educative and problem-solving approaches to nursing intervention is essential when working with families who are dealing with a chronic condition. They need increased knowledge to realistically evaluate the changes that are occurring and that may occur. These families also need to problem-solve in order to determine the most appropriate ways for them to adapt to changes, especially permanent ones. Chronic illness can be both emotionally and financially draining. Different coping mechanisms and resources must be mobilized to reduce tension and to maintain financial stability. The possibility of death may also be a matter for the nurse to work through with chronically ill adults and their families. Families should be encouraged to express their fears and, if the client's situation warrants it, to prepare for death. Reading materials written by Kubler-Ross (1974, 1975) can enhance a community health nurse's skill in working with clients who are dying.

The hospice movement is gaining popularity in this country (refer to Chapter 20). Hospice care is designed to keep the chronically ill person who is terminal at home as long as possible. It is a cost-effective and humane method of health care. A family-centered, multidisciplinary approach is followed, with an emphasis placed on improving the quality of life for both the client and the client's family during the final stages of dying. Community health nurses are regular participants on this interdisciplinary team and thus they must be prepared to deal with the concerns of dying clients and their families.

When working with any chronically ill adult, the community health nurse will more than likely use the referral process. There are a variety of community resources, such as the Lost Chord Club, the Multiple Sclerosis Association, the Cancer Society, Goodwill Industries, the division of vocational rehabilitation, and the department of social services, that will help clients and their families to adapt to chronic illness. Chapter 20 discusses support and education for the caregiver and the client in the home when chronic illness is present.

Men and Women with HIV/AIDS

HIV-related disease (human immunodeficiency virus) and AIDS (acquired immunodeficiency syndrome) are epidemic worldwide. Between 1981 and May 1990 AIDS was diagnosed in 136,000 persons, and more than three fifths of them have died. The World Health Organization estimates that 6 to 10 million people worldwide have been infected with HIV and that 15 to 20 million will be infected by the year 2000 (Rice, 1991, p. 300). People with HIV infection can develop AIDS, including severe opportunistic infections, Kaposi's sarcoma, tuberculosis, and multiple systems medical complications. Without treatment, about 50% of people develop AIDS within ten years of becoming infected with HIV, and another 40% or more develop other clinical illnesses associated with HIV infection (USDHHS, 1991, Healthy people, p. 74).

In the United States the end of 1993 saw 390,000 to 480,000 cases of AIDS. It has become the seventh leading cause of potential years lost in this country and costs to deal with it are enormous. Although some therapeutic agents extend survival, there is currently no treatment to prevent death among people with AIDS. Additionally, a recent study has shown that "for asymptomatic patients treated with 500 mg of zidovudine [AZT], a reduction in the quality of life due to severe side effects of therapy approximately equals the increase in the quality of life associated with a delay in the progression of HIV disease" (Lenderking, Gelber, Cotton, Cole, Goldhirsch, Volberding, and Testa, 1994, p. 738).

Table 16-9 depicts, according to age, sex, and race/ethnicity, deaths from AIDS occurring in 1990 and 1991, with cumulative totals reported through December 1992, for the United States. Deaths for women and children increased at or above the corresponding rate for their male counterparts: for women, about 70% of both reported cases and deaths from AIDS were among minorities. For children this same number was 75%.

The human immunodeficiency virus (HIV) responsible for AIDS was isolated in 1984. More recent information indicates that the virus is more complex than originally thought, and that the body's immune system becomes impaired soon after a person is infected (Hellinger, 1988, Forecasting, p. 309). AIDS cases are reported to the CDC based on a uniform case definition and case report form. The definition of AIDS was broadened in 1987 to incorporate a broader range of AIDS indicator diseases and conditions; the HIV diagnostic tests are used to improve the sensitivity and specificity of the diagnosis (CDC, 1989, HIV/AIDS, p. 15). The definition was again broadened in January 1993. HIV selectively infects and destroys cells that display a CD4 antigen on their surface, primarily T4 lymphocytes. The new definition includes, as an AIDS indicator, a CD count of 200 or fewer as opposed to the normal 600 to 1200 cells/mm^3 blood (CDC, 1992, HIV/AIDS, p. 3).

The time between infection with HIV and the onset of symptoms ranges from 6 months to 5 years or more. It appears that infection with the virus may not always lead to AIDS. About 78% of AIDS patients have one or both of two rare diseases: *pneumocystis carinii* pneumonia (PCP), a parasitic infection of the lungs; and a type of cancer known as Kaposi's sarcoma (KS) (USDHHS, 1987, Facts about AIDS, p. 4). Other opportunistic infections include unusually severe yeast infections, cytomegalovirus, herpes virus, and parasitism. The early signs and symptoms of AIDS are similar to those of a cold or flu and include fever, shaking, night sweats, enlarged lymph nodes, unexplained weight loss, yeast infections, persistent cough, persistent diarrhea, fatigue, and loss of appetite.

People who are HIV-infected are at high risk for developing active tuberculosis, particularly in settings where cough-inducing procedures (sputum induction and aerosolized pentamidine treatments) are being performed. At no time in history has tuberculosis been as great a concern as it is today (CDC, 1992, HIV/AIDS p. 5). The prevention of tuberculosis transmission in health-care settings requires that all of the following basic approaches be used: a) prevention of the generation of infectious airborne particle (droplet nuclei) by early identification and treatment of persons with tuberculous infection and active tuberculosis, b) prevention of the spread of infectious droplet nuclei into the general air circulation by applying source-control methods, c) reduction of the number of infectious droplet nuclei in air contaminated with them, and d) surveillance of health-care-facility personnel for tuberculosis (CDC, December 7, 1990, p. 1).

It is also imperative that patients be screened for tuberculosis and that treatment be started immediately when indicated. The Centers for Disease Control and Prevention have published excellent materials that describe who is at risk for tuberculosis and how they should be screened and treated (CDC, December 7, 1990).

AIDS initially appeared in men and many people still think that it is a disease of gay men. However, the number of AIDS cases due to heterosexual transmission rose by approximately one third from 1989 to 1990, and because of the rising incidence in this group the number of women and children dying of HIV infection and AIDS will continue to increase until the epidemic is brought under control (Noble, 1991, p. 609). The increase in deaths among women is alarming and only recently have the differences between men and women infected with HIV been studied (Smeltzer, 1992). For example, the incidence of Kaposi's sarcoma in men is 15%; in women it is 2%. *Pneumocystis carinii* pneumonia (PCP) is almost always the initial major opportunistic infection in males with HIV. In women esophageal candidiasis is the most common initial opportunistic infection (Smeltzer, p. 153). Further, cervical abnormalities ranging from abnormal Pap smears to carcinoma have been reported to occur more frequently in women who are HIV-infected. Lack of attention to AIDS in women leads to five outcomes (Smeltzer, p. 155): failure to counsel about risk reduction, delay in testing and pretest and posttest counseling, delay in treatment and exclusion from clinical drug trials, denial of social services, and a higher mortality rate.

Flaskerud (1992) has written a cogent article discussing HIV disease and levels of prevention that can

16-9 AIDS Deaths by Race/Ethnicity, Age at Death, and Sex, Occurring in 1990 and 1991, and Cumulative Totals Reported through December 1992, United States[1]

Race/ethnicity and age at death[2]	Males			Females			Both sexes		
	1990	1991	Cumulative total	1990	1991	Cumulative total	1990	1991	Cumulative total
White, not Hispanic									
Under 15	33	53	306	30	30	207	63	83	513
15-24	206	203	1,702	49	33	216	255	236	1,918
25-34	4,609	4,699	28,010	275	326	1,654	4,884	5,025	29,664
35-44	6,035	6,753	35,225	237	267	1,205	6,272	7,020	36,430
45-54	2,566	2,826	14,900	72	114	470	2,638	2,940	15,370
55 or older	1,134	1,188	7,129	140	124	895	1,274	1,312	8,024
All ages	14,583	15,722	87,382	803	894	4,656	15,386	16,616	92,038
Black, not Hispanic									
Under 15	108	88	608	109	97	594	217	185	1,202
15-24	170	186	1,316	74	100	479	244	286	1,795
25-34	2,334	2,417	14,410	691	760	4,021	3,025	3,177	18,431
35-44	2,813	3,194	16,047	683	719	3,448	3,496	3,913	19,495
45-54	924	1,100	5,414	154	233	881	1,078	1,333	6,295
55 or older	433	476	2,403	94	105	465	527	581	2,868
All ages	6,782	7,461	40,245	1,805	2,014	9,908	8,587	9,475	50,153
Hispanic									
Under 15	47	36	287	45	36	261	92	72	548
15-24	112	103	753	34	47	211	146	150	964
25-34	1,509	1,571	9,131	275	325	1,623	1,784	1,896	10,754
35-44	1,677	1,818	9,372	231	286	1,223	1,908	2,104	10,595
45-54	550	620	3,308	69	97	353	619	717	3,661
55 or older	237	284	1,341	30	41	174	267	325	1,515
All ages	4,132	4,432	24,223	684	832	3,855	4,816	5,264	28,078

[1]Data tabulations for 1990 and 1991 are based on date of death occurrence. Data for deaths occurring in 1992 are incomplete and not tabulated separately, but are included in the cumulative totals. Tabulations for 1990 and 1991 may increase as additional deaths are reported to CDC.

[2]Data tabulated under "All ages" include 232 persons whose age at death is unknown. Data tabulated under "All racial/ethnic groups" include 269 persons whose race/ethnicity is unknown.

From Centers for Disease Control and Prevention: *HIV/AIDS surveillance year end edition,* Atlanta, Ga., 1993, The Centers, p. 18.

be used by community health nurses in community education efforts. She emphasizes the three levels of prevention that guide practice and discusses two categories of cofactors that make AIDS a possibility. Exposure cofactors are those behaviors or situations that might affect acquisition of the infection (blood transfusions and anal receptive sex) and trigger cofactors that influence the extent of the disease. Trigger cofactors are noninfectious (for example, the client's nutritional state), as well as infectious. "Infectious co-factors can contribute to the progression from HIV infection to acquired immunodeficiency syndrome (AIDS) both from antigenic overload and stimulation, and from coincident immunosuppression" (Flaskerud, p. 138).

Following the principles of the three levels of prevention, primary prevention of exposure to HIV by clients who are HIV antibody–negative is carried out by avoiding behaviors associated with exposure to HIV: sexual, intravenous, and perinatal transmission.

16-9 AIDS Deaths by Race/Ethnicity, Age at Death, and Sex, Occurring in 1990 and 1991, and Cumulative Totals Reported through December 1992, United States—cont'd

Race/ethnicity and age at death	Males			Females			Both sexes		
	1990	1991	Cumulative total	1990	1991	Cumulative total	1990	1991	Cumulative total
Asian/Pacific Islander									
Under 15	1	—	10	1	1	3	2	1	13
15-24	—	3	16	—	1	3	—	4	19
25-34	44	71	283	3	4	24	47	75	307
35-44	69	80	398	5	6	33	74	86	431
45-54	31	32	186	2	6	18	33	38	204
55 or older	21	17	86	3	4	19	24	21	105
All ages	166	203	980	14	22	101	180	225	1,081
American Indian/Alaska Native									
Under 15	1	3	6	1	—	2	2	3	8
15-24	4	1	12	1	1	2	5	2	14
25-34	16	27	103	3	6	17	19	33	120
35-44	12	26	78	1	3	9	13	29	87
45-54	3	4	26	—	—	2	3	4	28
55 or older	2	5	13	—	—	1	2	5	14
All ages	38	66	238	6	10	33	44	76	271
All Racial/Ethnic Groups									
Under 15	191	180	1,218	186	164	1,069	377	344	2,287
15-24	492	497	3,802	158	182	912	650	679	4,714
25-34	8,522	8,794	51,998	1,250	1,421	7,346	9,772	10,215	59,344
35-44	10,624	11,903	61,241	1,160	1,282	5,925	11,784	13,185	67,166
45-54	4,084	4,591	23,874	298	451	1,728	4,382	5,042	25,602
55 or older	1,827	1,976	10,989	268	274	1,556	2,095	2,250	12,545
All ages	25,740	27,941	153,314	3,320	3,774	18,576	29,060	31,715	171,890

Abstinence, safe sex, testing all blood products, avoiding IV drug use, and prevention of pregnancy by women who are at high risk for HIV are all part of the primary prevention of AIDS. Secondary prevention focuses on those who are HIV antibody–positive. The secondary level of prevention stresses immediate management of infections and practicing excellent health habits. The third level of prevention stresses enhancing the immunocompetence one has and avoiding exposure to cofactors that would further compromise the individual. People with AIDS are well aware of the prejudice that has often surrounded the disease, and successful survivors with AIDS have discovered this is truly a "do it yourself" disease. A goal

for all community health nurses reading this text should be that their clients will never feel that their nurse does not support them. Our specialty area has the unique skills to help fight this terrible tragedy and we will all benefit when it is under control.

Clearly the emphasis with AIDS needs to be on prevention of disease. The development of a safe and effective HIV vaccine is a "high priority for the coming year although the prospects for the availability of such a vaccine are uncertain" (USDHHS, 1991, Healthy people, p. 74). The Health Status Objectives, the Risk Reduction Objectives, and the Services and Protection Objectives provide direction for health programming. They emphasize increased testing for HIV infection with counseling and follow-up accompanied by public education efforts on the risks and precautions needed to slow the spread of the disease.

The National League for Nursing has developed the *Caring for Persons with AIDS Test* to assist nurses in learning more about AIDS. This test is intended for nurses working in hospitals, long-term care facilities, home health agencies, and schools of nursing to measure the nurse's knowledge and ability to apply basic principles in AIDS patient care (NLN, 1989, p. 563). For more information about this test the National League for Nursing can be contacted at 1-800-NOW-1-NLN, or in New York City at 1-212-989-9393.

The National Center for Nursing Research (now the National Institute of Nursing Research) has awarded monies to promote research in nursing care of persons with AIDS (Research Reporter, 1989, p. 24). There are also resources at the federal level for AIDS education and information. The Centers for Disease Control and Prevention oversee the National AIDS Information Hotline (1-800-342-AIDS), which offers information and answers questions, and the National AIDS Information Clearinghouse (1-800-458-5231), which provides many of the same services as the Hotline but also is a direct source of free, government-approved educational materials such as brochures, posters, and displays.

A Spanish translator can be reached at 1-800-344-7432. The number for the hearing impaired is 1-800-343-7889. Orders for bulk quantities or single copies of publications can be placed through the Clearinghouse's toll-free number. The Centers for Disease Control and Prevention can be called for AIDS statistics at 1-800-342-2437. There are often community support groups available for the AIDS client.

Marital Crises

It is not uncommon for the community health nurse to encounter families who are experiencing some form of marital crisis. The divorce rate has increased dramatically in the past three decades. Between 1965 and 1980 the rate more than doubled. Although the upsurge in divorce has occurred among adults of all ages, it has been greatest among those under 45 years of age (Glick and Lin, 1986). Whereas there is some evidence to suggest that this trend is slowing down, marital crisis is still a major life stress for the adult population group. Between 1970 and 1992 the number of single-parent situations increased by 6.7 million

(U.S. Bureau of the Census, 1993). Reasons for this increase were divorce and separation, as well as a rise in the number of never-married parents.

Marital disenchantment, separation, and divorce occur throughout adulthood and are not a problem of youth alone. During middlescence, for instance, spouses find that they have more time together, and if they are unable to reestablish intimacy or reinforce it, they may become disenchanted with their marital relationship. In addition, the sexual changes (menopause and climacteric) that occur during middlescence can also adversely affect the way in which spouses relate in the marital relationship.

Disenchantment, separation, and divorce have an impact on all family members. Adults, as well as children, need to make major changes. Experiencing feelings of uncertainty, betrayal, insecurity, failure, and loss is common during this time. As with all crises, the primary focus of the community health nurse with clients who are experiencing marital stress is on helping them to achieve homeostasis and growth. Adaptation could require divorce or separation, but it also may occur through renegotiation and alteration of family patterns that are dysfunctional. A therapeutic approach that encourages problem-solving rather than blaming can best facilitate successful adaptation during this time of crisis.

Anticipatory guidance activities by the community health nurse may be instrumental in preventing marital crises. Preparing young adults to handle the stresses of parenthood or middlescent couples to deal with the conflicts during launching, for instance, may decrease the amount of distress experienced at these times.

Family Violence

"A person is more likely to be hit or killed in his or her own home by another family member than anywhere else" (Gelles and Straus, 1979, p. 115). Even as we write this section, a famous talk show host is interviewing a couple where the man has repeatedly hit and injured his spouse: "I love her very much. I just can't help myself—I hit her hard when I am angry." His wife states, "Even though he has broken my nose several times and each of my arms, I know he loves me. It is just his way." Intrafamilial violence is more prevalent than often recognized; Chapters 14 and 15 discussed the abuse and neglect of children. Studies also suggest that between 2 and 4 million women are physically battered each year by partners including

◀ *Summaries of Explanations of Violence* ▶

- **Biological**

  Aggression is an innate characteristic that is either an instinctual drive (the instinctivist school of thought) or neurologically based (neurophysiological theories). The latter examines how brain functioning and/or hormones influence degrees of aggressive tendencies and/or violent behaviors. Research evidence links increased testosterone levels to increases in aggression, but the studies do not indicate a causal relationship and factors such as mood, sampling difficulties, and environment must be considered as intervening characteristics.

- **Role of alcohol**

  Research indicates that alcohol seems to facilitate aggression because of the negative affect it has on conscious cognitive processing, yet violence occurs as frequently *without* the presence of alcohol. Alcohol is often used as an excuse or a justification for violence.

- **Psychoanalytical viewpoint**

  This position, espoused by Freud and followers, states that violence results from ego weaknesses and the internal need to discharge hostility. Frustration is the stimulus that leads to the expression of aggression. Catharsis or the expression of the aggression results in a decrease of subsequent aggressive behaviors.

- **Social-learning theory**

  Aggression and violence are learned responses and may be considered adaptive or destructive depending on the situation. The family, television, and environmental conditions serve as models for children to learn how to be aggressive and/or violent.

- **Cultural attitudes fostering violence**

  Tacit acceptance of violence as a means to resolve conflict. War and weapons are justified as protection. In everyday language, we jokingly threaten to "kill" people or "beat them up." We accept physical punishment as a way to discipline children under "certain circumstances." Pornographic depictions of women are legal and deemed as erotica.

- **Power and violence**

  Violence or its threat is often used as a method of persuasion, as in rape or incest. Fear of being a victim of violence keeps people, primarily women, in positions of submission.

- **Poverty**

  Being poor is a condition of oppression, and aggression and violence are methods of expressing such oppression. Poverty needs to be considered as a circumstance in which violence occurs rather than as factor causing such behaviors.

- **Subculture of violence**

  There is a theme of violence that permeates the life-style values of the individuals who are party of this "cultural group." Violence is a fairly typical method of resolving conflict.

From Hanrahan P, Campbell J, and Ulrich Y: Theories of violence. In Campbell J and Humphreys J, eds: *Nursing care of survivors of family violence,* St. Louis, 1993, Mosby, p. 6.

husbands, former husbands, boyfriends, and lovers. Between 21% and 30% of all women in the United States are estimated to have been beaten by a partner at least once. More than 1 million women seek help for injuries caused by battering each year and the vast majority of domestic homicides are preceded by episodes of violence (USDHHS, 1991, Healthy people, p. 61). Battering in lesbian and gay relationships has been reported in the literature; however, the theoretical and empirical studies conducted on heterosexuals cannot be assumed to translate to the experiences of homosexual couples (Campbell and Fishwick, 1993, p. 69).

Why violence is so pervasive in the family where bonds are often the strongest is difficult to understand. Hanrahan, Campbell, and Ulrich (1993) have summarized the explanations for violence in our society (refer to the box above). Different cultures have varying interpretations about what constitutes violence, and the nurse must consider others' views of violence from economic, kinship, and territoriality perspectives, as well as the influence of spiritual, moral, somatic, psychological, and metaphysical issues (Hanrahan, Campbell, and Ulrich, p. 30).

Family violence involves battering and verbal/emotional abuse (National Coalition Against Domestic Violence [NCADV], 1989, What is; NCADV, 1989, On verbal/emotional). Battering often includes an attack by one spouse on another—pushing, slapping, punching, kicking, knifing, shooting, or throwing an object—with intent to do bodily harm. Both men and women are victims of domestic violence, but the more frequently and seriously injured are women.

Domestic violence has serious ramifications for the individual, family, and community. It can result in physical and emotional injury, death, temporary or permanent separation of families, and financial hardship. U.S. statistics about domestic violence reflect its overwhelming scope:

- Over 50% of all women will experience physical violence during the course of an intimate relationship, and in 24% to 30% of these women battering will occur regularly (NCADV, 1989, What is).
- Every 15 seconds the crime of battering occurs (NCADV, 1989, What is), and it is the single largest cause of injury to women in the United States (NCADV, 1988).
- In 50% or more marriages, there has been at least one incident of battering or assault on the woman (Drake, 1982, p. 40).
- A National Crime Survey found that, over a 12-month period, at least 2.1 million married, divorced, or separated women were victims of rape, robbery, aggravated or simple assault by their partners; and that 32% of these women were victimized more than once (NCADV, 1988). Estimates of battering range as high as 3 to 4 million women annually.
- In 1986, 30% of female homicide victims were killed by their husbands or boyfriends (NCADV, 1988).
- In 36 states, under many circumstances it is legal for a husband to rape his wife (NCADV, 1988).

Although assault and assault with intent to commit murder are crimes, police agencies hesitate to get involved in situations involving domestic violence. Frequently police departments do not have uniform reporting procedures for domestic violence, and thus cases of domestic violence are not reported to the police. Police may treat domestic violence as more of a social problem than a criminal one. Police follow-up of incidents of domestic violence account for a high percentage of deaths and injuries to police officers.

There are no stereotypes of battered wives; they come from all educational, social, and economic backgrounds. Some characteristics that have been observed with consistency include an early exposure to violence as a child, economic dependence on one's partner, lack of awareness of alternatives, poor self-image, and inadequate support systems. Often friends and relatives of the battered woman find it easier to ignore the situation or even sanction the abuse. The battered partner may be kept from contact with others who could provide help. She may be depressed and may frequently mention minor somatic complaints when seen by health care personnel, and may or may not show obvious signs of physical injury. She often believes that her partner will reform if she can just "wait it out."

The partners may be characterized as angry, resentful, suspicious, jealous, tense, insecure, moody, and a "loser" (National Mental Health Association, 1988). They often feel guilty and remorseful following an episode of abuse, and things may calm down for awhile. However, it does not take much to trigger a new episode of abuse. In fact, the abuse is very likely to occur again, and it may become more severe. A violent relationship can easily go on to become a violent system.

Concrete linkages between battered wives and battered children have been demonstrated in some research literature (NCADV, 1988). When one occurs community health nurses should look for the other. Some studies have also shown that children who have seen their parents use violence are more likely to use violence themselves as adults (Drake, 1982; Kalmuss, 1984). Kaufman and Zigler (1987) found, however, after a critical review of the literature on intergenerational transmission of violence, that there is not a direct cause and effect relationship between a history of abuse and future abuse. They propose that multiple determinants such as stress, poverty, history of abuse, and lack of supportive relationships influence transmission of violence across generations. These findings suggest that the community health nurse could reduce future abuse through a preventive, supportive approach.

Humphreys (1993) believes that every family should be assessed for family violence. Table 16-10 lists the indicators of potential or actual wife abuse from history; Table 16-11 gives the indicators of wife abuse from physicial examination. Community health nurses can use these guides to assess women at risk for violence; assessment data are then used as a basis for nursing interventions including referral to community resources, when it is indicated.

The community health nurse is in a unique position to see the family at home and may be the first to observe an abusive relationship. The nurse can help clients to look at the situation and to see alternatives to

TABLE 16-10 Indicators of Potential or Actual Wife Abuse from History

Area of assessment	At-risk responses*
Primary concern/reason for visit	Unwarranted delay between time of injury and seeking treatment
	Inappropriate spouse reactions (lack of concern, overconcern, threatening demeanor, reluctance to leave wife, etc.)
	Vague information about cause of injury or problem; discrepancy between physical findings and verbal description of cause; obviously incongruous cause of injury given
	Minimizing serious injury
	Seeking emergency room treatment for vague stress-related symptoms and minor injuries
	Suicide attempt; history of previous attempts
Family health history	
Family of origin	Traditional values about women's role taught
	Spouse abuse or child abuse (may not be significant for wife but should be noted)
Children	Children abused
	Physical punishment used routinely and severely with children
	Children are hostile toward or fearful of father
	Father perceives children as an additional burden
	Father demands unquestioning obedience from children
Partner	Alcohol or drug abuse
	Holds machismo values
	Experience with violence outside of home, including violence against women in previous relationships
	Low self-esteem; lack of power in workplace or other arenas outside of home
	Uses force or coercion in sexual activities
	Unemployment or underemployment
	Extreme jealousy of female friendships, work, and children, as well as other men; jealousy frequently unfounded
	Stressors such as death in family, moving, change of jobs, trouble at work
	Abused as a child or witnessed father abusing mother
Household	Poverty
	Conflicts solved by aggression or violence
	Isolated from neighbors, relatives; few friends; lack of support systems
Past health history	Fractures and trauma injuries
	Depression, anxiety symptoms, substance abuse
	Injuries while pregnant
	Spontaneous abortions
	Psychophysiological complaints
	Previous suicide attempts
Nutrition	Evidence of overeating or anorexia as reactions to stress
	Sudden changes in weight
Personal/social	Low self-esteem; evaluates self poorly in relation to others and ideal self, has trouble listing strengths, makes negative comments about self frequently, doubts own abilities

*At-risk responses are derived from clinical experience and review of the literature.

From Campbell J, McKenna LS, Torres S, Sheridan D, and Landenburger K: Nursing care of abused women. In Campbell J and Humphreys J, eds: *Nursing care of survivors of family violence,* St. Louis, 1993, Mosby, pp. 255-256.

Continued

TABLE 16-10   Indicators of Potential or Actual Wife Abuse from History—cont'd

Area of assessment	At-risk responses
Personal/social—cont'd	Expresses feelings of being trapped, powerlessness, that the situation is hopeless, that it is futile to make future plans
	Chronic fatigue, apathy
	Feels responsible for spouse's behavior
	Holds traditional values about the home, a wife's prescribed role, the husband's prerogatives, strong commitment to marriage
	External locus of control orientation, feels no control over situation, believes fate or other forces determine events
	Major decisions in household made by spouse, indicates far less power than he has in relationship, activities controlled by spouse, money controlled by spouse
	Few support systems, few supportive friends, little outside home activity, outside relationships have been discouraged by spouse or curtailed by self to deal with violent situation
	Physical aggression in courtship
Sleep	Sleep disturbances, insomnia, sleeping more than 10 to 12 hours per day
Elimination	Chronic constipation, diarrhea, or elimination disturbances related to stress
Illness	Frequent psychophysiological illnesses
	Treatment for mental illness
	Use of tranquilizers and/or mood elevators and/or antidepressants
Operations/hospitalizations	Hospitalizations for trauma injuries
	Suicide attempts
	Hospitalization for depression
	Refusals of hospitalization when suggested by physician
Personal safety	Handgun(s) in home
	History of frequent accidents
	Does not take safety precautions
Health care utilization	No regular provider
	Indicates mistrust of health care system
Review of systems	Headaches, undiagnosed gastrointestinal symptoms, palpitations, other possible psychophysiological complaints
	Sexual difficulties, feels husband is "rough" in sexual activities, lack of sexual desire, pain with intercourse
	Joint pain and/or other areas of tenderness, especially at the extremities
	Chronic pain
	Pelvic inflammatory disease

their current lifestyle. This usually involves examining available community resources for both immediate and long-term assistance. Counseling services, shelters for battered women and their children, self-help programs, job training, and financial assistance are a few of the community services available to help domestic violence victims. Community health nurses provide supportive assistance when the client is using these community services. Community health nurses also facilitate comprehensive, ongoing care that is coordinated with other community groups and agencies, refer clients to safe houses, and serve as client advocates.

There are over 1400 shelters and safe homes for battered women servicing more than 375,000 women and children (NCADV, 1989, Statistics from). Increasingly, community health nurses are providing valuable services in shelters for battered women and their

16-11   Indicators of Wife Abuse from Physical Examination

Area of assessment	At-risk findings
General appearance	Increased anxiety in presence of spouse
	Watching spouse for approval of answers to questions
	Signs of fatigue
	Inappropriate or anxious nonverbal behavior
	Nonverbal communication suggesting shame about body
	Flinches when touched
	Poor grooming, inappropriate attire
Vital statistics	Overweight or underweight
	Hypertension
Skin	Bruises, welts, edema, or scars, especially on breasts, upper arms, abdomen, chest, face, and genitalia
	Burns
Head	Subdural hematoma
	Clumps of hair missing
Eyes	Swelling
	Subconjunctival hemorrhage
Genital/urinary	Edema, bruises, tenderness, external bleeding
Rectal	Bruising, bleeding, edema, irritation
Musculoskeletal	Fractures, especially of facial bones, spiral fractures of radius or ulna, ribs
	Shoulder dislocation
	Limited motion of an extremity
	Old fractures in various stages of healing
Abdomen	Abdominal injuries in pregnant women
	Intra-abdominal injury
Neurological	Hyperactive reflex responses
	Ear or eye problems secondary to injury
	Areas of numbness from old injuries
	Tremors
Mental status examination	Anxiety, fear
	Depression
	Suicidal ideation
	Low self-esteem
	Memory loss
	Difficulty concentrating

From Campbell J, McKenna LS, Torres S, Sheridan D and Landenburger K: Nursing care of abused women. In Campbell J and Humphreys J, eds: *Nursing care of survivors of family violence,* St. Louis, 1993, Mosby, p. 257.

children. They complete health assessments, make appropriate referrals to community resources, provide health counseling, conduct group health education sessions, and provide consultation to the shelter staff relative to the health aspects of operating a group home. In this type of setting community health nurses are active members of an interdisciplinary team and provide a unique perspective to the delivery of comprehensive health care. Their focus on preventive, as well as curative, services enhances the care provided to this population group. Because of the complex dynamics related to family violence, confidentiality in regard to the location of shelters for battered victims is maintained by health professionals throughout the community.

The nurse needs to be aware of these resources and refer families to them. Unfortunately, more than 40% of battered women and their children who need emergency housing are denied immediate shelter because of a lack of space (NCADV, 1989, Statistics from). Across the country domestic violence hotlines receive more than 2 million phone calls yearly, and the toll-free National Domestic Violence Hotline (1-800-333-SAFE) receives an average of 5000 calls every month (NCADV, Statistics from). The hotline is staffed 24 hours every day by people who respond to requests for information, discuss options, and provide shelter referrals. The National Coalition against Domestic Violence in Washington, D.C. (202-638-6388) is an excellent source of information and referral.

The Nursing Network on Violence against Women (NNVAW) was founded in 1985 during the first National Nursing Conference on Violence against Women, held at the University of Massachusetts at Amherst. The ultimate goal of NNVAW is to provide a nursing presence in the struggle to end violence in women's lives. NNVAW writes a quarterly column for *Response: To the Victimization of Women and Children,* a journal founded by and associated with the Center for Women's Policy Studies in Washington, D.C. NNVAW can be contacted by writing NNVAW, Dr. Karen Landenburger, University of Washington, School of Nursing SC-74, Seattle, Washington 98195. A book written specifically for nurses on family violence is *Nursing Care of Survivors of Family Violence* (1993) by Campbell and Humphreys. The book is an excellent, practical resource for clinicians, researchers, and teachers. These authors stress that preventive interventions at both the family and community level are essential to reduce future domestic violence.

Individuals Who Are Incarcerated

People who are in prison are generally underserved with their health care concerns because the general public has little sympathy for criminals and also because prisons are often located in isolated areas (Fontes, 1991). Further, data about the people in prisons show that they are represented by the poor, the minorities, the poorly educated, and the inner-city population. In a 1979 study of New York City prison inmates, 85% of the population were blacks and Hispanics. Of this population, 32.9% were unemployed and 64% could not raise a bond of $5000 or less (Alexander-Rodriguez, 1983).

Further illustrating the fact that prisoners are both underserved and unserved are that syphilis and tuberculosis, the "classic diseases of the nineteenth century,

remain the classic diseases of the late twentieth century in American prisons. The rate of syphilis in the prisoner population has been shown to be as high as 1,869/100,000 population, far greater than the rate of 12/100,000 in the U.S. population in 1980" (Alexander-Rodriguez, 1983, p. 116).

Chaisson (1981) called prisons the "last frontier of the health care system." Community health nurses have a remarkable history of care to underserved aggregates, demonstrated by Lillian Wald's work with immigrants in New York City. Furthermore, the profession of nursing is based on the philosophy that adequate and appropriate health care is to be available to all, regardless of the setting. Based on this philosophy, "Standards of Nursing Practice in Correctional Facilities" was developed by the American Nurses Association, Council of Community Health Nurses in 1985. The purpose of the document is to guide the professional nurse working in a correctional facility, including specialty facilities such as those for women, juveniles, and the mentally ill. The standards are to be used in conjunction with other publications of the American Nurses Association, including the *Standards for Clinical Nursing Practice* (1991); *Nursing: A Social Policy Statement* (1980); *Code for Nurses with Interpretive Statements* (1985); and *Standards for Organized Nursing Services* (1982). The American Public Health Association has also published *Standards for Health Services in Correctional Institutions* (1976).

The role of the nurse in the prison setting is generally to provide primary care services from the point of entry to transfer to other settings or release (ANA, 1985, Standards of nursing practice). Primary health services in this field include using the nursing process in screening, providing direct health care services, teaching, counseling, and assisting prisoners to manage their own health care. Alexander-Rodriguez (1983) writes that there is a basic conflict between the goals of correctional health care and correctional institutions. "The biggest challenge for a nurse working in a prison, is to remain true to the humanistic philosophy of nursing and not be slowly and imperceptibly converted to the role of prison keeper. When that happens it is time to get out of prison health care" (Alexander-Rodriguez, p. 116).

There is a steady increase in the number of women who are incarcerated: the number has more than doubled over the past 10 years (Desmond, 1991). This increase has societal implications because imprisonment affects not only the woman herself, but her family of origin and, most powerfully, her children.

Pregnant women in prison have additional concerns because women in federal prisons may not participate in the direct care of their infants after birth (Hufft, 1992). Thus the birth mother has the choice of either placing her infant for adoption or for guardianship. Care of pregnant women in prisons is complicated by stress, restrictive physical environments, alterations in social supports, and the displacement of the maternal role functions after birth (Hufft). Fogel and Martin (1992) have studied incarcerated women who are mothers and who are not mothers; both groups have high levels of depression that did not mitigate over time, but the mothers had high levels of anxiety that remained high.

Another high-risk aggregate in the group of those incarcerated is the older male prisoner. Although prisons have predominately younger males, the number of older prisoners (50 years and over) is increasing and now makes up 4% of the U.S. inmate population (Colsher, Wallace, Loeffelholz, and Sales, 1992). Table 16-12 presents the self-reported and physician-diagnosed illnesses of a number of inmates. Both modification of the environment and more nursing care may be indicated as these people age. Community placement issues upon release from prison are also major concerns for this aggregate at risk. Many of these older men no longer have ties with family and have chronic health problems that require professional care.

Prisons are used as clinical nursing laboratories in some universities (Fontes, 1991; Roell, 1985; Hall and Ortiz-Peters, 1986), which provides an opportunity for prospective prison nurses to identify the health needs of this aggregate. Increasingly, community health nurses are expanding their services to prisoners in city and county jails. In these settings the nurse may conduct health education programs, screen for and follow-up on sexually transmitted diseases, act as a health care resource to staff, assist prisoners in finding health care resources upon discharge, and provide supportive and problem-solving counseling.

Gays and Lesbians

Homosexual men and women played predominant roles in the news following President Clinton's inauguration after he promised to challenge the ban on homosexuals in the military. The New York Times Metro Report (Sunday, March 7, 1993, p. 37) reported: "For some homosexuals, the response is a boiling take-to-the-streets anger. For others, it is a visceral

TABLE 16-12 Percentage of Male Inmates with Lifetime History of Specific Self-Reported Physician-Diagnosed Illness

	Age, y		
	50–59 (n = 82)	>59 (n = 37)	Overall (n = 119)
Arthritis	40.2	56.8	45.4
Hypertension	36.7	45.9	39.7
Any venereal disease	21.5	21.6	21.6
Stomach or intestinal ulcers	18.3	27.0	21.0
Prostate problems	17.1	27.0	20.2
Myocardial infarction	17.7	21.6	19.0
Emphysema	14.6	27.0	18.5
Diabetes	10.1	13.5	11.2
Asthma	8.5	10.8	9.2
Stroke	3.8	16.2	7.8
Cancer	6.3	8.1	6.9
Cirrhosis or liver disease	4.9	2.7	4.2
Injury requiring medical care	78.5	73.0	76.7

From Colsher PL, Wallace RB, Loeffelholz PL, and Sales M: Health status of older male prisoners: A comprehensive survey, *Am J Public Health* 82(6): 882, 1992.

despair poured out to analysts and friends. Some are scared, others proud. A few are exhausted, burned out by a lifetime of fighting that began in adolescence with their own families." Lesbians are "invisible" women in society because they cannot be distinguished by appearance and because of the homophobic nature of our society. There are likely a significant number of lesbians in nursing (Eliason and Randall, 1991).

Eliason and Randall (1991) reported findings that lesbians are reluctant to seek care with their health concerns because of negative past experiences and even harm. Further, "research directed specifically toward lesbian health is remarkably new. Few of these studies have been focused on physical health needs" (Hitchcock and Wilson, 1992, p. 178).

If quality nursing care is to be given nonjudgmentally, nurses must recognize their own homophobias and identify their incorrect knowledge base. Nurses need not advocate lesbianism but rather understand that it is a healthy alternative way of living for many people over the world. Further, it is important that the health care needs of all persons be identified and, with health care planning and programming, then implemented.

The Health Care of Women

A careful reading of this chapter gives some indication that women are an aggregate at risk when health needs are examined. There has been a widespread view in science and medicine that there are few differences between men and women when health problems are addressed; women's health used to be synonymous with reproductive health. However, social, scientific, and political forces have united resulting in a clearer understanding that women's health is separate from the health of men. A crucial example is women with AIDS: it was first diagnosed as a man's disease, and it has been defined and treated in the manner that males respond to the disease. However, Smeltzer's work (1992), which was quoted earlier in this chapter, discusses the manner in which HIV infections affect women much differently than men. AIDS is now the leading cause of death for women between the ages of 20 to 40 in major cities and one of the top five causes of death for women nationally (Smeltzer, p. 152). Given these numbers, more attention must be paid to women infected with HIV.

Further indication of the at-risk status of women is the fact that, of the 3 million homeless people in this country, women and children are the fastest growing subgroup of this population (Hodnicki, Horner, and Boyle, 1992). The terrible results of homelessness for this aggregate have already been discussed. Other evidence of the vulnerability of this group is the fact that millions of women each year are battered and abused and that even health care professionals believe that "abuse cannot be that terrible or the woman would leave" (King and Ryan, 1989). In fact, King and Ryan report that perhaps nurses find it difficult to deal with abuse as a health issue because of personal experiences that they are trying to repress: in one study 18% of nurses questioned reported personal abuse and another 28% reported abuse of mothers, sisters, friends, neighbors, or co-workers.

The Jacob's Institute of Women's Health (4409 12th Street, SW, Washington, D.C. 20024-2188) is an organization committed to excellence in women health care. The Institute has published *The Women's Health Data Book: A Profile of Women's Health in the United States* (Horton, 1992), which compiles in a single publication much of the available national data on the issues central to an understanding of women's health. It is highly readable and uses charts and graphs. Readers concerned with this issue will find the source interesting and informative.

THE COMMUNITY HEALTH NURSE'S ROLE IN MAINTAINING THE HEALTH OF ADULT MEN AND WOMEN

Health is a blend of developmental, physiological, psychological, spiritual, and social factors. When one of these aspects of health breaks down, all are affected. Community health nurses take into consideration all these factors to develop intervention strategies that comprehensively address clients' needs. The implementation of comprehensive intervention strategies frequently requires interdisciplinary team work.

Health is affected by human development, but only limited nursing research has focused on the adult from a developmental framework (Stevenson, 1984, p. 55). Stevenson states that a foundation of nursing research about adult development in relation to health promotion, illness, and crisis situations is needed to develop nursing actions and activities. Without this knowledge, nursing must draw from the social and psychological sciences when incorporating individual and family development into health care.

Adults have a variety of health care needs but they are also busy people. They have responsibilities at home, at work, and in the community, and often spend so much time achieving and doing for others that their own health care needs are overlooked or neglected. It is not an easy task to motivate adults to participate in health activities, especially if they consider themselves to be well. Well adults do not always recognize or act on health needs, and may ignore primary prevention activities.

Various approaches are often needed to plan nursing interventions that address the health needs of well adults. The community health nurse implements interventions on all levels of prevention—primary, secondary, and tertiary. Use of the referral process (refer to Chapter 10) is an integral part of promoting the health of the adult. Nurses can help adults become aware of the available resources that meet their health care needs and refer them to these resources when appropriate. However, many health care resources are organized to deal with acute health care episodes rather than with preventive health care measures.

Health Promotion through Preventive Intervention

As discussed in earlier chapters, health promotion begins with people who are basically healthy and encourages the development of lifestyles that maintain and support health and well-being. Although little is known about how individuals and families move toward more optimal health and about what assists them in the process (Chalmers and Farrell, 1983, p. 62), a great deal is known about many health promotion activities, such as nonsmoking, that enhance a healthy lifestyle.

Some examples of health promotion activities that help adult clients to improve or maintain their well-being are displayed in the box at right. The adult will have more control over some of these activities than others. Some areas of health promotion, such as environmental health and occupational health and safety, are as much matters of legislation and enforcement as individual decision-making. Obtaining documented data about outcomes of health promotion and nursing interventions that facilitate improved health outcomes is critical while working toward influencing legislation and health policy. When encouraging health promotion activities, the nurse should remember that people bring their own beliefs, attitudes, and values to health care situations. Beliefs about individual and family susceptibility to illness, the severity of illness in terms of health and lifestyle disruption, the effectiveness of diagnostic and prevention measures, and barriers to care will affect the health promotion and prevention activities in which a person engages (Rosenstock, 1966).

Community health nurses carry out many primary prevention activities when helping adults to act on personal health risks. They are particularly interested in helping the adult to learn about preventable health problems and about health behaviors that can promote wellness. A major primary prevention activity with adults is health teaching and counseling about family and personal health risk factors, accident prevention and safety, nutrition, personal hygiene, health examinations, family planning, STDs, disease transmission, and immunizations. Such health teaching, with use of resources as appropriate, may help to prevent an illness or injury, dental caries, an unwanted

> ◀ *Healthy Adults: Selected* ▶
> *Activities and Decisions*
> *for Promoting Health*
>
> 1. Cessation of smoking
> 2. Not drinking to excess
> 3. Adequate nutritional intake
> 4. Control of environmental hazards
> 5. Promotion of worksite health and safety
> 6. Prevention and control of hypertension
> 7. Pap smear at least every 3 years
> 8. Regular self-examination of the breasts and testicles
> 9. Knowledge of and action on cancer warning signs
> 10. Counseling to promote mental health
> 11. Regular dental care
> 12. Regular health care
> 13. Regular exercise

Modified from USDHEW: *Healthy people: the Surgeon General's report on health promotion and disease prevention,* Washington, D.C., 1979, U.S. Government Printing Office, pp. 152-154.

pregnancy, marital disenchantment, a suicide attempt, a case of tetanus, a case of flu, an incident of child abuse, or an STD. Health teaching activities help the adult to look at health in relation to present and future functioning.

Primary prevention and health risk appraisal are major goals of health promotion, but are not always easily attainable. In recent years there has been increased emphasis on primary prevention; however, many preventive health care measures, such as yearly physical examinations, are not covered under many forms of health insurance and become out-of-pocket expenses for the client. Health screening programs can provide valuable health services to persons who otherwise would not obtain them.

The community health nurse can help clients to assess individual and family health risk factors on an informal basis and can encourage health actions which decrease these risks. Health risk appraisal can also be handled through an automated process in which an individual's health-related behaviors and personal characteristics are compared to mortality statistics and other epidemiological data. Relating individual and group data helps individuals to identify their risk of dying from a specific condition by a specified time and the amount of risk which could be eliminated by making appropriate behavioral changes in health practices. This automated approach is increasingly accessible to the general public and can have beneficial health consequences. However, the real challenge for health professionals is in assisting people to act on personal health risks.

Safety for the adult is a key factor to consider when developing health teaching and risk appraisal strategies. Accidents kill adults in astounding numbers and account for 45% of deaths in the 20 to 29 age group (refer to Table 16-3). Motor vehicle accidents make up a large portion of these deaths, but accidents also happen at home, at work, and in the community. The nurse can help the adult to assess for potential safety hazards and to identify ways to correct them. Suggestions on measures to promote safety, such as having stairway handrails, conveniently located electrical outlets, indirect nonglare lighting, and safe water and sewage disposal; keeping equipment in proper working order; providing easy entry to and exist from bathtubs and showers; maintaining stairs and landings free from clutter; and making sure that rugs are not loose can help to prevent accidents in the home.

Health teaching of the young adult should focus on violence in addition to accident prevention. Accidents, suicide, and homicide are the leading causes of death for persons 20 to 29 years of age. It is important to try to determine the nature and timing of critical precedents that place individuals at high risk for committing violent acts against themselves or others and to identify significant persons or groups in contact with high-risk individuals who could save the individual's life. White males are most at risk for committing suicide (refer to Table 16-3).

In order to prevent certain conditions, nurses can assist adults in looking at their own personal health habits and risk factors. Smoking, excessive intake of alcoholic beverages, lack of sufficient rest, and an inadequate diet all have an impact on present and future health status.

When nurses function from a prevention perspective they stress the importance of medical, dental, and ophthalmologic examinations for prevention, early diagnosis, and treatment of disease. Secondary preventive health measures for the adult include practicing self-examination of the breasts and testicles, yearly Pap smears, and adherence to prescribed medical and dental regimens. The adult should be assisted to see the value of monitoring and screening for conditions for which he or she has a familial or individual predisposition, such as cardiovascular accidents, diabetes, cancer, or hypertension. Appendix 16-1 sum-

marizes adult screening procedures used with adult clients and the age at which they should be done. Information in this table provides parameters for discussion when the community health nurse is carrying out health counseling.

Tertiary prevention health activities that the nurse may use with the adult are related to rehabilitation activities that minimize the degree of disability of the condition. These activities are discussed in Chapter 18, where the nurse's role in rehabilitation of the handicapped adult is covered. They involve interdisciplinary functioning and focus on encouraging client compliance with prescribed medical and dental regimens, as well as exploring ways to promote coping behaviors.

Pender, Barkauskas, Hayman, Rice, and Anderson (1992, p. 108) have described three points at which a person or a group may be highly receptive to input about health promotion and disease prevention. These three points result from the developmental framework of looking at people along with person-environment interactions that result in either normative stress or nonnormative stress. These three points include the following: age-specific times which are the same for most people including menarche, parenthood, and retirement; historically-specific times in the life of a society including changes in the roles of men and women and insecurity in the labor market; and finally, events that vary among individuals and families including death of a partner or geographic relocation.

This text is built upon a developmental framework; nurses can build their interventions with individuals and groups upon the expected and unexpected transitions in people's development. This principle is one of the contributions of nursing to the health of our nation.

The health risks and the morbidity and mortality for adults mandate that community health nurses continue their education lifelong. Family violence, homelessness, tuberculosis, HIV/AIDS, unemployment, chronic illness—these are topics that are overwhelming in scope and that can affect practitioners themselves. Dealing with them means that nurses be well-informed, that they build in supports, both informal and formal, for the stressful times in their lives, and that political involvement at some level is crucial. All citizens have the right to a home and to a basic minimum of health care. This can happen only when policies are implemented at a federal level.

Legislation Affecting Adult Health

The legislation that influences the adult also makes an impact on other age groups. The Social Security Act of 1935 and its amendments provide maternal-child health programs, which are discussed in Chapters 4 and 14. The Social Security Act also provides for Medicaid and Medicare, for which the medically indigent or terminally ill adult may qualify. The Public Health Service Act of 1944 and its amendments have helped to provide adult health care services. Health planning and environmental health legislation have also benefitted adult health (refer to Chapters 4 and 13).

Among legislation that specifically addresses the adult population is the Occupational Safety and Health Act of 1970, which is discussed in Chapter 17. It deals with maintaining the health of the adult in the workplace and focuses on maintaining wellness. Two pieces of legislation passed in the current decade, The Americans with Disabilities Act and The Family and Medical Leave Act, will also significantly influence the health of adults in the coming years. These acts are discussed in Chapter 4.

Summary

The breadth of the health issues affecting adult men and women is vast. Of all of the population groups presented in this text, adults have the greatest opportunity to improve their health status because they have monetary and physical independence. The fact that younger and older people depend on them can present burdens and challenges.

Adults who financially and emotionally support other age groups are vulnerable to unique pressures and stresses. It is often hard for them to admit that they have health problems or are experiencing stress.

The role of the nurse in helping adults achieve their developmental tasks is an important one. Understanding human development and its impact on health is essential. It is easier for adults to promote and to maintain health when they know about health behaviors that enhance wellness and prevent stress. Major goals of the community health nurse when working with adults are to increase health promotion, prevent illness, and promote self-care capabilities. To accomplish these goals nurses need a supportive work environment, engagement in the politics of health care, and a belief in lifelong learning.

◀ *An Exercise in Critical Thinking* ▶

Read the following scenario (Berne, Dato, Mason, and Rafferty, 1990, p. 11) and then write a paragraph describing your feelings and the course of action you would take in the next week. Do you believe that this situation could ever happen to you or someone that you know?

Imagine You Are Homeless . . .

Imagine you are a 33-year-old woman with three children. Your apartment burned down six months ago. You and your children had been living with your sister in her cramped apartment until she had another baby, and now there simply was not enough room for everyone.

You sleep in your car at night. During the day, you walk the streets with your children trying to find an apartment you can afford. Finally, you go to the department of social services to try to find shelter for the night and are told that your children may have to be placed in foster care if a place cannot be found for all of you. Knowing that the foster care system in this city is unreliable and sometimes unsafe, you agree to spend the first night in an overcrowded warehouse-type shelter, where you end up sleeping on the floor.

You and your children have no privacy here. Many of the children and adults have colds and you hear that tuberculosis has been an increasing problem among the homeless. When the opportunity arises, you agree to move into one of the single-room occupancy hotels that the city is using to house homeless families "temporarily." That temporary shelter becomes your home for 13 months.

The temporary shelter consists of one 10 by 10 ft. room. You have no kitchen, no refrigerator, no stove or cooking facilities. There is one bed for you and your three children.

You pull the mattress off the bed at night to make room for all of you to sleep and then pull the sheets off the bed in the day to eat on the floor.

You use running water to keep your baby's milk cool and you do the dishes in the tub where you bathe and store things.

There is no place for your children to play, no place to sit, no place to do homework. When they try to play in the hall, they are approached by drug dealers and sometimes even pimps.

This is what life is like for you and your children. Imagine the gradual dissipation of your own and your children's self-esteem and the isolation and depression that eventually overwhelm you. Imagine having a future without space, without privacy, without hope.

Screening Flow Chart for Health Promotion and Disease Prevention in Primary Care of Male and Female Adult Patients

I. Screening tests found to be effective

	20	21	22	23	24	25	26	27	28	29	30	31	32	33	34	35	36	37	38	39	40
Hx Data base, initial (subsequently update only)	□	□	□	□			□			□			□			□			□		
Alcohol use	□						□						□						□		
Smoking (nonsmokers)	□						□						□						□		
Rheumatic heart disease	□																				
PE Complete physical examination																					
Weight	□				□				□				□			□			□		
Blood pressure	□			□			□			□			□			□			□		
Mouth, neck exam	□			□			□			□			□			□			□		
Breast exam	□			□			□			□			□			□			□		
Testicular exam	□			□			□			□			□			□			□		
Prostatic exam	□			□			□			□			□			□			□		
Pelvic exam	□			□			□			□			□			□			□		
Lab Pap smear	□	□		□			□			□			□			□			□		
Stool guaiac																					
Mammography																□					
Sigmoidoscopy																					
DT booster	□										□								□		
Rubella titer	□																				
PPD	□									□									□		
VDRL	□						□						□						□		

II. Screening tests possibly effective

	20	21	22	23	24	25	26	27	28	29	30	31	32	33	34	35	36	37	38	39	40
Serum cholesterol	□																				
Tonometry																					

III. Teach, counsel re:

	20	21	22	23	24	25	26	27	28	29	30	31	32	33	34	35	36	37	38	39	40
Exercise	□				□				□			□				□			□		
Nutrition	□				□				□			□				□			□		
Stress reduction, life change events	□				□				□			□				□			□		
Seat belts	□				□				□			□				□			□		
Report mouth sores	□						□						□						□		
BSE	□						□						□						□		
Neck, testicular palpation	□						□			□			□			□					
Report postmenopausal bleeding																					
Obtain dental exam, dental prophylaxis	□				□				□			□				□			□		

The Screening Flow Chart. Taking into account the findings of major studies and the recommendations of significant authorities, a flow chart has been developed. It is designed to facilitate a comprehensive, cost-effective lifetime preventive screening program for each patient.

It can best be used by inserting it into the patient chart cover, at the time the individual enters the NP's practice. The date should be plotted above the appropriate column, based on the patient's age. All screening tests recommended for the 20-year-old, as well as those indicated at the patient's current age, should be accomplished. Normal test results can be indicated by placing a □ in the appropriate box. An ⊠ would signify an abnormal finding. Specific abnormal data could be recorded on an adjacent page. Subsequent visits could be planned for the asymptomatic, essentially healthy individual for the purpose of primary and secondary preventive screening at intervals, as indicated by the flow sheet.

41 42 43 44 45 46 47 48 49 50 51 52 53 54 55 56 57 58 59 60 61 62 63 64 65 66 67 68 69 70

This flow sheet should be regarded as a guideline, since ultimately each patient's prevention program should be tailored to individual needs, based on age, sex, risk factors, socioeconomic status, and mutual specific concerns of the patient and provider. It should be emphasized that these guidelines apply to asymptomatic persons. Patients with symptoms require a complete work up and persons at risk need a more intensive screening program.

From Lindberg SC: Periodic preventive health screening schedule for adult men and women: a guide for the primary care practitioner, *Nurse Practitioner* 5(5):9-13, 1980.

References

Adams PF and Benson V: *Current estimates from the National Health Interview Survey 1984,* 10(176), Hyattsville, Md., 1990, National Center for Health Statistics, Vital Health Statistics.

Adams PF and Benson V: *Current estimates from the National Health Interview Survey, 1984,* 10(181), Hyattsville, Md., 1991, National Center for Health Statistics, Vital Health Statistics.

Allen DG and Whatley M: Nursing and men's health: some critical considerations, *Nursing Clinics of North America* 21(1):3-13, 1986.

American Cancer Society: *Cancer facts and figures—1993,* Atlanta, Ga., 1993, The Society.

American Heart Association (AHA): *Fact sheet on heart attack, stroke, and risk factors,* Dallas, 1992, The Association.

AHA: *1993 heart and stroke fact statistics,* Dallas, 1992, The Association.

AHA: *1990 research facts,* Dallas, 1989, The Association.

AHA: *Research: the heart of it all,* Dallas, 1989, The Association.

Alexander-Rodriguez T: Prison health—a role for professional nursing, *Nurs Outlook* 31(2):115-118, 1983.

American Nurses Association: *Code for nurses with interpretive statements,* Kansas City, Mo., 1985, The Association.

American Nurses Association: *Nursing: a social policy statement,* Kansas City, Mo., 1980, The Association.

American Nurses Association: *Standards of clinical nursing practice,* Kansas City, Mo., 1991, The Association.

American Nurses Association: *Standards of nursing practice in correctional facilities,* Kansas City, Mo., 1985, The Association.

American Nurses Association: *Standards for organized nursing services,* Kansas City, Mo., 1982, The Association.

American Public Health Association (APHA): Anti-smoking effort for pregnant women lowers rates of low weight babies, *Nation's Health,* March 1984, p. 11.

APHA: *Standards for health services in correctional institutions,* Washington, D.C., 1976, The Association.

Bennett EG and Woolf DS: Current approaches to substance abuse and treatment. In Bennett EG and Woolf DS, eds: *Substance abuse,* Albany, N.Y., 1991, Delmar Publishers.

Berne AS, Dato C, Mason DJ, and Rafferty M: A nursing model for addressing the health needs of homeless families, *Image: J Nurs Scholarship* 22(1):8-13, Spring 1990.

Bowdler JE: Health problems of the homeless in America, *Nurse Pract* 14(7):44,47,50,51, 1989.

Bowdler JE and Barrell LM: Health needs of homeless persons, *Public Health Nurs* 4(3):135-140, 1987.

Byrd JC, Shapiro RS, and Schiedermayer DL: Passive smoking: a review of medical and legal issues, *Am J Public Health* 79:968-972, 1989.

Caldwell LR: Questions and answers about menopause, *Am J Nurs,* 85(9):968-972, 1982.

Campbell J and Fishwick N: Abuse of female partners. In Campbell J and Humphreys J, eds: *Nursing care of survivors of family violence,* St. Louis, 1993, Mosby.

Campbell JC and Humphreys JC: *Nursing care of survivors of family violence,* St. Louis, 1993, Mosby.

Campbell JC and Humphreys JC: *Nursing care of victims of family violence,* Norwalk, Conn., 1984, Appleton/Lange.

Campbell J, McKenna LS, Torres S, Sheridan D, and Landenburger K: Nursing care of abused women. In Campbell J and Humphreys J, eds: *Nursing care of survivors of family violence,* St. Louis, 1993, Mosby.

Centers for Disease Control and Prevention (CDC): *Guidelines for preventing the transmission of tuberculosis in health-care settings, with special focus on HIV-related issues, MMWR* 39:RR-17, December 7, 1990.

CDC: *HIV/AIDS Surveillance Report,* Atlanta, Ga., July 1992, The Centers.

CDC: *HIV/AIDS surveillance: AIDS cases reported through October 1989,* Atlanta, Ga., November 1989, The Centers.

CDC: *HIV/AIDS surveillance report,* Atlanta, Ga., September 1990, The Centers, pp. 1-18.

CDC: *HIV/AIDS surveillance year end edition,* Atlanta, Ga., 1993, The Centers.

CDC: *National action plan to combat multidrug-resistant tuberculosis, MMWR* 41:RR-11, June 19, 1992.

Chalmers K and Farrell PI: Nursing interventions for health promotion, *Nurse Pract* 8(11):62-64, 1983.

Chaisson G: Correctional health care: beyond the barriers, *Am J Nurs* 81:737-738, 1981.

Cigarette advertising—United States, 1988, *MMWR* 39(16):261-265, April 27, 1990.

Colsher PL, Wallace RB, Loeffelholz PL, and Sales M: Health status of older male prisoners: a comprehensive survey, *Am J Public Health* 82(6):881-883, 1992.

Cox J: Koop says up tax, cut liquor ads, *USA Today* June 1, 1989, p. A1.

Desmond AM: The relationship between loneliness and social interactions in women prisoners, *J Psychosocial Nurs* 29(2):5-9, 1991.

Division of Gerontology, The University of Michigan: *Aging in the modern world,* Ann Arbor, 1957, The University of Michigan.

Drake VK: Battered women: a health care problem in disguise, *Image* XIV (June):40-47, 1982.

Duvall EM: *Family development,* ed 2, New York, 1962, Lippincott.

Duvall EM and Miller BC: *Marriage and family development,* ed 6, New York, 1985, Harper & Row.

Eliason MJ and Randall CE: Lesbian phobia in nursing students, *Western J Nurs Research* 13(3):363-374, 1991.

Erikson EH: *Childhood and society,* ed 2, New York, 1963, Norton.

Erikson EH: *The life cycle completed: a review,* New York, 1982, Norton.

Ershoff DH, Mullen PD, and Quinn V: A randomized trial of serialized self-help smoking cessation program for pregnant women in an HMO, *Am J Public Health* 79(2):182-187, 1989.

Estes NJ, Smith-DiJulio K and Heinemann ME: *Nursing diagnosis of the alcoholic person,* St. Louis, 1980, Mosby.

Figley CR and McCubbin HI, eds: *Stress and the family,* vol 2, New York, 1983, Brunner/Mazel.

Fincer J: Sean Marsee's smokeless death, *Reader's Digest,* October 1985, pp. 107-112.

Flaskerud JH: HIV disease and levels of prevention, *J Community Health Nurs* 9(3):137-150, 1992.

Fogel CI and Martin SL: The mental health of incarcerated women, *Western J Nurs Research* 14(1):30-47, 1992.

Fontes HC: Prisons: logical innovative clinical nursing laboratories, *Nurs and Health Care* 12(6):300-303, 1991.

Friend T: High death rate among Blacks hard to explain, *USA Today,* February 9, 1990, p. 1D.

Gelles RJ and Straus MA: Violence in the American family, *J Social Issues* 35:113-117, 1979.

Glick PC and Lin SL: Recent changes in divorce and remarriage, *J Marriage Family* 48:737-748, 1986.

Hall C and Ortiz-Peters R: Faculty practice in a prison setting: implications for teaching, *J Nurs Educ* 25(7):306-309, 1986.

Hanrahan P, Campbell J and Ulrich Y: Theories of violence. In Campbell J and Humphreys J, eds: *Nursing care of survivors of family violence,* St. Louis, Mo., 1993, Mosby.

Havighurst RJ: *Developmental tasks and education,* New York, 1972, David McKay.

Heart attacks, *Newsweek,* February 8, 1988, pp. 50-54.

Hellinger FJ: Forecasting the personal medical care costs of AIDS from 1988 through 1991, *Public Health Rep* 103(3):309-319, 1988.

Hill J: The psychological impact of unemployment, *New Society* 43:118-120, 1978.

Himmelstein DU and Woolhandler S: *The national health program chartbook,* Cambridge, Mass., 1992, Center for National Health Program Studies.

Hitchcock JM and Wilson HS: Personal risking: lesbian self-disclosure of sexual orientation to professional health care providers, *Nursing Research* 41(3):178-183, 1992.

Hodnicki DR, Horner SD, and Boyle JS: Women's perspectives on homelessness, *Public Health Nurs* 9(4):257-262, December 1992.

Horton JA, eds: *The women's health data book: a profile of women's health in the United States,* Washington, D.C., 1992, The Jacob Institute of Women's Health.

Hough EE, Lewis FM, and Woods NF: Family response to a mother's chronic illness: case studies of well-and poorly adjusted families, *Western J Nurs Research* 13(5):568-596, 1991.

Humphreys J: Children of battered women. In Campbell J and Humphreys J, eds: *Nursing care of survivors of family violence,* St. Louis, 1993, Mosby.

Hufft AG: Psychosocial adaptation to pregnancy in prison, *J Psychosocial Nurs* 30(4):19-23, 1992.

Hypertension and strokes: a success story, *Newsweek,* February 8, 1988, p. 60.

Johnston LD, O'Malley PM, and Bachman JG: *Monitoring the future: 18th national high school senior survey,* news release, Ann Arbor, April 9, 1993, University of Michigan Institute of Social Research.

Kaforey EC: Crisis intervention and the new unemployed, *AAOHN* 32:154-157, 1984.

Kalmuss D: The intergenerational transmission of marital aggression, *J Marriage Family* 46:11-19, 1984.

Kaufman J and Zigler E: Do abused children become abusive parents? *Am J Orthopsychiatry* 57:186-193, 1987.

King MC and Ryan J: Abused women: dispelling myths and encourage intervention, *Nurse Pract* 14(5):47-48, 50, 53-54, 1989.

Kinzel D: Self-identified health concerns of two homeless groups, *Western J Nurs Research* 13(2):181-194, 1991.

Knafl KA and Grace HK: *Families across the life cycle.* Boston, 1978, Little, Brown.

Krystal E, Moran-Sackett M, and Cantoni L: Serving the unemployed, *Social Casework* 64(1):67-76, 1983.

Kubler-Ross E: *Questions and answers on death and dying,* New York, 1974, Collier Books.

Kubler-Ross E: *Death: the final stage of growth,* Englewood Cliffs, N.J., 1975, Prentice-Hall.

Lawrence RC, Hocberg MC, Kelsey JL, McDuffie FC, Medsger TA, and Felts WR: Estimates of the prevalence of selected arthritic and muscule skeletal diseases in the United States, *J Rheumatol* 16:427-441, 1989.

Lenderking WR, Gelber RD, Cotton DJ, Cole BF, Goldhirsch A, Volberding PA, and Testa MA, for the AIDS Clinical Trials Group: Evaluation of the quality of life associated with zidovudine treatment in asymptomatic human immunodeficiency virus infection, *N Engl J Med* 330:738-743, 1994.

Leslie AL and Swider MS: Changing factors and changing needs in women's health care, *Nursing Clinics North America* 21(1):111-123, 1986.

Lindberg SC: Periodic preventive health screening schedule for adult men and women: a guide for the primary care practitioner, *Nurs Pract* 5(5):9-13, 1980.

Lindsey A: Health care for the homeless, *Nurs Outlook* 37(2):78-81, 1989.

Madonia JF: The trauma of unemployment and its consequences, *Social Casework* 64:482-488, 1983.

Margolis LH and Farran DC: Unemployment: the health consequences in children, *NC Med J* 66:268-269, 1981.

McGrath E, Keita GP, Strickland BR, and Russo NF, eds: *Women and depression: risk factors and treatment issues,* Washington, D.C., 1990, American Psychological Association.

Mihaly LK: *Homeless families: failed policies and young victims,* Washington, D.C., 1991, Children's Defense Fund.

Moen P: Preventing financial hardship: coping strategies of the unemployed. In McCubbin HI, Cauble AE, and Patterson JM, eds: *Family stress, coping and social support,* 1983, Springfield, Ill.

Monmaney T: The fitness connection. Couch potatoes: off your duffs, *Newsweek,* February 8, 1988, p. 60.

Monmaney T, Springen K, Hager M, and Shapiro D: The cholesterol connection, *Newsweek,* February 8, 1988, pp. 56-58.

Murray R and Zentner J: *Nursing assessment and health promotion through the life span,* ed 6, Englewood Cliffs, N.J., 1989, Prentice-Hall.

National Association of Community Health Centers: *Community health centers: a quality system for the changing health care market,* McClean, Virg., 1986, National Clearinghouse for Primary Care Information.

National campaign aims to snuff out smokeless tobacco use by young folks, *Knoxville News-Sentinel,* February 22, 1990, p. A10.

National Cancer Institute: *Questions and answers about PDQ, the National Cancer Institute's Computerized Database for physicians,* Washington, D.C., 1989, The Institute.

National Coalition against Domestic Violence (NCADV): *NCADV statistics: May 1988,* Washington, D.C., 1988, The Coalition.

NCADV: *Statistics from 1987 NCADV domestic violence statistical survey,* Washington, D.C., 1989, The Coalition.

NCADV: *What is battering?* Washington, D.C., 1989, The Coalition.

NCADV: *On verbal/emotional abuse,* Washington, D.C., 1989, The Coalition.

National Institute for Disability and Rehabilitation Research: *Stroke: rehab brief,* Washington, D.C., 1989, U.S. Government Printing Office.

National League for Nursing: Caring for persons with AIDS test, *Nurs Health Care* 10(10):563, 1989.

National Mental Health Association: *Depression: what you should know about it,* Alexandria, Virg., 1988, The Association.

National Safety Council: *Accident facts, 1991 edition,* Chicago, 1991, The Council.

National Safety Council: *Accident facts, 1994 edition,* Chicago, 1994, The Council.

New pattern of birth defects linked to pregnant smokers, *Knoxville Journal,* October 12, 1985, p. A3.

Newman RB and Newman PR: *Development through life: a psychosocial approach,* Homewood, Ill., 1975, Dorsey Press.

New York Times: *For gay people, a time of triumph and fear,* Sunday March 7, 1993, p. 37.

Noble GR: How the response to the epidemic of HIV infection has strengthened the public health system, *Public Health Reports* 106(6):608-615, 1991.

Northouse L: The impact of cancer on the family: an overview, *International Psychiatry in Medicine* 14:215-242, 1984.

Office of Minority Health—Resource Center (OMH-RC): Cancer hits some minorities hard. In *Cancer and minorities: closing the gap,* Washington, D.C., 1989, Department of Health and Human Resources.

OMH-RC: *Cancer and minorities.* In *Cancer and minorities: closing the gap,* Washington, D.C., 1989, Department of Health and Human Resources, p. 1.

O'Hare WP: *The rise of poverty in rural America,* Washington, D.C., 1988, Population Reference Bureau.

Park PB: Health care for the homeless: a self-care approach, *Clinical Nurse Specialist* 39(4):171-174, 1989.

Pender NJ, Barkauskas VH, Hayman L, Rice VH, and Anderson ET: Health promotion and disease prevention: toward excellence in nursing practice and education, *Nurs Outlook* 40(3):106-113, 1992.

Public Health Foundation, Data for the healthy people 2000 objectives: *The public health foundation's new core data base,* Washington, D.C., July 1991, The Foundation.

Research Reporter: Rush College of Nursing Awarded $500,000 AIDS grant, *Nurs Res* 38(1):24, 1989.

Rice DP: Health status and national health priorities, *Western J Medicine* 154:294-302, March, 1991.

Robert Wood Johnson Foundation: *Challenges in health care: a chartbook perspective 1991,* Princeton, N.J., 1991, The Foundation.

Robertson MJ and Cousineau MR: Health status and access to health services among the urban homeless, *Am J Public Health* 76(5):561-563, 1986.

Roell S: Prison practicum scores points with students and inmates, *Nurs Health Care* 6(2):103-105, 1985.

Rosenstock I: Why people use health services, *Milbank Q* 44:94-127, 1966.

Ryan MT: Providing shelter. The homeless chronically mentally ill, *J Psychosocial Nurs* 27(6):14-18, 1989.

Sempos C, Fulwood R, Haines C, Carroll M, Anda R, Williamson DF, Remington P, and Cleeman J: The prevalence of high blood cholesterol levels among adults in the United States, *JAMA* 262(1):45-52, 1989.

Smeltzer SC: Women and AIDS: sociopolitical issues, *Nurs Outlook* 40(4):152-158, 1992.

Smith DE, Wesson DR, and Linda LK: Clinical approaches to acute and chronic interventions in the sedative-hypnotic abuser. In Einstein S, ed: *Drugs in relation to the drug user,* pp. 192-243, New York, 1980, Pergamon Press.

Sperling D: Alcohol is leading U.S. drug worry, *USA Today* January 24, 1990, p. D1.

Stern L: How to find a job: new ways of winning in today's tough market, *Modern Maturity* 36(3):25-28, 30, 32-34, 1993.

Stevenson JS: Adulthood: a promising focus for future research. In Werley HH and Fitzpatrick JJ, eds: *Annual review of nursing research,* vol I, New York, 1984, Springer.

Stevenson JS: *Issues and crises during middlescence,* New York, 1977, Appleton-Century-Crofts.

Swineburne P: The psychological impact of unemployment on managers and professional staff, *J Occup Psychol* 54:47-64, 1981.

Taylor C, Lillis C, and LeMone P: *Fundamentals of nursing: the art and science of nursing care,* Philadelphia, 1989, Lippincott.

Thompson JM, McFarland GK, Hirsch JE, & Tucker SM: *Mosby's Clinical Nursing,* ed 3, St. Louis, 1993, Mosby.

U.S. Bureau of Labor Statistics: *Employment and earnings,* 34(1):217, 1987.

U.S. Bureau of the Census: *Household and family characteristics, March 1988 concurrent population reports,* Series P-20, No 437, Washington, D.C., 1989, U.S. Government Printing Office.

U.S. Bureau of the Census: Population profile of the United States: 1993, Series P23-185, Washington, D.C., 1993, U.S. Government Printing Office.

U.S. Department of Health, Education and Welfare (USDHEW): *Smoking and health: report of the advisory committee to the Surgeon General of the Public Health Service,* Washington, D.C., 1964, U.S. Government Printing Office.

USDHEW: *Healthy people: the Surgeon General's report on health promotion and disease prevention,* Washington, D.C., 1979, U.S. Government Printing Office.

USDHEW: *Promoting health/preventing disease: objectives for the nation,* Washington, D.C., 1980, U.S. Government Printing Office.

U.S. Department of Health and Human Services (USDHHS): *The 1990 health objectives for the nation: a midcourse review,* Washington, D.C., 1986, U.S. Government Printing Office.

USDHHS: *Prevention '86/'87: federal programs and progress,* Washington, D.C., 1987, U.S. Government Printing Office.

USDHHS: *Facts about AIDS,* Washington, D.C., 1987, U.S. Government Printing Office.

USDHHS: *Health United States, 1983,* Washington, D.C., 1983, U.S. Government Printing Office.

USDHHS: Prevention '93/'94: Washington, D.C., in press, U.S. Government Printing Office.

USDHHS: *The Surgeon General's 1989 report on reducing the health consequences of smoking: 25 years of progress,* Washington, D.C., 1989, U.S. Government Printing Office.

USDHHS: *Healthy people 2000: national health promotion and disease prevention objectives, full report, with commentary,* Washington, D.C., 1991, U.S. Government Printing Office.

USDHHS: *Health status of the disadvantaged: chartbook 1990,* DHHS Pub No. (HRSA) HRS-P-DV 90-1, Washington, D.C., 1991, U.S. Government Printing Office.

USDHHS: *Health status of minorities and low-income groups,* ed 3, Washington, D.C., 1991, U.S. Government Printing Office.

USDHHS: *Women's health: report of the Public Health Service Task Force on Women's Health Issues,* DHHS Pub No. (PHS)85-5026, Washington, D.C., 1985, U.S. Government Printing Office.

U.S. National Center for Health Statistics: *Advance report of final mortality statistics, 1988,* Monthly Vital Statistics Report, Vol 39, No 7, Supplement, Hyattsville, MD, DHHS Pub No (PHS)91-1120, 1990, Table 4, p. 16.

U.S. National Center for Health Statistics: *Health, United States, 1991,* Hyattsville, Md., 1992, Public Health Service.

U.S. Preventive Services Task Force: *Guide to clinical preventive services: an assessment of the effectiveness of 169 interventions,* Baltimore, Md., 1989, Williams & Wilkins.

Voyanoff P: Unemployment: family strategies for adaptation. In Fibley CR and McCubbin HI, eds: *Stress and the family,* vol II, New York, 1983, Brunner/Mazel, pp. 90-102.

Warner KE: Smoking and health: a 25-year perspective, *Am J Public Health* 79 (12):141-142, 1989.

Williams GD, Stinson FS, Parker DA, Harford TC, and Noble JN: Demographic trends, *Alcohol Health Res World* 11(3):80-93, 1987.

With neither home nor health, *Emerg Med* 21(4):21-24, 27-28, 31-32, 35-36, 38, 43-44, 46, 1989.

Woolley AS: Challenging RN students: practicing assessment skills in an urban rescue mission, *Nurse Educator* May-June, 32-33, 1985.

Selected Bibliography

Allen DG and Whatley M: Nursing and men's health: some critical considerations, *Nurs Clin North Am* 21:3-13, 1986.

Andrews B and Brown GW: Marital violence in the community: a biographical approach, *J Psychiatry* 153:305-312, 1988.

Campbell JC and Sheridan DJ: Emergency nursing interventions with battered women, *J Emerg Nurs* 15:1, 12-17, 1989.

Campbell JC and Sheridan DJ: Women's responses to sexual abuse in intimate relationships, *Health Care Women Int* 10:335-346, 1989.

Campbell JC and Sheridan DJ: The dark consequences of marital rape, *Am J Nurs* 89:946-949, 1989.

Campbell JC and Sheridan DJ: A test of two explanatory models of women's responses to battering, *Nurs Res* 38:1, 18-24, 1989.

Cohen C, Teresi J, and Holmes D: The mental health of homeless men, *American Geriatrics Society* 36:6, 492-502, 1991.

Damrosch S and Strasser J: The homeless elderly in America, *Gerontolog Nurs,* 14:10, 26-29, 1988.

Duffy ME: Determinants of health promotion in midlife women, *Nurs Res* 37(6):358-362, 1988.

Flaskerud JH: Prevention of AIDS in Blacks and Hispanics: nursing implications, *J Community Health Nurs* 5:1, 49-58, 1988.

Francis M: Homeless families: rebuilding connections, *Public Health Nursing* 8(2):90-96, 1991.

Silverman MM, Lalley TL, Rosenberg ML, Smith JC, Parron D, and Jacobs J: Control of stress and violent behavior: midcourse review of the 1990 health objectives, *Public Health Rep* 103:1, 38-47, 1988.

Stuart EP and Campbell JC: Assessment of patterns of dangerousness with battered women, *Issues Mental Health Nurs* 10:245-260, 1989.

Talashek ML, Tichy AM, and Salmon ME: The AIDS pandemic: a nursing model, *Public Health Nurs* 6:182-188, 1989.

Tobacco and health, *Am J Public Health,* special issue, 79:2, 1989.

USDHHS: *Surgeon General's workshop on violence and public health,* Washington, D.C., 1984, The Department.

Women's health—report of the Public Health Service Task Force on women's health issues, *Public Health Reports* 100:73-106, 1985.

Wynder EL: Tobacco and health. A review of the history and suggestions for public health policy, *Public Health Rep* 103(1): 8-17, 1988.

Occupational Health Nursing

OBJECTIVES

Upon completion of this chapter, the reader should be able to:

1. Discuss the *Healthy People 2000* national health objectives for occupational health.
2. Summarize the purpose, intents, and mandates of the Occupational Safety and Health Act of 1970.
3. Discuss the evolution of occupational health nursing in the United States.
4. Describe recommended educational preparation and professional opportunities for the occupational health nurse.

5. Understand the objectives and functions of the occupational health nurse.
6. Discuss the 10 leading work-related diseases/injuries in the United States.
7. Discuss AIDS and hepatitis B as contemporary workplace health concerns.

Occupational health is the application of public health principles and medical, nursing and engineering practice for the purpose of conserving, promoting and restoring the health and effectiveness of workers through their place of employment.

MARY LOUISE BROWN, OCCUPATIONAL HEALTH NURSING, NEW YORK, 1956, SPRINGER, P. 1. USED BY PERMISSION.

The first census in 1790 revealed the United States to be an agricultural nation; however, the Industrial Revolution rapidly changed this. Between 1870 and 1910 the U.S. population rose 132%, whereas the number of persons working in industry rose almost 400% (Morris, 1976, p. 109). Today there are approximately 110 million workers in the United States (USDHHS, 1991, Healthy people, p. 65).

The working population is basically a well population, and maintaining its health is extremely important to the economic status of the nation. There is great diversity among our nation's workers representing all socioeconomic levels, ethnic and racial groups, and cultural and religious backgrounds. Occupational health professionals are involved in making the workplace a safe and healthy place to be, and emphasize primary prevention activities such as health protection and promotion. This chapter addresses the role of the occupational health nurse in promoting the health of workers and their families in the community.

OCCUPATIONAL HEALTH IN THE UNITED STATES

Work is a major means of establishing individual, family, and national economic security, but the workplace is not always a healthy place to be. By the mid 1800s many Americans worked under unsafe or unhealthy conditions, and workers rallied for shorter work days, health and safety measures, and child labor laws. At that time almost half of all employees in New England factories were children from 7 to 16 years of age. In 1836 Massachusetts became the first state to enact a child labor law (Felton, 1976, p. 809). In 1850 Massachusetts became the first state to study occupational health; in 1879, the first state to pass legislation requiring factory safety inspections; and in 1886, the first state to require reporting of industrial accidents.

Around the turn of the century, occupational medicine began to emerge in the United States. The Homestake Mining Company sponsored the first industrial medical department in the United States in 1887 (United States Department of Labor [USDL], 1977, p. 15). In 1888 Betty Moulder, a nurse, was hired by a group of Pennsylvania coal mining companies to care for the miners and their families, but little is known of her duties or accomplishments (Haag and Glazner, 1992, p. 56; Parker-Conrad, 1988, p. 156). At this time, public awareness of occupational health hazards also increased, and physicians began to write about occupational disease.

The federal government issued its first major report on occupational safety and health in 1903 (USDL, 1977, p. 15-16). It was at this same time that a pioneer in occupational medicine, Dr. Alice Hamilton, began her work. In 1910 she became the chair of the first Occupational Disease Commission in the United States in the state of Illinois; in 1911 she headed the newly formed Federal Occupational Disease Commission.

Dr. Hamilton achieved international recognition for her research and writings on occupational diseases and conditions, and she is considered by many to be the founder of occupational medicine in this country. Among her numerous publications are the classic *Industrial Poisons in the United States* (1925), and *Exploring the Dangerous Trades: the Autobiography of Alice Hamilton, M.D.* (1943). Dr. Hamilton lived a long and remarkable life. She died the year that the Occupational Safety and Health Act of 1970 was passed, at the age of 101.

During Dr. Hamilton's time the emergence of labor unions and the formation of the U.S. Department of Labor placed new emphasis on occupational health and safety. Although for different reasons, workers and employers agreed on the value of maintaining worker health. Workers were concerned about their health because if they were not healthy, their economic security was threatened. The employer wanted a healthy worker because an unhealthy one threatened the economic stability of the workplace. A major point of difference between employers and workers was what happened when an employee died or became ill, injured or disabled due to work-related conditions. At the time it had to be proven that the employer was negligent before the worker could receive financial compensation for medical care or lost wages. When compensation was granted to workers it was usually minimal.

Selected Legislation and Events in Occupational Health in the United States—1936 to Present

◀   ▶

1936   *Walsh-Healy Act* sets occupational safety and health standards and minimum age limitations for workers employed in government contract work.

1938   *Fair Labor Standards Act* sets a minimum age for child labor: 16 years old for general work and 18 years old for hazardous work, applicable to most industrial settings. Also establishes maximum hours and minimum wages for interstate commerce workers.

1939   American Industrial Hygiene Association established.

1941   *Federal Mine Inspection Act* passes, helping to ensure greater safety in the mining industry.

1946   American Academy of Occupational Medicine established. It merges with the American Occupational Medicine Association to form the American Academy of Occupational and Environmental Medicine in 1988.

1948   All states have enacted *Workers' Compensation* acts.

1952   *Coal Mine Safety Act* is passed, ensuring greater coal mine safety.

1966   *Mine Safety Act* is passed, requiring mandatory inspections and health and safety standards.

1969   *Coal Mine Health and Safety Act* is passed, setting mandatory health and safety standards for underground mines.

1970   *Occupational Safety and Health Act of 1970* is passed. It is the most significant piece of occupational safety and health legislation in the U.S., establishing the Occupational Safety and Health Administration (OSHA) and the National Institute of Occupational Safety and Health (NIOSH).

1972   *Black Lung Benefits Act* provides benefits to black lung victims.

1977   *Federal Mine Safety and Health Act* is passed, consolidating all existing mine legislation into one act.

1979   *Healthy People* is published by the U.S. Public Health Service, establishing occupational health as a national health priority area, and national health objectives are developed for occupational safety.

1990   The *Americans with Disabilities Act* is passed, safeguarding the rights of the disabled worker.

1991   *Healthy People 2000* is published by the U.S. Public Health Service, continuing occupational health as a national health priority area.

1993   *Family Leave Act* provides protection from loss of employment when time is needed by an employee to care for ill children, spouse, parent or the employee's own illness—employees are entitled to up to 12 weeks unpaid leave during the year.

In the early 1900s workers began to take a firm stand on the right to be compensated for job-related illness, injury, or disability, and state workers' compensation legislation began to develop. The first workers' compensation acts met with much resistance from employers and many were ruled to be unconstitutional. In 1911 New Jersey passed the first workers' compensation act to be upheld by the courts. Other states quickly followed, with nine more acts in 1911; 11 in 1912; and 11 in 1913 (USDL, 1977, p. 77). This legislation signaled the development of industrial health services in the workplace (Haag and Glazner, 1992, p. 56). However, the primary function of these services was often to provide emergency care for on-the-job illness and injury.

This period saw much happening in occupational health. Cornell University Medical College established an occupational disease clinic in 1910, and others soon opened around the country (Felton, 1976,

p. 814). The U.S. Department of Labor was elevated to a cabinet-level position in 1913. The Office of Industrial Hygiene and Sanitation in the U.S. Public Health Service, and the Industrial Hygiene Section of the American Public Health Association were both established in 1914 (Felton, p. 812). In 1916 the American Association of Industrial Physicians and Surgeons (AAIPS) was organized in Detroit, Michigan (Felton, p. 813).

Almost 25 years after workers' compensation began to be legislated, the *Social Security Act of 1935* helped to provide for worker economic security through programs such as unemployment insurance. The act also made available funds that helped to enable the creation of divisions of industrial hygiene in several states and local health departments in industrial areas (McGrath, 1945, p. 123). Significant legislation and events in occupational health in the United States since 1935 are given in the box above.

◀ *Occupational Safety and Health:* Healthy People 2000 *Objectives* ▶

Health Status Objectives

1. Reduce deaths from work-related injuries to no more than 4 per 100,000 full-time workers.
2. Reduce work-related injuries resulting in medical treatment, lost time from work, or restricted work activity to no more than 6 cases per 100 full-time workers.
3. Reduce cumulative trauma disorders to an incidence of no more than 60 cases per 100,000 full-time workers.
4. Reduce occupational skin disorders or diseases to an incidence of no more than 55 per 100,000 full-time workers.
5. Reduce hepatitis B infections among occupational exposed workers to an incidence of no more than 1,250 cases.

Risk Reduction Objectives

6. Increase to at least 75 percent the proportion of worksites with 50 or more employees that mandate employee use of occupant protection systems, such as seatbelts, during all work-related motor vehicle travel.
7. Reduce to no more than 15 percent the proportion of workers exposed to average daily noise levels that exceed 85 dBA.
8. Eliminate exposures which result in workers having blood lead concentrations greater than 25 ug/dL of whole blood.

9. Increase hepatitis B immunization levels to 90 percent among occupationally exposed workers.

Services and Protection Objectives

10. Implement occupational safety and health plans in 50 states for the identification, management, and prevention of leading work-related diseases and injuries within the State.
11. Establish in 50 States exposure standards adequate to prevent the major occupational lung diseases to which their worker populations are exposed (Byssinosis, asbestosis, coal workers' pneumoconiosis, and silicosis).
12. Increase to at least 70 percent the proportion of worksites with 50 or more employees that have implemented programs on worker health and safety.
13. Increase to at least 50 percent the proportion of worksites with 50 or more employees that offer back injury prevention and rehabilitation programs.
14. Establish in 50 States either public health or labor department programs that provide consultation and assistance to small businesses to implement safety and health programs for their employees.
15. Increase to at least 75 percent the proportion of primary care providers who routinely elicit occupational health exposures as a part of patient history and provide relevant counseling.

From USDHHS *Healthy people 2000: health promotion and disease prevention objectives for the nation, full report, with commentary,* Washington, D.C., 1991, U.S. Government Printing Office, pp. 298-308.

OCCUPATIONAL HEALTH AND THE *HEALTHY PEOPLE 2000* OBJECTIVES FOR THE NATION

Healthy People 2000: Health Promotion and Disease Prevention Objectives for the Nation (1991) is the latest in a series of "Healthy People" documents (refer to Chapter 5). Occupational health is a priority area in *Healthy People 2000,* and the occupational health objectives of this document are listed in the box above. These national objectives address the areas of improving health status, reducing risk factors and improving services/protection, and targeting reduction of work-related death, injuries, cumulative trauma disorders, back injury, skin disorders, lead poisoning, lung disease, hearing loss, and communicable diseases. One objective, "to implement state occupational safety and health plans for the identification, management, and prevention of leading work-related diseases and injuries in all 50 states," was an especially aggressive undertaking since only 10 states had such programs in 1990 (A Public Health Service, 1992). However, by 1992, 32 states had such plans in place (A Public Health Service).

To date, progress on achieving national occupational health objectives is mixed. Progress has been reported on reducing work-related injury deaths; however, increases have occurred in the incidence of nonfatal work-related injuries (notably among nurses and personal care workers), cumulative trauma disorders such as carpal tunnel syndrome, occupational skin disorders, and hepatitis B infections among occupationally exposed workers (A Public Health Service, 1992). Accomplishment of these objectives will be facilitated by the implementation of occupational safety and health education; occupational safety and health activities by state public health or labor departments; and increasing the number of primary care providers, such as nurses, who routinely elicit occupational health histories and provide appropriate follow-up.

OCCUPATIONAL HEALTH LEGISLATION IN THE UNITED STATES

The box on p. 668 presents an overview of significant legislation and events in occupational health in the United States over the last 60 years. In comparison with other industrial nations, the United States was slow to enact occupational safety and health legislation. By 1884 Germany had already enacted a law that provided for a comprehensive system of occupational health, including compensation for occupational illness, injury, or disability irrespective of who was responsible for the occurrence of the condition (McCall, 1977, p. 21).

For years occupational health nurses, occupational physicians, and countless workers stressed the hazards in the American workplace. In 1968 the Surgeon General, Dr. William Steward, told Congress that U.S. Public Health Service studies showed that 65% of industrial workers were exposed to toxic or harmful substances or conditions in their place of employment (Stellman and Daum, 1973, pp. xiii-xiv). The same year an occupational health law was defeated by Congress.

Many Americans thought that legislation in the workplace would endanger the free enterprise system. However, with the support of workers and labor unions, the Occupational Safety and Health Act of 1970 was passed, making the United States the last major industrial nation to enact such legislation. The Occupational Safety and Health Act of 1970 is the most significant piece of occupational safety and health legislation in the United States (Babbitz, 1992, p. 12).

Occupational Safety and Health Act of 1970

The Occupational Safety and Health Act of 1970 (Public Law 91-596) made the health of workers a public concern and made a national commitment to maintaining worker health and preventing work-related disease, disability, and death. At the time the law was passed more than 14,000 American workers were being killed at the workplace each year, over 2 million suffered disabling injuries, and millions more were dying from job-related illnesses and conditions (Bingham, 1992, p. 1325).

Intents and Mandates of the Act

The intents of this act were to (1) prevent placing toxic substances in the workplace, (2) regulate exposure to toxic and dangerous substances already in the workplace, and (3) compensate workers for occupational illness and injury. To carry out these intents, the act had specific mandates:

1. Formation of the:
   a. *Occupational Safety and Health Administration (OSHA).* Sets and enforces standards for occupational safety and health. Under the jurisdiction of the Department of Labor.
   b. *National Institute for Occupational Safety and Health (NIOSH).* Researches and recommends occupational safety and health standards to OSHA and carries out training programs. Under the jurisdiction of the Department of Health and Human Services, the Centers for Disease Control and Prevention offers a toll-free number for public information (1-800-35-NIOSH).
   c. *Occupational Safety and Health Review Commission.* A quasijudicial agency charged with ruling on cases forwarded to it by the Department of Labor when disagreements arise over the results of safety and health inspections performed by the Department's Occupational Safety and Health Administration. Review of a commission decision can be obtained in the U.S. Court of Appeals.
   d. *National Advisory Council on Occupational Safety and Health.* A consumer and professional council to make occupational safety and health recommendations to OSHA and NIOSH.
   e. *National Commission on State Workers' Compensation Laws.* A temporary evaluative commission to study and make recommendations on the adequacy of state workers' compensation laws to the President. *Official termination date: October 30, 1972.*
2. Establishment of federal occupational safety and health standards.

3. Imposition of fines and sentences for violation of federal occupational safety and health regulations.

The act also requires employers to keep records of work-related deaths, injuries, and illnesses for OSHA review. Under the act, states can develop their own occupational safety and health administrations as long as the state standards meet or exceed the federal standards.

Some Problems with the Act

There have been a number of problems with the act, including the following areas:

Funding. Funding for the act has been grossly inadequate, and has affected the ability of OSHA to carry out its intents and mandates. According to the *Budget of the United States, Fiscal Year 1994, Appendix,* estimated funding is set at approximately $294 million for OSHA with an additional $68 million available in grants to states for the cost of their OSHA programs, and $112 million to NIOSH. This amounts to less than $2 per citizen per year in federal occupational safety and health spending.

Coordination of Services. OSHA and NIOSH are under the jurisdiction of two different federal departments. OSHA is under the Department of Labor and NIOSH is under the Department of Health and Human Services, and their resources and services have not always been well coordinated. NIOSH researches occupational safety and health standards and OSHA has the authority to set and enforce them. Interagency problems have also existed. Until recently, OSHA records were kept by the Bureau of Labor Statistics in the Department of Labor; now OSHA has its own office of Recordkeeping and Data Analysis (McNeely, 1992, p. 21).

Fines and Sentences. Extremely low fines and sentences were set by the original provisions of the act. Even though recent increases have been made, they may still not serve as incentives to employers to improve working conditions. OSHA can now levy fines for each willful or repeated violation of the act up to $70,000 (increased from $10,000) and $7,000 for serious violations of the act (increased from $1,000) (McNeely, 1992, p. 21). Fines can be discounted in negotiations between OSHA and the company (McNeely, p. 21).

Economic Impact Statements. Economic impact statements became policy in 1975. They are an occupational cost analysis study of a proposed OSHA standard or regulation. If a company can show that it would not be economically feasible to comply with a standard or regulation, it can appeal the proposed regulation.

Scope of the Problem. There are hundreds of thousands of workplaces covered under the act. Added to this is the fact that there are more than 80,000 chemicals in the workplace (Greaves, 1992, p. 1333), and thousands of these chemicals are considered to be toxic or carcinogens. The immensity of problems such as work-related injuries, illness, disability, and death add to the scope. A look at the 10 leading causes of work-related illness later in this chapter helps to illustrate the enormity of the problem.

Legal Challenges. In the first year of the act approximately 100 bills were introduced in Congress to amend or repeal it (McNeely, 1992, p. 19). Almost every occupational health standard established by OSHA has been challenged in the courts, leading to costly and time-consuming delays in establishing standards (McNeely, p. 19). Legal arguments challenging the right of OSHA to set and enforce occupational safety and health standards continue.

Lack of Trained Personnel. There are severe shortages of occupational health nurses and other occupational health professionals. NIOSH Educational Resource Centers are making strides to train and educate professionals in the field. The American Public Health Association (APHA) and The American Association of Occupational Health Nurses (AAOHN) advocate educational programs that prepare health professionals in occupational health and safety. With its present workforce, OSHA can inspect only about 2% of the nation's workplaces in any given year (McNeely, 1992, p. 20). It has been noted that there are more park rangers than OSHA inspectors, and that typical workplaces will see an inspector once every 77 years—about as often as we see Halley's Comet! (McNeely, p. 20)

Rule-Making Process. The rule-making process of OSHA is cumbersome and time-consuming. In its first 13 years OSHA issued only 11 new or revised health standards, one standard on exposure to noise, and 26 new or revised safety standards (Office of Technology Assessment, 1985, p. 22). In the OSHA rule-making process there must be public hearings held on proposed OSHA standards, with the burden of proof for justification of the standard resting on OSHA. Before these hearings advance notice of the proposed standard must be given and a pre-hearing public comment period provided. After the hearing there is a post-hearing public comment period before final rule is posted.

The Occupational Safety and Health Act and the Occupational Health Nurse

The provisions of the Occupational Safety and Health Act of 1970 affect occupational health nursing practice. The nurse needs to have a knowledge of the standards established under the act and make certain that the workplace is in compliance with the act's rules and regulations. The nurse will often participate in OSHA on-site visits to the workplace and assist workers in understanding their rights under the act. The nurse uses NIOSH educational materials and training programs.

OCCUPATIONAL HEALTH NURSING IN THE UNITED STATES

In her classic text *Occupational Health Nursing,* Mary Louise Brown defined occupational health nursing as "The application of nursing and public health procedures for the purpose of conserving, promoting and restoring the health of individuals and groups through their places of employment" (Brown, 1956, p. 15). Today's occupational health nurses continue to practice these concepts and principles, as well as others that have evolved over time.

It should be noted that occupational health nurses originally were called *industrial nurses.* As the scope of the practice broadened the title was changed. The box on p. 673 gives a chronological overview of occupational health nursing in the United States. The evolution of occupational health nursing closely follows advances in public health and occupational health and its history is interesting. In 1895 the woman considered by many to be the first occupational health nurse in the United States, Ada Mayo Stewart, was hired by the Vermont Marble Company. Much has been written about Miss Stewart. Her sister Harriet, also a nurse,

worked with her during the first year of her practice (Parker-Conrad, p. 156).

The Vermont Marble Company was ahead of its time. It provided worker benefits such as housing, a library, profit-sharing, general accident insurance, and a company store (Felton, 1988; Pinkham, 1988, p. 20). When the company decided to offer nursing services Ada Mayo Stewart was an outstanding candidate for the job. She had studied the classics, history, mathematics, English, and Latin, and had graduated from Waltham Training School for Nurses where she had received training in "district nursing" (refer to Chapter 1) (Pinkham, p. 20).

Miss Stewart was employed as a visiting nurse who gave care in the home to sick company employees and family members, and went into the schools to teach health practices to the children of employees. She often traveled through town on bicycle and "conversed" in a form of sign language with many non–English speaking residents (Markolf, 1945, p. 127). In addition to her other nursing responsibilities she learned about the health care customs of the native countries of the people she cared for, and taught health education in the schools (Markolf, pp. 127-128), making her an early practitioner of both transcultural and school nursing. The March 1945 issue of *Public Health Nursing* celebrated the 50th anniversary of Miss Stewart's work. For that issue Miss Stewart, now Ada Markolf, wrote an article entitled "Industrial Nursing Begins in Vermont." This interesting article was written in third person, as she told the story of the "first" occupational health nursing experience in the United States (Brown, 1988, p. 434).

In the early part of the twentieth century many significant events occurred in occupational health nursing. At this time retail stores, cotton mills, and the mining industry began to have programs staffed by nurses (Gardner, 1916, p. 301; Waters, 1919, p. 728; McGrath, 1946, Felton, 1976, p. 814). Florence S. Wright wrote the first book on industrial nursing in 1919. In 1920 the National Organization for Public Health Nursing established an Industrial Nursing Section that defined industrial health nursing (Brown, 1988, p. 435; Pravikoff, 1992, p. 532). The National Organization for Public Health Nursing later became the National League for Nursing.

In 1942 the American Association of Industrial Nurses (AAIN) was founded with Catherine Dempsey as the first president. The new association published the journal *Industrial Nursing.* At its foundation the AAIN had annual membership dues of 50 cents

An Overview of Occupational Health Nursing in the United States

1895 Ada Mayo Stewart (Markolf) is hired by the Vermont Marble Company.

1897 Anna B. Duncan is hired by the Benefit Association of John Wanamaker Company (New York).

1913 First registry for industrial nurses originates in Boston.

1915 Boston Industrial Nurses' Club organized.

1916 Factory Nurses' Conference organized (forerunner of the American Association of Industrial Nurses).

1917 First training course to educate occupational health nurses: *Industrial Service for Nurses,* offered at Boston College.

1919 Florence S. Wright writes *Industrial Nursing.*

1920 The National Organization for Public Health Nursing (NOPHN) establishes an Industrial Nursing section.

1942 American Association of Industrial Nurses is founded (becomes the American Association of Occupational Health Nurses in 1977).

1945 *Industrial Nursing* journal begins publication (1945-1949).

1946 Bertha McGrath writes a manual on industrial nursing, *Nursing in Industry,* in collaboration with the National Organization for Public Health Nursing.

1953 *American Association of Industrial Nurses Journal* established (Changing to *Occupational Health Nursing* in 1969 and *AAOHN Journal* in 1986).

1956 Mary Louise Brown writes the classic book *Occupational Health Nursing.*

1970 *Occupational Safety and Health Act of 1970* passes, having numerous implications for occupational health nursing practice.

1971 American Board of Occupational Health Nurses (ABOHN) formed to establish certification standards and examinations; first examination given in 1974.

1979 *Healthy People* establishes occupational health as a national health priority area, and national health objectives are developed for occupational safety.

1981 American Association of Occupational Health Nurses (AAOHN) establishes a research committee.

1982 First research session held at the annual AAOHN Conference.

1990 AAOHN established priority research areas in occupational health nursing (refer to box on p. 681).

1991 *Healthy People 2000* continues occupational health as a national health priority area.

1994 Dr. Bonnie Rogers writes *Occupational Health Nursing.*

(Parker-Conrad, 1988, p. 158), and its membership numbered approximately 300 nurses from 16 states (Martin, 1977, p. 10). On January 1, 1977, the AAIN changed its name to the American Association of Occupational Health Nurses (AAOHN). Today AAOHN has chapters in every state and a membership of more than 12,500 nurses.

American Association of Occupational Health Nurses

The AAOHN is a professional association for registered nurses involved in occupational health. It works in close cooperation with the American Nurses Association (ANA), its membership, and the 23,000 occupational health nurses that are practicing in the United States.

The mission of AAOHN is to promote occupational health nursing, maintain professional integrity, and enhance its professional status (AAOHN, 1989, A commitment). AAOHN has divisions of professional affairs, governmental affairs, public affairs, and membership. The association establishes standards of occupational health nursing practice, assists nurses in providing quality care, and serves as an advocate for occupational health and occupational health nursing (AAOHN, A commitment).

AAOHN is actively involved in occupational health legislation and reform (Babbitz, 1992, p. 14), and assisted in developing the *Healthy People 2000* occupational health objectives. The association was instrumental in having occupational health nurses placed on the staff of OSHA in 1988 (Barlow, 1992, p. 465; Haag and Glazner, 1992, p. 59). The *AAOHN Journal* is published by the association. This outstanding journal regularly publishes clinical articles, research studies, and continuing education units. For further information on the association contact the American Association of Occupational Health Nurses at 50 Lenox Pointe, Atlanta, Georgia 30324 (404-262-1162).

Occupational Health Nursing Education

Occupational health nursing integrates public health and nursing theory, with an emphasis on community health nursing. In the United States integration of occupational health nursing theory and concepts into undergraduate nursing education has been very limited. Historically, short courses were a primary form of instruction in occupational health nursing (Rogers, 1991, p. 101). One of the first such courses was offered by Boston University College of Business Administration in 1917 (Barlow, 1992, p. 464; Parker-Conrad, 1988, p. 159). It consisted of 10 lectures per week for 16 weeks, a 2-week practicum, and assistance with job placement (Parker-Conrad, p. 159). Early course content frequently focused on industrial injuries and medical problems common to the worksite (Barlow, p. 464; Rogers, p. 101).

Discussions on integrating occupational health nursing content into baccalaureate curricula have been under way for almost 50 years. In 1945 the National Organization for Public Health Nursing and the American Association of Industrial Nurses took a position that *specific* courses in industrial nursing should not be a part of the undergraduate nursing program, and *specialty education* was recommended at the graduate level (AAIN, 1976; Olson and Kochevar, 1989, p. 33). However, these organizations recommended that schools of nursing place more emphasis on examining industrial influences on the health of workers and their families, and advised *integration* of this content throughout the student's educational program (Markolf, 1945, p. 129). In a study done by Rogers (1991) of baccalaureate schools of nursing in the United States, 58% of the responding schools indicated they had integrated curricular content on worker health and 47% had integrated content on basic occupational health nursing services. In an AAOHN membership survey 90% of the respondents believed that the association should encourage implementation of occupational health nursing content in undergraduate nursing curricula (Rogers, 1991, p. 102). The USDHHS has recommended that the professional education of all primary health care providers should include appropriate instruction in occupational safety and health (USDHHS, 1991, Healthy people, p. 297).

The purpose of integrating occupational health content in baccalaureate programs is not to prepare occupational health nurses at the undergraduate level, but to prepare nurses to have an understanding of the relationship between work and health and to be able to practice in a variety of health care settings. This content helps the nurse to function more safely and effectively in the work environment. Graduate education in the specialty area of occupational health nursing is available in several universities across the country.

Graduate Education

The National Institute for Occupational Safety and Health Educational Resource Centers (NIOSH ERCs) offer graduate and continuing education in occupational health and safety for health professionals. They operate under federal grants, and student stipends are often available.

Currently there are 14 such centers at major universities across the nation (a list of these centers can be obtained by contacting NIOSH at 513-533-8225). All of these ERCs have a nursing component and four offer doctoral education in nursing (Pravikoff, 1992, p. 533). Graduate education in occupational health nursing, especially on the doctoral level, is in its infancy.

Many occupational health nurses cannot take advantage of graduate education because they are not prepared at the baccalaureate level. A study by Lusk, Disch, and Barkauskas (1988) showed that approximately 65% of the respondents were prepared at the associate degree or diploma level, 13% had a baccalaureate degree in nursing, 17% had a baccalaureate degree in another field, and 2% had a master's degree in nursing. A significant role of an OHN leader at the worksite is to help nursing staff to advance their practice through education.

Qualifications of the Occupational Health Nurse

AAOHN supports the baccalaureate degree in nursing as basic preparation for entry into occupational health nursing practice (AAOHN, 1986). In addition, coursework in occupational health nursing theory and practice, health care administration, epidemiology, toxicology, safety, environmental health, health education, rehabilitation, industrial health, ergonomics, and business psychology is recommended (Babbitz

> ◀ *Staffing Recommendations for an Effective Occupational Health Nursing Program* ▶
>
> - One occupational health nurse for up to 300 employees in an industrial setting and up to 750 in a nonindustrial setting
> - Two or more occupational health nurses for up to 600 industrial employees
> - Three or more occupational health nurses for up to 1,000 employees in an industrial setting
>
> - One occupational health nurse for each additional 1,000 employees in either setting
> NOTE: Larger and more hazardous occupational settings require more nursing personnel. Smaller organizations can implement an effective program with part-time nursing services.

From American Association for Occupational Health Nurses: *Occupational health nursing: the answer to health care cost containment,* Atlanta, Ga., 1991, The Association.

and Bodnar, 1989). Knowledge of individual and group skills is also beneficial.

AAOHN recommends a minimum of 2 years of professional nursing experience in a primary care setting, such as community health, ambulatory care, emergency, or critical care units before entering occupational health nursing practice (AAOHN, 1986). Additional experience in areas such as mental health, rehabilitation, and medical-surgical nursing is desirable.

Certification of the Occupational Health Nurse

Certification for occupational health nurses (OHNs) has been available since 1974. It involves a combination of work experience, coursework, and written examination. Areas involved in certification testing include knowledge of toxicology, treating chemical exposures, ergonomics, the Occupational Safety and Health Act and workers' compensation legislation, and competence in physical assessment (Maciag, 1993, p. 39). In 1996 a baccalaureate degree will be required for OHN certification (Maciag, p. 39).

Standards of Practice

Standards of practice are a baseline against which nursing actions can be measured. AAOHN (1988, Standards) has developed standards for occupational health nursing practice. These standards address policy, personnel, resources, nursing practice, and evaluation, and can be obtained through AAOHN. They are periodically revised to reflect the changing scope and essence of practice (AAOHN, Standards).

Objectives of Occupational Health Nursing

Primary objectives for the occupational health nurse are to:

1. Protect the worker from occupational safety and health hazards
2. Promote a safe and healthful workplace
3. Facilitate efforts of workers and workers' families to meet their health and welfare needs
4. Promote education and research in the field

Occupational safety and health is an interdisciplinary team effort, and the nurse must work cooperatively with the worker, his or her family, and the community to accomplish occupational safety and health objectives. The nurse realizes that successful fulfillment of these objectives will promote high-level wellness, enhance quality of life, increase job productivity, and produce a safer work environment.

The number of nurses required to implement these objectives is determined by the size of the company, the type of workplace, the number of employees, employee health status, and actual, as well as potential, health and safety problems (AAOHN, 1991, Occupational health nursing). Close to two thirds of all occupational health nurses work alone, often without direct medical supervision. This high level of autonomy and independence makes this specialty area of nursing distinctly different from many other areas of nursing practice. Staffing recommendations for an effective occupational nursing program are given in the box above. If these minimal staffing recommendations are not met it can be extremely difficult to implement nursing roles and responsibilities. To accomplish these objectives the occupational health nurse carries out specific functions. These functions are broad, comprehensive, and complex.

◄   *The Five Most Frequently Selected Current and Future Activities*   ►

Current

1. Care of illness and emergencies

2. Counsel on health risks
3. Follow up workers' compensation claims

4. Perform periodic health assessments

5. Evaluate return to work

Future

1. Analyze trends in health promotion, risk reduction and expenditures
2. Develop special health programs
3. Recommend more efficient and cost-effective operation
4. Conduct research to determine cost-effective alternatives
5. Meet with other health disciplines to solve problems

From Lusk SL: Corporate expectations for occupational health nurses' activities, *AAOHN* 38(8):373, 1990. Reprinted by permission of the American Association of Occupational Health Nurses, *AAOHN,* Volume 38, Issue 8.

Functions of the Occupational Health Nurse

The functions of the occupational health nurse are oriented heavily toward prevention, protection, and health promotion (Barlow, 1992, p. 464). These functions focus on keeping the worker healthy. Occupational health nursing functions can be classified into the categories of administration and management, environmental surveillance, direct nursing care, health education, counseling, and research.

Confidentiality and ethics play an important role in all occupational health nursing functions. The AAOHN (AAOHN, 1991, Code) has published a *Code of Ethics* for occupational health nurses to help guide them in this important area of nursing practice. Ethical issues confronting the occupational health nurse include such things as informed consent, confidentiality of health care records, resource allocation, drug testing in the workplace, right-to-know issues, and concerns related to AIDS. The AAOHN code of ethics stresses the need to protect and promote the health and safety of the worker while at the same time safeguarding the worker's rights.

The confidential treatment of health information and records and the worker's right to privacy are considered professional obligations of the occupational health nurse. To protect employees from unauthorized or indiscriminate access to health information, it is recommended that written policies and procedures be developed on record access; that educational activities be carried out to let employees, employers, and other health care providers know about policies in regard to record access; and that legal counsel be sought by the nurse in instances of unclear or questionable practice situations (AAOHN, 1988, Confidentiality).

The following describes the specific roles and activities of the occupational health nurse. It should be noted that many of these roles and responsibilities overlap, and that the nurse's functions reflect emphasis on primary prevention.

Administration and Management

In performing these functions OHNs are involved in many activities ranging from health promotion to rehabilitation. Research by Lusk (1990) examined corporate expectations for the occupational health nurses' activities. Lusk noted that expansion of the occupational health nurse's role was expected and that many of the desired future activities selected by management were related to cost-containment activities. The most frequently selected current and future occupational health nursing activities, as reported in this study, are given in the box above. The operation of the occupational health service at the workplace is a major part of the nurse's administrative and management function and involves numerous activities. A major purpose of an occupational health service is to optimize the health of the worker through preventive and curative services within a framework of caring (Rogers, Winslow, and Higgins, 1993, p. 59).

Administration and management functions include managing the occupational health service, keeping an up-to-date occupational health nursing policy and procedure manual, training and supervision of auxiliary health personnel, cooperation with federal and state occupational health regulatory bodies, maintenance of occupational health records, student supervision, community resource collaboration, and quality assurance activities. Publications are available from

AAOHN to assist the nurse in establishing an occupational health service.

Recordkeeping is an important administrative function. Just as she or he does in the hospital setting, the nurse has both legal and professional responsibilities to keep accurate, comprehensive, up-to-date written records (Ossler, 1988, p. 8). Laws regulating medical documentation exist and the nurse must adhere to them.

Occupational health nursing records must conform to company policy, OSHA regulations, and nursing standards. Records should note all employee contacts with the health service, beginning with the preemployment physical and interview. They should include the reason for the visit, nursing plans of care, results of screening procedures, periodic health appraisals, health risk assessments, rehabilitation activities, community referrals, and worksite educational programs in which the worker has participated. *These records are confidential.*

Student supervision/education is a significant administrative responsibility. The nurse is involved in the educational programs of nursing students and may be involved in the educational programs of other disciplines, such as occupational safety and health, social work, vocational rehabilitation, toxicology, public health, and audiology. The occupational health nurse also helps to supervise physicians involved in occupational medicine residency programs (Bertsche, Sanborn, and Jones, 1989).

One "uncharted" educational area that occupational health nurses can develop is that of educating school children about occupational safety and health. Such education can encourage future workers to be informed about occupational health and serve as a recruitment tool through which children become interested in occupational health and occupational health nursing. Comprehensive school health education curricula that incorporate concepts of occupational health were recommended a decade ago in the document *Promoting Health, Preventing Disease: Objectives for the Nation* (USDHHS, 1980, p. 42). To date, little progress has been made in this endeavor.

Community resource collaboration is crucial to providing comprehensive care to workers and their families. Developing collaborative networks with community resources is an important administrative function. The nurse needs to be knowledgeable about community resources in order to use them effectively (refer to Chapter 10). Resources of particular interest to the occupational health nurse include state and local health departments, vocational rehabilitation agencies, counseling services for problems such as alcoholism, drug abuse, and domestic violence, and voluntary organizations such as the American Heart Association, American Lung Association, American Diabetic Association, and American Cancer Society.

Quality assurance and accountability is an essential administrative activity. Chapter 23 presents concepts of quality assurance that can be applied in all aspects of community health nursing practice. Figure 17-1 presents interacting elements in accountability and quality care in occupational health nursing. It illustrates the importance of research, theory, and education working together to define the scope of nursing practice. It also depicts the significance of using the nursing process and legal mandates to guide practice. Standards of practice assist the OHN in providing quality nursing care and in assuring accountability for nursing functions (Randolph, 1988, p. 167).

Quality assurance activities include such activities as peer review, self-evaluation and audit, and overall program evaluation (refer to Chapter 23). Part of the quality improvement process is anticipating problems before the delivery of care (Widtfeldt, 1992, p. 329). However, if a quality improvement program is not in place, there is no reason such a program cannot be developed for the occupational health service (Widtfeldt, p. 328). One measure of quality of care is employee satisfaction with the services (Rogers, Winslow, and Higgins, 1993, p. 64). Research has indicated that employees are generally satisfied with the occupational health nursing services (Rogers, Winslow, and Higgins, p. 61).

As nurses implement quality assurance activities, they will often find themselves advocating for more comprehensive occupational health services. Chapters 13 and 24 discuss this function and the process of establishing health services in a variety of settings. Chapter 23 expands on how to address issues of quality in community health nursing practice.

Environmental Surveillance

The nurse continuously surveys the work environment for health hazards and works to establish cause and effect relationships between workplace hazards and occupational health conditions. These surveillance activities are implemented with other members of the occupational health team: members of management, occupational safety personnel, industrial hy-

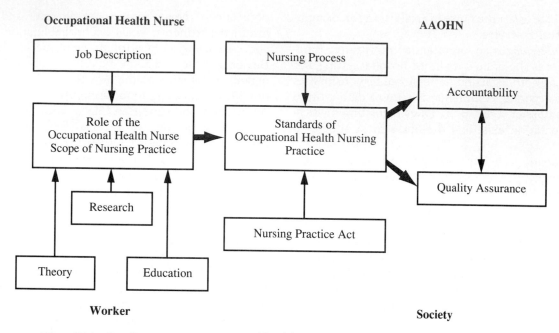

Figure 17-1   Quality care in occupational health nursing. (From Randolph SA: Occupational health nursing: a commitment to excellence, *AAOHN J* 36:166, 1988.)

gienists, and physicians. Surveillance activities may sometimes be carried out in conjunction with OSHA visits and inspections at the workplace.

Environmental surveillance involves evaluating in which area of the workplace illness or injury occurs or is likely to occur, what kinds of illness or injuries occur, the timing of incidents (e.g., frequency and intervals), and the possible etiology. Potential stressors, hazardous equipment, and known and suspected irritants should be routinely and regularly recorded and monitored. An example of this process is illustrated in the following situation.

▶ An occupational health nurse suspected that one area of the plant in which she worked had a higher-than-average noise area. After obtaining permission from the plant management to do periodic audiometric testing on the workers in this area in combination with testing on a control group, she began to collect data to confirm her hypothesis. Employees in both areas were tested every 6 months. Over a period of time the nurse was able to show that the workers in this one area had increasingly abnormal audiograms and that the control group had consistently normal ones. The workers themselves had not noticed any change in hearing, but the audiograms told a different story. As a result of the study corrective measures were taken. In this example, the nurse's actions assisted in facilitating the health of the workers.

Appendix 17-1 represents an assessment guide that assists occupational health nurses in systematically completing an environmental survey. Environmental surveillance is essential for an accurate diagnosis of safety and health problems in the workplace and is an important primary prevention activity. Occupational health nurses apply the principles of epidemiology and community assessment when implementing surveillance activities at the worksite (refer to Chapters 11 and 12).

Direct Nursing Care

The direct nursing care given by the occupational health nurse ranges from assessment to rehabilitation. The direct nursing care activities of the OHN include, but are not limited to, physical assessment and screening, rehabilitation, communicable disease control, emergency care, treatment of nonoccupational injuries and illnesses, and treatment of acute and chronic conditions. The nurse will use many health education strategies and community resources in these endeavors.

Occupational health disorders can be life-changing in magnitude. It is estimated that as many as 100,000 deaths occur each year as a direct result of occupational disease and illness (USDHHS, 1986, p. 109). An incalculable number of diseases and illnesses occur as well. Each year more than 10 million traumatic injuries occur on the job, with over 3 million of these being classified as severe (USDHHS, 1991, Healthy people, pp. 296, 299). Although fatal occupational injuries have gradually declined, injuries resulting in permanent disabilities are increasing. More than 1.8 million occupational injuries result in permanent disabilities each year in the United States (USDHHS, Healthy people, pp. 296, 299).

The nurse is in an excellent position to promote health in the workplace. Workers often comply with nursing plans of care and view the nurse as someone who is concerned about them. The direct nursing care functions of the occupational health nurse are diverse and demand a high level of nursing skill, professional flexibility, and independence. To carry out these functions, the nurse must be able to assess both the worker and the workplace.

Physical assessment and screening procedures are done on a regular basis. The nurse needs to be skilled in physical assessment of the well adult, and often does employment and return-to-work physicals. The nurse does selected screening procedures on an ongoing basis during the employee's term of employment. These screening measures involve periodic blood pressure measurement, urinalysis, hematocrit and hemoglobin testing, audiometrics, electrocardiograms, vision screening, and pulmonary function analysis. Such screening measures are important because they provide baseline and subsequent data for the study of occupational injury and illness and contribute to a comprehensive health history. Many worksites offer special training to enable the occupational health nurse to implement such screening activities (e.g., audiometrics and pulmonary function). The nurse frequently conducts health risk appraisals (refer to Chapter 9). These appraisals help nurses to identify major health risks in the aggregate being served, counsel workers about potential health problems, and assist in establishing sound worker educational programs. For example, when analyzing the results of health risk data the nurse may find that over 70% of the workers smoke. The nurse may explore the possibility of providing a "Smokebusters Program" to reduce the incidence and prevalence of smoking in this at-risk aggregate and to help prevent heart disease and cancer.

Rehabilitation services are another direct nursing care function. The nurse will often be involved in developing and implementing employee rehabilitation plans and activities. Rehabilitation activities should begin as soon as possible, and many of these activities will be carried out in the workplace. Rehabilitation planning should incorporate the worker and his or her family in addition to other occupational health personnel and community resources. Following rehabilitation, the nurse may be involved in assessing and facilitating the employee's ability to return to work. Other components of the nurses role in rehabilitation are discussed in Chapter 18.

Communicable disease control is becoming a more prominent concern for the OHN. Numerous communicable diseases exist in the workplace, including influenza, the common cold, hepatitis B, and AIDS. The nurse treats and attempts to prevent these diseases. Statistics show that more than 15 million work days are lost each year due to influenza alone (Murphy, 1989). Approximately 300,000 new cases of hepatitis B are reported each year. It is estimated that as many as 80% of American adults are not fully immunized. The workplace can serve as a setting to maintain appropriate immunization schedules (Murphy). Permanent immunization records on employees need to be kept and updated. The occupational health nurse uses the epidemiological process described in Chapter 11 to prevent and control communicable disease at the worksite.

Emergency care is probably the most dramatic of the occupational health nurse's direct care functions. The nurse must be skilled in cardiopulmonary resuscitation, first aid, and emergency care techniques. The nurse is often the first health professional in the workplace to have contact with the ill or injured worker, and often has to make a decision and take action immediately.

Nonoccupational illness and injuries are also part of the nurse's direct care function. Although these are incurred outside the workplace, they have an effect on work and the work setting. The occupational health nurse will treat these conditions initially and will refer the client as necessary to community agencies.

Among the nonoccupational conditions the nurse should be aware of are alcoholism and drug abuse. If an employee comes to work under the influence of drugs and/or alcohol and the employer allows the individual to remain, workers' compensation laws in many states would rule in favor of the worker in the event of occupational injury. For the safety of the worker, and to protect the employer from liability, employees who are unfit to work should not be permitted at the worksite. In some cases the worker's supervisor will make the decision regarding fitness for work, and in other cases the nurse will. The challenge for the occupational health nurse is to influence management to initiate effective treatment programs dealing with all health problems of employees.

Acute and chronic conditions are treated on a daily basis by the nurse. These conditions range from the common cold to the crippling effects of arthritis or work-related injuries. As the U.S. population ages and the incidence of chronic conditions increases, the nurse will become more involved in providing care for people with these conditions. Many community agencies (e.g., American Heart Association, American Lung Association) provide excellent services and information in relation to chronic conditions. Agencies in the community that may be useful to the nurse in this effort are discussed in Chapters 18 and 20.

Health Education and Health Promotion

These activities focus on promoting wellness, and there is unlimited opportunity to implement them in the workplace. The OHN is interested in these programs because they help to promote the workers' right to health and improve the quality of life. Employers are often interested in such activities from the standpoint of cost containment and public relations, believing that such programs can enhance company image, reduce workers' compensation costs, result in fewer medical benefits being used, result in less time lost from work, and enhance productivity.

Employers realize that it can cost them less to educate workers about health care risks than to pay the high cost of illness, injury, and disability. For example, each employee who smokes costs his or her employer $960 per year in excess illness costs (Sorensen, Lando, and Pechacek, 1993, p. 121). If successful smoking cessation programs can be implemented in the workplace, this cost can be greatly reduced.

The National Survey of Workplace Health Promotion Activities (USDHHS, 1987), conducted by the U.S. Department of Health and Human Services, showed that 66% of worksites having more than 50 employees sponsored at least one health promotion activity each year; the larger the worksite the more likely it

was to have such activities, and many of these activities were developed and implemented by worksite staff. The most frequently cited programs were smoking control (35.6%), health risk assessment (29.5%), back care (28.6%), stress management (26.6%), and exercise/fitness (22.1%). Other worksite health promotion programs included blood pressure control, weight control, nutrition education, and lifestyle and behavioral change. Employers are quick to use nurses in such health education programs (Davidson, Widtfeldt, and Bey, 1992, p. 181).

The Occupational Safety and Health Act of 1970 requires that workers have the right to know the health hazards they are exposed to in the workplace. Making the worker aware of these hazards is frequently a role of the occupational health nurse. Another important aspect of health education and health promotion is the interpretation of health and welfare benefits to the employee. This means interpreting benefits offered through the employer, as well as providing information about available community resources and services.

Finding time at the workplace to implement health education activities can be a challenge because employers may not be willing to grant work time and employees have little free time on the job except for lunch and coffee breaks. Distributing educational materials in the lunchroom or in pay envelopes and using posters, fliers, and short videos are examples of efficient and effective methods of health education in the worksite. The nurse can also coordinate health education activities in the workplace with those going on in the community. For example, if the community is celebrating health and fitness week, or having a smoking cessation activity such as a "Smokebusters Program," the nurse can build on these activities in the workplace.

Counseling

Health counseling is an important occupational health nursing function. Counseling issues often focus on normal growth and development, family health, workplace stressors, at-risk health behaviors, and results of tests and screenings. If the counseling required is beyond the scope of the nurse and the client is in agreement, a referral can be made to a counseling resource in the community.

Research

"Not all nurses need to conduct research but all nurses need to use research findings in their practice"

> ◀ **American Association of Occupational Health Nurses:** ▶
> **Research Priorities in Occupational Health Nursing**
>
> - Effectiveness of primary health care delivery at the worksite
> - Effectiveness of health promotion nursing intervention strategies
> - Methods for handling complex ethical issues related to occupational health (e.g., confidentiality of employee health records, truth telling)
> - Strategies that minimize work related health outcomes (e.g., back injuries)
> - Health effects resulting from chemical exposures in the workplace
> - Occupational hazards of health care workers
> - Factors that influence worker rehabilitation and return to work
>
> - Mechanisms to assure quality and cost effectiveness of occupational health programs (e.g., effects of employee assistance programs or health surveillance programs on improving employee health)
> - Effectiveness of occupational health nursing programs on employee productivity and morale
> - Factors that contribute to behavioral changes among health care workers for self-protection from occupational hazards (e.g., HIV/AIDS)
> - Factors that contribute to sustained risk reduction behavior related to lifestyle choices (e.g., smoking, substance abuse, nutrition)
> - Effectiveness of ergonomic strategies to reduce worker injury and illness

From American Association of Occupational Health Nurses (AAOHN): *AAOHN research priorities in occupational health nursing,* Atlanta, Ga., February, 1990, The Association. Used with permission of the author.

(Lusk, 1993, p. 153). Research links theory, education, and practice (LoBiondo-Wood and Haber, 1994, p. 6). Further, research tests theory, builds a knowledge base in the field, and serves as the basis for practice in the profession. Nurse researchers, management, and practicing nurses need to work collaboratively to use research findings in nursing practice (Rogers, 1992, Research utilization, p. 41).

The National Center for Nursing Research was established in 1986 and in 1993 became the National Institute for Nursing Research (NINR) (refer to Chapter 1). This institute has assisted nursing researchers in making significant strides. In 1981 the AAOHN established a research committee for the purpose of promoting occupational health nursing research. At its 1982 annual conference the first research session on occupational health nursing studies was held (Silberstein, 1983, p. 9). In 1990 research priorities were established by AAOHN. These research priorities are given in the box above.

Vigorous strides have been made in occupational health nursing research over the last decade. The *AAOHN Journal* regularly publishes research articles and information, and AAOHN offers research awards in occupational health nursing (Rogers, 1992, Clinical, p. 352). Occupational health nursing roles, education, scope of practice, and programmatic activities are frequent research topics (Rogers, 1990, p. 541). Recent topics in occupational health nursing research include functions, stress, management, health promotion, smoking, occupational disease exposure, back injury, and hypertension (Atkins and Magnuson, 1990, p. 563).

Work as a Developmental Task

Work is an activity carried out by people to provide economic and social security. Society expects that adults will work and be self-sufficient; often, being out of work carries with it many negative societal connotations. Our nation sanctions work and promotes the work ethic.

Work is a point of social contact and of personal growth and expression. People identify closely with work, and their personal identity is focused around their work life. Work has been described as a developmental task for the American adult (Duvall and Miller, 1985; Stevenson, 1977). The developmental tasks of work are carried out simultaneously with family and individual developmental tasks across the life cycle. Duvall and Miller (1985) see the young adult as facing the work-related task of selecting and training for an occupation, the adult and middlescent as carrying out a socially adequate worker role and creating a balance between family, community, work, and leisure, and the aged adult as adjusting to retirement.

Stevenson (1977) describes the developmental

tasks of the young adult as integrating personal values with career development and socioeconomic constraints; the early-middle-years adult as developing socioeconomic consolidation and assuming responsible positions in occupational activities; the late-middle-years adult as maintaining flexible views in occupational positions, preparing for another career when feasible, and preparing for retirement; and the adult in late adulthood as pursuing a second or third career and/or adjusting to retirement. If these work-related developmental tasks are left undone or are interrupted, sequential development can be affected and stress can occur.

OCCUPATIONAL HEALTH STRESSORS AND WORKER HEALTH

Most occupational illnesses and injuries are preventable. The *stressors* in the workplace that cause occupational illness and injury are extensive and diverse. They can be categorized (with examples) as:

1. *Chemical:* liquids, gases, dusts, particles, fumes, mists, and vapors
2. *Physical:* electromagnetic and ionizing radiation, noise, pressure, vibration, heat, and cold
3. *Biological:* insects, mold, fungi, and bacteria
4. *Ergonomic:* monotony, fatigue, boredom, stress; the effects of the environment on humankind

It is often difficult to formulate cause-and-effect relationships between occupational stressors and specific illnesses and conditions. A primary problem in formulating cause-and-effect relationships is that no immediate, observable effect of the stressor may be apparent. Long latency periods may exist between contact with the stressor and stressor effects. For example, occupational cancers usually do not become evident until 5 to 40 years after the initial exposure to the carcinogen (CDC, March 9, 1984, p. 127). Asbestosis often has a 30-year or longer latency period. In diseases and conditions with long latency periods, the worker may already have left the job where contact occurred by the time the condition is apparent, making it increasingly difficult to identify and trace the stressor.

The influence of multiple stressors is another factor which affects cause-and-effect relationships. A victim may have been occupationally, environmentally, and personally exposed to many stressors, the interactions between them may greatly increase the risk of contracting the condition, and their effects may not be easily separated (CDC, March 9, 1984, p. 126). It may also become difficult to ascertain which stressor caused the problem. How can the miner with emphysema prove that mine work rather than a heavy smoking habit was the primary factor in the causation of the disease?

The fact that valid, comprehensive occupational health statistics are often not readily available further complicates the situation (USDHHS, 1991, Healthy people, p. 309). Better data collection systems are needed for work-related disease, injury, and death.

Birth and death certificates are commonly used in this country to obtain health statistics, but occupational information such as job and place of employment are generally missing or incomplete. However, in an attempt to develop preventive strategies for conditions such as low-birth-weight infants, to determine teratogens, and to decrease the incidence of infant mortality, parental employment has become a part of the standard *U.S. Fetal Death Certificate.*

The national health objectives in *Healthy People 2000* addressed the need for primary care health professionals to routinely elicit occupational health exposures as part of a client's health history. Health professionals need to collect and analyze work-related injury and illness data from primary care visits, workers' compensation claims, and hospital discharge and admission data. These data would need to include known or potential stressors that the worker was exposed to in the workplace. Until occupational health data are routinely collected and analyzed it will be difficult to formulate cause-and-effect relationships and develop effective prevention plans.

Educating the worker to the hazards of the workplace and actions that can be taken to minimize them is a critical step in illness and injury reduction. One problem related to this can be the difficulty of overcoming the attitudes and actions of the workers themselves. Many people who are exposed to occupational hazards deny the risks of working around such hazards and do not take steps to lessen their chances of developing health problems. It may also be difficult to get the worker to realize that a stressor exists, especially if the stressor is invisible to the human eye (e.g., gases, asbestos). People are less suspicious of, and tend to minimize the effects of, hazards they cannot see.

TABLE 17-1 The 10 Leading Work-Related Diseases and Injuries—United States

Diseases/conditions	Examples
1. Occupational lung diseases	Asbestosis, byssinosis, silicosis, coal workers' pneumoconiosis, lung cancer, occupational asthma
2. Musculoskeletal injuries	Disorders of the back, trunk, upper extremity, neck, lower extremity; traumatically induced Raynaud's phenomenon
3. Occupational cancers (other than lung)	Leukemia, mesothelioma; cancers of the bladder, nose, and liver
4. Traumatic injury and death	Amputations, fractures, eye loss, lacerations
5. Cardiovascular diseases	Hypertension, coronary artery disease, acute myocardial infarction
6. Disorders of reproduction	Infertility, spontaneous abortion, teratogenesis
7. Neurotoxic disorders	Peripheral neuropathy, toxic encephalitis, psychoses, extreme personality changes (exposure-related)
8. Loss of hearing	Noise-induced hearing loss
9. Dermatological conditions	Dermatoses, burns (scaldings), chemical burns, contusions (abrasions)
10. Psychological disorders	Neuroses, personality disorders, alcoholism, drug dependency, stress reactions

From Centers for Disease Control and Prevention: Leading work-related diseases and injuries—United States (occupational lung diseases), *MMWR*, p. 25, January 21, 1983; and USDHHS: *Healthy people 2000: health promotion and disease prevention objectives for the nation, full report, with commentary,* Washington, D.C., 1991, U.S. Government Printing Office.

LEADING CAUSES OF WORK-RELATED DISEASES AND INJURIES

In 1983 NIOSH developed a list of the 10 leading work-related diseases and injuries in the United States. Problems were placed on the list because of the frequency of their occurrence, severity of effect, and the likelihood that preventive strategies could be developed and implemented (List of ten, 1988). NIOSH research is focusing on these problem areas, and national strategies to prevent these diseases and injuries have been developed in conjunction with Schools of Public Health and community health organizations across the country. This list of work-related diseases and injuries has been integrated into *Healthy People 2000* and objectives have been developed to reduce the incidence of the conditions.

Occupational disease and injury are significant national concerns; they impact on the quality of life for individuals, families and communities. In addition to their potential for causing serious physical illness and injury, occupational stressors also have a negative impact on the worker's psychosocial well-being. They can elicit anxiety, depression, irritability, personality changes, and role changes.

From a financial standpoint it is estimated that billions of dollars are lost annually due to work-related diseases and injuries through wages, medical expenses, insurance claims, and production delays. Millions of workdays are lost each year to work-related illness and absenteeism. For personal, societal, and economic reasons there is a great need to reduce the incidence of work-related injury, disease and death in the United States. Table 17-1 lists the 10 leading work-related diseases and injuries in the United States. These conditions are diverse and extensive and include physical and psychosocial problems.

Occupational Lung Diseases

Occupational lung diseases encompass a number of pulmonary diseases including byssinosis (brown lung), asbestosis, coal workers' pneumoconiosis (black lung), and silicosis. These diseases were specifically addressed in the *Healthy People 2000* objectives by calling on every state to develop exposure standards adequate to prevent these major occupational lung diseases. Earlier national health objectives that had targeted the elimination of these diseases were not achieved. Other occupational lung diseases include lung cancer, emphysema, asthma, and chronic industrial bronchitis.

The potential is high for workplace exposure to

substances causing these diseases. Annually more than 1.2 million workers are exposed to silica dust and more than 500,000 are exposed to cotton dust (NIOSH, 1986, Occupational lung, p. 1). The illness, disability, and death caused by these diseases is enormous, and early recognition of these diseases is often difficult due to long latency periods before the diseases are detectable. Two occupational lung diseases with exceptionally long latency periods are silicosis (latency period of approximately 15 years) and asbestosis (latency period of approximately 30 years). Once long periods of time have elapsed it becomes increasingly difficult to link the occupational stressor to the occupational disease. Other factors, such as smoking, can contribute to the disease process and obscure the link between disease and toxic exposure at work.

Prevention strategies for occupational lung disease include stricter standards and regulations, increased surveillance of regulation compliance by employers, hazard removal, health education and training, and technology such as engineering designs for better ventilation and substance isolation (NIOSH, 1986, Occupational lung, pp. 4-7; USDHHS, 1991, Healthy people, p. 306).

Musculoskeletal Injuries

Factors that contribute to musculoskeletal injuries in the workplace are *environmental hazards; human biological factors* such as size, strength, or range of motion; *behavioral or lifestyle factors* such as insufficient sleep, mental lapses, and lack of adequate fitness; and *inadequacies in health care diagnosis and treatment* (NIOSH, 1986, Musculoskeletal injuries, pp. 1-2). Musculoskeletal workplace hazards are called workplace *traumatogens* (NIOSH, p. 1). A traumatogen is a source of biomechanical stress stemming from job demands that exceed the worker's strength and/or endurance, such as heavy lifting or repetitive, forceful manual twisting (NIOSH, p. 1). Although these injuries result in few work-related deaths, they account for a great amount of human suffering and loss of productivity.

Impairments to the musculoskeletal system are estimated to affect more than 24 million persons (Brisson, Nordin, and Zetterberg, 1992, p. 715). The workplace is estimated to account for more than 20% of all back sprains and injuries reported to medical authorities (USDHHS, 1987, p. 73). Back injuries are associated with improper handling of materials, re-

petitive motion, and vibration injuries. Prevention measures include health education, employer compliance with regulations, improved equipment design, limiting biomechanical stresses on the worker, and rotation of workers to jobs with different physical demands (CDC, 1983, musculoskeletal injuries). Occupational health nurses play an active role in implementing these control measures and prevention of musculoskeletal injuries.

Occupational Cancers

More than 200 years have passed since Sir Percivall Pott, a physician, linked cancer of the scrotum in chimney sweeps to their occupational exposure to soot (NIOSH, 1986, Occupational cancers, p. 1). Estimates of the percentage of cancers related to the workplace are as high as 20%. The incidence rate of some cancers among occupational groups is obvious and significant (e.g., cancer of the bone in radium dial workers, mesothelioma in asbestosis workers) (USDHHS, 1987, p. 73); however, some occupationally induced cancers such as mesothelioma can appear decades after exposure to the carcinogen. Table 17-2 lists some occupational cancers and carcinogens by industry and occupation. The occupational health team needs to develop strategies that will prevent unnecessary deaths from occupational cancers.

Problems in documenting occupationally induced cancers can obscure important epidemiological associations and considerations. Some of these problems are described below (CDC, March 9, 1984).

1. Errors in diagnosis and classification of cancers can occur, and unusual neoplasms are often misdiagnosed.
2. There is a lack of meaningful occupational histories. In only a few states is information collected on the work histories of cancer victims; hence, crucial associations with occupational carcinogens are often missed.
3. Precise measurements of levels and duration of exposures have not been generally available, resulting in an inability to delineate dose-response relationships in a consistent manner.
4. The occupational etiology of a very rare cancer due to a specific agent, such as hemangiosarcoma of the liver to vinyl chloride, is much more readily documented than the occupational etiology of cancer caused by several factors.

TABLE 17-2 Selected Occupational Cancers

Cancer	Industry/occupation	Agent
Hemangiosarcoma of the liver	Vinyl chloride polymerization	Vinyl chloride monomer
	Industry vintners	Arsenical pesticides
Malignant neoplasm of nasal cavities	Woodworkers, cabinet/furniture makers	Hardwood dusts
	Boot and shoe producers	Unknown
	Radium chemists, processors, dial painters	Radium
	Nickel smelting and refining	Nickel
Malignant neoplasm of larynx	Asbestos industries and utilizers	Asbestos
Mesothelioma	Asbestos industries and utilizers	Asbestos
Malignant neoplasm of bone	Radium chemists, processors, dial painters	Radium
Malignant neoplasm of scrotum	Automatic lathe operators, metalworkers	Mineral/cutting oils
	Coke oven workers, petroleum refiners, tar distillers	Soots and tars, tar distillates
Malignant neoplasm of bladder	Rubber and dye workers	Benzidine, alpha and beta naphthylamine, auramine, magenta, 4-aminobiphenyl, 4-nitrophenyl
Malignant neoplasm of kidney	Coke oven workers	Coke oven emissions
Lymphoid leukemia, acute	Rubber industry	Unknown
	Radiologists	Ionizing radiation
Myeloid leukemia, acute	Occupations with exposure to benzene	Benzene
	Radiologists	Ionizing radiation

From Centers for Disease Control and Prevention: Leading work-related diseases and injuries—United States (occupational cancers other than lung), *MMWR*, p. 126, March 9, 1984. Modified from Rutstein DD, Mullan RJ, Frazier TM, Halperin WE, Melius JM, and Sestito JP: Sentinel health events (occupational): a basis for physician recognition and public health surveillance, *Am J Public Health* 73:1054-1062, 1984.

5. Highly significant differences in the rates of cancer among small subgroups of a population may be overlooked because these rates affect the overall rate for cancer in the larger study population only slightly, if at all. This creates what has been called the "dilution factor."

There are thousands of suspected carcinogens in the workplace that are not regulated. Exposure to carcinogens does not always cause cancer, and not everything is a carcinogen. *The dose, frequency of exposure, and duration of contact are often the key to the toxicity of a substance.* For example, many chemicals such as zinc, nickel, tin, and potassium are essential for health in small quantities but are toxic in larger quantities.

Traumatic Injury and Death

Traumatic injuries include amputations, fractures, lacerations, eye loss, acute poisonings, burns and death. The *Healthy People 2000* occupational health objectives address the need for reduction of deaths from work-related injuries; reducing work-related injuries that require medical treatment, lost time from work, or restricted work activity; reducing cumulative trauma disorders; and increasing the number of worksites that offer back injury prevention and rehabilitation programs.

As previously discussed, NIOSH estimates that at least 10 million traumatic injuries occur on the job each year, about 3 million of which are severe (USDHHS, 1991, Healthy people, p. 299), and approximately

10,600 workers die annually in the United States from work-related injury (Skovron, 1992, p. 725). Occupational trauma is second only to motor vehicle accidents as a reported cause of unintentional death in the United States (NIOSH, 1986, Severe occupational trauma, p. 1). Although work-related deaths are gradually declining, nonfatal work-related injuries are on the rise (A Public Health Service progress report, 1992). Work-related injuries are costly in terms of human suffering and in dollars and cents. The total cost of work-related accidents is approximately $47 billion each year (National Safety Council, 1990).

Construction workers, nursing and personal care workers, and farm workers have some of the highest rates of work-related injury in the United States (USDHHS, 1991, Healthy people, p. 299). Of special interest to nurses is the fact that reports of injuries among nursing home workers and other personal caregivers have also increased in recent years. Back injuries account for 40% of the injuries occurring in these workers (USDHHS, Healthy people, p. 299).

Cumulative trauma disorders are on the rise in the workplace, almost doubling between 1987 (100 cases per 100,000 workers) and 1989 (192 cases per 100,000 workers) (A Public Health Service progress, 1992). These disorders often occur as a result of repetitive motion and repeated pressure in the workplace. Repetitive motions may lead to disorders such as carpal tunnel syndrome, tendinitis, ganglionitis, and bursitis, as well as damage to muscles, tendons, ligaments, and joints. The prevention of traumatic injury is related to implementing engineering controls, practicing safe work habits, using personal protective equipment, and monitoring the workplace for emerging hazards (USDHHS, 1991, Healthy people, p. 300). As discussed in Chapter 2, engineering strategies focus on environmental modifications for the purpose of eliminating or managing environmental factors that affect healthy living. The occupational health nurse assumes an important role in assessing and reinforcing the need for such measures and helping to implement them in the workplace.

Cardiovascular Disease

Cardiovascular diseases are the leading cause of death in the United States. Although personal risk factors play an important role in developing these diseases, factors in the workplace such as stress and exposure to cardiotoxins also contribute their effects (USDHHS, 1987, p. 74). The acute cardiac effect of carbon monoxide is well known, and research has also linked workers exposed to carbon disulfide with cardiovascular symptoms and arteriosclerotic heart disease (Fine, 1992, p. 593-594). An association between acute episodes of anginal pain, myocardial infarction, and even cardiovascular death from occupational exposures to nitroglycerine and other aliphatic nitrates has been shown (Fine, p. 594). Other occupational exposures that may increase the risk of cardiovascular disease include cobalt, lead, antimony, and cadmium (NIOSH, 1986, Occupational cardiovascular diseases, p. 2). The effects of passive inhalation of smoke in relation to cardiac disease has also been documented. Environmental smoke in the workplace needs to be considered in relation to cardiovascular disease, and many workplaces are placing restrictions on smoking or prohibiting it all together.

Control of cardiovascular disease is addressed in the *Healthy People 2000* occupational health objectives under implementation of programs on worker health and safety. The worksite is an excellent location for teaching individuals about positive health practices and addressing and implementing preventive programs on personal risk factors such as such as smoking cessation, proper diet, blood pressure control, exercise, and stress reduction. An increasing number of workplaces have established health promotion and wellness programs designed to prevent premature deaths related to cardiovascular disease. These programs often work in partnership with community resources such as the American Heart Association and refer employees to community resources when indicated.

Reproductive Disorders

In the late 1800s unusually high rates of infertility, spontaneous abortion, stillbirth, neonatal death, and macrocephaly were noted in European lead-working communities and a link was made between industrial chemicals and reproductive disorders (LeMasters, 1992, p. 151). Contemporary research has shown that exposure to specific occupational stressors can cause reproductive disorders. Maternal exposure to some toxicants can cause infertility, menstrual disorders, illness during pregnancy, chromosome or breast milk alteration, early onset of menopause, and libido suppression (LeMasters, p. 153). Fetal exposure to some toxicants can result in preterm delivery, fetal death, low birth weight, congenital malformation, and developmental disabilities (LeMasters, p. 153). Paternal exposure to some toxicants has been linked to sterility and chromosomal alteration (NIOSH, 1988, Disorders of reproduction, p. 1). Research has shown sterility in male dibromochloropropane workers, impotence in workers exposed to specific neurotoxins, increased birth defects among children born to female pharmaceutical workers, and excessive spontaneous abortions and chromosomal alterations among health care personnel exposed to anesthetic gases (USDHHS, 1987, p. 74; NIOSH, Disorders of reproduction, p. 1). These mutagenic and teratogenic effects can affect several generations (Sax and Lewis, 1989, vol I, p. 7).

Neurotoxic Disorders

Disorders of the nervous system that result from toxic exposures in the workplace have been recorded throughout history. As early as the first century AD palsy in workers exposed to lead dust was noted (NIOSH, 1988, Neurotoxic disorders, p. 1). More than 850 chemicals in the American workplace have been identified as toxic to the central nervous system, and the number of workers exposed to neurotoxic chemicals has been estimated at 8 million (USDHHS, 1987, p. 74). *Healthy People 2000* addresses worker exposure to neurotoxins.

Peripheral neuropathy, characterized by numbness and tingling in the feet or hands followed by clumsiness and/or incoordination, is one of the most common and serious problems in workers exposed to neurotoxins. These workers may find their ability to work impaired on either a temporary or permanent basis. Behavioral neurotoxicity and changes in behavior resulting from chemical exposure can also occur. Chemicals well known for causing neurotoxic symptoms include arsenic, carbon disulfide, carbon monoxide, kepone, lead, manganese, and mercury. The Mad Hatter of Lewis Carroll's *Alice in Wonderland* was not purely a figment of Carroll's imagination. In Carroll's time hatters used mercury in hatmaking and many of them went mad due to mercury poisoning. Workers exposed to neurotoxic agents need screening programs to detect the early symptoms of central nervous system damage (Baker, 1992, p. 570).

Psychological Disorders

Psychological disorders in the workplace include affective disturbances such as anxiety, depression, and job dissatisfaction; maladaptive behavioral or lifestyle patterns; and chemical dependencies and alcohol abuse (NIOSH, 1988, Psychological disorders, p. 2). Psychological disturbances can be brought on by anxiety, boredom, stress, monotony, and fatigue. They are heavily concentrated among workers with lower income, lower education, fewer skills, and less prestigious jobs (NIOSH, p. 4). Workers who are balancing the responsibilities of employment and family caregiving are also at risk for experiencing psychological stress (McGovern and Matter, 1992, p. 35).

Psychological stressors are present on all jobs. At any one time, an estimated 8% to 10% of the work force is suffering from a disabling emotional or psychological condition (USDHHS, 1987, p. 75). Stress-related symptoms contribute to absenteeism and lost productivity, and company health care expenses for psychological conditions are estimated to cost $75 billion annually (USDHHS, p. 75).

Jobs designed to improve working conditions, surveillance of psychological disorders and work factors, education and training, and increased psychological health services for workers are prevention strategies for work-related psychological disorders (NIOSH, 1988, Psychological disorders, p. 7). The occupational health nurse should be sensitive to the fact that family members are often the victims of the effects of work stress and psychological disturbance. Group sessions on stress awareness and management may be especially helpful for workers and their families. The nurse should refer workers to community mental health resources when appropriate and resources in the community that may be able to assist the worker in balancing the responsibilities of caregiving and work.

One interesting work-related psychological phenomenon is *mass psychogenic illness,* which occurs when a number of workers simultaneously experience similar symptoms seemingly contagious in nature but whose etiology can only be linked to a psychological stressor. Symptoms of mass psychogenic illness often include, headaches, nausea, chills, blurred vision, muscular weakness, and difficulty breathing (Colligan and Stockton, 1978; Moss, p. 671). The illness is frequently linked with workers being overcome by strange odors (Colligan and

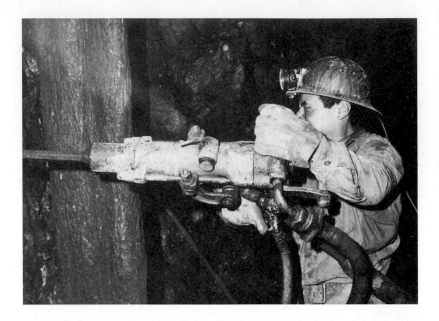

Figure 17-2 Many American workers are exposed to dangerous levels of noise. (Courtesy World Health Organization.)

Murphy, 1979; Moss, p. 671). Epidemics of mass psychogenic illness typically occur in controlled social settings such as workers on a factory assembly line (Moss, p. 671). It has been routinely linked with stressful job situations.

When such outbreaks do occur it is recommended that symptomatic persons be removed to a quiet, out-of-the-way area and that the situation be handled as quietly as possible to prevent mass spread of the symptoms (CDC, 1983, Epidemic). The nurse must be sensitive to the needs of the worker while maintaining a focus on the reality of the situation. It is important to remember that the symptoms are real to those who are experiencing them. Talking openly with workers about the phenomena may be the most effective means of ending an epidemic. *The nurse must be careful not to diagnosis all such occurrences as mass psychogenic illness; each situation should be carefully evaluated, since there may actually be a hazardous occupational stressor present.*

Hearing Loss

Approximately 10 million American workers are exposed to potentially harmful noise levels (McCunney, 1992, p. 1121) (refer to Figure 17-2). Noise is a physical stressor that can result in hearing loss. Noise-induced hearing loss in the workplace was recognized in the early 1700s by Bernardo Ramazzini in his writings on the diseases of occupations. By the early

twentieth century boilermakers' deafness, caused by riveting inside metal boilers, was an occupational hazard of considerable magnitude (NIOSH, 1988, Noise-induced hearing loss, p. 1). Federal efforts to regulate occupational noise began in 1955. Noise-induced hearing loss is one of the most common and preventable occupational problems. Research studies indicate that worker hearing loss is directly related to worker noise exposure levels (McGuire, 1991, p. 211).

Hearing loss due to industrial noise is often represented on audiograms by a notch at approximately 4000 Hz (refer to Figure 17-3). This notch is often referred to as the industrial noise trauma notch. The person suffering from such a hearing loss may initially complain of *tinnitus,* which is a ringing sound in the ear. The onset of hearing loss can be gradual, and people may be unaware of initial hearing loss. Most workers are unaware of hearing loss until the damage is severe or affects communication.

The occupational health nurse plays a key role in an industrial hearing conservation program and often has significant responsibility for the implementation, coordination, and continuing administration of the hearing conservation program (McGuire, 1991, pp. 233, 239). A successful industrial hearing conservation program complies with the OSHA hearing conservation program regulations and plant site regulations. Some activities implemented by the nurse in these programs are given in the box on p. 690.

The nurse obtains the workers' medical and occu-

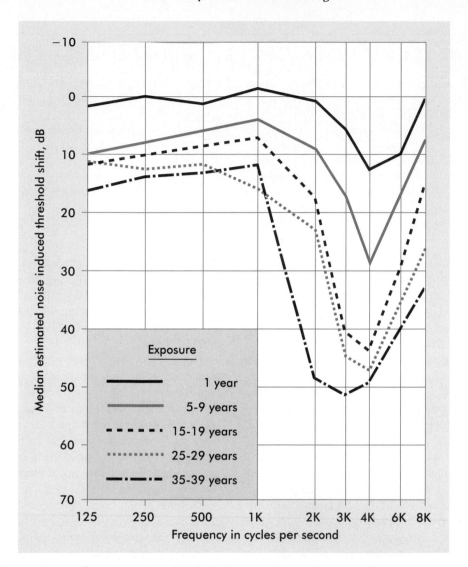

Figure 17-3   Median permanent threshold shifts in hearing levels as a function of exposure years to jute weaving noise. (Data taken from Taylor WA, Mair A, and Burns W: Study of noise and hearing in jute weaving, *Acoustical Society of American* 48:524-530, 1965, as cited in USDHHS: *NIOSH publications on noise and hearing: criteria for a recommended standard—occupational exposure to noise,* Cincinnati, Oh., 1991, NIOSH, p. 511).

pational histories, carries out audiometric testing, refers employees with hearing complaints or questionable audiograms to a physician, educates and counsels employees about industrial noise, supplies employees with appropriate hearing protection devices, and encourages employees to wear these devices in and outside of the work environment. Activities to prevent work-related hearing loss include the development of new technology to make work processes quieter and attenuate workplace noise sources, the application of effective hearing conservation pro-

grams, the use of hearing protection devices by workers, and additional research on noise-induced hearing loss (NIOSH, 1988, Noise-induced hearing loss).

Dermatological Disorders

Reduction of dermatological disorders is one of the *Healthy People 2000* occupational health objectives. Occupational skin disorders are on the increase and are the most prevalent causes of occupational illness and lost time from work (A Public Health Service

◀ *Nursing Activities in Hearing Conservation Programs* ▶

- Assesses the workers' environment for noise exposure and coordinates with management work areas where hearing protection should be worn.
- Determines employees who may be predisposed to hearing loss.
- Performs audiometric testing on prospective employees, continues to measure employees' hearing periodically, and examines audiometric data for accuracy and reliability.

- Provides effective hearing protection for employees, including individually fitting employees for such hearing protection.
- Provides ongoing educational programs on hearing conservation and noise abatement in the workplace.
- Assists in implementing administrative and engineering controls to reduce noise levels and prevent noise in the workplace.

progress, 1992). An estimated 34% of all occupational illnesses are dermatological (NIOSH, 1988, Dermatological conditions, p. 3).

Large surface areas of the skin are directly exposed to the environment, making this organ especially vulnerable to occupational diseases (NIOSH, 1988, Dermatological conditions, p. 1). Dermal absorption of some chemicals may be more serious than absorption by inhalation. Occupational dermatoses can be divided into four major categories: 1) mechanical—friction and pressure, 2) chemical, 3) physical—heat, cold, radiation, and 4) biological—viruses, bacteria, fungi, and parasites (Tucker and Key, 1992, p. 557).

Workers in agriculture are at four times greater risk of contracting skin disease than workers in other industries (Moses, 1989, p. 118). This is largely due to their exposure to pesticides and chemicals. The most effective prevention measures are health education activities, engineering controls that eliminate skin exposure through isolation, containment or redesign of the industrial process, personal protective clothing, and the use of less toxic chemicals in the workplace (USDHHS, 1991, Healthy people, p. 301). Dermatological conditions are usually amendable to early diagnosis and treatment.

HEPATITIS B IN THE WORKPLACE

The *Healthy People 2000* occupational health objectives specifically addressed reducing the risk of exposure to hepatitis B virus (HBV) and the incidence of hepatitis B in the workplace. However, hepatitis B infections are on the rise in the workplace (A Public Health Service progress, 1992). As health care workers, nurses are at a much higher risk for exposure to HBV than the general public. Each year approximately 12,000 health care workers become infected with

HBV, resulting in 6200 clinical HBV infections, 600 hospitalizations, and 1200 people becoming carriers (USDHHS, 1991, Healthy people, p. 301). Hepatitis B is responsible for approximately 200 deaths annually among health care workers (Garibaldi and Janis, 1992, p. 607).

Blood is the single most important source of HBV transmission in the workplace, and vaccination is recommended for all health care workers who have regular contact with blood. Federal legislation has made HBV vaccine available at no cost to employees who are occupationally at risk for the disease. Unfortunately, fewer than 40% of health care workers nationwide have been immunized for hepatitis B (Garibaldi and Janis, 1992, p. 607).

Prevention measures include health education, vaccination against the disease, and safe work practices such as the use of gloves, masks, and protective clothing; proper handling of blood products; and adequate disposal of contaminated waste. The nurse can assist the worker in seeing the value of such preventive measures.

AIDS IN THE WORKPLACE

The acquired immunodeficiency syndrome (AIDS) epidemic is a rapidly growing threat to the health of the nation. A separate priority area in *Healthy People 2000* was devoted to HIV infection. Since there is no known cure for AIDS, the first priority of the public health system must be to prevent its spread (USDHHS, 1991, Healthy people, p. 480) (refer to Chapters 11 and 16 for further information on AIDS).

At least 1 million people in the United States are infected with HIV and therefore at risk for developing AIDS (USDHHS, 1991, Healthy people, p. 480). The number of people diagnosed with AIDS in the United

States rises daily and has increased from under 100 in 1981 to 289,320 by March 1993 (CDC, 1993, HIV/AIDS, p. 3). This is almost a 3000% increase in 12 years.

The AIDS epidemic is being felt everywhere, including the workplace. AAOHN has published the *AAOHN Resource Guide, HIV Infection/AIDS in the Workplace.* The resource guide includes 1) definitions, 2) HIV infection/AIDS information, and 3) resource information, and addresses topics such as worker surveillance, counseling, policy development, research, ethics, confidentiality, and the right to work. AAOHN has recommended that workers with AIDS be employed for as long as possible, confidentiality of HIV testing results and records be maintained, management take aggressive action to establish AIDS policy and education at the workplace, and discrimination against the HIV-positive employee be discouraged (AAOHN, 1989, A year).

Many people who are infected with HIV are asymptomatic and may not be aware that they are infected. In the absence of symptoms, there is no indication that these persons are less capable of performing on the job than noninfected workers (Jaffe and Schmitt, 1992, p. 693). In the workplace the risk of HIV infection is directly related to potential exposures to blood or body fluids from coworkers or clients (Jaffe and Schmitt, p. 693).

Research by Hansen, Booth, Fawal, and Langer (1988) showed that most workers held some negative attitudes and myths about HIV-positive coworkers. There is a great need for health education programs to educate workers and employers about AIDS and to dispel myths. Research by Nyamathi and Flaskerud (1989) revealed statistically significant improvements in AIDS knowledge following an AIDS education program with employees.

The occupational health nurse has been, and will likely continue to be, a key figure in AIDS policy development and educational programming (Harris, 1990, p. 11). It is frequently the nurse who implements AIDS education in the workplace and refers workers to community resources and programs. This requires that the nurse keep up-to-date with rapidly changing AIDS research, information, and statistics.

OCCUPATIONAL HEALTH AND MINORITY WORKERS

Employment in hazardous occupations is much more common among minority workers (blacks, Hispanics, Asians, and Native Americans) than their white counterparts. This results in a disproportionate number of occupational diseases, injuries, and deaths within these population groups. These workers are less likely to receive adequate health care and are often not even properly diagnosed (Friedman-Jimenez, 1989, p. 70). Nurses need to consider this in their plans of care and when implementing health education and safety programs.

Black and Hispanic workers tend to be underrepresented in low-risk occupations and highly overrepresented in dangerous high-risk ones (Morris, 1989, p. 53; Friedman-Jimenez, 1989, p. 65). Fifteen percent of the 7 million black workers are permanently disabled from work-related causes, compared to 10% of white workers. Blacks have a 37% greater likelihood of suffering work-related illness or injury and a 20% greater likelihood of dying from a job-related condition than whites (Morris, p. 53). Hispanics are heavily represented in the hazardous occupations of farm work and manufacturing. Farm work is the most hazardous occupation in the United States, with more than 1600 deaths annually and 160,000 disabling injuries (Ubell, 1989, p. 5). Many of these deaths and injuries occur among seasonal, migrant farm workers, and it was for this reason that migrant farm work has been selected for further discussion in this text. Many of the areas of concern discussed in the following section apply at least in part to other minority workers in other work settings.

Migrant Farm Workers

There are approximately 4.2 million migrant farm workers and their dependents in the United States (CDC, June 5, 1992, p. 2). Migrant workers face numerous health hazards (refer to Figure 17-4) and are not protected by many of the laws which govern the health and welfare of other workers. Farm workers are excluded completely or partially from federal laws including the National Labor Relations Act (which guarantees the right to join a union and bargain collectively), the Fair Labor Standards Act (which governs minimum wage and child labor), the Occupational Safety and Health Act (which governs standards of health and safety in the workplace), and state workers' compensation laws and unemployment insurance laws (Moses, 1989, p. 115). Family-owned farms are often excluded from government safety supervision and inspection (Ubell, 1989, p. 5).

Some states have made provisions for the migrant worker, but these provisions are sparse, and the mi-

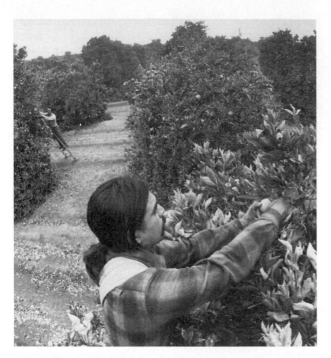

Figure 17-4   Migrant farm workers are exposed to many health risks. (Courtesy U.S. Department of Agriculture.)

grant worker has little legislative protection. Migrant farm workers face many problems including financial instability, child labor, poor housing, lack of education, and impaired access to health and social services.

Financial Stability

Migrant farm workers represent a large, mobile supply of cheap labor. Their work is characterized by low wages, long hours, few benefits, and poor working conditions. They are the working poor, without many of the health and welfare benefits that other workers have. Many migrant farm families have incomes below the poverty level and live in chronic poverty.

Child Labor

Child labor has all but disappeared from U.S. industry, except in the agricultural sector. Many migrant children work because it brings in additional family income. Growers continue to use child labor because it is inexpensive and available. Migrant children who work are subject to the same job hazards and health risks as adults, including long hours and hazardous or faulty equipment and chemicals. They show increased incidence of accidental injury on the job. Working often keeps migrant children from school and other normal childhood activities.

Housing

Migrant farm workers often live in substandard housing (Watkins, Larson, Harlan, and Young, 1990, p. 567). Housing is generally crowded and inadequate, and living conditions are not safe or sanitary. Migrant housing has been compared to slave quarters: horrible and dehumanizing, without adequate heat, light, or ventilation, and often without plumbing or refrigeration (Goldfarb, 1981, p. 42). These unsanitary and unsafe housing conditions are breeding grounds for diseases, disability, hopelessness, and death.

Education

Many migrant children never enter high school and, of those who do, few graduate. It is not that migrant families do not want an education for their children; they just have great difficulty obtaining it. Their mobility and the seasonal nature of farm work necessitate frequent school change and absences. School officials are frequently lax in enforcing school attendance and other regulations for migrant children. Migrant children may be labeled slow, retarded, uncooperative, or uninterested when actually the situation is more a social problem than a question of the children's educational ability or attitude.

The aspirations of migrant families that their children receive a good education go unfulfilled. As long as migrant children are poorly educated, it will be difficult for them to escape their present living conditions.

Access to Services

These workers and their families face language, cultural, financial, immigration, educational, and other barriers to obtaining necessary health and welfare services (CDC, June 5, 1992, p. 2). Although migrant workers may qualify for federal aid programs and services, they may not be aware of them, and restrictive local and state policies may limit access to them. In 1969 a Supreme Court decision (Shapiro v. Thompson, 394 U.S. 618) ruled that a state could not exclude persons from welfare benefits because they were not residents of that state or had not resided in that state for a specific period of time. As a result of this ruling many migrant workers are now eligible for services such as Aid to Families with Dependent Children, food stamps, WIC, and Medicaid.

Communities may be indifferent to issues of migrant health and welfare. Migrant workers generally have no voice in community planning and decision-making and often do not feel a sense of belonging to the communities in which they work.

Health

Migrant farm workers are historically found in rural communities where there are fewer health services to begin with. The transient nature of their work makes it difficult to provide continuous, comprehensive health services; many migrant workers are uninsured; and many are not aware of the health care services available to them.

Many migrant families do not have a regular source of primary health care, have numerous and complex health problems, and evidence higher rates of diseases and conditions than other Americans. In relation to the general population, migrant workers have higher incidence of tuberculosis, parasitic diseases, communicable diseases, diabetes, hypertension, malnutrition, high-risk pregnancies, and infant mortality (CDC, June 5, 1992, p. 2). They have high rates of digestive diseases and inadequate diets, high incidence of hospitalization and chronic illness in children, and low rates of childhood immunization (Watkins, Larson, Harlan, and Young, 1990, p. 568). Although they have a higher incidence of high-risk pregnancy, migrant women are less likely to have adequate prenatal care than their white counterparts. Migrant workers are six times more likely to develop tuberculosis than other employed adults (CDC, p. 1). Research has shown that migrant workers are at high risk for developing malignant lymphoma, leukemia, multiple myeloma, testicular cancer, and cancer of the gastrointestinal tract (Moses, 1989, pp. 121-122). Goldfarb (1981) found that the average life expectancy for the migrant worker was 49 years, while the average life expectancy for the nation as a whole was 74 years. This figure is statistically and *morally* significant. Migrant health is an important area that needs to be addressed in the United States.

Migrant farm work is one of the most hazardous occupations in the United States. A major problem with estimating occupational injury among migrant farm workers is that few reliable statistics are kept. Two well-documented occupational health hazards for the migrant farm worker are injuries from farm machinery and exposure to agricultural chemicals such as pesticides.

Thousands of farm workers are affected each year from exposure to pesticides. Acute health effects from exposure to pesticides range from eye infections, upper respiratory tract irritability, and contact dermatitis to systemic poisoning that can result in death (Moses, 1989, p. 117). The primary route of exposure to pesticides, except for fumigants, is through the skin, and they may persist on the skin for several months (Moses, p. 116). Few studies have been done on the chronic health problems related to pesticide exposure, and surveillance and record-keeping on these exposures is lacking.

An important source of health care for the migrant family is the Migrant Health Center. There are more than 100 such centers in the United States. Service areas for these centers include mental health, substance abuse, transportation, pharmacy, dental, emergency, environmental health, prenatal, pediatric, and social services (National Association of Community Health Centers, 1991, p. 19). Preventive services provided by these centers include health education and counseling, immunizations, blood lead screening, antepartal care, developmental and physical assessments, hearing exams, and the supplemental food program for Women, Infants, and Children (WIC) (National Association of Community Health Centers, p. 19). Approximately 500,000 migrant workers are served by these centers each year (CDC, June 5, 1992, p. 2). The nurse plays a major role in service provision in these centers. Many services are provided by primary care nurses.

The stresses the migrant worker must face such as poor working conditions, problems with access to health services, decreased educational opportunities for themselves and their children, and low wages all contribute to poverty and poor health beyond what most Americans will ever experience. Because the migrant worker is often concerned with immediate, day-to-day survival, planning for the future can be difficult.

The nurse working with migrant families can facilitate their efforts in obtaining health care. In doing so, the nurse needs firsthand knowledge of community resources, health care facilities, and occupational hazards. The nurse may need to assume the role of client advocate. Helping to assure the health of migrant workers is a challenging endeavor, as well as a social and professional responsibility that cannot be overlooked.

A LOOK TO THE FUTURE

More than any other health profession, the nurse has been at the forefront of occupational health in the

---

◀ *An Exercise in Critical Thinking* ▶

Nurses are workers. What are some of the occupational stressors that nurses are exposed to in the workplace? What are some primary prevention activities to protect nurses from the effects of these stressors? What are some of the occupational stressors you are concerned about in your nursing career?

United States. Our national health agenda is now emphasizing community-based care and preventive health services. The occupational health nurse has historically been involved in these activities and will be able to assist other health professionals in their achievement. Nurses will be called on to develop, implement, and evaluate worksite health programs.

Occupational health nurses are conducting research, developing educational programs, and advocating for legislative change. The American Association of Occupational Health Nurses (AAOHN) has made a firm commitment to research. Educational opportunities will increase in occupational health nursing, with a significant number of occupational health nurses holding masters or doctorate degrees in the future. In addition, the education of school children and the general public about occupational health will be part of the nurse's agenda.

AAOHN was instrumental in the development of the *Healthy People 2000* occupational health objectives and continues to play an active role in the nation's occupational health agenda and legislation. Through such political activities there will be more complete disclosure of harmful agents in the workplace, more effective legislation, and higher levels of worker and community health. By continuing to monitor the social, economic, and political forces affecting the nation's health, the nurse will be able to help shape these forces to meet occupational health needs.

Ethical issues will increase in scope and individual nurses, as well as their professional organizations, will need to monitor them closely. Issues such as AIDS and hepatitis B in the workplace, confidentiality, right-to-know, and cost containment that may adversely affect expense worker health will remain significant.

Summary

Occupational health influences not only the status of the individual worker but also the health of society as a whole. Maintaining the health of the working population is an important task of all health professionals. Historically, nursing has been at the forefront of occupational health activities and has served as a role model to other professions in the field.

This chapter has addressed many occupational health concerns of workers, their families, and the community, illustrating that occupational health is a rapidly emerging and changing field. It is notable that there have been more advances in the protection of workers from occupational health hazards in the United States in the last 25 years than in the entire history of the nation. Our country now has federal and state legislation to protect the health and safety of the worker, occupational health is a national health priority, and national occupational health objectives are being implemented. It is hoped that nursing students will look at occupational health nursing as a potential area of study and practice. Occupational health nursing will be an important part of the nursing of the future; it is an exciting, challenging field with unlimited potential.

References

American Association of Industrial Nurses: *The nurse in industry,* New York, 1976, The Association.

A Public Health Service progress report on Healthy People 2000: *Occupational Safety and Health,* Washington, D.C., 1992, Centers for Disease Control and Prevention.

American Association of Occupational Health Nurses (AAOHN): *AAOHN code of ethics and interpretive statements,* Atlanta, Ga., 1991, The Association.

AAOHN: *Occupational health nursing: the answer to health care cost containment,* Atlanta, Ga., 1991, The Association.

AAOHN: *AAOHN research priorities in occupational health nursing,* Atlanta, Ga., 1990, The Association.

AAOHN: *A commitment for excellence,* Atlanta, Ga., 1989, The Association.

AAOHN: A year of progress..... American Association of Occupational Health Nurses 1988 Annual Report, *AAOHN J* 37(4), 1989.

AAOHN: *Confidentiality of health information* (position statement), Atlanta, Ga., 1988, The Association.

AAOHN: *Standards of practice,* Atlanta, Ga., 1988, The Association.

AAOHN: *Educational preparation for entry into professional practice* (position statement), Atlanta, Ga., 1986, The Association.

Ashford NA: *Crisis in the workplace,* Cambridge, Mass., 1976, MIT Press.

Atkins J and Magnuson N: Occupational health nursing research June 1984 to June 1989, *AAOHN J* 38(12):560-566, 1990.

Babbitz MA: Approaching the 21st century: congressional agenda for health care and occupational health, *AAOHN J* 40(1):12-15, 1992.

Babbitz MA and Bodnar EM: *Promote wellness at the worksite: become an occupational health nurse,* Atlanta, Ga., 1989, American Association of Occupational Health Nurses.

Baker EL: Neurologic disorders. In Rom WR: *Environmental and occupational medicine,* ed 2, Boston, 1992, Little, Brown, pp. 561-572.

Barlow R: Role of the occupational health nurse in the year 2000, *AAOHN J* 40(10):463-467, 1992.

Bertsche PK, Sanborn JS, and Jones ER: Occupational medicine residency training programs: the role occupational health nurses play, *AAOHN J* 37:316-320, 1989.

Bingham E: The occupational safety and health act. In Rom WR: *Environmental and occupational medicine,* ed 2, Boston, 1992, Little, Brown, pp. 1325-1332.

Brisson PM, Nordin M, and Zetterberg CL: The musculoskeletal system and occupational syndromes. In Rom WR: *Environmental and occupational medicine,* ed 2, Boston, 1992, Little, Brown, pp. 715-724.

Brown ML: *Occupational health nursing,* New York, 1956, Springer.

Brown ML: An historical perspective: one hundred years of industrial or occupational health nursing in the United States, *AAOHN J* 36(10):433-435, 1988.

Budget of the United States government FY 1994, Washington, D.C., 1993, U.S. Government Printing Office.

Centers for Disease Control and Prevention (CDC): Leading work-related diseases and injuries—U.S. (occupational lung diseases), *MMWR* pp. 24-27, January 21, 1983.

CDC: Leading work-related diseases and injuries—U.S. (occupational cancers other than lung), *MMWR* pp. 125-128, March 9, 1984.

CDC: Leading work-related diseases and injuries—U.S. (musculoskeletal injuries), *MMWR* pp. 189-190, April 15, 1983.

CDC: Epidemic psychogenic illness in an industrial setting—Pennsylvania, *MMWR* pp. 189-190, June 10, 1983.

CDC: Prevention and control of tuberculosis in migrant farm workers, *MMWR* pp. 1-15, June 5, 1992.

CDC: *HIV/AIDS surveillance report: first quarter edition* 5(1), May 1993, The Centers.

Colligan MJ and Murphy LA: Mass psychogenic illness in organizations: an overview, *J Occup Psychol* 52:77-90, 1979.

Colligan MJ and Stockton W: The mystery of assembly-line hysteria, *Psychology Today,* June 1978, pp. 93-99, 114-116.

Cox AR: Planning for the future of occupational health nursing. Part II: comprehensive membership survey, *AAOHN J* 37:356-360, 1989.

Davidson G, Widtfeldt A, and Bey J: On-site occupational health nursing services. Estimating the net savings: part I, *AAOHN J* 40(4):172-181, 1992.

Duvall EM and Miller BC: *Marriage and family development,* ed 6, New York, 1985, Harper and Row.

Felton JS: The genesis of American occupational health nursing: part II, *AAOHN J* 34:31-35, 1988.

Felton JS: 200 years of occupational medicine in the U.S., *J Occupat Med* 28:809-814, 1976.

Fine LJ: Chapter 44: Occupational heart disease. In Rom WR: *Environmental and Occupational Medicine,* ed 2, Boston, 1992, Little, Brown, pp. 593-600.

Friedman-Jimenez G: Occupational disease among minority workers: a common and preventable public health concern, *AAOHN J* 37:64-70, 1989.

Gardner, MS: *Public health nursing,* New York, 1916, MacMillan.

Garibaldi R and Janis B: Occupational infections. In Rom WR: *Environmental and occupational medicine,* ed 2, Boston, 1992, Little, Brown, pp. 607-618.

Goldfarb RL: *Caste of despair,* Ames, IA, 1981, Iowa University Press.

Greaves WW: The Toxic Substances Control Act. In Rom WR: *Environmental and occupational medicine,* ed 2, Boston, 1992, Little, Brown, pp. 1333-1338.

Haag AB and Glazner LK: A remembrance of the past, an investment for the future, *AAOHN J* 40(2):56-60, 1992.

Hamilton A: *Exploring the dangerous trades: the autobiography of Alice Hamilton, M.D.,* Boston, 1943, Little, Brown.

Hamilton A: *Industrial poisons in the United States,* New York, 1925, McMillan.

Hansen B, Booth W, Fawal HJ, and Langer RW: Workers with AIDS: attitudes of fellow employees, *AAOHN J* 36:279-283, 1988.

Harris J: AIDS policy and education in the workplace, *AAOHN J* 38:6-11, 1990.

Including industrial nursing in basic curriculum, *Pub Health Nursing* 37:129, 1945.

Jaffe HA and Schmitt J: AIDS in the workplace. In Rom WR: *Environmental and occupational medicine,* ed 2, Boston, 1992, Little, Brown, pp. 685-713.

LeMasters G: Occupational exposures and effects on male and female reproduction. In Rom WR: *Environmental and occupational medicine,* ed 2, Boston, 1992, Little, Brown, pp. 147-170.

List of ten leading work-related diseases and injuries, Atlanta, Ga., 1988, NIOSH.

LoBiondo-Wood G and Haber J: *Nursing research: methods, critical appraisal, and utilization,* ed 3, St. Louis, 1994, Mosby.

Lusk SL: Linking practice and research, *AAOHN J* 41(3):153-157, 1993.

Lusk SL: Corporate expectations for occupational health nurses' activities, *AAOHN J* 38(8): 368-374, 1990.

Lusk SL, Disch JM, and Barkauskas VH: Barriers to advanced education for occupational health nurses, *AAOHN J* 36(11):457-463, 1988.

Maciag ME: Occupational health nursing in the 1990s: a different model of practice, *AAOHN J* 41(1):39-45, 1993.

Markolf AS: Industrial nursing begins in Vermont, *Pub Health Nursing* 37:125-129, 1945.

Martin G: New roles for the occupational health nurse, *Job Safety and Health* 5(4):9-15, 1977.

McCall B: How West Germany protects its workers, *Job Safety and Health* 5(7):21-25, 1977.

McCunney RJ: Occupational exposure to noise. In Rom WR: *Environmental and occupational medicine,* ed 2, Boston, 1992, Little, Brown, pp. 1121-1132.

McGovern P and Matter D: Work and family: competing demands affecting worker well being, *AAOHN J* 40(1):24-35, 1992.

McGrath BJ: *Nursing in commerce and industry,* New York, 1946, The Commonwealth Fund.

McGrath BJ: Fifty years of industrial nursing in the United States, *Publ Health Nursing* 37:119-124, 1945.

McGuire JL: Hearing conservation and employee conservation. In Hansen DJ, ed: *The work environment: occupational health fundamentals,* volume 1, Chelsea, Mich., 1991, Lewis, pp. 209-240.

McNeely E: Tracking the future of OSHA, *AAOHN J* 40(1):17-23, 1992.

Morris LD: Minorities, jobs, and health, *AAOHN J* 37:53-55, 1989.

Morris R: *The American worker,* Washington, D.C., 1976, U.S. Government Printing Office.

Moses M: Pesticide related health problems and farm workers, *AAOHN J* 37(1)115-130, 1989.

Moss L: Mental health and the changing workplace environment. In Rom WR: *Environmental and occupational medicine,* ed 2, Boston, 1992, Little, Brown, pp. 667-684.

Murphy DC: The primary care role in occupational health nursing, *AAOHN J* 37:470-474, 1989.

National Association of Community Health Centers, Inc.: *Community and migrant health centers: a key component of the U.S. health care system—overview and status report 1991,* Washington, D.C., 1991, The Association.

National Institute of Occupational Safety and Health (NIOSH): *The national survey of workplace health promotion activities,* Washington, D.C., 1987, NIOSH.

NIOSH: *Proposed national strategies for the prevention of leading work-related diseases and injuries: occupational lung diseases* (NIOSH Publication No. 89-128), Cincinnati, Oh., 1986, NIOSH Publications.

NIOSH: *Proposed national strategies for the prevention of leading work-related diseases and injuries: musculoskeletal injuries* (NIOSH Publication No. 89-129), Cincinnati, Oh., 1986, NIOSH Publications.

NIOSH: *Proposed national strategies for the prevention of leading work-related diseases and injuries: occupational cancers* (NIOSH Publication No. 89-130), Cincinnati, Oh., 1986, NIOSH Publications.

NIOSH: *Proposed national strategies for the prevention of leading work-related diseases and injuries: severe occupational traumatic injuries and diseases* (NIOSH Publication No. 89-131), Cincinnati, Oh., 1986, NIOSH Publications.

NIOSH: *Proposed national strategies for the prevention of leading work-related diseases and injuries: occupational cardiovascular diseases* (NIOSH Publication No. 89-132), Cincinnati, Oh., 1986, NIOSH Publications.

NIOSH: *Proposed national strategies for the prevention of leading work-related diseases and injuries: disorders of reproduction* (NIOSH Publication No. 89-133), Cincinnati, Oh., 1988, NIOSH Publications.

NIOSH: *Proposed national strategies for the prevention of leading work-related diseases and injuries: neurotoxic disorders* (NIOSH Publication No. 89-134), Cincinnati, Oh., 1988, NIOSH Publications.

NIOSH: *Proposed national strategies for the prevention of leading work-related diseases and injuries: noise-induced hearing loss* (NIOSH Publication No. 89-135), Cincinnati, Oh., 1988, NIOSH Publications.

NIOSH: *Proposed national strategies for the prevention of leading work-related diseases and injuries: dermatological conditions* (NIOSH Publication No. 89-136), Cincinnati, Oh., 1988, NIOSH Publications.

NIOSH: *Proposed national strategies for the prevention of leading work-related diseases and injuries: psychological disorders* (NIOSH Publication No. 89-137), Cincinnati, Oh., 1988, NIOSH Publications.

National Safety Council: *Work injury and illness rates 1989,* Chicago, Ill., 1990, The Council.

Nyamathi A and Flaskerud JH: Effectiveness of an AIDS education program on knowledge, attitudes and practices of state employees, *AAOHN J* 37:397-403, 1989.

Office of Technology Assessment: *Preventing illness and injury in the workplace* (OTA Pub No OTA-H-257), Washington, D.C., 1985, U.S. Government Printing Office.

Olson DK and Kochevar L: Occupational health and safety content in baccalaureate nursing programs, *AAOHN J* 37:33-38, 1989.

Ossler CC: Record keeping, *AAOHN J* 36:8-14, 1988.

Parker-Conrad J: A century of practice: occupational health nursing, *AAOHN J* 36:156-161, 1988.

Pinkham J: 100 years of industrial nursing has vastly improved workplace safety, *Occup Safety Health* 57(4):20-23, 1988.

Pravikoff DS: General nursing and occupational health nursing, *AAOHN J* 40(11):531-537, 1992.

Prestholdt C and Holt BA: Balancing baccalaureate student nursing education, *AAOHN J* 37:465-469, 1989.

Randolph SA: Occupational health nursing: a commitment to excellence, *AAOHN J* 36:166-169, 1988.

Rogers B: Research corner: clinical and research awards given at AOHC, *AAOHN J* 40(7): 352-354, 1992.

Rogers B: Research corner: research utilization, *AAOHN J* 40(1):41, 1992.

Rogers B: Occupational health nursing education: curricular content in baccalaureate programs, *AAOHN J* 39(3):101-108, 1991.

Rogers B: Occupational health nursing practice, education and research: challenge for the future, *AAOHN J* 38(11):536-543, 1990.

Rogers B: Establishing research priorities in occupational health nursing, *AAOHN J* 37:493-500, 1989.

Rogers B, Winslow B, and Higgins S: Employee satisfaction with occupational health services, *AAOHN J* 41(2):58-65, 1993.

Rutstein DD, Mullan RJ, Frazier TM, Halperin WE, Melius JM, and Sestito JP: Sentinel health events (occupational): a basis for physician recognition and public health surveillance, *Am J Public Health* 73:1054-1062, 1984.

Sax NI and Lewis RJ: *Dangerous properties of industrial materials,* ed 7, vol 1, New York, 1989, Van Nostrand Reinhold.

Serafini P: Nursing assessment in industry, *Am J Public Health* 66(8):755-760, 1976.

Silberstein C: Nursing research in occupational health, *AAOHN J* 31:9, 1983.

Skovron ML: Epidemiology of occupational injury. In Rom WR: *Environmental and occupational medicine,* ed 2, Boston, 1992, Little, Brown, pp. 725-731.

Sorensen G, Lando H, and Pechacek TF: Promoting smoking cessation at the workplace: results of a randomized controlled intervention study, *J Occ Med* 35(2):121-126, 1993.

Stellman JM and Daum DM: *Work is dangerous to your health,* New York, 1973, Vintage Books.

Stevenson JS: *Issues and crisis during middlescence,* New York, 1977, Appleton-Century-Crofts.

Taylor WA, Mair A, and Burns W: Study of noise and hearing in jute weaving, *Acoustical Society of America* 48:524-530, 1965.

Tucker SB and Key MM: Occupational skin disease. In Rom WR: *Environmental and occupational medicine,* ed 2, Boston, 1992, Little, Brown, pp. 551-560.

Ubell E: How dangerous is your job? *Parade* January 8, 1989, pp. 4-7.

U.S. Department of Health, Education and Welfare: *Healthy People,* Washington, D.C., 1979, U.S. Government Printing Office.

U.S. Department of Health and Human Services (USDHHS): *Promoting health, preventing disease: objectives for the nation,* Washington, D.C., 1980, U.S. Government Printing Office.

USDHHS: *Promoting health/preventing disease: a midcourse review,* Washington, D.C., 1986, U.S. Government Printing Office.

USDHHS: *The national health survey of workplace health promotion activities,* Washington, D.C., 1987, U.S. Government Printing Office.

USDHHS: *Healthy People 2000: health promotion and disease prevention objectives for the nation, full report, with commentary,* Washington, D.C., 1991, U.S. Government Printing Office.

USDHHS: *NIOSH publications on noise and hearing: criteria for a recommended standard—occupational exposure to noise,* Cincinnati, Oh., 1991, NIOSH.

U.S. Department of Labor: *Labor firsts in America,* Washington, D.C., 1977, U.S. Government Printing Office.

Waters Y: Industrial nursing, *Publ Health Nursing* 11:728-731, 1919.

Watkins EL, Larson K, Harlan C, and Young S: A model program for providing health services for migrant farmworker mothers and children, *Pub Health Reports* 105(6):567-576, 1990.

Widtfeldt AK: Quality and quality improvement in occupational health nursing, *AAOHN J* 40(7):326-332, 1992.

Wright FS: *Industrial nursing,* New York, 1919, MacMillan.

Selected Bibliography

Brodeur P: *Expendable Americans,* New York, 1974, Viking.

Brown ML: *Occupational health nursing: principles and practice,* New York, 1981, Springer.

Brown ML and Meigs JW: Occupational health nursing services, *Industrial Medicine and Surgery* 24:84-88, 1955.

Charley IH: *The birth of industrial nursing,* Baltimore, 1954, Williams and Wilkins.

Felton JS: Teaching occupational health at the secondary level, *J Occup Med* 23:27-29, 1981.

Finn PL Occupational safety and health education in the public schools: rationale, goals, and implementation, *Preventive Med* 7(3):245-249, 1978.

Garvey J: At the workplace: the OHN and hearing conservation, *Nurs Times* 79:25-27, October 5, 1983.

Goldstein DH: The occupational safety and health act of 1970, *Am J Nurs* 71:1535-1538, 1971.

Goldwater LJ: From Hippocrates to Ramazzini, *Annals of Medical History* 8:27, 1936.

Hart BG: The aging work force: challenges for the occupational health nurse, *AAOHN J* 40(1):36-40, 1992.

Lee JA: *The new nurse in industry* (NIOSH Pub), Washington, D.C., 1978, U.S. Government Printing Office.

Page JA and O'Brien MW: *Bitter wages,* New York, 1973, Grossman.

Scott R: *Muscle and blood,* New York, 1974, Duncan.

Selleck CS, Sirles AT, and Newman KD: Health promotion at the workplace, *AAOHN J* 37:412-422, 1989.

Sluchak TJ: Ergonomics: Origins, focus and implementation considerations, *AAOHN J* 40(3): 105-112, 1992.

U.S. Department of Labor: *Important events in American labor history, 1778-1975,* Washington, D.C., 1976, U.S. Government Printing Office.

APPENDIX 17-1

Assessment Guide for Nursing in Industry: a Model

1. Community in which industry is located

    a. Description of the community
       (1) Size in area and population

       (2) Climate, altitude, rainfall

       (3) Pollution (noise, radiation, etc.)

       (4) Housing

       (5) Transportation

       (6) Schools

1. Just as industry affects the community, so the community affects industry.

    a. Use three or four key descriptive words.
       (1) How far do the employees travel to work and are the workers neighbors?

       (2) Are there times or seasons that are more hazardous than others?

       (3) Can the workers' dermatitis or hearing loss be attributed to the community or is it work related?

       (4) Is there adequate, safe housing in the area? Must the worker spend too great a percentage of his or her salary on housing?

       (5) Is there safe, adequate transportation to work as well as to a hospital or school?

       (6) Do children have to be bused to school or attend overcrowded classes?

Continued

Assessment Guide for Nursing in Industry: a Model—cont'd

(7) Sanitation

(8) Protection: fire, police, etc.

(9) Trends

b. Population

    (1) Age distribution

    (2) Sex distribution

    (3) Ethnic and religious composition

    (4) Socioeconomic characteristics

c. Health information

    (1) Vital statistics

    (2) *Disease incidence and prevalence*

    (3) *Health facilities available*

    (4) Community resources

2. The company

a. Historical development

b. Organizational chart

c. *Policies*

    (1) Length of the work week

    (2) Length of work time

    (3) *Sick leave*

    (4) *Safety and fire provisions*

d. Support services (benefits)

    (1) Insurance programs

    (2) Retirement program

    (3) Educational support

    (4) Safety committee

---

(7) Are roaches and rats common to the area?

(8) Are the workers and the industry protected?

(9) Is the area becoming more urban? Residential? Rundown? Deserted?

b. How alike or different is the population of the industry from that of the community?

    (1) Are the families of child-rearing age or of retirement age?

    (2) Are there more men or more women?

    (3) Are there certain customs or languages that are predominant in the community?

    (4) What is the level of education of the community? What is the mean community income?

c. Is it an ill or well community?

    (1) What is the infant mortality rate, birth rate, average life expectancy? Usually the local health department has this information.

    (2) *What are the leading causes of morbidity and mortality?*

    (3) *What physical facilities and professional services are available?*

    (4) Are there day-care centers, drug rehabilitation facilities, Alcoholics Anonymous groups, etc.?

2. The official name and address of the company.

a. Get a perspective on how, why, and by whom the company was founded and compare it with the present situation.

b. What is the formal order of the system and to whom will the nurse be responsible?

c. *If there is a policy manual, try to obtain a copy. Are the workers aware of the manual?*

    (1) How many days a week does the industry operate?

    (2) Are there several shifts? Breaks? Is there paid vacation?

    (3) Is there a clear policy, and do the workers know it?

    (4) Is management aware of situations or substances in the plant which represent danger? Are there organized fire drills? *The Federal Register* is the source of information for federal standards and serves as a helpful guide.

d. What is the attitude of management concerning worker benefits?

    (1) *Is there a system for health insurance and life insurance, and is it compulsory?* Does the company pay all or part? *Who fills out the necessary forms?*

    (2) Are the benefits realistic?

    (3) Can the worker further his or her education? Will the company help financially?

    (4) The programmed Red Cross First Aid course is excellent. For information consult your Red Cross. *If there is no committee, do certain people routinely handle emergencies?*

Assessment Guide for Nursing in Industry: a Model—cont'd

(5) Recreation committee

e. Relations between worker and management

f. Projection for the future

3. The plant

a. General physical setting
   (1) The construction

   (2) Parking facilities and public transportation stops
   (3) Entrances and exits

   (4) Physical environment

   (5) Communication facilities
   (6) Housekeeping
   (7) Interior decoration

b. The work areas

   (1) Space
   (2) Heights: workplace and supply areas

   (3) Stimulation
   (4) Safety signs and markings
   (5) Standing and sitting facilities

   (6) Safety equipment

c. Nonwork areas
   (1) Lockers

   (2) Hand-washing facilities

   (3) Rest rooms

   (4) Drinking water

   (5) Recreation and rest facilities

(5) Do the workers have any communication with or interest in each other outside the work setting?

e. This is difficult information to get, but it is important to know how each perceives the other.

f. If the company is growing, workers may see themselves as having a secure future; if not, they may be worried about their job security. How will plant expansion affect the need for nursing services?

3. Draw a small map to scale, labeling the areas. When an accident occurs, place a pin in the exact location on your map. Different-color pinheads can be used for keeping statistics.

a. What is the gross appearance?
   (1) What is the size and general condition of buildings and grounds?
   (2) How far does the worker have to walk to get inside?

   (3) How many people must use them? How accessible are they?
   (4) Comment on heating, air conditioning, lighting glare, drafts, etc.
   (5) Are there bulletin boards, newsletters?
   (6) Is the physical setting maintained adequately?
   (7) Are the surroundings conducive to work? Are they pleasing?

b. Get permission to examine them. Use *The Federal Register* as a guide.
   (1) Are workers isolated or crowded?
   (2) *Falls and falling objects are dangerous and costly to industry.*
   (3) Is the worker too bored to pay attention?
   (4) Is danger well marked?
   (5) Are chairs safe and comfortable? Are there platforms to stand on, especially for wet processes?
   (6) Do the workers make use of hard hats, safety glasses, face masks, radiation badges, etc.? Do they know the safety devices the OSHA regulations require?

c. Where are they located? Is there easy access?
   (1) If the work is dirty, workers should be able to change clothes. Are they taking toxic substances home?
   (2) If facilities and supplies are available, do workers know how and when to wash their hands?
   (3) How accessible are they and what condition are they in?
   (4) Can a worker leave the job long enough to get a drink of water when he or she wants to?
   (5) Can a worker who is not feeling well lie down? Do workers feel free to use the facilities?

Continued

(6) Telephones

(6) Can a worker receive or make a call? Does a working mother have to stay home because she can't be reached at work?

(7) Ashtrays

(7) Are people allowed to smoke in designated areas? Is it safe?

4. The working population

4. Include worker and management, but separate data for comparison.

  a. General characteristics

  a. Be as accurate as possible, but estimate when necessary.

    (1) *Total number of employees*

    (1) Usually, if an industry has 500 or more employees, full-time nursing services are necessary.

    (2) General appearances

    (2) Heights, weights, cleanliness, etc.

    (3) *Age and sex distribution*

    (3) Certain screening programs are specific for young adults whereas others are more for the elderly. Some programs are more for women; others are more for men. Is there any difference between day and evening shift? Are the problems of the minority sex unattended?

    (4) Race distribution

    (4) Does one race predominate? How does this compare with the general community?

    (5) Socioeconomic distribution

    (5) Great differences in worker salaries can sometimes cause problems.

    (6) Religious distribution

    (6) Does one religion predominate? Are religious holidays observed?

    (7) Ethnic distribution
    (8) Marital status

    (7) Is there a language barrier?
    (8) Widowed, single, divorced people often have different needs.

    (9) *Educational backgrounds*
    (10) Life-styles practiced

    (9) *Can all teaching be done at approximately the same level?*
    (10) Are certain life-styles frowned upon?

  b. Type of employment offered

  b. What percentage of the work force is blue-collar and what percentage is white-collar?

    (1) Background necessary

    (1) What educational level is required? Skilled vs. unskilled?

    (2) Work demands on physical condition
    (3) Work status

    (2) Stength needed: sedentary vs. active.
    (3) Part-time vs. full-time; overtime?

  c. Absenteeism

  c. Is there a record kept? By whom? Why?

    (1) *Causes*
    (2) Length

    (1) *What are the five most common reasons for absence?*
    (2) Absenteeism is costly to the employer. There is some difference between one 10-day absence and ten 1-day absences by the same person.

  d. Physically handicapped

  d. Does the company have a policy about hiring the handicapped?

    (1) Number employed
    (2) *Extent of handicaps*

    (1) Where do they work? What do they do?
    (2) Are they specially trained? Are they in a special program? Do they use prosthetic devices?

  e. Personnel on medication
  f. Personnel with chronic illness

  e. Know what medication and where the employee works.
  f. At what stage of illness is the employee? Where does the employee work? Will he or she be able to continue at this job?

5. The industrial process
  a. Equipment used
    (1) General description of placement

5. What does the company produce and how?
  a. Portable vs. fixed; light vs. heavy.
    (1) Mark each piece of large equipment on the scale map.

    (2) Type of equipment

    (2) Fans, blowers, fast moving, wet or dry.

Assessment Guide for Nursing in Industry: a Model—cont'd

b. Nature of the operation

    (1) *Raw materials used*

    (2) Nature of the final product

    (3) Description of the jobs
    (4) Waste products produced

c. *Exposure to toxic substances*

d. Faculties required throughout the industrial process

6. The health program

  a. Existing policies
    (1) Objectives of the program
    (2) *Preemployment physicals*

    (3) First-aid facilities
    (4) *Standard orders*

    (5) *Job descriptions for health personnel*
  b. Existing facilities and resources

    (1) Trained personnel
    (2) Space

    (3) *Supplies*
    (4) *Records and reports*

  c. *Services rendered in the past year*
    (1) Care needed
    (2) Screening done
    (3) Referrals made
    (4) Counseling done
    (5) Health education

  d. *Accidents in the past year*

  e. *Reasons employees sought health care*

b. Get a brief description of each state of the process so that you can compare the needs and abilities of the worker with the needs of the job.

    (1) *What are they and how dangerous are they? Are they properly stored?* Check *The Federal Register* for guidelines on storage.
    (2) Can the workers take pride in the final product or do they make parts?
    (3) Who does what? Where? Label the map.
    (4) What is the system for waste disposal? Are the pollution control devices in place and functioning?

c. *Describe the toxins to which the worker is exposed and the extent of exposure.* Include physical and emotional hazards. Remember that chronic effects of industrial exposure are subtle; a person often gets used to having mild symptoms and won't report them. *The Federal Register* contains specifications for exposure to toxins and some states issue state standards.

d. The need for speed, hearing, color vision, etc., can help determine the types of screening programs necessary.

6. Outline what is actually in existence as well as what employees perceive to be in existence.
  a. Are there informal, unwritten policies?
    (1) Are they clear?
    (2) Are they required? Are they paid for by the company? Is the information used to deselect?
    (3) What is available? What is not available?
    (4) Is there a company physician who is responsible for first aid or emergency policy? If so, work closely with him or her in planning nursing services.
    (5) If there are no guidelines to be followed, write some.

  b. Sometimes an industry that denies having a health program has more of a system than it realizes.
    (1) *Who responds in an emergency?*
    (2) Where is the sick worker taken? Where is the emergency equipment kept?
    (3) *Make a list and describe the condition* of each item.
    (4) What exists? The Occupational Safety and Health Act requires that employers keep three types of records: a log of occupational injuries and illnesses, a supplemental record of certain illnesses or injuries, and an annual summary (forms 100, 101, and 102 are provided under the act). Good records provide data for good planning.

  c. Describe as specifically as possible.
    (1) Chronic or acute? Why?
    (2) Where? By whom? Why?
    (3) By whom? To whom? Why?
    (4) Often informal counseling goes unnoticed.
    (5) What individual or group education was offered by the company?

  d. Including those occurring after work hours, as some of these accidents may be directly or indirectly work-related.

  e. List the five major reasons.

From Serafini P: Nursing assessment in industry, *Am J Public Health* 66(8):755-760, 1976. (Author's name is now P. Serafini Blanco.)

The Adult Who is Handicapped

OBJECTIVES

Upon completion of this chapter, the reader should be able to:

1. Summarize five national health objectives for chronic disabling conditions.
2. Distinguish between the terms *chronic condition, disability,* and *handicap.*
3. Discuss the concepts of normalization and mainstreaming.
4. Explain individual, family, and societal variables that influence adaptation to a handicap.
5. Discuss the grieving process in relation to chronic conditions.
6. Identify the critical elements of chronic sorrow.

7. Describe areas of major concern for persons with a handicap.
8. Discuss the role of community health nurses when working with adults who are handicapped.
9. Identify community resources that provide services to people who are handicapped.
10. Identify legislation that provides health care resources and services for adults who are handicapped.

When one is working with people who are handicapped, it must be remembered that first they are people and, secondary to that, they have a handicapping condition.

From early in recorded time people have noted the handicapping conditions among them. Handicapping conditions were recorded as early as the fourth century BC (Buscaglia, 1983, p. 152). Hippocrates, Aristotle, Galen, and other ancient Greeks studied such conditions and sought explanations for their existence. In early times many people who were handicapped died in childhood and few lived to adulthood.

Throughout history societies have dealt in various ways with members who were handicapped. Attitudes toward the handicapped have ranged from acceptance to rejection and from understanding to fear. The Elizabethan Poor Law of 1601 (refer to Chapter 4) equated handicapping conditions with crime and under this law people who were handicapped were often disenfranchised, publicly punished, and imprisoned (Sussman, 1966, p. 3). The classic story of the *Hunchback of Notre Dame* illustrates society's reaction to disfigurement during the eighteenth century.

Today being handicapped is no longer considered criminal. However, people who are handicapped may arouse anxiety and discomfort in others and be socially stigmatized and isolated. Like other minority groups, people who are handicapped have been subjected to various forms of social prejudice and discrimination.

The World Health Organization estimates that 10% of the world's population, 400 million people, are disabled (Frye, 1993, p. 43). It is estimated that there are 43 million disabled Americans (USDHHS, 1991, p. 40). Malnutrition, communicable diseases, inadequate prenatal care, untreated trauma, and genetic, environmental, and personal risk factors all play a role in the etiology of disabilities (Frye, p. 43-44).

Approximately 10% of Americans are limited in activity because of a disabling condition (USDHHS, 1991, p. 40). Figure 18-1 shows that, although the prevalence of disabling conditions increases with age, these conditions occur across the lifespan. Chronic disabling conditions are a serious health problem for Americans, and preventing these conditions is part of the *Healthy People 2000* national health objectives.

HEALTHY PEOPLE 2000 AND CHRONIC DISABLING CONDITIONS

Of the 10 leading causes of death in the United States, eight of them are chronic disabling conditions or have potential to cause such conditions. *Healthy*

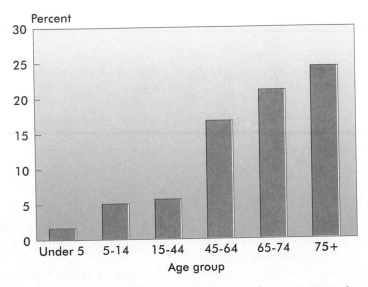

Figure 18-1 Percentage of people experiencing limitation of major activity due to disability. (From USDHHS: *Healthy People 2000: national health promotion and disease prevention objectives, full report, with commentary,* Washington, D.C., 1991, U.S. Government Printing Office, p. 41.)

◀ Healthy People 2000: *Chronic Disabling Conditions* ▶

1. Increase years of healthy life to at least 65 years.
2. Reduce to no more than 8 percent the proportion of people who experience a limitation in major activity due to chronic conditions.
3. Reduce to no more than 90 per 1,000 people the proportion of all people aged 65 and older who have difficulty in performing two or more personal care activities, thereby preserving independence.
4. Reduce to no more than 10 percent the proportion of people with asthma who experience activity limitation.
5. Reduce activity limitation due to chronic back conditions to a prevalence of no more than 19 per 1,000 people.
6. Reduce significant hearing impairment to a prevalence of no more than 82 per 1,000 people.
7. Reduce significant visual impairment to a prevalence of no more than 30 per 1,000 people.
8. Reduce the prevalence of serious mental retardation in school-aged children to no more than 2 per 1,000 children.
9. Reduce diabetes-related deaths to no more than 34 per 100,000 people.
10. Reduce the most severe complications of diabetes as follows:

End-stage renal disease	1.4/1,000
Blindness	1.4/1,000
Lower extremity amputation	4.9/1,000
Perinatal mortality	2%
Major congenital malformations	4%

11. Reduce diabetes to an incidence of no more than 2.5 per 1,000 people and a prevalence of no more than 25 per 1,000 people.
12. Reduce overweight to a prevalence of no more than 20 percent among people aged 20 and older and no more than 15 percent among adolescents aged 12 through 19.
13. Increase to at least 30 percent the proportion of people aged 6 and older who engage regularly, preferably daily, in light to moderate physical activity for at least 30 minutes per day.
14. Increase to at least 40 percent the proportion of people with chronic and disabling conditions who receive formal patient education including information about community and self-help resources as an integral part of the management of their condition.
15. Increase to at least 80 percent the proportion of providers of primary care for children who routinely refer or screen infants and children for impairments of vision, hearing, speech and language and assess other developmental milestones as part of well-child care.
16. Reduce the age at which children with significant hearing impairment are identified to no more than 12 months.
17. Increase to at least 60 percent the proportion of providers of primary care for older adult who routinely evaluate people aged 65 and older for urinary incontinence and impairments of vision, hearing, cognition, and functional status.
18. Increase to at least 90 percent the proportion of perimenopausal women who have been counseled about the benefits and risks of estrogen replacement therapy for prevention of osteoporosis.
19. Increase to at least 75 percent the proportion of worksites with 50 or more employees that have a voluntary established policy, or program for the hiring of people with disabilities.
20. Increase to 50 the number of States that have service systems for children with or at risk of chronic and disabling conditions.

From USDHHS: *Healthy People 2000: national health promotion and disease prevention objectives, full report, with commentary,* Washington, D.C., 1991, U.S. Government Printing Office, pp. 445-468.

People 2000 has objectives that specifically address chronic disabling conditions; these objectives are given in the box above. Preventive measures to limit the occurrence of these conditions are essential to maximize the potential of the individual, family, community, and society.

CHRONIC AND HANDICAPPING CONDITIONS: RELATED BUT DISTINCT PHENOMENA

People under the age of 18 are most likely to have disabilities associated with mental impairment, asthma, mental illness, deafness, hearing disorders, and speech impairments; young adults are more likely to have orthopedic and back impairments; and at older ages degenerative diseases such as arthritis and heart disease are prevalent (USDHHS, 1992, p. 23). It is important to remember that *not* all chronic conditions are handicapping. Chronic and handicapping conditions are related yet distinct phenomena.

Chronic Conditions

From a classic perspective, chronic conditions were defined in Chapter 11 as impairments or deviations from normal that have at least one of the following characteristics: permanency, residual disability, irreversible pathological causation and alteration, need for special rehabilitation and training, and need for a period of long-term supervision and care (Commission on Chronic Illness, 1957, p. 4). Chronic conditions include diseases such as cancer, heart disease, diabetes, cerebral palsy, deafness, speech or visual impairment, drug addiction, alcoholism, epilepsy, spinal cord injury, mental or emotional illness, mental retardation, multiple sclerosis, muscular dystrophy, orthopedic impairment, and perceptual handicaps such as dyslexia, brain dysfunction, and developmental aphasia.

Chronic conditions can cause functional limitations and adversely affect an individual's ability to carry out one or more major life activities such as communication, ambulation, self-care, socialization, education, vocational training, transportation, housing, and employment. Chronic conditions often become disabling, and heart disease, orthopedic conditions, arthritis, emphysema, and mental retardation are chronic conditions with high rates of disability (refer to Table 18-1). Chronic conditions may become handicapping conditions, according to the following schema of disease (WHO, 1981, p. 8):

Disease/condition → impairment →
disability → handicap

A chronic condition becomes a handicap based on the *level of disability* it imposes on an individual.

What is Disability?

The World Health Organization (1981, p. 8) has defined a disability as any restriction or lack of ability to perform an activity in the manner, or within the range, considered to be normal for a human being. In 1990 the *Americans with Disabilities Act (ADA)* defined a

disability as a physical or mental impairment that substantially limits one or more of an individual's major life activities. Included in this definition are individuals who have a record of an impairment or are regarded as having such an impairment. Chronic conditions can encompass the entire range of disability. For example, the person with cerebral palsy may evidence functional abilities ranging from independence to total dependence. Figure 18-2 illustrates some functional limitations of adults with disabilities.

The level of disability is determined by combining the results of multiple assessment, including clinical evaluation, use of standardized performance tests and scales, assessment of client and family perceptions and knowledge, and measurement of ability to carry out activities of daily living (ADL). While definitions for levels of disability vary among disciplines, the majority of these definitions include ADL and employment abilities. Below are four general levels of disability, taking into consideration ADL and employment abilities:

Level I: Partial disability characterized by slight limitation in one or more of the major life activities; able to take part in school, competitive employment, and self-care

Level II: Partial disability characterized by moderate limitation in one or more of the major life activities; generally able to attend school, work regularly or part-time (but the employment may need to be modified); may need assistance with self-care

Level III: Partial disability characterized by severe limitation in one or more of the major life activities; usually unable to attend school or work regularly (considered occupationally disabled); often requires assistance with self-care

Level IV: Total disability characterized by complete, or almost complete, dependency on others for activities of daily living, self-care, and economic support; usually unable to work or attend regular school

When a chronic condition becomes severely disabling and it substantially limits an individual's ability to carry out normal life functions, it becomes a handicapping condition.

Handicapping Conditions

A *handicap* is a condition that *substantially* limits one or more of an individual's major life activities and

18-1   Conditions with Highest Risk of Disability

Chronic condition	Number of conditions (1,000s)	Percent causing activity limitation	Rank	Percent causing major activity limitation	Rank	Percent causing need for help in basic life activities	Rank
Mental retardation	1,202	84.1	1	80.0	1	19.9	9
Absence of leg(s)	289	83.3	2	73.1	2	39.0	2
Lung or bronchial cancer	200	74.8	3	63.5	3	34.5	4
Multiple sclerosis	171	70.6	4	63.3	4	40.7	1
Cerebral palsy	274	69.7	5	62.2	5	22.8	8
Blind in both eyes	396	64.5	6	58.8	6	38.1	3
Partial paralysis in extremity	578	59.6	7	47.2	7	27.5	5
Other orthopedic impairments (not in back or extremities)	316	58.7	8	46.2	8	14.3*	12
Complete paralysis in extremity	617	52.7	9	45.5	9	26.1	6
Rheumatoid arthritis	1,223	51.0	10	39.4	12	14.9	11
Intervertebral disk disorders	3,987	48.7	11	38.2	14	5.3	—
Paralysis in other sites (complete/partial)	247	47.8	12	43.7	10	14.1*	13
Other heart disease/disorders†	4,708	46.9	13	35.1	15	13.6	14
Cancer of digestive sites	228	45.3	14	40.3	11	15.9*	10
Emphysema	2,074	43.6	15	29.8	—	9.6	15
Absence of arm(s)/hand(s)	84	43.1	—	39.0	13	4.1*	—
Cerebrovascular disease	2,599	38.2	—	33.3	—	22.9	7

*Figure has low statistical reliability or precision (relative standard error exceeds 30 percent).
†Heart failure (9.8%) valve disorders (15.3%), congenital disorders (15.0%), all other and ill-defined heart conditions (59.9%).
NOTE: Data are estimates (annual averages) based on household interviews of the civilian noninstitutionalized population.
From National Health Interview Survey, 1983-1986. As cited in Disability risks of chronic illnesses and impairments, *Disability Stat Bull* 2(Fall):2, 1989.

fulfillment of normal roles (President's Committee on Employment of the Handicapped, 1978; WHO, 1981). A handicap will often cause physical and emotional pain, discomfort, and expenditure of a great deal of time, effort, and money (Buscaglia, 1983, p. 14). The level of disability caused by a handicapping condition is used to determine client needs, intervention strategies, and appropriate community resources. Individuals with handicapping conditions have complex social, emotional, physical, educational, and financial needs that may involve redefining family and community roles, relationships, and responsibilities.

Mainstreaming and Normalization

When discussing the person who is handicapped the concepts of mainstreaming and normalization are used. Recent legislation, such as the Americans with Disabilities Act of 1990, has helped to assure the rights of Americans with disabilities and has assisted them in living as normal a life as possible in the community.

Mainstreaming refers to integrating the person who is handicapped into the everyday life of the community. The person functions in the "mainstream" of the community and is not separated from it. Many people who are handicapped are already in the mainstream of the community and are difficult to distinguish from the community's nonhandicapped members. For others, special efforts need to be taken for this integration to occur.

Normalization refers to assisting persons who are handicapped to live as normal a life as possible. Normalization assists people in participating in the same activities of daily living as other members of the

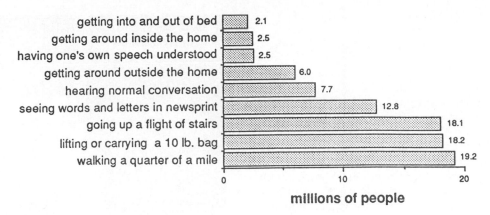

Figure 18-2   Functional limitation of adults with disabilities. (From Kraus LE and Stoddard S: *Chartbook on disability in the United States, an InfoUse Report,* Washington, D.C., 1989, National Institute on Disability and Rehabilitation Research, p. 3.)

community such as employment, home maintenance, school, and social and recreational activities.

Mainstreaming and normalization focus on maximizing the strengths of people who are handicapped and enhancing their quality of life. Successful implementation requires interdisciplinary planning, care management, appropriate community resources, and recognition that people who are handicapped are entitled to the same rights and respect as everyone else. Normalization and mainstreaming reinforce the philosophy that people who are handicapped are "people first," and that secondarily they have a handicapping condition.

ADAPTATION TO A HANDICAP

Adaptation to a handicap is a complex process and is influenced by individual, family, community, and societal variables. How these variables interact with each other will determine how well the individual and family adapts to the handicap.

Societal Attitudes toward People Who Are Handicapped

Society creates handicaps (Buscaglia, 1983), and societal attitudes toward people who are handicapped play a major role in individual and family adaptation to the handicapping condition. In fact, the debilitating aspects of a handicap result not so much from the condition itself but from the manner in which others

define and respond to it (Hahn, 1988). Societal attitudes often make people uncomfortable in communicating with people who are handicapped (Penrose, 1983; University of Michigan, 1981), which increases their social isolation.

Many societal attitudes toward people who are handicapped are negative and nonfacilitative. Lack of knowledge and misconceptions about the etiology, treatment, and prognosis of handicapping conditions can lead to such attitudes. People who are handicapped are often characterized as being helpless, suffering, dependent, and emotionally unstable, and may be held at least partially responsible for their disability (Seifert, 1981). Buscaglia (1983) described an interesting study in relation to such attitudes. In the study, nonhandicapped people were viewed in two different situations: 1) in a wheelchair or with leg braces, giving the impression of being handicapped, and 2) without the wheelchair or leg braces in a normal situation. In the first instance the individual was described as helpless, hopeless, and of decreased value; however, the same person in the second situation was described positively. Studies have shown that even people with handicapping conditions have negative attitudes toward people who are handicapped (Dixon, 1977, p. 308), and that handicapping conditions pose a serious threat to one's self-image.

Societal attitudes have been described as "invisible barriers" (Kendrick, 1983, p. 17). The impact of these barriers is seen in the quote from Deborah Kendrick, a mother who is blind:

Figure 18-3 Societal attitudes influence how individuals, families, and groups perceive differences among individuals in a society and can either facilitate or inhibit individual growth and development. (Courtesy Donald Sims and photographer H. Morgan Smith, Explorations, Brigade Quartermasters. Morgan Smith has more than 30 years membership in the Explorers Club, is an honorary member of the Choco Indian tribe, and is an anthropologist and naturalist who has conducted numerous archeological excavations.)

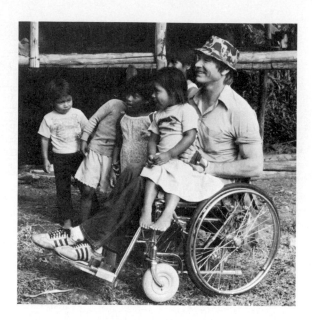

The difficulty is neither in being blind nor in being a mother. It is in the attitudes of others, the *invisible barriers* which can separate me from other mothers and my children from their children. (Kendrick, p. 18)

Handicapping conditions are viewed differently by various cultures, as is shown in the example of Donald Sims (refer to Figure 18-3), who has impaired functioning of his lower extremities following a motorcycle accident. He found that when he visited the Choco Indians in Panama his strengths were respected and his differences accepted. The attitudes of the Choco Indians helped him to realize his potential, and Sims stated:

An unbelievable experience! They treated me as though I was no different—I was accepted as a person—a people, a culture with no concept of handicapped. I did what I could, they did their thing, and we all worked and played together. No one shied away from the chair. The Choco Indians made my Panama trip the most wonderful experience since my accident. They helped reinstate my faith in people, life itself, and a positive attitude toward all things.

Safilios-Rothschild (1982), in her classic work on the handicapped, identified a number of variables that affect the attitudes a society has toward people who are handicapped. These variables are presented in the box on p. 709; people who are handicapped have many negative societal attitudes to overcome. Societal attitudes have a significant impact on the residential, educational, occupational, health, and/or social ser-

vices available to the person who is handicapped in the community.

Too often people look at individuals who are handicapped in terms of their limitations, not their strengths. The nurse can facilitate building on these strengths and assist the community in gaining a realistic understanding of handicapping conditions through health education activities in settings such as schools and workplaces. For example, it is not uncommon for children in classroom settings to encounter peers who deviate from what is defined as "normal." A sensitive teacher and school nurse can help children to accept peers who are different, understand why these differences exist, and promote normalization and mainstreaming. Nurses can help to facilitate more positive societal attitudes toward people who are handicapped, serve as client advocates, and be instrumental in the passage of disability legislation.

Individual and Family Variables Influencing Adaptation to a Handicap

In addition to societal variables, individual and family variables also affect adaptation to a handicap. Because these variables interact, it is difficult to separate the effects of one from another.

The Family with a Handicapped Member

The family plays a key role in rehabilitation outcomes (Reeber, 1992, p. 332; Watson, 1992, p. 51;

Variables Affecting Societal Attitudes toward People Who Are Handicapped

Beliefs regarding the value of physical and mental integrity

The value a society places on physical and mental integrity will greatly affect societal acceptance of people who are handicapped and the scope of services offered to them. If a society highly values physical and mental integrity and "devalues" people who are handicapped, they may experience prejudice, discrimination, and be isolated from the mainstream of society in placements such as institutions for the mentally ill and mentally retarded and other long-term care facilities.

Beliefs in relation to illness

In most societies, people who are acutely ill are usually allowed to be "sick" for the duration of their illness. However, once the condition becomes chronic the person may be expected to "adjust," and may even be expected to perform "normally" in relation to societal roles and expectations, even when achieving such behavior may be difficult.

Beliefs regarding condition occurrence

If it is believed that the individual had a high degree of responsibility in the occurrence of the condition, less aid and assistance may be given. Obesity, alcoholism, mental illness, AIDS, domestic violence, and drug abuse are examples of this.

The role of the government in alleviating social problems

If a society does not believe that the government should assume an active role in alleviating social problems, there may be little public assistance or social support for people who are handicapped.

Beliefs regarding the origins of poverty

Many people who have handicapping conditions live in poverty. If a society believes that poverty is generally a matter of self-will, there may be less willingness to assist people who are handicapped.

The rate of unemployment and economic development

When unemployment is high and/or the economy is unstable, people who are handicapped may be at a disadvantage in hiring and employment practices; and there may also be less inclination to financially subsidize those who are handicapped.

Modified from Safilios-Rothschild C: *The sociology and social psychology of disability rehabilitation,* New York, 1982, University Press of America, p. 4.

Youngblood and Hines, 1992, p. 325). A nursing assessment that examines the needs of the entire family unit (refer to Chapters 7 and 9) and the family's perception of the disability needs to be done. The family assessment process should include family characteristics and family perceptions of roles, disability, health care, coping skills, and support systems (Youngblood and Hines, p. 325). The box on p. 710 presents some questions that aid in determining family strengths and the family's perception of the disability. Each family will adapt and cope differently. As indicated in Chapter 8, some families are more vulnerable to stress than others, and handicapping conditions can produce stress for the entire family.

When persons become disabled they and their families experience stress (Winterhalter, 1992, p. 23). Research has found that families of persons who are handicapped may be treated as if they are different from other families or somehow to blame for the handicap (Buzinski, 1980). This creates even more

stress and can make it more difficult for families to adjust.

A handicapping condition requires that a family make many decisions regarding family goals and priorities, division of labor, use of time, family roles, allocation of financial resources, and caregiving. For example, parents of handicapped children may not go through "launching" when the child reaches adulthood, and may need to reexamine the goals they had for themselves and their children. Also, families are often forced to organize priorities around the needs of the handicapped member and, frequently, the financial demands of the condition place economic hardships on the family. The availability of appropriate community resources can assist the family in adapting to the handicap and prevent family burnout.

In addition to caring for a handicapped family member, families are expected to carry out other life activities and responsibilities such as school, work, and household maintenance. Despite all this, many

◀ *Assessment of Family's Perception of Disability* ▶

I. Family Characteristics
- What are the biological characteristics of each family member?
- What is the family's cultural/ethnic background?
- What are the socioeconomic resources available to family members?
- What are the personality characteristics of each family member?

II. The Family's Perception of Rules and Roles
- What are the rules that govern family interactions?
- How do family members interact with each other?
- What is the structure of the family unit?
- How are rules and roles assigned?
- What events cause rules and/or roles to change?

III. The Family's Perception of the Disability
- What meaning does the disability have for each family member?
- What responsibility does each member have for the management of the disability?
- How are decisions made about the management of the disability?

- How are family interactions affected by the disability?

IV. The Family's Perception of Health Care
- What experiences have family members had with healthcare systems?
- What experiences with healthcare systems have resulted from the disability?
- What expectations do family members have in regard to the management of the disability?
- How do family members expect to interact with healthcare professionals?

V. The Family's Perception of Coping Skills and Support Systems
- How have family members reacted to crisis in the past?
- What information does the family need about the disability?
- What resources are available to family members?
- What support systems are available to family members?

From Youngblood NM and Hines J: The influence of the family's perception of disability on rehabilitation outcomes, *Rehabilitation Nursing* 17(6):325, 1992. Reprinted from *Rehabilitation Nursing,* Volume 17, Issue 6, with permission of the American Association of Rehabilitation Nurses, 5700 Old Orchard Road, First Floor, Skokie, Ill. 60077-1057. Copyright © 1992 American Association of Rehabilitation Nurses.

families remain the primary caregivers for their handicapped members. As discussed in Chapter 8, this is often stressful to families because they may be required to compromise or accept less than a perfect solution in order to adapt to the situation (McCubbin and McCubbin, 1993). Family caregivers do experience considerable stress, and if the stress becomes too great they may decide to place the handicapped family member outside the home.

Studies have shown that families are more likely to place handicapped members outside the home when the following variables exist: the person is severely disabled; the family structure is incapable of providing adequate time, care, and resources; there is a high level of family conflict and discord, such as marital dissatisfaction; and community support systems are insufficient (Sherman and Cocozza, 1984; Giele, 1984). Supportive interventions can help to alleviate some of the stress the family is experiencing as a result of such variables.

In recent years greater emphasis has been placed on identifying strategies to promote family stability and growth after a handicapping condition has been diagnosed. The *Beach Center on Families and Disabilities* is sponsored by the National Institute on Disabilities and Rehabilitation Research (NIDRR). Its research focuses on individualizing services to families, enhancing family capabilities, and providing advocacy services. For further information contact Beach Center on Families and Disabilities, University of Kansas, Bureau of Child Research, 3136 Haworth Hall, Lawrence, Kansas 66045 (903-864-7600 or 800-854-4938).

Variables Influencing Adaptation

The impact of a handicapping condition on the individual and family is influenced by a number of variables. These variables are listed in the box on p. 711 and discussed here. The variables are not prioritized as this will vary with each family and situation.

◀ *Variables Affecting* ▶
Adaptation to a Handicap

The stage of grief and mourning
Age at which the handicapping condition occurred
Age-appropriateness of the handicap
Rapidity of onset of the handicap
Level of disability caused by the handicap
Visibility of the handicap
Value of the handicapped area
Attitudes regarding self
Attitudes of significant others
Community resources available and used
Coping mechanisms used
Prognosis and/or expected duration of the handicap

◀ *Critical Attributes* ▶
of Chronic Sorrow

There is a perception of sorrow or sadness over time
in a situation that has no predictable end.
The sadness or sorrow is cyclic or recurrent.
The sorrow or sadness is triggered either internally or
externally and brings to mind the person's losses,
disappointment or fears.
The sadness or sorrow is progressive and can intensify
even years after the initial sense of disappointment,
loss or fear.

From Lindgren CL, Burke ML, Hainsworth MA, and Eakes GG:
Chronic sorrow: a lifespan concept, *Scholarly Inquiry for Nursing
Practice: An International Journal* 6(1):31, 1992. Used by permission
of Springer Publishing Company, Inc., New York, 10012.

The *stage of grief and mourning* the individual and family have reached in relation to the handicap is important. The person and family experiencing a handicap have definitely suffered a loss. This loss may take many forms, such as loss of health, independence, control over life, privacy, body image, personal relationships and roles, social status, financial stability, material possessions, and self-fulfillment (Lewis, 1983). It may be compounded by the fact that there may be no immediate end in sight and the individual is grieving personally while experiencing the effects of significant others grieving also (Werner-Beland, 1980). Until grieving has been successfully carried out, rehabilitation and adaptation cannot be fully successful. Unresolved grief can seriously alter and affect interpersonal relationships and family functioning.

Community health nurses play a major role in helping families to experience a healthy grieving process. Being able to accept the fact that *grief is normal* helps the nurse to assist families in working through the process in a constructive manner.

The stages in the grief and mourning process in relation to a handicap closely resemble the stages discussed by Kubler-Ross (1969) when looking at death and dying. The following list describes the grief and mourning process that a person and family go through when adapting to a handicapping condition:

Denial. The individual/family is not prepared to accept the reality and ramifications of the handicap and deny that it is occurring.

Awareness. The individual/family realizes that the handicap is real, the loss becomes real, and feelings of hostility, bitterness, and anger can arise in response to it.

Mourning. The individual/family actively grieves for the loss that has occurred.

Depression. The individual/family realizes the permanency, long-term nature, or other ramifications of the condition and experiences feelings of rejection, helplessness, altered self-esteem, and despair. This is often a very encompassing and time-consuming stage.

Adaptation. The individual/family becomes capable of coping with the handicap. Although periods of depression may occur periodically, the goal of this stage is equilibrium and rehabilitation.

Related to the grieving process is the concept of *chronic sorrow.* Chronic sorrow is a term used to describe the long-term periodic sadness and depression the client and family experience in relation to chronic illness (Lindgren, Burke, Hainsworth, and Eakes, 1992, p. 27). Chronic sorrow is a form of unresolved grieving and its critical attributes are given in the box above. Although it is natural for some chronic sorrow to occur, the nurse should work with the client and family to help achieve grief resolution and promote successful coping and adaptation.

The *age* at which a handicapping condition occurs and the *age-appropriateness* of the condition are also critical to adaptation. Handicapping conditions that occur after the development of personal self-image frequently cause more difficulty with coping and adaptation. A child born without an arm will have a different adjustment process than the child who loses an arm at age 5 or the adult who loses an arm at 50. The internalized body image of the adult makes it difficult to accept, much less incorporate, drastic alterations of body structure (Safilios-Rothschild, 1982, p. 80). An age-appropriate handicap is more easily accepted than one not commonly found among individuals of a particular age group. For example, an elderly person with a hearing impairment or arthritis is often more readily accepted than is a preschooler with the same conditions.

The *rapidity of a condition's onset* is also critical to adjustment. If a condition develops gradually, as does rheumatoid arthritis, the adjustment time is lengthened and there is an opportunity to develop skills, resources, support systems, and coping mechanisms. If the occurrence is sudden, as with traumatic injury, there is little or no adjustment time. Any person needs time to adapt to a condition, and rehabilitation techniques may need to be delayed until adaptation can take place. Sudden change is often difficult to incorporate into one's body image (Safilios-Rothschild, 1982, p. 88). Similarly, a sudden alteration in the image of oneself held by others is difficult to absorb.

The *level of disability* associated with a condition will have a great deal to do with the adjustment the individual/family is able to make. Generally, the higher the level of disability, the more difficult it is to adjust. An individual with a paralyzed hand will likely have less difficulty in adjustment than a paraplegic or a person who is severely mentally retarded. The level of disability will be a major determinant of the functional capacity the individual is able to attain.

The level of disability has an impact on the person's ability to accomplish the age-specific developmental tasks discussed throughout this text. They include such things as establishing an occupation and a companionship lifestyle, utilizing leisure time, and taking part in civic activities. The person who is handicapped is often impeded in accomplishing developmental tasks.

The *visibility* of the condition affects the adjustment made to it. People generally have stronger reactions to visible than to invisible signs and symptoms. Any visible condition will generally elicit more discriminating individual and societal responses than a nonvisible or slightly visible condition.

The *value of the handicapped part* is of major importance. A person becomes more upset when something happens to a part of the body that is highly valued. The value placed on body parts will vary from individual to individual; however, some parts seem to have a higher value than others. Facial disfigurement illustrates well the value placed on certain body parts. Although facial disfigurement causes few physical limitations, it is one of the most difficult handicapping conditions to adjust to because of the high value placed on facial characteristics (Safilios-Rothschild, 1982, p. 126). Conditions that create sexual handicaps are also difficult for most people to accept. The social value placed on body parts or functions significantly affects the type and degree of stigma attached to the handicap.

Attitudes regarding self and the attitudes about oneself held by significant others are critical to the outcome of a handicapping condition. If such attitudes are negative, their impact can be detrimental to the outcome of the condition. Community health nurses, and others in therapeutic roles, should build upon the positive attitudes found and help the client and significant others to analyze why negative attitudes exist. Since attitudes have an important effect on an individual's social and psychological adjustment to his or her handicap, it is crucial for the community health nurse to identify attitudes that may hamper successful adaptation.

Community resources play a key role in handicap outcome. Handicap adjustment is impeded if rehabilitation services are not available, appropriate, or accessible. Rehabilitation is an extremely important concept and will be discussed in a separate section of this chapter.

Coping abilities of the individual and family are very important, and how well the family is able to cope with the handicapping condition will influence the client's recovery and adaptation (Reeber, 1992, p. 333). Using effective coping strategies can moderate the psychological impact of the condition (Miller, 1992, p. 19). Effective coping helps to reduce tension and maintain equilibrium, promote family growth, enhance sound decision-making, maintain autonomy, avoid the use of negative self-evaluation, and control potential stressors before they become a problem (Miller, p. 21). Having good community support systems and appropriate community resources aids the family in successful coping.

The *prognosis* of the condition is an important variable in adaptation. If the long-term prognosis does not show much hope of cure or recovery it can be discouraging, and even devastating, to the client and

◀ ▶ *Some Areas of Concern for the People Who Are Handicapped*

Education
Financial stability
Employment
Access to service
Health care
Social and recreational opportunities
Sexuality
Guardianship
Community residential opportunities
Attendant services
Respite care

family. Conditions where the prognosis is more encouraging make it easier for the family to cope and adapt.

SOME AREAS OF CONCERN FOR PEOPLE WHO ARE HANDICAPPED

Some areas of concern to the person who is handicapped are listed in a box above and discussed here. The degree to which these concerns are evidenced is highly individual.

Education

Historically, people who are handicapped have been at an educational disadvantage in the United States. It was not until 1975 that the federal government enacted a mandatory education law for people who were handicapped. Before this time, if a person did not "fit" into existing local school district programs, the school district was not responsible for the person's education, and many people who were handicapped were denied an education unless their families could afford to send them to private schools. The Education for All Handicapped Children Act of 1975 changed this by providing for educational services for people who are handicapped from the ages of 3 to 21. The law gave parents the right to participate in the educational plan developed for their child. However, once the age of 21 is reached educational opportunities are limited, and this can pose a special hard-

ship for families, especially families with handicapped members who may not be eligible for other training, higher education, or employment (e.g., people who are mentally retarded).

By law the handicapped adult who applies for college entrance, job training, or adult basic education must be considered on academic records and cannot be discriminated against because of the handicap. Also, educational programs cannot limit the number of handicapped students admitted and are required to accommodate the student who is handicapped (e.g., provision of access, translators for the deaf).

Some people who are handicapped utilize homebound instruction to learn a skill or become educated for a career. The U.S. Department of Education recognizes the National Home Study Council (1601 Eighteenth Street, N.W., Washington, D.C. 20009; phone 202-234-5100) and its *Directory of Accredited Home Study Schools* as a resource for locating quality schools of home study. Also, the National Library Service for the Blind and Physically Handicapped has a network of libraries throughout the United States that produce, distribute, and loan educational materials.

Some companies offer educational assistance programs to people who are handicapped. Two such programs are offered through Apple Computer and International Business Machines (IBM). Apple Computer established the *Disability Solutions Group* to help make computers more accessible to people with disabilities and provide a database that describes adaptive devices, software programs, disability-related organizations, publications, and networks. To receive more information on Apple services contact Apple Computer, Inc. Disability Solutions Group, 20525 Mariani Avenue, Cupertino, Calif. 95014 (408-996-1010). IBM offers educational assistance to people with disability through the IBM *Independence Series Information Center.* This center helps individuals learn how health technology and computers can improve the quality of life for the person with disabilities at school, home, and work. To receive more information contact IBM Independence Series Information Center, P.O. Box 1328, Boca Raton, Fla. 34429.

Financial Stability

Financial stability is a major concern for people who are handicapped. An adult who is handicapped is financially responsible for himself or herself. While many adults who are handicapped are financially

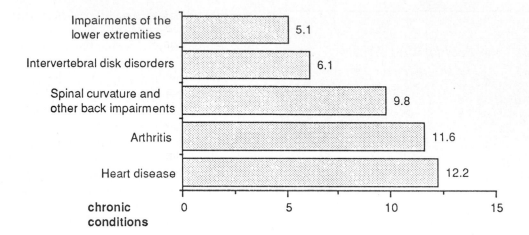

percent of all conditions causing work limitation

Figure 18-4 The five leading chronic conditions causing work limitation. (From Kraus LE and Stoddard S: *Chartbook on disability in the United States, an InfoUse Report,* Washington, D.C., 1989, National Institute on Disability and Rehabilitation Research, p. 42.)

independent, some are unable to achieve this independence and must rely on assistance programs for financial support. Many families with a handicapped member have financial problems as a result of the condition.

Financial assistance programs for the adult who is handicapped are offered through the state department of human or social services (DHS or DSS) or the federal Social Security Administration (SSA) (refer to chapter 4). Under the Social Security Administration the person who is handicapped may be eligible for Social Security Disability Insurance benefits or Supplemental Security Income (SSI). Social Security Disability Insurance may be paid to a disabled worker under 65 and his or her family when earnings are lost or reduced due to the worker's disability. SSI makes monthly payments to qualified children and adults who are disabled and have limited income and resources. Under DHS/DSS the person may be eligible for all forms of aid such as General Assistance and Aid to Families with Dependent Children (AFDC). Private disability insurance programs also offer benefits to the person who is handicapped. The nurse should encourage the adult who is handicapped, and his or her family, to explore the different employment and funding possibilities available.

Employment

Many chronic conditions limit a person's ability to work (refer to Figure 18-4). The President's Committee on Employment of the Handicapped was established by President Harry Truman in 1947 to facilitate employment of handicapped war veterans and other handicapped Americans. The name of the committee has since been changed to the *President's Committee on Employment of People with Disabilities* (1331 F. Street, 3rd Floor, Washington, D.C. 20004-1107, 202-376-6200). The committee sponsors the *Job Accomodation Network* that assists employers in accomodating the workplace to the handicapped worker; has publications dealing with employment opportunities and issues; and takes part in public education and affirmative action. In addition, many states have a *Governor's Committee on Employment of People with Disabilities.* Across the nation there are state *Employment Service* (ES) Offices that are mandated by law to employ a specialist trained in working with people who are handicapped and assist the handicapped job seeker in finding employment. A publication, *Careers and the Handicapped,* helps to provide information on employment needs for people with handicaps and is published by Equal Opportunity Publications, 150 Motor Parkway, Suite 400, Greenlawn, New York 11740.

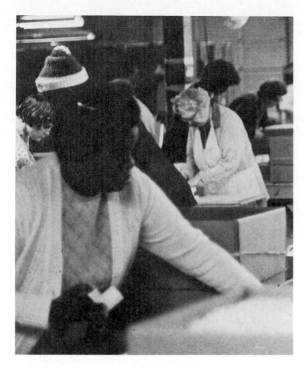

Figure 18-5 The great majority of adults who are handicapped can achieve skills that permit them to be gainfully employed. Sheltered workshops provide job training and placement services that enhance an individual's abilities to function in competitive as well as noncompetitive work environments. (Courtesy of Sunshine Industries, a nonprofit voluntary agency, sponsored by the Association of Retarded Citizens/ Knox County, Tennessee, and Mary Louise Peacock, photographer.)

Adults who are handicapped are found in competitive, modified, and sheltered employment. *Competitive employment* is work with nonhandicapped members of the workforce on an equal basis, such as a job on the assembly line at an automotive factory. *Modified employment* is work done with nonhandicapped members of the workforce to meet the needs of the handicapped workers. *Sheltered employment* (refer to Figure 18-5) is work that is available specifically for people who are handicapped and is done under direct supervision and guidance. Private organizations such as Associations for Retarded Citizens and Goodwill Industries frequently sponsor such employment, and legislation provides for special preference being given in bidding on government contracts to workplaces offering sheltered employment.

As a result of the *Americans with Disabilities Act* (ADA) employers are prohibited from discriminating against any qualified individual with a disability in terms of job hiring, training, compensation, and advancement (Mirone, 1993, p. 36). Employers cannot ask job applicants about the existence, nature, or severity of a disability; medical history; health insurance claims; or work absenteeism (Reno, 1993, p. 9A). Employers who discriminate against the handicapped face legal action, fines, and penalties.

People who are handicapped have proven to be loyal, trustworthy, capable, dependable employees who are willing to work, have good job performance, and reliable attendance records. Our country's work ethic makes employment a central part of life. It is a societal expectation that people will work and be self-sufficient. Work has a great deal to do with how people identify themselves, as well as how they are identified by others. Employment offers the possibility of improving an individual's and family's quality of life and increasing self-esteem.

Access to Resources and Services

A major barrier to employment and other life activities for the handicapped person is limited access to community services, resources, and employment. Aids such as ramps, elevators, wide aisles and doorways, and modified transportation assist people who are handicapped in gaining access to resources, services, and employment.

Accessible transportation is a critical component of independence and self-sufficiency. Many people who are handicapped are either unable to drive or cannot afford a car. Provisions of the Americans with Disabilities Act have provided for accessibility to intracity rail and bus transportation for the handicapped; however, air travel and long-distance bus travel are not addressed in the law (Watson, 1990, p. 326). Other countries have made much greater strides with transportation needs of handicapped persons than has the United States. In Sweden all public vehicles are accessible to the handicapped. France has a rail system that has specially equipped cars for the handicapped, Japan has a totally accessible rail system, and Great Britain requires that all taxis be accessible (Dietl, 1983).

In the United States a shortage of available and reliable public transportation prevents people who are handicapped from taking part in employment and many other activities and necessitates heavy reliance on friends, relatives, Dial-A-rides, and other voluntary transportation services. Medicaid may provide transportation to medical appointments. To assist the person who is handicapped in independent driving, the American Automobile Association (AAA) publishes *The Handicapped Driver's Mobility Guide.*

Health Care

People with handicapping conditions require more health care services than the general population. Many are eligible for the state and federally funded programs of Medicaid and Medicare. However, these programs may not provide for assistive devices and other necessary health care. Private health insurance is often difficult for handicapped persons to obtain because the condition precedes their insurance application—called a preexisting condition—or because they are considered high risk. Many people who are handicapped do not have health insurance that adequately meets their needs.

People who are handicapped often have difficulty gaining access to health care. They report that they cannot afford regular medical care; many doctors refuse to take Medicaid or Medicare; transportation to health care is often difficult to arrange; facilities may not be handicap accessible; and assistive devices are often too expensive or not available (deBalcazar, Bradford, and Fawcett, 1988, pp. 30, 32, 34). During health care procedures personal dignity and privacy need to be taken into consideration, and special positioning and comfort measures may be necessary. People who are handicapped report that they often do not use health care services because of professionals who are insensitive and unaware of the special needs imposed by a disability (deBalcazar, Bradford, and Fawcett).

Social and Recreational Opportunities

Few social and recreational programs are designed for people who are handicapped, and they may have difficulty accessing existing social and recreational programs in the community. Some adults who are handicapped, especially those who are mentally retarded, often find great enjoyment in participating in social and recreational activities planned especially for them (e.g., parties, camp, athletic activities). Others, such as the severely diabetic, may readily integrate into existing community activities. Whatever the level

of disability, people should have social and recreational opportunities available to them.

The Itinerary, a magazine for travelers with disabilities, specializes in helping people who are handicapped know about "accessible" vacations. To make national parks more accessible, the National Park Service has travel guides for people who are handicapped. The *Society for the Advancement of Travel for the Handicapped* (SATH) represents the interests of disabled travelers, provides a clearinghouse on travel for the disabled throughout the world, offers travel tips, and has listings of travel agents who are experienced in dealing with people who are handicapped. SATH can be reached at 347 Fifth Avenue, Suite 610, New York, New York 10016 (212-447-SATH).

Sexuality

Many myths and misconceptions surround the sexuality of people who are handicapped, and they are often treated as if they were asexual or as if sex were inappropriate for them. Being disabled does not change a person's need for intimacy, even though it may alter the experience of sexual fulfillment (Cole and Cole, 1981, p. 279). Achievement of intimacy with a partner often leads to increased self-esteem and fulfillment. Adults who are handicapped may find that health care professionals ignore, or view as unimportant, the sexual aspects of their disability.

The person who is handicapped needs the same knowledge about love and caring, sexual functioning, intimacy, and sexual responsibility that other people need. It cannot be expected that individuals will make informed, appropriate decisions if they do not have the information needed to make them.

Like the rest of the population, people who are handicapped may have sexual problems at some time or another, and medical evaluation and sexual counseling is often helpful. If sexual dysfunction exists, the person can be helped to find avenues of sexual expression and fulfillment. Like other persons, individuals who are handicapped should be made aware of community resources such as sexual counseling and family planning services. Unfortunately, the lack of counseling resources and the reluctance of professionals to deal with the topic can leave the client with little assistance in working out sexual problems and concerns.

Nurses have recognized and written about sexuality concerns and needs of people who have chronic and handicapping conditions (Hahn, 1989; Burgener, 1989). In general, health care professionals need to look closely at their own attitudes about sexuality and the person who is handicapped. Preconceptions about what is sexually appropriate can deny, limit, or inhibit the person from sexual expression and fulfillment; and even an unconscious gesture can convey negative meaning to handicapped persons and affect how they feel about themselves and their sexuality. Bibliographical materials on sexuality and disability are periodically published by the *Sex Information and Education Council United States* (SIECUS) and offer the health care professional some insightful readings.

Guardianship

Many people who are handicapped do not need guardians and are able to go through their entire life making their own decisions. This is especially true of people who are physically handicapped. Guardianship is often considered for individuals who are severely disabled, especially those who are mentally ill or mentally retarded. Guardianship can be either plenary (complete) or partial. Partial guardianship implies that the person is able to carry out some functions independently but needs assistance in carrying out other functions. If no guardian is appointed the person is responsible for making his or her own decisions.

Parents are "natural" guardians of their own minor children and can make legal decisions for them. Parents are *not* natural guardians of their adult offspring who are handicapped and cannot make their legal decisions without having guardianship. Once the age of majority is reached, a person is legally responsible for himself or herself unless a legal guardian has been appointed by the court. Many parents are unaware of this fact, which can present a problem when their adult offspring need medical care or other services. Anticipatory guidance in relation to guardianship needs is helpful.

Handling guardianship issues is difficult for many families. Families who have handicapped adult offspring frequently experience a crisis when they realize that their offspring are not able to make rational decisions at the age of maturity. Parents at this point can no longer avoid the reality that their offspring may never develop the skills to function independently, and feelings of sadness and hopelessness are not uncommon. It is crucial for health care professionals to recognize the distress these parents are experiencing and provide support during this critical period. Helping families to identify the strengths their adult offspring have, and the potential they have for benefitting from experiences that are developmentally within their reach, can reduce parents' anxiety and increase their ability to plan for the future.

With some families siblings, relatives, or friends may be asked to assume guardianship responsibility for an adult who is handicapped, which may not be a feasible or practical solution to the situation. The nurse can assist the family in looking at guardianship options and analyzing what is best for everyone involved.

At times community health nurses have found that families assume that adults who are handicapped are unable to care for themselves just because they are handicapped. It is important to remember that not all adults who are handicapped need guardians. In fact, most of them do not.

Community Residential Opportunities

It is the right of persons who are handicapped to live their lives as normally and independently as possible in the mainstream of the community. Many people who are handicapped do not require any specialized form of housing and live independently in the community. For some people who are handicapped, especially those with mobility limitations or those who are wheelchair bound, adaptations need to be made to make housing accessible.

The nation's *Independent Living Centers* help people who are handicapped to live independently by providing services such as wheelchair repair, training of attendants, and referrals for employment and housing (Robert Wood Johnson Foundation, 1992, p. 76). A publication, *Independent Living,* assists people who are handicapped with independent living needs and is available through Equal Opportunity Publications, 150 Motor Parkway, Suite 400, Greenlawn, New York 11740.

People with handicaps who need to adapt their homes may be eligible for home improvement loans insured by the Department of Housing and Urban Development (HUD). The HUD-insured loan can be used to remove architectural barriers or hazards in the home and make home adaptations. They may also be eligible for rental assistance through HUD.

Accessible housing is essential if people with handicaps are to be able to live independently in the community. Builders and contractors are often unaware of modifications or regulations involving handicap accessibility. The *Center for Accessible Housing,* the nation's first research and training center focusing on making housing accessible and available to people with handicaps, is funded by the National Institute on Disability and Rehabilitation Research (NIDRR) of the U.S. Department of Education. The center offers design solutions (including floor plan designs), training, information, referral, and technical assistance to improve the quality and availability of residential environments for people with disabilities. For further information about the center contact Center for Accessible Housing, North Carolina State University, P.O. Box 8613, Raleigh, North Carolina, 27695-8613 (919-515-3082).

Community living arrangements should meet the needs of the individual. These placements include nonmodified independent living, modified independent living, living in the household of another, foster care, group homes, long-term care facilities such as nursing homes, and state residential facilities. When selecting a residential placement, objectives for the individual should be established and the facility carefully evaluated.

The funding and monitoring of residential placements will vary from state to state. People looking for specific placements can check with local departments of human or social services, departments of mental health, HUD, or specialty agencies dealing with the conditions involved. Some examples of such agencies are the local Association for Retarded Citizens, the National Association for Multiple Sclerosis, and associations for the blind. These agencies are often aware of community placement opportunities and can refer people to appropriate resources.

In many areas restrictive zoning regulations do not allow group homes for people who are handicapped. Restrictive zoning policies have led to the clustering of community residential facilities for people who are handicapped, especially people who are mentally retarded, in areas where zoning regulations were not restrictive. These are often less desirable residential areas.

In recent years there has been a return to the community of people who resided in institutional settings, particularly those who are mentally handicapped. For example, the number of psychiatric mental hospital residents has decreased from 560,000 in 1955 to less than 125,000 (Shadish, Lurigio, and Lewis, 1989, p. 2). People who are leaving institutional settings need to be prepared to return to the community and the community needs to be prepared for their return. When this preparation is not done many problems can arise. If not adequately prepared the individual will have difficulty adapting to this new setting; if the community is not prepared it will not facilitate the individual's adjustment. Many communities have gone to court to prevent, remove, or restrict residences for the handicapped.

Families, like the handicapped adult and the community, need assistance in dealing with the deinstitutionalization process. Frequently they need help to reestablish their relationship with their adult offspring, especially if this individual has been institutionalized for several years and they have had limited contact with him or her. Often families must reevaluate all the decisions that were made in relation to the future of an adult who is handicapped. If the handicapped member returns home, the family may again have to decide how to ensure adequate care, as well as deal with increased physical, mental, social, and economic responsibilities. If he or she returns home or to another setting in the community, such as an adult foster care home, the family may have to deal with feelings of guilt and inadequacy in regard to the original placement, concern regarding financial and parental responsibility, and uncertainty as to the appropriateness of the placement. An example of the dilemma that this transition from institution to community can pose with a family is seen with Mrs. Bartel.

▶ **Mrs. Bartel, a 75-year-old widow receiving Social Security, was being seen by the community health nurse for hypertension. Mrs. Bartel's blood pressure was unusually high on this home visit and she seemed troubled. When the nurse asked her if something was upsetting her, she began crying and stated that John, her 52-year-old son, who was moderately retarded and had been in a local institution for 35 years, was now being considered for community placement in an adult foster care home. She had received a letter inviting her to a case conference to discuss this placement, but she had no way to get there. Mrs. Bartel was worried that her son was not being appropriately placed and that she would be expected to pay for the community placement. With Mrs. Bartel's permission, the nurse contacted the case conference coordinator** and shared Mrs. Bartel's concerns. It was established that the nurse on the community placement team would visit with Mrs. Bartel and the community health nurse to discuss the situation.

The nurse visited and explained the process of community placement to Mrs. Bartel. She arranged for her to visit John's tentative foster home so that she could meet the people who would be responsible for John's care. She assured Mrs. Bartel that John's needs would be met and that there would be no charge to her for the placement. The nurse assured Mrs. Bartel that she would be able to visit John, that his placement would be regularly monitored, and that a change in placement would be made if necessary. After visiting the adult foster home, Mrs. Bartel said, "I wish I had had this choice 35 years ago. I would never have placed John in the institution. I know I cannot take care of him, but here it is more like a home. He will have a more normal life and I am happy for him. I will be able to die in peace."

The community health nurse, using available resources, was able to help ease this transition for Mrs. Bartel and aid in her adjustment to her son's deinstitutionalization. Concerns like Mrs. Bartel's are not uncommon.

The community health nurse can do much to help educate the community and its leaders regarding the needs of a person who is handicapped. Actively participating on community advisory boards established to facilitate community placement programs provides many opportunities to influence community leaders and to educate the public.

Attendant Services

The person who is handicapped may not be able to carry out all the activities of daily living. When this happens the person can benefit from attendant services. The attendant assists the person in such activities as maintaining personal appearance and hygiene (e.g., feeding, dressing, grooming), mobility, household maintenance, safety, companionship, and resource utilization. It is estimated that more than 850,000 Americans currently use some form of community-based attendant services (Litvak, Zukas, and Heumann, 1987; Consumer management, 1988) and that at least 7.7 million noninstitutionalized Americans age 15 and above have personal care limi-

tations and need personal assistance to carry out activities of daily living (Kraus and Stoddard, 1989, p. 5). This means that four out of five Americans who need attendant services are not receiving them. Personal care limitations are assessed using one of two scales: activities of daily living (ADLs) and instrumental activities of daily living (IADLs). ADLs include bathing, dressing, eating, walking, and other personal activities, whereas IADLs encompass preparing meals, shopping, using the phone and communicating, doing laundry, and other measures of being able to live independently (Kraus and Stoddard, 1989, p. 5).

For many people who are handicapped the unavailability of attendant services is a major determinant to their ability to live independently and to obtain employment (Opie and Miller, 1989, p. 196; Kafka, 1993, p. 14). Without these services, people who are handicapped may be needlessly placed in nursing homes and other institutional settings (Kafka, p. 14).

Unfortunately, there is a lack of adequate attendant services in the United States; no comprehensive, uniform system for providing such services exists; and services vary greatly from state to state. These services are sometimes obtainable through Medicaid, Department of Human Services (Social Services Block Grant Title XX), Older Americans Act provisions, Veterans Administration, and various state and locally funded programs. The community health nurse can be instrumental in helping clients to obtain such services.

Respite Care

It is unfair to expect the caretakers of persons who are handicapped to provide 24-hour-a-day care and to assume all the burden for this care. However, this frequently happens and, increasingly, caretakers are experiencing burnout.

Respite care is one solution to the problem of caretaker overload. It provides short-term, 24-hour-a-day placement, including, but not limited to, the following settings: nursing homes, clients' homes, private homes, foster care, group homes, hospitals, and institutions. Respite care provides relief for the caretaker and may avoid institutionalization. It is also successful in decreasing stress and increasing coping ability, attitudes, and adaptability (Sherman and Cocozza, 1984). A caretaker may request respite care for personal reasons such as illness, vacation, or mental health. Whatever the reason, it is legitimate for the caretaker to request time away.

Most people are unfamiliar with the concept of respite care, and in the United States it is difficult to obtain. When it exists privately, the costs are often prohibitive. Some families and organizations have developed respite co-op groups where they exchange periods of time in caring for their respective handicapped family members. The Omnibus Budget Reconciliation Act of 1981 allowed Medicaid waivers for reimbursement of respite care if the cost is the same or less than institutional care.

When assisting a client in looking for respite care, agencies that deal with the specific condition(s) involved should be contacted, along with the local department of social or human services. The community health nurse can be instrumental in advocating respite care services for clients and in making this very important need known to the community. If only from a cost-effectiveness standpoint, the community should be interested. It is more economical to finance respite care services than it is to provide institutional care or long-term care. The humane reasons for providing such care cannot be measured.

LEGISLATION

An overview of federal legislation and voluntary efforts which facilitate service provisions for persons with disabilities is presented in Appendix 18-1. Major pieces of legislation have provided the mechanisms for meeting many of the needs of people who are handicapped. Some of these pieces of legislation include the following:

Developmental Disabilities Act (1971)
Rehabilitation Act of 1973
Developmental Disabilities and Bill of Rights Act (1975, 1984)
Education for All Handicapped Children Act (1975)
Mental Health Systems Act (1980)
Civil Rights of Institutionalized Persons Act (1980)
Protection and Advocacy for Mentally Ill Individuals Act (1986, 1988)
Americans with Disabilities Act (1990)

The most significant piece of legislation addressing the needs of Americans who are disabled is the Americans with Disabilities Act of 1990 (Public Law 101-336). This act helped to ensure the civil rights of persons who are handicapped; empower them; and offer them opportunities, promise, and dignity. The act is designed to provide a clear mandate to end discrimination against individuals with disabilities and deals with issues such as housing, employment, public transportation, and communication services. As a result of this legislation, all across America ramps are being installed, doorways and aisles are being widened, interpreters are being provided, workplaces are accommodating the handicapped, and there is greater access to public transportation. These things are helping to make a difference in the lives of people who are handicapped. The act calls on everyone to remove barriers to access (Reno, 1993). According to Attorney General Janet Reno, this law is helping to break down not only physical barriers but social barriers as well, and has helped people with and without handicaps to work together to eliminate the barriers that have kept our worlds separate and prevented people from being treated equally (Reno).

The nurse needs to be knowledgeable about legislation that affects people who are handicapped and to advocate for necessary legislation. The nurse needs to be able to assist clients in knowing their rights under the law and how to procede when these rights are violated.

REHABILITATION

Rehabilitation is the process of restoring an individual to the fullest physical, mental, social, vocational, and economic usefulness possible. Major goals of rehabilitation are to integrate the individual into society and provide as normal a life as possible. A key component of many rehabilitation programs is vocational rehabilitation. Here, a chief goal is to place a client in a job with a stable employer and good benefits (Handicapper small business, 1989, p. 18). Vocational rehabilitation efforts frequently involve assessment of the client's work potential, vocational education and training, purchase of the assistive devices necessary for employment, vocational counseling and employment placement, evaluation, and follow-up. Many vocational rehabilitation services are provided for under the Rehabilitation Act of 1973 through its state-federal vocational rehabilitation programs. In order to qualify for these programs a person must be at least 16 years old, have a physical or mental disability that constitutes an employment handicap, and be able to become employable as a result of the education, training, and rehabilitation. To apply for rehabilitation services the person should contact the local office of the state Department of Education, Division of Vocational Services. Other rehabilitation programs are offered through hospitals, long-term care facilities, and outpatient settings.

Rehabilitation is important since cures do not exist for many chronic and handicapping conditions. Comprehensive programs are multidisciplinary and combine medical treatment with physical and occupational therapy, as well as sociological, psychological, and economic counseling and services. Rehabilitation is a comprehensive, long-term process and demands a high level of commitment.

Federal Government Rehabilitation Resources

The U.S. Department of Education offers many services to people who are handicapped. The address for the U.S. Department of Education is Mary E. Switzer Building, Room 3024, 330 C. Street SW, Washington, D.C. 20202 (202-205-5482).

The department houses the Clearinghouse on Disability Information (202-205-8241). The Clearinghouse was established in 1975 to respond to inquiries from handicapped people and serves as a resource to organizations and professionals who supply information to people who are handicapped.

The department's Office of Special Education and Rehabilitative Services Administration administers vocational, educational, and rehabilitation programs, publishes the quarterly periodical *American Rehabilitation,* and houses the *National Institute on Disability and Rehabilitation Research* (NIDRR) [U.S. Department of Education, 400 Maryland Avenue S.W., Washington, D.C. 20202-2572, (202-205-9151)]. The department provides financial and leadership support to the states for vocational rehabilitation services; however, programs are administered by each state and will vary greatly from one state to another.

NIDRR sponsors Rehabilitation Research and Training Centers (RRTCs), Rehabilitation Engineering Centers, Regional Disability and Business Technical Training Centers, and research, contributing to the independence of people with disabilities by seeking improved services, products, and rehabilitation practices. NIDRR also gathers disability data and publishes the *Disability Statistics Bulletin, Disability Statistics Abstracts,* and *Disability Statistics Reports.* These publications are available from the Disability Statistics Project of the Institute for Health and Aging, University of California, 201 Filbert Street, Suite 500, San Diego, California 94133-3203 (415-788-8916).

The *National Rehabilitation Information Center* (NARIC) (800-34-NARIC) was established in 1977 and is a library and information center funded by NIDRR. It collects and disseminates the results of federally funded research projects. NARIC publishes the *NARIC Quarterly, NARIC Guide to Disability and Rehabilitation Periodicals, The Directory of National Information Sources on Disabilities,* and *Resource Guides* on selected rehabilitation topics. NARIC's online computerized databases are REHABDATA, ABLEDATA, and ABLE INFORM. REHABDATA (800-346-2742) contains bibliographical information on the NARIC library; ABLEDATA (800-227-0216) provides information about commercial rehabilitation products; and ABLE INFORM (301-589-3563) is an electronic bulletin board of assistive technology, disability, and rehabilitation information maintained by NARIC and ABLEDATA.

The Rehabilitation Process

Rehabilitation programs involve casefinding; interdisciplinary assessment, planning, intervention, and evaluation; vocational rehabilitation, counseling, and placement; restorative services; and retraining. The process follows the same steps as the nursing process (refer to Chapter 9). It involves data gathering, formation of diagnosis and rehabilitation prognoses, goals, plans, follow-up, and evaluation. Records are kept and discharge planning is done (refer to Chapter 10).

Rehabilitation activities should begin as soon as possible to minimize the consequences of the condition. There is a direct correlation between the time the injury or illness occurred, when the rehabilitation referral was made, and the success of the rehabilitation program. The longer the time lapse between the condition occurring and the referral for rehabilitation care, the greater the chance that rehabilitation efforts will not be effective (Donnelly, 1983, p. 40).

Family involvement in the process is important, and if the family is supported during the initial phase of rehabilitation they are often more effective in supporting the client and have better long-term adaptation to the disability (Winterhalter, 1992, p. 23). Once immediate care needs are met, the nurse helps to coordinate activities, maintains communication with the client and family, and assists in community resource utilization.

The rehabilitation plan of care is done in conjunction with the client and family; family involvement is critical in the rehabilitation process. When a crisis such as a disability strikes one family member, all members are affected, and family variables such as coping patterns, knowledge of the condition, expectations, and economic status will affect the family's ability to adapt (Watson, 1989, p. 318). Adaptation is crucial to successful rehabilitation outcomes. Factors related to adaptation have been previously discussed in this chapter.

The rehabilitation process is often under the control of professionals rather than the client and family (Walkover, 1988). This fosters client and family dependence and can inhibit the rehabilitation process. There is a need to shift the responsibility for achieving rehabilitation goals to the client and family and to focus on self-management and self-care (Sawyer and Crimando, 1984).

Self-management techniques are directed toward developing the capacity in clients to make appropriate decisions about their life and health care. Self-management has been shown to increase motivation toward achievement of rehabilitation goals, which is critical to the successful outcome of the rehabilitation process (Sawyer and Crimando, 1984). Motivation is increased if the client believes that the rehabilitation program is realistic and will result in increased independence and quality of life.

The client must be willing to participate in the demanding process of rehabilitation and realize many major life changes may need to occur. The client must make the effort necessary to improve his or her condition, endure the therapeutic procedures, and adjust to assistive devices.

The problems do not end with rehabilitation. In fact, rehabilitation may often accentuate some of them because it will restore the person to a level where it will be necessary to deal with the nonhandicapped population on his or her own. The person often needs help in seeing the value of becoming part of the mainstream. This may be a difficult task, especially if society is not willing to accept the person who is handicapped socially or emotionally even after successful rehabilitation.

THE COMMUNITY HEALTH NURSE'S ROLE WITH THE ADULT WHO IS HANDICAPPED

Community health nurses carry out many roles with adults who are handicapped. These include roles as resource coordinator, counselor, casefinder, advocate, health educator, direct care provider, and health planner. When implementing these roles, community health nurses use the nursing process and are involved in primary, secondary, and tertiary preventive activi-

ties. A deterrent to primary prevention is that the etiology of many chronic and handicapping conditions is unknown. Due to the long-term nature of handicapping conditions, the client is likely to be involved in rehabilitation activities for extended periods of time.

When working with the adult who is handicapped, the community health nurse must include the caretakers in establishing, implementing, and evaluating the plan of care. Caretakers should be helped to use anticipatory guidance, plan for the long-term implications associated with the condition, set realistic expectations, and use self-management techniques. Health care professionals can provide support, guidance, knowledge, and assistance, but only the client and his family can evoke change.

Allowing for meaningful expression of feelings that may range from despair and hopelessness to unrealistic optimism is one of the most significant functions of a community health nurse when working with individuals who are handicapped (Safilios-Rothschild, 1982, p. 90). The nurse must be equipped to deal with this range of feelings.

Nurses have a variety of personal feelings that can inhibit or enhance their ability to function effectively. When working with clients who are handicapped, professionals must be careful not to temper their empathy for clients with patronization and encouragement of dependency (Peters, 1982, p. 36). Because of the complexities of providing therapeutic services to people who are disabled, community health nurses have found it beneficial to have peer collaboration in which they have the opportunity to examine their feelings in relation to clients' needs and nursing interventions.

Community Resource Utilization

Crucial to the successful adaptation to chronic and handicapping conditions is the utilization of community resources. (Holmes, Karst, and Kuehn, 1992, p. 23). The knowledgeable community health nurse refers clients to community resources as appropriate (refer to Chapter 10), because clients often are not aware of the resources available to them or how to work with these resources.

Some excellent resources were noted previously under federal government rehabilitation resources. Many resources are available, but often it is difficult for the client to locate them. The nurse can help the client and family be aware that they need to be persistent when exploring resources and not become discouraged and give up too easily. Searching out available resources can be a trying experience even for the experienced health care professional. Often word of mouth or other people with the same condition can make the client aware of resources. Self-help groups can provide clients with valuable information about community resources.

The search for resources can be harrowing. The nurse may want to make telephone or direct contacts on behalf of the client, because this can both help to avoid client discouragement and can make the nurse more aware of community resources. Resources others take for granted, such as appropriate clothing and household furnishings, tools, and appliances, can be difficult to obtain for the person who is handicapped.

Another helpful publication is *Health Information Resources in the Federal Government.* This publication is available from the Office of Disease Prevention and Health Promotion (Contact: National Health Information Center, U.S. Department of Health and Human Services Public Health Service, P.O. Box 1133, Washington, D.C. 20013-1133). The magazine *Exceptional Parent* publishes an annual directory of organizations that provide services to people who have handicaps. It is available from Exceptional Parent Magazine, 1170 Commonwealth Avenue, Boston, Mass. 02134 (617-730-5800). Also, the National Spinal Cord Injury Association (800-962-9629) publishes a *National Resource Directory* that provides resource information and is available through the Association.

Not to be forgotten, the local telephone directory is a valuable source of information. Some directories include specific sections on community resources. Many agencies are located under the governmental phone listings, or under specific headings in the yellow pages such as hospitals, hospital equipment, rehabilitation, and mental health. Local health departments and departments of human or social services, federal Social Security Administration offices, state Developmental Disability Councils, United Way, and public libraries are all valuable sources of information.

Nurse's Responsibility In Rehabilitation

The community health nurse is in a key position to help the client and family accept and implement the rehabilitation program. A nursing organization, the *Association of Rehabilitation Nurses* (ARN), is an excellent

---

◄ *Nursing Diagnoses Used Most* ►
Frequently in Rehabilitation
Nursing Practice

*Impaired physical mobility
*Self-care deficit
*Alteration in urinary elimination pattern
*Impaired skin integrity
*Alteration in bowel elimination pattern
*Potential for physical injury
*Knowledge deficit
*Impaired verbal communication
*Decreased activity tolerance
  Alterations in comfort
  Impaired thought process
  Ineffective family coping
  Noncompliance
  Body image disturbance
  Self-esteem disturbances
  Alteration in nutrition: Less than required
  Health management deficit
  Impaired home maintainance management
  Sensory perception alterations
  Uncompensated swallowing impairment

*Top 9 diagnoses.
From Sawin KJ and Heard L: Nursing diagnoses used most frequently in rehabilitation nursing practice, *Rehabilitation Nursing* 17 (5):257, 1992. Reprinted from *Rehabilitation Nursing,* Volume 17, Issue 5, with permission of the American Association of Rehabilitation Nurses, 5700 Old Orchard Road, First Floor, Skokie, IL. 60077-1057. Copyright 1992 American Association of Rehabilitation Nurses.

---

resource on rehabilitation programs and activities. The association has published the document *Rehabilitation Nursing: Scope of Practice; Process and Outcome Criteria for Selected Diagnoses* in conjunction with the American Nurses Association (American Nurses Association and Association of Rehabilitation Nurses, 1988). These diagnoses evolved from a research study to determine the most frequently used diagnoses by rehabilitation nurses (Sawin and Heard, 1992, p. 256), and are given in the box above. ARN offers continuing education and training in rehabilitation nursing and is focusing on research-based rehabilitation practice and determining the research interests of its members (Hoemann, Dayhoff, and Thompson, 1993, p. 40). ARN has developed standards of rehabilitation nursing practice and a certification program that has been offered through the Rehabilitation Nursing Certification Board since 1984. The association publishes the journals *Rehabilitation Nursing and Rehabilitation Nursing Research.* For further information the association can be contacted at ARN, 5700 Old Orchard Road, Skokie, Illinois 60077-1057 (708-966-3433).

The community health nurse frequently works with clients who have chronic disabling conditions with rehabilitation needs. Adherence to recommended therapeutic regimes is a major problem among persons with these conditions (Redeker, 1988, p. 31). Careful assessment, including assessment of client and family health beliefs, may assist the nurse in helping the client to plan for care that clients will accept (Redeker, p. 34).

The nurse collaborates with other members of the rehabilitation team and promotes a multidisciplinary treatment approach. The nurse assists in helping the client and family to adjust to the changes imposed by the condition (Power, 1989, p. 73), and assists families to enhance their abilities to cope, grow, and adapt. Nurses also coordinate community resources, provide support and encouragement, implement care management activities, and facilitate program evaluation.

Evaluating the client's rehabilitation regime is an important role for the nurse. Use of a client satisfaction survey can be an effective method of evaluation. This process can provide data about client perceptions of their care, serve as a basis for decision-making about patient care, and can help to show clients and families that their opinions are valued (Courts, 1988, p. 79). Sample items for such a survey are given in Figure 18-6.

Nurses need to look at their attitudes in regard to people who are handicapped. Numerous studies have shown that health care providers have many inaccurate perceptions and negative attitudes about people who are disabled (Lindgren and Oermann, 1993, p. 121). Lindgren and Oermann conducted a study to examine the attitudes of nursing students toward the disabled and to determine the effect of an educational program on these attitudes. Study results showed that students had significantly higher scores and more positive attitudes following the education program. Each nurse needs to assess his or her attitudes and become more knowledgeable in the area of disability.

The nurse's role in rehabilitation is varied and comprehensive. She or he will need to be flexible and adaptable in implementing rehabilitation care and sensitive to the needs of the client and family. The nurse needs to work in close collaboration with other members of the rehabilitation team.

The Nurse, Affirmative Action, and Advocacy for the Person Who Is Handicapped

The nurse is the health professional most familiar with the health care system in its totality, including its gaps and inequities. Sometimes the gaps and inequities in the system can be managed, but sometimes they need to be challenged.

The person who is handicapped is at risk in the system and often finds it difficult to advocate for herself or himself. It is frequently someone other than that person who is in the best position to advocate change.

Client advocacy among health professionals is a recent phenomenon. Many health professionals hesitate to put themselves in client advocacy positions for the following reasons:

1. *Advocacy is an unfamiliar role.* Professionals have generally not been trained to be advocates and are not used to undertaking such a role. The person assuming an advocacy role is not conforming to the established system and may be pressured to conform. The advocate may find advocacy difficult, awkward, and uncomfortable.

2. *Fear of reprisal.* An individual can be punished for advocacy actions in many ways. Often, the greater the impact of the advocacy action, the greater the risk of reprisal. The advocate must be aware of the possibility of reprisal and must decide the possible outcomes of his or her behavior.

3. *Role conflict.* It can be difficult for the professional to remain separate from the professional role and place himself or herself in the role of advocate, especially if the advocate role is in conflict with the professional one. It is difficult to take stands contrary to the stand of other professionals in the field or contrary to the organization for which one works.

4. *Apathy.* Some will choose to be apathetic and not be involved. If one is not personally or directly affected, this role may be assumed.

5. *Lack of support.* If one finds oneself standing alone, or almost alone, it is often difficult to take a firm stand on any position. If one lacks the support of significant others, the stand also becomes difficult.

Preadmission information
How did you find out about the rehabilitation unit? (Check one)
☐ Doctor
☐ Nurse
☐ Other health person
☐ Friend
☐ Other (please name) _____
Did the nurse or doctor talk to you before you came?   ☐ Yes   ☐ No
If yes, did you get your questions answered?   ☐ Yes   ☐ No
If yes, did you understand what the unit was like?   ☐ Yes   ☐ No
What should patients know about the rehabilitation unit before coming to the unit?

About your care	**Always**	**Often**	**Sometimes**	**Rarely**	**Never**	**NA**
I was included in planning my care.	☐	☐	☐	☐	☐	☐
The staff listened to my problems.	☐	☐	☐	☐	☐	☐
Questions about sex were answered.	☐	☐	☐	☐	☐	☐
My call light was answered quickly.	☐	☐	☐	☐	☐	☐
I learned about my medications.	☐	☐	☐	☐	☐	☐
Nurses explained things to be done to me.	☐	☐	☐	☐	☐	☐
Therapists explained things to be done to me.	☐	☐	☐	☐	☐	☐
Family						
My family was included in planning my care.	☐	☐	☐	☐	☐	☐
My family was taught how to care for me.	☐	☐	☐	☐	☐	☐
My family had their questions answered.	☐	☐	☐	☐	☐	☐
My family went to family support group.	☐	☐	☐	☐	☐	☐
My family rate this group as helpful.	☐	☐	☐	☐	☐	☐
If you had speech problems, please answer the following:						
Therapist helped me learn to talk.	☐	☐	☐	☐	☐	☐
My speech improved.	☐	☐	☐	☐	☐	☐
Staff understood my speech problem.	☐	☐	☐	☐	☐	☐
I learned to talk with the staff.	☐	☐	☐	☐	☐	☐
Family was taught to understand my speech.	☐	☐	☐	☐	☐	☐

Results and evaluation
Did you have special things to learn before you came?   ☐ Yes   ☐ No
Did you learn what you wanted to learn?   ☐ Yes, definitely.   ☐ Yes, I think so.   ☐ No, I don't think so.   ☐ No, definitely not.
If needed, would you return to the unit?   ☐ Yes   ☐ Probably   ☐ No
Would you tell others to come to the unit?   ☐ Yes   ☐ Probably   ☐ No
What I liked most about the rehabilitation center:

_____
_____

What I liked least about the rehabilitation center:

_____
_____
_____

Figure 18-6   Sample items on a patient satisfaction survey. (From Courts NF: A patient satisfaction survey for a rehabilitation unit, *Rehab Nurs* 13(2):80, 1988. Reprinted from Rehabilitation Nursing, Volume 13, Issue 2, with permission of the American Association of Rehabilitation Nurses, 5700 Old Orchard Road, First floor, Skokie, Ill. 60077-1057. Copyright 1988 American Association of Rehabilitation Nurses.)

6. *Change implications.* Professionals realize the implications of changing a situation. To encourage change, to take a stand, is often to encourage stress. Are we willing to give up a system, possibly a stable one, to invoke an unstable one?

Health professionals and the organizations they represent may hesitate to advocate on behalf of the client for a variety of reasons. Concerns such as not enough time, not enough money, no one to help, not wanting to get involved on an emotional level, and the system not being ready for such a change all are common. It is easy to feel empathy with these concerns as most of us have probably voiced them at one time or another. Taking an advocacy stand requires time and a commitment to the belief that all clients have a right to essential health care services. Clients also have the right to be treated with respect and dignity when using these services. If one believes people have these rights, the question of advocating or not advocating becomes almost secondary whenever one sees an individual's rights being violated or ignored.

The impact that a nurse can have on the system as an advocate should not be underestimated. An example of this is the case of a nurse working with a local association of parents of retarded children.

The parents in a local association for retarded citizens were increasingly aware of instances of suspected abuse to their children in the institutional setting in which they resided. The parents had talked with the institution administration and felt that they were not receiving adequate information; some of the parents felt intimidated. The parents were concerned about the implications of their actions on their institutionalized children. If they continued to press for information, they were worried about reprisals. If they did not press for information, they were worried that the situation would get worse. A nurse who was a member of the association was able to take action because she did not fear reprisal and she had the support of the parent group.

The nurse met with the parents and the institution administration. After assessing and concluding that there was a problem and that the administration was resistant to change, the nurse examined the laws of the state regarding child abuse. One section of the law clearly stated that an institution must be independently investigated when there were suspected cases of child abuse or neglect. The nurse knew that state institutions were not adhering to that section of the law. By obtaining legal counsel, and working with the established grievance procedure for state mental health clients, the community health nurse was able to help effect change in the system. The state now has impartial investigations of all cases of child abuse in state institutions, and parents or guardians have access to the results.

The advocacy efforts of this community health nurse (one of the authors of this text) had many positive effects. Reporting procedures for institutional cases of suspected abuse and neglect were clearly written and implemented in that state. The state legislature appropriated a large sum of money to be used in further protection and advocacy services for people who are developmentally disabled. In addition, the general public became increasingly aware of the needs of people who are mentally handicapped.

Nurses are in a position to correct public misconceptions about people who are handicapped. They can work to gain greater acceptance of individuals who are handicapped in whatever setting they reside. The nurse can be instrumental in promoting a positive attitude toward the handicapped by the general public.

Summary

The number of individuals in society who are accurately characterized as disabled can be expected to increase and demand for services to these individuals will increase concomitantly.

Adults who are handicapped are confronted with adapting to their handicaps amidst societal, family, and individual variables, which influence adaptation and growth-promoting activities. Many handicapping conditions are long-term and require ongoing use of a number of community resources. The need for better communication, coordination, and cooperation among these resources is great, as is the need for greater accessibility to services and greater availability of attendants for handicapped people.

Community health nurses are in a unique position to assist clients who are handicapped to obtain services that will enhance adaptation and promote growth. They assist clients with rehabilitation and work cooperatively with the clients and their families to establish plans of care. A sensitivity to the needs of this population group and an awareness that there are individual differences among clients who are handicapped are both essential for the community health nurse to function effectively with clients who have special needs.

Increasingly, health care professionals are becoming actively involved in advocacy for this population group. Advocacy has been critical in the procurement of many essential services for these clients. While legislation in the last decade has reflected a more positive attitude toward people who are handicapped, there remain numerous unmet needs. Professionals must continue to facilitate public awareness about handicapping conditions and the needs of people who are experiencing them. Adults who are handicapped are at risk and deserve their share of the country's health resources.

References

American Nurses Association and Association of Rehabilitation Nurses: *Rehabilitation nursing: scope of practice; process and outcome criteria for selected diagnoses,* Kansas City, Mo., 1988, American Nurses Association.

Burgener S: Sexuality concerns of the post-stroke patient, *Rehab Nurs* 14(4):178-181, 1989.

Buscaglia LF, ed: *The disabled and their parents: a counseling challenge,* ed 2, Thorofare, N.J., 1983, Slack.

Buzinski P: Groups for brothers and sisters of developmentally disabled children: one component of a family-centered approach, *Issues Compr Pediat Nurs* 4(1):45-50, 1980.

Cole TM and Cole SS: Sexual adjustment to chronic disease and disability. In Stolov WC and Clowers MR, eds: *Handbook on severe disability,* Washington, D.C., 1981, U.S. Government Printing Office, pp. 279-288.

Commission on Chronic Illness: *Chronic illness in the United States, vol I: Prevention of chronic illness,* Cambridge, Mass., 1957, Harvard University Press.

Consumer management of attendant services: benefits and obstacles, *NARIC Q* 1(2):1, 6-14, 1988.

Courts NF: A patient satisfaction survey for a rehab unit, *Rehab Nurs* 13(2):79-81, 1988.

deBalcazar YS, Bradford B, and Fawcett SB: Common concerns of disabled Americans: issues and options, *Social Policy* 19(2):29-35, 1988.

Dietl D: The phoenix: from the ashes and looking to the ultimate barrier: our own attitude, *J Rehab* 49(3):12-17, 1983.

Disability risks of chronic illnesses and impairments, *Disability Stat Bull* 2(Fall):1-2, 4, 1989.

Dixon JK: Coping with prejudice: attitudes of handicapped persons toward the handicapped, *J Chron Dis* 30:307-321, 1977.

Donnelly DC: Rehabilitation and the occupational health nurse, *Occupational Health Nursing* 31(8):39-42, 1983.

Frye BA: Review of the World Health Organization's report on disability prevention and rehabilitation, *Rehabilitation Nursing* 18(1):43-44, 1993.

Giele JZ: A delicate balance: the family's role in the care of the handicapped, *Family Relations* 33(1):85-94, 1984.

Goldman CE: Advocacy in the '80's, *Disabled USA* 1:21-23, 1984.

Hahn H: Can disability be beautiful? *Social Policy* 18(3):26-32, 1988.

Hahn K: Sexuality and COPD, *Rehab Nurs* 14(4):191-195, 1989.

Handicapper small business association provides assistance, *J Rehab* 55(2):18, 1989.

Hoemann SP, Dayhoff NE, and Thompson TC: The initial ANF research survey: rehabilitation nursing research interests of ARN members, *Rehabilitation Nursing* 18(1):40-41, 1993.

Holmes GE, Karst RH, and Kuehn MD: Community resource utilization in rehabilitation: the shape of the future, *American Rehabilitation* 18(3):23-25, 1992.

Kafka B: A civil rights or interdependence perspective on attendant services, *Rehabilitation Gazette* 33(1):13-14, 1993.

Kendrick D: Invisible barriers: how you can make parenting easier, *Disabled USA* 1:17-19, 1983.

Kraus LE and Stoddard S: *Chartbook on disability in the United States, an InfoUse Report,* Washington, D.C., 1989, National Institute on Disability and Rehabilitation Research.

Kubler-Ross E: *On death and dying,* New York, 1969, Macmillan.

Lewis KS: Grief in chronic illness and disability, *J Rehab* 29(3):8-11, 1983.

Lindgren CL, Burke ML, Hainsworth MA, and Eakes GG: Chronic sorrow: a lifespan concept, *Scholarly Inquiry for Nursing Practice: An International Journal* 6(1):27-40, 1992.

Lindgren CL and Oermann MH: Effects of an educational intervention on students' attitudes toward the disabled, *J Nursing Ed* 32(3):121-126, 1993.

Litvak S, Zukas H, and Heumann J: *Attending to Americans: assistance for independent living,* Berkley, Calif., 1987, World Institute on Disability.

McCubbin MA and McCubbin HI: Families coping with illness: the resiliency model of family stress, adjustment, and adaptation. In Danielson CB, Hamel-Bissell B, and Winstead-Fry P, eds: *Families health and illness: perspectives on coping and intervention,* St. Louis, 1993, Mosby.

Miller JF: *Coping with chronic illness: overcoming powerlessness,* ed 2, Philadelphia, Penn., 1992, F. A. Davis.

Mirone JA: Understanding the Americans with Disabilities Act, *Healthcare Trends and Transitions* 4(5):36-38, 1993.

Opie ND and Miller ET: Attribution for successful relationships between severely disabled adults and personal care attendants, *Rehab Nurs* 14(4):196-199, 1989.

Penrose J: Double handicap. Does he take sugar? *Nurs Times* 79:52-54, 1983.

Peters L: Women's health care: approaches in delivery to physically disabled women, *Nurse Pract* 7:34-37, 48, 1982.

Power DW: Working with families: an intervention model for rehabilitation nurses, *Rehab Nurs* 14:73-79, 1989.

President's Committee on Employment of the Handicapped: *Affirmative action to employ handicapped people,* Washington, D.C., 1978, U.S. Government Printing Office.

Redeker NS: Health beliefs and adherence in chronic illness, *IMAGE* 20(1):31-34, 1988.

Reeber BJ: Evaluating the effects of a family education intervention, *Rehabilitation Nursing* 17(6):332-336, 1992.

Reno J: Disability law will be enforced, *USA Today,* Monday, July 26, 1993, p. 9A.

Robert Wood Johnson Foundation: *Challenges in health care,* New York, 1992, The Foundation.

Safilios-Rothschild C: *The sociology and social psychology of disability rehabilitation,* New York, 1982, University Press of America.

Sawin KJ and Heard L: Nursing diagnoses used most frequently in rehabilitation nursing practice, *Rehabilitation Nursing* 17(5):256-262, 1992.

Sawyer HW and Crimando W: Self-management strategies in rehabilitation, *J Rehab* 50(1):27-30, 1984.

Seifert KH: The attitudes of working people toward disabled persons, especially in regard to vocational rehabilitation. In Spiegel AD and Podair S, eds: *Rehabilitating people with disabilities into the mainstream of society,* Park Ridge, N.J., 1981, Noyes Medical.

Shadish WR, Lurigio AJ, and Lewis DA: After deinstitutionalization: the present and future of mental health long-term care policy, *J Social Issues* 45(3):1-15, 1989.

Sherman BR and Cocozza JJ: Stress in families of the developmentally disabled: a literature review of factors affecting the decision to seek out-of-home placements, *Family Relations* 33(1):95-103, 1984.

Sussman MB, ed: *Sociology and rehabilitation,* Washington, D.C., 1966, American Sociological Association.

United States Department of Health and Human Services (USDHHS): *Healthy People 2000: national health promotion and disease prevention objectives, full report, with commentary,* Washington, D.C., 1991, U.S. Government Printing Office.

USDHHS: *Health United States 1991,* Washington, D.C., 1992, U.S. Government Printing Office.

University of Michigan: Toward a barrier-free society; breaking the isolation of handicap, *Research News* 22, November-December 1981.

Walkover M: Social policies: understanding their impact on families with impaired members. In Chilman CS, Nunally EW, and Cox F, eds: *Chronic illness and disability,* Newbury Park, Calif., 1988, Sage, pp. 220-247.

Watson PG: Indicators of family capacity for participating in the rehabilitation process: report on a preliminary investigation, *Rehab Nurs* 14(6):318-322, 1989.

Watson PG: The Americans with Disabilities Act: more rights for people with disabilities, *Rehabilitation Nursing* 15(6):325-328, 1990.

Watson PG: Family issues in rehabilitation, *Holistic Nurs Pract* 6(2):51-59, 1992.

Werner-Beland JA: *Grief responses to long-term illness and disability,* Reston, Virg., 1980, Reston.

Winterhalter JG: Group support for families during the acute phase of rehabilitation, *Holistic Nurs Pract* 6(2):23-31, 1992.

World Health Organization (WHO), Expert Committee on Disability Prevention and Rehabilitation: *Disability prevention and rehabilitation,* Technical Report Series 668, Geneva, 1981, The Organization.

Youngblood NM and Hines J: The influence of the family's perception of disability on rehabilitation outcomes, *Rehabilitation Nursing* 17(6):323-326, 1992.

Selected Bibliography

Acorn S and Bampton E: Patients' loneliness: a challenge for rehabilitation nurses, *Rehabilitation Nursing* 17(1):22-25, 1992.

Ayrault EW: *Sex, love, and the physically handicapped,* New York, 1981, Continuum.

Biordi B and Oermann MH: The effect of prior experience in a rehabilitation setting on student's attitudes toward the disabled, *Rehabilitation Nursing* 18(2):95-98, 1993.

Carling PJ: Access to housing: cornerstone of the American dream, *J Rehab* 55(3):6-8, 1989.

Cornelius DA: Who cares? A handbook on sex education and counseling service for disabled people, ed 2, Baltimore, Md., 1982, University Park Press.

Derstine JB: The rehabilitation clinical nurse specialist of the 1990s: roles assumed by recent graduates, *Rehabilitation Nursing* 17(3):139-140, 1992.

Gordon S: Sexuality and the disabled, *Aust J Sex Marriage Family* 2(4):157-164, 1981.

Haber LD: Identifying the disabled: concepts and methods in the measurement of disability, *Social Sec Bull* 51(5):11-28, 1988.

Hoeman SP: Community-based rehabilitation, *Holistic Nurs Pract* 6(2):32-41, 1992.

Kirk K: Chronically ill patients' perceptions of nursing care, *Rehabilitation Nursing* 18(2):99-104, 1993.

Lavallee DJ and Crupi CD: Rehabilitation takes to the road, *Holistic Nurs Pract* 6(2):60-66, 1992.

Leahy MJ, Habeck RV, and VanTol B: Doctoral dissertation research in rehabilitation: 1980-1989, *Rehabilitation Counseling Bull* 35(4):253-288, 1992.

Makas E: Positive attitudes toward disabled people: disabled and nondisabled persons' perspectives, *J Social Issues* 44(1):49-61, 1988.

Peterson Y: The impact of physical disability on marital adjustment: a literature review, *Family Coordinator* 28(1):47-51, 1979.

Reed KL: History of federal legislation for persons with disabilities, *Am J Occ Therapy* 46(5):397-408, 1992.

Rothenberg RB and Koplan JP: Chronic disease in the 1990s, *Annual Rev Public Health* 11:267-296, 1990.

The Americans with Disabilities Act questions and answers, Washington, D.C., 1991, U.S. Equal Employment Opportunity Commission and U.S. Department of Justice Civil Rights Division.

Topolnicki DM: The gulag of guardianship, *Money* 18(3):149-152, 1989.

Weiss DV: Accessible vacations, *J Rehab* 54(3):8-9, 1988.

An Overview of Legislation and Voluntary Efforts for the Handicapped in the United States

1798   U.S. Congress establishes a marine hospital to provide for disabled seamen (England had established such a facility in 1588).

1902   Goodwill Industries is originated by a minister, Dr. Edgar Helms, to provide employment opportunities for people who are handicapped.

1918   Federal Board of Vocational Rehabilitation established to provide vocational rehabilitation services to the disabled veterans of World War I.

Massachusetts becomes the first state to establish public provisions to aid in the vocational rehabilitation of disabled citizens.

1920   The first Vocational Rehabilitation Act (Public Law 565) is passed. Services under the act were primarily for physically disabled military personnel. This act was administered by the Vocational Rehabilitation Administration.

1935   Social Security Act is passed, resulting in increased federal appropriations to states for vocational rehabilitation with direct relief provided for the disabled. Amendments to this act have povided for SSI, Disability Insurance, Medicare, and Medicaid.

1943   Amendments to the Vocational Rehabilitation Act of 1920 broaden vocational rehabilitation services to include facilitating a disabled person to engage in competitive employment and include such services as diagnosis, medical and surgical treatment, prescriptions, hospitalization, books, tools, and occupational equipment.

Baruch Committee on Physical Medicine is established by the son of Dr. Simon Baruch, a confederate army surgeon and pioneer in the field of physical medicine. The committee supports research and scholarship in physical medicine.

1944   The Public Health Act of 1944 (Public Law 78-410) provides for professional education, training, and research on many handicapping conditions.

1945   Joseph Bulova School of Watchmaking establishes a training program in watchmaking for people who are handicapped. Forerunner of many companies offering employment and training opportunities to the handicapped.

1946   National Mental Health Act (Public Law 79-487) authorizes extensive federal support for mental health research, diagnosis, prevention, and treatment, establishing the National Institute of Mental Health and state grant-in-aid programs for mental health under the U.S. Public Health Service.

1947   The Department of Rehabilitation and Physical Medicine is started at New York University College of Medicine at Bellevue Hospital under the direction of Dr. Howard Rusk. The first comprehensive program in rehabilitation at Bellevue was made possible by a grant from the Baruch committee. This department served as a model for the development of rehabilitation centers all over the world.

1953   Establishment of the Department of Health, Education, and Welfare with the Office of Vocational Rehabilitation as a part.

1954   Federal provisions made to support training and education programs for professional rehabilitation personnel in the form of scholarships, stipends, research, and construction grants.

1956   Amendments to the Social Security Act give benefits to workers and their families during periods of extended disability.

The Mental Health Study Act (Public Law 84-812) authorizes grants to facilitate a program of research into resources and methods of care for the mentally ill. The act authorized grants for participation in a national study and reevaluation of the human and economic problems of mental illness.

1963   Mental Retardation Facilities and Community Mental Health Centers Construction Act of 1963 (Public Law 88-164) provides assistance in combating mental retardation through grants for construction of research centers and facilities for people who are mentally retarded. It provides assistance in improving mental health services through construction of community mental health centers.

1965   Amendments to the Vocational Rehabilitation Act of 1920 provide for increased flexibility in financing and administrating state rehabilitation programs and for assisting in the expansion and improvement of rehabilitation services financed by a state-federal payment sharing plan. The word *handicapped* was substituted for *physical disability*. The Federal Board of Vocational Education is established.

Medicaid and Medicare are established by federal law. Both programs provide essential health and health-related services for individuals who are handicapped (refer to Chapter 4).

The Mental Retardation Facilities and Community Mental Health Centers Construction Act Amendments of 1965 (Public Law 89-105) authorize assistance in meeting the initial cost of professional and technical personnel for comprehensive community mental health centers.

1968   Architectural Barriers Act (Public Law 90-480) is passed. The act mandated that almost any public building constructed or leased by federal funds must be accessible to the physically handicapped, and that

Continued

An Overview of Legislation and Voluntary Efforts for the Handicapped in the United States—cont'd

all construction after 1968 using federal funds ensure building accessibility to handicapped persons with no exceptions allowed. The act affected many educational settings and was enforced by the Architectural Barriers Compliance Board. However, the mandates of this law were ignored, and in 1978 Congress created a compliance board to enforce the law (Goldman, 1984).

1971   Developmental Disabilities Act* (Public Law 91-517) is passed. The act states that each state would receive federal funds to establish and maintain services that are required by developmentally disabled children and adults. These services include diagnosis, evaluation, treatment, personal care, special living arrangements, training, education, sheltered employment, recreation, counseling, protective and sociolegal services, information services, transportation services, and follow-up services.

Urban Mass Transportation Act (Public Law 91-453) is passed. The act states that special efforts would be made in federally funded mass transportation to include usage by persons who are handicapped.

1973   Rehabilitation Act of 1973* (Public Law 91-453) is a landmark piece of legislation that replaced the 1920 act. It authorizes vocational rehabilitation services: emphasizes services to those with severe handicaps, expands the federal role in service and training programs, defines services necessary for rehabilitative programs, establishes the National Architectural and Transportation Barriers Board, and begins affirmative action programs to facilitate employment of the handicapped. This act is the basis for rehabilitation services and programs.

Social Security Act of 1935 amendments eliminate previous categories of Aid to the Blind, Aid to the Aged (Old Age Assistance), and Aid to the Disabled under which direct financial assistance was given to people who were handicapped. Supplemental Security Income is established as of January 1, 1974, under which the aged, blind, and disabled could qualify.

1974   Rehabilitation Act Amendments of 1974 (Public Law 93-576) authorizes the White House Conference on the Disabled.

Numerous transportation legislation including the following:
1. Amtrak Improvement Act (Public Law 93-140) stated that the Amtrak corporation must ensure that the handicapped would not be denied trans-

portation because of the handicap. Provisions did not apply to commuter and short-haul service.
2. Federal Aid Highway Act (Public Law 93-87) stated that funding could not be approved for any state or federal highway not granting reasonable access for the movement of the physically handicapped across curbs.
3. National Mass Transportation Act (Public Law 93-503) stated that mass transit funds could not be approved unless the rates charged persons who are handicapped were reduced rates from regular fare.
4. Federal Bus Act (Public Law 93-37) stated that all federally funded projects to improve bus transportation must include plans to facilitate usage by people who are handicapped.

1975   Developmental Disabilities Assistance and Bill of Rights Act* (Public Law 94-103) creates a system of advocacy on the state level to pursue legal and other actions necessary to eliminate the problems facing citizens with mental retardation, epilepsy, autism, and cerebral palsy and also expands the national effort to protect the rights of the developmentally disabled.

Education for All Handicapped Children Act (Public Law 94-142) passes. Enabled by September 1, 1980, a free, appropriate public education to all persons aged 3 to 21 years old regardless of handicapping condition involved. Recently the federal government has tried to deregulate the act, but proposed changes created such a furor among the disabled, their families, and advocates that the changes were withdrawn.

1977   Reorganization of the Department of Health, Education, and Welfare with creation of the Office of Human Development. The Administration for Handicapped Individuals (AHI) is under the Office of Human Development and oversees (1) Rehabilitation Services Administration, (2) President's Committee on Mental Retardation, (3) Architectural and Transportation Barriers Compliance Board, (4) White House Conference on Handicapped Individuals, (5) Developmental Disabilities Office, and (6) Office of Handicapped Individuals.

Federal Aviation Act of 1958 amends (Public Law 95-163) to provide special rates (reduced) on a space-available basis to persons with severe visual or hearing impairments and other physically or mentally handicapped people as defined by the Civil

*NOTE: Laws that have had, or have the potential for having, major impact on the person who is handicapped are indicated by an asterisk.

An Overview of Legislation and Voluntary Efforts for the Handicapped in the United States—cont'd

Aeronautics Board, as well as any attendant required by such persons.

1978 Rehabilitation Act Amendments establishes the Council on the Handicapped to function as a steering committee to make recommendations to the President concerning the needs of disabled individuals, and establishes the National Center for Rehabilitation Research.

1980 Mental Health Systems Act* (Public Law 96-398) gives the states more authority to plan community mental health centers, to increase the quality of mental health services, and to reach more people. Includes advocacy provisions and a Bill of Rights of Mental Health.

Civil Rights of Institutionalized Persons Act* (Public Law 96-247) authorizes actions for redress in cases involving deprivations of rights of institutionalized persons that were secured or protected by the Constitution of the United States. The act states that when an action has been commenced in any court of the United States seeking relief from conditions that deprive persons residing in such institutions of any rights, privileges, or immunities secured or protected by the Constitution or laws of the United States that causes them to suffer grievous harm, the Attorney General of the United States may intervene.

1982 Telecommunications for the Disabled Act (Public Law 97-140) amends the Communication Act of 1934 to provide that persons with impaired hearing are insured reasonable access to telephone service by requiring that all coin-operated telephones, telephones frequently used by hearing-impaired persons, and emergency telephones provide an internal means of coupling with hearing aids. Retrofitting could be required on coin-operated and emergency telephones.

The Surface Transportation Assistance Act (Public Law 97-424) encourages removal of architectural barriers.

1984 Rehabilitation Amendments (Public Law 98-221) modifies the definition of severely disabled and places the age limit for disability benefits at 16 years. Made the National Council on the Handicapped an agency independent from the Department of Education.

Developmental Disabilities Assistance and Bill of Rights Act (Public Law 98-527) formally establishes a Bill of Rights for the developmentally disabled.

1986 Protection and Advocacy for Mentally Ill Individuals Act of 1986* (Public Law 99-319) establishes protec-

tion and advocacy services for individuals who are mentally ill. Restated the Bill of Rights for mental health patients. Promotes the establishment of family support groups for the families of people with Alzheimer's disease.

Education of the Deaf Act (Public Law 99-371) consolidates several free-standing statutes relating to federally supported educational institutions for the deaf into one effective piece of legislation.

Rehabilitation Amendments (Public Law 99-506) emphasize the rehabilitation needs of disabled Native Americans, provide funding for disability technology, and expand the influence of the National Council on the Handicapped.

Employment Opportunities for Disabled Americans Act (Public Law 99-643) amends the Social Security Act to improve employment opportunities for disabled Americans.

Air Carrier Access Act of 1986 greatly improves access to air transportation for people who are handicapped.

1988 Numerous pieces of technology-related legislation including:
1. Hearing Aid Compatibility Act of 1988 (Public Law 100-394) requires telephones manufactured or imported into the United States after August 16, 1989 be hearing-aid compatible.
2. Technology-Related Assistance for Individuals with Disabilities Act of 1988 (Public Law 100-407) establishes a competitive grant program to enable participating states to develop and implement programs to promote technology-related assistance to individuals with disabilities.
3. Telecommunications Accessibility Act (Public Law 100-542) ensures that the federal telecommunication system is fully accessible to hearing-impaired persons who use telecommunications.

Protection and Advocacy for Mentally Ill Individuals Amendments Act of 1988 (Public Law 100-509) amends the 1986 act to reauthorize the act and to establish a governing authority for protection and advocacy in each state.

1990 The Americans with Disabilities Act* (Public Law 101-336) was passed. A landmark piece of legislation designed to provide a clear and comprehensive mandate to end discrimination against individuals with disabilities. It addresses such issues as housing, employment, public transportation, and communication services.

The Well Elderly: Needs and Services

OBJECTIVES

Upon completion of this chapter, the reader should be able to:

1. Construct a personal philosophy of aging.
2. Discuss societal values and attitudes in relation to aging.
3. Discuss the *Healthy People 2000* initiative in relation to aging.
4. State major causes of mortality and morbidity for the elderly.
5. Discuss health promotion and wellness activities for the elderly.
6. Identify significant legislation in relation to older Americans.
7. Describe barriers to health care for the elderly.
8. Conceptualize the community health nurse's role in promoting healthy aging.

There's no shame in growing old—we're all doing it. Age is, after all, the one thing we all share.

MAGGIE KUHN

Meet Art Johnson, a retired school principal from Waterford, Michigan. At 80 years of age he taught adult education at a local high school, golfed competitively, continued postgraduate education, and helped with coaching Little League Baseball. He was known and loved in his community.

Meet Hattie Harris of Rochester, New York, where the city declared a "Hattie Harris Day." At 91 years of age she was described as the "elder statesman of the Republican Party" and the "Mayor of Strathallan Park." In those positions she advised political candidates, sought financial backing from business leaders, and set up neighborhood political rallies.

Meet Herbert Kirk of Bozeman, Montana. In 1993, at 97 years of age, he received his bachelor's degree from Montana State University. At the graduation ceremony Mr. Kirk received a standing ovation from the thousands of people gathered at the university fieldhouse. Part of the ceremony included the reading of a congratulatory letter sent by President Bill Clinton. Mr. Kirk is the oldest living naval aviator in the United States and, in 1992, won two gold medals in the International Track Athletic Congress in Finland.

Individuals like Art Johnson, Hattie Harris, and Herbert Kirk can be found in any American community. They are examples of older Americans who have lived life to its fullest and best. They exemplify successful aging!

AGING DEFINED

Aging and "old age" are relatively contemporary phenomena. The average Stone Age human lived 15 years. By the late 1700s people lived into their 30s, and the life expectancy for turn-of-the-century Americans was slightly less than 50 years (Painter, 1993, D1).

Aging is a natural and lifelong process of growing and developing. Everyone is aging! Aging is a *universal phenomenon* that begins at birth and continues throughout life, as well as an *individual process* that incorporates personal life experiences. In most societies terms such as *aged, old,* and *elderly* are used to describe persons who have achieved a certain chronological age. This chronological age varies among nations. In the United States the age of 65 is often used to designate old age.

It is interesting to note that the designation of old age in the United States is primarily legislatively determined. The Social Security Act of 1935 set eligibility for federal "old age" retirement benefits at age 65, and this became what our society views as "old age." Americans are now living longer than they did in 1935, and old age is being redefined both socially and politically.

SOME PERSPECTIVES ON AGING

Throughout history aging persons have been portrayed in literature and art as wise individuals, strong in character, and leaders of their people. Older people are the gatekeepers of the nation's history, values, culture, and traditions. The vigor and productiveness of individuals such as Art Johnson, Hattie Harris, and Herbert Kirk should be usual for Americans, and nursing needs to facilitate such healthy, active aging. The box on p. 734 highlights a number of older people.

American Attitudes Toward Age and Aging

America is an ageist society. Robert Butler, a renowned gerontologist, coined the term *ageism* in 1968 and defined it as a process of systematic stereotyping of, and discrimination against, people because they are old (Sheppard, 1990, p. 4). The Gray Panthers (Figure 19-1), an organization that staunchly advocates the rights of older people, views ageism as the use of age to define capability and role. The costs of ageism are great: as with other forms of prejudice it is dehumanizing and inhibits people from maximizing their potential.

Biases against aging are so deeply ingrained in our society that they unintentionally surface in everyday life—in writing, films, and even conversation—denying older persons their individuality and the opportunity to maximize their potential (American Association of Retired Persons [AARP], 1984, pp. 3, 6). Descriptors such as vigorous, active, attractive, and independent are often used to describe a person of 20, 30, or 40, but rarely one of 60, 70, or 80.

In general, Americans are not educationally, socially, or emotionally prepared for old age (McGuire, 1987, p. 174) and many myths and misconceptions about aging exist. The box on p. 735 looks at some common myths about aging. People need to become

◀   *Go For It—Healthy, Active Aging*   ▶

Mary Baker Eddy directed the Christian Science Church at 89.

Harold and Bertha Soderquist joined the Peace Corps and learned a foreign language when he was 80 and she was 76.

Thomas Edison, the inventor of the electric light bulb, filed for his 1033th patent at the age of 81.

Albert Schweitzer was in charge of an African hospital at 89 and helped build a half-mile road near the hospital at 87.

George Bernard Shaw was writing at 91.

Claude Pepper served as a U.S. Congressman at 88.

Ronald Reagan served as President of the United States in his 70s.

Maggie Kuhn headed the Gray Panthers at 88.

Anna Mary Moses, better known as Grandma Moses, illustrated an edition of *'Twas the Night Before Christmas* when she was 100.

Frank Lloyd Wright began his most creative and prolific work at the age of 69 and was active until his death at 91.

Herbert Kirk graduated from Montana State University in 1993 at age 97. The university was 100 years old that year.

Excerpts from Harris DK: *Sociology of Aging,* ed 2, New York, 1990, Harper and Row; and Comfort A: *Say yes to old age: developing a positive attitude toward aging,* New York, 1990, Crown.

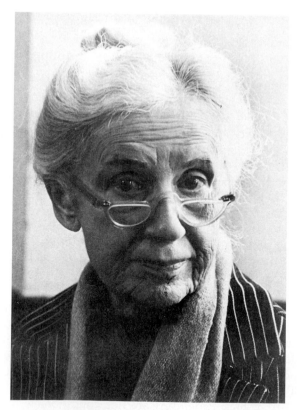

Figure 19-1   Maggie Kuhn, founder of the Gray Panthers. (Courtesy Julie Jensen, Photographer.)

knowledgeable about the aging process; develop realistic, positive attitudes toward aging; and realize that older people are valuable and contributing members of society (McGuire, 1993b, Promoting positive attitudes, p. 5). Nurses need to evaluate their attitudes about age and aging and how these attitudes affect nursing care, along with engaging in activities that promote healthy aging and enhance the quality of life for the elderly.

Community health nurses have unique opportunities to facilitate healthy aging. For example, they can implement aging education programs in schools, teach elderly clients about available resources in the community, work with area agencies on aging to enhance service provision to the elderly (e.g., Senior Centers, local Offices on Aging, senior apartments), provide direct nursing care, and engage in implementing health education activities and programs. Innovative nurses have developed nurse-run clinics for senior citizens that provide essential health services; developed community aging education programs; and participated in community planning activities for the elderly.

Cross-Cultural Aging

Six percent of the world's population, 332 million people, are older than 65, and over one half of the world's elderly population live in developing nations (U.S. Bureau of the Census, 1992, p. v). By the year 2000 there will be more than 426 million elderly in the world (U.S. Bureau of the Census, p. v). Of all coun-

Myths About Aging

All Older People Are Alike

Fact: Older people are uniquely individual.

Most Older People Live in Institutional Settings

Fact: Only 5% of older people are in institutional settings.

The Majority of Older People are Lonely and Isolated From Their Families

Fact: The majority of older people live in a family setting. Many older people live near their children and have regular contact with friends and family.

Older People Cannot Learn

Fact: Older people are capable of learning and enjoy learning. The senior "Elderhostel" program is a good example of this.

The Majority of Older People View Themselves as Being in Poor Health

Fact: The majority (71%) of older people report their health as being good or excellent.

Older People Cannot Work

Fact: Approximately 3.6 million older Americans are in the labor force.

The Majority of Older People Have Incomes Below the Poverty Level

Fact: Only 20% of older Americans are classified as poor or near-poor.

Most Older People Have no Interest in Sexual Activity

Fact: The need for sexual activity does not stop with old age.

Old Age Begins at 65

Fact: In this country 65 was legislated as the age for Social Security Retirement benefits; but when "old age" begins is very individual.

Excerpts from Harris DK: *Sociology of Aging,* ed 2, New York, 1990, Harper and Row, p. 5; and American Association of Retired Persons: *A profile of older Americans 1993,* Washington, D.C., 1993, The Association.

tries, Sweden has the largest proportion of people over age 65 (U.S. Bureau of the Census, 2-19). Various countries and cultures differ in how they view and define elderly.

In some cultures elderly people are given elevated status and treated with great respect. Unfortunately, individuals from such cultures (e.g., Asian) may lose the advantageous position of older people seen in their society when their families emigrate to a Western culture such as the United States (Chen, 1987). The box on p. 736 illustrates some of the cultural and ethnic diversity in the elderly population in the United States.

Cultural sensitivity helps the nurse to elicit cultural values, attitudes, and health practices that affect how clients respond during times of stress and illness and aids in developing and implementing effective health promotion strategies. The cultural assessment guide found in Appendix 7-1 assists the community health nurse in obtaining cultural data. Understanding different cultural values and attitudes in relation to aging and health is essential for community health nurses to develop strategies that enhance the quality of life for the aged.

Developmental Tasks of Aging

Aging is a stage of human development, and all stages of human development are interrelated and have specific *developmental tasks.* Accomplishing developmental takes assists the individual in self-fulfillment and personal growth (refer to Figure 19-2). A number of developmental tasks exist for the elderly person, including establishing appropriate and satisfying living arrangements, adjusting to retirement and retirement income, establishing comfortable routines, safeguarding physical and mental health, adjusting to changes in health status, remaining in touch with family members and friends, continuing a supportive relationship with spouse or significant other (including a satisfying sexual relationship), keeping active and involved (including involvement in community activities), developing a personal philosophy of life, and having a sense of worth as a person (Duvall and Miller, 1985, p. 318; Murray and Zentner, 1989, pp. 525-526). According to Erikson (1982), older persons are faced with resolving the psychological conflict of *integrity versus despair,* with the successful accomplishment of integrity occurring when individuals review

◀ *A Look at Cultural/Ethnic Diversity in the Elderly—U.S.* ▶

Racial diversity within the elderly population is increasing in the U.S. Presently, 1 in 10 elderly are of races other than White, and by 2050 this is expected to increase to 2 in 10.

Black (2.5 million) and Hispanic (1.1 million) elderly Americans are the most heavily represented ethnic groups among the aged.

Between 1990 and 2050 the number of Black elderly is expected to quadruple and the Hispanic elderly population is expected to be seven times larger.

There is a *disparity in longevity* between ethnic groups. Life expectancy at birth is 79 years for White females, 74 years for Black females, 73 years for White males, and 65 years for Black males. However, longevity is increasing in U.S. ethnic groups. (About one-fifth of elderly Blacks and elderly Hispanics were 80+ in 1990 and this is expected to increase to one-third by 2050).

There is *economic disparity* between ethnic groups. Approximately 34 percent of elderly Blacks, 23 percent of elderly Hispanics and 10 percent of elderly Whites live in poverty. The lifetime employment earnings for elder Whites are significantly higher than the earnings for elder Blacks and Hispanics. This implies fewer retirement resources for Blacks and Hispanics.

From U.S. Bureau of the Census: *Sixty-five plus in America,* Washington, D.C., 1992, U.S. Government Printing Office, p. v, pp. 2-10 to 2-12.

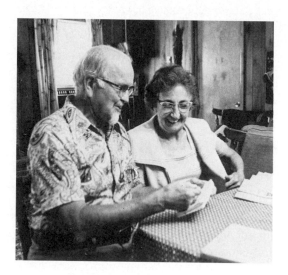

Figure 19-2 An aging couple.

their life activities, accept what they have done, and feel satisfied with what they have accomplished. Accomplishing developmental tasks often involves role reorientation when children are launched from the home, assuming caregiver roles with elderly parents, and changing work and leisure roles.

DEMOGRAPHY OF AGING PERSONS

In colonial times in the United States, half the population was under age 16 and only a few people lived to the age of 65 (U.S. Bureau of the Census, 1992, p. 2-1). Today less than 25% of Americans are under age 16, and 12.5% of the population, more than 31 million people, are over 65.

Since 1900 there has been a tenfold increase in older people (from 3 million to 31 million), and the percentage of Americans 65 and older has tripled (from 4% to 12%). Figure 19-3 illustrates this "aging" of America, how it is expected to continue, and how the "population pyramid" in the United States is changing. Analysis of this figure shows that by 2030 there will be as many people 65 and older in the United States as there are people under the age of 20. The box on p. 746 gives some descriptive information on aging and the elderly in the United States.

Of particular interest is the expanding age group of people 85 years and older. Figure 19-4 displays the growth of this age group in the United States from 1900 to 2050. In the 85 and older age group there are almost 36,000 centenarians, people who are 100 years old or older. The U.S. Bureau of the Census predicts there will be at least 1 million centenarians by 2080, and there could be as many as 5 million (U.S. Bureau of the Census, 1992, p. 1). This increase in the number of "oldest old" has significant implications for nursing and health care.

HEALTHY PEOPLE 2000 AND AGING

Healthy People 2000 (USDHHS, 1991) addressed the health of older Americans and formulated a national health goal to increase the span of healthy life for

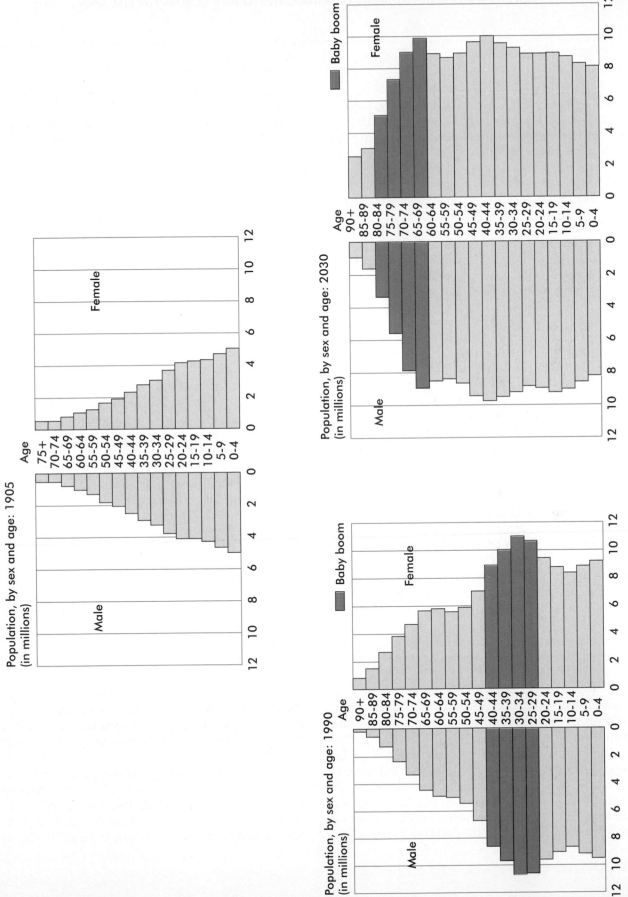

Figure 19-3 Population characteristics by age and sex, United States: 1905, 1990, and 2030. (From U.S. Bureau of the Census: *Sixty-five plus in America*, Washington, D.C., 1992, U.S. Government Printing Office, pp. 1-2, 2-4, 2-9.)

◀ *Aging in the United States* ▶

A child born today can expect to live to be 75+ years of age, compared to age 47 for a child born in 1900.

The elderly population increased more than 20% over the last decade. (Among American elderly, 18 million are age 65 to 74, 10 million are age 75 to 84, and 3 million are 85+.)

From 1980 to 1990 America's "oldest old", those 85+, increased almost 38% and is the most rapidly growing segment of our population.

The centenarian population, people 100+, doubled during the 1980s and 79% are female.

From 2010 to 2030 the elderly population is expected to **increase** 73% while the population under age 65 would **decrease** almost 3%. By 2040 we could have more people aged 65 or older than we have persons under 20 years of age.

More than half of the elderly live in the nine states of California, New York, Florida, Pennsylvania, Texas, Illinois, Ohio, New Jersey, and Michigan. Each of these states has more than 1 million elderly residents, and California has the largest number (3.1 million) while Florida has the largest proportion (18.4%).

Elderly women outnumber elderly men three to two.

Only 5% of American elderly reside in institutional settings such as nursing homes.

The majority of noninstitutionalized elderly (67%) live in a family setting, and about 31% live alone.

Data from American Association of Retired Persons: *Profile of older Americans 1993,* Washington, D.C., 1993, The Association; and U.S. Bureau of the Census: *Sixty-five plus in America,* Washington, D.C., 1992, U.S. Government Printing Office, pp. v, 1-1 to 1-2).

Americans (USDHHS, 1991, p. 6). Almost 30 specific national health objectives for the elderly are integrated throughout the document and given in Appendix 19-1 (USDHHS, pp. 589-591). These objectives illustrate the course of action the federal government is taking in providing health services to the elderly. The nurse should be familiar with these objectives, understand how they impact on nursing care, and be at the forefront of working to ensure they are met.

According to *Healthy People 2000,* the most important aspect of health promotion activities for older people is to maintain health and functional independence, and a significant number of the health problems evidenced with aging are either preventable or can be controlled by preventive activities (USDHHS, 1991, pp. 24, 587). In addition to primary prevention activities strong social support and regular primary care services are important in promoting the health of older adults (USDHHS, p. 587).

Unfortunately, many older people are not adequately participating in preventive health activities in relation to exercise, nutrition, immunizations, and health care visits. According to *Healthy People 2000,* less than a third of the noninstitutionalized elderly report participation in moderate physical activity, such as walking and gardening on a regular basis; less than 10% routinely engage in vigorous physical activity; only 10% receive pneumococcal vaccine and 20% receive influenza vaccines; and many do not have adequate nutritional intake or regular physical examinations and screenings. Nurses can encourage elderly clients to take part in preventive health activities. For the elderly, changing certain risk behaviors into healthy behaviors can improve health and reduce the likelihood of disability (USDHHS, 1991, p. 587). Today's Americans have the opportunity to stay healthy and active for longer than ever before!

Morbidity and Mortality

Most older people generally view their health positively. More than 70% of older people living in the community describe their health as excellent, very good, or good (AARP, 1993, p. 12). There was little difference between the sexes on their rating of health; however, older blacks were much more likely to relate their health as fair or poor (44%) than older whites (28%) (AARP, p. 12).

Major causes of death among people aged 65 and older are heart disease, cancer, stroke, chronic obstructive pulmonary disease, pneumonia, and influenza (National Center for Health Statistics [NCHS], 1992, pp. 19-20; USDHHS, 1991, p. 587). The most frequently occurring chronic problems for people 65 and older are arthritis (48%), hypertension (37%), hearing impairments (32%), heart disease (30%), orthopedic impairments (18%), cataracts and sinusitis (14% each), and diabetes (10%) (AARP, 1993, p. 13). Other

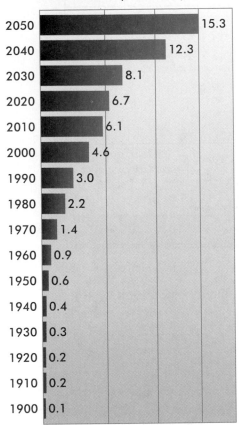

Population 85 years and over:
1900 to 2050 (in millions)

2050	15.3
2040	12.3
2030	8.1
2020	6.7
2010	6.1
2000	4.6
1990	3.0
1980	2.2
1970	1.4
1960	0.9
1950	0.6
1940	0.4
1930	0.3
1920	0.2
1910	0.2
1900	0.1

Figure 19-4 U.S. population 85 years and over: 1900 to 2050. (From U.S. Bureau of the Census: *Sixty-five plus in America,* Washington, D.C., 1992, U.S. Government Printing Office, p. 2-10.)

the effects of chronic conditions, is an important part of health promotion for older adults (NCHS, p. 19). The number of days in which usual activities are restricted because of illness or injury increases with age. Older people average 34 days a year of this restricted activity (AARP, 1993, p. 12).

Health Care Expenditures

Although the 65 and older age group represents 12% of the U.S. population, it accounts for 36% of total personal health care expenditures. This amounts to $5360 per older person per year and includes $72 billion in Medicare expenditures and $20 billion in Medicaid expenditures (AARP, 1993, p. 14). About $1500 of these expenditure came from direct payment "out-of-pocket" expenditures by the elderly individual (AARP, p. 14). These expenditures are more than four times the amount spent by younger persons on personal health care (AARP, p. 14).

Hospital expenses (42%) are the largest part of health expenditures for the elderly, followed by physicians (21%) and nursing home care (20%) (AARP, 1993 p. 14). Older people account for 35% of all hospital stays and 47% of all hospital days (AARP, p. 14).

Mental Health

Mental health is an important aspect of healthy aging. The United States has failed to ensure older persons access to community mental health services, and many older persons have unmet mental health needs (USDHHS, 1991, p. 26). Depression is considered to be a significant problem for the elderly, and 30% to 50% will experience depression severe enough to interfere with activities of daily living (Harper, 1989). Signs and symptoms of depression in the elderly often do not follow the patterns seen in younger individuals (Salamon, 1989). The elderly frequently describe physical rather than emotional manifestations of illness, and as a result depression often goes undetected by families and health professionals (USDHHS, p. 26). Unresolved depression can result in elder suicide, which is a major mental health concern among the elderly.

Men aged 65 through 74 have the highest rate of suicide in the United States (USDHHS, 1991, p. 26). *Healthy People 2000* has set a national objective to reduce suicides in this aggregate (USDHHS, p. 588).

chronic conditions include osteoporosis, incontinence, digestive disorders, constipation, chronic pain, sleep disturbance, Alzheimer's disease, and dementia.

Chronic conditions can have a great impact on quality of life and a person's ability to carry out activities of daily living (NCHS, 1992, p. 20). As discussed in Chapter 18, the incidence of chronic conditions increases with age, and these conditions can significantly affect physical functioning and activities of daily living (refer to Figure 19-5). Elderly persons most affected by health limitations are women, the poor, and minorities. However, income has a greater effect than race and sex on activity limitation. Improving functional independence in late life, and limiting

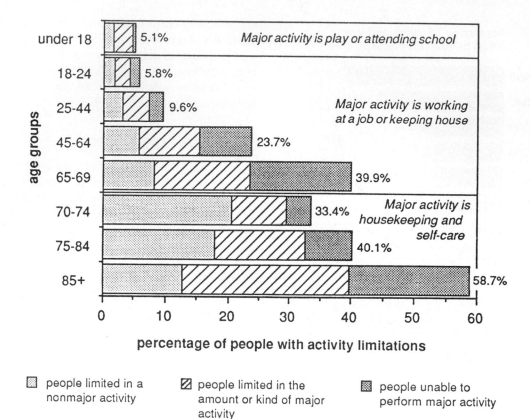

Figure 19-5 Activity limitations of all degrees by age groups. (From Kraus LE and Stoddard S: *Chartbook on disability in the United States, an InfoUse Report,* Washington, D.C., March 1989, U.S. National Institution on Disability and Rehabilitation Research, p. 10.)

The American Association for Retired Persons (AARP, 1989) has published *Elder Suicide: A National Survey of Prevention and Intervention Programs* to increase understanding among the general public about this problem. Among Americans 65 and older, the suicide rate is 50% higher than that of the general population (AARP). A research study by Meehan, Saltzman, and Sattin (1991) demonstrated that the rate of elder suicide has increased in recent years. Important high-risk indicators for suicide include social isolation and loneliness; pain and illness; status changes in employment, income, and independence; a sense of hopelessness; and previous suicide attempts. There are few suicide prevention and intervention programs which specifically target older persons, and few professionals are specifically trained in elder suicide prevention and counseling (AARP).

Health professionals "need to consider how current approaches to suicide prevention can better reflect the special circumstances of older persons" (Meehan, Saltzman, and Sattin, 1991, p. 1200). Nurses and other

health professionals need to recognize the clinical symptoms and risk factors for depression—bereavement, loneliness, and low self-esteem; assist in preventing depression; and assist in obtaining early diagnosis and treatment when depression occurs (USDHHS, 1991, p. 26).

SOME CONSIDERATIONS IN HEALTH PROMOTION OF THE AGED

A medical model focusing on secondary and tertiary prevention and disease pathology has historically been used in provision of health services to the elderly. Instead, health care that focuses on primary prevention and health promotion needs to be used. The *Healthy People 2000* age-related objectives are a move in this direction, and focus on health promotion activities.

Nurses need to be educated in gerontology and the health promotion needs of the elderly. It is interesting to note that education in gerontology is frequently lacking in the educational programs of health care professionals, and no health profession has claimed service to the elderly as its unique task. In a 1980 position paper the World Health Organization (WHO) recommended that nurses be the primary health care workers responsible for providing comprehensive health care to the elderly (WHO, 1980). Challenging and enriching opportunities exist for community health nurses in implementing health care for the elderly. Nurses need to be educated about aging and be familiar with the aging process. Nurses can use this knowledge in health promotion activities with the elderly, including health education activities to assist the elderly client in understanding the normal changes of aging.

Normal Changes of Aging

Aging is a natural and lifelong process that begins at the moment of birth. As we age, physical, psychosocial, and emotional changes occur. The physical, mental, and psychological changes associated with aging occur very gradually and are highly individual (e.g., less than 1% of the physical function an individual has at age 30 is lost each succeeding year). Normal body changes are associated with the aging process. Listed in Table 19-1 are some physical changes that occur with aging along with their implications. Elderly people, as well as nurses, must take these changes into account if the client's potential for health and wellness is to be maximized and changes of aging are to be accommodated. For instance, smooth muscle weakness and muscle atrophy often lead to constipation with older people. However, diet can be changed to help overcome this problem so that the client may not need other treatments.

Another change that comes with aging is thinning of the vaginal walls and atrophy of the testes. As a result, sexual experiences are different from those of earlier years but can still be fulfilling and pleasurable. Sexuality is often overlooked in care of the aging client. The community health nurse can help older clients to obtain the information and counseling they need to fulfill their sexuality.

Health care professionals tend to ignore death as a health education topic, but it is a topic that needs to be discussed. The end result of the aging process is death, and nurses, the aged, and their families must come to terms with helping the client and family work through this final stage of life and growth. Nurses should evaluate their own feelings and thoughts about death and dying in order to enhance client care.

Numerous books have been written that address elderly people who wish to remain healthy and enjoy old age. The noted psychologist B.F. Skinner has written (with M.E. Vaughn) *Enjoy Old Age: A Program of Self Management* (1983) out of his own life experience; Maggie Kuhn has written *Maggie Kuhn on Aging* (1977); and Alex Comfort has written *Say Yes to Old Age: Developing a Positive Attitude Toward Aging* (1990). A common theme in all of these books is that aging is individual, can be modified, and can be enjoyable.

The changes of aging listed in Table 19-1 do occur. However, aging can be enjoyed, the quality of life can be improved, and aging can be a time of great personal and family growth and fulfillment. Americans are fortunate to live in a country where they are able to grow old. They need to take advantage of, and look forward to, this opportunity for a long and active life.

Health Promotion and Wellness

Nursing efforts need to focus on health promotion with the elderly and facilitation of wellness and healthy aging. Health promotion and wellness activities have the potential to facilitate wellness, reduce premature death and disability, maintain health and functional independence of older adults, and improve the overall quality of life (USDHHS, 1991, p. 24, 587). Health promotion activities can assist in changing or eliminating risk factors such as lack of exercise, cigarette smoking, passive inhalation of smoke, excessive alcohol intake, obesity, high cholesterol diets, and environmental exposures that can lead to chronic diseases and conditions. Health promotion activities can help to postpone or avoid chronic diseases and conditions. *Healthy People 2000* has set an objective to increase to at least 90% the proportion of people aged 65 and older who have the opportunity to participate in at least one organized health promotion program through a senior center, lifecare facility, or other community-based setting that serves older adults each year (USDHHS, p. 589).

However, many older people are familiar with a health care system that has not encouraged or provided preventive health activities. Studies have shown that older people go to the doctor primarily when something is wrong; have trouble with the idea of

19-1 Physical Changes with Age

Change	Implications
Skeletal System	
1. Calcification of vertebral ligaments; drying out of invertebral discs	1. Postural change, decreased stature
2. Fibrocartilaginous atrophy; muscle atrophy	2. Loss of muscle power; contractures; paralysis; decreased respiration efficiency
3. Osteoporotic bone change	3. Decreased bone mass resulting in diminished weight bearing; spontaneous fractures
4. Ossification of joint cartilage	4. Joint stiffness; ankylosis
Gastrointestinal System	
1. Atrophy of mucosal linings; diminished production of hydrochloric acid (achlorhydria)	1. Delayed gastric emptying; decreased secretion of enzymes; impaired absorption; diminished food appeal
2. Smooth muscle weakness; muscle atrophy	2. Decreased excretory efficiency; incontinence; constipation; diminished peristalsis
Respiratory System	
1. Increase in residual lung volume	1. Distressed breathing; fear, anxiety; CO_2 retention; limited mobility
2. Muscle atrophy	2. Impaired ventilation, reduced ability to cough or deep breathe
3. Thickened membranes, alveoli, and capillaries	3. Impaired diffusion of O_2; diminished lung resiliency; impaired circulation
Neurologic System	
1. Atrophy of brain surface and brain cells	1. Behavioral changes: diminished emotions; disrupted self-image; less adaptability; confusion; disorientation; narrowing of interests
2. Atrophy of tendon reflexes	2. Stimuli-response change
3. Spinal cord synapse degeneration	3. Diminished overall coordinntion of neuromuscular, circulatory, glandular systems; increased susceptibility to shock
4. Optic and auditory nerve changes	4. Diminished vision and hearing
Genitourinary System	
1. Muscle weakness; muscle atrophy	1. Retention; guilt or embarrassment; incontinence
2. Kidney: reduced filtration; reduced blood flow; atrophy of glomeruli, tubules, nephrons; interstitial fibrosis	2. Urine retention; infection; pain, fear, anxiety; urinary stones; polyuria; nocturia; diminished excretion of toxic substances; diminished bladder capacity
3. Increasd bladder-urethra infection	3. Urinary stasis
4. In females, atrophy of ovarian, uterine, vaginal tissues; thinning of vaginal walls	4. Decreased lubrication; loss of fertility; need for increase in stimulation time
5. In males diminished spermatogenesis; decreased number of sperm; atrophy of testes; enlargement of prostate	5. Increased time for erection; reduced intensity of sensation; reduced volume and viscosity of seminal fluid; reduced force of ejaculation

NOTE: Listed in the left-hand column are major physical changes associated with normal aging; among these are changes often compounded by chronic disease. In the right-hand column are listed implications of these changes. It is often helpful to take these implications into account when providing care to older persons.

19-1 Physical Changes with Age—cont'd

Change	Implications
Nutrition and Metabolism	
1. Vitamin deficiencies: lack of vitamin B, inflammation of mucous membranes of the mouth; lack of vitamins C and K, capillary fragility	1. Discomfort; decreased food appeal; multiple bruises; disturbed self-image; fear, anxiety
2. Metabolic rate decrease—estimated at 1 percent per year after 25	2. Changes in nutrition, drug reaction, hypothermia
3. Depletion of water	3. Increased stress in excretion; constipation
4. Increased proportion of body fat	4. Less muscle mass, weakness; storage of nutrients in body fat
5. Mineral intake deficiency	5. Malnutrition; bone demineralization
6. Teeth: diseases, lost, ill-fitting dentures	6. Dehydration, malnutrition
7. Decreased digestive enzymes, gastric acidity, saliva	7. Impaired digestion; swallowing stress; cracking of mucous membranes of the mouth
Cardiovascular System	
1. Protein degeneration; lipofuscin accumulation	1. Diminished cardiac output—decreased blood flow to brain, heart, kidneys, liver
2. Fibrosis of blood vessel lumen; calcification of arteries; elongation of arteries	2. Increased systolic blood pressure; vasal sluggishness
3. Thickening of vessel membranes; slight thickening of the left ventricular wall	3. Impaired tissue nourishment; impaired removal of waste; edema
4. Increased perivascular fibrosis tissue	4. Increased peripheral resistance to blood flow; edema
Skin and Cutaneous Tissue	
1. Atrophy of sweat glands, hair follicles, subcutaneous tissue	1. Decreased perspiration; balding; increased susceptibility to trauma, abrasions, bed sores; inability to regulate body temperature
2. Deposits of melanin	2. "Age spots" occur and blemishes and growths are more frequent
3. Thickening of connective tissue	3. Finger and toenail thickening and hardening
4. Epidermal atrophy	4. Wrinkling of skin, fragility and dryness, decreased elasticity and slower wound healing
Immune System	
1. Decreased ability to make antibodies	1. Increased risk of infections
Sensory	
1. Lens becomes opaque and rigid	1. Decreased ability to focus on near objects
2. Yellowing of lens	2. Increased difficulty with color discrimination
3. Peripheral vision decreased	3. Lessened field of peripheral vision
4. Taste buds atrophy	4. Decreased sense of taste and appetite

From Linda David, Institute of Gerontology, as Consultant to Relocation Preparation Program, Pennsylvania Department of Public Welfare. Reference utilized: Rossman I: Human aging changes. In Burnside IM ed., *Nursing and the aged,* New York, 1976, McGraw-Hill; Kimmel DC.: Biological and intellectual aspects of aging. In Kimmel DC, ed: *Adulthood and aging,* New York, 1974, Wiley, chap 8, pp. 369-376; Jennings M, Nordstorm M, and Schumake N, Physiologic functioning in the elderly, *Nurs Clin North Am* 7(6):237-246, June 1972; Cameron M: *Views of aging: a teacher's guide,* Ann Arbor, 1967, Institute of Gerontology, University of Michigan-Wayne State University, pp. 146-148; Heckheimer EF: *Health promotion of the elderly in the community,* Philadelphia, 1989, Saunders.

having tests done when they have no symptoms; rely on health care professionals to recommend preventive tests or screenings; and do not know when to request tests or what to expect from them (AARP, 1991, p. 15). Getting older people to take part in health promotion activities can be a challenging but rewarding experience. The nurse can help the elderly client to see that "an ounce of prevention is worth a pound of cure." Community health nurses can assist people in taking responsibility for maintaining their health and promote healthy aging.

When implementing health promotion and wellness activities for the elderly client, community health nurses emphasize primary prevention activities but use secondary and tertiary prevention activities as well (refer to Chapter 11). Examples of *primary prevention interventions* that the community health nurse may implement include health education measures in relation to the normal changes of aging; need for preventive medical care (e.g. regular physical exams, receiving immunizations for pneumonia and influenza); proper exercise, nutrition, and oral health; safety measures; and health assessment. These activities also include anticipatory guidance that can help prepare the individual and family for significant life changes such as retirement. Predisposition to conditions such as coronary artery disease can be altered with a preventive program of exercise, good nutrition, avoidance of smoking, and protection from stress.

Primary prevention is integrally linked with health promotion and wellness. A goal of primary prevention activities is to help the elderly to maintain physical functioning and independence as long as possible (Alford and Futrell, 1992, p. 221; USDHHS, 1991, p. 587). Wellness programs for seniors are often located in local senior centers, churches and fitness organizations.

Secondary prevention activities involve early diagnosis and treatment, including encouraging and facilitating regular medical and dental care and periodic screening for conditions (e.g., hypertension and diabetes); encouraging adherence to medical treatment regimens; carrying out self-monitoring activities such as breast and testicular self-exams; and assessing for the warning signs of cancer. *Tertiary prevention* involves rehabilitative and restorative activities and include physical, occupational, recreational, and speech therapy and adjusting to activities of daily living in relation to changing levels of functioning.

The National Council on the Aging (NCOA) sponsors the *Health Promotion Institute.* This institute works to promote the ongoing development of primary, secondary, and tertiary prevention services that will help older Americans to achieve a higher quality of life and that will enhance awareness among older Americans of the importance of health promotion activities.

The American Association of Retired Persons (AARP) sponsors the *National Eldercare Institute on Health Promotion* that works to promote wellness among older Americans and to stimulate development of health promotion programs. It offers publications and materials on health education for seniors and serves as a resource center. Its publication *Healthy Older Adults* (1991) discusses topics such as good nutrition, exercise, injury prevention, health of older women, mental health, alcohol abuse, smoking, oral health, and osteoporosis. The Institute also offers a health calendar for seniors.

Health promotion for the elderly is multifaceted. Preventive interventions in relation to exercise, safety, elder abuse and neglect, nutrition, physical examinations, medications, employment, income, and housing are discussed here and illustrate select nursing activities possible with elderly clients and their families.

Exercise

Regular exercise helps optimize physical and mental health throughout life. Physiological decline associated with aging may actually be the result of inactivity, and older people can obtain significant benefits from exercise (USDHHS, 1991, p. 24; Rosenburg, 1993, p. 3). A survey by the National Center for Health Statistics showed that exercise can help prevent disease and extend and improve the quality of life; however, only one fourth of older Americans exercise regularly (National Resource Center on Health Promotion and Aging (NRCHPA), 1991, p. 11). Increased levels of physical activity are associated with reduced incidence of coronary heart disease, hypertension, colon cancer, depression, and anxiety (USDHHS, p. 24). Exercise can also help to prevent or alleviate low back pain and reduce the pain of arthritis. *Healthy People 2000* has set objectives to increase the proportion of elderly people who engage regularly in light to moderate physical activity (USDHHS, p. 589).

Many older people report that they are unsure of what types of exercise they should be doing and the duration of such exercise. In research by O'Neill and Reid (1991) 87% of the elderly in the study perceived that they had at least one major barrier that prevented their involvement in physical activity, such as an existing health problem or lack of knowledge about exercise resources and regimes (refer to Figure 19-6).

As with everyone else, older people with existing diseases and conditions should consult a physician before engaging in an exercise program. Many communities have YMCAs, YWCAs, and other fitness centers that offer senior exercise programs. There are many publications on exercise targeted for seniors and each person will want to assess what best meets his or her needs.

Safety

Accidents are one of the leading causes of death among the elderly. Physiological factors that contribute to accidents are weakness, slowed reaction time, uncertain gait, and changes in hearing and vision. Falls are the leading cause of accidental death in those 65 and older and each year more than a half-million elderly Americans are treated in the emergency room for falls (Heckheimer, 1989, p. 353). *Healthy People 2000* has numerous objectives that address the need to reduce accidental injuries from falls, motor vehicle accidents, and fires in older adults (USDHHS, 1991, p. 588). Many accidents occur in the home and could be prevented if people followed simple safety rules and eliminated hazards in the home environment. The nurse can assist the client in learning about such safety precautions.

Fear of falls and their resultant injuries limits the activities of many older people. Since most falls occur in or around the home, the home should be assessed for safety hazards and made as safe as possible. Stairs and bathrooms are the most dangerous locations for falls. Stairs need to be adequately lighted, free of clutter, and be equipped with handrails and nonskid surfaces whenever possible. It may be helpful to outline the edge of each step with a luminescent or contrast tape or color and to paint top and bottom steps so that they are easily noticed. Bathrooms should have hand rails, nonslip adhesive surfaces in tubs and showers, and nonslip flooring.

Other safety precautions around the home include having enough light; having light switches within easy reach; using a light when getting up at night; using nonskid soles on shoes; eliminating throw rugs, cast-

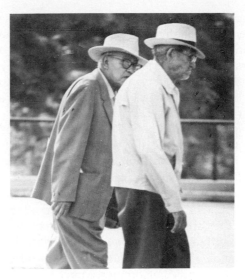

Figure 19-6 Nurses should stress the benefit of exercise to health. Exercising with a friend battles loneliness. (Courtesy of Ken Yamaguchi. In Castillo HM: *The nurse assistant in long-term care: a rehabilitative approach,* St. Louis, 1992, Mosby.)

ers on chairs, and extension cords; avoiding sedation; and placing distinct labels on medications and toxic substances. Smoking in bed should be eliminated. To avoid accidental scaldings and burns, lowering hot water heater temperatures and labeling hot and cold water facets is helpful. Accidental hypothermia or hyperthermia (heat stress) may occur in the elderly. Older people need to be encouraged to dress warmly during cool months, not stay outside for a long time during periods of extreme heat or cold, and keep their homes adequately heated in the winter and cooled in the summer. In many communities the poor elderly can obtain financial assistance from local resources to adequately heat their homes during the winter. Area Offices on Aging are knowledgeable about such resources.

Having a telephone in the home is an important safety measure. The telephone and emergency numbers should be in a convenient, accessible location— often at the bedside. Telephone services such "Friendly Caller" programs help to give the elderly contact with the outside world in case of an emergency and should be considered for the frail or isolated elderly. Use of a personal medical emergency response system helps to ensure the safety and independence for frail, chronically ill, or homebound elderly (Heckheimer, 1989, p. 354).

The nurse can be of assistance in making seniors aware of the health risks of accidents and in helping to prevent them. The nurse can also help older adults understand that safety is an area over which they have control and that safety precautions can help to promote health and maintain quality of life. Older adults owe it to themselves to "play it safe."

Crime and the elderly is another safety concern. Contrary to popular belief, the elderly have the lowest victimization rates of any age group in our society except for "personal larceny with contact" (i.e., purse snatching and pickpocketing) (Harris, 1990, p. 400). However, when crimes are committed against the elderly they are often more serious than for other age groups, and research shows that the elderly rank fear of crime as a major concern (Harris, p. 401; Heckheimer, 1989, p. 371). Common crimes experienced by the elderly are purse snatchings, fraud, theft, vandalism, and harassment (Heckheimer, p. 371). Some characteristics of the elderly that make them more vulnerable to crime are decreased physical strength, decreased sensory perception, and living alone. Fraud in the form of consumer fraud, confidence games, and medical quackery is a major form of crime against the elderly (Harris, p. 406). Fear of crime may add to the social isolation of elderly people.

Elder Abuse and Neglect

It has been estimated that more than 1,000,000 older Americans are abused and neglected each year (Heckheimer, 1989, p. 375). These mistreated elders are often frail, dependent, over age 70, and women. Abuse may be *physical* (e.g., beating, murder), *psychological* (e.g., intimidation, fear), or *financial/material* (e.g., misuse or misappropriation of funds or property). Neglect can be either passive or active. *Passive neglect* is the unintentional failure to fulfill a caretaking obligation due to things such as ignorance or lack of ability. *Active neglect* is an intentional failure to fulfill a caretaking obligation. Examples of neglect are nonprovision of food or health-related services, deprivation of dentures or eyeglasses, and abandonment (Douglass, 1988). A new form of abandonment has been dubbed "granny dumping," and often involves an elderly person being left at a hospital emergency room by caretakers (Hey and Carlson, 1991, p. 1). They are abandoned by children, family, or friends who no longer want or can handle the responsibility of caregiving and who are relinquishing this responsibility (Hey and Carlson, p. 1).

Each state has some kind of elder abuse legislation, similar to child abuse legislation, to protect the elderly (Miller, 1990). According to Miller, elder abuse is seldom reported to appropriate protective agencies (p. 603). As with other forms of family violence, authorities may hesitate to become involved.

Signs and Symptoms of Abuse and Neglect

Detecting elder abuse is not always easy (Ashley and Fulmer, 1988). Murray and Zentner (1989, p. 503) state that signs and symptoms of elder abuse include bruises, fractures, malnutrition; undue confusion not attributable to the physiological consequences of aging; conflicting explanations about the elder's condition; unusual fears exhibited by the elder; a report of the daily routine that contains many gaps; apparent impaired functioning or abnormal behavior by the caregiver; and indifference or hostility displayed by the caregiver in response to questions. Avoidance of questions and vague responses may also indicate risk of neglect or abuse. A recent, unexpected change in the financial status of the caregiver can be a sign of financial abuse. A number of factors play a part in elder abuse, including crowded or inadequate family living conditions, marital problems in the caregiving family, insufficient income, increasing dependency needs of the elderly, pathological parent-child relationships (e.g., children who were mistreated by parents now mistreating parents), pathological caregivers, and functional impairment of caregivers (Harris, 1990, p. 409). Lack of knowledge regarding elderly persons health needs can also lead to neglect. Also, many caretakers are elderly themselves and have difficulty taking care of their own needs, much less the needs of another family member.

Documentation and Reporting

According to Miller (1990, pp. 628-629), in assessing cases of suspected abuse or neglect the health professional should document (1) background data (e.g., client's name, address, phone number, caregiver name, documentation of previous maltreatment); (2) any signs of abuse or neglect (e.g., bruises, welts, burns, broken bones, hunger); (3) severity of symptoms; (4) indicators of maltreatment intentionality (e.g., caregiver will not allow nurse to be alone with client); (5) symptoms of acute or chronic illness (e.g., incontinence); (6) functional incapacity (e.g., an inability to dress or toilet without assistance); (7) aggravating social conditions (e.g., client lives alone and is isolated); (8) source or information (e.g., agency referral); and (9) recommendations (e.g., opening the case for home health care services). If the nurse suspects abuse or neglect she or he is usually mandated by state law to report it to the appropriate agency, often the state department of human or social services.

Prevention

Prevention is the key to resolving the serious problem of elder abuse. Primary prevention activities include encouraging people to plan for future care needs while they are healthy and capable of making such decisions, providing adequate community resources to prevent caregiver burnout (e.g., respite care, financial aid, counseling), fostering personal self-esteem, and promoting positive attitudes about aging. Secondary prevention efforts focus on early casefinding and treatment (e.g., crisis intervention, Neighborhood Watches and "buddy" systems). Tertiary prevention interventions involve family and caregiver rehabilitation activities in relation to counseling and care management, and in some cases the removing of the elderly person from the setting. However, the community placement options for such elders are often limited.

Nutrition

Nutrition is an important aspect of health across the lifespan. Researchers have estimated that 15% to 50% of those age 65 and older have poor nutrition or are malnourished (Greely, 1991). Many older persons have at least one chronic condition that could improve with proper nutrition. Poor nutrition among older people occurs due to a number of problems such as illness, lack of proper hydration, oral health problems, poverty, medications, social isolation, and mobility limitations (Malnutrition, 1993, p. 4). Although inadequate nutrition is usually evidenced in various forms of malnutrition, overnutrition can also be a problem. *Healthy People 2000* has set an objective to increase to at least 80% the receipt of home food services by people aged 65 and older who have difficulty in preparing their own meals or are otherwise in need of home-delivered meals (USDHHS, 1991, p. 589).

The *Nutrition Screening Initiative* is a program sponsored by the American Academy of Family Physicians, American Dietetic Association, and the National Council on the Aging and funded in part by Ross Laboratories. It is committed to the identification of nutritional problems in older persons, improved elder nutrition, and improved delivery of nutrition services to the elderly. The Initiative has developed a checklist that can be helpful to the nurse when initiating discussion about diet and nutrition (refer to Figure 19-7). The Initiative can be contacted at 1010 Wisconsin Avenue NW, Suite 800, Washington, D.C., 20007 (202-625-1662).

Nutrition plays an important part in maintaining health, independence, and quality of life for older Americans. The aging process can actually be slowed down through eating well (Greely, 1991). Eating the proper foods can help older Americans to lower their risks of health problems such as high blood pressure, osteoporosis, diabetes, heart disease, and cancer (NRCHPA, 1991, p. 9). Early diagnosis and treatment of nutritional problems can improve the management of chronic conditions in older people.

Deficiencies in intake of protein, calcium, iron, and vitamins C and A are common among elderly persons. Foods such as cheeses, yogurt, and buttermilk may help to meet these deficiencies and are good sources of protein. Some suggestions for a longer, healthier life through good nutrition are given in the box on p. 749.

In general, people should eat a variety of foods; maintain a desirable weight; avoid fried and fatty foods; eat an adequate amount of fiber-rich foods; and avoid too much sugar and starch (Greely, 1991). A dietary daily regimen for the elderly is given in the box on p. 749. If a person is not getting adequate nutrition from their daily diet then supplements should be taken (Greely).

Adequate water intake is an essential part of good nutrition. Fluid intake is often less because the aging process may reduce the thirst sensation, and some aging persons limit fluid intake to ease problems with urinary incontinence (Murray and Zentner, 1989, p. 509). Fluids are necessary to maintain kidney function, aid in the absorption of medications and high fiber foods, decrease side effects of some medications, aid in expectoration, soften stools, and prevent dehydration.

Getting Seniors to Eat Well

The community nurse plays an important role in senior nutrition counseling, helping elders to realize that their physical, emotional, and economic status all play a part in good nutrition. Getting seniors to eat well and pay attention to nutrition is a complex challenge. Problems such as ill-fitting dentures, loss of teeth, and periodontal disease make chewing painful and can make it difficult to maintain good nutrition. Also, a decreased sense of smell directly affects the

The warning signs of poor nutritional health are often overlooked. Use this checklist to find out if you or someone you know is at nutritional risk.

Read the statements below. Circle the number in the *yes* column for those that apply to you or someone you know. For each *yes* answer score the number in the box. Total your nutritional score.

DETERMINE YOUR NUTRITIONAL HEALTH

	Yes
I have an illness or condition that made me change the kind and/or amount of food I eat.	2
I eat fewer than 2 meals per day.	3
I eat few fruits or vegetables, or milk products.	2
I have 3 or more drinks of beer, liquor, or wine almost every day.	2
I have tooth or mouth problems that make it hard for me to eat.	2
I don't always have enough money to buy the food I need.	4
I eat alone most of the time.	1
I take 3 or more different prescribed or over-the-counter drugs a day.	1
Without wanting to, I have lost or gained 10 pounds in the last 6 months.	2
I am not always physically able to shop, cook, and/or feed myself.	2
	Total

Total your nutritional score. If it's —

0-2   **Good!** Recheck your nutritional score in 6 months.

3-5   **You are at moderate nutritional risk.** See what can be done to improve your eating habits and lifestyle. Your office on aging, senior nutrition program, senior citizens center or health department can help. Recheck your nutritional score in 3 months.

6 or more   **You are at high nutritional risk.** Bring this checklist the next time you see your doctor, dietitian or other qualified health or social service professional. Talk with them about any problems you may have. Ask for help to improve your nutritional health.

These materials developed and distributed by the Nutrition Screening Initiative, a project of:

American Academy of Family Physicians

The American Dietetic Association

National Council on the Aging, Inc.

Remember that warning signs suggest risk, but do not represent diagnosis of any condition.

Figure 19-7   Nutrition Screening Checklist. (From *Nutrition Screening Initiative, 1992,* Washington, D.C., a cooperative effort of the American Dietetic Association, the American Academy of Family Physicians, and the National Council on Aging. Used with permission.)

◀ *Suggestions for a Longer, Healthier Life through Good Nutrition* ▶

Establish good eating patterns now and stick to them. The quality of your diet becomes even more important as you age and is critical in your later years.

To strengthen your body's ability to combat infection and chronic disease, make sure you eat food containing immune-friendly nutrients such as vitamins E and B_6 and the mineral zinc.

To prevent your bones from becoming porous and brittle, choose food rich in vitamin D and calcium.

To ensure your digestive system stays healthy, active and regular, include at least 20 grams of fiber in your diet every day.

To safeguard your vision and help delay later-life problems such as cataracts, increase your intake of vitamins C, E, and betacarotene.

To reduce your risk of cardiovascular disease, limit fat, dietary cholesterol and sodium and focus on sources high in vitamins B_6, B_{12} and folate as well as soluble fiber, calcium and potassium.

To help keep your mind alert and your nervous system performing at its best, vitamins B_6, B_{12} and folate should be in your diet.

To maintain your idea body weight and keep excess fat off, stay active and choose a diet low in fat, high in complex carbohydrates and dietary fiber.

To keep your appetite hearty and your muscles healthy, mix aerobic exercises (walking or swimming) with simple activities that strengthen muscle.

From Rosenburg IH: As you age: 10 keys to a longer, healthier, more vital life, *Worldview* 5(2):2-3, 1993.

elderly person's ability to taste and enjoy food, and certain medications can depress appetite or taste sensations. Other factors, such as diminished efficiency of the digestive and excretory systems, reduced income, and loneliness and depression affect nutritional status.

Older people living alone are especially vulnerable to the problems of inadequate nutrition, often losing interest in meal planning and preparation. Eating with others helps to make mealtimes more enjoyable (Promoting, 1993, p. 9). The frail elderly may lack the dexterity and energy to feed themselves and thus pose a unique nutritional challenge.

The nurse should implement a nutritional assessment such as a 3-day diet recall to assist in evaluating a client's nutritional status and needs. Such a recall can lead to discussions of food preparation and preferences, buying habits, and eating problems and can be an excellent teaching tool. Older persons have developed a lifetime of food practices, and the nurse needs to remember that nutrition habits are not easy to change. Also, cultural, ethnic, religious beliefs, and income strongly influence nutritional practices (refer to Figure 19-8).

"Spending down" for food is difficult when food prices keep increasing and senior income remains relatively constant. The nurse can assist in low-cost food buying and preparation. Ingenuity in using dried legumes, beans, whole cereal grains, poultry, fish,

◀ *Daily Dietary Regimen* ▶
for the Person 65+

2 to 3 half-cup servings of milk, cheese or yogurt for men

4 half-cup servings of milk, cheese or yogurt for women

6 or more servings of whole-grain breads or cereals

3 to 4 half-cup servings of fruits

3 to 5 half-cup servings of vegetables

2 to 3 servings (approximately 5 to 7 ounces) of protein such as lean meat, poultry, fish, and alternatives such as eggs, nuts, and dried beans and peas

From Greely A: *Nutrition and the elderly,* Washington, D.C., 1991, Publication No. (FDA) 91-2243, United States Department of Health and Human Services.

dried fortified milk, and less expensive cuts of meat is often helpful. Although not always inexpensive, foods such as low-fat cheeses and yogurt are good sources of protein and keep well when refrigerated.

Many seniors are not aware of the meal programs in the community that can help to stretch the food budget such as Food Stamps, Meals on Wheels, and meals at senior centers. Alternating meal preparation with someone else, and "Meal Clubs," where meal

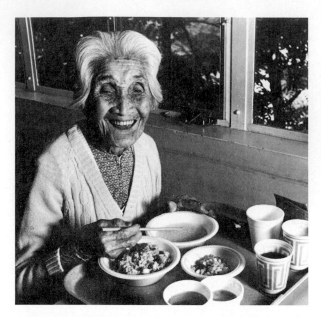

Figure 19-8   Chopsticks and oriental food make the meal enjoyable for this elderly Japanese lady. (Courtesy Ken Yamaguchi. In Castillo HM: *The nurse assistant in long-term care: a rehabilitative approach,* St. Louis, 1992, Mosby.)

preparation responsibilities are shared, can help to curb food costs, offer variety to meals, and provide companionship. Cooking in larger quantities and freezing foods may be a helpful idea. Many local restaurants offer senior discounts and local churches frequently sponsor meals for seniors.

Serving foods in an attractive, pleasant manner often enhances appetite. Fixing foods with different textures and aromas and using flavor boosters such as commercially prepared flavor enhancers and spices can enhance appetite (Promoting, 1993, p. 9). Switching around from food to food during meals (after three bites) helps to prevent sensory adaptation in which the palate becomes less sensitive to taste and food becomes less tasty (Promoting, p. 9). Also, eating each food separately, rather than mixing them, helps to increase the ability to taste the food (Murray and Zentner, 1989, p. 509). Good oral hygiene should be encouraged and helps to promote appetite.

Physical barriers to proper nutrition need to be considered. Lack of transportation to well-stocked and cost-efficient grocery stores, restaurants, and food programs can pose a nutrition problem. Physical disabilities such as orthopedic problems and poor vision can inhibit the ability to shop. Shopping assistance may be available through local homemaker services,

senior centers, or friends and family. Some grocery stores are now providing electric shopping carts that could be useful to the older shopper.

On a national level numerous resources on nutrition and the elderly exist, such as the U.S. Administration on Aging's National Eldercare Institute on Nutrition, which conducts research and provides information on nutrition for the elderly, American Dietetic Association Gerontological Nutritionist Practice Group, and National Meals on Wheels Foundation, which was created to promote public awareness and financially support senior meal programs. These organizations can assist the nurse in obtaining nutrition resources. Local nutritional services to the elderly are often coordinated through senior centers and Area Offices on Aging. When the nutrition problems of the client are beyond the scope of the nurse, a nutritionist or physician should be contacted. Many local health departments have nutritionists on the staff; nutritionists are also available through local hospitals and county extension services.

Physical Examinations

Regular physical and dental examinations need to continue throughout old age. They can help to detect conditions early, minimize their effects, and help to prevent further complications. Without these examinations problems that could be prevented or treated might go undetected and develop into serious conditions. For example, a sigmoidoscopy can detect polyps that 10 years later might become cancer of the colon, and early detection of diabetes can help to keep the disease under control. Health habits regarding sleep, exercise, alcohol, and cigarette consumption can be discussed with clients at the time of such examinations. Health risk appraisals (refer to Chapter 9) can be done and used to assist the professional in preventive counseling activities. A schedule of when periodic health examinations should be done is given in Figure 19-9.

Medications

The elderly account for 32% of all prescription drug use—400 million prescriptions a year (National Resource Center on Health Promotion and Aging [NRCHPA], 1991, p. 5). By the year 2000 the elderly are expected to account for more than half of the prescription drugs dispensed (NRCHPA, p. 5). They also take a significant number of over-the-counter medications.

Periodic health examination protocol						
Age	20	30	40	50	60	70+
Physical exam and health risk assessment	Every 5 years		3 years	Every 2 years		Yearly
Blood pressure	Yearly					
Cholesterol	Every 5 years					
Breast and pelvic exam	Every 3 years		Yearly			
Pap smear	Yearly					
Mammography		Baseline at 35	2 years	Yearly		
Stool for blood			3 years	Yearly		
Proctosigmoidoscopy				Every 3 years (after 2 yearly negatives)		
Immunizations	Tetanus/diphtheria—every 10 years Influenza—yearly after age 65 Pneumovax—at age 65					

Figure 19-9 Periodic health examinations. (From Annual checkups—who needs them, *Aging* 365:2, 1993.)

At least 25% to 50% of the elderly in the community make errors in their medication regimens (Palmieri, 1991, p. 34), and tend to self-medicate in terms of increasing or decreasing prescribed medication dosages. About 25% of hospital admissions of older Americans result from taking prescriptions incorrectly, and almost one fourth of all nursing homeadmissions result from older adults being unable to take their medications properly (NRCHPA, 1991, p. 5). *Healthy People 2000* has an age-related objective to increase to at least 75% the number of primary health care providers who routinely review with their patients aged 65 and older all prescribed and over-the-counter medicines they are taking each time a new medication is prescribed (USDHHS, 1991, p. 590). When assessing drug use it is important to note the amount being taken in addition to what has been prescribed.

Some older Americans do not take their medications because they cannot afford to buy them, and Medicare does *not* pay for the cost of prescription drugs. A common practice among some elderly is to take less than the prescribed medication dosage to decrease cost.

The physiological changes that come with aging alter how older adults distribute, metabolize, and excrete drugs; make them particularly susceptible to adverse drug effects; and cause increased plasma levels of drugs. Decline in the function of the kidney is the single most important reason for this altered responsiveness (Palmieri, 1991, p. 33). The elderly do not actually achieve therapeutic effects at lower doses than younger adults (Palmieri, p. 33). Among the elderly, changes in behavior and mental status may be attributed to senility and depression, and a drug reaction many go unsuspected and unrecognized. There is an extensive list of medications that cause psychiatric symptoms (Medical Letter, Inc., 1993).

Older people frequently have chronic disease conditions that require long-term multiple-drug therapy. Research studies have revealed that the longer older people take a prescription, and the more drugs they take, the greater the chance they will not take them as prescribed (NRCHPA, 1991, p. 5). These same studies show that older people are often confused about the medicines they take.

Health professionals need to be careful in explaining medication regimens to older people. The community health nurse is in an excellent position to help clients avoid medication errors and comply with medication regimens. During home visits a medication history is essential. This can be initiated with questions such as "Let's take yesterday, starting with when you woke in the morning. What was the first medicine you took? How much of the medicine do you take? How many times a day do you take the medication? What do you take the medicine for?" and repeating such questions for all medications involved. Checking a client's medication and assessing for side effects needs to be done on each visit. Alcohol intake of the elderly person should be assessed in relation to the effect it can have on medication and drug interactions. Appendix 19-2 provides a guide to use when doing a medication assessment with elderly persons. A medication assessment should be completed on a regular basis because factors that effect drug use can change dramatically in a very short time period.

Employment and Retirement

Millions of senior citizens have retired from the workplace. However, over 3 million older Americans are working and approximately half of these workers are employed part-time (U.S. Bureau of the Census, 1992, pp. 4-5). The National Council on the Aging (NCOA) offers the *Senior Community Service Employment Program* and works with employers in helping them to see the advantages of hiring older workers and keeping older workers in the workplace.

Retirement is a contemporary phenomenon. Before the passage of the retirement provisions of the Social Security Act of 1935 (refer to Chapter 4), few Americans retired or could afford to retire. Most people worked until they were too ill or disabled to work, and really could not enjoy their retirement years. With the advent of retirement benefits people were able to retire from work, and a new developmental task was created.

Today many people are able to retire from work while they are still in good health. Some people retire early, many retire between the ages of 60 and 70, and some never completely retire. Retirement is looked forward to by some and dreaded by others. The span of one's life that is spent in retirement has grown from 3% in 1900 (Growing old, 1985) to more than 20% today.

Many older people continue to work after retirement in part-time or voluntary positions. *Retired Senior Volunteer Programs* (RSVP) are active in many communities. The *Service Corps of Retired Executives* (SCORE) is a well-known volunteer effort sponsored by the U.S. Small Business Administration that matches retired

executives with businesses that can use their services. Senior citizens can be found volunteering their time in all aspects of community life; it has been estimated that one in four older Americans performs volunteer community services.

A strong correlation exists between successful retirement and retirement planning. The nurse can be instrumental in helping people recognize the need for retirement planning, can assist persons in seeing the options open to them, make them aware of community resources, and offer support and encouragement during this stage of transition.

The National Council on the Aging (NCOA) and the American Association of Retired Persons (AARP) have information available that assists in planning for retirement, and many workplaces have retirement planning programs available. Planning for retirement is more than just financial planning; it is planning for the entire retirement experience. It is a time for role restructuring and major decisions such as choosing where one will live, deciding on a new or part-time career, determining educational, recreational and leisure pursuits, addressing relationships with friends and family, and reassessing finances. For many, retirement is the first time when they have significant amounts of time for leisure and recreational pursuits.

Income

Income security is a major issue for everyone throughout life. Without adequate financial security the older person may neglect many important health services and quality of life will be impaired. In old age, especially after retirement, many Americans live on relatively fixed incomes. The median income of older persons is approximately $14,000 a year for men and $8,000 for women, and the majority of people age 75 and older who live alone have incomes below $10,000 (NCOA, 1993, p. 10). Almost 4 million older Americans live in poverty and another 2 million are classified as "near-poor" (having incomes between 100% to 125% of the poverty level) (NCOA, p. 11). Older women, minorities, and the "oldest old" (those 85 and older) are more likely to live in poverty (USDHHS, 1992, *Income of the Aged Chartbook*).

The major source of income for Americans is Social Security; nine out of ten aged households receive Social Security benefits (USDHHS, *Income of Aged Chartbook,* 1992, p. 8). Only 7% of the elderly receive public assistance, and 5% receive Veteran's benefits

(USDHHS, *Income of Aged Chartbook,* p. 8). Social Security Act programs for the elderly person in relation to income were discussed in Chapter 5 and include Old Age, Survivors and Disability Insurance (OASDI) and Supplemental Security Income (SSI). OASDI is the largest entitlement program in the United States today. Refer to Chapter 5 for specific information on these programs.

Private employee pension programs are another form of retirement income. These plans, like OASDI, are paid into during the person's working years and benefits are paid out during retirement. Such pension plans provided approximately 9% of the income of those 65 and older in 1990 (NCOA, 1993, p. 15), with less than half of the elderly receiving such pensions (USDHHS, 1992, *Income of Aged Chartbook,* p. 8).

Housing and Living Arrangements

Housing is a major health concern for the elderly. Some housing options for the elderly include independent living, congregate housing, assisted living, and shared housing, in settings such as apartments, condominiums, duplexes, mobile homes, single-family homes, and retirement communities. Innovative housing ideas for the elderly are being developed, including home sharing, home equity conversion, group homes, "granny flats," and home renovations that suit the individual's changing needs. The Center for Independent Living discussed in Chapter 18 helps to develop innovative floor plans and interior designs that aid the elderly person in independent living.

Many older Americans live in their own homes. However, housing for the elderly is generally older (many live in units that are more than 30 years old), less adequate, and less well maintained than for other age groups. For elderly men, 76% live with a spouse, 7% live with relatives, and 17% live alone or with nonrelatives; and for elderly women 41% live with a spouse, 16% live with relatives, and 43% live alone or with nonrelatives (AARP, 1993, pp. 3-4).

The National Council on the Aging (NCOA) has a national goal of decent, affordable, safe, and appropriate housing for senior citizens (NCOA, 1993, p. 18). However, an 80% decline over the past decade in federal spending for housing and community development has placed 800,000 older adults on waiting lists for subsidized housing and is making this goal difficult to achieve (NCOA, p. 18). Appropriate and affordable housing helps to provide security and com-

fort, encourages socialization, and prevents or delays the costly alternative of institutionalization (NCOA, p. 18). Whether to live in their own homes or apartments, live with relatives, or live in a long-term care facility are just some of the many issues that confront the elderly. No one housing alternative is the single best choice for all older persons (NCOA, p. 40).

Rural Elderly

According to the 1990 census, 25% of older Americans, 7.7 million people, live in a rural setting, and the number continues to grow (Profile, 1993, p. 11). In many cases the elderly in these rural towns are the "oldest-old", those 85 and older. The health promotion needs of the rural elderly are extensive. The rural elderly have a greater incidence of chronic health conditions such as arthritis, cardiovascular disease, and diabetes than elderly living in metropolitan areas (Growing old, 1993, p. 19). Minority rural elders have poorer health than other rural elders (Growing old, p. 19).

The elderly in rural America are often isolated from access to health care services and have inadequate health care. Between 1981 and 1988 190 rural hospitals closed, and more continue to close (Where doctors, 1993, p. 13). Many rural areas have a shortage of health care professionals; studies have shown that rural areas have almost 44% fewer physicians than metropolitan areas (Where doctors, p. 13) and many do not have a drugstore. Rural elderly often lack access to public transportation and may not have transportation to get to necessary health care services. These same elderly may live in isolated areas and have to travel 5 miles or more to a main road (Growing old, 1993, p. 23). The 1992 reauthorization of the Older Americans Act addressed health and welfare issues of the rural elderly (NCOA, 1993, p. 36).

NCOA's National Center on Rural Aging (NCRA) advocates for the rights of the rural elderly and works with federal and national organizations that provide funds, develop policies, and provide services for this at-risk aggregate. The National Resource Center for Rural Elderly (University of Missouri, Kansas City, Missouri) focuses on service provision, housing, and health care for the elderly and serves as a clearinghouse for information. Community health nurses need to help link the rural elderly to the services that are available and advocate further services for them. For example, elderly persons who belong to AARP can obtain prescribed medications at a reduced cost by mail if there is no drugstore in their community.

SIGNIFICANT LEGISLATION

Two extremely significant pieces of legislation for the elderly are the Social Security Act of 1935 and the Older Americans Act of 1965. The Social Security Act was discussed in Chapter 4 and the Older Americans Act is presented here.

Older Americans Act

Under President Lyndon B. Johnson, Congress passed the Older Americans Act (OAA) of 1965, which gave national attention to the needs of the elderly and authorized the Administration on Aging within the Department of Health and Human Services. It funded research and training in gerontology, facilitated development of regional, state, and local programs on aging, and was an effort to assist older Americans in achieving:

- An adequate retirement income
- The best possible physical and mental health available
- Suitable, affordable housing
- Necessary restorative services
- Employment without age discrimination
- Retirement in health, honor, and dignity
- Meaningful activity within the widest range of civic, cultural, and recreational opportunities
- Provision of efficient and coordinated community services
- Benefits from research knowledge that can sustain and improve health and quality of life
- Freedom, independence, and the free exercise of individual initiative in planning and managing their own lives

Over the years the act has been amended to include the establishment of area agencies on aging, multipurpose senior centers (discussed later in this chapter), senior employment and volunteer programs, senior nutrition programs, health education and preventive health activities, senior transportation services, and in-home health care. Under provisions of the act the next White House Conference on Aging will be held in 1994—this conference was last held in 1981. The act is a major piece of legislation relating to services for older Americans. Appendix 19-3 presents some significant amendments to the act.

Social Security Act of 1935

The Social Security Act of 1935 mandates many programs that serve elderly people. The main provisions of the act that affect older Americans are the income support programs of Old Age, Survivors and Disability Insurance (OASDI) and Supplemental Security Income (SSI), and the health components of Medicare and Medicaid. Refer to Chapter 4 for a discussion of these programs and Appendix 4-1 for amendments to the Act.

Other Legislation

Several other pieces of legislation have helped to improve the quality of life for the elderly. Examples of this legislation include the Age Discrimination in Employment Act of 1967, which prevented age discrimination in employment and protected workers from forced retirement, the Rehabilitation Act of 1973, which provided for rehabilitation services to Americans, the Research on Aging Act of 1974, which created the National Institute of Aging in the National Institutes of Health, and the Americans with Disabilities Act of 1990, which assured the rights of Americans with disabilities. These pieces of legislation have helped to provide important services to older Americans.

SELECTED RESOURCES ON AGING

There are many resources for older Americans in both the public and private sectors. Public sector resources are supported by tax dollars and exist on the federal, state, and local levels. Private sector resources will vary greatly from community to community and are both voluntary (nonprofit) or proprietary (for-profit) in nature.

Governmental/Public Resources

The U.S. Department of Health and Human Services (USDHHS) is the major federal agency involved in providing services to older people, and detailed information on this department can be found in Chapter 5. Within this department are agencies that provide extensive services to elderly Americans including the Social Security Administration, Administration on Aging, and the National Institute on Aging. Senior Centers across the country are a resource that receives significant funding through the provisions of the Older Americans Act of 1965.

The *Administration on Aging* (202-619-0724) is the principal agency charged with carrying out the provision of the Older Americans Act. The Administration publishes *Aging* magazine. Each year in May the Administration sponsors Older American's Month. The Administration helped to fund a recent Public Broadcasting System (PBS) documentary entitled *Our Nation's Health . . . Healthy Aging* that is available from Healthy Aging, Box 306, Coventry, CT 06238 (203-834-9888).

The *National Institute on Aging* (301-496-4000) was established to conduct and support biomedical and behavioral research and training related to the aging process for the purpose of increasing knowledge about aging and the associated physical, psychological, and social factors resulting from advanced age. It publishes *Resources for Women's Health and Aging* and has fact sheets on aging. Free copies of these publications can be obtained by calling 800-222-2225.

The *Social Security Administration* (SSA) was discussed in Chapter 5. It administers the Social Security Act programs of Old Age, Survivors and Disability Insurance, "Social Security," and Supplemental Security Income (SSI) that are used extensively by senior citizens. Branches of Social Security Administration offices can be found in the local telephone directory under federal government listings.

Numerous other federal agencies provide assistance to the elderly. The Department of Agriculture offers many food and nutrition programs. The Department of Housing and Urban Development subsidizes low-cost public housing for the elderly. The Department of the Treasury offers assistance with income tax problems and filing taxes through the Internal Revenue Service. The Department of Labor enforces the Age Discrimination in Employment Act. The Department of the Interior issues Gold Age Passports (free) and Golden Eagle Passports (low-cost) for the federal park system to senior citizens. The Department of Transportation underwrites funding to assist in providing mass transportation that services the elderly. The Department of Defense offers programs for retired veterans, often through Veteran's Administration hospitals. The U.S. Small Business Administration sponsors the SCORE program discussed earlier in this chapter.

ACTION is an independent federal agency that administers volunteer programs. Its purpose is to mobilize Americans for voluntary service throughout the United States through programs that help meet basic human needs and support self-help efforts of low-income families and impoverished communities. ACTION offers Foster Grandparents, Retired Senior Volunteers Program (RSVP), and Senior Companions, and many older Americans are volunteers in these programs.

The Older Americans Act of 1965 provides funding to states to establish state and local agencies on aging. These agencies plan and coordinate programs for older people. Local agencies on aging can be located by calling the Federal Information Center or by checking the local telephone directories under county or city government listings.

The Older Americans Act of 1965 also provides funding for senior centers. These centers provide social, recreational, educational, and nutritional services to senior citizens. The first senior center was the William Hodson Senior Center established by the New York City Department of Welfare in 1943 (The First Half-Century, 1993, p. 2). Today there are more than 12,000 senior centers across the nation serving more than 7 million Americans (The First Half-Century, p. 2). The passage of the Older Americans Act of 1965 provided ongoing funding for such centers and designated them as the primary organizations for service delivery to the elderly in the community (The National Institute, 1993, p. 10). In 1970 the National Institute of Senior Centers was formed (The National Institute, p. 10). Today senior centers continue to provide valuable services for aging citizens; information about them is often found under local governmental listings in the phone book.

Private/Voluntary Resources

Private/voluntary resources are numerous and will vary from community to community. On a national level two private, voluntary agencies that work actively for the elderly are the National Council on the Aging (NCOA) and the American Association for Retired Persons (AARP). These two groups, along with the activist Gray Panthers and other groups on aging, have lobbied for legislation, resources, and services for older persons.

National Council on the Aging (NCOA)

Established in 1950, the NCOA is a private, nonprofit organization that serves as a national resource for information and consultation and sponsors publications, special programs, advocacy activities, research, and training to meet older persons' needs and improve their lives. NCOA forms cooperative relationships with government and private agencies to educate the public and professionals about the aged and to provide services to the aged.

In 1987 NCOA was cofounder with the Child Welfare League of America of Generations United, a coalition of more than 100 national organizations dedicated to linking the needs and resources of generations. Generations United focuses on themes and programs that help to bring young and old together. NCOA also works closely with the Center for Understanding Aging (P.O. Box 246, Southington, CT 06489-0246) and Generations Together (University of Pittsburgh, 811 William Pitt Union, Pittsburgh, PA 15260) to promote aging education and intergenerational activities. Such affiliations have been successful in developing programs such as the Senior Center/ Latchkey program that links seniors with young children home alone after school. NCOA is headquartered at 409 Third Street SW, Washington, D.C. 20024 (202-479-1200).

American Association of Retired Persons (AARP)

The AARP was established in 1958 by Dr. Ethel Percy Andrus, founder of the National Retired Teachers Association. AARP today has over 30 million members across the United States in almost 4000 local chapters and is the largest nonprofit, nonpartisan membership organization in the world.

The purposes of AARP are to enhance the quality of life for older persons; promote independence, dignity, and purpose for older persons; provide leadership in determining the role of older persons in society; and improve the image of aging. Membership in the group is limited to those aged 50 years and older.

AARP publishes a bimonthly magazine, *Modern Maturity,* that offers retirement advice, travel ideas, and health tips, and also publishes the monthly *AARP News Bulletin.* It sponsors a tax assistance program to help older taxpayers, provides leadership in legislative issues, and is an advocate for the elderly. It is headquartered at 601 E Street, Washington, D.C. 20049 (202-434-2277).

Other community resources include senior centers, adult day care programs, home care agencies, family service agencies, geriatric counselors, health care professionals, churches, community service groups, and caregiver support groups. Listings for many agencies

can be found in the local telephone directory or can be obtained through local health departments or United Community Service agencies. The nurse needs to be aware of resources and services for the elderly in the community and refer clients to them when appropriate. The nurse can be an advocate for necessary community services.

BARRIERS TO HEALTH CARE

Societal attitudes are barriers to all care, including health care. These attitudes often inhibit healthy aging, affecting resource availability and care given.

Major barriers to health care for the elderly are access to health services and the cost of health services. A major access barrier is that of transportation. There is little public transportation in the United States, so the elderly person may have to rely on friends and family, a taxi, Dial-a-Ride, and church or volunteer groups for transportation services. Seniors living in rural areas are especially affected by the problems of transportation and access to service. As a result of the Americans with Disabilities Act of 1990 buildings are now becoming more accessible for people who need to use wheelchairs, walkers, and other mobility appliances, but "accessibility" remains a problem.

Cost is another major barrier to health care. Many health care services are costly and may not be covered under private insurance, Medicare, or Medicaid. If services are too expensive the elderly may not use them. For example, Medicare does not pay for prescription drugs, and if an elderly person does not have these drugs paid for by private insurance or Medicaid he or she may not purchase them. The prices of food, medicine, doctors' visits, and gas continually rise, yet many older people live on a fixed income and cannot afford the services they need.

THE NURSING ROLE

As early as 1925 an editorial in the *American Journal of Nursing* alerted nurses to the increasing need to prepare for care of the elderly (Editorial, 1925). The American Nurses Association (ANA), National League for Nursing (NLN), National Gerontological Nursing Association (NGNA), and the National Conference of Gerontological Nurse Practitioners (NCGNP) have helped to keep nurses aware of educational opportunities in gerontology and issues relevant to the health

◄ *Standards of Gerontological Nursing Practice* ►

Standard I. Organization of Gerontological Nursing Services

All gerontological nursing services are planned, organized, and directed by a nurse executive. The nurse executive has baccalaureate or master's preparation and has experience in gerontological nursing and administration of long-term care services or acute care services for older clients.

Standard II. Theory

The nurse participates in the generation and testing of theory as a basis for clinical decisions. The nurse uses theoretical concepts to guide the effective practice of gerontological nursing.

Standard III. Data Collection

The health status of the older person is regularly assessed in a comprehensive, accurate, and systematic manner. The information obtained during the health assessment is accessible to and shared with appropriate members of the interdisciplinary health care team, including the older person and the family.

Standard IV. Nursing Diagnosis

The nurse uses health assessment data to determine nursing diagnoses.

Standard V. Planning and Continuity of Care

The nurse develops the plan of care in conjunction with the older person and appropriate others. Mutual goals, priorities, nursing approaches, and measures in the care plan address the therapeutic, preventive, restorative, and rehabilitative needs of the older person. The care plan helps the older person attain and maintain the highest level of health, well-being, and quality of life achievable, as well as a peaceful death. The plan of care facilitates continuity of care over time as the client moves to various care settings, and is revised as necessary.

Standard VI. Intervention

The nurse, guided by the plan of care, intervenes to provide care to restore the older person's functional capabilities and to prevent complications and excess disability. Nursing interventions are derived from nursing diagnoses and are based on gerontological nursing theory.

Standard VII. Evaluation

The nurse continually evaluates the client's and family's responses to interventions in order to determine progress toward goal attainment and to revise the data base, nursing diagnoses, and plan of care.

Standard VIII. Interdisciplinary Collaboration

The nurse collaborates with other members of the health care team in the various settings in which care is given to the older person. The team meets regularly to evaluate the effectiveness of the care plan for the client and family and to adjust the plan of care to accommodate changing needs.

Standard IX. Research

The nurse participates in research designed to generate an organized body of gerontological nursing knowledge, disseminates research findings, and uses them in practice.

Standard X. Ethics

The nurse uses the code for nurses established by the American Nurses' Association as a guide for ethical decision making in practice.

Standard XI. Professional Development

The nurse assumes responsibility for professional development and contributes to the professional growth of interdisciplinary team members. The nurse participates in peer review and other means of evaluation to assure the quality of nursing practice.

Reprinted with permission from ANA: *Standards and scope of gerontological nursing practice,* Kansas City, Mo., 1987, The Association. Copyright 1987, American Nurses Association.

care of older people (Johnson and Connelly, 1990, iv).

The role of the nurse in working with the elderly client has been discussed throughout this chapter in reference to healthy aging, health promotion, and concerns of the elderly. The nurse may assume the role of advocate for the elderly client, assist the client in using community resources, coordinate and manage care, and assist in helping the client maintain independence.

Graduates of nursing programs are entering practice where the majority of clients are over age 65 and many over 85 years old (Small, 1993, p. 27). Nurses need to be able to provide quality care to elderly clients by understanding the aging process; common problems of aging; functional abilities associated with aging; public policy and economics; health maintenance and promotion; long-term care needs; ethics and attitudes; and cultural variations and opportunities for professional development (Johnson and Connelly, 1990, p. 3). A knowledge of community resources for the elderly is essential for the nurse.

ANA's (1987) *Standards of Gerontological Nursing Practice* are presented in the box on p. 757. These standards address the application of the nursing process to gerontological nursing, interdisciplinary collaboration, and the integration of theory and research in practice. The ANA established certification of gerontological nurses in 1973; as of January 1992 there were almost 10,000 certified gerontological nurses (LeSage, 1993, p. 19). The ANA's Council on Gerontological Nursing has been involved in many important gerontological nursing initiatives (LeSage, p. 17). The National League for Nursing (NLN) is committed to the improvement of education and practice in gerontological nursing and to the provision of quality long-term care (Waters, 1993, p. 23).

Summary

Aging is a universal phenomena—everyone is aging. It is important to remember that the elderly person is a unique individual with unique health care needs. Our societies' ageist attitudes often become self-fulfilling prophecies in old age and inhibit healthy aging. Nurses need to be aware of their own attitudes about aging and how these attitudes affect nursing care and caring.

Healthy People 2000 has addressed health needs of the elderly and established numerous national health objectives for this aggregate. Nurses frequently provide care to elderly clients and need to be aware of national health objectives, health concerns of the elderly, the physiological changes of aging, legislation that has an impact on the elderly, and community resources. Nurses are advocates for health care resources and services for the elderly and work to minimize barriers to care such as societal attitudes, inadequate resources and services, problems of accessibility, and transportation and limited income.

The expected growth of the population over 65 signals an expanding nursing role and opportunity to work with older people. Nurses need to be educated in gerontology; nursing has the opportunity to be the leader in the delivery of health care services to the elderly. Planning and impelementing policy for the elderly client is a significant challenge for community health nurses.

◀ *An Exercise in Critical Thinking* ▶

After reading this chapter you are aware of the *Healthy People 2000* national health objectives for older people and numerous needs, resources, and services in relation to the elderly client. What do you see as the greatest major health care concern for today's older Americans? What can nurses in your community do to help meet this health care need?

Healthy People 2000 National Health Objectives Targeting Older Adults

Health Status Objectives:

Reduce suicides among white men aged 65 and older to no more than 39.2 per 100,000.

Reduce deaths among people age 70 and older caused by motor vehicle crashes to no more than 20 per 100,000.

Reduce deaths among people aged 65 through 84 from falls and fall-related injuries to no more than 14.4 per 100,000.

Reduce deaths among people aged 85 and older from falls and fall-related injuries to no more than 105 per 100,000.

Reduce residential fire deaths among people aged 65 and older to no more than 3.3 per 100,000.

Reduce hip fractures among people aged 65 and older so that hospitalizations for this condition are no more than 607 per 100,000.

Reduce to no more than 20 percent the proportion of people aged 65 and older who have lost all of their natural teeth.

Increase years of healthy life to at least 65 years.

Reduce to no more than 90 per 1,000 people the proportion of all people aged 65 and older who have difficulty in performing two or more personal care activities, thereby preserving independence.

Reduce significant hearing impairment among people aged 45 and older to a prevalence of no more than 180 per 1,000.

Reduce significant visual impairment among people aged 65 and older to a prevalence of no more than 70 per 1,000.

Reduce epidemic-related pneumonia and influenza deaths among people aged 65 and older to no more than 7.3 per 100,000.

Reduce pneumonia-related days of restricted activity for people aged 65 and older.

Risk Reduction Objectives:

Increase to at least 30 percent the proportion of people aged 65 and older who engage regularly, preferably daily, in light to moderate physical activity for at least 30 minutes per day.

Reduce to no more than 22 percent the proportion of people aged 65 and older who engage in no leisure-time physical activity.

Increase immunization levels for pneumococcal pneumonia and influenza immunization among institutionalized chronically ill or older people to at least 80 percent.

Increase to at least 40 percent the proportion of adults aged 65 and older who have received, as a minimum within the appropriate interval, all of the screening and immunization services and at least one of the counseling services appropriate for their age and gender as recommended by the U.S. Preventive Services Task Force.

Services and Protection Objectives:

Increase to at least 80 percent the receipt of home food services by people aged 65 and older who have difficulty in preparing their own meals or are otherwise in need of home-delivered meals.

Increase to at least 90 percent the proportion of people aged 65 and older who had the opportunity to participate during the preceding year in at least one organized health promotion program through a senior center, lifecare facility, or other community-based setting that serves older adults.

Increase to at least 30 the number of States that have design standards for signs, signals, markings, lighting, and other characteristics of the roadway environment to improve the visual stimuli and protect the safety of older drivers and pedestrians.

Increase to at least 75 percent the proportion of primary care providers who routinely review with their patients aged 65 and older all prescribed and over-the-counter medicines taken by their patients each time a new medication is prescribed.

Extend to all long-term institutional facilities the requirement that oral examinations and services be provided no later than 90 days after entry into these facilities.

Increase to at least 60 percent the proportion of people aged 65 and older using the oral health care system during each year.

Increase to at least 80 percent the proportion of women aged 40 and older who have ever received a clinical breast examination and a mammogram, and to at least 60 percent those aged 50 and older who have received them within the preceding 1 to 2 years.

Increase to at least 95 percent the proportion of women aged 70 and older with uterine cervix who have ever received a Pap test, and to at least 70 percent who received a Pap test within the preceding 1 to 3 years.

Increase to at least 50 percent the proportion of people aged 50 and older who have received fecal occult blood testing within the preceding 1 to 2 years, and to at least 40 percent those who have ever received proctosigmoidoscopy.

Increase to at least 40 percent the proportion of people aged 50 and older visiting a primary care provider in the preceding year who have received oral, skin, and digital rectal examinations during one such visit.

Increase to at least 60 percent the proportion of providers of primary care for older adults who routinely evaluate people aged 65 and older for urinary incontinence and impairments of vision, hearing, cognition, and functional status.

Increase to at least 90 percent the proportion of perimenopausal women who have been counseled about the benefits and risks of estrogen replacement therapy.

From USDHHS: *Healthy People 2000, full report, with commentary,* Washington, D.C., 1991, U.S. Government Printing Office, pp. 588-590.

Kent County Health Department: Seniors Substance Abuse Project

ASSESSMENT FORM

Name _____ ID# _____

Occupation _____

Language in the home _____

Current living arrangements _____

_____

Number of children _____

Significant others _____

_____

RELEASE OF INFORMATION

I, _____ , agree to participate in a Seniors Substance Abuse Project conducted by the Kent County Health Department. I authorize Donna Spruit, R.N., from the Kent County Health Department to release information regarding my medication and health status to _____

_____
(doctor or agency).

I also authorize _____ (doctor or agency) to give information regarding my medication and health status to Donna Spruit, R.N.

Recipients of substance abuse services have rights protected by State and Federal Law and promulgated rules. For information, contact Seniors Project Supervisor, Kent County Health Dept., 700 Fuller, N.E., GR, MI., 49503, 774-3040 or the Office of Substance Abuse Services, Recipient Rights Coordinator, P.O. Box 30035, 3500 North Logan, Lansing, MI 48909.

   Client's signature _____

   Date _____

   Witness _____

   Relationship to Client _____

Interviewer's name_____ Date _____

Site of interview _____

APPENDIX 19-2
Kent County Health Department: Seniors Substance Abuse Project—cont'd

page 2
Seniors Project Questionnaire

ID # _____

Date _____

KNOWLEDGE OF MEDICATIONS

List each medication (including over-the-counter and home remedies) the client is taking in the left-hand column. In the right-hand column, write down what the client says is the reason [for] taking this drug. Include how much and how often he [or she] claims to take each. Use the client's words if possible. It is important that the *client's perceptions* be recorded, not the interviewer's.

Name of drug	Reason for taking	Amount of frequency (with meals/ without meals)

Continued

Kent County Health Department: Seniors Substance Abuse Project—cont'd

---

KENT COUNTY HEALTH DEPARTMENT SENIOR SUBSTANCE ABUSE QUESTIONNAIRE MEDICATION USE/MISUSE

Risk factor Analysis: Date: _____ ID # _____

Evaluate the status of risk factor and circle the number on the left which best describes the client's risk. 0 for not-at-all to 5 for very much a problem. On the right of each risk factor write in any comments which may help clarify the specific situation, e.g., "diet implications"— *special weight reduction 1500 cal. diet. lo Na lo chol.;* "side effects"—*C/O dry mouth, excessive tiredness;* "sensory deprivation"—*poor vision, cataracts both eyes.*

0 1 2 3 4 5   Cost _____

0 1 2 3 4 5   Confusion _____

0 1 2 3 4 5   Diet implications _____

0 1 2 3 4 5   Difficulty opening safety closures _____

0 1 2 3 4 5   Depression _____

0 1 2 3 4 5   Drug intolerance _____

0 1 2 3 4 5   Forgets to take medication _____

0 1 2 3 4 5   Fear of taking medication _____

0 1 2 3 4 5   Inappropriate storage:

                ____ temperature, humidity_____

                ____ removal from original container _____

                ____ medication stored at bedside _____

0 1 2 3 4 5   Language barrier _____

0 1 2 3 4 5   Lack of knowledge regarding meds _____

0 1 2 3 4 5   Living alone _____

0 1 2 3 4 5   Multiple prescriptions _____

0 1 2 3 4 5   Multiple pharmacies _____

0 1 2 3 4 5   Multiple physicians _____

0 1 2 3 4 5   Physician hopping _____

0 1 2 3 4 5   Outdated medications _____

0 1 2 3 4 5   Over-the-counter use _____

0 1 2 3 4 5   Reading disability _____

0 1 2 3 4 5   Sensory deprivation _____

0 1 2 3 4 5   Side effects _____

0 1 2 3 4 5   Stopping medication _____

0 1 2 3 4 5   Stretching medication _____

0 1 2 3 4 5   Sharing medication _____

0 1 2 3 4 5   Not following prescribed regimen _____

0 1 2 3 4 5   Transportation difficulty _____

0 1 2 3 4 5   Use of household remedies (i.e., baking soda) _____

0 1 2 3 4 5   Mood-altering drugs _____

0 1 2 3 4 5   Use of alcohol _____

0 1 2 3 4 5   Other (list):

                                                       _____

0 1 2 3 4 5   _____

0 1 2 3 4 5   _____

0 1 2 3 4 5   _____

Total Risk Factor Score _____

Interviewer's Signature

Kent County Health Department: Seniors Substance Abuse Project—cont'd

KENT COUNTY HEALTH DEPARTMENT
Seniors Substance Abuse Questionnaire Guide
Risk Factor Analysis

Review each risk factor with client and determine applicability. Rate the risk factor from 0 (not applicable, no risk) to 5 (high risk), and circle the appropriate number. This analysis requires your professional judgment and is based upon your assessment of the client and his personal situation.

Cost

The client may consider some of his medications to be very costly. If his income level is low and/or fixed, he may not be able to afford these medications. Determine his priority for expenses—medications may not be high priority, and therefore, the risk of omission is increased.

Confusion

Rate this according to how well oriented the client sems to be. Does he relate approrpriately to time and place, etc.?

Diet Implications

Is the client on a special diet such as low sodium, low cholesterol, weight reduction, diabetic? Some medications contain sodium, i.e., Mylanta, Maalox. Some medications are to be taken on an empty stomach, while others are to be taken with meals. Milk is to be avoided with certain drugs. It is important to determine whether the client adheres to these recommendations.

Difficulty Opening Safety Closures

Patients with arthritis may have increased difficulty opening safety caps. They may omit a dose just because of the hassle or worse yet, they may transfer drugs to an unmarked container. (See inappropriate storage.) Determine how likely this risk is. Client may be unaware that easy-open caps are available from the pharmacy.

Depression

Is the client now depressed or does he have a history of depression? Because of the many losses suffered by the elderly, some degree of depression is fairly common. Depression may influence adherence to a medical regimen. Likewise, depression may be a side effect of some drugs.

Drug Intolerance or Allergy

History of intolerance or allergy would have implications for current drug use. It would be important that this information be readily available in case of emergency. Rate this risk according to the severity and likelihood of recurrence.

Forgets to Take Medication

Does the client state that he sometimes forgets to take medication? Determine how likely this is. This risk may go hand-in-hand with confusion, or it may stand alone. Not all persons who forget to take medication are confused. They may be overwhelmed by the number of medications they are to take or they may be distracted by other activities. Listen for key phrases like, "Don't know if I remembered."

Client may be threatened or embarrassed to admit forgetfulness. Good, non-threatening interviewing will be helpful here.

Fear of Taking Medication

Some clients are reluctant to take drugs, even those that are prescribed. Determine if the client has any such reluctance. Some clients may be very open and verbal about this fear. Rate this risk according to how likely it is that the client would not take needed medication.

Inappropriate Storage

Temperature, Humidity: Medications are subject to deterioration in certain temperature extremes and high humidity. Storage in the bathroom is undesirable. Storage in the refrigerator is required for certain drugs and contraindicated for others. Check labels or check with pharmacist if necessary.

Removal from Original Containers: Many clients are tempted to put all pills together in one container, especially when they travel. This is a very unsafe practice. All medications should remain in the original containers until needed. It is considered safe to place medications in special dispensers. These are best when divided by time of day they are to be taken. This helps the problem of forgetfulness. However, a list of what each drug is should be available nearby for emergency information, especially if traveling.

Medication Stored at Bedside: Although this may seem like a very convenient storage site, it runs the risk of error if the client should happen to take medications when not fully awake. Also, too easy access may make over-using certain medications more likely, such as pain medication or mood-altering drugs. Having to go to the storage site allows a more purposeful effort and hopefully a more accurate dosage.

Language Barrier

Labels and directions written in a language not understood by a client could lead to misuse. Also, if the client does not understand verbal instructions given by the doctor or pharmacist, there is increased potential for misuse.

Lack of Knowledge Regarding Medications

See first part of Questionnaire, "Knowledge of Medications." How well does the client understand what the medications he/she is taking are for, how to take them, how much to take, and how often?

Living Alone

This may or may not be a risk factor, depending on how well the client has adapted to living alone. Living alone can be a problem if there is no support system to encourage the client to take good care of himself. Motivation to comply with a medical regimen will be affected in some cases.

Continued

APPENDIX 19-2
Kent County Health Department: Seniors Substance Abuse Project—cont'd

KENT COUNTY HEALTH DEPARTMENT
Seniors Substance Abuse Questionnaire Guide
Risk Factor Analysis

Multiple Prescriptions

The more medications the clients are taking, the more likely they are to have a problem with adverse drug interactions, side effects, inclusion about dosage and schedule, etc.

Multiple Pharmacies

Going to more than one pharmacy to have prescriptions filled is undesirable. The pharmacist may be unaware of other drugs being taken by the client and he/she will be hampered in his/her ability to do a drug profile and advise the client on possible incompatibility of certain drugs.

Multiple Physicians

Since the elderly tend to have a number of chronic illnesses, they frequently find themselves being treated by a number of specialists, i.e., internist, rheumatologist, cardiac specialist, gastroenterologist. This is sometimes unavoidable, and it is important that each physician be aware of what drugs the other has prescribed. The client has responsibility for conveying that information.

Physician Hopping

This is different from "multiple physicians." Here clients go from one doctor to another within a short span of time because they are not satisfied with their care. This can be a dangerous and fruitless practice and frequently results in multiple prescriptions for similar drugs, i.e., mood-altering drugs, antibiotics, pain medication. The client rarely informs the new doctor of his recent previous visits to other doctors. There are clients who have gotten three prescriptions for the same drug from three different doctors and ended up taking all three, and therefore, three times the desired dosage.

Outdated Medication

All drugs should be discarded once they are outdated. *Saving drugs* is a potentially dangerous practice because they can change in composition and may be harmful if used. Also their presence in the medicine chest could result in someone accidentally taking the old drug instead of the desired one. The risk factor can be most accurately evaluated by a home visit where the medicine chest can be viewed or by asking the client to bring all drugs to the next visit.

Over-the-Counter Use

Clients who regularly use over-the-counter drugs run the risk of drug interactions, especially if they are taking other prescription medication. Sometimes clients do not count over-the-counter drugs as "real" drugs. They do not realize that these drugs also have side effects and contraindications. The more over-the-counter drugs used by the client and the greater the frequency, the higher the risk rating they would receive from this risk factor.

Reading Disability (Comprehension)

This is not be to confused with the "language barrier" problem. What is considered here are perceptual difficulties that could be the result of a stroke (aphasia) or possibly a life-long condition. If a client is unable to read and understand the information on the label, it would signal a risk of misuse.

Sensory Deprivation

Visual, auditory, or other sensory-related problems that may influence the client's ability to follow directions or correctly self-administer medications, i.e., reduced vision or blindness, loss of feeling in fingertips, deafness.

Side Effects

Undesirable effects caused by the drug may influence a client to avoid taking a needed drug, i.e., disagreeable taste, dry mouth, dizziness, nausea, drowsiness, lingering bad taste in mouth, impotence.

Stopping Medication

When the client stops taking a prescribed drug before the desired therapeutic results are obtained, this is a medication misuse. This risk factor could occur as a result of unpleasant side effects, cost, emotional reasons, denial of illness, symptoms reduction (blood pressure medication, antibiotics), embarrassment.

Stretching Medication

The client tries to make the medication last longer by skipping doses or taking less than the prescribed dose. This is usually done for financial reasons or because the client desires to minimize the amount of drugs he is taking.

Sharing Medication

Usually a misplaced friendship gesture. The friend tells the client that this drug worked for him, "why doesn't he take one." A very dangerous practice.

Not Following Precribed Regimen

This may or may not be a *deliberate* act on the part of the client. It could be the result of "confusion," "forgetfulness," or "stretching medication." Adjusting dosage schedules ad lib can be potentially hazardous depending upon the drug and its intended action.

Transportation Difficulty

This may not be a problem unless it results in not getting a prescription filled or related effect such as not making a follow-up visit to the doctor, which might be a necessary component in monitoring a drug's effectiveness.

Use of Household Remedies

The use of such items as baking soda for upset stomach could be a problem if the client were on a low sodium diet and/or hypertensive, since baking soda is high in sodium.

APPENDIX 19-2

Kent County Health Department: Seniors Substance Abuse Project—cont'd

KENT COUNTY HEALTH DEPARTMENT
Seniors Substance Abuse Questionnaire Guide
Risk Factor Analysis

The household remedy would need to be evaluated as to the contents, amount taken, and frequency.

Mood-Altering Drugs

This category of drug runs a risk of its own because of the nature of the drug and the condition it is intended to alleviate. These drugs may be habit forming. A depressed client may overdose himself.

Use of Alcohol

Some drugs interact or are increased by the use of alcohol. It would be important to determine how much and how often the client utilized alcohol. A history of alcohol abuse would be significant.

Asking the following questions developed by John A. Ewing, Director for the Center for Alcohol Studies at the University of North Carolina may be helpful:

1. Have you felt the need to cut down your drinking?
2. Have you ever felt annoyed by criticism of your drinking?
3. Have you had guilty feelings about drinking?
4. Do you ever take a morning eye-opener?

If two or three questions receive a positive response, the likelihood that the person is an alcoholic is high.

Add up the total risk factor score and place in the designated space. By looking over the form, you can determine which risk factors you can help eliminate or reduce through intervention. Write up a plan with the client. After six to eight weeks, readminister the tool and determine if the total risk factor score has been lowered.

Reproduced by permission of the Nursing Division, Kent County Health Department, Grand Rapids, MI; Wanda Bierman, RN, MS, Family Health Services Supervisor and Donna Spruit, RN, Geriatric Services, Principal Developers.

The Older Americans Act of 1965: Significant Amendments and Changes

1967 *Older Americans Act; Amendments of 1967 (Public Law 90-42)*—Authorized studies to look at the availability and adequacy of training resources in gerontology and to evaluate present and future trends and needs for such personnel and programs. Resulted in increased funding and training in the field of gerontology. Placed new emphasis on providing services to seniors.

1969 *Older Americans Act; Amendments of 1969 (Public Law 91-69)*—Mandated increased state planning for act programs through state agencies on aging. Increased the emphasis on coordination with local programs and program evaluation. Authorized grants to states and communities for model projects on services to the elderly. Established the National Older Americans Volunteer Program (NOAVP). NOAVP's main purpose was to help retired persons avail themselves of opportunities for voluntary service in their communities and helped to subsidize this through provision of transportation, meals, and other necessary services needed for them to participate. Major components of NOAVP were: (1) *Retired Senior Volunteer Program (RSVP)* and (2) *Foster Grandparents*.

1972 *Older Americans Act; Amendments of 1972 (Public Law 92-258)*—Amended the act to provide grants to states for the establishment, maintenance, operation, and expansion of low-cost meal projects, nutrition training, and education, as well as opportunity for social contacts for the elderly. Established the Nutrition Program for the Elderly and brought the nutrition of the elderly into the national limelight. From this legislation sprang many senior nutrition services.

1973 *Older Americans Act; Comprehensive Amendments of 1973 (Public Law 93-29)*—Established the Federal Council on Aging and the National Information and Resources Clearinghouse for the Aging. Required that a sole state agency administer the provisions of the act in conjunction with local agencies on aging. Established Multipurpose Senior Centers and Older Readers Services. These multipurpose centers combined social, recreational, health, and nutrition aspects for seniors into one accessible program. These centers also placed a new and increasing emphasis on the social needs of seniors and attempted to decrease social isolation for seniors through a community-based program.

1974 *Older Americans Act; Amendments of 1974 (Public Law 93-351)*—Provided for increased funding for transportation for the elderly, especially transportation services that facilitated the elderly in using the nutrition programs and multipurpose centers already designated under the act. The transportation needs of the elderly living in rural areas were explored. This same year a separate presidential proclamation declared May to be Older Americans Month, and this tradition has been carried on by a presidential proclamation each year since.

1975 *Older Americans Act; Amendments of 1975 (Public Law 94-135)*—Established social services programs especially for seniors. A significant part of these amendments involved two separate acts: *Age Discrimination Act of 1975* and *Older Americans Community Service Employment Act of 1975*. Both of these acts carry the same public law number as the amendments and are incorporated into the amendments. The Age Discrimination Act prohibited discrimination on the basis of age, largely in relation to employment. The Community Service Employment Act section of the amendments provided for community service employment for seniors where they were eligible to receive a wage. Most employment programs under the act, before this time, had involved voluntary employment for seniors. These amendments also attempted to attract more qualified people into the field of gerontology through increased funding for training.

1978 *Comprehensive Older Americans Act; Amendments of 1978 (Public Law 95-478)*—The Amendments of 1978 were extensive and provided for improved and increased programs for older Americans. These amendments called for a great reduction in the paperwork necessary to run the program; increased planning, coordination, evaluation, and administration efforts; and facilitated the quality of programs. They also established the Advisory Council on Aging; provided for area agencies on aging to contract for legal services and to carry out demonstration projects on the legal services necessary for older Americans; provided for exploring alternative work modes for older Americans such as the Senior Environmental Protection Corps with the Environmental Protection Agency (EPA); provided for grants to Indian tribes for older American services to tribes members; set up a White House Conference on Aging for 1981 (there had previously been such conferences in 1961 and 1971); provided for a study of racial and ethnic discrimination in programs for

The Older Americans Act of 1965: Significant Amendments and Changes—cont'd

older Americans; and outlined the programs of (1) *Congregate Nutrition Services* and (2) *Home Delivered Nutrition Services for the Elderly.* In addition, these amendments mandated development and implementation of national labor policy for the field of aging; discussed the concept of "preretirement" education and planning services; authorized special projects on long-term care and alternatives to institutionalization such as adult day care, supervised living in public or nonprofit housing, family respite, preventive health services, home health and homemaker services, home maintenance programs, and geriatric health maintenance organizations; and authorized demonstration projects for community model programs to improve and expand social services, and nutrition services, and to promote the well-being of older Americans. High priority for placement of these demonstration projects was given to rural areas and rural agencies on aging.

1981 *Older Americans Act; Amendments of 1981 (Public Law 97-115)*—Emphasized the provision of nutritional programs in congregate settings and facilitated access to such programs. These amendments also encouraged the formation of university-affiliated and other multidisciplinary centers on aging as well as long-term care projects, and brought migrant and seasonal farm workers and organizations more in line with the provisions of the act.

1984 *Older Americans Act; Amendments of 1984 (Public Law 98-459)*—Often referred to as the Older Americans Personal Health Education and Training Act. Provided for a comprehensive array of community-based, long-term care services to appropriately sustain older people in their communities and homes. Authorized the designing of a uniform, standardized *program of health education and training* for older Americans with direct involvement of graduate educational institutions of public health in the design of such a program and direct involvement of graduate education institutions of public health, medical sciences, psychology, pharmacology, nursing, social work, health education, nutrition, and gerontology in the implementation of such a program. Planned for such education and training programs to be carried out in multipurpose senior centers as already provided for under the act.

1986 *Older Americans Act; Amendments of 1986 (Public Law 99-269)*—Amended the Older Americans Act to in-

crease the federal contribution to senior nutrition programs covered under the act to about 57 cents per meal. Mandated that the Secretary of Agriculture and the Secretary of Health and Human Services jointly disseminate to state agencies, area agencies on aging, and providers of nutrition services covered under the act information concerning the existence of *all* federal commodity processing programs in which they would be eligible to participate, and the procedures necessary to participate in such programs.

1987 *Older Americans Act; Amendments of 1987 (Public Law 100-175)*—Often referred to as the Health Care Services in the Home Act of 1987. Established grants to states for *in-home health care services* for the frail elderly, for periodic *preventive health* services to be provided at senior centers or appropriate alternative sites, and to implement programs with respect to the prevention of abuse, neglect, and exploitation of the elderly. Authorized a 1991 White House Conference on Aging, and reauthorized the Act through fiscal year 1991. Required a direct reporting relationship between the Commissioner on Aging and the Secretary of Health and Human Services; added an outreach program on Supplemental Security Income, food stamps, and Medicaid-benefits; increased funds for administration of area agencies on aging and community service employment projects; added a Demonstration Project Authority in areas of health education and promotion, volunteerism, and consumer protection from home care services; and added a program for grants to assist older Hawaiian natives.

1992 *Older Americans Act; Amendments of 1992 (Public Law 102-375)*—A four-year reauthorization of the Older Americans Act that established a study committee to look at the quality of home care services for older adults; established funding for in-school intergenerational activities where older adults could serve as tutors, teacher aides, living historians, speakers, playground supervisors, lunchroom assistants, and other roles; directed more services to minorities and rural elderly; placed increased emphasis on health promotion for the elderly; increased funding for senior nutrition programs and added supportive services for family caregivers of the frail elderly; and authorized a White House Conference on Aging before December 31, 1994.

References

Alford DM and Futrell M: AAN working paper: wellness and health promotion of the elderly, *Nurs Outlook* 40(5):221-226, 1992.

American Association of Retired Persons (AARP): *A profile of older Americans 1993*, Washington, D.C., 1993, The Association.

AARP: *Healthy older adults*, Washington, D.C., 1991, The Association.

AARP: *Truth about aging: guidelines for accurate communications*, Washington, D.C., 1984, The Association.

AARP: *Elder suicide: a national survey of prevention and intervention programs*, Washington, D.C., 1989, The Association.

American Nurses Association: *Standards and scope of gerontological nursing practice*, Kansas City, Mo., 1987, The Association.

Annual checkups who needs them, *Aging* 365:2-3, 1993.

Ashley J and Fulmer T: No simple way to determine elder abuse, *Geriatric Nurs* 9(3):286-288, 1988.

Cameron M: *Views of aging: a teacher's guide*, Ann Arbor, 1967, Institute of Gerontology, University of Michigan—Wayne State University.

Castillo HM: *The nurse assistant in long-term care: a rehabilitative approach*, St. Louis, 1992, Mosby.

Chen M: Older Asians, *J Gerontological Nurs* 13(11):18-25, 1987.

Comfort A: *Say yes to old age: developing a positive attitude toward aging*, New York, 1990, Crown.

Douglass RL: *Domestic mistreatment of the elderly—towards prevention*, Washington, D.C., 1988, AARP.

Duvall EM and Miller BC: *Marriage and family and family development*, ed 6, New York, 1985, Harper and Row.

Editorial, *Am J Nurs* 25(5):394, 1925.

Erikson EH: *The life cycle completed: a review*, New York, 1982, Norton.

Greely A: *Nutrition and the elderly*, Washington, D.C., 1991, Publication No. (FDA) 91-2243, U.S. Department of Health and Human Services.

Growing old in America: an ABC News closeup, *TV Guide*, December 28, 1985.

Growing old in rural America: new approach needed in rural health care, *Aging* 365:18-25, 1993.

Harper MS: Depression, suicide significant risks in elderly, *Mental Health Suppl Rep to AAHA Provider News*, Washington, D.C., February 24, 1989, American Association of Homes for the Aging.

Harris DK: *Sociology of aging*, 2 ed, New York, 1990, Harper and Row.

Heckheimer EF: *Health promotion of the elderly in the community*, Philadelphia, 1989, Saunders.

Hey RP and Carlson E: "Granny dumping": new pain for U.S. elders, *AARP Bull* 32(8):1, 16, 1991.

Jennings M, Nordstorm M, and Schumake N: Physiologic functioning in the elderly, *Nurs Clin North Am* 7(6):237-246, 1972.

Johnson MA and Connelly JR: *Nursing and gerontology: status report*, Washington, D.C., 1990, Association for Gerontology in Higher Education.

Kimmel DC: Biological and intellectual aspects of aging. In Kimmel DC, ed: *Adulthood and aging*, New York, 1974, Wiley.

Kraus LE and Stoddard S: *Chartbook on disability in the United States, an InfoUse Report*, Washington, D.C., March 1989, U.S. National Institute on Disability and Rehabilitation Research.

Kuhn ME: *Maggie Kuhn on aging*, Philadelphia, 1977, Westminister.

LeSage J: Initiatives in gerontological nursing education: the role of the American Nurses' Association's Council on Gerontological Nursing. In Heine C, ed: *Determining the future of gerontological nursing education*, New York, 1993, National League for Nursing Press, pp. 17-22.

Malnutrition: tackling a major problem, *Worldview* 5(2):4, 1993.

McGuire SL: Aging education in schools, *J School Health* 57(5):174-176, 1987.

McGuire SL: Promoting positive attitudes toward aging: literature for young children, *Childhood Education*, Summer 1993a, pp. 204-210.

McGuire SL: Promoting positive attitudes through aging education: a study with preschool children, *Gerontol Geriatrics Ed* 13(4):3-12, 1993b.

Medical Letter, Inc.: Drugs that cause psychiatric symptoms, *The Medical Letter on Drugs and Therapeutics* 35(901):65-70, 1993.

Meehan P, Saltzman L, and Sattin R: Suicides among older United States residents: epidemiologic characteristics and trends, *Am J Public Health* 81(9):1198-1200, 1991.

Miller C: *Nursing care of older adults: theory and practice*, Glenville, Ill., 1990, Scott, Foresman/Little, Brown Higher Education.

Murray RB and Zentner JP: *Nursing assessment and health promotion strategies throughout the life span*, ed 4, Norwalk, Conn., 1989, Appleton & Lange.

National Center for Health Statistics: *Health United States 1991 and prevention profile*, Hyattsville, Md., 1992, Public Health Service.

National Council on the Aging (NCOA): Public policy agenda 1993-1994, *Perspect Aging* 22(1):1-46, 1993.

National Resource Center on Health Promotion and Aging (NRCHPA): *Medications and the elderly*, Washington, D.C., 1991, U.S. Government Printing Office.

Nutrition Screening Initiative, a cooperative effort of the American Dietetic Association, American Academy of Family Physicians, and National Council on Aging, Washington, D.C., 1992, Nutrition Screening Initiative.

O'Neill K and Reid G: Perceived barriers to physical activity by older adults, *Can J Public Health* 82(6):392-396, 1991.

Painter K: Better care and plain old luck are keys, *USA Today* April 7, 1993, pp. D1-2.

Palmieri DT: Clearing up the confusion: adverse effects of medications in the elderly, *J Gerontolog Nurs* 17(10):32-35, 1991.

Promoting elderly appetites: a feast for the senses, *Worldview* 5(2):9, 1993.

Profile of the Rural U.S., *Aging* 365:10-11, 1993.

Rosenburg IH: As you age: 10 keys to a longer, healthier, more vital life, *Worldview* 5(2):2-3, 1993.

Rossman I: Human aging changes. In Burnside IM, ed: *Nursing and the aged*, New York, 1976, McGraw-Hill.

Salamon MJ: Wide variety of treatable mental disorders seen among elderly, *Mental Health, Suppl. Rep. to AAHA Provider News*, Washington, D.C., February 24, 1989, American Association of Homes for Aging.

Sheppard HL: Damaging stereotypes about aging are taking hold: how to counter them? *Perspect Aging* 19(1):4-8, 1990.

Skinner BF and Vaughn ME: *Enjoy old age: a program of self-management*, New York, 1983, Norton.

Small NR: National consensus conference on gerontologic nursing competencies. In Heine C, ed: *Determining the future of gerontological nursing education*, New York, 1993, National League for Nursing Press, pp. 27-31.

The first half-century of senior centers charts the way for decades to come, *Perspect Aging* 22(2):2-6, 1993.

The National Institute of Senior Centers and the senior center field: a chronology, *Perspect Aging* 22(2):10-11, 1993.

U.S. Bureau of the Census: *Sixty-five plus in America,* Washington, D.C., 1992, U.S. Government Printing Office.

U.S. Department of Health and Human Services (USDHHS): *Income of the Aged Chartbook 1990,* Washington, D.C., 1992, U.S. Government Printing Office.

USDHHS: *Healthy People 2000, full report, with commentary,* Washington, D.C., 1991, U.S. Government Printing Office.

Waters V: National League for Nursing: initiatives in gerontological nursing education. In Heine C, ed: *Determining the future of gerontological nursing education,* New York, 1993, National League for Nursing Press, pp. 23-26.

Where doctors are few and far between, *Aging* 365:12-17, 1993.

World Health Organization (WHO): *Draft position paper on health care of the elderly,* Geneva, October, 1980, The Organization.

Selected Bibliography

Advice to elders: drink up for health, *Worldview* 5(2):5, 1993.

American Association for Retired Persons (AARP): *Growing together: an intergenerational sourcebook,* Washington, D.C., 1986, The Association.

Brower HT and Crist MA: Research priorities in gerontologic nursing for long-term care, *Image* 17(1):22-27, 1985.

Brower HT and Yurchuck ER: Teaching gerontological nursing in southern states, *Nurs Health Care* 14(4):198-205, 1993.

Conn VS: Self-management of over-the-counter medications by older adults, *Pub Health Nurs* 9(1):29-36, 1992.

Hawranik P: Clinical possibility: preventing health problems after the age of 65, *J Gerontolog Nurs* 17(11):20-25, 1991.

Kubler-Ross E: *On death and dying,* New York, 1969, Macmillan.

Lank NH and Vickery CE: Nutrition education for the elderly: concerns, needs and approaches, *J Applied Gerontolog* 6(3):259-267, 1987.

McGuire SL: Promoting positive attitudes toward aging among children, *J School Health* 56(8):322-324, 1986.

Nutrition: Rx for chronic disease, *Worldview* 5(2):7, 1993.

Richardson JL: Perspective in compliance with drug regimens among the elderly, *J Compliance Health Care* 1(1):33-45, 1986.

Shaw B and Cristol J: Bridges: intergenerational approaches to health promotion for the well elderly, *Public Health Rep* 104(1):91-93, 1989.

Standards and Guidelines Committee of the National Institute of Senior Centers: Standards and guidelines help centers do their work better for more people; accreditation now a likely next step, *Perspec Aging* 22(3):16-19.

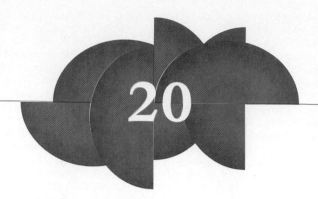

20

Clients with Long-Term Care Needs: Home Health, Hospice, and Other Services

OUTLINE

OBJECTIVES

Upon completion of this chapter, the reader should be able to:

1. Describe the factors influencing the growing need for long-term care.
2. Discuss population groups at risk for needing long-term care services.
3. Identify the settings where long-term care services are provided.
4. Discuss the concept of home care and the range of home care services available in the community.
5. Summarize governmental financing for long-term care.
6. Explain legislation influencing long-term care service delivery.
7. Discuss barriers to the provision of community-based long-term care and methods for improving long-term care service delivery.
8. Analyze the role of the community health nurse in long-term care.

770

Like good cheese
She sits idly waiting to be
*   selected or needed*
But the ugly mold of age
Repels life's amateurs
And turns them away
Ignorant of the quality inside

RUTH NAYLOR

This text stresses the importance of working with aggregates at risk in the community in order to prevent major community health problems. Of all the groups discussed, none is growing more rapidly or has more primary, secondary, and tertiary prevention needs than the population that requires long-term care: the elderly, the chronically ill, and the disabled across the life span. Members of these groups are often ignored by society because their qualities are not recognized.

Multiple institutional and community settings provide long-term care services for individuals across the life span. While this chapter focuses on the role of the community health nurse in providing services at home for people who have long-term care needs, community health nurses must be critically aware of the role institutional settings play in long-term care. Institutional settings provide the most extensive, formal long-term care services and consume a major portion of the long-term health care dollar.

An inevitable result of the current financing of health care for many Americans is to be made powerless by sickness and poverty (Getzen, 1988). This occurs because often dependent individuals must deplete their life savings to pay for extended institutional long-term care. A significant amount of the funds for long-term care comes from consumers: "the elderly currently pay, on the average, more than 18 percent of their annual income out-of-pocket for health insurance premiums, deductibles, co-payments, balance billings from physicians, and non-covered services, such as long term care. Many pay more" (Robert Wood Johnson Foundation, 1991, p. 825). In 1989 44% of long-term institutional care in nursing homes was paid out-of-pocket by individuals and families (Robert Wood Johnson Foundation, p. 86).

Long-term care is a significant women's issue. Older women are twice as likely as older men to be institutionalized. The person most likely to enter a nursing home is the oldest-old female; one in four women 85 years of age or above resides in a nursing home, compared to one in seven men in this age group (Hing, 1987). Although they use institutional services more frequently, women often do not have the financial resources to pay for them. Women constitute 72.4% of the elderly poor (Ross, Danzinger, and Smolensky, 1987). A significant number of older women who reside in nursing homes are impoverished either upon entering the institution or sometime during the nursing home stay (Sekscenski, 1987). Further, since women are the traditional caregivers in our society, they experience social, emotional, and physical burdens related to long-term care in addition to financial ones. Stone, Cafferata, and Sangl (1987) found, in a national sample of informal caregivers who were assisting frail elderly persons, that the majority of these caregivers (71.5%) were female. Caregiving responsibilities can place an individual at risk for social isolation and physical or emotional health problems (Deimling and Bass, 1986; Pruchno and Resch, 1989).

Since there is a growing demand for long-term care, the focus in this chapter is on examining the role of the community health nurse in this area of practice. Emphasis is placed on identifying current long-term care resources, gaps in the present system, and future needs of this rapidly growing population.

DEFINING LONG-TERM CARE

Approaches and attitudes to caring for the aging and for the chronically ill in the United States are changing rapidly. Long-term care today implies a continuum of health and social services and includes both institutional and noninstitutional care. Broadly defined, long-term care services

are those typically needed by persons in declining health or by those suffering from chronic or terminal illnesses. These services include homemaker, chore, and social services; nutrition and health education; personal care aid; occupational, physical and speech therapy; and skilled nursing. Individual requirements may vary from minor personal care or homemaker services in normal housing to a full range of nursing, rehabilitative, and personal services that can be provided only in an institutional setting. The distinction

We thank Judith Harris, RN, MPH, Vice President, Nursing Services, Visiting Nurse Association of Greater Philadelphia, for her expert review of this chapter.

between long-term care and acute care lies in whether the primary reason for the service is to diagnose or treat an illness or to assist an individual whose capacity for functioning has been impaired by illness or age. (Congressional Budget Office, Technical Analysis Paper, 1977, p. 1.)

The General Accounting Office has defined long-term care as

one or more services provided on a sustained basis to enable individuals whose functional capacities are chronically impaired to be maintained at their maximum levels of psychological, physical, and social wellbeing. The recipients of services can reside anywhere along a continuum from their own homes to any type of institutional facility (GAO, 1983, p. 1).

Although long-term care entails a variety of institutional and community-based services, public programs disproportionately support institutional care. In 1987 66% of Medicare funds were used to purchase hospital care; 72% of Medicaid funds were used for institutional services (evenly split, 36% each, between hospital and nursing home care) that same year (Letsch, Levit, and Waldo, 1988). A very small portion of public funds are spent on home-based services. Medicare expenditures for home health care services account for about 3% of total Medicare outlays (Rivlin and Wiener, 1988): Medicare primarily covers acute care and is not intended to provide coverage for the long-term care needs of the dependent elderly (GAO, 1988). Although Medicaid funds about 50% of nursing home care, it funds only approximately 12% of home-based services (GAO, 1988).

A crisis exists in the long-term care system because financing for services has not kept pace with the growing need for services (Getzen, 1988). The present system requires significant out-of-pocket spending for nursing home care and other long-term care services that had not been anticipated by its users. Consequently, incomes are strained, life savings are used up, and an increasing number of individuals are becoming dependent on welfare funding for services. Being dependent on welfare assistance is degrading for many elderly persons (Rivlin and Wiener, 1988). Consumer inability to pay for extended care has created a two-class system of long-term care, one for the poor and one for the wealthy. This has, in turn, stimulated concerns about quality of care, especially in relation to the delivery of nursing home services. Nursing homes that accept only private-pay patients generally provide higher-quality care than those dependent on Medicaid patients (Rivlin and Wiener).

FACTORS INFLUENCING THE GROWTH OF LONG-TERM CARE SERVICES

Six factors in American society have influenced the need for increasing organized long term care services: epidemiological conditions, changes in informal support systems, sociodemographic factors, consumer preference, and increasingly sophisticated medical technology. Medicare had a powerful effect on these factors when it was created in 1965.

Epidemiological Conditions

Americans are living longer, the causes of death are changing, chronic illness is increasing, and the gap between male and female longevity is widening. It is crucial to the subject of long-term care to recognize that the rise in numbers and percentages of people in this country is among the very groups who need long-term care services the most. As medical technology and public health practice have advanced, an increasing number of vulnerable infants and disabled children and adults have been saved and life expectancy has risen dramatically, causing a significant expansion in the numbers of people 65 years of age and older. Persons in these population groups often have multiple chronic conditions and frequently require institutional or community-based long-term care services. Home health and other long-term care services are primarily delivered to the aging and the chronically ill (Robert Wood Johnson Foundation, 1991).

Not all elderly are at risk for long-term care. As studies of functional dependency and chronic illness consistently indicate, those most vulnerable are among the subgroup 85 years of age and older. Although only a small number (5%) of the elderly are in institutional settings, nearly 25% of the oldest-old (persons aged 85 and over) reside in nursing homes (U.S. Bureau of the Census, 1992.) This segment of the elderly population is growing the fastest and is illustrated in Figure 20-1. Between 1960 and 1987 the oldest-old increased from 5.6% to 9.6% of the elderly. By the year 2050 the number of persons aged 85 and over is projected to be 15.3 million, or 23.8% of the elderly population (U.S. Bureau of the Census, 1989, p. 40).

Although several factors (age, poverty, health status, sex, and living arrangements) have been associated with the use of health care services, data suggest that the key variables are poverty, age, and health

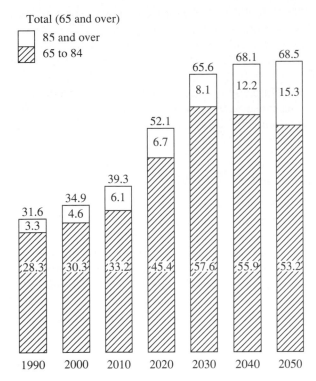

Figure 20-1   Projections of the elderly population, by age, for 1990 to 2050. (middle series projections in millions). (From U.S. Bureau of the Census: *Population profile of the United States: 1989,* Current Population Reports, Series P-23, No. 159, Washington, D.C., 1989, U.S. Government Printing Office, p. 40.)

status. Data from the National Medical Care Expenditure Survey (NMCES) related to the use of home health care show that the poor and near-poor are about twice as likely as the nonpoor to receive these services. These data also reflected that persons with activity limitations and those who consider themselves as having a poor health status are much more likely to use home health care services than the nonlimited and individuals who consider themselves as having a good health status. However, the elderly with activity limitations and poor health status are more likely to use home health services than either the younger limited population (6.7% versus 3.3%) or the nonelderly with poor health status (6.9% versus 1.5%). The elderly in this study also use home health care much more intensively than younger home health care users. Although elderly women are more likely than elderly men to use home health services, women less than 65 years of age did not use more home health services than nonelderly men. Individu-

als living alone use more health services than persons living with their spouses (2.4% versus 1.5%) or children or other relatives (2.4% versus 0.7%) (Berk and Bernstein, 1985). Among the elderly, women are more likely than men to live alone: in this country 80% of the 8.8 million elderly persons who live alone are women. Elderly persons living alone are almost five times as likely to be poor as elderly couples and are twice as likely as other aging persons to have no children. Children are a major source of care and assistance for the elderly person (Commonwealth Fund Commission on Elderly People Living Alone, 1987).

People are living longer because they are dying of different diseases now than 80 years ago. Infectious diseases are no longer the leading cause of death as was the case in the early 1900s (refer to Chapter 1). Cancer, heart disease, and stroke are now the chief killers, and they are often degenerative and chronic. As previously mentioned, individuals affected by these conditions usually require long-term care services. It is clear that epidemiological factors and demographic changes will make significant demands upon the long-term care delivery system in the near future. It is estimated that the number of older persons in nursing homes will nearly double, to about 2.2 million residents, by the year 2000 (Burke, 1988, December).

Informal Supports

The availability of informal supports is one of the prime keys to disabled people living in the community. Over 4%, or 7.7 million persons age 15 and above among the noninstitutionalized population, need assistance with daily activities. Of these, more than 5 million need help with instrumental activities of daily living (IADLs) (e.g., meal preparation, shopping, and doing laundry), and 2.5 million need assistance with activities of daily living (ADLs) (e.g., bathing, dressing, eating, and toileting) (Kraus and Stoddard, 1989, p. 5). Many individuals with IADL and ADL dependencies could not reside in the community without assistance from informal supports.

The family is the primary source of care for the disabled and the frail elderly (Doty, 1986; Kraus and Stoddard, 1989; OTA, 1987). Close to 80% of the 13.3 million persons of working age who have a work disability live with their families (Kraus and Stoddard, 1989; Robert Wood Johnson Foundation, 1991). About 75% of the disabled older persons residing in the community rely solely on family and friends, and most of the remainder depend upon a combination of family care and paid help (Liu, Manton, and Liu, 1986; Soldo, 1983). In 1982 about 2.2 million informal caregivers were providing unpaid assistance to 1.2 million noninstitutionalized, functionally impaired, elderly persons who reported problems with at least one ADL. A significant number of informal caregivers also provide assistance to elderly persons who have problems with IADLs but who are not ADL-dependent. Informal caregivers for the elderly are predominantly female, with adult daughters providing about one third of the long-term care (Stone, Cafferata, and Sangl, 1987, pp. 10-11).

Sanger (1983) states that four consequences of industrialization—geographical mobility, rising incomes, urbanization, and careers for women—have all changed the ability of families to provide informal support. Although the mobility rate has been declining in the past several decades, a large number of people move from one residence to another and many move significant distances. Of the 45.1 million persons who moved between March 1990 and March 1991, 7.1 million, or 17%, moved from one state to another (U.S. Bureau of the Census, 1993, p. 10).

Rising incomes allow people to live apart and to negate the dependence families have on one another. Small urban homes are not designed for intergenerational families. The average number of persons per household in 1992 was 2.62 people (U.S. Bureau of the Census, 1993). Industrialization has made it both possible and necessary for women to take on a career outside the home. During recent decades females have increasingly joined the paid labor force. This will make it more difficult for them to provide informal care for elderly relatives (Scanlon, 1988). It is anticipated that work obligations may conflict with caregiving responsibilities to a greater extent in the future than they do now (Stone, Cafferata, and Sangl, 1987).

Sociodemographic Factors

There are three sociodemographic factors that have increased the need for people to use formal long-term care services. Sanger (1983) lists these as the decline in the number of children a family chooses to have, the aging of the providers of care, and the increasing rates of divorce and remarriage. Simply summarized, there are fewer children to care for parents who are living longer lives. These children are also older when they are required to care for their parents. Data from the

1982 National Long-Term Care Survey showed that the average age of the caregivers assisting the disabled and/or frail elderly was 57.3 years (Stone, Cafferata, and Sangl, 1987). Further, divorce may change the bonds of affection and obligation, and children and stepchildren may face extremely difficult decisions about those for whom they should care. Aging persons themselves may be alone as the result of divorce or death.

Consumer Preference

Work by Lerman (1987) and others (McAllister, 1986) provides validation to the commonsense idea that people want to be treated and cared for at home rather than in institutional settings. Home has the advantage of providing security and familiarity and it also reduces exposure to iatrogenically induced problems of hospitals and nursing homes. Costs are less and the client and family are able to be in charge of the client's care.

Medical Technology

What's new in home care? In the words of Judith P. Harris, Vice President of Patient Services for the Visiting Nurse Association of Greater Philadelphia, it is

high technology. Just look at what is available in the home today that even a few years ago seemed an impossibility: some of the more progressive home care agencies offer services so patients can remain at home on ventilators. Home intravenous therapies now include total parenteral nutrition (TPN), hydration, antibiotics, pain management, chemotherapy, and drugs to treat AIDS-related infections. Specialty infusions include Lasix, Dopamine/Dobutamine, Desferoxamine and Neupogen. Patients may receive all types of gastro-intestinal tube feedings. PICC lines (peripherally-inserted central catheters) can stay in place for a long time and reduce the number of times a patient needs to be stuck with a needle during the course of therapy (Harris, 1992, p. 15).

The Creation of Medicare

Medicare was signed into law in 1965 by President Lyndon Johnson. It was created to cover the health care costs, including home care, for the elderly. By 1985 the number of Medicare-certified agencies providing home health care had climbed from 1800 to 5700. Concomitantly, expenditures for home health care services jumped from $46 billion in 1967 to $2.3 billion in 1987 to $3.8 billion in 1991 (George, 1992, p. 30). Table 20-1 depicts the growth in home health agencies providing Medicare services from 1979 to 1990; most of the growth occurred among for-profit freestanding and hospital-based home health agencies due to changes in governmental regulations. The traditional nonprofit providers, including visiting nurse associations and governmental agencies, deceased in number (GAO, 1992, p. 2). Details of how Medicare finances home health care services are presented later in this chapter.

PROFILE OF THE LONG-TERM CARE POPULATION

Certain population groups are at risk for needing long-term care services, and in the minds of many people the category of people at greatest risk is the elderly. There is no question that the elderly population experiences more chronic illness, physical functional limitations, and activity limitation than younger age groups. However, not all elderly are disabled and the aged alone are not the only individuals needing long-term care services: more than 660,000 persons aged 25 to 44 years need assistance in IADL and another 250,000 individuals in this age category need help in ADL. The number of persons 45 to 64 years of age needing assistance in IADL is close to 1.4 million and 540,000 more need help with ADL. The percentage of people in any age group needing assistance with ADL and IADL is relatively small (under 10%) until advanced age (Kraus and Stoddard, 1989, p. 29).

Several groups of nonaged people who use long-term care services are easily identified: the physically and mentally disabled and the mentally ill. In recent years the deinstitutionalization of clients with chronic conditions such as mental illness, mental retardation, and immobilizing physical problems has resulted in a significant increase in the number of individuals of all ages who need long-term care resources in their local communities, including home care.

The Physically and Mentally Disabled

Approximately 13.6 million noninstitutionalized people in the United States over the age of 15 report severe functional limitations. An estimated 13.3 million noninstitutionalized persons, accounting for

TABLE 20-1 Growth in Home Health Agencies Providing Medicare Services from 1979 to 1990

HHA type	1979 Number	1979 Percent	1990 Number	1990 Percent
Provider-based:				
Hospitals	349	12.2%	1,508	26.4%
Other	17	0.6	110	1.9
Free-standing:				
For-profit	165	5.8	1,918	33.5
Private nonprofit	443	15.5	710	12.4
Government	1,274	44.6	952	16.6
VNA	511	17.9	478	8.4
Other	99	3.4	45	0.8
Total	**2,858**	**100.0%**	**5,721**	**100.0%**

From General Accounting Office—Report to the Chairman, Subcommittee on Health and Long-Term Care, Select Committee on Aging, House of Representatives: *Medicare: rationale for higher payment for hospital-based home health agencies,* Washington, D.C., 1992, U.S. Government Printing Office, p. 2.

8.6% of the working-age population (16 to 64 years old), have a work disability. Of those with work disability it is estimated that 7.25 million have a disability that severely limits work ability. Work disabilities for institutionalized people (2.5 million persons) are more pervasive and usually are severe enough to prevent them from working (Figure 20-2). A high percentage of people with work disabilities is found among persons of working age receiving care in mental hospitals and residential treatment centers (81.8%), in homes for the aged (93.8%), homes and schools for the mentally handicapped (94.5%), and homes for the physically handicapped (91.1%) (Kraus and Stoddard, 1989).

Although many elderly are included in the figures for functional limitations, a significant number of Americans age 64 and under are functionally limited or mentally disabled. About 20% of people under 65 who earn less than $10,000 annually have disabilities, compared to only 7% to 8% of people earning at least $30,000 per year (Robert Wood Johnson Foundation, 1991, p. 72). About 9% of families care for a chronically ill family member at home, and close to one third of these individuals are adults (Figure 20-3) in the

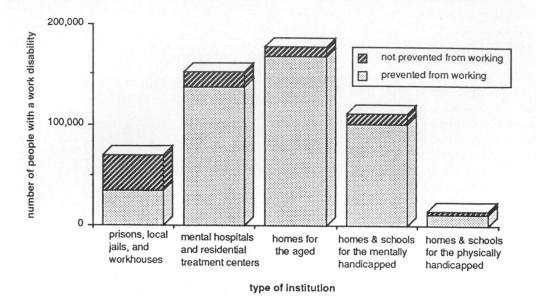

Figure 20-2 Number of working-age persons with work disabilities in institutions, by setting. (From Kraus LE and Stoddard S: *Chartbook on disability in the United States, an InfoUse report,* Washington, D.C., 1989, National Institute on Disability and Rehabilitation Research, p. 47.)

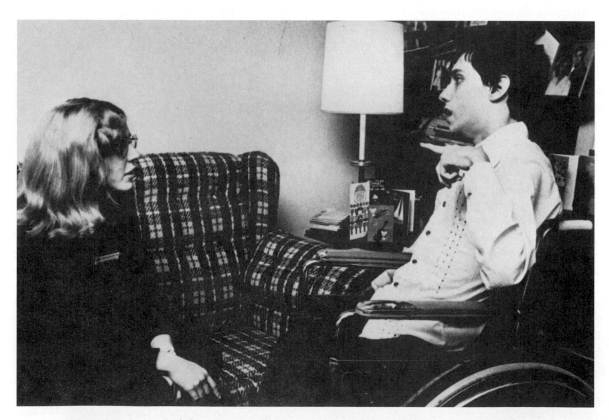

Figure 20-3 Young adults who are physically disabled frequently have extended health care needs that cannot be overlooked when planning long-term care services. These young people often can become productive members of society if they have social and community supports that help them handle their disabling conditions. (From Genesee Region Home Care Association, Rochester, NY.)

prime of life (Robert Wood Johnson Foundation, 1984, p. 16).

The chronically ill experience a variety of health problems that can cause activity limitations. Chronic health conditions that most often cause activity limitations of any kind include multiple sclerosis, paralysis of extremities, emphysema, intervertebral disk disorders, and epilepsy (Kraus and Stoddard, 1989, p. 24). These conditions mandate changes in lifestyle and careers and alter family functioning (Pitzele, 1986).

Children, as well as adults, have activity limitations and disability. Over 3.2 million children under the age of 17 have limitations in activity and about 2 million children under the age of 18 have a physical, mental, or emotional disability. Among this population males, blacks, and the poor are more highly represented (Kraus and Stoddard, 1989, p. 31). The types of chronic handicapping conditions causing disability in childhood are presented in Table 15-2.

Children who have functional disabilities often need a complex array of long-term care services. Appendix 10-1 presents a case history of one such child and vividly illustrates that young and aging Americans are highly dependent on our long-term health care system.

The profile of the mentally disabled or retarded population is not clear because estimates of their percentage range from 0.67% (1.6 million people) to 3% (6.5 million people). Of these individuals, approximately 89% are mildly retarded, 6% are moderately retarded, 3.5% are severely retarded, and 1.5% are profoundly retarded (Kraus and Stoddard, 1989, p. 6). Individuals moderately to profoundly retarded (176,000 to 715,000 people) usually need ongoing long-term care. The long-term care services needed by the mentally retarded are discussed in Chapter 18.

The Mentally Ill

An estimated 23 million adults currently suffer from a major mental or behavioral disorder other than substance abuse and about twice that number experience mental illness sometime throughout their lives (USDHHS Public Health Service, 1989). Mental illness cost the public billions of dollars annually, yet a significant number of individuals in need of mental health services are not receiving them. Those at risk are the disadvantaged, women, aged, and handicapped (Belk, 1987; NCOA, 1986; President's Commission on Mental Health, 1978; Weissman, 1987).

Among the mentally ill the most neglected and most needy are the chronic mentally ill. It is estimated that about 2.8 million adults in the United States have severe and persistent mental disorders; of these, 2 million suffer schizophrenia. Whereas anxiety and depression are the most common of the major mental disorders, schizophrenia is the one most likely to result in functional disabilities (USDHHS Public Health Service, 1989). The majority of individuals with chronic mental illness, roughly 59%, reside in the community as a result of the deinstitutionalization trend of the early 1970s (Robert Wood Johnson Foundation, 1991). A comprehensive and accessible array of biopsychosocial and supportive long-term services is needed to address the needs of the chronic mentally ill. Individuals among this population group frequently have multiple and complex physical and mental difficulties and a broad range of functional problems such as impaired capacity to work in competitive employment, problems with basic tasks of daily living, difficulty coping with stress and minor everyday issues, and inability to seek out sustained assistance.

A significant number of people who receive and require mental health assistance need long-term care services. Chapter 18 discusses in greater detail the service needs of people who are physically and mentally disabled. When working with the chronic mentally ill in the community it is important not to overlook their physical health problems, because often these problems greatly limit their functional abilities.

The Aging

The only universal feature of the older population is age. Most aging people are leading healthy, independent lives. The poverty rate among the elderly declined from 35.2% in 1959 to 12.4% in 1991 (U.S. Bureau of the Census, 1993, p. 43). "The great majority of elderly Americans are the wealthiest, best fed, best housed, healthiest, most self-reliant older population in our history" (Fowles, 1983, p. 6). However, a large number of individuals in this population group have difficulty functioning independently because of poor health and lack of money, transportation, employment, and social interaction. The elderly from minority groups, aging individuals over 85, and aging women are affected by these problems to a greater degree than other elderly groups. In 1991 elderly women (15.5%) were almost twice as likely to be poor as elderly men (7.9%), with black women having

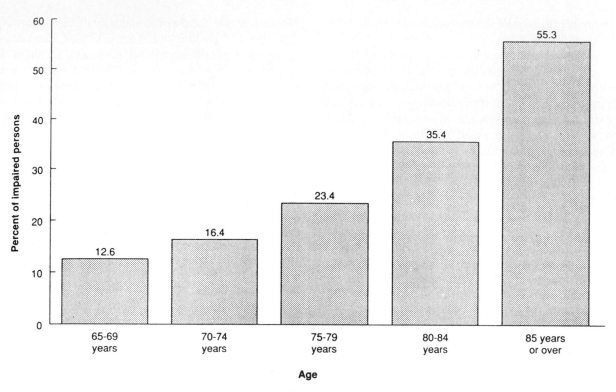

NOTE: IADL is instrumental activities of daily living; ADL is activities of daily living.

Figure 20-4   Effect of age on the probability of risk of IADL or ADL impairment, 1984-85. (From Scanlon WJ: A perspective on long-term care for the elderly, *Health Care Financ Rev*, 1988 Annual Suppl., December 1988, p. 9.)

the highest poverty rate, 39.3%. In this same year 25.6% of elderly black men were poor, and 15.4% of elderly Hispanic men and 24.5% of elderly Hispanic women were poor (U.S. Bureau of the Census, p. 43).

It has consistently been identified that the needs of older people increase with age. The young-old, or individuals 65 to 74 years of age, are generally able to remain functionally independent. Those above 75 want to be independent but often need much more help to do so. The aged above 85 represent, however, the greatest concern: the proportion of the aged dependent in 1984 ranged from 18 to 48 per 1000 for persons 65 to 74 years of age, from 37 to 97 per 1000 for persons 75 to 84 years of age, and from 90 to 286 per 1000 for persons 85 years of age and older. These data reflect that the proportion dependent among persons 85 years of age and over is from double to triple the proportion dependent among persons 75 to 84 years of age (Fulton, Katz, Jack, and Hendershot, 1989, p. 10).

Approximately 7 million elderly people need some type of care assistance, ranging from need for help with ordinary household tasks to need for total assistance in every activity of daily living. Approximately 30%, or 2 million, older persons needing long-term care assistance have only limited long-term care dependencies. However, a significant number (20%, or 1.4 million) of aging persons needing long-term help are almost totally dependent (Scanlon, 1988, p. 7). The need for assistance with ADLs and IADLs increases markedly in the old-old or fragile-elderly age group (Figure 20-4). Among the young-old population, only about 13% need help with long-term care, but among the oldest-old 55% require assistance (Scanlon, p. 7).

Those with Chronic or Acute Conditions

Most older people have at least one chronic condition and many have multiple conditions. The most frequently occurring chronic conditions for the elderly

65 and older are arthritis (48%), hypertension (37%), hearing impairments (32%), heart disease (30%), orthopedic impairments (18%), cataracts and sinusitis (14% each), and diabetes (10%) (AARP, 1993, p. 13).

The major causes of hospitalization of elderly people include the following (May, Kelly, Mendlein, and Garbe, 1991):

- Acute ischemic heart disease
- Cerebrovascular disease
- Congestive heart failure
- Pneumonia
- Chronic ischemic heart disease
- Cardiac dysrhythmias
- Hip fracture
- Fluid/electrolyte imbalance
- Hyperplasia of prostate

In the age group 85 years and older, septicemia and gastrointestinal hemorrhage rose to the final positions on this list.

Dementia

The notion that dementia among the elderly is inevitable and affects the majority of older people is not supported by statistical data. The prevalence of severe dementia among elderly subgroups ranges from 1% (ages 65 to 74) to 7% (ages 75 to 84) to 25% (above age 85); an estimated 1.5 million Americans suffer from severe dementia and require constant care. Between 1 million and 5 million others have mild or moderate dementia. Dementia places a person at risk of requiring institutionalization. It is estimated that at least half of nursing home residents in the United States have dementia (OTA, 1987).

Although a relatively small percentage of the elderly suffer from dementia, interest in this condition as a significant health problem is growing for a number of reasons. One major reason is the anticipated increase in the number of persons with dementia. It is estimated that by the year 2040, 7.4 million Americans will be demented, which is five times as many persons as today. Concern about dementing illnesses is also rising because financial costs and personal stresses related to these conditions are great. From a financial perspective, it costs billions of dollars each year to care for these individuals (OTA, 1987, p. 5). The fact that caregivers of persons with dementia experience burdens and stresses related to their caregiving obligations is well documented (Eagles, Beattie, Blackwood, Restall, and Ashcroft, 1987; Fitting,

Rabins, Lucas, and Eastham, 1986; George and Gwyther, 1986; OTA, 1987; Zarit, Todd, and Zarit, 1986). It has also been demonstrated that caregiving places individuals at risk for developing health problems (George and Gwyther, 1986; Haley, Levine, Brown, Berry, and Hughes, 1987; OTA, 1987).

Dementia designates a group of illnesses characterized by a progressive and usually irreversible loss of mental function (Prochazka, Henschke, Skinner, and Last, 1983, p. 1). Some 70 conditions can cause dementia (refer to box on pp. 780 and 781). The diseases classified as degenerative are those whose progression cannot be arrested. Alzheimer's disease is the most common degenerative dementing illness, found in 66% of all cases (OTA, 1987, p. 12).

Alzheimer's Disease

Alzheimer's disease (AD) was named for Alois Alzheimer, a German doctor who in 1907 accurately described the typical brain alterations related to morphological, neurochemical, and physiological dysfunction. These alterations are irreversible. The cause is unknown; nevertheless, distinctive alterations in and loss of nerve cells are detectable in the brain tissue of affected persons. It is believed that Alzheimer's disease is actually a group of related disorders distinguished by their symptoms, rate of progression, inheritance patterns, and age of onset. Researchers are exploring genetic and environmental causes, as well as defects in the immune system, as explanations for the disease. Until the cause is known, treatment can be only symptomatic (Burns and Buckwalter, 1988; OTA, 1987).

Affected people manifest various stages as the disease progresses, from forgetfulness with long-term and short-term memory, to confusion and finally to dementia. These stages differ in length and intensity from one person to another. The symptoms include a decline in mental status involving changes in memory, language, praxis, mood, concentration, cooperation, thought process, and perception, with progressive deterioration. Mood changes occur until finally the person becomes completely passive. During the end stages help is needed with the simplest activities of daily living, and the person commonly assumes the fetal position (Buckwalter, Abraham, and Neuendorger, 1988).

The onset of symptoms is usually noticed first by the affected person, family, friends, or peers at work, rather than by health care professionals. The person

◀ *Disorders Causing or Simulating Dementia* ▶

Disorders Causing Dementia
Degenerative Diseases

Alzheimer's disease
Pick's disease
Huntington's disease
Progressive supranuclear palsy
Parkinson's disease (not all cases)
Cerebellar degenerations
Amyotrophic lateral sclerosis (ALS) (not all cases)
Parkinson-ALS-dementia complex of Guam and other island areas
Rare genetic and metabolic diseases (Hallervorden-Spatz, Kufs', Wilson's, late-onset metachromatic leukodystrophy, adrenoleukodystrophy)

Vascular Dementia

Multiinfarct dementia
Cortical micro-infarcts
Lacunar dementia (larger infarcts)
Binswanger disease
Cerebral embolic disease (fat, air, thrombus fragments)

Anoxic Dementia

Cardiac arrest
Cardiac failure (severe)
Carbon monoxide

Traumatic Dementia

Dementia pugilistica (boxer's dementia)
Head injuries (open or closed)

Infectious Dementia

Acquired immunodeficiency syndrome (AIDS) AIDS dementia
  Opportunistic infections
Creutzfeldt-Jakob disease (subacute spongiform encephalopathy)
Progressive multifocal leukoencephalopathy
Post-encephalitic dementia
Behcet's syndrome
Herpes encephalitis
Fungal meningitis or encephalitis
Bacterial meningitis or encephalitis
Parasitic encephalitis
Brain abscess
Neurosyphilis (general paresis)

Normal Pressure Hydrocephalus (communicating hydrocephalus of adults)

Space-Occupying Lesions

Chronic or acute subdural hematoma
Primary brain tumor
Metastatic tumors (carcinoma, leukemia, lymphoma, sarcoma)

Multiple Sclerosis (some cases)

Auto-Immune Disorders

Disseminated lupus erythematosus
Vasculitis

Toxic Dementia

Alcoholic dementia
Metallic dementia (e.g., lead, mercury, arsenic, manganese)
Organic poisons (e.g., solvents, some insecticides)

Other Disorders

Epilepsy (some cases)
Post-traumatic stress disorder (concentration camp syndrome—some cases)
Whipple disease (some cases)
Heat stroke

Disorders That Can Simulate Dementia
Psychiatric Disorders

Depression
Anxiety
Psychosis
Sensory deprivation

Drugs

Sedatives
Hypnotics
Antianxiety agents
Antidepressants
Antiarrhythmics
Antihypertensives
Anticonvulsants
Antipsychotics
Digitalis and derivatives
Drugs with anti-cholinergic side effects
Others (mechanism unknown)

◀   *Disorders Causing or Simulating Dementia—cont'd*   ▶

Disorders That Can Simulate Dementia—cont'd

Nutritional Disorders

Pellagra (B_6 deficiency)
Thiamine deficiency (Wernicke-Korsakoff syndrome)
Cobalamin deficiency (B_{12}) or pernicious anemia
Folate deficiency
Marchiafava-Bignami disease

Metabolic Disorders (usually cause delirium, but can be difficult to differentiate from dementia)
Hyper- and hypothyroidism (thyroid hormones)

Hypercalcemia (calcium)
Hyper- and hyponatremia (sodium)
Hypoglycemia (glucose)
Hyperlipidemia (lipids)
Hypercapnia (carbon dioxide)
Kidney failure
Liver failure
Cushing syndrome
Addison's disease
Hypopituitarism
Remote effect of carcinoma

Modified from Katzman R, Lasker B, and Bernstein N: Accuracy of diagnosis and consequences of misdiagnosis of disorders causing dementia. Contract report prepared for the Office of Technology Assessment, U.S. Congress. In Office of Technology Assessment: *Losing a million minds: confronting the tragedy of Alzheimer's disease and other dementias,* Washington, D.C., 1987, U.S. Government Printing Office, pp. 13-14.

usually hides early symptoms such as memory loss and decreased mental ability, possibly for years. Progression is insidious, with a diagnosis frequently made more than 4 years after the onset of symptoms. The average duration of Alzheimer's disease is 8.1 years, but duration is unpredictable: in some people it has remained as long as 25 years. The individuals usually die from other illness such as pneumonia, heart disease, or kidney failure (OTA, 1987).

Alzheimer's disease causes mental anguish for the affected person and for the significant others. Caring for the individual places a constant burden on families and taxes their resources. Community health nurses play a major role in helping afflicted persons and their families to obtain appropriate care. A mental health model that focuses on adapting to the individual's behavior appears to benefit them more than a medical model focused on correcting a disability. A specific pattern of care that emphasizes medical evaluation and drug management, combined with mental health care in nursing homes and day care centers that coordinate their services with social and aging services, is emerging (OTA, 1987, p. 43).

A variety of social and aging services are frequently available in the community to assist demented persons and their families to enhance the quality of their lives (refer to box on p. 782). Community health nurses are often in a unique position to help families obtain needed services. The Alzheimer's Disease and Related

Disorders Association (ADRDA) is a valuable resource for both health care professionals and clients. This association provides resource materials that help families to establish an effective management program at home, offers group support services for families experiencing related stresses, and assists families in identifying community resources skilled in working with affected persons. However, many health care services do not address the needs of individuals with dementia. Persons especially likely to be unable to obtain adequate services are those without families, individuals from minority and ethnic groups, individuals experiencing disease onset in middle age, individuals residing in rural areas, veterans, and the poor (OTA, 1987, p. 45).

Support for informal caregivers is essential. The problems faced by families dealing with dementia are complex and very stressful and place them at high risk for experiencing financial difficulties in addition to health problems. "The primary needs of informal caregivers are respite care, information on the diseases and care methods, information about services, and a broadened range of services" (OTA, 1987, p. 63). The range of services for persons with dementia and their families is very limited in many communities.

Kohlman, Wilson, Hutchinson, and Wallhagen (1991) have synthesized the knowledge about Alzheimer's disease and family caregiving published over the last 10 years. Community health nurses working with

◀   *Care Services for Individuals with Dementia*   ▶

Adult day care	Information and referral to services	Physician services
Case management	Legal services	Protective services
Chore services	Mental health services	Recreational services
Congregate meals	Occupational therapy	Respite care
Dental services	Paid companion/sitter	Skilled nursing
Home delivered meals	Patient assessment	Speech therapy
Home health aide services	Personal care	Supervision
Homemaker services	Personal emergency response systems	Telephone reassurance
Hospice services	Physical therapy	Transportation

From Office of Technology Assessment (OTA): *Losing a million minds: confronting the tragedy of Alzheimer's disease and other dementias,* Washington, D.C., 1987, U.S. Government Printing Office, p. 36.

clients who have this diagnosis will find helpful resources and directions for research in this reference. An example of the material available to community health nurses working with Alzheimer's patients and their families in the home setting is the August 1991 issue of the *Journal of Home Health Care Practice* (Parsick and Triebsch, editors). This journal provides the home health care professional with current information regarding the needs of the AD patient and caregivers and includes nursing problems such as communication, nutrition, disorientation, ethical decisions, and respite for families.

There is no question that long-term care resources must be expanded. Statistical data show that the number of persons needing long-term services will increase dramatically in the next several decades. Defining at-risk aggregates in the community and subgroups within these aggregates who need these services, and pinpointing exactly at what intensity they need the services, will be the future challenge of health care providers.

DEFINING FORMAL HOME CARE SERVICES

The founder of modern community health nursing, Lillian Wald, was introduced in the first chapter of this text. Wald and her contemporaries nursed the sick of all ages in their homes and also provided instructions to reduce illness and to promote health. The goal of these early home health care visits was to care for the sick, teach the family how to care for the ill person, and above all to protect the public from the spread of disease (Buhler-Wilkerson, 1991, p. 7). Wald's work with the Metropolitan Life Insurance Company to

provide home health services was also described in Chapter 1; she was instrumental in developing a plan to extend nursing care to the Metropolitan's industrial policyholders during illness. The experiment was tremendously successful because the nurses, at a cost of five cents per policy, reduced the number of death benefits paid and also created the public image of a concerned humanitarian institution for the "Met." To provide this care across the country the organization used both existing visiting nurse associations and their own nurses. "For many visiting nurse associations, this new business partnership meant that without additional fund-raising, they could extend their services to more of the working class. Only three years later, Metropolitan Life Insurance Company was paying for one million nursing visits each year at a cost of roughly $500,000 per year. By 1916, the Metropolitan visiting nurse service was available to 90% of its 10.5 million policyholders living in 2,000 United States and Canadian cities" (Buhler-Wilkerson, p. 7-8) (refer to Figure 20-5).

By the 1920s, twenty years later, care of ill people in their homes by nurses had declined. Infectious diseases such as smallpox and yellow fever were no longer the leading causes of death and chronic diseases, much less dramatic in their impact, generated public concern. Further, patients of all classes began to seek hospital-based care since practitioners in this setting were better prepared than previously. Despite these changes, home care has been reaffirmed as an essential community service from a public health perspective throughout this century (Administration of Home Health Nursing, 1945; ANA, 1992; Bedside nursing care, 1945; Haupt, 1953; Olson, 1986).

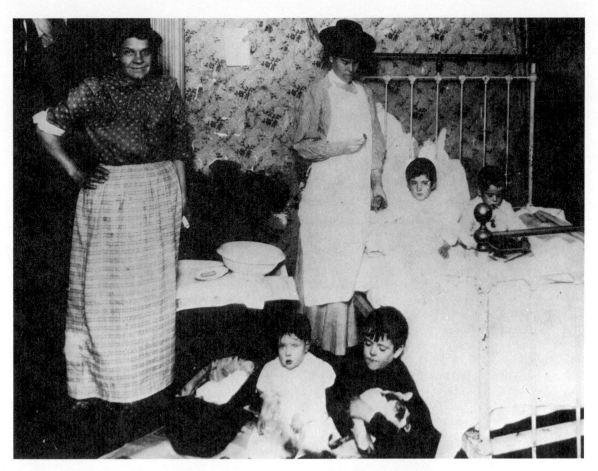

Figure 20-5   The increased emphasis being placed on home health care is not new. Home health care services have been provided by public health nurses in the United States since the late 1800s. Individuals across the life span benefit from these services. (Courtesy Metropolitan Life Insurance.)

Today home health care services are the fastest-growing industry in the United States. The dramatic change in the development of home-based health services shows little indication of slowing. This chapter discusses reasons for this resurgence of interest in the home setting for the provision of services, the role of the nurse in this setting, reimbursement issues, family concerns, and the future for home health care. The philosophy of hospice care of the dying is also presented.

In 1992 the ANA further refined the concept of home health nursing in its document *A Statement on the Scope of Home Health Nursing Practice.* This document defined home health nursing as a "synthesis of community health nursing and selected technical skills from other specialty nursing practices" (ANA, 1992, p. 5), such as medical-surgical nursing, gerontological nursing, and parent-child nursing. The health care deficits of the client determine the appropriate augmentation of other specialty skills with community health nursing practice. As discussed in Chapter 2, the home health nurse who practices within a community health nursing framework provides specialty focused skilled care beyond the individual and family. Nursing care from this perspective directs attention to aggregate needs, "with the predominate responsibility for care to the population as a whole" (ANA, p. 5). In line with this philosophy the home health nurse's role as a multidisciplinary care coordinator is important in facilitating the goal of care (ANA, p. 6). The Webster case situation in Chapter 2, p. 53, illustrates the importance of the care coordinator role in facilitating the goal of care beyond the individual family.

Home care includes a broad range of homebased

TABLE 20-2 Types of Home Health Care Agencies in the United States*

Type of agency	Description of agency
Official	A governmental or public agency, usually a local health department, which is supported by state and local taxes. Official agencies are mandated by law to provide certain specific services, such as communicable disease follow-up. They provide health promotion and disease prevention services as well as home health care.
Voluntary	A private, nonprofit agency whose operating funds come largely from individual contributions, fees-for-service, united community funds, contracts for service, grants, and other nonofficial sources of funding. Voluntary agencies are governed by a board of directors. These agencies are not required by law to provide specific types of services; they primarily, but not exclusively, provide home health care services. The visiting nurse associations traditionally have been the major voluntary organizations which provide home health care services in a local community.
Combination	A combined governmental (a local health department) and voluntary agency (a VNA), whose operating funds came from both official and nonofficial sources. This organizational structure was promoted for the purposes of preventing duplication of services, decreasing continuity of care difficulties and reducing the cost of delivering local health care services. A combination agency provides both health promotion/disease prevention and home health care services.
Private, nonprofit	A privately owned agency which is tax exempt because of its nonprofit status. Unlike voluntary agencies, these agencies are governed by the owner(s) of the organization. Their major source of revenue is fee-for-service. Private nonprofit agencies are usually established to provide home health care services only.
Proprietary	A private agency established to make a profit. These agencies are not eligible for tax exemption. They are governed by their owner(s), who are increasingly large corporations. Their major source of revenue is a fee for service. Like the private, nonprofit agencies, proprietary agencies are usually established to provide home health care services only.
Hospital-based	A home health care agency run and governed by a hospital. Sources of revenue and tax status vary depending on the type of hospital (governmental, voluntary, private, nonprofit, or proprietary) which has established the home health care agency. It is predicted that the numbers of hospital-based home health care agencies will increase dramatically in the next decade.

*Refer to Chapter 5 for further discussion of official and voluntary agencies.
From Health Care Financing Administration: *Medicare program: home health agencies—conditions of participation and reductions in recordkeeping requirements,* 42 CFR, Part 484, Sections 484.1 through 484.52, Washington, D.C., October 1989, U.S. Department of Health and Human Services; and Hirsh L, Klein M, and Marlowe G: *Combining public health nursing agencies: a case study in Philadelphia,* New York, 1967, Department of PHN, NLN, p. 3.

health and social services such as home management assistance, personal care, consumer education, and financial counseling services. Social home care services are covered under Title XX of the Social Security Act for clients who qualify for Title XX assistance (Title XX is discussed later in this chapter). These services are provided by diverse community agencies such as local departments of social service, family service organizations, and councils on agencies.

During the past 10 years demonstration projects have experimented with different approaches for delivering home care. One approach has been to mix formal (professionally directed) services with informal supports (family and friends). Others extend the informal system with homemaker services and Meals on Wheels. Another approach has been to place nursing home candidates in foster homes; the paid caregiver in the foster home provides a private room, meals, laundry, assistance with ADLs, and 24-hour assistance. A community health nurse provides nurs-

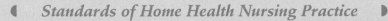

◀ *Standards of Home Health Nursing Practice* ▶

Standard I.   Organization of Home Health Services

All home health services are planned, organized, and directed by a master's-prepared professional nurse with experience in community health and administration.

Standard II.   Theory

The nurse applies theoretical concepts as a basis for decisions in practice.

Standard III.   Data Collection

The nurse continuously collects and records data that are comprehensive, accurate, and systematic.

Standard IV.   Diagnosis

The nurse uses health assessment data to determine nursing diagnoses.

Standard V.   Planning

The nurse develops care plans that establish goals. The care plan is based on nursing diagnoses and incorporates therapeutic, preventive, and rehabilitative nursing actions.

Standard VI.   Intervention

The nurse, guided by the care plan, intervenes to provide comfort, to restore, improve, and promote health, to prevent complications and sequelae of illness, and to effect rehabilitation.

Standard VII.   Evaluation

The nurse continually evaluates the client's and family's responses to interventions in order to determine progress toward goal attainment and to revise the data base, nursing diagnoses, and plan of care.

Standard VIII.   Continuity of Care

The nurse is responsible for the client's appropriate and uninterrupted care along the health care continuum, and therefore uses discharge planning, case management, and coordination of community resources.

Standard IX.   Interdisciplinary Collaboration

The nurse initiates and maintains a liaison relationship with all appropriate health care providers to assure that all efforts effectively complement one another.

Standard X.   Professional Development

The nurse assumes responsibility for professional development and contributes to the professional growth of others.

Standard XI.   Research

The nurse participates in research activities that contribute to the profession's continuing development of knowledge of home health care.

Standard XII.   Ethics

The nurse uses the code for nurses established by the American Nurses Association as a guide for ethical decision making in practice.

From American Nurses Association: *Standards of home health nursing practice,* Kansas City, Mo., 1986, The Association, pp. 5-19. Reprinted with permission from *Standards of Home Health Nursing Practice.* © 1986, American Nurses Association, Kansas City, Mo.

ing care, education of the caregiver, and ongoing assessment. The life satisfaction scores of people in foster home settings such as these have been high (Oktay and Volland, 1987).

A very important component of home care is home *health* care. Based on materials prepared by multiple professional organizations such as the National Association of Home Health Agencies, the ANA, and the NLN, the Department of Health, Education and Welfare (now the Department of Health and Human Services) defined home health care as (Warhola, 1980, p. 9).

that component of a continuum of comprehensive health care whereby health services are provided to individuals and families in their places of residence for the purpose of promoting, maintaining or restoring health, or of maximizing the level of independence, while minimizing the effects of disability and illness, including terminal illness. Services appropriate to the needs of the individual patient and family are planned, coordinated, and made available by providers organized for the delivery of home health care through the use of employed staff, contractual arrangements, or a combination of the two patterns.

Home health services are made available based upon patient care needs as determined by an objective patient assessment administered by a multidisciplinary team or a single health professional. Centralized professional coordination and case management are included. These services are provided under a plan of care that includes, but is not limited to appropriate service components such as medical, dental, nursing, social work, pharmacy, laboratory, physical therapy, speech therapy, occupational therapy, nutrition, homemaker–home health aide service, transportation, chore services, and provision of medical equipment and supplies.

Multiple types of agencies (refer to Table 20-2) provide home health care services. Both the government and private sectors of our health care delivery system are active in delivering home health services. The number and types of home health care agencies have proliferated in the past two decades, mainly due to the passage of the Medicare health insurance program for the elderly and the Medicaid health program for the poor in 1965. Both programs established mechanisms for reimbursing home health services and provided an impetus for the expansion of these services across the country. Proprietary and institutional affiliated agencies (hospital and skilled nursing facilities) are growing the most rapidly.

The proliferation of home health care agencies provided an impetus for the development in 1986 of *Standards of Home Health Nursing Practice* by the American Nurses Association. These standards guide agencies and nurses in providing care of the highest quality for home health care clients and are presented in the box on p. 785.

Presented below and on p. 787 are four case histories that represent the type of care offered by home health agencies across the country. The case studies illustrate the direct service role, as well as the care coordinator role, of the home health care nurse. The Visiting Nurse Service of the Toledo District Nurse Association, the agency that published these case histories, has been caring for elderly and disabled persons for more than 83 years. Throughout these years this organization has provided millions of home visits to needy persons (Visiting Nurse Service, 1984, p. 57.)

These case histories clearly illustrate that individuals across the life-span need community-based home care services. They also reflect the increasing complexity of client care demands and the need for coordinated, multidisciplinary home health services. Most importantly, they show that skilled home-based nursing services can make a difference; they help families to strengthen their coping abilities and they assist disabled persons to improve their functional capabilities and avoid unnecessary institutionalization.

VNS CARING IN TOLEDO, OHIO: FOUR CASE EXAMPLES*

CASE EXAMPLE ONE

Sixteen-year-old boy run over by train which inflicted massive trauma resulting in amputation of left hindquarter, amputation of arm, multiple pelvic fractures, fracture of transverse process, avulsion of urethra-prostate-testes and L-sileium exposing peritoneal sac, laceration L. ureter and L. iliac arteries, resulted in colostomy, supra-pubic cystotomy, hemipelvectomy, bilateral orchiectomy, skin grafts to hip sockets, etc.

After only five weeks in the hospital, client was allowed to go home (on Coordinated Home Care, saving over 30 hospital days) with a 24″ × 24″ graft in L pelvic area with open draining area. The VNS Home Care Coordinator managed this complex referral, coordinated arrangements for special dressing sup-

*From Visiting Nurse Service (VNS) of Toledo: Eighty-three years of caring, *Caring* 3:61, 1984. Case examples were written by Janet Blaufuss, RN, former Executive Director of the Visiting Nurse Service of the Toledo District Nurse Association, Toledo, Ohio, 1984.

plies and equipment and facilitated care throughout the period of need. The case nurse said, "The coordinator made it all come together and work." Clearly, the value of the coordinator having home care experience and familiarity with agency operations was evident.

Nursing visits were daily for two weeks, then reduced to three times a week as the family became more confident in care. Nursing activities included aseptic wound care, supervision of colostomy care, suprapubic catheter care, observation for complications with prompt intervention, instruction of family in all aspects of care and encouraging this adolescent to become independent in ADL's. To promote usual family activities, the nurse supported their decision to go on a weekend camping trip within the first two weeks and arranged to make visits at the local campsite.

Physical and occupational therapy services were provided for ADL's, gait training, transfers, strengthening and stump wrapping. Since this boy was left-dominant, he had to relearn all activities one-handed

with the nondominant side. When a left arm prosthesis was secured, the OT (who herself has an upper extremity prosthesis) resumed visits to aid in learning its use.

A total of 129 home health visits were provided over a nine-month period to aid in his excellent recovery, and he has now returned to school.

Although several intervening hospitalizations were required for re-evaluations and surgical revisions, none were necessary for complications, e.g., infection.

This example of teamwork included various surgery specialists, numerous VNS staff, and, of course, the family.

CASE EXAMPLE TWO

A 70-year-old patient who had transhepatic biliary disease, probably cancer of head of pancreas and a history of cancer of gallbladder was admitted to service after insertion of a transhepatic ring catheter which allows bile to drain from the common duct to the duodenum.

The patient and family were quite anxious re: involved procedures. The visiting nurse instructed the family in home care including such things as withdrawing of bile, irrigating ring catheter technique, dressing changes using aseptic technique, changing catheter plug, and teaching of signs of complications, in addition to monitoring hypertension status, nutrition/hydration, reactions to x-ray treatment, medications and pain control.

After verbal and demonstrative teaching, the family was able to provide the necessary care and patient was discharged in stabilized condition.

CASE EXAMPLE THREE

A 5-month-old infant who had been normal at birth developed pneumococcal meningitis with resulting hydrocephalus, severe neurologic deficits and seizure disorders. The mother, who was single and 16 years old, wanted to care for the child at home as long as possible so a referral was made to VNS.

At the time of hospital discharge, the child was totally unresponsive and had no purposeful movements, was on continuous gastric tube feedings with a Kangaroo pump, and required a suction machine and vaporizer. Nursing care consisted of providing and teaching re: dressing changes around the G-tube, tube irrigation, frequent repositioning, ROM, skin care and hygiene, relaxation and stimulation techniques, and use of Kangaroo pump. Additionally, the home care nurse assessed neurological and respiratory status and provided frequent intervention related to medication regimen, irritability, and seizure control. A home

health aide assisted the mother with care, bathing and stimulation techniques. A total of 54 home health visits were provided over a five-month period.

The Maternal Child Health nurse supported this young mother in her difficult decision to place the child in an extended care unit for the developmentally disabled at one year of age (where she visits frequently and takes her home every other weekend) so she could return to school.

At the time of discharge from VNS, this young child could take water orally, respond to the mother and had some purposeful movement.

CASE EXAMPLE FOUR

A 76-year-old client had a long history of Crohn's disease and malabsorption syndrome, and after multiple admissions for weight loss, malnutrition and dehydration, a permanent subclavian line was inserted in early summer of 1981 for total parenteral nutrition. It became apparent that adequate nutrition could only be attained through TPN and she would need regular infusions of amino acids, electrolytes, minerals and, eventually, fatty acids through this subclavian line. VNS nurses worked closely with physicians, hospital nurses, nutritionists, pharmacists, social workers, and patient's family in planning for adequate predischarge teaching and adequate home support for this patient. Through a joint effort between VNS and the community hospital, the patient's elderly brother has been successfully managing her four-times-a-week home TPN infusion, and once-a-week lipid infusion. This patient has the original subclavian line in place (for over two years) and it has remained free of any signs and symptoms of infection for over two years. In addition to care for the subclavian line and TPN infusions, VNS has helped the brother learn to care for the patient's permanent colostomy and chronic abdominal fistula.

Patient's condition has deteriorated gradually over the last two years; she now has an indwelling foley catheter and is essentially bed bound, requiring the services of a home health aide. Patient appears to have suffered at least one CVA and has been hospitalized for erratic blood sugars, and abnormal blood values which reflects the necessary and frequent nursing intervention. Nutritionally she has remained stable, demonstrating a weight gain of sixteen pounds over two years (originally weight was 88 pounds and now is 104 pounds).

Through the joint efforts of VNS, the community hospital, and the family, this patient has been able to go home and remain at home, without serious nutritional compromise, over the last two years.

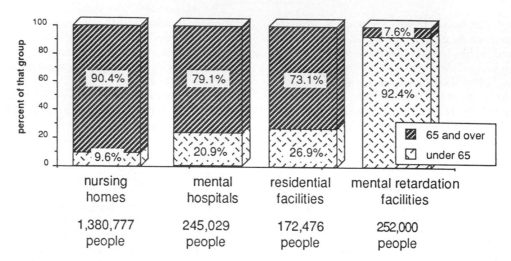

Of the more than 2 million people served in institutions many are over the age of 65.

Figure 20-6   Number of residents in long-term care institutions and percentage of residents in each type of facility by age. (From Kraus LE and Stoddard S: *Chartbook on disability in the United States, an InfoUse report,* Washington, D.C., 1989, National Institute on Disability and Rehabilitation Research, p. 21.)

ANALYSIS OF OTHER LONG-TERM CARE SETTINGS

Contrary to popular belief, long-term care services are provided by diverse institutional and community-based settings rather than only by large state hospitals and county facilities. In fact, focus has been placed on developing a wide variety of alternative community-based services for all at-risk aggregates who need long-term care resources.

Institutional Settings

Figure 20-6 displays the types of institutions that provide long-term care services. By far the largest number of institutionalized residents who require long-term care are served by various types of nursing homes: skilled nursing facilities, intermediate care facilities, and personal care facilities. The majority of residents in nursing homes (90.4%), mental hospitals (79.1%), and residential facilities (73.1%) are elderly. However, in facilities for mentally retarded persons, almost all (92.4%) are under the age of 65; 76% are between 22 and 64 years of age (Kraus and Stoddard, 1989, p. 21).

As a result of the projected aging of the U.S.

population and societal trends that bear on the availability of informal caregivers, there is a growing concern about access to long-term care services. It is anticipated that the elderly long-term care population will increase from an estimated 6.2 to 6.5 million in 1985 to about 14.3 million in 2020. During this same time period the nursing home population is expected to increase to about 4.2 million because the most rapidly growing segment of the disabled elderly is the extremely dependent—those with five or more ADL limitations (GAO, 1988). ADL dependency dramatically increases a person's risk of being institutionalized: 5% of dependent elderly with only IADL limitations and approximately 12% of those with only one or two ADL dependencies reside in nursing homes; however, 50% of the aged with five or six ADL limitations reside in nursing homes (Scanlon, 1988, p. 7). Severely dependent elderly have difficulty obtaining nursing home care (GAO, 1988). It is unlikely that this situation will improve because the increase in nursing home beds has not kept pace with the aging of the American population. This has occurred because states have vigorously attempted to control Medicaid costs by limiting the supply of nursing home beds (Scanlon, p. 9).

During the 1970s and early 1980s focus was placed

on determining whether dependent elderly could be cared for in the community at a lower cost than in nursing homes. Medicare and Medicaid waiver programs and demonstration projects were established that allowed a percentage of the funds (less than the cost of nursing home care) that would normally have been used for nursing home care to be used for community-based services (Kemper, Applebaum, and Harrigan, 1987). Under those programs case management mechanisms were established to ensure that individuals who could receive appropriate care at less cost in their own home or other settings could obtain the assistance needed to do so. However, because of the difficulty in identifying at-risk individuals who were likely to enter a nursing home, few of these projects demonstrated that this process and expanded community services decreased overall health care expenditures (Hughes, 1985; Kane, 1988; Weissert, Cready, and Pawelak, 1988). In spite of this finding, the case management model for delivering services to long-term care populations continues to be advocated, because some projects have demonstrated cost effectiveness and many persons with long-term care needs prefer to remain in their homes as long as possible (Capitman, 1988; GAO, 1988; Zawadski and Eng, 1988).

Defining who does and who does not need nursing home care is difficult, because nursing home need is a product of complex interactions among individual, medical, social, and economic circumstances. For example, individuals whose medical problems limit their functional abilities but who have available support systems are less likely to enter a nursing home than individuals with the same type of medical problems and functional difficulties who have no support systems to provide ongoing assistance.

Estimates of the number of persons likely to use nursing home care are based on characteristics of people who have used nursing homes in the past. On the basis of a study that merged data files estimating these characteristics for both the institutionalized and noninstitutionalized populations, the major predictors of nursing home use among the elderly are (GAO, 1983, p. 38):

- Whether they are dependent in the basic activities of daily living for eating, toileting, bathing, and dressing
- Whether they are mentally ill or have received a diagnosis of injury, cancer, or digestive, metabolic, blood, or genitourinary disorders

- How old they are (young-old or old-old)
- Whether, with these characteristics, they live alone or have help from spouse, family, or friends

Recent studies reflect similar characteristics among nursing home residents (GAO, 1988; Scanlon, 1988).

The importance of informal support networks in preventing institutionalization cannot be overestimated. As previously discussed, about 75% of the dependent elderly are cared for in their homes. Most families want to care for their disabled family members and keep them at home as long as possible. Often in doing so these families experience extreme financial costs and stress and place themselves at risk for experiencing health problems (OTA, 1987). Families usually opt for institutional care as a solution for dealing with their stress only after their personal resources for coping have become exhausted (Johnson and Johnson, 1983; Pallett, 1990; Zarit and Zarit, 1982).

When visiting in the home environment community health nurses should assess characteristics that place people at risk for requiring nursing home placement and should work with the client and family to explore other long-term care options. Adult day care programs, respite care, alternative family care homes, residential care facilities, and domiciliary care facilities are a few examples of such options.

Community health nurses play a crucial role in assessing the level of care needed by clients who require long-term care services. Reducing inappropriate use of nursing home beds by people who are capable of living at home—a "gatekeeping mechanism"—can save costly and scarce health care resources and can better meet clients' physical and emotional needs.

Community-Based Settings

Community-based and home care settings are becoming increasingly important sites for the provision of long-term and acute-care services. Escalating health care expenditures in the early 1980s provided the impetus for refocusing health care delivery patterns; outpatient ambulatory care and office settings now provide many services once performed only in the inpatient setting, and home health care is increasingly being used to reduce the length of hospital stays. As a result of these trends, a new subindustry—the walk-in clinic—for providing acute care has arisen, home health care is increasing at an estimated average annual rate of 20% to 25%, and new methods for financing and delivering long-term care have emerged (GAO, 1988; Waldo, Levit, and Lazenby, 1986).

There are a variety of formal community settings that provide long-term care services including, but not limited to, board and care facilities, continuing care retirement communities, social/health maintenance organizations, adult day care, community mental health and senior centers, outpatient facilities and clinics, sheltered workshops, and numerous voluntary organizations such as the Alzheimer's Disease and Related Disorders Association. However, the majority of the dependent disabled are cared for in their homes by informal caregivers (GAO, 1988; OTA, 1987). Formal community-based and home care services are usually used only when the informal care system breaks down or informal supports are not available (OTA), and to supplement the care of informal providers.

GOVERNMENTAL LONG-TERM CARE FINANCING

The Health Care Financing Administration (HCFA) is the primary source of funding for long-term services. The major portion of public expenditures for long-term care services goes to institutional care, with the Medicaid program being the principal payor for this type of care. The Medicaid program pays for over half of all nursing home expenditures. It supports long-term institutional care in a variety of facilities, including skilled nursing facilities (SNFs), intermediate care facilities (ICFs), intermediate care facilities for the mentally retarded (ICFs/MR), and mental hospitals. The Medicare program pays for skilled and complementing skilled (home health aide services) home health care services, and care in skilled nursing facilities during acute phases of illness. This program does not support long-term care in nursing homes and other facilities providing unskilled or custodial services (GAO, 1988).

Noninstitutional long-term care or home care is currently funded by four federal programs—Title XVIII (Medicare), Title XIX (Medicaid), and Title XX (block grants to states for social services) of the Social Security Act, and Title III of the Older Americans Act (O'Shaughnessy, Price, and Griffith, 1985, October 17, pp. XI-XII). The basic characteristics of each of these

programs were discussed in Chapter 4. The type of home care services financially supported by each program is presented below.

Medicare (Title XVIII)

The largest governmental expenditures for home health care services are made by Medicare. Medicare expenditures for home health care are increasing dramatically: between 1968 and 1985, Medicare spending for home health care had an annual growth rate of 24%. Medicare expenditures for home health care in 1968 were $60 million and in 1985 were $2.3 billion. It is anticipated that Medicare outlays for home health care will increase significantly because of the aging of the population (Waldo, Levit, and Lazenby, 1986, p. 11). It has been estimated that individuals 65 years of age and above receive 85% to 90% of the home health services provided in the United States (Cassak, 1984; Ginzberg, Balinsky, and Ostow, 1984).

Both Part A (hospital insurance) and Part B (supplemental medical insurance) of Medicare include provisions for home health care. Medicare reimburses a home health care agency for the following services (HCFA, 1989, Medicare program; HCFA, 1991):

- Part-time or *intermittent* skilled nursing services provided by or under the supervision of a registered nurse
- *Intermittent* physical, occupational, or speech therapy provided by or under the supervision of a qualified therapist
- *Intermittent* medical social services provided by or under the supervision of a qualified social worker
- *Intermittent* home health services provided by a home health aide who has completed a competency evaluation program and is supervised by a registered nurse who possesses a minimum of 2 years of nursing experience, at least 1 year of which must be in the provision of home health care, and who has supervised home health aide services for at least 6 months
- Medical supplies (other than drugs and medications) and the use of medical appliances
- Hospice services including short-term inpatient care, nursing care, therapy services, medical social services, home health aide services, physician services, and counseling.

Provisions of the Omnibus Budget Reconciliation

Act of 1980 (Public Law 96-499) expanded the home health benefits offered by Medicare so that beneficiaries are permitted unlimited home health visits without the requirement for a prior hospital stay or payment of a deductible amount. To qualify for those benefits, Medicare beneficiaries must be *homebound;* the services must be prescribed and periodically reviewed by a physician (at least once every 60 days); and the client must need part-time or *intermittent, skilled* nursing care and/or therapy services (physical, occupational, or speech therapy). When home health aide services are needed, the registered nurse, or appropriate professional staff member if only therapy services are provided, must make supervisory visits (refer to Table 20-4) to the client's residence on a regular basis (HCFA, 1991).

Landmark changes in the Medicare program have occurred as a result of a lawsuit brought against Medicare by the National Association for Home Care (NAHC) in the late 1980s. The suit contained two essential claims: (1) the challenge to the part time or intermittent policy for length of care allowed clients, and (2) how "medical necessity" is interpreted to qualify a client for care. The successful conclusion to the lawsuit did not change Medicare regulations but did change HCFA's interpretation of them, so that more services could be provided. Several of these changes are noteworthy (Staggers' Lawsuit, 1988, pp. 1-3):

1. Clients are considered homebound if they attend adult day care centers, renal dialysis clinics, or outpatient radiation or chemotherapy facilities when the purpose is to receive medical care. Regarding adult day care patients, it is the agency's responsibility to demonstrate that attendance at the day center is for the purpose of receiving medical care.
2. A new skilled service is described—skilled nursing management and evaluation of a patient care plan—that allows coverage for nurses who need to manage certain complex unskilled care cases.
3. Specific coverage standards are set out for venipuncture in stable and unstable patients. For example, a client receiving prothrombin whose blood test results indicate stability within the therapeutic range will qualify for a skilled nursing visit once a month to continue appropriate monitoring.
4. A client cannot be denied solely on the basis of having a chronic disease or terminal illness.
5. An order for "personal care" of a home health aide is allowed, with the boundaries of that personal care to be determined by the nurse following a care plan rather than by a physician.
6. Coverage of family counseling is specifically recognized as part of the function of a medical social services visit, in which family counseling is incidental to beneficiary counseling and designed to remove an impediment to the delivery of safe and effective care.

The *Medicare Home Health Agency Manual,* known as HIM 11 (HCFA, 1989), has been rewritten to address these changes. It contains many case examples clarifying coverage criteria and is useful on a daily basis for the staff nurse.

With its statutory emphases on part-time acute and postacute treatment of illness, the Medicare program does not adequately address the long-term care needs of the aging population (GAO, 1988). The homebound and the part-time or intermittent skilled nursing criteria for eligibility make it impossible for many chronically ill or disabled aging persons to qualify for Medicare home health care benefits. With public expenditures on health care rising dramatically, it is unlikely that the Medicare program will be expanded to cover additional long-term care services for the aged. Finding new approaches for meeting the long-term care needs of the elderly is a growing challenge for health care providers.

Managed health care systems are emerging as a way of financing home health care. Managed care controls, monitors, reviews, and directs health care in the most efficient manner and recommends the most appropriate treatment in the most efficient environment. The client's symptoms are usually controlled by the payor in a way that does not overuse the delivery system.

Managed systems include health maintenance organizations (HMOs) and preferred provider organizations (PPOs). Home health agencies have developed relationships with HMOs because the federal government has encouraged Medicare beneficiaries to join HMOs. Under a managed care system community health nurses have greater control placed on the delivery of home care services so that the care plan is well organized. Usually an assessment visit is authorized; following the nursing assessment, the plan of care is discussed with the system reviewer, who then gives authorization for care, usually 1 week at a time. The goal is cost containment and systematic allocation of resources (Daniels, 1988; McNiff, 1988; St. Armand, 1988).

Medicaid (Title XIX)

The current Medicaid statute provides states with the authority to include a variety of home and community-based services in their Medicaid programs. Medicaid programs can cover case management, personal care services, day care, private duty nursing, and home health services (GAO, 1988). Unlike the requirements of the Medicare program, home health under Medicaid includes *skilled* and *unskilled* services. To qualify for home care benefits under Medicaid clients must meet income eligibility requirements, have the services ordered by a physician, and have the plan of care reviewed by a physician every 60 days. Clients do not need to be homebound to receive Medicaid benefits.

Since Medicaid is a state-administered program, the range of home care benefits offered varies from state to state. However, in order to be federally subsidized under Medicaid, a state must provide at least home health services. Personal care services are not mandated by the federal government (Federal Register, 1985). States also have the freedom to determine eligibility requirements and the amount of service they will reimburse under Medicaid. Some states extend home care benefits to the "medically needy," those persons who do not qualify for regular Medicaid benefits but who have inadequate financial resources to meet health care costs.

Section 2176 of the Omnibus Budget Reconciliation Act of 1981 (Public Law 97-35) expanded the range of long-term services that can be offered by the Medicaid program; this act established the Medicaid Waiver Authority to implement 2176 Waiver programs of home- and community-based care. "Under these programs, states can provide a comprehensive array of medical and social services including case management, homemaker and home health aides, personal care, adult day care, habilitation care and respite care to avoid more costly institutional care" (U.S. Senate, Committee on Finance, 1984, p. 78). These programs serve individuals in the community who would require the level of care provided in a skilled nursing facility or intermediate care facility if they did not receive 2176 Waiver services. The costs of the community-based waiver services cannot exceed the cost of institutional care.

Although the major portion of public expenditures for long-term care for poor people is provided under the Medicaid program, many low-income persons still have unmet long-term care service needs. In some states home health agencies are finding it increasingly difficult to serve Medicaid clients, because they are often reimbursed for their services at a cost less than the true cost of providing the service. In other states eligibility requirements are restrictive and the range of services offered by the Medicaid program is inadequate. Such discrepancies can prevent a large number of people from receiving needed long-term care.

Social Services Block Grants to States (Title XX)

The Title XX program was established by the 1975 Amendments to the Social Security Act. The Omnibus Budget Reconciliation Act of 1981 (Public Law 97-35) altered Title XX, reformulating it as a federally funded Social Services Block Grant (Blancato, 1986). The Social Services Block Grant, like other block grants, provides the states freedom in determining the populations to be served and the types of services to be offered. The Social Services Block Grant program provides funding for a comprehensive array of social services directed toward the following goals (GAO, 1986, Community):

- Achieving or maintaining economic self-support to prevent, reduce, or eliminate financial dependency
- Achieving or maintaining self-sufficiency, including reduction or prevention of dependency for daily care
- Preventing or remedying neglect, abuse, or exploitation of children and adults unable to protect their own interests, or preserving, rehabilitating, or reuniting families
- Preventing or reducing inappropriate institutional care by providing for community-based care, home-based care, or other forms of less intensive care
- Securing referral or admission for institutional care when other forms of care are not appropriate, or providing services to individuals in institutions

A broad range of home-based services can be provided by the states under Title XX, including homemaker, home health aide, home management, personal care, consumer education, and financial counseling services. As with Medicaid, the benefits offered under this program vary from state to state. In order to qualify for Title XX services, clients must meet income eligibility requirements.

In order for states to participate in the Title XX program, they must establish a Comprehensive Annual Service Program plan that outlines the services they will provide, to whom, and by what methods. Federal spending under Title XX is capped, and funds are allocated among states on the basis of their populations. Social Services Block Grant funds aid states in meeting local needs not met by other social service agencies in the community (GAO, 1986, Community). However, the limited funding for this program does not allow states to expand home care services significantly.

Title III under the Older Americans Act of 1965

The Older Americans Act of 1965 established the Administration on Aging in the Department of Health, Education, and Welfare and authorized a variety of health and social services projects for aging citizens (refer to Chapter 5). In 1978 amendments to the Older Americans Act consolidated several existing titles (Titles III, V, and VII) of the original act and revised and expanded Title III. Title III is now designed to encourage and help state and local agencies to concentrate resources on developing a comprehensive and coordinated system to serve elderly citizens age 60 and over (House Select Committee on Aging, 1985).

Title III mandates a broad range of social services for the elderly, including but not limited to home health, home health aide, homemaker, and nutritional services. The only eligibility requirement for participation in the Title III program is that clients must be at least age 60. Unlike Medicare, clients do not need to be homebound and do not need skilled nursing care in order to qualify for home health benefits.

Title III is a state-administered program, carried out under the direction of the Department of Health and Human Services. Federal expenditures under Title III are capped. In fiscal 1985 appropriations for Title III totaled $785 million. Of these funds, $265 million were allocated for supportive services and $68 million for home-delivered nutrition services. A significant amount ($336 million) of these monies was also appropriated for congregate nutrition services. Recently emphasis has been placed on using OAA mon-

ies for home care and supportive services because of the increasing number of the oldest-old. These fragile elderly frequently find it difficult to use community-based services. Legislation allows states to transfer a percentage of their OAA allocation among funding categories and increasingly states are doing so in order to expand homecare services (Senate Special Committee on Aging, 1985). The 1987 Amendments to this act authorized nonmedical in-home services (e.g., in-home respite, telephone and visiting reassurance, and chore maintenance) for the *dependent* elderly (GAO, 1988, p. 287).

Displayed in Table 20-3 is a comparison of the essential characteristics of the four governmental funding programs just described.

Increasingly, federal and state governments are focusing attention on in-home services under all of their programs in order to reduce inappropriate, costly institutional care. As this shift occurs, emphasis is being placed on evaluating the cost effectiveness of community-based services. There is concern that increasing the numbers of people eligible for home care and liberalizing coverage of services would increase the overall national health bill (Rivlin and Wiener, 1988). The cost effectiveness of community alternatives to institutionalization has not yet been conclusively proved (U.S. Senate, Committee on Finance, 1984; GAO, 1988).

As this chapter is written, President Clinton's Health Security Act of 1993 is being presented to the country in preparation for debate regarding its merits and costs on Capitol Hill. The proposed legislation includes an increase in Medicare premiums for new prescription drug coverage, as well as a benefit that would help the elderly and disabled younger Americans with coverage for long-term care. The proposed program would help those qualifying to obtain services at home or in the community to avoid institutionalization. However, the costs of both of these programs is in the billions and there is doubt about their inclusion in the final legislation that will emerge.

LEGISLATION INFLUENCING LONG-TERM CARE SERVICE DELIVERY

In addition to the legislation that authorizes funding for long-term home care services, several other pieces of federal legislation influence long-term care service delivery. Some of this legislation is discussed in the following section.

TABLE 20-3 Comparison of Essential Characteristics of Four Governmental Programs Funding In-home Services

	Social Security Act			Older Americans Act
	Title XVIII	Title XIX	Title XX	Title III
Services Authorized				
Nursing	Yes	Yes	No	Yes
Therapy	Yes	Yes	No	Yes
Home health aide	Yes	Yes	Yes	Yes
Homemaker	No	No	Yes	Yes
Chore	No	No	Yes	Yes
Medical supplies and appliances	No	No	Yes	Yes
Program Eligibility				
Client must meet age requirement	Yes	No	No	Yes
Client must meet income requirement	No	Yes	Yes	No
Client must need part-time or intermittent skilled nursing care	Yes	No	No	No
Client must be homebound	Yes	No	No	No
Services to client must be authorized by a physician in accordance with a plan of care	Yes	Yes	No	No
Services must be included in state plan	*	Yes	Yes	Yes
Administration	Federal	State	State	State
Funding	Open ended	Open ended	Capped	Capped

*Federally administered program—no state plan required.

From General Accounting Office (GAO): *Improved knowledge base would be helpful in reaching policy decisions on providing long-term, in-home services for the elderly,* HRD-82-4, Washington, D.C., October 1981, U.S. Government Printing Office, p. 26.

Omnibus Budget Reconciliation Act (OBRA) of 1980

In December 1980 President Jimmy Carter signed into law the Omnibus Budget Reconciliation Act of 1980. Included in this law are provisions relating to home care benefits under Title XVIII (Medicare). The emphasis of the act was to encourage the use of noninstitutional services such as home health care to fight escalating health care costs.

The amendments relating to home health care were as follows:

1. Unlimited home health visits would be available under parts A and B of the Medicare program.
2. The existing 3-day prior hospitalization requirement for home health benefits under part A would be eliminated.
3. The $60 deductible, which home health benefits under part B are subject to, would be eliminated.
4. The need for occupational therapy would be added to the list of qualifying criteria for home health benefits.
5. The elimination of the requirement that proprietary (for-profit) home health agencies have state licenses to participate in the Medicare home health program.

OBRA legislation since 1980 has in some years contained amendments that expand or restrict long-term care services. For example, as discussed previously in this chapter, this legislation in 1981 created a Social Services Block Grant and 2176 Medicaid Waivers. The latest OBRA Act (OBRA-89) increased Medicare and Medicaid payments for hospice care but froze fees for durable medical equipment (DME) (NAHC,

1989, December). Omnibus Budget Reconciliation legislation needs to be monitored carefully by health professionals because amendments significantly influence the type of long-term care/services funded by the federal government.

Diagnostic-Related Groups

Another piece of legislation has significantly challenged the long-term care system. On April 20, 1983, President Reagan signed Public Law 98-12, which included the establishment of a prospective payment system (PPS) based on the 467 diagnostic related groups (DRGs) that allow pretreatment diagnosis billing categories for almost all hospitals reimbursed by Medicare. "Culminating a series of hospital billing and reimbursement reforms that were initiated decades ago, these changes will permanently alter the nature of health care delivery as we have known it" (Shaffer, 1983, p. 388).

The importance of prospective payment for hospital discharges is that health care providers are paid at rates that are set in advance and fixed for certain periods. Thus if a hospital treats a client for less than the amount fixed under the DRG, it can keep the profit; if it charges more, it must absorb the loss. Greater efficiency in client care becomes imperative; under the traditional system, the more a hospital spent, the more it was paid by Medicare.

DRGs have influenced hospital care in two ways: patients are experiencing much shorter hospital stays and they are being discharged sicker than before the advent of DRGs ("quicker and sicker"). These changes have influenced the complexity and quantity of community health nursing services; there are more requests for service and the requests are technically more complicated (Kornblatt and Fisher, 1985). Further, community health nurses are spending more time teaching the family to care for the ill members—families are learning to work with complex equipment such as morphine pumps, hyperalimentation lines, and Hickman catheters. Nurses with critical care and "high tech" skills are moving from the hospital setting to the home. Community-based nurses are updating their technical expertise and are learning to administer total parenteral nutrition, intravenous antibiotic therapy, intravenous chemotherapy, oxygen, and feeding tubes. Blood level testing for cholesterol, glucose, and clotting factors is also routine, as are blood pressure monitoring, apnea monitoring, cardiac pacing, rate and rhythm, and fetal monitoring.

One development that vividly demonstrates the growth of high technology in home care is pediatric home care, which is the fastest-growing segment of the home care field (Laxton, 1989). This growth is occurring because of a recent phenomenon in childbirth—infants born with the human immunodeficiency virus infection or anomalies requiring complex care. Another reason for growth is that home care is less costly than institutional care. Neonatology has made tremendous advances in the past few years, and babies who would have died are now living. Nationally there are about 2000 children whose respiratory function depends daily on the assistance of mechanical ventilators. Thousands more depend on parenteral nutrition, intravenous drugs, and other advanced devices. Helping parents deal with these issues on a daily basis has made unprecedented demands on both professionals and the lay public (Lidke 1989). Many children would remain in the hospital if pediatric home care services were not available. Thus pediatric home care is becoming a subspecialty in the home care field.

Prospective payment for home health services is "an idea whose time has come" (Lorenz and Meeker, 1992, p. 10). Since this system of payment became a reality for inpatient hospital services, Congress has been considering its extension to home health care agencies. Like DRGs in the hospital setting, prospective reimbursement means that an agency will know, before any services are given, how much it will be paid for them. The Health Care Financing Administration is currently studying two methods for prospective reimbursement: One is based on a per-visit payment unit and the other is based on a per-episode payment unit. Whatever unit is used, prospective payment will demand that agencies use the most effective methods possible to reach goals that are appropriate and desirable for clients and families.

Balanced Budget and Emergency Deficit Control Act of 1985 (Gramm-Rudman-Hollings Act)

Signed into law on December 12, 1985, this act mandated that the federal budget be balanced (have a $0 deficit) by 1991. To accomplish this goal, stipulations were established to reduce the federal deficit by a specified amount each year for a 6-year period beginning in 1986. The General Accounting Office (GAO) had the responsibility of analyzing federal spending to determine whether the deficit reduction targets could be met. If they could not be met, across-the-board reduction sufficient to bring the deficit in line with the targeted goal of the Gramm-Rudman-Hollings Act was to be made in domestic spending programs. Selected antipoverty programs (e.g., Medicaid and AFDC) were exempt from cuts, and health programs such as Medicare and Migrant Health Centers could be reduced by no more than 2% per year.

Although the U.S. Supreme Court declared the Gramm-Rudman-Hollings Act unconstitutional on July 7, 1986, members of Congress indicated at that time their intention to rectify the constitutional shortcomings of this act to achieve a balanced federal budget (Spiegel, 1987, p. 404). Gramm-Rudman-Hollings reduction is now addressed in the OBRA legislation. The 1989 OBRA contained reduction stipulations for part A and part B Medicare payments (NAHC, 1989). Achieving a balanced federal budget is necessary and long overdue. The federal deficit is creating a crisis. However, legislation that mandates across-the-board cuts, regardless of worth, is not a sound way to address this crisis.

BARRIERS TO ADEQUATE COMMUNITY-BASED LONG-TERM CARE

Various problems in the community and in the health care delivery system make it difficult for clients who have long-term care needs to avoid unnecessary institutionalization. These problems can be summarized under four categories: (1) lack of community resources, (2) acute-focused reimbursement mechanisms, (3) fragmentation and lack of coordination, and (4) family burnout.

Lack of Community Resources

A significant factor preventing many of the chronically disabled from obtaining adequate long-term care is the scarcity of formal alternatives to institutionalization (GAO, 1988; NCOA, 1986; OTA, 1987). After it is ascertained by caregivers and families that an individual cannot live at home without support or health care, staying in the community depends upon social supports, adequate financial resources, and the availability of health and social services.

Many older people, especially those older than 75, have characteristics that place them at risk for being institutionalized. Unfortunately, the very dependent elderly often find it difficult to obtain needed services in the home. Data from the 1982 National Long-Term Care Survey showed that 5% (168,000 aging persons) of the dependent elderly needed more help with ADLs and 34% (1.1 million persons) were not receiving the help they needed with IADLs (GAO, 1986, *Medicare*, p. 50).

The lack of adequate housing (and especially supportive congregate or domiciliary housing for people who live alone) for the frail elderly and disabled is a major barrier to community long-term care services. One problem with current housing arrangements is affordability: fuel prices, interest rates, and construction costs have all made housing costs difficult to manage on a limited income. Another problem is that households are becoming smaller; while rents are increasing, the number of people paying rent is decreasing as a result of increasing divorce rates and increasing numbers of aged and deinstitutionalized people living alone. In large cities single room occupancy (SRO) hotels, formerly a source of housing for many, are being converted into condominiums.

In some communities innovative housing programs sponsored by the Department of Housing and Urban Development have provided suitable alternatives to institutionalization. The National Housing Act, Section 202, provides a direct loan program based on the current securities marketed by the Treasury Department. The level of these interest rates makes housing projects attractive to builders; they are financially sound as well. Section 8 of the same act provides for direct subsidies to individuals who occupy Section 8 housing. The sponsors of such housing, usually non-profit organizations, receive full market rent. However, the federal government pays a portion of the rent.

Acute-Focused Reimbursement Mechanisms

Another barrier to effective long-term care is inadequate financial coverage for needed long-term care services. The Medicare program was specifically designed to provide protection for acute-care needs (Rivlin and Wiener, 1988). Once a client's condition becomes stable or once skilled services such as nursing, speech, or physical therapy are no longer needed, Medicare coverage for home health care ceases. Medicare specifically prohibits payment for custodial care. According to the Official *Medicare Manual,* "Care is considered custodial when it is for the purpose of meeting personal needs and could be provided by persons without professional skill or training; for example, help in walking, getting in and out of bed, bathing, eating, dressing, and taking medicine" (HCFA, 1989, October). These are precisely the functions needed by many clients with long-term care needs.

Other problems with Medicare home health benefits are that housekeeping and food services arrangements are not covered. One of the most serious problems is that services must be *intermittent* to be covered. For example, home health aides, in conjunction with other services and for a finite period of time, may work only a few hours a day, several days a week, and their hours may not exceed 32 per week. This type of care is often inadequate when a client needs help with activities of daily living on a constant basis.

Private insurance plans offer little or no coverage for long-term care. Most major medical insurance plans exclude nursing home or home health care or cover only private duty nursing in the home. In 1987 private insurance paid for only 1% of all nursing home costs and even a smaller fraction of home care (U.S. Bureau of the Census, 1992).

Medicaid, the assistance program for the very poor, does cover long-term care, but clients must deplete their own resources to qualify as "medically needy" in order to receive these funds. However, for persons who meet the eligibility requirements, the Medicaid program more effectively meets the long-term care needs of clients than does Medicare. Services do not have to be skilled (a client may have custodial needs met) and the services may be delivered by a person who has received some training for personal care services.

Medicaid expenditures for home care remain small (Rivlin and Wiener, 1988). Because Medicaid is a state-administered program, services vary considerably from state to state. In some states participation is limited in home and community-based services because these states view the services as (1) potentially costly and difficult to manage and (2) not permitting targeting of services to address the specific long-term care needs of the elderly (Justice, 1988, p. 121). States are unable to target specific population groups because Medicaid requirements mandate that all eligible recipients in the state must have access to available services developed with Medicaid financing (GAO, 1988, p. 27).

Fragmentation and Lack of Coordination

It has consistently been documented that fragmentation and lack of coordination in the long-term care system make it extremely difficult for clients to obtain needed long-term care services (OTA, 1987; Rivlin and Wiener, 1988). Consequently, a significant number of the noninstitutionalized population need but do not receive long-term care.

Existing formal long-term care services are provided by an array of state and local agencies that have differing eligibility requirements and finance mechanisms. Clients who have multifaceted needs frequently find it difficult, if not impossible, to identify the appropriate service provider. Most communities have no central organization or professional that assists the chronically impaired client in locating and coordinating needed long-term care services (Rivlin and Wiener, 1988).

Obtaining needed long-term care services often places unnecessary hardships on the client. It is not unusual for clients to have to make separate trips to several agencies in order to arrange a comprehensive package of services. An aged client, for example, may have to apply separately for Medicaid, Meals-on-Wheels, transportation services, Title XX homemaker services, and home nursing services.

Fragmentation and lack of coordination have left many gaps in the long-term care delivery systems. Thus unnecessary institutionalization among high-risk groups continues and the costs for long-term care services are rising dramatically. Efforts to develop comprehensive, coordinated systems for delivering community-based services must be expanded.

Family Burnout

An estimated 60% to 85% of all disabled or impaired people are helped by the family in a significant way. It has been demonstrated over the years that the family is the primary source of care for the frail elderly in the community (Callahan, Diamond, Giele, and Morris, 1980; Doty, 1986; Stone, Cafferata, and Sangl, 1987). Family caretakers play a pivotal role in helping chronically disabled family members to avoid institutionalization. Caring for impaired family members, however, can place a heavy and expensive burden on the family, especially when care is required for an extended period of time. Many chronically impaired persons have been placed in nursing homes because their families are unable to bear the emotional, physical, and financial strain of providing home care in the absence of support from community programs (Kane and Kane, 1987).

Currently only a few community resources provide temporary relief for family caregivers. Where community resources do exist, eligible families often lack adequate knowledge of long-term care options. In a caregiver survey conducted for the U.S. Congress Office of Technology Assessment (OTA), the majority of the respondents who listed respite care as "essential" either knew these services were not available or did not know whether they were available (OTA, 1987, p. 63).

In order for long-term care programs to be effective, the needs of family caregivers, as well as dependent family members, must be addressed. As discussed previously, caregivers of the dependent disabled need respite care, information about services, a broad array of community- and home-based health and social services, and knowledge about health conditions and care methods (OTA, 1987).

METHODS FOR IMPROVING THE LONG-TERM CARE SYSTEM

With population estimates that project dramatic increases in the over-75 age group and with health care costs expanding, it is obvious that the present system is not meeting and will not in the future meet the need for long-term care services. A number of methods for improving the system have been suggested, including:

1. Expansion of noninstitutional forms of long-term care while developing disincentives to construction of more institutional capacity
2. Emphasis on appropriate discharge planning
3. Effective gatekeeping and initial placement of clients assessed as appropriate for institutionalization
4. Targeting home care services to the people who need them the most

Discharge planning has been discussed in Chapter 10 and thus will not be expanded on here. It is important to remember, however, that chronically ill and disabled clients often need extensive discharge planning services.

Expansion of Noninstitutional Alternatives

A number of demonstration projects have been funded at the state and federal level to evaluate the appropriateness of expanding noninstitutional alternatives and decreasing capacity levels in institutional settings. In the state of New York, for example, the Nursing Home Without Walls program was initiated in 1978 to encourage noninstitutional alternatives as an appropriate cost-effective policy for long-term care of the elderly (Lombardi, 1987). Four components of the program included (1) intervention in the actual process of nursing home placement so that clients are exposed to home care before a nursing home placement decision is made, (2) cost containment with a limit set on the per capita cost of services, (3) case management of services so that social and medical services are integrated into the system, and (4) waivered services so that services not included in the Medicaid law, such as respiratory therapy and home improvement, can be offered to those needing them.

Another demonstration of the expansion of noninstitutional forms of long-term care is Enriched Housing (Nursing home without walls, 1982, p. 107). Enriched Housing serves that portion of the population who is able to live independently but needs some help with personal care, meal preparation, housekeeping, shopping, laundry, heavy cleaning, transportation, and 24-hour emergency coverage. The typical person entering this program does not have an informal support network to help him or her to live independently. The program differs from the Nursing Home Without Walls program in that the client must also need housing. In this program the person enters the housing secured by the program, usually a portion of a rent-subsidized building. Payment is generally through SSI.

Adult foster care is another mandated service in many states for people over 18 who are socially, mentally, or physically handicapped. Its purpose is to provide the opportunity for normal family and community life and help with problems. A foster home for adults is usually operated by individuals in their own homes and provides room, board, housekeeping, personal care, and supervision to four or fewer adults on a 24-hour basis. Those eligible for the program include people who receive AFDC (Aid to Families with Dependent Children) or SSI. Talmadge and Murphy (1983) found that both patients and their families can benefit from well-planned foster home placements.

Economical shared or sheltered housing for the elderly and disabled deserves greater effort. Improved federal funding of long-term care services should accompany efforts to use volunteer efforts on behalf of this population. One mutual aid scheme involving the exchange and banking of time in long-term care could be centered on congregate housing developments or similar concentrations of older citizens. These would ordinarily be built without adequate service supports. Residents could be admitted initially across a range of ages and disabilities. When able, they could be encouraged to help care for one another in a variety of ways. Those on waiting lists for apartments could be encouraged to help as well. In exchange, residents subsequently would receive aid from new and more able helpers. These exchanges are in existence today and can probably be increased in number and intensity by a mild effort to back them publicly. People who help others would be guaranteed help in return. If no one volunteered to provide that subsequent help, it would be financed publicly and delivered by paid workers. Time devoted to helping others would be backed hour for hour by the full faith and credit of the United States—probably the best form of currency since the silver certificate. In this way we could build faith in a currency of altruism (Sanger, 1983, p. 104).Adult day care centers are another noninstitutional alternative for people and families needing help. Day care centers provide assistance for adults who cannot be left alone during the day yet do not require 24-hour nursing care in an institution. A wide variety of services, including nutritious lunches, medical and social services, occupational, speech, and physical therapy, and health screening, are often available to clients. Those who profit from this kind of service are persons with Alzheimer's disease, the physically impaired with diagnoses such as arthritis or stroke, the mentally impaired, and the socially impaired or isolated individual. Candidates are evaluated in their homes before enrollment and the daily attendance fee is usually based on a sliding scale fee schedule.

Developing Effective Gatekeeping Mechanisms

Developing models, such as local area management organizations (LAMOs) and social–health maintenance organizations (S/HMOs), are another solution for dealing with the problems in the long-term care system (Ruchlin, Morris, and Eggert, 1982). Both are methods of financing and organizing health care for the elderly and are variations of the health maintenance organizations (HMOs) described in Chapter 5. Funding for LAMOs and S/HMOs comes from all public monies currently designated for short-term and

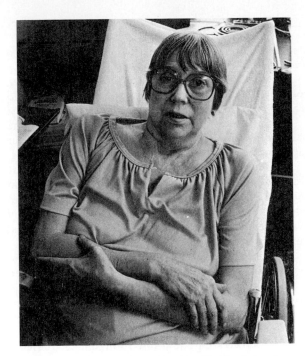

Figure 20-7 Jane Richards, who has lost both her legs to gangrene and circulation problems, lives at home rather than in a nursing home. (Anne Lennox/Times-Union.)

long-term medical care, rehabilitation, and custodial services. The LAMO enrolls all people with functional deficits and provides the services necessary to help them at home, utilizing informal supports whenever possible. The S/HMO enrolls all elderly people, anticipating that low use of services by the relatively well elderly compensates for extensive use by the vulnerable and severely ill. Both models function as gatekeepers into the long-term care system; case managers function as brokers for the services needed by the elderly population served, and they also certify the level of care needed. ACCESS in New York is a LAMO that has been successful in saving millions of dollars, primarily through the reduction of acute hospitalizations (Eggert and Brodows, 1982).

The story of ACCESS client Jane Richards (refer to Figure 20-7 and p. 808) made newspaper headlines when the public heard what the agency had to offer (Eisenberg, 1983).

When examining various ways for expanding noninstitutional long-term care alternatives, community health nurses must understand that although the demand for home care services is likely to grow, home health care does not necessarily ensure cost reduction.

A WOMAN IS RESCUED FROM A NURSING HOME

Henrietta homemaker Jane Richards lost a leg to gangrene in June 1978.

But Mrs. Richards, then a 63-year-old widow, convinced herself that life would go on, that she would learn to get around again through physical therapy.

By the time she had mastered solo trips to the bathroom, her circulation problem flared again. Four months after her first operation, she lost her other leg.

She recalls being devastated. Where would she go? How would she take care of herself? To whom could she turn? There seemed no good answers for a woman who was still relatively young, still lively, still involved in the world around her and yet trapped in a helpless, immobile body.

After she spent 10 months in the extended care facility of Genesee Hospital, a social worker suggested a possible answer: round-the-clock skilled nursing care at home, arranged by ACCESS, a federal demonstration project, run by Monroe County Long-Term Care Inc., an independent non-profit corporation.

ACCESS is testing the assumption that encouraging long-term care at home and in nursing homes will cut medical costs, relieve the backup of patients waiting to leave hospitals, and also provide more comfortable, humane medical care for the elderly, Executive Director, Gerald M. Eggert said.

Its goal is to help people who need long-term health care receive it in the least costly setting appropriate to their needs, he said.

Mrs. Richards believes ACCESS liberated her. After undergoing a battery of medical, financial and social evaluations arranged through the program, a caseworker found her an apartment accessible to a wheelchair-bound tenant, and supplied equipment, such as a hospital bed, trapeze and a specially designed wheelchair.

Bills were paid primarily through Medicaid, the government's health program for the poor.

Finally, in October 1979, after 1½ years in various medical institutions, Mrs. Richards went home. At first, she depended on help from around-the-clock aides. Two years later, that care was reduced to eight hours a day, four hours in the morning and four in the evening, where it remains today.

"I've been very pleased with what they've done for me," she said, chatting in her sun-drenched living room. "I'd recommend it to anybody. I'd have nothing left, no spirit if they put me in a nursing home. I would figure they had stuck me in a nursing home to die."

Until a few years ago, programs aimed at keeping the elderly and chronically disabled out of nursing homes were rare. If Mrs. Richards lost her legs a decade ago, chances are she would have spent the rest of her life in a nursing home.

Today, however, she is among hundreds of Monroe County residents who, despite serious disabilities and handicaps, live at home rather than in hospitals or nursing homes, and who stress the personal and economic advantages of that decision.

Since its 1977 start, ACCESS has received 19,558 referrals from families, physicians, community health nurses and agencies and hospital discharge staff members in Monroe County, said Belinda S. Brodows, deputy director.

ACCESS works like a broker, assessing patients' needs, arranging home health aides, social workers and other services through existing private agencies and conducting periodic follow-ups.

But its key feature is the authority to approve Medicaid and Medicare payments for long-term care services. Since November, the program has been authorized to approve Medicare benefits for 100 days of home health care and nursing home care without the usual requisite three-day hospital stay.

In the past, Eggert said, a major obstacle to encouraging long-term health care was the tilt in government health insurance programs toward acute-care coverage, which encouraged people to go to hospitals or nursing homes.

As a result of ACCESS, increasing numbers of chronically ill or disabled people in Monroe County are getting medical care and living at home: Between 1978 and 1982, the percentage of hospital patients referred to ACCESS—patients who were assessed as needing skilled nursing level care and who returned home—increased to 61 percent from 19 percent.

The percentages are higher for patients referred from the community: In 1978, 81 percent of the patients assessed at home stayed at home; the percentage rose to 96 percent in 1982.

At a time when rising health care costs and the burgeoning population of elderly are threatening Medicare's solvency, many doctors, geriatric specialists, and policy-makers believe programs like ACCESS may be the wave of the future.

From Eisenberg C: A woman is rescued from a nursing home, *Times-Union,* May 3, 1983, Rochester, NY, p. 8.

A study carried out by the Government Accounting Office (GAO, 1982) showed that when expanded home health care services were made available to those in need of long-term care services, client satisfaction improved. However, those services did not reduce nursing home, hospital, or total service costs. The study concluded that the focus of research should be on how to provide services most effectively and efficiently in various health care settings. Researchers in the study agreed that *targeting* services to people in the community in the most cost-effective manner was crucial. Simply expanding home health care to all those in need of long-term care was neither efficient nor cost-effective (Capitman, 1988).

Targeting Services

When they think of targeting long-term care services, community health nurses must know that a relatively small group of elderly are extremely high users of medical care. In Colorado, 0.5% of Medicare beneficiaries who were enrolled continuously for 4 years accounted for 57% of the acute hospital use, and 18% accounted for 88% of overall Medicare use (McCall and Wai, 1983). This pattern is part of a larger phenomenon known as Pareto's law that has been recognized in the business world for many years:

The fact that a small number of people account for a disproportionate share of activities is common knowledge among management experts. There is a basic phenomenon that is encountered in many human activities. It is couched in these general terms. In a given activity, only a few of the actors contribute to (account for) a major and disproportionate share of the action. This distribution is variously called the Pareto Law (after the noted Italian economist who recognized the universality of the phenomenon); the Lorenz curve (after an economist who applied it to distributions of family incomes); the A-B-C curve where the "A" items are the small number accounting for the major share of the activity while the "C" items, large in number, account for a small percentage of the activity, whereas the "B" items are intermediate; the 80-20 curve since 20% of the items accounting for 80% of the activity is a common distribution (Gavett, 1983).

Targeting needed services to the 20% of the long-term care population who use 80% of the resources is the key to effective and efficient use of services. The choice should not be between institutional and non-institutional care but between acceptable and unacceptable care. Hospice programs, for example, focus on helping families to care for ill family members by providing services that are most appropriate for each individual family.

HOSPICE CARE

Hospice is a humanistic approach to the care of the dying. One of the three main diagnoses of home care clients is cancer. This disease is a chronic one that requires services much more important than medical care. For the elderly, cancer often progresses slowly and thus leads to a longer period of home care than other diseases. Hospice presents a solution to many of the needs of this population group, as well as to clients across the life-span who are dealing with the difficulties associated with cancer.

The hospice concept is an approach to providing care for terminally ill clients and their families: it is a way of dying rather than a place where dying people receive care. It focuses on helping people to die with dignity and on assisting families with the grieving process. It emphasizes relieving psychological and physical distress.

The hospice movement developed from the work of Cicely Saunders, a physician from England. She founded St. Christopher's Hospice in 1960, which became a model for similar programs in the United States. In the early 1970s the first American hospice was organized in New Haven, Connecticut.

The development of the hospice movement in the United States is relatively recent, beginning only 25 years ago. However, the growing number of aging people as already discussed, the tremendous growth in medical technology that extends life, the growing awareness and fear of cancer, and the involvement of educated consumers who desire a voice in treatment have led to rapid growth in this movement in recent years. Further, cost containment has been another important issue since caring for the terminally ill in the cure-focused setting of a high-technology hospital is more expensive and less comfortable than the home setting. Since the inception of the movement the number of hospices has expanded significantly.

Hospice is a movement that emphasizes the following ideals (ANA, 1987):

- Help in dealing with emotional, spiritual, and medical problems
- Support for the entire family
- Keeping the patient in his or her home for as long as appropriate and making his or her re-

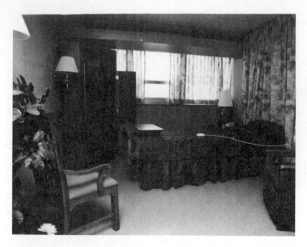

Figure 20-8 The homelike atmosphere of the inpatient hospice unit of Genesee Region Home Care complements the services provided by the home hospice program. (Used with permission of Genesee Region Home Care Association, Rochester, N.Y.)

maining life as comfortable and as meaningful as possible
• Centrally coordinated home care, inpatient, acute, and respite care, and bereavement services
• Professional services from a health care team supplemented by volunteer services, as appropriate to individual circumstances
• Relief of pain and other symptoms

Organizations providing hospice services vary, ranging from small homes run by church groups to hospitals or home health agencies. There are five models: the free-standing hospice, the hospital-affiliated free-standing hospice, the hospital-based hospice including either a centralized team or a specialized hospice team, the hospice within an extended care facility, and finally, home care programs that are hospital-, community-, or nursing-based (ANA, 1987). Figure 20-8 depicts the inpatient hospice unit of Genesee Region Home Care. It complements the home hospice program of this agency and provides terminally ill patients help with pain control, gives their families respite for short periods, and teaches families how to deal with the signs of terminal illness in the home setting.

Hospice programs that meet the standards of care developed by the National Hospice Organization are medically directed by a qualified physician and provide both inpatient and home-based care as needed. Care is provided by an interdisciplinary team 24 hours

a day, 7 days a week. Volunteers are an integral part of this team. The patient and his or her family are the central figures on the team, as well as the unit of service, and as such are actively involved in developing the management plan. Plans of care address pain and symptom management, psychosocial and spiritual difficulties, coping with dying, and bereavement. Support services for staff are an essential component of a hospice, as staff members must be able to deal with the grieving process first in order to assist the families.

Under Medicare, hospice is a comprehensive home care program that provides all the reasonable and necessary medical and support services for the management of a terminal illness. Medicare covers physician and nursing services, medical appliances and supplies, outpatient drugs for symptom management and pain relief, short-term respite care in an inpatient setting, home health aide and homemaker services, nutrition counseling, medical social services, physical and occupational therapy, and speech and language pathology services. Medicare clients receive hospice benefits when the physician certifies that they are terminally ill and when the client chooses hospice care for terminal care rather than standard Medicare benefits. Care must also be provided by a Medicare-certified hospice. At the end of this chapter is the story of one family's experience with hospice; it depicts the focus on the family, comfort in dying, and the interdisciplinary nature of hospice care.

In 1987 The American Nurses Association developed *Standards and Scope of Hospice Nursing Practice.* The section on standards includes the rationale for each standard and lists criteria for measuring achievement of the standard, with the criteria being divided into structure, process, and outcome components. Also included in the document is historical material on the development of hospice and the roles and responsibilities of hospice nurses. The standards of hospice nursing practice are presented in the box on p. 803.

THE ROLE OF THE COMMUNITY HEALTH NURSE IN LONG-TERM CARE

If current demographic trends continue, we will clearly be faced with increased numbers of people at advanced ages. The unknown variable will be the health of this group. If the health of this group in the future is not considerably different from the health of the present cohort, a huge proportion of

◀ *Standards of Hospice Nursing Practice* ▶

Standard I.   Organization of Hospice Services

The hospice program identifies and meets the needs of terminally ill clients and their families. The program is centrally administered by an executive officer who may be a nurse.

Standard II.   Interdisciplinary Collaboration

The nurse collaborates with other members of the hospice interdisciplinary team, including the client, family, physician, other nurses, social worker, volunteer, and clergy. The team is coordinated by a qualified health care professional from the discipline most appropriate in each case. The team meets regularly to develop and maintain an appropriate plan of care for the client and family.

Standard III.   Data Collection

The nurse systematically collects data that are comprehensive and accurate.

Standard IV.   Nursing Diagnosis

The nurse uses assessment data to determine nursing diagnoses.

Standard V.   Planning

The nurse participates in the development of the interdisciplinary team's plan of care for each client and family. The nurse's input into the plan is based on nursing diagnoses and is congruent with the hospice philosophy, hospice policies, interdisciplinary concepts, and an appreciation of the importance of the client's and family's participation in developing the plan.

Standard VI.   Intervention

The nurse, guided by the interdisciplinary care plan, provides effective nursing care to maximize the quality of the client's life by providing pain and symptom control measures and by facilitating the client's and family's progress toward the goals they set.

Standard VII.   Evaluation

The nurse continually evaluates the client's and family's responses to the interdisciplinary team's interventions.

Standard VIII.   Continuity of Care

The nurse, as a member of the interdisciplinary team, assures continuity of care for the terminally ill client and family.

Standard IX.   Ethics

The nurse uses the American Nurses Association's Code for Nurses and other appropriate resources, such as "Deciding to Forego Life-sustaining Treatment" as guides for ethical decision making in practice.

Standard X.   Theory

The nurse applies theoretical concepts as a basis for decisions in practice.

Standard XI.   Research

The nurse participates in research activities that contribute to the profession's continuing development of knowledge about hospice nursing care.

Standard XII.   Professional Development

The nurse participates in peer review and other means of evaluation to assure the quality of nursing practice. The nurse assumes responsibility for professional development and contributes to the professional growth of the interdisciplinary team members.

From American Nurses Association: *Standards and scope of hospice nursing practice,* Kansas City, Mo., 1987, The Association, pp. 3-15.

the population will be suffering from chronic diseases. Today, health-care resources are stretched to the point at which federal entitlement programs for the health care of the elderly have become a major political issue. Increased pressures on the limited resources of our society will require difficult decisions in terms of the quantity and quality of health care for older Americans. The only approach that can forestall these consequences of increased life expectancy is for substantial inroads to be made in the prevention, treatment, or management of the common chronic diseases of aging (Schneider and Brody, 1983, p. 855).

Nurses are increasing their involvement with this growing at-risk long-term care population and are becoming leaders in caring for people who have long-term needs. In fact, long-term care is very likely to become a key growth area for professional nursing (Reif and Estes, 1983, p. 149). Nurses already represent the largest number and percent of professional workers involved in long-term care; however, estimates suggest that there is a growing shortage of nurses in the areas of long-term care and gerontology.

There are seven areas on which community health nurses should focus to provide more adequate long-term care. These are prevention at all three levels among people across the life span, functional independence for clients rather than a cure, families' coping abilities, care management, interdisciplinary functioning, evaluation of services, and responsible public policy making.

Use Levels of Prevention

Throughout this text the concepts of disease prevention and health promotion have been stressed. The importance of these concepts cannot be overemphasized, especially when one examines the problems encountered by long-term care population groups. In order to decrease the number of people needing long-term care, it is essential to concentrate our efforts on the primary prevention of chronic problems.

Since the prepathogenesis period of disease (refer to Chapter 11) begins early in life, primary prevention and health promotion activities that address many problems encountered by chronically disabled persons and the aged must be introduced when working with young people. Health education programs that address such matters as lifestyle modification, stress management, and retirement planning, and counseling services that help individuals to develop a risk profile, are examples of such activities. Other examples are integrated throughout Chapters 14 through 19.

Community health nurses are uniquely able to apply the concepts of prevention as they work with clients who need long-term care. Primary, secondary, and tertiary preventive activities are commonly implemented by nurses who provide home health care services. Examples of primary prevention activities include accident prevention education and teaching about infection control. Helping a client with diabetes to learn how to self-administer insulin injections and to handle postsurgical wound care are examples of secondary prevention activities.

Tertiary prevention, continuing care and rehabilitation, is frequently carried out with people who need long-term care. These people often need help with physical, occupational, and/or speech therapy to return to or maintain their optimal level of functioning. The challenge facing the community health nurse at the tertiary level of prevention is how to maintain an ongoing working relationship with clients so that the care plan can be adjusted in response to the client's and family's changing circumstances and conditions. Strategies that community health nurses can use to help clients manage chronic diseases include medical record coauthoring, self-monitoring, educational support groups, family involvement, and telephone or postcard contact with clients. Excellent literature is available that describes how to use these strategies (American Hospital Association, 1982).

Help Families to Cope

The family is the primary support system for the elderly person residing in the community (U.S. Bureau of the Census, 1992). It has long been recognized that the family is also the primary resource in maintaining the aged in the community when chronic illness and functional decline begin to appear.

Approaches to develop long-term care services should first seek ways to buttress the family and its competence and capacity to cope with the increasing demands and strains, then augment the family resources with community services that permit the family to maintain its supportive involvement (Koff, 1982, p. 16).

Most aging people have some informal support systems that provide assistance with activities of daily living when necessary (Stone, Cafferata, and Sangl, 1987). Community health nurses should not, however, expect families and other informal supports to do the impossible—to provide care with no relief over long periods of time. Helping families to cope and not burn out is crucial. One way for informal supports to be strengthened is to provide for respite care, or time off, from caring for a chronically disabled family member. *Respite care* is a pioneering field in the United States, and unfortunately relatively few programs are available that clients can afford (Hildebrandt, 1983; Lawton, Brody, and Saperstein, 1989).

There is no one model for respite care. Some bring caregivers to clients, paying for aide service in the home. Others bring clients to hospitals and other facilities.

Respite care is a wise financial investment. Evidence shows that this type of care can delay nursing home admission, keep families together, and keep public expenditures at a minimum (Ellis and Wilson, 1983).

Helping families to find an affordable respite program, and helping a community to initiate a home or institutional respite program, are very significant community health nursing functions. The Omnibus Budget Reconciliation Act of 1981 allows Medicaid waivers for reimbursement of respite care if the cost is the same as or less than institutional care. Also, the Tax Equity and Fiscal Responsibility Act of 1982 includes a hospice benefit provision that allows money to be used for respite care if the client is terminally ill. OBRA legislation has been increasing these benefits since 1982.

Family members and other informal supports need to be nurtured. Supportive counseling helps families to deal with feelings of guilt and frustration that arise when caring for an ill family member. When they provide care for a chronically disabled person, community health nurses must focus attention on the needs of the family, as well as the client. Ignoring the family may result in the client not getting the assistance that he or she needs.

A review of the literature on the informal caregiver of clients in the home setting reveals four major areas of published information (Horning, 1991): characteristics of the informal caregiver, assessment of the client-caregiver dyad, education and support for the client-caregiver dyad, and caregiver stress. The author designed an inservice project for a visiting nurse association to prepare community health nurses to care for client-caregiver dyads: professionals concerned with this subject will find this an important resource.

The Pennsylvania Department of Aging has published *Caregivers Practical Help,* a manual for family caregivers of older Pennsylvanians. It is a readable and practical book that is free to families in the state. Area Agencies on Aging throughout the country publish similar articles of assistance for families.

Focus on Functional Independence

Clients with long-term care needs often have conditions that cannot be cured. The goal for their care is to help them to maintain quality in their lives and to continue to function at the highest possible level. With the cure orientation that pervades our health care system, this can be a difficult orientation for a community health nurse to develop and maintain. This orientation becomes easier to handle as one sees through practice that clients can live satisfying lives even when they have not been cured. The story of Jane Richards, discussed earlier in this chapter, is an example of a client who was not cured but yet is able to function independently and peacefully in the community. Community health nurses play a significant role in assisting clients to achieve greater functional independence.

The recently created National Eldercare Institute on Health Promotion can be a valuable resource for nurses who are assisting clients to achieve greater functional independence. The American Association of Retired Persons is the lead organization for the Institute; Meharry Medical College will focus efforts of the Institute on outreach to minority elders. The principal objectives and activities of this institute are presented in a box on p. 806.

Managed Care

Historically, care management has been an integral part of community health nursing practice. Renewed focus on this process has developed because dramatic changes in the health care delivery system have increased the complexity of client care issues and the need for increased community resources to address client needs. Care management is being advocated as a means to improve client access to health care resources and the effective and efficient use of these resources. As discussed earlier in this chapter, care management projects have emerged to address the needs of special population groups or aggregates such as the frail elderly and the mentally ill. Care management should be integrated into every nurse's practice. Most clients using long-term care services need assistance in dealing with the multiple resources required to meet their needs.

Care management is an essential component of comprehensive health care in all client settings. It is a problem-solving process that involves the assessment of the client's and family's total health care needs; coordination of resources and the delivery of health care services; and the continual monitoring of client and family progress (ANA, 1986). A major component of care management involves making decisions about which health care professional or community resource can best meet current client needs and what plan of care is the most appropriate to address these needs. Use of the nursing process (discussed in Chapter 9) and the referral process (discussed in Chapter 10) aids the community health nurse in making these decisions.

Use All Members of the Health Care Team

No one discipline can address the array of needs experienced by long-term care clients. The problems

◀ *National Eldercare Institute on Health Promotion* ▶

Principal Objectives of the Insitute Include:

- Serving as a knowledge base and program resource on health promotion, disease, and disability prevention for vulnerable older persons and their caregivers;
- Promoting the effective transfer, dissemination, and utilization of relevant information on health promotion to audiences across the continuum of care; and
- Providing training and technical assistance on health promotion and aging, focusing on agencies and organizations comprising the national, state, and community Eldercare coalitions.

Activities of the Institute Will Include:

- Linkages with other organizations and institutions

through task forces, for example, with federal agencies and researchers;
- A library and database to respond to written and phone inquiries;
- Outreach to elders-at-risk through the development of program guides, publications, and audiovisual materials;
- Publication of the Institute newsletter, *Perspectives in Health Promotion and Aging;*
- Development of resource lists on health promotion topics for older adults;
- Training and technical assistance to professionals in the fields of health promotion and aging; and
- National conferences on health promotion and aging.

From National Eldercare Institute on Health Promotion: *Perspectives in Health Promotion and Aging* 7(1), Washington, D.C., 1992, American Association of Retired Persons.

involved with long-term care demand that all members and levels of health care providers be involved. The community health nurse must be attuned to drawing on the health care team's sources whenever possible. Jane Richards' care plan, for example, used a physical therapist, an occupational therapist who carried out an assessment of the environment, a vendor of medical supplies and equipment who ordered materials including a wheelchair specifically prepared for her, a rehabilitation home economist who taught her to be self-sufficient in her kitchen, and a social worker who helped her to think through long-range plans and to find housing. In addition, she received daily ongoing personal care from a home health aide. Many of these people continue to be involved at intervals.

The community health nurse often functions as the coordinator of the health care team, an extremely important role which must not be neglected. The client can easily feel that care is fragmented if no one person has overall responsibility for complete care. Understanding the roles of each team member (refer to Table 20-4) can facilitate planning and coordination. The role definitions presented in Table 20-4 should be regarded only as a starting point for developing effective team relationships. When entering any new service agency, spend time with each member of the team to determine how they function.

The central figures on any long-term health care team must be the client and his or her family. In order to achieve the highest level of functioning possible for

the client, the client must be actively involved in establishing a plan of care appropriate to his or her needs. Engaging families in the therapeutic process is essential because often they have needs of their own that must be addressed. In addition, families are frequently participants in the rehabilitation process and provide continuing support for disabled family members after health care providers leave the home environment.

Evaluate Services

An integral part of working in any health care setting is evaluation. The evaluation process helps health care professionals to determine whether they are providing appropriate and quality services in an effective and efficient way. In this era of decreasing resources it is essential for community health professionals to monitor carefully how they use available resources. The needs of at-risk aggregates, such as those composing the long-term care population, can only be met if resources are allocated and used in a responsible manner.

Community health nurses at all levels must assume responsibility for evaluating the way in which nursing services are delivered. While nursing administrators have the overall task of seeing that evaluation is done, staff-level professionals must be accountable for assessing their own practice. They must also supervise the care they have delegated to others, such as home

20-4 Role Descriptions for Select Members of the Long-term Health Care Team*

Discipline	Role description
Community health nurse†	*An essential professional member of the health care team*—The professional nurse utilizes the nursing process to determine client needs, to establish a plan of care in conjunction with the client, to provide skilled nursing services, and to evaluate care delivered by the nursing team. Traditionally, the professional nurse has assumed a case management role on the health care team. As a care manager, the community health nurse focuses on determining the comprehensive needs of the client and the client's family, makes referrals to appropriate community resources as needed, and coordinates care among the multiple agencies providing services to a family.
Homemaker–health aide	*A paraprofessional who is trained to assist clients with personal care and light household tasks*—According to the Medicare conditions of participation for home health agencies, a home health aide's "duties include the performance of simple procedures as an extension of therapy services, personal care, ambulation and exercise, household services essential to health care at home, assistance with medications that are ordinarily self-administered, reporting changes in the patient's condition and needs, and completing appropriate records" (HCFA, 1989, October). Home health aides providing only personal care must be supervised by professional nurses via supervisory visits to the client's home at least every *2 weeks* if skilled nursing or therapy service is also needed by the client. If the client needs only custodial care, home health aide supervisory visits must be made once every 60 days (HCFA, July 1991).
Nutritionist	*A professional team member who assists clients in meeting their basic nutritional needs*—The nutritionist assesses a client's nutritional status, helps the client to plan an adequate and appropriate dietary intake, suggests ways to plan economical nutritious meals, helps clients to learn about therapeutic diets, and teaches about food purchasing and preparation. These professionals are often used as resource persons by other members of the health care team.
Physician	*A professional team member who is either a doctor of medicine or osteopathy*—The Medicare conditions of participation for home health agencies specify that the physician must establish and authorize the client's plan of treatment in writing and must review this treatment plan at least once *every 60 days* to determine if care is appropriate and necessary (HCFA, 1989, October). In addition to establishing a plan of treatment, the physician evaluates the client's medical status and provides medical care as needed. A physician also serves on a home health agency's professional advisory committee.

*The central figures on any long-term health care team must be the client and his or her family.
†In order to be certified for Medicare and Medicaid funding, a home health agency must provide nursing services.
From Health Care Financing Administration (HCFA): *Medicare program: home health agencies—conditions of participation and reductions in recordkeeping requirements,* 42 CFR, Part 484, Sections 484.1 through 484.52, Washington, D.C., 1989, U.S. Department of Health and Human Services; and Health Care Financing Administration: Medicare program: home health agencies-conditions of participation, 42 CFR, Part 484, *Federal Register* 56:32967-32975, 1991, July 18.

Continued

20-4   Role Descriptions for Select Members of the Long-term Health Care Team—
cont'd

Discipline	Role description
Social worker, medical	*A professional member of the home health care team who works with clients who are experiencing significant psychosocial, financial, or environmental difficulties*—Medical social workers apply the principles of social case work to help clients to enhance their emotional and social adjustment and to adapt to change. The primary purpose of their intervention is to reduce psychosocial, financial, and environmental barriers which are adversely affecting a client's health status or response to health care. Medical social workers provide direct counseling services, refer clients to community resources, assist clients in attaining needed social and health care services, and help plan for institutional community placements such as nursing home or extended-care facility placements. They also serve as resource persons for other members of the health care team who are dealing with difficult psychosocial, financial, or environmental problems.
Therapists, occupational	*Professional members of the team who work with clients that have difficulty carrying out activities of daily living*—After determining the self-care activities most important to the client, the occupational therapist assesses the environment to identify safety hazards and barriers to self-care, recommends environmental modifications which would help the client to increase independence and to prevent accidents, and assists the client in learning techniques, such as the use of simple eating and dressing devices which promote effective and efficient client functioning. The occupational therapist focuses on helping the client to improve motor coordination and muscle strength so that the client can reach his or her maximum level of functioning.
Therapists, physical	*Professional members of the team who work with clients who have functional impairments related to neuromuscular problems*—After assessing the client's functional abilities, phsyical therapists help clients to preserve, restore, and improve neuromuscular functioning and to increase their self-care capabilities. Physical therapists carry out a broad range of activities to help clients reach their maximum level of functioning. Performing needed range-of-motion, strengthening, and coordination exercises; recommending the use of appropriate orthopedic and prosthetic devices; and teaching clients ambulation techniques and how to use assistive appliances are a few examples of the activities performed by physical therapists.
Therapists, speech-language	*Professional members of the team who work with clients who have communication problems*—After assessing the client's speech, language, and hearing abilities, speech therapists concentrate on helping clients to increase their functional communication skills. Based on client needs, the speech therapist may initiate exercises to increase functional speaking skills, teach esophageal speech, recommend the use of communication appliances such as intraoral devices or hearing aids, identify barriers in the environment which inhibit effective communication, and teach significant others in the environment how to communicate with the client.

health aides and homemakers. When community health nurses delegate or assign tasks to others, they are responsible for seeing that these tasks are performed in an acceptable way.

A variety of direct and indirect measures are currently used by community health nurses to evaluate the delivery of nursing services, such as direct observation of care, case management conferences, annual performance evaluations, and record reviews. The Standards of Home Health Nursing Practice (ANA, 1986) referred to earlier in this chapter should guide the development of an evaluation plan that includes criteria for measuring quality and methods for assuring that care is consistent with professional standards (refer to Chapter 23). Requirements of reimbursement sources must also guide the development of evaluation measures. Community health nurses in home health agencies must, for example, fulfill the following evaluation requirements in order to receive Medicare reimbursement for health services provided by their agency (HCFA, 1989, Medicare program; HCFA, 1991):

- Conduct an overall evaluation of the agency's total program at least once a year to examine to what extent the agency's program is *appropriate, adequate, effective,* and *efficient*
- Establish a professional *advisory* group that includes at least one physician, one registered nurse, one member who is neither an owner nor an employee of the agency, and appropriate representatives of other professional disciplines, such as social work, physical therapy, and speech therapy, who are providing service for the agency; the group must meet frequently to advise agency staff on professional issues and to participate in overall agency evaluation
- Review with the patient's physician the appropriateness of the plan of treatment as often as the severity of the patient's condition requires but at *least once every 60 days.*
- Have the registered nurse, or appropriate professional staff member, if other services are provided, make a supervisory home health aide visit *at least every 2 weeks* if skilled nursing or therapy services are needed by the client or *once every 60 days* if only custodial care is needed
- Conduct a clinical record review on active and closed records *at least quarterly* to ensure that established policies are followed in providing services
- Employ only those home health aides who

have completed a competency evaluation program

Two types of record reviews are conducted in the home health setting: quality care audit and utilization review. During the *quality care audit* process, health care providers focus on appraising the quality of care received by clients using predetermined standards of care, as evidenced by documentation in the client's record (refer to Chapter 23). During a *utilization review* the client's records are assessed for the purposes of evaluating the appropriateness of the client's admissions and discharges; the appropriate and adequate use of personnel; and over- and underutilization of services (Koch and Fairly, 1993).

Staff-level community health nurses can play a very important role in all evaluation review procedures. Staff involvement in evaluation processes helps administrators to obtain a clearer picture about service delivery issues. As case managers, staff-level nurses are in a unique position to identify gaps in service and deficiencies of care.

Work toward Responsible Public Policy

Thus far in this chapter, ample evidence has been presented to demonstrate that public policy for long-term care in this country is inadequate. Carolyn Williams, a leader in community health nursing, writes:

It is important that nurses—particularly those who consider themselves community health nursing specialists—assign a high priority to participation in the formation of health policy and broader public policy (1983, p. 225) . . . primarily because this is a crucial modality for influencing the health of defined populations (p. 228).

Involvement in forming public policy can be at any one of a number of levels. These levels range from apathy and no participation to voting to holding public office. All levels require knowledge of the issues; community health nurses in long-term care possess this as an outcome of their experience.

Involvement in the political arena is both fun and professionally rewarding. Working with professional organizations such as the National Association for Home Care and the American Public Health Association is a good way to get started in the political arena. These organizations are making a concerted effort to analyze key health care issues and to promote strategies that may resolve some of the current health care delivery problems.

FACTORS INFLUENCING ETHICAL DECISION-MAKING IN THE HOME

A number of factors make an impact on the ethical dilemmas and decisions that caregivers in the home environment encounter. Since home health care is the most rapidly growing segment of the health care industry, nurses will continue to be more frequently challenged by the ethical dilemmas confronting them. Burger, Erlen, and Tesone (1992) discuss the five factors that influence ethical decisions:

1. *Time.* Home nurses visit the family and client on an intermittent basis and thus have to quickly assess and determine what has value and meaning to those involved and need to establish plans of care within the first few visits.
2. *Involvement.* Patients and caretakers are active partners in care and must assume responsibility for treatments when professionals are not present.
3. *Interdisciplinary communication.* The home setting presents limited opportunities for direct communication between professionals involved in the client's and family's care.
4. *Support system.* The accessibility, availability, and affordability of a caretaker affects options the client has. Without an appropriate caretaker there are few alternatives; financial constraints, time, and ability are other concerns.
5. *Ethics committee.* Ethics committees available in many hospitals are less available in the home setting and, thus, families, clients, and professionals can feel alone. It is recommended that home health care personnel be educated in ethical decision-making, that an ethicist be consulted to help both clients and professionals with these problems, and, finally, that counselors be available to assist caregivers with stress management.

Increasingly, state home health organizations are focusing on developing guidelines to facilitate ethical decision-making in practice. The ANA Center for Ethics and Human Rights also assists practitioners and administrators in dealing with ethical issues encountered in the clinical setting. This center can be reached by phone at 202-554-4444, ext. 293 or 294.

Summary

Increasing numbers of people across the life span have long-term care needs that must be addressed by local communities throughout our nation. Elderly persons, who constitute the most rapidly growing population group in America, are particularly at risk for needing long-term care services. Although most elderly people experience good health, certain chronic, disabling illnesses do increase with aging.

The fastest-growing component of the United States health care delivery system is long-term care. Diverse and multiple social, health-related, and health care organizations deliver a variety of long-term care services to people in need. Despite the dramatic growth in the long-term care industry, many chronically disabled persons still do not receive the services they need. Developing strategies to eliminate barriers to adequate community-based, long-term care must receive greater attention by health care providers in this decade. There is no question that the aging of the American population will increase the need for long-term care services in the future.

Long-term care presents challenges and opportunities for the community health nurse. Developing solutions to overcome the deficiencies and to fill the gaps in the long-term care system will require major policy changes at all three levels of government. However, community health nurses at all levels of practice can be instrumental in effecting change in the health care delivery system. Innovative projects that more adequately address the needs of at-risk long-term care populations are beginning to emerge across the country.

◀ *An Exercise in Critical Thinking* ▶

The story in Appendix 20-1 recounts how three different families have coped with terminal illnesses using the hospice program (Fine, 1990, Section I). Think about how the goals of nursing care differ for these people as compared to a well-baby or school population. What interventions does the community health nurse in a hospice setting use as compared to those used in a well-baby clinic? How do you evaluate the importance of interdisciplinary functioning in the hospice setting? Would you consider having a career in hospice nursing? Discuss why you would or would not become a hospice nurse.

APPENDIX 20-1

—————————————————— HOME AS HOSPICE ——————————————————

The Terminally Ill Can Find Help for Themselves and Their Family

Once she accepted the truth, once her options were gone, Peg Johnson looked at the finite future—too short, too soon—and chose to face it at home. There, in her brave, new world, she took some small measure of control over what remained of her life in the ever-present shadow of death.

Johnson, dwarfed by the corduroy lounge chair in which she sat, spoke about her choice one recent afternoon. As she sat, pale and thin, feet elevated, the bulge of her belly prominent beneath a pale blue coverlet, she seemed at ease. Her spirit seemed strong.

"So far," she said. "I'm not saying that I'm going to be this way always. But I believe in God, and I think that helps."

Linda Trout helps, too. A nurse, she is the coordinator of the hospice program at Taylor Hospital in Ridley Park; Johnson has been a patient at the hospital on and off since she was diagnosed with colon cancer two years ago. Trout visits Johnson at her home in Prospect Park to treat, to advise, to talk, to listen.

In a sense, hospice is an old story made new.

"In the first part of the century, most people died at home," said Andrew Parker of the National Hospice Organization (NHO). "There was caring, there was comfort, there were people around. And then we moved into an era where most people die in a hospital . . . isolated and abandoned."

The recent hospice movement, begun in England in the 1960s, is a coordinated program of care—medical, psychological, social and spiritual—for the terminally ill and their families. Although hospice care sometimes is delivered in a separate facility, often it permits people to live, and die, in their own homes, cared for by their own families, surrounded by their own things. Since the first hospice opened in this country—in 1974, in Connecticut—the movement has expanded steadily to the present 1,700 hospices nationwide.

"Hospice makes two promises," Parker said. "You won't die alone, and you won't die in pain. And it delivers."

•

It was a terrible year, 1989.

In January, Helen Margaret Johnson, known as Peg—67 years old, mother of a grown son and daughter, widow for 13 years—underwent colostomy surgery. In April, she had heart surgery, a valve replacement. Chronic lymphocytic leukemia, diagnosed in 1982, remained a complication.

With all that, she carried on: "And I was doing pretty good, but they told me in the beginning that the cancer had spilled over to the pelvic area. I must have resigned myself, because nothing has been that difficult."

Her hospice care began on Oct. 3.

Hospice generally means several things: that the patient has six months or less to live, that treatment is often palliative or centered on pain control, and that family members assume much of the care. It isn't for everyone, said Toni McClay, who runs Taylor's program: Some families simply cannot accept that a patient is beyond the point where recovery is possible.

That was not the case with Johnson. She has made her funeral arrangements, paid for her casket. Even so, she has not entirely given up: "I have friends of many faiths praying for me. Methodist. Presbyterian. Baptist. Episcopalian." A smile, wry and brief, crosses her lips. "It can't hurt."

On one visit, midafternoon on a Thursday, the affection between nurse and patient was evident. Trout bent to kiss Johnson's cheek, then sat down to talk with her and her daughter, Cathy Giarrusso, 44, who was visiting from Georgia. Two or three times a week, Trout, 37, makes house calls to Johnson, each visit lasting an hour or more. A social worker comes about twice a month, Johnson said, and the conversations "get some of the miseries off your mind." Taylor's three dozen hospice volunteers, who work with the staff of five nurses, make themselves available as needed.

Half an hour of breezy chitchat passed before Trout segued gracefully from social topics to medical ones.

"How's your appetite?" she asked gently.

"Not terrific," Johnson replied.

Persistent, painful sores in Johnson's mouth and throat had improved, but drinking citrus juices—once her favorite, now too acidic—still hurt. Trout recommended a "homemade mouthwash" of Epsom salts and peroxide.

Trout knelt at Johnson's side, took her blood pressure, dressed the site of a small skin cancer, inquired about her weight. (About 114, Johnson said, "but most of that is tumor.") Giarrusso reported her mother's temperature to be 99.3.

Johnson's forthrightness about her illness, her approaching death, had surprised Giarrusso. Such openness once was uncharacteristic of her mother, she said, but she is grateful for it—"It's easier to deal with someone who knows they're dying, rather than you know and they don't"—and thinks she knows its source.

Her mother, trying to protect her, had been evasive about her father's condition before his death in 1976. "So when I came here," Giarrusso recalled, "it was not quality time I had with him. He was in a coma and died three days after I got here."

This time, she and her mother have said what they wanted and needed to say to each other. During a visit in June, they even chose the casket together. Her brother, David—who lives in Philadelphia with his own family but stays with his mother one or two nights a week—found funeral-planning morbid and excluded himself from it.

According to Parker of the NHO, hospice care helps families get through the grieving process—partly by counseling and partly by their involvement in a family member's care.

"There's healing (of grief) going on when you're serving a loved one," Parker said. Most hospices also operate bereavement programs for the surviving family members, he said, because "loss is something that our culture doesn't deal with well."

Peg Johnson chose hospice care for the comfort of being at home, where she can set her own schedule for eating and sleeping, sitting up and lying down.

When her doctor suggested the hospice program, she was initially hesitant. "At the time, I thought it was a little soon," she said, "but it wasn't. You always think it's too soon."

•

Not every patient wants to know as much as Peg Johnson knows.

Anna Mills is one who doesn't.

Sunlight filters through the lace curtains of her living room and onto the hospital bed where she lies beneath a crocheted comforter. A large yellow cat named Mikey is asleep beside her.

Mills is chatty, smiling, uncomplaining and, at 85, dying of breast cancer. Since June, Linda Trout has been visiting the two-story brick twin that Mills shares with her daughter, Ann Bevan, and her niece, Anna Mae Happersett.

The house is homey and welcoming, overflowing with a lifetime's collection of dolls—"My babies," Mills calls them—baby dolls with china hands, fashion dolls in elaborate gowns, a Princess Di bought in the Bahamas.

Twice a week, Trout is greeted at the Ridley Park home like family. When Mills speaks of "my girls," the words encompass Ann and Anna Mae and Trout. As much as possible, Trout makes the visit appear to be a social call. When Mills admires the cameo brooch at Trout's throat, she and Trout discuss a shared love of antiques.

Trout is fond of the women, admiring of their closeness, respectful of Mills' choices.

"She is not aware of her diagnosis," Trout said, although the hospice worker suspects that Mills really knows the truth. "She has chosen not to recognize it," Trout said. "She thinks she's sick because she fell three years ago, and she thinks the pain she is having is from that."

Mills' evasion of the truth is explained by family history, Happersett said: "She's seen her husband go (from cancer). And she won't take needles . . . she's seen them give him needles constantly and torture him." Such avoidance can make home care a challenge—Mills will not enter the hospital, wear a catheter, accept injections—for both hospice workers and family members.

But denial is not uncommon, hospice workers agree. Most, however, say that their mission is to make patients and families as comfortable as possible, not to force them to confront unhappy truths.

"We respect people's right to be who they are, to have their own defenses," said Karen Neyer, 39, a hospice social worker at Lankenau Hospital on the Main Line. "We do not impose our standards on other people. We use the language they use. As we form a relationship, if there's a space to challenge, to open doors, we knock on them."

For Linda Trout, triumph meant finding a long-acting morphine pill that seems to be controlling the pain in Anna Mills' right leg, a result of her disease spreading to the bone.

In the kitchen, out of earshot, Trout calls Bevan at work to discuss the possibility of catheterizing Mills for bladder control, to spare her daughter and niece having to change absorbent bed pads numerous times a day.

"But, of course, if it causes her mental anguish, it's no good," Trout said into the telephone. "Whatever is best for her."

Bevan has agreed to discuss the matter with her mother, however, and Trout packs her carryall to depart. She bends to kiss Mills and straighten her yellow-flowered sheets. Mills beams.

"I love her," she said of Trout. "I love my girls."

Outside, in her car, Linda Trout reflects on the emotional nature of nursing patients who will all die.

"It's OK for me to cry," she said quietly. "And I do. It's a relationship for me that's gone. I get in my car and cry."

She began studying nursing only seven years ago and, then, only because her husband was diagnosed with leukemia. She wanted to learn how to care for him. At some point, however, it became her calling, her profession, and after his death, she found herself drawn to the terminally ill. This has remained true, even though she has since remarried.

"Disease has been here since the dinosaurs, and I can't change that," she said. "But if I can make it better . . . I don't think anyone should live in pain. Or die in pain."

She said that her work had changed her in subtle ways. "Probably, I live one day at a time now," she said. "And my friendships and family are more cherished."

●

For the Rev. Wesley K. Meixell, minister and widower, it is all over now, except for the memories—and the continuing support of the hospice program at Taylor Hospital.

His wife, Lorna, died on Oct. 22, 1988, after 35 years of marriage. The final seven months were a tumultuous time filled with fear and hope, pain and despair.

Lorna Meixell, an advertising artist at Franklin Mills, began suffering dizziness, weakness and loss of peripheral vision early in 1988. On March 23, she learned why: The diagnosis was glioblastoma, a rare and fatal brain tumor.

"The doctor told me no one survives that unless it's a miracle," Meixell recalled. He is pastor of Norwood United Methodist Church—and he put his faith in a miracle.

It was not to be. His wife's deterioration was gradual but steady. He remembered all the parishio-ners he had visited in hospitals over the years and their wishes to be at home. Right after Labor Day, his wife began receiving hospice care.

"She just felt better, being at home," he said. The hospice team was "very compassionate, very caring, all of them."

It began with a home-health aide, two hours a day, five days a week. By the end, a nurse was taking care of her eight hours a day. The Meixells' combined insurance paid for it all, 100 percent, he said. Most hospice care—65 to 70 percent—is covered by Medicare, the rest by private insurance or Medicaid; many hospice programs absorb the cost for uninsured patients.

"We do not turn anyone away," said Taylor's Toni McClay.

And after a patient's death, hospices do not abandon the survivors. Meixell still attends a monthly bereavement support group, most of whose members also lost spouses and understand the truth of Meixell's painfully learned knowledge: "Even if you're prepared for (death), it's still very hard to accept."

During his wife's illness, at the time of her death and afterward, the hospice team offered comfort and support, he said; "When she died, in those months—and even now—they said, 'If you're having trouble dealing with the loss, call us. Any time. Twenty-four hours a day.'"

From Fine MJ: Home as hospice: the terminally ill can find help for themselves and their families, *The Philadelphia Inquirer,* Section I, 1990, January 28, 1990, p. 6.

References

Administration of Home Health Nursing: care of the sick by health departments, *Public Health Nurs* 37:339-342, 1945.

Aging America: trends and projections—1987-88 ed, Washington, D.C., 1987, U.S. Special Committee on Aging.

American Association of Retired Persons (AARP): *A profile of older Americans: 1993,* Washington, D.C., 1993, The Association.

American Hospital Association: *Strategies to promote self-management of chronic disease,* Chicago, 1982, The Association.

American Nurses Association: *Standards of home health nursing practice,* Kansas City, Mo., 1986, The Association.

American Nurses Association: *Standards and scope of hospice nursing practice,* Kansas City, Mo., 1987, The Association.

American Nurses Association: *A statement on the scope of home health nursing practice,* Kansas City, Mo., 1992, The Association.

Bedside nursing care by official agencies, *Public Health Nurs* 37:333-334, 1945.

Belk J: Federal policy and disabled people, *Caring* 6(8):6-9, 52-54, 1987.

Berk ML and Bernstein A: Use of home health services: some findings from the National Medical Care Expenditure Survey, *Home Health Care Serv Q* 6(1):13-23, 1985.

Blancato R: The Older American Act as a vehicle, *Pride Institute J Special Issue,* 29-32, 1986.

Buckwalter KC, Abraham IL, and Neuendorger MM: Alzheimer's disease: involving nursing in the development and implementation of health care for patients and families, *Nurs Clin North Am* 23(1):1-9, 1988.

Buhler-Wilkerson K: Home care the American way: an historical analysis, *Home Health Care Service Quarterly,* 12(3):5-17, 1991.

Burger AM, Erlen JA, and Tesone L: Factors influencing ethical decision-making in the home setting, *Home Healthcare Nurse* 10(2):16-2-, March-April 1992.

Burke TR: Long-term care: the public role and private initiatives, *Health Care Financ Rev,* 1988 Annual Suppl, pp. 1-5, December 1988.

Burns EM and Buckwalter KC: Pathophysiology and etiology of Alzheimer's disease, *Nurs Clin North Am* 23(1):11-29, 1988.

Callahan JJ, Diamond LD, Giele JZ, and Morris R: Responsibilities of families for their severly disabled elders, *Health Care Financ Rev* 1:29-49, 1980.

Capitman JA: Case management for long-term and acute medical care, *Health Care Financ Rev,* 1988 Annual Suppl, pp. 53-56, 1988.

Cassak D: Hospitals in home health care: an industry in transition, *Health Industry Today* 47(7):16-28, 1984.

Commonwealth Fund Commission on Elderly People Living Alone: *Old, alone and poor: a plan for reducing poverty among elderly people living alone,* Baltimore, Md, 1987, The Commission.

Congressional Budget Office, Budget Issue Paper: *Long-term care for the elderly disabled,* Washington, DC, February, 1977, U.S. Congress.

Congressional Budget Office, Technical Analysis Paper: *Long-term care actuarial cost-estimates,* Washington, D.C., 1977, U.S. Congress.

Daniels K: Will nurses control care at home? *Home Healthcare Nurse* 6(2):18-23, 1988.

Deimling GT and Bass DM: Symptoms of mental impairment among elderly adults and their effects on family caregivers, *J Gerontol* 41:779-784, 1986.

Doty P: Family care of the elderly: the role of public policy, *Milbank Q,* 64:34-75, 1986.

Eagles JM, Beattie JAG, Blackwood GW, Restall DB, and Ashcroft GW: The mental health of elderly couples: 1. The effects of a cognitively impaired spouse, *Brit J Psychiat* 180:299-303, 1987.

Eggert G and Brodows B: The access process: assuring quality in long-term care, *Quality Rev Bull* 8(2):10-15, 1982.

Eisenberg C: A woman is rescued from a nursing home, *Times Union,* May 3, 1983, Rochester, NY, p. 8.

Ellis V and Wilson D: Respite care in the nursing home unit of a veteran's hospital, *Am J Nurs* 83(10):1433-1434, 1983.

Federal Register: Medicaid program: home and community-based services, *Final Rule* 50(49):10013-10028, March 1985.

Fine MJ: Home as hospice: the terminally ill can find help for themselves and their families, *The Philadelphia Inquirer,* Section I, January 28, 1990.

Fitting M, Rabins P, Lucas MJ, and Eastham J: Caregivers for dementia patients: a comparison of husband and wives, *Gerontologist* 26:248-252, 1986.

Fowles D: The changing older population, *Aging* 339:6-11, 1983.

Fulton JP, Katz S, Jack SS, and Hendershot GE: *Physical functioning of the aged, 1984,* Series 10: Data from the National Health Survey, No 167, DHHS Pub No (PHS) 89-1595, Hyattsville, Md., USDHHS, March 1989.

Gavett J: *Hospital experimental program high cost patient study,* Rochester, N.Y., 1983, University of Rochester School of Management, unpublished study.

General Accounting Office (GAO): *Improved knowledge base would be helpful in reaching policy decisions on providing long-term, in-home services for the elderly,* HRD-82-4, Washington, D.C., October 1981, U.S. Government Printing Office.

GAO: *The elderly should benefit from expanded home health care but increasing these services will not insure cost reductions,* Washington, D.C., December 1982, U.S. Government Printing Office.

GAO: *Medicaid and nursing home care: cost increases and the need for services are creating problems for the states and the elderly* (GAO IPE-84-1), Washington, D.C., October 1983, U.S. Government Printing Office.

GAO: *Community services: block grant helps address local social service needs,* Pub No HRD 86-91, Washington, D.C., May 1986, U.S. Government Printing Office.

GAO: *Medicare: need to strengthen home health care payment controls and address unmet needs,* Pub No HRD-87-9, Washington, D.C., December 1986, U.S. Government Printing Office.

GAO: *Long-term care for the elderly: issues of need, access and cost,* Washington, D.C., November 1988, U.S. Government Printing Office.

GAO—Report to the Chairman, Subcommittee on Health and Long-Term Care, Select Committee on Aging, House of Representatives: *Medicare: rationale for higher payments for hospital-based home health agencies,* Washington, D.C., 1992, U.S. Government Printing Office.

George J: Heat's on the home health-care business, *Philadelphia Business Journal,* October 7-13, pp. 29-30, 1992.

George LK and Gwyther LP: Caregiver well-being: a multidimensional examination of family caregivers of demented adults, *Gerontologist* 26:253-259, 1986.

Getzen TE: Longlife insurance: a prototype for funding long-term care, *Health Care Financ Rev* 10(2):47-55, 1988.

Ginzberg E, Balinsky W, and Ostow M: *Home health care: its role in the changing health services market,* Totowa, N.J., 1984, Rowman and Allanheld.

Haley WE, Levine EG, Brown SL, Berry JM, and Hughes GH: Psychological, social, and health consequences of caring for a relative with senile dementia, *J Am Geriat Soc* 35:405-411, 1987.

Harris JP: High tech is a boost to home health care, *Special Advertising Section: Health Care Career Forum, Philadelphia Inquirer,* September 16, 1992, p. 15.

Haupt AC: Forty years of teamwork in public health nursing, *Am J Nurs* 1:53, 1953.

Health Care Financing Administration (HCFA): *Medicare home health agency manual, HIM 11,* Washington, D.C., 1989, USDHHS.

HCFA: *Medicare program: home health agencies—conditions of participation and reductions in recordkeeping requirements,* 42 CFR, Part 484, Sections 484.1 through 484.52, Washington, D.C., October 1989, USDHHS.

HCFA: Medicare program: home health agencies—conditions of participation, 42CFR, Part 484, *Federal Register* 56:32967-32975, 1991, July 18.

Hildebrandt ED: Respite care in the home, *Am J Nurs* 83(10):1428-1430, 1983.

Hing E: Use of nursing home by the elderly: preliminary data from the 1985 national Nursing Home Survey, *Advance Data from Vital and Health Statistics* No. 142, USDHHS Pub No(PHS) 87-1250, Hyattsville, Md., 1987, Public Health Service.

Hirsh L, Klein M, and Marlowe G: *Combining public health nursing agencies: a case study in Philadelphia,* New York, 1967, Department of PHN, NLN.

Horning JC: Support and education for the caregiver and client in the home: an inservice project for community health nurses, *J Commun Health Nursing* 8(3):155-161, 1991.

House Select Committee on Aging: *Building a long-term policy: home care data and implications,* Pub. No. 98-484, Washington, D.C., 1985, U.S. Government Printing Office.

Hughes SL: Apples and oranges? A review of evaluations of community-based long-term care, *Health Serv Res* 20:460-488, 1985.

Johnson CL and Johnson FA: A micro-analysis of "senility": the response of the family and the health professionals, *Culture Medicine Psychiat* 7:77-96, 1983.

Justice D: *State long-term care reform: development of community care systems in six states,* Washington, D.C., April 1988, National Governors Association.

Kane RA: The noblest experiment of them all: learning from the national channeling evaluation, *Health Serv Res* 23:189-198, 1988.

Kane R and Kane R: *Long-term care: principles, programs, and policies,* New York, 1987, Springer.

Kemper P, Applebaum R, and Harrigan M: Community care demonstrations: what have we learned? *Health Care Financ Rev* 8:87-100, 1987.

Koch MW and Fairly TM: *Integrated quality management: the key to improving nursing care quality,* St. Louis, 1993, Mosby.

Koff T: *Long-term care: an approach to serving the frail elderly,* Boston, 1982, Little, Brown.

Kohlman GF, Wilson HS, Hutchinson SA, and Wallhagen M: Alzheimer's disease and family caregiving: critical synthesis of the literature and research agenda, *Nurs Res* 40(6):331-337, 1991.

Kornblatt E and Fisher M: The impact of DRGs on home health nursing, *Quality Rev Bull* 11(10):290-294, 1985.

Kraus LE and Stoddard S: *Chartbook on disability in the United States, an InfoUse report,* Washington, D.C., 1989, National Institute on Disability and Rehabilitation Research.

Lawton MP, Brody EM, and Saperstein AR: A controlled study of respite service for caregivers of Alzheimer's patients, *Gerontologist* 29(1):8-16, 1989.

Laxton CE: Editorial introduction, *Caring* 8(5):2, 1989.

Lerman D: *Home care: positioning the hospital for the future,* Chicago, 1987, American Hospital Publishing.

Letsch SW, Levit KR, and Waldo DR: National health expenditures, 1987, *Health Care Financ Rev* 10(2):109-122, 1988.

Lidke K: Technology-dependent children: addressing problems that arise from success, *Advance,* Fall 1989, Ann Arbor, University of Michigan Medical Center, pp. 2-15.

Liu K, Manton K, and Liu BM: Home care expenses for noninstitutionalized elderly with ADL and IADL limitations, *Health Care Financ Rev* 7(2):52, 1986.

Lombardi T: Nursing home without walls, *Caring* 6(5):4-9, 1987.

Lorenz BR and Meeker AB: Prospective payment: an idea whose time has come, *Caring* 10-13, July 1992.

May DS, Kelly JJ, Mendlein JM, and Garbe PL: Surveillance of major causes of hospitalization among the elderly in 1988, *MMWR* 40(SS-1):7-21, 1991.

McAllister JC: Controversial issues in home health care: a roundtable discussion, *Am J Hosp Pharm* 43:933-946, April 1986.

McCall N and Wai H: An analysis of the use of medical services by the continuously enrolled aged, *Med Care* 21(6):1983.

McNiff ML: Impact of managed care systems on home health agencies, *Home Health Nurs* 6(2):10-13, 1988.

National Association for Home Care (NAHC): *Home care and hospice provisions contained in the Omnibus Budget Reconciliation Act of 1989,* HR3299 Special Rep No 341a, Washington, D.C., December 1989, The Association, pp. 1-3.

National Council on Aging (NCOA): Public policy agenda 1986-1987, *Perspect Aging* 15(2):1-64, The Council, 1986.

National Eldercare Institute on Health Promotion: *Perspectives in health promotion and aging* 7(1), Washington, D.C., 1992, American Association of Retired Persons.

Naylor R: *Christian living,* March-April 1983, p. 21.

Nursing home without walls: its progress and future—summary of proceedings of meeting, Albany, NY, June 22-23, 1982, New York State Senate Health Committee.

Office of Technology Assessment (OTA): *Losing a million minds: confronting the tragedy of Alzheimer's disease and other dementias,* Washington, D.C., 1987, U.S. Government Printing Office.

Oktay J and Palley H: Home health and in-home service programs for the chronically limited elderly: some equity and adequacy limitations, *Home Health Care Serv Q* 2(4):5-28, 1981.

Oktay JS and Volland PJ: Foster home care for the frail elderly as an alternative to nursing home care: an experimental evaluation, *Am J Public Health* 77(12):1505-1510, 1987.

Olson HH: Home health nursing, *Caring* 5(8):53-61, 1986.

O'Shaughnessy C, Price R, and Griffith J: *Financing and delivery of long-term services for the elderly,* Pub No 85-1033, Washington, D.C., October 17, 1985, Congressional Research Service, Library of Congress.

Pallett PJ: A conceptual framework for studying family caregiver burden in Alzheimer's type dementia, *Image: J Nurs Schol* 22(1):52-58, 1990.

Parsick J and Triebsch HC, eds: *J Home Health Care Practice* 3(4):1-80, August 1991.

Pennsylvania Department of Aging: *Caregivers practical help,* 231 State Street, Harrisburg, Penn., 17101, The Department.

Pitzele SK: *We are not alone: learning to live with chronic illness,* New York, 1986, Workman.

President's Commission on Mental Health: *Task panel reports submitted to the President's Commission on Mental Health, vol III,* Washington, D.C., 1978, U.S. Government Printing Office.

Prochazka Z, Henschke P, Skinner E, and Last P: *Memory loss and confusion: dementia, a guide for caring people,* Adelaide, Aust., 1983, Health Promotion Services, South Australian Health Commission.

Pruchno RA and Resch NL: Husbands and wives as caregivers: antecedents of depression and burden, *Gerontologist* 29:159-165, 1989.

Reif L and Estes C: Long-term care: new opportunities for professional nursing. In Aiken L, ed: *Nursing in the 1980s: crises, opportunities and challenges,* Philadelphia, 1983, Lippincott.

Rivlin AM and Wiener JM: *Caring for the disabled elderly,* Washington, D.C., 1988, Brookings Institution.

Robert Wood Johnson Foundation: *Annual report 1983,* New York, 1984, The Foundation.

Robert Wood Johnson Foundation: *Challenges in health care: a chartbook perspective 1991,* Princeton, N.J., 1991, The Foundation.

Ross C, Danzinger S, and Smolensky E: The level and trend in poverty in the United States, 1939-1979, *Demography* 24, 1987.

Ruchlin H, Morris J, and Eggert G: Management and financing of long-term care services, *New Engl J Med* 306:101-106, 1982.

Sanger AD: *Planning home care with the elderly—patient, family, and professional views of an alternative to institutionalization,* Cambridge, Mass., 1983, Ballinger.

Scanlon WJ: A perspective on long-term care for the elderly, *Health Care Financ Rev,* 1988 Annual Suppl, December 1988, pp. 7-15.

Schneider EL and Brody JA: Sounding board: aging, natural death, and the compression of morbidity—another view, *New Engl J Med* 309:854-856, 1983.

Sekscenski ES: Discharged from nursing homes: preliminary data from the 1985 National Nursing Home Survey, *Advance Data from Vital and Health Statistics,* No 142, USDHHS Pub No (PHS) 87-1250, Hyattsville, Md., 1987, Public Health Service.

Senate Special Committee on Aging: *Developments in aging: 1984,* vol 1, Report 99-5, Washington, D.C., February 1985, U.S. Government Printing Office.

Shaffer FA: DRGs: history and overview, *Nurs Health Care* 4:388-396, 1983.

Soldo B: The elderly home care population: national prevalence rates, selected characteristics, and alternative sources of assistance, *Working Paper* 1466-29, Washington, D.C., 1983, Urban Institute.

Spiegel AD: *Home health care,* ed 2, Owings Mills, Md., 1987, Rynd Communications.

St. Armand L: Managed care: fitting pieces of the puzzle together, *Home Health Nurse* 6(2):14-17, 1988.

Staggers' Lawsuit: *Part II, NAHC Report,* No 275, Washington, D.C., August 12, 1988, National Association for Home Care, pp. 1-3.

Stone R, Cafferata GL, and Sangl J: *Caregivers of the frail elderly: a national profile,* Washington, D.C., 1987, U.S. Government Printing Office.

Stone RI: The feminization of poverty among the elderly, *Women's Stud Q* 17(1,2):20-34, 1989.

Talmadge H and Murphy D: Innovative home care program offers appropriate alternative for elderly, *Hosp Progr* 50-51, 72, 1983.

U.S. Bureau of the Census: *Population profile of the United States: 1989,* Current Population Rep, Series P-23, No 159, Washington, D.C., 1989, U.S. Government Printing Office.

U.S. Bureau of the Census: *Sixty-five plus in America,* Current population reports, Special studies, pp. 23-178, Washington, D.C., 1992, U.S. Government Printing Office.

U.S. Bureau of the Census: *Population profile of the United States: 1993,* Current population reports, series P23-185, Washington, D.C., 1993, U.S. Government Printing Office.

USDHHS, Public Health Service: *Promoting health/preventing disease: year 2000 objectives for the nation, draft for public review and comment,* Washington, D.C., September 1989, U.S. Government Printing Office.

U.S. Senate, Committee on Finance: *Long-term health care: hearing before the subcommittee on health of the committee on finance,* United States Senate, ninety-eighth Congress, Washington, D.C., 1984, U.S. Government Printing Office.

Visiting Nurse Service of Toledo—eighty-three years of caring, *Caring* 3:57-61, 1984.

Waldo DR, Levit KR, and Lazenby H: National health expenditures, 1985, *Health Care Financ Rev* 8(1):1-22, 1986.

Warhola C: *Planning for home health services: a resource handbook,* Department of Health and Human Services, DHHS Pub No HRA 80-14017, Washington, D.C., 1980, U.S. Government Printing Office.

Weissert WG, Cready CM, and Pawelak JE: The past and future of home- and community-based long-term care, *Milbank Q* 66:309-390, 1988.

Weissman MM: Advances in psychiatric epidemiology: rates and risks for major depression, *Am J Public Health* 77(4):445-451, 1987.

Williams CA: Making things happen: community health nursing and the policy arena, *Nurs Outlook* 31:225-228, 1983.

Zarit SH, Todd PA, and Zarit JM: Subjective burden of husbands and wives as caregivers: a longitudinal study, *Gerontologist* 26:260-266, 1986.

Zarit SH and Zarit JM: Families under stress: interventions for caregivers of senile dementia patients, *Psychother Theory Res Practice* 19:461-471, 1982.

Zawadski RJ and Eng C: Case management in capitated long-term care, *Health Care Financ,* 1988 Annual Suppl, pp. 75-82.

Selected Bibliography

Brechling BG and Kuhn D: A specialized hospice for dementia patients and their families, *Am J Hospice Care* 6(3):27-30, 1989.

Dush D: Trends in hospice research and psychosocial palliative care, *Hospice J* 3(4):13-28, 1988.

Hollingsworth C: *Clinical procedure manual for home health care,* ed 2, Baltimore, Md., 1990, Williams & Wilkins.

Home health and hospice manual: regulations and guidelines, Owings Mills, Md., 1988, National Health Publishing.

Jones ML: *Home care for the chronically ill child,* New York, 1985, Springer.

Kalnins I: Home health agency preferences for staff nurse qualifications, and practices in hiring and orientation, *Public Health Nurs* 6(2):55-61, 1988.

Keating SB and Kelman GB: *Home health care nursing concepts and practice,* Philadelphia, 1988, Lippincott.

McNeil JM: Americans with disabilities: 1991-1992, U.S. Bureau of the Census, Current population reports, P 70-33, Washington, D.C., 1993, U.S. Government Printing Office.

Pasquale DK: Characteristics of Medicare-eligible home care clients, *Public Health Nurs* 5(3):129-134, 1988.

Pawling-Kaplan M and O'Connor P: Hospice care for minorities: an analysis of a hospital-based inner city palliative care service, *Am J Hospice Care* 6(4):13-21, 1989.

Ryan MA: Education and service collaboration in hospice, *Am J Hospice Care* 6(6):23, 1989.

Shamansky SL, ed: Home health care, *Nurs Clin North Am* 23(2):1988.

Shuster GF and Cloonan PA: Home health nursing care: a comparison of not-for-profit and for-profit agencies, *Home Health Care Services Q* 12:23-36, 1991.

Stiller SB: Success and difficulty in high tech home care, *Public Health Nurs* 5(2):68-75, 1988.

Turner-Henson A, Holaday B, and Swan JH: When parenting becomes caregiving: caring for the chronically ill child, *Fam Community Health* 15:19-30, 1992.

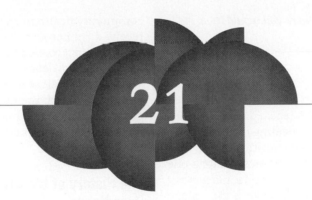

21

Aggregate-Focused Interventions: Group Work, Clinics, and Nursing Centers

---

OBJECTIVES

Upon completion of this chapter, the reader should be able to:

1. Discuss the advantages and disadvantages of using the group approach to promote the health of population groups.
2. Describe six ways that groups can meet health needs of clients.
3. Discuss how a group is formed and the functions of the community health nurse as a group leader.
4. Summarize the phases in the life of a group.
5. Discuss how developments in society have contributed to the development of clinic and ambulatory care services.
6. Explain how community health nurses establish and maintain clinic services.
7. Describe the role of the community health nurse in the clinic setting.
8. Define the term *nursing center*.
9. Describe the services offered by a nursing center.
10. Describe parish nursing and block nursing.

In every enterprise consider where you would come out.

PUBLIUS SYRUS

"There are many ways to skin a cat" is one way of saying that a goal can be reached by numerous routes. This axiom applies to meeting the health care needs of people in community health nursing. The nurse who visits people in their homes is taking one route. As discussed in Chapters 14 and 19, nurses visit parents of newborns to help them with the unique tasks that accompany parenthood and visit aging people to help them with changing developmental tasks. Other routes, explained in Chapters 15 and 17, are the school nursing role and the occupational health nursing role.

In this chapter three more methods of meeting people's health care needs are presented: group work, clinic services, and nursing centers. These methods can be used by nurses to provide primary, secondary, and tertiary preventive services to groups and aggregates so that they achieve their maximum level of functioning. The methods focus on groups of people rather than on the nurse-to-family approach used in home visits. Clients come to the nurse rather than the nurse serving the family members in their own personal environment.

GROUP WORK IN COMMUNITY HEALTH NURSING

Community health nurses have long worked with groups of people to meet health care needs effectively. In this context *group* is defined as a gathering of people who are together for a specific reason. An example of the use of group work in community health nursing practice is a parent effectiveness training class. Parents in this situation come together to discuss ways to rear children effectively. A gathering of people at a bus stop does not meet the definition of a group.

Community health nursing agencies frequently use the group intervention strategy. Community health nurses focus on delivering services to populations in census tracts and on caseloads rather than on individual clients only. Thus needs common to an area are more readily apparent, particularly if caseload analyses and a community assessment are done. One community health nurse realized that she continually received numerous referrals from the intermediate school district to visit families with children who had developmental delays, and that many of these families were clustered close together. To help meet the needs of these families, the nurse formed a parent support group to serve the many primary and secondary health needs of this population.

The History of the Group Approach to Health Care Needs

Kurt Lewin is generally considered to be the founder of modern group process. His research during World War II was aimed at increasing work production and changing food consumption patterns. Lewin found that group discussion and decision helped people to change their ideas much more effectively than lectures or even individual instruction (Lewin, 1947). Giving people information alone did not motivate them to change personal attitudes and behavior. Rather, discussion in groups helped persons to become involved, conceptualize ideas, and take health action. Group participants learned something about their own behavior in group settings, and the information gained was relevant to their personal lives.

Another development in the group approach to health was *group psychotherapy.* It became a part of the treatment plan of psychologists and psychiatrists in the 1920s and 1930s, but it was not until the 1960s that group process and group psychotherapy came together (Loomis, 1979, p. 5). During the decade of the 1960s the *encounter group* movement proliferated, and the differences between sensitivity groups and psychotherapy groups blurred. It was realized that everyone, not just "sick" people, could benefit from group process.

The terms *group process, group dynamics,* and *group interaction* all refer to the way groups work and provide methods to assess and observe group functioning. Groups are formed for a variety of psychological, social, and educational purposes such as losing weight, controlling drug usage and smoking, and giving support during divorce and death. Nurses are part of a group on the health team and in professional associations, in choirs, parent-teacher organizations, League of Women Voters, and synagogues. Clearly group work is an integral part of life in the United States today.

Advantages and Disadvantages of the Group Approach

The definition of community health nursing states that promoting and preserving the health of populations is its goal. Thus, nurses are constantly viewing ways of helping people to look critically at their own health behavior.

Telling people about healthy behavior is not enough—the low immunization levels of preschool children discussed in Chapter 14 is verification of that statement. There must be a way of helping people to value preventive health practices so that they will change their health behavior. Lewin's work, among that of many others, gives evidence that groups can help to accomplish this. A major reason for using the group approach is that different kinds of people with similar concerns can work on these concerns together. Feelings of isolation and aloneness that are so often a part of crisis can be worked through. "I'm not the only one who feels this way, and that's a relief" becomes a frequent comment.

It must be emphasized that the group approach will not meet all clients' health needs. Some people will never feel secure enough to leave their own familiar surroundings, to find transportation, to have the needed energy and skill, or even want to become part of a group. There are people who lack the social expertise, experience, and motivation required to become involved in a group. This behavior can be learned, but it requires patience and skill on the part of the nurse to teach it. An overwhelmed 17-year-old single mother with two children under 2 years of age who has exhibited poor bonding behaviors with her newborn probably needs an intense one-to-one relationship with a nurse before she can profit from a group discussion about parenting.

Nurses gain valuable information about a family when they see individual family members interacting in their own surroundings. A data base on the family system as discussed in Chapter 7 is very difficult to collect when the client is a member of a larger group. Situations that warrant a family-centered nursing approach are best handled in the home environment.

Some people like to function in groups; others do not. These differences need to be respected because an individual's attitude and beliefs regarding the group experience will have an effect on group learning and outcomes.

Luft (1970, p. 30), in his classic writings on group process, summarized the advantages of group versus individual productivity and problem-solving:

1. There are definite advantages and disadvantages to group versus individual problem-solving and productivity.
2. When a problem demands a single overall insight or an original set of decisions, an individual approach may be best.
3. Problems calling for a wide variety of skills and information or the cross-checking of facts and ideas seem to call for a group approach. Feedback and free exchange of thinking may stimulate ideas that would not have emerged by solo effort.
4. If goals are shared, then there is greater likelihood for cooperative effort; when the group goal is not shared by members, morale and productivity may suffer. Consequently, when the goal is decided upon by group discussion and participation, there is greater likelihood of full member involvement.
5. The greater the group members' desire for individual prominence and distinction, the lower will be their friendly sharing or group morale.
6. When members decide on the need for group effort, the smaller the size of the group the better it will function, provided that the necessary diversity of skills and group maintenance resources are present.
7. A group may be a source of strong interpersonal stimulation; a group will also generate its own conformity pressures. In order to decide between group and individual work, these two sets of forces (stimulating and binding) should be kept in mind.
8. A society that places highest value on the worth and freedom of the individual also encourages the strongest independent thought, independent work, and independent responsibility. An inherent goal of a sound group in such a society is the reaffirmation of true independence while meeting group needs concerning tasks and morale.

How Community Health Nurses Use the Group Approach

Loomis (1979, pp. 3-11) has discussed six ways that groups can be used to meet the biopsychosocial health needs of clients: support, task accomplishment, socialization, learning–behavior change, human relations training, and psychotherapy–insight and behavior change.

Support. This text focuses on the developmental needs of clients throughout the life cycle. Many people are healthy, but during periods of rapid development and change they need help to manage the maturational and situational crises that can occur. La Leche League groups, classes of expectant parents, and widow-to-widow programs come under this category. Primary prevention of problems is the thrust of support groups because they help those participating to develop healthy methods of dealing with potentially difficult situations.

Because of limited resources, a recognition of the value of support group interaction, and the complex nature of current health problems, community health nurses are increasingly initiating support groups for at-risk clients and/or their families. Support groups are established in a variety of settings including schools, clinics, industries, neighborhood centers, and other community facilities. They are developed for multiple purposes, such as to promote self-esteem among elderly clients (Janosik and Miller, 1982); to help role-reversal couples to adjust to changes in their lifestyles (Moch, 1988); to assist families in dealing with the burden of caregiving (Schmitt, 1982; Watson, 1987); and to help families deal with grief (Demi, 1984). The support group intervention strategy can be a cost-effective and efficient way to meet the needs of at-risk groups. Community health nurses who guide these types of group experiences find them to be rewarding and meaningful.

Task Accomplishment. Large complex tasks need more than one person to carry them out. The interdisciplinary team of a health department that includes nurses, physicians, environmentalists, nutritionists, and physical therapists is one example of how meeting the health care needs of people is accomplished by a group.

Clients in a group can help each other to accomplish goals as well. One large senior citizen's center uses retired volunteer physicians, nurses, and laypersons to carry out monthly health screening. The workers are needed and *feel* needed, and the clients screened feel that they are helped "by people who understand them."

On a larger scale, community action groups or coalitions have been developed to address major health problems in society. One significant example of this type of group is the national Healthy Mothers, Healthy Babies Coalition, which has affiliated coalitions in the majority of the states. This coalition is a cooperative venture of 80 national voluntary, health professional, and governmental organizations established to accomplish the specific task or goal of improving maternal and infant health through education (Arkin, 1986). Public health leaders believe that coalition-building is essential in order to deal with the public health needs evident in our nation (Institute of Medicine, 1988). Community action groups are being developed on national, state, and local levels and are becoming powerful in influencing health care delivery issues. These groups are involved in areas such as fund-raising for innovation health planning activities, informing the public about major health problems, and influencing public policy by developing relationships with legislators and other public officials. All of these are important activities for community health nurses and enhance the effectiveness of clinical practice.

Socialization. Situational and maturational crises such as death, divorce, and retirement can produce pain and isolation. Parents Without Partners, Welcome Wagon Clubs, and senior citizens' activity clubs provide fellowship for those experiencing common needs. As with support groups, clients can learn to develop new ways of dealing with crises through socialization.

Learning–Behavior Change. Having a new colostomy and coping with a new diagnosis of diabetes or leukemia are situational crises common to the community health nurse. Clients must learn completely new methods of functioning and living with irrigations, diet, and approaching death. Groups composed of clients with common problems provide support in addition to teaching new methods of coping. Ostomy clubs, Weight Watchers, and Parents Anonymous are examples of learning–behavior change groups.

Group learning–behavior change sessions should be carefully planned and related to the purpose of the group experience. The community health nurse may focus on providing information unknown to group participants, such as when the nurse is working with a group of expectant parents who want to learn about labor and delivery processes. At other times the community health nurse focuses on the facilitator role, especially when group members are learning how to cope with changes in their lifestyle.

When establishing a learning–behavior change group, it is essential for the nurse to obtain baseline data about what is already known by the group, as well as the interests and needs of individual group members. This data base can help the nurse to select appropriate content, educational materials, and educational strategies.

Major functions of community health nurses are health education and problem-solving with groups and with individuals. Current practice trends emphasize group intervention when appropriate, to reach the greatest number while containing costs. Community health nurses make significant contributions to public health through group work. Research has demonstrated that group health educational experiences can effect changes in health-related knowledge, practices, and attitudes (Centers for Disease Control and Prevention, 1986).

Human Relations Training. The National Training Laboratory (now the NTL Institute for Applied Behavior Science) was established in Maine in 1947 to look at informal experimental methods of teaching group process (Luft, 1970, p. 4). It was designed as a 3-week workshop for professional people who wanted to deal more effectively with coworkers. T-groups or skills-training groups grew from the NTL. The subsequent encounter group movement was another later outgrowth. The purpose of these human relations groups is education. Such groups usually meet for a specific number of hours with the purpose of learning cognitively and affectively about human relations. Assertiveness training, body workshops, emotive therapy, and sexuality workshops are all kinds of human relations training groups. They have grown rapidly and their effectiveness depends greatly upon the skills of the leader. Before community health nurses refer clients to them or attend them, they should investigate the quality and preparations of the leader.

Psychotherapy–Insight and Behavior Change. Therapy groups are conducted to treat clients, usually people who are discontented and want to change something about their lives. Such groups are usually led by people with graduate degrees in nursing, medicine, or psychology. This group classification is different from the other five because it focuses on the goal-directed alteration of how the client relates to himself and others in an overall way. Psychotherapy may include

altering specific behaviors or learning new ways of relating to other people, but it also includes specific assistance with how one feels about oneself (Loomis, 1979, p. 11). Staff-level community health nurses usually do not conduct these types of groups. If clients need psychotherapy, they are referred by the community health nurse to a mental health specialist.

Developing a Group

Before nurses think about using the group approach to meeting health needs, they must be familiar with the policies of their employing agency. Some agencies will not permit nurses to form groups under their auspices. Others will actively support group efforts if they are compatible with agency philosophy and resources. The nurse must also know whether or not her or his workload can support the added responsibility of group work. This can be ascertained by discussion with the nurse supervisor. Chapter 22 deals more fully with this aspect of the nurse's role, that is, dealing with caseload management issues.

Since community health nurses work with populations such as a county, a city, or a township, common needs that can be met by a group may be expressed by clients, staff nurses, or others (for example, school officials). If the client and the nurse are so inclined, almost any health need can be met by the group process except those for which clients need one-to-one relationships (Loomis, 1979, p. 19). The very young single mother referred to earlier is a client whose needs may not be met by the group process. Frequently it can be useful to combine group and individual intervention strategies. For example, one nurse had a family in her caseload that included a child with spina bifida and resultant paraplegia. The nurse visited the home to assess family functioning and the environment, as well as to help the mother with the child's daily routine. The nurse also referred the parents to a parent group at the intermediate school, where they received support from families with similar problems.

Once a need common to a number of people has been established, the potential group members need to be contacted. The nurse should discuss with them the objectives that can be accomplished in a group. The important principle involved is that the nurse must have objectives in mind for the group, the clients must have needs in mind, and the two should be congruent. This principle is also valid when the nurse is considering a referral to an already established group; it must meet the needs of the client. For example, a support group for new parents would probably not be helpful for a client with severe postpartum depression.

To facilitate this principle, contracting is suggested when working with groups. A contract is a written statement of the mutual expectations of both client and nurse for each other. Chapter 9 discusses contracting with families; the same principles can be applied to groups. Contracts provide a basis for evaluation of the progress that takes place; the key question to consider is whether you have met the objectives you set out to achieve.

The setting plays a crucial role in groups. Several questions, such as those below, should be asked in order to determine whether a particular setting is appropriate.

- Is the group meeting in a place that is easily accessible, that can be reached by public transportation or personal cars easily?
- Is the meeting place near the population being served?
- Is the location of the meeting place safe after dark?
- Does the meeting room provide privacy and warmth?
- Do seating arrangements facilitate group interaction?
- Will the facility be consistently available?

Besides the setting, there are many other factors to consider when developing a group. The size of the group is a major consideration. Though there are no clear rules, a group of five to 15 people usually facilitates good communication. When the group should meet is another important variable. If it is composed of unemployed persons, mornings may be fine. Wage earners, on the other hand, are likely to be free only in the evenings. The frequency and length of meetings and child care arrangements are other issues that need to be decided by nurse and clients. If small children are to be brought along with clients, there needs to be a place with equipment and a caretaker provided. None of these details have "right" and "wrong" answers, but it is essential that clients know them and help to plan them.

Many nurses are hesitant to use the group approach to nursing care because they lack experience with this intervention strategy. Careful planning, staff development activities that facilitate the understanding of group dynamics, and guidance from professionals comfortable with this process will reduce fear.

The Life of a Group

It is helpful for nurses who lead groups to understand that a group goes through phases that include the initiation phase, the working phase, and the termination phase (Knopke and Diekelmann, 1978, p. 135). During the initiation phase the group is oriented to its goals and purposes. Included in this information are the time limitations and behavior expected of group members. The working phase encourages problem-solving through discussion. The final phase, termination, encourages expressions of warmth, anger, and depression as distancing devices for the final separation that will occur as part of the group process.

The Functions of the Community Health Nurse as Group Leader

Effective leadership is fundamental to a positive group experience; there are four functions that are appropriate for nurse group leaders (Marram, 1978, pp. 124-127):

1. The leader facilitates benefits of group membership. People join groups for the reasons discussed earlier and the leader can help the group to meet expected objectives by outlining a direction for the group and interpreting group objectives.
2. The leader maintains a viable group atmosphere by keeping relationships within the group pleasant or relatively secure. Group members need to feel free to be present and to be able to discuss their concerns. Being able to experience new behaviors is also important to growth.
3. The leader oversees group growth by keeping members attuned to the objectives and by clarifying issues in terms of how they relate to the objectives. The leader also needs to periodically help the group evaluate the progress made toward their objectives.
4. The leader regulates individual members' growth within the group setting. People will move toward objectives at different speeds and some members may need more specific objectives than others. The leader is concerned not only with the progress of the group toward objectives but also with the growth of individuals within the group.

To succeed in implementing leadership responsibilities in a group, a nurse must have an awareness of how people interact with each other. Community health nurses must use basic interviewing and communication skills in all settings, and group work is no exception. People want to be able to communicate and this can be facilitated by asking open-ended questions, asking direct questions, and using other techniques such as reflection and role-playing. Games and audiovisual aids are different methods that can be used to stimulate interaction between group members.

Table 21-1 is a summary of the interventions that community health nurses use when they are group leaders. The table presents the types of interventions used, along with end goals of each intervention. Having an awareness of group intervention strategies and why they are used helps one to effectively guide the group process and to develop criteria for evaluating group dynamics.

Abraham, Niles, Thiel, Siarkowski, and Cowling (1991) describe how the group process was used with elderly people and demonstrated how principles of group work and specific group interventions can be adapted for use with the depressed elderly, including those who have functional and cognitive impairments. They carried out group work in addition to group therapy and emphasize that even though education groups focus on learning and discussion instead of therapy, both are equally therapeutic.

It is unrealistic to expect that participants (in a group) will limit themselves to these (educational) topics and that no personal issues will emerge. The key in education groups is how to handle such personal issues. This is done best by having the group leader use interpersonal (rather than therapeutic) skills, such as active and sensitive listening.

Education groups need as much structuring by the leader as therapy groups. Not only does this facilitate group activity, it also introduces a sense of safe group environment that is key to active participation. A sense of safety also encourages members to bring up topics of discussion that are personally relevant and important to them. In our groups, over the course of several meetings, topics became progressively more personal and pertinent to the concerns and fears that are so typical of long-term care residents. Whereas earlier subject material was safe and did not involve feelings and conflicts, this was not the case for later topics.

It is the succession of topics as well as their content that creates the group process. For instance, by having group members share their favorite poems, they were given a safe avenue for sharing what is important to them, what beauty means to them, as well as some feelings. In turn, this encouraged group interaction. Similarly, discussing Alzhei-

mer's disease, expressing fears of developing the disease, and expressing concerns about residents with Alzheimer-type symptoms opened the way for personalizing specific concerns about growing old in later sessions (Abraham, Niles, Thiel, Siarkowski, and Cowling, 1991, p. 641).

Nurses who are interested in working with groups but who have never done so should ask for supervision and a preceptor to help them with the process. Effective communication with group members and agency personnel, careful scheduling, and attention to small details of organizing the group can help this to be a successful experience. Review of the literature is also helpful when community health nurses consider developing groups in the clinical setting. Zander (1982) has written a readable practical book for neophytes who are concerned about creating a group and practicing group process skills.

THE EVOLUTION OF CLINIC SERVICES AND NURSING CENTERS

Community health nurses have long worked in clinics. Beginning with the era of Lillian Wald, they have had to assume a considerable amount of responsibility, make independent judgments, and use skill in teaching clients. These competencies especially fitted them to work in the relatively independent clinic setting.

Early efforts at the beginning of the century to improve maternal-child health and to control communicable disease frequently resulted in the development of clinic services for underserved aggregates. For example, between 1900 and 1930 many milk dispensaries evolved into preventive health centers.

In her history of the origins of nursing centers, Glass (1989, p. 21) begins with the work of Lillian Wald and also describes the endeavors of Mary Breckinridge with the Frontier Nursing Service in Hyden, Kentucky (Figure 21-1); Margaret Sanger, the pioneer birth control activist in Europe and the United States; and a nurse settlement house in Orange, New Jersey. The three women named were pioneer feminists well-known to activists working for the health of women today. Wald's accomplishments with nursing clinics are detailed in Chapter 1. In 1923 Breckinridge used the principles of program planning, described in Chapters 12 and 13, to determine where nursing services were needed in rural mountainous Kentucky. After surveying a three-county area covering 1000 square

21-1   A Summary of Leader Interventions

Type of intervention	Goals of intervention
Support	Provides supportive climate for expressing ideas and opinions, including unpopular unusual points of view.
	Facilitates members continuing with their ongoing behavior.
	Helps reinforce positive forms of behavior.
	Creates a climate in which silent members may feel secure enough to participate.
Confrontation	Aids in growth and development; helps unfreeze members from being stuck in one mode of functioning.
	Helps reduce some forms of disruptive behavior.
	Helps members deal more openly and directly with each other.
Advice and suggestions	Shares expertise, offers new perspectives.
	Helps focus group on its task and goals.
Summarizing	Helps keep group on its task by reviewing past actions and by setting agenda for future sessions.
	Brings to focus still unresolved issues.
	Organizes past in ways that help clarify; brings into focus themes and patterns of interaction.
Clarifying	Helps reduce distortion in communication.
	Facilitates focus on substantive issues rather than allowing members to be sidetracked into misunderstandings.
Probing and questioning	Helps expand a point that may have been left incomplete.
	Gets at more extensive and wider range of information.
	Invites members to explore their ideas in greater detail.
Repeating, paraphrasing, and highlighting.	Helps members continue with their ongoing behavior, invites further exploration and examination of what is being said.
	Clarifies and helps focus on the specific, important, or key aspect of a communication.
	Sharpens members' understanding of what is being said or done.
Reflecting: Feelings	Orients members to the feelings that may lie behind what is being said or done.
	Helps members deal with issues they might otherwise avoid or miss.
Reflecting: Behavior	Gives members the opportunity to see how their behavior appears to others and to see and evaluate its consequences.
	Helps members to understand others' perceptions and responses to them.
Interpretation and analysis	Renders behavior meaningful by locating it in a larger context in which a causal explanation is provided.
	Helps members understand both the likely bases of their behavior and its meaning.
	Summarizes a pattern of behavior and provides a useful way of examining it and working to modify it through the insights gained.
Listening	Provides an attentive and responsive audience for those who participate.
	Models a helpful way for members to relate to one another; gives a feeling of sharing and mutual concern.
	Helps members sharpen their own ideas and thinking as they realize that indeed others are listening and concerned about what they are saying.

From Sampson E and Marthas M: *Group process for the health professions,* New York, 1981, Wiley, pp. 258-260. Reprinted by permission of John Wiley and Sons, Inc.

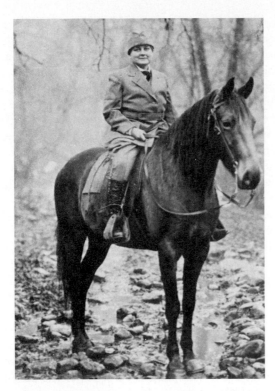

Figure 21-1 Mary Breckinridge founded the Frontier Nursing Service in Lexington, Kentucky. Her nurses used horses to service families in the hills of Kentucky. (Reprinted by permission of the Frontier Nursing Service, Wendover, Ky.)

miles she concluded that a decentralized system of health care was essential. Based on her study, The Kentucky Committee for Mothers and Babies opened their first nursing center in Hyden, Leslie County, in September 1925. By 1930 there were six nursing centers, each serving a five-mile radius, with the objectives of providing the following: skilled care for the sick of all ages and women in childbirth, the health education of the population, social services, and the advancement of economic independence.

Margaret Sanger (1870-1966) began her career as a visiting nurse in New York City; her work with poor women and children stimulated her interest in birth control and women having control over their own bodies. Because the Comstock Act of 1873 declared birth control material as obscene and prohibited the mailing of it, Sanger travelled to France to obtain information. She opened the first birth control clinic in America in 1916 in Brooklyn; she was shortly arrested and spent the first of her many sentences in jail. The

establishment of today's Planned Parenthood Federation is to her credit and her contributions to the health of women is inestimable.

These are dramatic, wonderful examples of the beginnings of nursing centers as we know them today. Additionally, large scale demonstration projects were sponsored by the Metropolitan Life Insurance Company to combat tuberculosis and other communicable diseases, and included programs of mass screening and health assessment, as well as community education activities (Kalisch and Kalisch, 1986).

By the 1930s child health conferences and maternity conferences or clinics were well established. Books on public health nursing practice written at this time addressed the role of the nurse in the clinic and stressed the need for conferences to achieve a well-balanced child welfare program (Gardner, 1928; National Organization for Public Health Nursing, 1939).

Clinic services were developed in the beginning of the century because a significant number of families could not afford other types of care. They were also established to reach a large number of individuals very quickly during epidemics of communicable diseases. These services have been maintained over the century because early efforts dramatically demonstrated their effectiveness in improving maternal-child health and in combating communicable diseases.

The nurse practitioner movement of the 1960s and 1970s significantly altered the role of nurses in community-based clinics. This movement evolved because the needs of disadvantaged aggregates across the life span were neglected. It was believed that well-trained nurses with expanded skills could help to eradicate the problem of inaccessible and fragmented health care services, especially in underserved areas. Increasingly, local health departments and other community health clinics are using nurse practitioners to provide comprehensive services for at-risk aggregates (Lawler and Valand, 1988, pp. 187-188).

During the 1980s and the early 1990s there was tremendous growth in ambulatory care or clinic services, particularly because of the introduction of the prospective payment system for Medicare-sponsored hospital stays. As the length of hospital stays has decreased, patient acuity at discharge has increased. This has resulted in the need for increased continuing care after discharge and has shifted the responsibility for patients' care to their families and community-based providers. Further, to increase cost-efficient care, insurers have encouraged people to have preadmission testing done on an outpatient basis and have moved many surgeries such as lens implantation to an outpatient basis. As a result, the number of days being spent in community hospitals is decreasing significantly while the number of outpatient visits is rising dramatically. In fact, ambulatory care is one of the fastest growing specialties in nursing.

USING CLINIC SERVICES IN COMMUNITY HEALTH NURSING

Clinics, often called *ambulatory health services,* are centers that examine and treat ambulatory clients on an outpatient basis. They are frequently operated under the auspices of a larger institution such as a hospital, medical school, group practice, HMO, health department, church, or community organization. Defining their services is difficult because they vary from one institution to the next.

The clinic setting offers a wide range of preventive health services. Clinics may provide only primary intervention; this is usually the main focus in immunization clinics. Or clinics may provide screening, diagnosis, and treatment services, such as those provided by clinics treating sexually transmitted diseases, which identify the disease, administer appropriate treatments, and locate contacts of the infected client for screening.

Clinics may serve only specific populations. Well-baby clinics usually provide assessment services for children from birth to 5 years of age, and family planning clinics usually serve females of childbearing age. Other clinics may serve anyone who comes at any time with any problem, as do walk-in clinics of large teaching hospitals and neighborhood health care centers. Emergency rooms function as ambulatory clinics in many towns where there are no other resources.

The majority of official local health agencies provide preventive clinic services on a continuing basis for selected population groups. It is common to find Well-child, EPDST, WIC, immunization, and communicable disease (e.g., sexually transmitted diseases and tuberculosis) clinic services provided on a regular basis in most health departments. Many also provide family planning, prenatal, dental health, primary care, and multiphasic diagnostic clinic services on an ongoing basis. The high pregnancy rate among adolescents provided an impetus for initiating comprehensive health services to youth through school-based health clinics (Dryfoos, 1985; Hirsch, Zabin, Streett, and Hardy, 1987). The St. Paul Maternal and Child Health

Program, one of the oldest school-based clinic projects, offers a wide range of services to students during school hours, such as immunizations, mental health counseling, prenatal care, family planning, and support groups (Maternal and Child Health Program, undated). Other significant health problems have also provided the stimulus for the development of clinic services by private and official community health agencies. For example, an increasing number of official health departments are providing primary health care services for the homeless and other medically indigent groups.

As discussed in Chapter 16, community health centers (CHCs) are also emerging across the country to assist medically underserved aggregates. These centers, federally supported under Section 330 of the Public Health Service Act, are located in every territory and state except Wyoming. They are located in both urban and rural settings and serve persons with special needs, such as coal miners with respiratory and pulmonary impairments, the elderly, people who are confined to their homes, and migrant and seasonal farmworkers. Most migrant health centers are operated together with CHCs. Data reveal that these centers have significantly influenced the health status of the population groups they are serving. Clients served by a CHC have a lower incidence of hospitalization than clients cared for in other health care settings. Studies have also shown a dramatic reduction in infant mortality in specific regions of the country after the establishment of a CHC: in the rural south, infant mortality decreased by 50%, and in Denver's CHC program it decreased by 25% (National Association of Community Health Centers, Inc., 1986).

The type of care provided through clinics may be episodic, in which only the immediate needs of the clients are handled, or comprehensive, providing all levels of preventive services: primary preventive, diagnostic, therapeutic, and rehabilitative services. Primary preventive and diagnostic services (e.g., screening for communicable diseases or health risks such as high blood cholesterol) are frequently the focus in clinics sponsored by official health agencies.

The Development of Nursing Centers

A number of terms are used to refer to nursing centers, including *nurse-managed care, community nursing center* or *organization,* or *nurse-run clinic.* These terms refer to organizations where nurses control practice and patient care and where education and research are paramount (Riesch, 1992, p. 16). Riesch reviewed the literature about nursing centers and defined them by three criteria: direct access by client/patient to the nurse, a nursing model of care, and holistic reimbursed services. Aydelotte and Gregory (1989) reported that, at the Second National Conference on Nursing Centers in 1984, the participants defined a nursing center as follows:

Nurse-Managed Centers are organizations that provide direct access to professional nurses who offer holistic, client-centered health services for reimbursement. With the use of nursing models of health, professional nurses in NMC's diagnose and treat human responses to potential and actual health problems. Examples of professional nursing services include health education, health promotion, and health-related research. Services are targeted to underserved individuals and groups. An effective referral system and collaboration with other health care professionals are an integral part of NMC's. As models of professional nursing practice and research, NMC's are ideal sites for faculty and student practice. They are administered by a professional nurse (Fehring, Schulte, and Riesch, 1986, p. 63).

Nursing centers first appeared in the literature in 1963 when Lydia Hall established the Loeb Center in New York (Riesch, 1992). The Center was described as being "close to public health nursing in an institutional setting "(Riesch, p. 16). During the 1970s and 1980s nursing centers grew for several reasons: nursing faculty identified underserved populations and realized that these groups could serve as learning experiences for students. Further, monies from federal and state legislatures and private foundations and professional organizations assisted in the development of the concept (Riesch, pp. 17-18). The Community Nursing Organizations Bill, signed into law in 1987, provided direct Medicare reimbursement to nurses and permitted the development of ten demonstration sites. "Nursing education has been the pacesetter in the development of nursing centers" (Courney, 1992, p. 1). The section at the end of the chapter, entitled "An Exercise in Critical Thinking," showcases two academic nursing centers that demonstrate the variety of services delivered by nursing centers and give some evidence of how students learn about models of care delivery that they can use in their own practice.

Nursing centers are growing rapidly: an estimated 250 were in place across the country, serving 118,000 Americans in 1990 (News, 1992, p. 70). About half were freestanding; others were affiliated with a hos-

pital, a public health or home health agency, or a retirement community. Those not freestanding were usually housed in a school of nursing where students were assigned to the center for clinical experience (News, p. 70).

Services Offered by Nursing Centers

Care offered by nursing centers usually focuses on health promotion activities such as health education classes, health screenings, and physical assessments (Holman, 1990, p. 6). "Some span the whole range of primary care: ambulatory and outpatient, physicals and check-ups, immunization and infusion therapy. One in five emphasizes assessment and screening; 21%, education or counseling; 11%, consultation; 3%, home health care" (News, 1992, p. 70).

Care in nursing centers is reimbursed in several ways: "Slightly more than a quarter of their services were paid for out of pocket while 19% were covered by private insurance and 24% by Medicare or Medicaid. The centers reported that 13% of care was uncompensated and that 17% was reimbursed by other methods" (News, 1992, p. 71).

Establishing and Maintaining Clinic Services and Nursing Centers

Community health nurses frequently assume a major role in planning, implementing, and evaluating services for aggregates with unmet needs. When establishing new health care service, the nurse uses the health planning process described in Chapter 13. Some specific factors to consider when setting up clinic services follow.

Determining the need for clinics and centers is the first responsibility of a health care professional interested in developing such services. Factors to consider during this process are the health status, lifestyle patterns, and demographic characteristics of the population being studied; community resources available to the population under consideration; health care use patterns; and health care accessibility variables such as location of resources and client referral processes. Chapter 12 describes how and where community health nurses obtain these data. When analyzing these data, it is important to examine trends over time and to identify strengths as well as limitations in the health care delivery system. The goal is to determine if services are lacking or if services are adequate but not used because of unique characteristics of the population being served or service delivery problems. For example, community health nurses may find that clients do not use clinic services because their location makes them inaccessible or clients are unaware they exist. If a need is verified, careful planning should take place before starting a clinic.

Several organizational activities need to be accomplished in order to ensure effective and efficient service delivery. Establishing specific objectives helps the nurse to determine what types of services to offer and what resources are needed to provide them. For example, the resources needed to staff a comprehensive child health conference would be significantly greater than those needed to staff an immunization clinic. Prospective clients should be part of the planning team to help ensure that clients' needs can be met through the proposed clinic.

Other organizational activities include determining the location for the clinic or center, securing necessary equipment and supplies, organizing facilities to ensure client privacy and effective and efficient service delivery, establishing procedures such as follow-up policies that promote quality care, obtaining adequate professional staff with the skills needed to manage client health needs, securing and training volunteers, and developing marketing strategies. All of these activities require careful thought and planning and include several components. For example, securing necessary equipment and supplies involves such things as identifying what is needed, determining where to purchase it, and establishing appropriate storage procedures for vaccines and other medications.

Determining a site requires special attention because location of a clinic or center influences the way it will be used. Some clients are affected more than others by the location, namely, the poor and the aged. Difficulty and expense of access are important, so a knowledge of the possible transportation alternatives is important. Accessibility also involves appointment delay time, waiting time, clinic or center hours, services offered, health care given, and client/professional relationships.

During the organizational phase evaluation procedures should be established. If this activity is neglected during the initial development phase, procedures will not be established to ensure collection of data needed to complete an evaluation once the clinic or center has been in operation. An overall evaluation of operations should occur at least once a year, but evaluation is an ongoing process that needs attention throughout the year. Procedures need to be established to evaluate overall operations and usage patterns. Questions for planners to consider when evaluating services are shared in a later section of this chapter.

Callan (1992) presents guidelines for nurses who are establishing and managing hospital-affiliated primary care clinics. Methods of determining services, staffing needs, and office, administrative, and facility requirements are also discussed. The guidelines are applicable to other ambulatory care setting as well.

Chapter 13 presented the need to empower an aggregate or a community if the health needs of that group were to be met. Buchanan and Gerrity (1989) describe how a nursing center in Philadelphia uses the collaboration of community leaders and the nursing profession to empower young families to address their health care needs. To be empowered "is to have control over the conditions that make action possible, thus to be able to do and have what one needs and wants" (Buchanan and Gerrity, p. 113). Creating healthy public policy, supportive environments, strong communities, and interpersonal skills are means to empowerment.

The importance of adequate planning when establishing and maintaining a clinic or center cannot be overstressed. Neglecting significant details during the planning phase can result in poor use of services. For example, one health department decided to open a well-baby clinic because it was determined that a rural portion of a large county was underserved. The first decision made was to send a staff nurse to school for preparation as a pediatric nurse practitioner. However, steps of the planning process were not logically followed after preparing this staff nurse for new role responsibilities. Thus, even though there were no other facilities for well-child care in the area, the clinic closed because of lack of clients. It was isolated with no public transportation available, so clients could not use the service.

The Role of the Community Health Nurse in the Clinic and Nursing Center

The community health nurse can function in various ways to meet the health needs of aggregates. As previously discussed, the expanded role of the nurse has aided community health nurses in more adequately meeting the health care needs of people in

---

Taxonomy of Ambulatory Care Nursing Activities

Patient Counseling

Client advocacy
Terminal/chronic illness
General support
Clinic procedures

Health Care Maintenance

General assessment
Preventive care instruction
Provide information
Follow-up assessment

Primary Care

Referral
Physical
Triage
History
Protocol care

Patient Education

General instruction
Standardized instruction
Plan of care
Illness/condition program
Individual instruction
Health care maintenance program

Therapeutic Care

Surgical preparation
Applications
Appliances
Noninvasive IV medications
Irrigations
Specimens
Recovery
Dressings
Blood therapy
Respiratory treatments
Measurement
Invasive medications
IV therapy

Normative Care

Directing
Chaperoning
Documents coordination
Transporting
Assisting
System
Communication
Preparation
Comfort

From Verran JA: Testing a classification instrument for the ambulatory care setting, *Research Nurs Health* 9:280, 1986.

---

clinics and nursing centers. The client population being served in many clinics has become more complex and acute. Nurses no longer serve as schedulers and receptionists. Their roles have enlarged to include management of clients with both acute and long-term care needs, handling of complex treatments and procedures, client counseling, and health education. In addition, nurses are often the primary providers for many clients and their families. Verran (1986), when studying the nursing care requirements of ambulatory clients attending a hospital-based ambulatory care center, developed a taxonomy that clearly illustrates the extensive range of activities assumed by nurses in clinic settings (refer to box above). Verran's taxonomy identifies six major responsibility areas that are assumed by ambulatory care nurses and activities to fulfill these responsibilities. Verran's taxonomy has been widely used and referenced in the development

and application of tools for primary care (Schroeder, 1987; Smyth, 1987).

The range of activities implemented by a nurse in a clinic setting or nursing center will vary based on its objectives and the needs of clients. Common roles assumed by the nurse in most community health settings are discussed below.

Manager

The role of manager was the main nursing function in clinics for many years. Nurses attended to the many details necessary in order for clinics to run smoothly: distributing client caseload, following up on clients with problems, bringing needed reports to physicians, preparing clients physically for examinations, performing procedures, supervising aides and practical nurses, and carrying out clerical work. Although all this is necessary, the nurse should perform *nursing* activities, that is, helping clients when they are unable to help themselves. The nurse should supervise other members of the health team as described in Chapter 22 so that they can carry out the functions that do not require the professional skills of a registered nurse. This means that the nurse will understand the different levels of functioning of team members and use them appropriately. Clerks and aides, as well as volunteers, can be valuable assets in the clinic. They can weigh and measure babies, file and pull records, label and carry specimens to the laboratory, act as receptionists, and take temperatures. Smooth flow of clients from waiting to examining rooms is important and can be facilitated by aides. As a manager, the community health nurse must understand that she or he is responsible for the care that these team members give. The nurse's supervision of team members is fundamental to the care given clients in the clinic setting.

Group Leader and Teacher

Many clinics and nursing centers have as one of their most important functions group sessions in which information is discussed that is designed to promote health. One example is an ostomy information clinic that disseminates information and helps clients to cope with problems related to their ostomies. Another example is a prenatal education program in a hospital setting in which the community health nurse meets with clients before appointments to share information about pregnancy, childbirth, child care, and role transition concerns. The concepts presented earlier in this chapter on developing and leading a group are applicable to the nurse's role in clinics as group leader and teacher.

Practitioner

The expanded role of the nurse has provided nurses with physical assessment and client management skills. Practitioners are able to identify the current health status of clients, including emotional and physical components, and to plan interventions that meet clients' needs. Practitioners carry out a variety of functions in both adult and child health clinics. Providing physical, mental, social, and emotional support, educating clients about their health conditions, and referring clients to needed community resources are examples of functions implemented by the practitioner. Practitioners often work with an interdisciplinary team and actively participate in client care conferences. They provide a continuum of nursing services, especially for clients who

have chronic health conditions or preventive health needs.

Evaluator

An integral part of working in these settings is evaluation. This process was discussed in depth in Chapter 13. Some specific questions to ask when evaluating services include the following: Are the objectives of the clinic or nursing center being met? If this is the immunization clinic in Smith County, for example, are children completely immunized upon school entrance (at age 6)? Are the numbers of clients being served increasing or decreasing? If the number of clients being served is changing, is it because the health service area population is changing or because clients feel that they are not being served adequately? The way clients feel about the care they receive determines whether or not they will use the health facility. Some method of client contact on a regular basis, either questionnaire or interview, provides data concerning this factor. Knowing who is served also means that a record system will be in operation so that number and kinds of visits can be tabulated easily. A good record system will also provide for continuity of care from one visit to the next and yet not be overly time-consuming.

PROMOTING THE COMMUNITY HEALTH NURSE PHILOSOPHY

Increasingly, community health nurses are working in nontraditional public health clinic settings such as nursing centers, or with ambulatory care health providers who do not share the same orientation to practice as theirs. This is occurring because health care delivery trends emphasize the provision of ambulatory care services, while funding sources do not reimburse primary prevention efforts. Thus focus is on developing a comprehensive package of services, including preventive and curative services, that will be reimbursed by third-party payors. To achieve this focus, a team of health providers, with various backgrounds and skills, is often involved in many clinic settings. A large role for community health nurses on these teams is to promote the philosophy of community health practice: orientation to wellness rather than illness; family-centered versus individual-centered practice; continuity rather than episodic intervention; and population-based or community health planning. Regardless of where community health nurses function, these concepts should be central to their practice. As was discussed in Chapter 2, it is *the nature of the practice—not the setting*—that distinguishes community health nursing from other specialty nursing areas. The concepts of community health nursing greatly enrich service delivery and nursing care in any clinic setting.

Community health professionals are developing creative approaches for providing and obtaining funding for essential clinic services. The state of Missouri, for example, is demonstrating that it is possible to coordinate primary care that focuses on the population as a whole, as well as on the health of individuals within the community (Riner, 1989, pp. 224-228). This state uses three levels of community health nurses: (1) the *generalist nurse,* whose role responsibilities include clinical nursing, general in nature, epidemiological follow-up, case management, community resource coordination, and home health care; (2) the *mastery nurse,* who has had special training for performing a complete physical examination, which increases early diagnosis and treatment through casefinding; and (3) the *advanced practice nurse,* a category that includes certified nurse practitioners, nurse midwives, and clinical nurse specialists. These nurses collaborate to promote a continuum of nursing services. Table 21-2 delineates the different role responsibilities of a CHN generalist and the advanced practice nurse when providing prenatal clinical nursing service in the Missouri system. In this system, the services provided by all three levels of nursing are reimbursed by third-party payors. The case management activities of the generalist are reimbursed through Medicaid. Medicaid also funds services provided by the mastery nurse because of the difficulty in recruiting physicians for underserved areas. Payment for nurse practitioners comes from a variety of sources, such as federal block grant monies, special state grants, and Medicaid.

Developing new ways of providing services for at-risk aggregates is essential in this era of cost containment. In order to handle the demands in the health care delivery system and the changing nature of current health problems, coordinated, community-wide approaches must be emphasized. Community health nurses have unique skills and knowledge to deal with these challenges.

Block Nursing and Parish Nursing

Two other nontraditional and creative settings where community health nurses serve at-risk aggregates are with the roles of block nursing and parish

TABLE 21-2	Collaboration of Community Health Nurse and Nurse Practitioner in Prenatal Care
Community health nurse	**Advanced practice nurse**
Client and family history	Review data
Current health status	Risk assessment
Screenings	Physical examination
Weight, blood pressure	Pap smear and pelvic
Laboratory work	examination
Urinalysis, blood	Fetal heart tones
Diet review	Fundal height
Danger signs	Education
Education	Referral
Case management	

From Riner MB: Expanding services: the role of the community health nurse and the advanced nurse practitioner, *J Commun Health Nurs* 6:227, 1989.

nursing. Both roles fill in gaps of the formal health care system, usually with older clients or those confined to the home.

Jamieson (1990) described *block nursing* as nursing on the block where the nurse lives, making services available based on need rather than reimbursement eligibility. Professional and volunteer community members, an informal network of family, friends, neighbors, church and civic groups, and service groups such as Boy and Girl Scouts, and people who are part of the neighborhood, provide many of the services needed. This include shopping, running errands, and providing respite care to relieve caregivers. Funding to pay for client assessments and direct care provided by aides/homemakers and nurses has come from sources such as grants, client fees, and demonstration projects. One block nurse program prevented hospitalization in 25% of its clients.

Parish nursing meets many of the same needs as block nursing; however, churches and synagogues provide the system whereby the services are offered.

Churches and synagogues have been promoting health and wholeness for centuries through the ministries of worship, music, sharing and caring. A new dimension is the addition of the nurse to the ministry team. For the past dozen years, nurses across the state and across the country have been using their nursing skills to demonstrate religious witness.

Some are volunteers; some are paid; some just get mileage. Some train volunteers; others actually staff the program. Some minister to their congregations only; others reach out into their communities. *Parish nursing* takes many forms, depending on each congregation—its needs, visions, and resources (Parish nursing, 1993, p. 1).

Both block and parish nursing use the informal health care system to meet needs not met by the formal health care system. Both also build on the concept of nursing neighbors in one's community. Likely not even the best national health care package will meet everyone's needs; the idealism of these services should continue to be a part of community health nursing because they can be a guide to caring for others in unique ways.

A FINAL COMMENT ON GROUP WORK, CLINIC SERVICES, AND NURSING CENTERS

As adequate finances for health care delivery become a scarcer commodity, health care agencies are moving in the direction of using clinics, nursing centers, and groups to meet the needs of people. One large health department in the midwest uses clinics almost exclusively; home visits to families are a rare occurrence. At a time when each home visit is costing taxpayers up to $100, it is not difficult to see why alternatives to home visiting are being considered.

It is important to remember that no one method will meet everyone's health needs and that nurses need "in every enterprise to consider where you would come out." Families generate, as well as help to solve, health problems, and this important aspect can be lost in group and clinic work. However, group and aggregate-focused interventions do have a place in health care, and each will increase in number. Remember, though, to start with the needs of clients to decide which route to use to assist them. This kind of choice contributes to the challenge, excitement, and creativity of community health nursing.

Summary

Nurses can use many routes to meet the health care needs of clients. Group work, clinic services, and nursing centers are possible routes. Advantages and disadvantages of the group approach are many and nurses need to be familiar with them. Understanding the methodology followed to develop a group, the phases of a group, and the functions of the nurse as a group leader is essential if the nurse is going to function effectively in a group setting.

Clinics have long been a place where community health nurses have served varied populations. The location aspect of clinic facilities plays an important part in how well they are utilized. Clinic services need to be well planned if they are to be effective. Thus it is crucial for the community health nurse to be familiar with the planning process.

Community nursing centers are gaining ground rapidly as one solution to the health care issues of this era. They are demonstrating that they cut the cost of care by keeping people healthy. Dealing with the anxieties of pregnant women and new parents, as well as preventing rehospitalizations of the elderly and frail, are methods of achieving this goal. Nursing centers are truly community health–focused, providing services to underserved aggregates and emphasizing education and prevention.

The community health nurse carries out multiple roles and functions in the clinic and nursing center setting—manager, group leader and teacher, practitioner, and evaluator. The nurse's major function is to assist clients to help themselves. Nurses must learn to appropriately delegate tasks to other members of the health care team so that they have sufficient time to work with clients.

Increasingly, health care agencies are using creative ways to meet the needs of aggregates in the community. However, a more effective and efficient health care delivery system must be established if the needs of all are to be met. Nurses must become involved in planning for the future so that a viable role for nursing is maintained in the evolving health care system.

◀   *An Exercise in Critical Thinking*   ▶

Appendix 21-1 contains descriptions of two academic nursing centers, demonstrating the variety of services offered by this segment of the health care delivery system. Think about the services that are offered and how they differ from the traditional clinic services that are part of many neighborhoods. What do you find attractive about learning in such an environment? Would you like to learn in a setting such as this? If so, why?

Nursing Center Models: Case Studies in Success

Southern Illinois University at Edwardsville Community Nursing Services

By Barbara C. Martin, EdD, RNC, Jacalyn Ryberg, MA, RNC, and Jacquelyn Clement, PhD, RN

The Southern Illinois University at Edwardsville (SIUE) Community Nursing Services provides an ideal setting for a community health experience. In this primarily black, inner city community, a clinical practicum for senior nursing students was developed with the local Head Start program in 1989.

Students were originally involved with case management for children with identified health problems. They worked with families to assure that the children had access to appropriate care. Working with families provided an excellent community health experience for nursing students and resulted in faster, more comprehensive resolution of health problems for Head Start children.

The program later expanded to include health screening services. The nursing students set up screening sites, collect blood samples, operate the screening test machines, identify health problems, and keep records.

As the students and faculty identify health problems, there is an increased opportunity to speak with the teachers, and on occasion parents. This dialogue facilitates information sharing and early intervention for the children.

In the summer of 1989, an elderly component was added to the practicum. In conjunction with the local housing authority, the students began to collect emergency data on a *Health Alert Form.* This form helps keep all pertinent data on the elderly residents of public housing in one accessible place.

The form is maintained in an opaque sleeve on the back of each apartment hall door. It is available to emergency teams, family members, and health care workers assuring continuity of care. Students visit the elderly in their homes, interview them, fill out the forms, and identify problems. In follow-up visits they do basic health education and medication teaching. They are also able to relate to problems of independent living that commonly occur upon hospital discharge.

Students appreciate the opportunity for practical application of the cultural concepts they learn in class as they are exposed to multigenerational families, elders in independent living settings, and accessing limited resources for those with limited financial assets.

As the nursing center grows, the educational experience opportunities for the students will expand. The potential benefits to clients, the community, the students, and the center are only limited by imagination.

University of Texas Nursing Services—Houston

By Glenda C. Walker, DSN, RN

In February 1991, The University of Texas School of Nursing at the Health Science Center in Houston (UTNS-H) opened an ambulatory nursing service center. The purposes of the UTNS-H were to provide educational and research opportunities for students and faculty.

At UTNS-H categories or clinical services include: high risk screening, health education, well child care, and home infusion therapy. Other services currently under development include: geriatric nursing care, women's health care, and psychiatric health care. When deviations from normal are found, patients are referred to either their private physician or the UT Family Practice clinic. When the patient needs follow-up monitoring and/or educational services, they are referred back to UTNS-H. This type of arrangement allows for cost-effective services delivered by the most appropriate provider with an emphasis on continuity of care.

UTNS-H also provides health education seminars on such topics as chronic disease, healthy life styles, stress management, and safety in the work place. In addition, ongoing health education classes are provided for patients who are referred to UTNS-H needing health education counseling, such as nutritional management of diabetes. UTNS-H encourages consumer/patient responsibility and accountability for the management of their health care.

Well child services provided by UTNS-H include: well baby exams (EPSDT), immunizations, TB skin tests, school physicals, and parenting classes. These services are provided at a variety of settings with an emphasis on easy access. For example, the UTNS-H pediatric nurse practitioner has provided EPSDT screenings at the City of Houston housing project apartments. In addition, a UTNS-H pediatric nurse practitioner provides well child services at a community-based health clinic five mornings a week. A collaborative agreement with UT Department of Pediatrics allows for supervision of the medical protocols, consultation regarding cases, and referrals to the department for those patients needing more extensive care.

UTNS-H provides home IV infusion services for patients who need continuing care within the home environment. A case management approach is utilized to meet the physical and emotional needs of the family and patients. It is believed that this approach will strengthen the coping resources of the family thereby minimizing costly rehospitalization.

As nursing embraces and lobbys for *Nursing's Agenda for Health Care Reform,* it is important for nursing centers to analyze how their activities correlate with that agenda. An initial analysis of UTNS-H activities and the agenda has proven successful for our current path.

From National League for Nursing, Council for Nursing Centers: *Connections,* New York, Winter 1992, The League, p.2.

References

Abraham IL, Niles SA, Thiel BP, Siarkowski KI, and Cowling WR: Therapeutic group work with depressed elderly, *Nurs Clin North America* 26(3):635-650, 1991.

Arkin EB: The Healthy Mothers, Healthy Babies Coalition: four years of progress, *Public Health Rep* 101:147-156, 1986.

Aydelotte MK and Gregory MS: Nursing practice: innovative models. In *Nursing centers: meeting the demand for quality health care,* Pub No. 21-2311, New York, 1989, National League for Nursing (NLN).

Buchanan M and Gerrity PL: Community wellness outreach: family health through empowerment. In *Nursing centers: meeting the demand for quality health care,* Pub No. 21-2311, New York, 1989, NLN.

Callan ME: Nurse practitioner management of hospital-affiliated primary care centers, *Nurse Practitioner* 17(8):71-74, 1992.

Centers for Disease Control and Prevention (CDC): The effectiveness of school health education, *MMWR* 35(38):593-595, September 26, 1986.

Courney D: Information sharing is the key, *Connections, National League for Nursing's Council for Nursing Centers,* 1-4, Winter 1992.

Demi AS: Hospice bereavement program: trends and issues. In Schraff SH, ed: *Hospice: the nursing perspective,* New York, 1984, NLN.

Dryfoos J: School-based health clinics: a new approach to preventing adolescent pregnancy? *Family Planning Perspect* 17(2):70-75, 1985.

Fehring R, Schulte J, and Riesch S: Toward a definition of nurse-managed centers, *J Commun Health Nursing* 3:2, 59-67, 1986.

Gardner MS: *Public health nursing,* ed 2, New York, 1928, Macmillan.

Glass LK: The historic origins of nursing centers. In *Nursing centers: meeting the demand for quality health care,* Pub No 21-2311, New York, 1989, NLN.

Hirsch MB, Zabin LS, Streett RF, and Hardy JB: Users of reproductive health clinic services in a school pregnancy prevention program, *Public Health Rep* 102:307-316, 1987.

Holman E: Nursing centers—state of the art and future initiatives: services and marketing strategies. In *Perspectives in nursing 1989-1991,* Pub No. 41-2281, New York, 1990, NLN.

Institute of Medicine: *The future of public health,* Washington, D.C., 1988, National Academy Press.

Janosik EH and Miller JR: Group work with the elderly. In Janosik EH and Phipps LB, eds: *Life cycle group work in nursing,* Monterey, Calif., 1982, Wadsworth.

Jamieson MK: Block nursing: practicing autonomous professional nursing in the community, *Nurs Health Care,* 11(5):250-253, May 1990.

Kalisch PA and Kalisch BJ: *The advance of American nursing,* ed 2, Boston, 1986, Little, Brown.

Knopke HJ and Diekelmann NL: *Approaches to teaching in the health sciences,* Reading, Mass., 1978, Addison-Wesley.

Lawler TG and Valand MC: Patterns of practice of nurse practitioners in an underserved rural region, *J Commun Health Nurs* 5:187-194, 1988.

Lewin K: Group decision and social change. In Newcomb TM and Hartley EL, eds: *Readings in social psychology,* New York, 1947, Holt.

Loomis ME: *Group process for nurses,* St. Louis, 1979, Mosby.

Luft J: *Group process: an introduction to group dynamics,* ed 2, Palo Alto, Calif., 1970, Mayfield.

Marram GP: *The group approach in nursing practice,* ed 2, St. Louis, 1978, Mosby.

Maternal and Child Health Program: *St. Paul Adolescent Health Services Project,* St. Paul, Minn., undated, St. Paul-Ramsey Medical Center.

Moch SD: Promoting health with role-reversal couples, *J Commun Health Nurs,* 5:195-202, 1988.

National Association of Community Health Centers, Inc.: *Community health centers: a quality system for the changing health care market,* McLean, Virg., 1986, National Clearinghouse for Primary Care Information.

National League for Nursing, Council for Nursing Centers: *Connections,* New York, 1992, Winter, The League.

National Organization for Public Health Nursing: *Manual of public health nursing,* ed 3, New York, 1939, Macmillan.

News, community nursing centers gaining ground as solution to health issues, *AJN* 92(7):70-71, 1992.

Parish nursing, *Pennsylvania Nurse* 48:1, July 1993, Pennsylvania State Nurses Association.

Riesch SK: Nursing centers: an analysis of the anecdotal literature, *J Professional Nurs,* 8(1):16-25, 1992.

Riner MB: Expanding services: the role of the community health nurse and the advanced nurse practitioner, *J Commun Health Nurs* 6:223-230, 1989.

Sampson E and Marthas M: *Group process for the health professions,* New York, 1981, Wiley.

Schmitt MH: Groups for the chronically ill. In Janosik EH and Phipps LB, eds: *Life cycle group work in nursing,* Monterey, Calif., 1982, Wadsworth, pp. 266-290.

Schroeder MA: Computers in nursing: applications for ambulatory care, *Nurs Econ* 5(1):27-31, 1987.

Smyth K: Justice and cooperation: moving ambulatory care practice into the 21st century, *J Ambulatory Care Manage* 10(3):76-81, 1987.

Verran JA: Testing a classification instrument for the ambulatory care setting, *Res Nurs Health* 9:279-287, 1986.

Watson WL: Intervening with aging families and Alzheimer's disease. In Wright LM and Leaher M, eds: *Families and chronic illness,* Springhouse, Pa, 1987, Springhouse, pp. 381-404.

Zander A: *Making groups effective,* San Francisco, 1982, Jossey-Bass.

Selected Bibliography

Bull CN and Bane SD: Growing old in rural America: new approach needed in rural health care, *Aging* 365:18-25, 1993.

Chamberlin RW: *Beyond individual risk assessment: community wide approaches to promoting the health and development of families and children,* Washington, D.C., 1988, National Center for Education in Maternal and Child Health.

Hatch JW and Voorhorst S: The church as a resource for health promotion activities in the black community. In National Institutes of Health: *Health behavior research in minority populations: access, design, and implementation,* NIH Pub. No. 92-2965, Washington, D.C., 1992, The Institutes.

Henshaw SK, Kenney AM, Somberg D, and Van Vort J: *Teenage pregnancy in the United States: the scope of the problem and state responses,* New York, 1989, Alan Guttmacher Institute.

Kinney CK, Mannetter R, and Carpenter MA: Support groups. In Bulechek GM and McCloskey JC: *Nursing interventions: essential nursing treatments,* ed. 2, Philadelphia, 1992, W.B. Saunders, pp. 326-339.

Oda DS and Boyd P: The outcome of public health nursing service in a preventive child health program: phase 1, health assessment, *Public Health Nurs* 5:209-213, 1988.

Redman B: *The process of patient education,* ed. 7, St. Louis, 1993, Mosby.

Schank MJ: Responsiveness of the well elderly to healthcare education programs, *Home Health Care Nurse* 10:47-52, 1992.

Selby ML, Riportella-Muller R, Sorenson JR, and Walters CR: Improving EPSDT use: development and application of a practice-based model for public health nursing research, *Public Health Nurs* 6:174-181, 1989.

Stimson DH, Charles G, and Rogerson CL: Ambulatory care classification systems, *Health Serv Research* 20(6):683-703, 1986.

The Medicaid Access Study Group: access of Medicaid recipients to outpatient care, *N Engl J Med* 330(20):1426-1430, 1994.

Thibodeau JA and Hawkins J: Evolution of a nursing center, *J Ambulatory Care Manage* 10(3):30-39, 1987.

Thornton J: Developing a rural nursing clinic, *Nurse Educator* 7(2):24-29, 1983.

Zuvekas A: Community and migrant health centers: an overview, *J Ambulatory Care Manage* 13:13-21, 1990.

Unit Six

Management of Professional Commitments

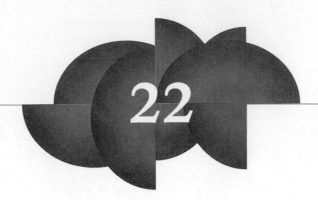

Utilizing Management Concepts in Community Health Nursing

OBJECTIVES

Upon completion of this chapter, the reader should be able to:

1. Explain how a staff-level community health nurse uses management skills in the practice setting.
2. Distinguish between the informal and formal structure of an organization.
3. Describe the five management functions used by community health nurses.
4. Discuss the elements involved in analyzing a caseload and a client care situation.
5. Differentiate between the terms *team nursing, primary nursing,* and *case management.*

6. Describe factors to consider when scheduling community health nursing activities.
7. Explain factors that affect priority determination and intensity of community health nursing service in caseload management.
8. Describe the use of delegation in community health nursing practice.
9. Identify select ANA standards that can guide management practice in a community health nursing setting.

The old scientific management was about ensuring control. The new will be about making sense out of chaos.

D.H. FREEDMAN

The community is an exciting setting that provides challenging opportunities for community health nurses. An outstanding characteristic of community health nursing is the independence of its practitioners. In any one day, a community health nurse may decide what families to visit and in what order they will be visited. During that day the nurse may make a nursing diagnosis and carry out nursing interventions without nursing supervision, without a doctor's order, or without even talking to another nurse. That day, he or she may also receive new referrals and make decisions on their priority. Furthermore, the nurse may be carrying out nursing care indirectly through delegation to registered nurses, licensed practical nurses, or home health aides. When these health personnel are caring for clients under the nurse's supervision, the nurse is responsible for the care given by them.

This independence and delegation in community health nursing practice must be accompanied by knowledge of management concepts. Knowledge of management concepts helps the community health nurse to provide care, directly and indirectly, to families and aggregates and to evaluate the quality of health services that the client receives. Available resources, such as finances and personnel, need to be managed so that maximum productivity, efficiency, and quality of care are achieved.

Managing the extensive amounts of data that community health nurses must collect and use is increasingly complex. Computerized management information systems are crucial for today's community health nurse manager: these systems are being used by CHN agencies across the country to facilitate effective and efficient resource management. Staff nurses use these systems as well to schedule and document client care and to communicate with members of the health care team.

Whatever role a nurse assumes in the community setting, be it staff nurse, supervisor, or administrator,

the nurse will participate in leadership and management functions to some degree. Community health nursing, like the management process, is a logical activity that helps clients, families, and aggregates to make goal-directed changes. The nurse facilitates these changes through the work of others. Thus a conscious application of the management process to nursing care at any level can make the nurse more effective in arranging his or her own personal workload, as well as in functioning within a larger system.

This chapter briefly analyzes concepts of management and then examines how the community health nurse can use them. A limited discussion of the historical development of management thought is also shared. Knowledge of the evolution of management concepts provides the information an individual needs to formulate a personal philosophy of management.

THE HISTORICAL DEVELOPMENT OF MANAGEMENT CONCEPTS

There are numerous leaders in the field of management who contributed to its development. To list them all here would be an almost impossible task. When reviewing the development of management thought, however, one can see that modern concepts of management have evolved over time. Historically, emphasis was placed on analyzing the functions and processes of management tasks, without taking into consideration the needs of the worker (see Chapter 17). Today, the trend is for managers to apply systems concepts (refer to Chapter 7) in the work environment in order to determine how to maintain employee satisfaction and to increase productivity and efficiency.

Frederick Taylor is the founder of the scientific management movement. His belief was that the planning of tasks needs to be separated from their performance. In relation to this thought, he felt that managers should be responsible for the planning and controlling of tasks and that employees should assume responsibility for production. He conducted time and motion studies to determine the best way to accomplish tasks, to develop work standards, and to identify how to divide the work between managers and employees. Taylor's book, *The Principles of Scientific Management,* was published in 1911.

Henri Fayol expanded on Taylor's thoughts by identifying a composite of well-defined functions and

We thank Judith Harris, RN, MPH, Vice President, Nursing Services, Visiting Nurse Association of Greater Philadelphia, for her assistance with this chapter.

tasks for managers. In 1916 he published his ideas about management, which were that managers have five basic functions: planning, organizing, commanding, coordinating, and controlling (Koontz, O'Donnell, and Weihrich, 1986, p. 11). With some minor changes, these functions are still used by most authorities on management.

Significant criticism of management occurred during the first half of the twentieth century, because managers emphasized task performance without looking at worker satisfaction. As a result of this criticism, modern management trends that stress the importance of examining employee needs emerged. The classic Hawthorne experiment conducted by Elton Mayo clearly demonstrated to management the value of looking at employees as people.

The Hawthorne studies of the Western Electric Company during the 1920s and 1930s applied the principles of psychology, social psychology, and sociology to the understanding of organizational behavior. The researchers of this study began by investigating the relationship between physical conditions of work and employee productivity; however, they found that social variables were much more important to productivity. The outgrowth of the Hawthorne study was the development of the concept of human relations, or the study of human behavior for the purposes of attaining higher production levels and personal satisfaction (Koontz, O'Donnell, and Weihrich, 1986, p. 13). The human relations concept has expanded into the behavioral science approach to management. A trend toward emphasizing employee satisfaction to increase production on the job is still visible. Employee motivation, the workplace as a social system, leadership within the organization, communication within the system, and personal and professional employee development are five major areas of concern to managers who use behavioral science methods and principles. Writings by Chris Argyris, Chester Barnard, Douglas McGregor, Kurt Lewin, Rensis Likert, Robert Tannenbaum, and others give a more in-depth perspective on the behavioral science movement.

The systems approach to management was another development among management concepts. With the systems approach, both the structure and the processes of an organization are analyzed. Emphasis is placed on examining how all the parts of an organization interact and interrelate to achieve the goals of the organization. Systems managers recognize that a change in one part of the organizational system affects all the other parts, just as practitioners using a systems approach recognize that a change (illness) in the family unit affects all other members of the family system (refer to Chapter 7).

Changing the manner in which systems are explored has been described by Gleick (1987) in his book *Chaos,* which examines "the science of the global nature of systems" (p. 5). In contrast to Taylor's work and the work of others who followed him in developing the science of management, Gleick examines systems holistically. Taylor and those who followed him used a reductionistic approach: complex phenomena could be understood by reducing them to their basic building blocks and looking at the mechanisms through which they interacted. For example, a health care agency would be analyzed department by department for its effectiveness under the science of reductionism. The sum of how each department functioned would result in the effectiveness of the organization. The science of chaos examines the system holistically and focuses on the dynamics of the overall system and the order that comes from the interactions of the parts of the whole. A basic tenet of the science of chaos is that the tiniest change in a system, be it the water dripping from a faucet or people working in an agency, causes profound changes in the system. "The simplest systems are now seen to create extraordinarily difficult problems of predictability" (Gleick, pp. 7-8). Further, though the conditions that bring about change and the change itself appear to be random, there is order in the chaos created in systems by miniscule changes (Gleick, pp. 7-8).

The importance of the science of chaos for managers, leaders, and all employees is discussed by Freedman (1992) who bases his thoughts on the work of both Gleick (1987) and Senge (1990). Managers think that they know their organizations because they believe in the reductionistic theory of cause and effect. If the workers for whom they are responsible carry out their job descriptions, the objectives of the organization will be reached. However, the relationship between cause and effect is much more complicated than many people understand. People working in an organization, when asked what they do, describe the daily tasks that they do rather than the system in which they work. Frequently workers believe that they have little impact on this system. The science of chaos tells managers that their tiniest actions, along with the smallest thoughts and actions of employees, make a dramatic impact on the agency system. Senge (1990) reports that managers who master systems thinking have "learning organizations" (p. 37). Such organizations are highly decentralized and decision-making at the department level maintains order throughout to constantly adjust to change.

Today community health nurses work in complex systems. To function effectively in these modern health care systems, the community health nurse must know not only nursing theory but management theory as well. Traditionally, management concepts were not emphasized during a nurse's academic study, even though nurses were expected to carry out management responsibilities in practice. Now it is recognized that the task of organizing health care delivery can be made easier and more powerful with knowledge of management concepts. That is why principles of management are covered during a nurse's basic educational preparation.

THE ORGANIZATIONAL STRUCTURE OF HEALTH CARE DELIVERY

The number of health care delivery systems in which community health nurses may work is increasing. They work in diverse health and health-related organizations, each of which may have a differing organizational structure and way of delivering nursing services.

Nurses must know the organizational structure of their employing agencies so that they can determine how to use agency resources and to identify appropriate ways to effect change within the organization. Organizational structure encompasses the formal and informal patterns of behavior and relationships in an organization. This includes both formal and informal position allocations, as well as the chain of command and the channels of communication.

The Informal Organizational Structure

The informal organizational structure refers to the personal and social relationships of people who work together. Informal relationships have no formal power. However, they can have a major impact on the organization and its management. The way in which a manager is viewed by the staff does influence the manner and effectiveness of her or his management.

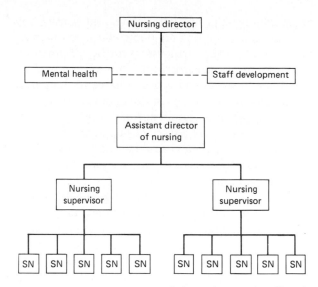

Figure 22-1   An organizational chart showing staff and line positions.

The Formal Organizational Structure

Formal organizational structure defines which people will do which tasks so that the objectives of the organization can be accomplished. It is the power structure of the organization. The rules, policies, procedures, control mechanisms, and financial arrangements of the organization are all part of the formal structure. The schematic organization is part of this formal structure and can be seen in an organizational chart.

Organizational Chart

An organizational chart diagrams the relationship among members of the organization and indicates the structure of authority, formal lines of communication, and levels of management and delegation. These all interrelate to accomplish the goals of the organization. An example of an organizational chart is presented in Figure 22-1.

An organizational manual supplements an organizational chart by supplying information about the requirements of the various job positions represented on the chart. Organizational charts and manuals are useful tools that describe the formal relationships in a particular organization. They do not show the informal relationships that exist.

Usually there are two types of positions in an

organization: *staff* and *line*. Figure 22-1 shows how staff and line positions are depicted on an organizational chart. The line structure is the basic framework of an organizational structure. The staff nurse is in a direct line position and is accountable to the person directly above him or her on the organizational chart. The term *staff nurse* should not be confused with *staff personnel*. The staff personnel supplement the line personnel in an advisory capacity. They are extensions of the administrator but usually have no authority to direct the actions of persons in the line position. Authority can, however, be delegated in several directions from both staff and line positions.

The line organization is characterized by a direct flow of authority from top to bottom. Each position has general authority over the one directly below it. Authority is inherent in line positions. For example, the assistant director of nursing has authority over the nursing supervisor, who in turn has authority over the staff nurse. Persons in staff positions, on the other hand, are delegated authority by top-level administrators (nursing director) to carry out specific tasks and responsibilities. Authority is not inherent in staff positions.

A manager must have a basic understanding of organizational power relationships in order to manage effectively. Four types of power relationships evolve in any organization:

1. Authority: the power to direct the actions of others
2. Responsibility: the obligation to carry out or perform tasks in an acceptable way
3. Accountability: the obligation to answer for one's actions
4. Delegation: assigning and empowering one person to act for another with the responsibility for the act remaining with the person who assigned it

Organizational structure and resulting power relationships in a health care agency assist personnel in all positions to carry out effectively the functions of management. It would be impossible to manage if such a structure did not exist. Effective and efficient management can occur only when personnel understand what they are responsible for and to whom they are accountable. Ignoring the power relationships in an organization can create real difficulties. Illustrative of this are the actions taken by the community health nurse in the following situation.

A community health nurse identified a need for a family planning program in two of the census tracts she served. Knowing that the county health department did not include these services, she independently arranged a group meeting in the clubhouse at a local park to discuss the need for these services with the people of the community. This was done without discussing the action with her supervisor.

Twenty community members attended the meeting. They quickly became emotionally involved in the issue and wanted immediate action taken by the health department to initiate such a service. The nurse became uncomfortable because she recognized that she did not have the power to make a definite commitment regarding the establishment of a new program. The community members became frustrated with the nurse's lack of action.

Had proper channels within the agency power structure been utilized, this situation would probably have been handled differently.

While examining this situation, the following questions quickly become obvious: Did the nurse have the authority to organize this meeting, and was she acting in a responsible and an accountable manner? What were her objectives for the meeting and did she clarify them for herself and the group?

When planning a meeting with a group such as the one above, it is crucial to seek the advice of individuals within the organization who have the authority to make decisions. When this is not done, it can result in stress and frustration for all parties involved. If the nurse had gone to her supervisor before the meeting, she would have been aware of the types of commitments she could make during the meeting. If, for instance, the health department did not have adequate resources to staff a family planning clinic, the group goal might be to look at alternative ways to obtain funding for family planning services in the community, rather than discussing only how the health department might provide these services.

Organizational Policies

Another component of the formal organization structure that maximizes functioning is organizational policies. Policies define the limits of acceptable activities and provide structure and guidelines for employee decision-making. They are generally developed to handle situations that occur consistently in daily practice. Policies that address how to handle referrals (refer to Chapter 10), when and how to conduct nursing audits (refer to Chapter 23), and benefits staff will have, such as travel allowance, are a few examples of policies commonly found in a community health agency. These types of policies provide direction for decision-making.

When policies are absolute, with no flexibility, they are considered *rules*. Rules are usually established in order to ensure client and staff safety and quality of care. The following are examples of rules:

- "No home visits are to be made at night in census tract 3 without an escort."
- "No immunizations are to be given until an allergy history has been taken."
- "Every fifth record closed to service must be audited."

When nurses accept employment within a health setting, it is assumed that they accept responsibility for following, enforcing, and informing others about agency policies. This means that the conditions of employment should be clearly understood before the nurse accepts a position within an organization. Otherwise the nurse may end up in a situation where it is necessary to follow certain policies that are inconsistent with her or his philosophy of practice.

Nursing personnel at all levels may be involved in writing policies. Policy statements should include the following items:

1. Reason for establishing the policy (philosophy behind the policy)
2. Actual policy statement
3. Guidelines for implementing the policy
4. Lead persons or department interpreting the policy
5. Persons affected by the policy

If used effectively, policies can increase the efficiency and ease with which individuals carry out their functions within an organization. Difficulties with implementing a policy will occur, however, if employees do not understand the reason for the policy, if employee input is not obtained when the policy is being formulated, if the policy is not clearly written, or if policies become numerous and prevent necessary flexibility for nursing practice.

ANA STANDARDS FOR PRACTICE

The American Nurses Association (1991) has developed "Standards for Organized Nursing Services and Responsibilities of Nurse Administrators Across All Settings." The standards (refer to box on p. 844) provide guidance to nurse administrators in addressing the rapid changes sweeping all settings where nursing care is delivered. For each of the nine standards there is a rationale and criteria. Neophyte and experienced nurses can use the standards to make decisions about the most effective employment opportunities, and both experienced and inexperienced students and nurses need assistance in how to use them. Agencies that follow these standards or similar ones are likely to promote organizational and staff growth and provide direction for the delivery of quality nursing services as well.

DEFINING MANAGEMENT LANGUAGE

Management is the planning, organizing, directing, coordinating, and controlling of activities in a system so that the objectives of that system are met. For community health nurses, that system may be represented by any number of settings in which the nurse practices, such as a public health agency, ambulatory care setting, a school, an industrial plant, or a home care organization.

Administration is a term that is often mistakenly used interchangeably with *management*. The principles of management and administration are the same, but the scope of functioning for managers and administrators varies. For instance, both administrators and managers set goals, but the administrator sets goals for a department, whereas a staff nurse sets personal goals when managing her or his workload responsibilities.

Leadership is influencing others to reach desired goals. Any organization has both formal (appointed) leaders and informal (those chosen by the group) leaders. "A leader is able to command trust, commitment, and loyalty of followers. Most work is done by people who do not have a formal leadership position. Many of these people are leaders who take responsibility for reaching group goals. A leader is the person who communicates ideas to others and influences their behavior to reach an objective" (Douglass, 1988, p. 3). Thus effective nurses at any organizational level use leadership and management skills: they positively influence those about them to promote the common

---

◀ *ANA Standards for Organized Nursing Services and Responsibilities of Nurse Administrators Across ANA Settings* ▶

Standard I. Philosophy and Structure

Organized nursing services have a philosophy and structure that ensure the delivery of effective nursing care.

Standard II. Nurse Administrator

Organized nursing services are administered by qualified and competent nurse administrators.

Standard III. Fiscal Resource Management

The nurse executive determines and administers the fiscal resources of organized nursing services. The nurse executive has an interactive role in the determination of the organization's fiscal resource requirements and their acquisition, allocation, and utilization.

Standard IV. Nursing Process

Within organized nursing services, the nursing process is used as the framework for providing nursing care to recipients.

Standard V. Environment for Practice

An environment is created within organized nursing services that enhances nursing practice and facilitates the delivery of care by all nursing staff.

Standard VI. Quality Assurance/Improvement

Organized nursing services have a quality assurance/improvement program.

Standard VII. Ethics

Organized nursing services have policies to guide ethical decision making based on the code for nurses.

Standard VIII. Research

Within organized nursing services, research in nursing, health, and nursing systems is facilitated; research findings are disseminated; and support is provided for integration of these findings into the delivery of nursing care and nursing administration.

Standard IX. Cultural, Economic, and Social Differences

Organized nursing services provide policies and practices that address equality and continuity of nursing services, and that recognize cultural, economic, and social differences among recipients served by the health care organization.

From American Nurses Association: *Standards for organized nursing services and responsibilities of nurse administrators across all settings,* Washington, D.C., 1991, The Association, pp. 3-10. Reprinted with permission of the American Nurses Association.

good and they apply management principles to their practice.

THE MANAGEMENT FUNCTIONS OF THE COMMUNITY HEALTH NURSE

The five management functions carried out by the community health nurse are planning, organizing, directing, coordinating, and controlling. These management functions help to link the entire organizational system together and assist the nurse in effectively managing workload responsibilities. Managing is done on many levels by nurses, depending upon their place in the organizational structure and their interest, skills, and educational background.

The director of nursing in an agency will probably spend more time managing than the staff nurse, at a level that affects all staff members. Staff nurses must,

however, use management functions to deliver nursing services. They can also influence how a director of nurses carries out management functions.

Management is a process that has both interpersonal and technical aspects and that uses human, physical, and technological resources to achieve well-defined goals (Koontz, O'Donnell, and Weihrich, 1986). Figure 22-2 depicts all the variables that influence how the manager implements the five functions of management. It also illustrates the cyclical nature of the management process (planning, organizing, directing, coordinating, and controlling); the functions overlap and do not always follow a sequential pattern.

Planning

Planning assists an organization in establishing a vision for the future. It means deciding in advance

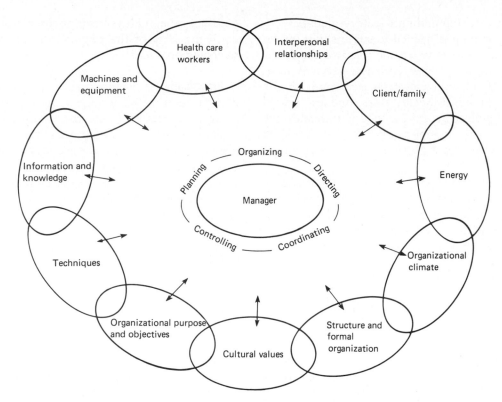

Figure 22-2 The manager links together subsystems of the organization. (From Clark CC and Shea CA: *Management in nursing: a vital link in the health care systems,* New York, 1979, McGraw-Hill, p. 9.)

what must be done and what the organization wants to achieve. Without planning, no set goals will be accomplished.

Planning gives purpose and direction to the decision-making process. It is the management function most often neglected because of the emphasis placed on carrying out day-to-day activities, the attitude that planning takes too much time, and the tendency for individuals to resist change. Planning is an important activity because it helps the organization to remain dynamic, to identify standards, and to determine what or who requires organization or direction. It increases the likelihood that activities will be orderly, predictable, and less costly. Most important, planning improves the quality and effectiveness of nursing care. Although planning does not guarantee the quality of outcomes, the evaluation aspects of this process help a manager to identify strengths and needs within the organization.

Health care planning should include both the provider and the consumer. Emergencies may necessitate individual decision-making and planning. In these situations it is important for the decision maker to explain to others involved in the process the circumstances and reasons for the emergency decision.

Planning uses past, present, and future information to project what services should be provided. Currently, the impact of political, social, economic, and technical forces is directly influencing the types of services provided by community health agencies and the type of personnel needed to implement these services. For instance, in health departments that provide bedside care, money allocated from taxes is increasingly scarce and third-party payments for home health care are an increasingly larger part of the health department budget. This budget change comes about because of demographic changes in the population, as well as social and political policy about the appropriateness of tax money for tertiary health care. Some of the results of these changes include a greater emphasis on delivering home health care, greater use of ancillary personnel such as home health aides, and a greater focus on older people who need "hands-on" care rather than on clients who need health teaching and anticipatory guidance.

Careful planning is needed to successfully implement nursing services when the focus of these services has changed. Activities such as in-service education for staff, planning for increased time for the supervision of home health aides, and the added paperwork involved in carrying out a home health care program are a few examples of factors that should be considered when one is planning for increased home health services.

An example of a staff nurse putting the planning process into action would be when working with the nursing supervisor to establish a clinic for the homeless in the staff nurse's area. Together they would develop a written plan that might include the following:

1. Specific, measurable objectives related to establishment of the conference
2. Time schedule for achieving objectives
3. Process for carrying out the objectives, including necessary resources
4. Evaluation methods to measure the success of the plan in relation to completion of objectives
5. Timetable for periodic evaluation

A staff community health nurse also implements the planning function when structuring the workday and when carrying out caseload management activities. The data gathering, diagnosis, and goal-setting phases of the nursing process are used for activities such as those described above.

During planning, many needs and goals may be identified and priorities for them must be set. The following points should be considered when priorities are being set.

Economic Impact. Considering the results if something is or is not done is crucial. Although an immunization campaign against rubella may be costly, it is much less expensive socially and economically than paying for the care of children who have congenital deformities resulting from in utero rubella. The cost-benefit aspect must also be considered. In one community, for instance, the health department discontinued a screening clinic for the geriatric population because it was not cost effective. It cost the health department $40 per client to do the screening, and 90% of those screened had recently received the same screening from their private physicians and planned to do so again in the future. This was duplication of services at a high cost to the health department.

Methods other than a screening clinic could be used to reach the 10% of the population not receiving the screening privately.

Practicality. Is the program necessary? What is being done currently? Will enough people benefit from it to make it worthwhile? Are there sufficient resources available, such as work force and money, to accomplish the stated goals? Is there enough organizational and community support to carry out the program? Does it meet the needs of the community? All of these are questions to be answered in relation to the practicality of the program.

Feasibility. Does the program fit the organization's policies and priorities? Are the resources available to carry out the program?

Legal Requirements. The organization must follow its legal mandates. The official health department, for example, has a legal mandate to control communicable disease. Home health agencies have regulations imposed by funding agencies; an example is Medicare, which mandates that home health aides have at least 12 hours of in-service education on a yearly basis. Thus an agency using home health aides would need to carefully plan its staff development program so that this requirement was met.

Urgency of the Situation. An emergency situation is usually given top priority. In one urban community, for instance, a large Mexican restaurant used home-canned chili peppers that were improperly prepared. Many of the restaurant's patrons developed botulism. This produced an emergency health situation that required urgent action to pinpoint the source of the poisoning and all patrons affected by the botulism agent. The county health department launched an immediate epidemiological investigation to pinpoint the cause. Many other health department activities were stopped or modified so that this serious problem could be given top priority. Once priorities are established, a manager must organize activities so priority goals can be implemented.

Increasingly there are competing priorities and demands for the available resources in any one health care organization. Nurses need to be able to defend their request for new or enlarging programs; they also should be able to see the "larger picture" for the total organization and perhaps defer to another colleague or discipline when requests or priorities conflict.

Organizing

Organizing determines how a manager implements planning to achieve stated goals. The organizational structure, as previously discussed, facilitates decision-making and assigning of tasks. There are three principal components of any organizational structure: people, work, and relationships. The interrelationship of these three variables is analyzed during the organizing phase to determine the best way to organize activities. A manager's major concerns when organizing are fourfold:

1. *Analysis of the system:* identifying strengths and needs of the present system in order to make it more effective and efficient in the future. Comparing present staff capabilities to the needs evidenced by clients being served is one example of how a system is analyzed.

2. *Analysis of functions:* defining all the tasks that are involved in a particular job and determining the relationships between various jobs. A nurse and supervisor analyzing a staff nurse's responsibilities when she or he has a caseload of eight bedside care clients, 40 families needing health supervision, and work in six schools and two clinics weekly is an example of this principle.

3. *Assigning job responsibilities:* grouping tasks to minimize duplication of effort and assigning responsibilities to individuals who have the knowledge and competence to carry out the job. Responsibility and authority limits should be clearly defined. Again, work with clients who need bedside care illustrates this principle. The home health aide should be assigned only basic physical care and the community health nurse should assess and supervise the care given by the home health aide. If the health care organization has a union, labor agreements may dictate the extent to which managers can expand or contract a role. The agreement may also stipulate who can be selected for a particular position and can impose limitations on innovation and deployment of personnel to carry out assignments.

4. *Implementation:* developing an atmosphere that allows for successful completion of the work to be done by identifying the structure of authority and support mechanisms in the system. Team meetings that provide support, case consultation, and identification of needs illustrate this concept.

Organizing requires a cooperative effort by a health care team working together to achieve the goals of the organization. This managerial function is familiar to community health nurses because they must organize the care of a family around the family's expressed needs and the resources of the health team working with them.

Directing

Effective programs and organizations include all levels of staff in the planning process so that information is disseminated by peers, at least in part, and "topdown" directing is minimized. The purpose of directing is to convey to workers what has occurred during the planning and organizing phases of management. The activities of directing include order giving, direction, leadership, motivating, and communicating.

Order giving involves helping an employee to identify what needs to be done in a way that fosters understanding and acceptance. A community health nurse who clearly and completely tells an aide the details of the physical care needed by a client with a cerebrovascular accident and also allows the aide to ask questions and provide input illustrates how effective order giving can be accomplished.

Direction refers to the effort made in an organization to ensure that all the work is done. Personal and professional guidance for people is basic to the concept of direction. In the community health setting, work activities are focused on the provision of services both to families and to the community. Thus the focus of direction should include guidance that helps staff to effectively intervene both with families and with the community. This helps staff to provide the services and the agency to achieve stated goals.

Employees are more likely to carry out directions if they assist in setting the goals and designing the interventions to reach them. When they are able to understand the justification for organizational goals and the strategies for meeting these goals, and when there is no doubt regarding what is expected of them, employees are able to carry out responsibilities without constant supervision. This, in turn, leaves more time for staff and supervisors to work on career development plans that focus on staff growth and challenging opportunities in the work setting. Most staff members desire these types of opportunities; however, supervision of home health paraprofessionals is frequently overlooked (Gilbert, 1992).

Leadership is the ability to influence and inspire others to reach the objectives of the organization. Success in leadership is the result of interaction between a leader and those for whom the leader is responsible in a work situation. No single type of leadership is always successful. Rather, a successful leader chooses a method that works for her or him in a particular situation. Leadership is critical to the climate of the organization. Leaders can command people to do things, but the most effective style is to lead so that people want to reach organizational objectives. A successful leader develops a style that fits him or her and the situation. A nursing leader, for instance, may be directive (authoritative or dictatorial) with new nursing staff members because they need more structure in an unfamiliar work environment and democratic with more experienced staff members because they need less direction. Both of these styles can be appropriate. The leader must decide what style to use and when. Each person in a leadership position should analyze her or his own assumptions and develop a style that is comfortable, meets the needs of the situation, and provides motivation for staff. This is defined as leadership and management by situation.

Motivating focuses on analyzing the needs of individual workers. Maslow's hierarchy of needs can provide a theoretical framework for examining worker needs. Maslow has developed a priority schema based on a continuum of needs beginning with those that are physiological and ending with self-actualization. He believes that a worker must satisfy lower-level needs (physiological) before the higher-level ones (self-actualization) become significant (Maslow, 1954). When working with other employees or when analyzing one's own behavior in the job setting, it may be found that work is not satisfying because lower-level needs are not being met. If this is the case, an effective manager attempts to build into the management system rewards that will help the employee to meet these basic human needs.

McGregor's (1960) classic work on management attitudes and employee motivation has promoted a philosophy of management that encourages staff growth and a rewarding environment for employees. His studies have provided the X and Y theories of motivation. Theory X illustrates a negative attitude in its assumptions about human nature, and Theory Y reflects positive attitudes about human nature (McGregor, pp. 33-35, 45, 49).

Theory X makes the following assumptions:

1. The average human being has an inherent dislike of work and will avoid it if at all possible.
2. Most people must be coerced, controlled, directed, or threatened with punishment to get them to put forth adequate effort toward achievement of organizational objectives.
3. The average human being prefers to be directed, wishes to avoid responsibility, has relatively little ambition, and wants security above all.

Theory Y makes the following assumptions:

1. The expenditure of physical and mental effort is as natural as play or rest.
2. A person will exercise self-direction and self-control in the service of objectives to which that person is committed.
3. Commitment to objectives is a function of the rewards associated with their achievement.
4. The average human being learns, under proper conditions, not only to accept but to seek responsibility.
5. The capacity to exercise a relatively high degree of imagination, ingenuity, and creativity in the solution of organizational problems is widely, not narrowly, distributed in the population.
6. Under the conditions of modern industrial life, the intellectual potential of the average human being is only partially utilized.

McGregor promoted Theory Y for the development of a directing style that would motivate employees. It is a more positive approach to working with people. McGregor's theories, like Maslow's framework, can be used as guidelines for managers.

Theory Z was published in 1981 (Ouchi, 1981). It expanded Theory Y and the democratic approach to leadership and focused on developing better ways to motivate and satisfy workers with the goal of increasing productivity. Based on successful Japanese organizations, Theory Z is a participative mode of decision-making that involves everyone who is affected by a decision.

Quality circles, a philosophy of management encouraging employee participation, use the concepts of Theory Z. Quality circles have three major determinents: administrative support, member training, and voluntary participation. They are based on the management belief that workers have abilities that can be used to solve problems that affect their work. Though quality circles have been employed in the acute care setting, they have been little used in community health settings (Schmele, Allen, Butler, and Gresham, 1991).

When using any set of guidelines to develop a management style, remember that work is more satisfying when workers are able to meet their own needs in the work situation. The nurse gives care to, and cares about, clients daily, and this is emotionally taxing. The needs of the nurse must also be met in the work setting.

Communicating with workers is crucial. The manager must be able to convey what is to be done, how it is to be done, who is to do it, and why it is to be done and to provide feedback on the activity. This feedback should emphasize the strengths, as well as the weaknesses, inherent in the employee's activity.

Communication implies a two-way process. The manager uses skill to convey what needs to be done. Noticing staff members' responses, both verbal and nonverbal, is a critical part of the process. If the person does not hear what has been said, appropriate communication has not occurred. The interviewing skills that are a primary tool of community health nurses should be used in communicating with health care workers. These skills will help the manager to direct, coordinate, and control activities within the organization.

Coordinating

Coordination links people on the health care team together to function in such a way that objectives are achieved. A problem arises when health care workers look at objectives in different ways. One nurse may consider nursing in the school setting as a low priority. The supervisor may think it a high priority. Thus coordinating can mean managing conflict. Conflict can promote growth but it can also reduce productivity. Effective coordination reduces and prevents growth-restricting conflict.

Controlling

Controlling is a process that measures and corrects the activities of people and establishes standards so that objectives are reached. The controlling function has three steps: establishing standards, measuring performance criteria, and correcting deviations from normal. The nursing audit, described in Chapter 23, is an example of a controlling function, as is a supervisory or evaluation conference between a staff nurse and a supervisor.

The following are the six characteristics of effective control:

1. *Adjustability.* A control mechanism must be flexible enough to respond to changing situations.
2. *Purposefulness.* A control measure should focus on a specific problem area, not an entire system.
3. *Practicality.* A control measure should not be instituted until it can be implemented reasonably.
4. *Meaningfulness.* A control measure must give direction to other controls and activities, not work against them.
5. *Enforceability.* A control measure should not be instituted until it is possible to put it into effect and to carry out the mandates of the control.
6. *Congruence.* The control measure should be consistent with other control measures and allow the manager to perform other responsibilities and activities.

The staff nurse who delegates care to a home health aide can use these characteristics of control so that quality care is given consistently. The nurse and aide must be flexible in their expectations of each other; an aide who has an ill child at home may not work as well on that day as on another. If the nurse is concerned about a particular client care problem, such as the aide's lack of understanding about maintaining skin integrity, she or he can use conference time to discuss that problem but should not bring all other concerns to the conference. The nurse needs the supervisor's support when working with the home health aide so that the solutions to the nurse's concerns are enforceable and not opposed by the supervisor.

The controlling function can provide direction for growth and thus should be considered a positive function. It is important to examine *strengths* of workers, as well as areas of concern, when implementing the controlling function of management.

MANAGEMENT INFORMATION SYSTEMS (MIS)

Processing data and using information efficiently and effectively is vital in any health care organization.

Appropriate data and information management can facilitate decision-making and increase productivity. With the current emphasis on cost containment, and the highly competitive nature of today's health care market, there is no question that methods must be identified to improve productivity, to enhance decision-making processes, and to use resources more effectively. One such method, the use of computerized information systems, is being advocated across the country. Community health agencies using computer-based processing systems are finding that these systems can be invaluable. The San Bernardino County Public Health Department found, for example, that a computerized format of the nursing process decreased charting time by 50% (Buelow, 1983, p. 1). A copy of one of this agency's computerized records is found in Appendix 22-1. It is revised periodically to reflect changes.

Computerized management information systems are being developed to support the management functions of planning, organizing, controlling, and evaluating. These systems enhance long-range planning processes and assist in resource allocation, personnel management, policy making, and client care documentation. Another primary function of such systems is to provide information needed to ensure efficient personnel performance (Parks, 1982, p. 6). They also provide a systematic generation and distribution of billing, financial, and statistical reports (Harris, 1990).

Management information systems provide systematic, comprehensive information that supports day-to-day activities and future planning. Information is more than raw data or facts that describe places, things, or events. Information is "data that has been processed into a form that is meaningful to the recipient and is of real or perceived value in current or prospective decisions" (Davis, 1974, p. 33). Computer software packages convert data into information.

Management information systems are currently being used by numerous community health care agencies. In 1983 the National Association for Home Care sent a computer services survey to all its members. Of those agencies responding, 72.9% were using computer services (NAHC, 1983, p. 14). One of the best-known management information systems for community and home health care is the one developed by the Visiting Nurse Association of Omaha, Nebraska. This system uses a classification scheme for client problems in community health nursing, that adapts easily to a computerized system of record keeping

(Simmons, Martin, Crews, and Scheet, 1986). As was previously discussed in Chapter 9, this scheme provides a very useful framework when developing nursing diagnoses for community-based practice.

Nationally there is a movement which supports the development of computerized nursing information systems (NIS). In 1982 a group of health care leaders met in Cleveland, Ohio, to discuss issues related to the development of an NIS. It was believed by this group that an NIS could advance nursing knowledge, develop nursing practice, and improve patient care. The NIS study group stressed that, in order for an NIS to be valuable to the nursing profession, it must provide nursing practice information in addition to management data. The study group identified several functions for which nursing practice information is needed. These functions are presented in Table 22-1 (Study Group on Nursing Information Systems, 1983, pp. 101 and 104).

Developing an MIS which meets the information needs of nurses takes careful planning and input from nurses. Computer experts can provide technical knowledge, skill, and advice about appropriate computer packages. However, in order for computer experts to select computer equipment, nurses must be able to identify the information they need for decision-making, as well as the nursing activities that must be supported by specific information sets. Information frequently needed by nurses in community health agencies, and why the information is important, is presented in Table 22-2.

Available computer systems for community health nursing settings still overwhelmingly support billing and the collection of demographic statistics. The fundamental need for rapid and accurate billing and the collection of fees is the reason for this fact. Further, nurses in the community setting are only now becoming computer literate. One large Visiting Nurse Association received a foundation grant to develop a "fully integrated computer system that would increase the cost economics that voluntary, not-for-profit home health care providers require to survive in the extremely competitive home health care market" (Visiting Nurse Association of Greater Philadelphia, 1990-1992, p. 2). During the first three years of the grant, the project developed and demonstrated a computerized voice messaging system for field and office staff to communicate with each other about patient care and defined a comprehensive system for the development of care plans which could be computerized. The final year the grant developed a philosophy for satisfying the information needs of such an agency, produced a methodology for the identification of an agency's information management requirements, produced a methodology for the evaluation and selection of commercially available software, confirmed "open" architecture as the desired bridge between acquired software and internally developed systems, and developed several applications that track and control agency programs.

When developing an MIS, nurses must take into consideration nursing ethics. They must ensure that the rights of both client and staff are protected when information is computerized. Nurses must carefully monitor access to client and personnel data; usually these types of data have limited access requirements placed on them when entered into an MIS.

The development of an MIS can create stress within an organization, especially when staff members have not previously worked with computers. When experiencing this stress, it helps to focus on what can be achieved long range through the use of an MIS. Initially it takes additional time out of one's schedule to become knowledgeable about the functioning of this type of system. However, a new system can, if used effectively, help an agency to improve the delivery of client care services and can reduce indirect service time.

APPLYING MANAGEMENT CONCEPTS IN COMMUNITY HEALTH NURSING

In the community health nursing setting nurses have multiple responsibilities. They may have a large number of families in their caseload, as well as a number of other nursing services to be performed. In addition, community health nurses need to develop collaborative relationships with other disciplines in order to coordinate family care and to establish priorities for home visits and other activities, such as school and clinic services. Community health nurses must also learn how to effectively delegate tasks to other nursing personnel.

Organizing and scheduling community health nursing activities is not an easy task for an experienced practitioner and, therefore, it is often overwhelming to a new staff member. These activities are easier to handle, however, if a new staff member applies management concepts while carrying out daily responsibilities.

TABLE 22-1	1982 Study Group on Nursing Information Systems: Functions for which Nursing Information is Needed

Nursing functions	Activities under each function
Patient care	Making nursing diagnoses
	Setting nursing care goals
	Choosing nursing actions
	Monitoring the quality of care
	Supporting patient education
Resource allocation	Nurse staffing
	Nurse scheduling
	Nursing care demand
Personnel management	Individual nurse-employee data on date of hire, work availability, performance capability, benefits received, experience, education, length of service, salary, etc.
Education	Patients
	Employees
	Students
Planning and policy making	Reports on care provided, resources used and outcomes achieved
	Nursing care cost (patient charges and revenue production)
	Institutional financial management
Investigations	Clinical evaluation
	Nursing research

From Study Group on Nursing Information Systems: Computerized nursing information systems: an urgent need, *Res Nurs Health* 6:104, 1983.

Using Planning Functions of Management as a Staff Nurse

The nurse can more readily carry out responsibilities if the following planning activities of management are used.

Scheduling Regular Conferences with the Nursing Supervisor

Scheduling regular conferences with the nursing supervisor can assist the nurse in analyzing her or his caseload responsibilities and in establishing priorities

22-2   Information Needs of Community Health Nurses: Areas of Computerized Data Collection, Contra Costa County Health Department

Information needs	Purposes for obtaining information
Knowledge of Health Needs of Those Served	
Identity	Provides a baseline for program development or deletion.
Place of residence	Provides a sampling for the correlation of services in any one group.
Family size	
Age groups	Provides a comparative sampling of services needed in a given area.
Socioeconomic levels	
Cultural background	Assists in the evaluation of the validity of ongoing programs.
Kinds of services given	
Nursing Personnel Statistical Requirements	
Actual nurse work hours available for service	If we commit our division to deliver skilled nursing to meet the nursing commitments of a great variety of medical programs, community developments, and research and study projects, we need to be sure we have access to funding and recruitment of the required skills, so that we can adequately meet our commitment.
Variety of referrals and problems handled by nurse	
Distribution of services per nurse	
Correlation of use of nurse work hours with known priority needs	
Variety of work load by nurse, by area	
Ratio of population to nurse coverage	Data provide information about the resources and skills presently available as well as baseline information with which to project skills, time and materials that will be needed in the future to meet new or changing programs and/or changing priorities for unchanging programs.
Ratio of supervision to nurses	
Review for nurse staff evaluation	
Departmental Needs from Nursing Statistics	
Profile of persons receiving nursing service	Provide appropriating bodies with a meaningful description of nurse activity and levels of operation.
Profiles of services given family, clinic and community	
Profile of community itself	Provide agency personnel with a better understanding of community needs.
Supplemental reporting of personal observations, and knowledge of person giving the specific service	Provide mandatory statistical reports for state and federal agencies (e.g., such as funded medical programs and home health agency reports).
Adequacy of service and pertinency of service in relation to agency expectations	

From Keyes G: Why we need nursing statistics. In *Management information systems for public health/community health agencies,* NLN Pub. No. 21-1506, New York, 1974, National League for Nursing, pp. 56-57.

for service (Figure 22-3). With the supervisor's help, the nurse should do both a case analysis of each family that is being seen and a caseload analysis of all the work that is being done.

Case Analysis. The nurse should learn to "diagnose" each case by answering questions such as the following:

1. What are the health problems of this family as viewed by the family and the nurse?

2. What resources does the family have for meeting these problems?
3. What movement does the family wish to make?
4. What resources are there in the community for meeting these needs?
5. What nursing activities are needed to contribute to the solution of the problems and to bring family and community resources into proper relationship with family needs?

6. Are there some parts of the problems or needs which cannot be met at present with the resources available?
7. What has the family done to work toward solving the problem?
8. How effective have nursing interventions and family actions been in resolving current health problems?

This case analysis should be done on a periodic basis, at least every 60 days, so that families who do not wish to make progress can be closed to service until such time as they again wish to work on an area of need. In addition, case analysis helps nurses to look at their approach to families and alter it so that they can be more effective. A written summary, as well as supervisory conferences, facilitates case analyses. A written summary of work with a family, after a given number of visits in a specified time frame, helps nurses to organize their care and their work. In general, nurses find it valuable to summarize a family record after 10 visits have been made or after they have seen the family for 6 months. The controlling function of management is in effect when case analysis is done because work with clients is being measured and corrected.

Caseload Analysis. Study of the caseload will also improve the planning ability of the nurse and will reveal gaps in service. A caseload analysis differs from a case analysis in that it focuses more on examining the quantity of work the nurse is responsible for and the multiple activities assigned than on the needs of individual families. Caseload analysis is done to determine whether a nurse has sufficient time to implement all assigned responsibilities, to ascertain whether time is being used effectively and efficiently, and to identify whether the needs present in a caseload of families reflect the needs of the population being served. Analysis of the caseload may be in relation to many aspects of service—the types and numbers of cases carried, the complexity of problems in the cases visited, the age groups served, the proportion of new referrals received, and the number of emergency or crisis situations, such as individuals with sputum testing positive for tuberculosis. In addition, it examines all the other activities a nurse engages in, such as school visits, clinic services, group work, committee meetings, coordination with other community agencies, and recording and planning time. When the caseload is studied, it is wise to graph or tabulate the

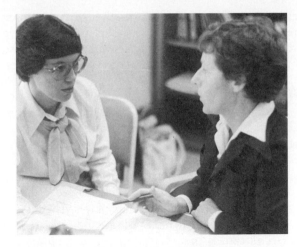

Figure 22-3   A staff nurse and supervisor in conference. Nurse/supervisor conferences are a common occurrence in community health nursing practice. Community health nurses find it helpful to meet with their supervisors on a regular basis to discuss caseload management and staff development issues.

findings so that they may be readily used and compared with caseloads in other areas or with the same area over time.

Simultaneous caseload study by several nurses may be encouraged occasionally to give a general picture of the services provided by the health agency and to allow for comparisons between nurses. When this was done in one health department, it was found that two of 15 census tracts had a disproportionate number of referrals. The result was that workload assignments were reallocated so that work was more evenly divided. The strength of such a procedure is its usefulness in helping the individual nurse to identify the uniqueness of cases in her or his own area and to examine whether there is adequate time to handle the demands of the workload. Freeman (1949, p. 358), in her classic writings on public health nursing supervision, stressed that nurses should not try to develop an "average" in the caseloads they carry but should develop a caseload pattern that will provide optimum community service. This is a key principle to follow today because of the diverse health problems in society and the dramatic changes in the population structure of the United States. When making comparisons, nurses must keep in mind that caseloads should reflect community needs and population characteristics (refer to Chapter 12 for the method of determining these needs and characteristics). One nurse may have a higher geriatric clientele than another nurse because of the uniqueness of the census tract she or he serves.

Use a Tickler System

A tickler system is a card file wherein each family in the nurse's caseload has an identification card displaying data such as name, address, telephone number, and service classification. It assists in scheduling family visits and determining what families need service and when, as well as the type of service needed. When a nurse makes a home visit, the date of this visit and the month and day for the next visit are indicated on the card. The card is then placed under the appropriate month in an index file box. If a tickler system is used effectively, a new nurse can quickly identify priorities for home visiting by noting how frequently the previous nurse visited a family and when the nurse planned the next visit. When a staff nurse has a caseload of families, an organized method such as a tickler file for determining when to see whom is essential.

Set Priorities

This allows the nurse to put activities in their order of importance or caseload priority. The following should be considered when establishing priorities:

Nursing Knowledge. The nurse has a strong theoretical background on which to base priorities for nursing service. This knowledge helps the nurse to analyze the nursing service needs of families who have particular types of problems and direct interventions as well. The developmental framework discussed in Chapters 13 through 19 of this book, along with the nurse's knowledge of crisis theory, for instance, helps a nurse to identify problems across the life span that present stress and, in some cases, crisis. For example, a single, pregnant adolescent may receive higher priority than a 25-year-old pregnant married person. The first client is dealing with the developmental tasks of two age periods—the adolescent and the young adult—and thus is more likely to experience a crisis than the 25-year-old, who is dealing with developmental tasks of only one age period.

Third-party Payors. To be reimbursed by third-party payors for nursing services, the community health nurse must follow established guidelines. For instance, Medicare requires that nursing care be given to clients who need skilled care and are homebound. If these conditions are not met and substantiated by documentation in the client record, Medicare will not pay for nursing services. Nurses do need to consider the financial constraints of their organization so that they meet the requirements established by funders. An organization cannot run without adequate funding. Medicare determines reimbursement for home health agencies via review of the Plan of Treatment which can be sent electronically to the agencies.

Community Needs. Statistical data, input from consumers, and reports from other professionals can often alert the community health nurse to critical community problems or lack of health services in certain areas. For example, if the herd immunity for measles is 10% in a certain section of a county, the community health nurse needs to spend time planning for the provision of immunization service to the total population in this section. This may leave the nurse less time for home visiting. In the long run, however, an immunization campaign could reduce the time the nurse needs for home visits. It takes far more time to individually contact families who need to update their immunization status than to conduct a mass campaign that alerts the total community to the need for immunization protection.

Agency Policies and Priorities. A community health nurse is responsible for following agency policy. Some agency policies read: "Premature infants should be seen weekly for 6 weeks" or "All newborns in the community are to be visited once." If the nurse finds, after analyzing the caseload, that it is impossible to implement an agency policy, she or he should not ignore the policy, but rather should take concrete action to see that it is changed. Many agencies, for instance, have recently found that it is impossible to visit all newborns because of the multiple needs present in the community. Unfortunately, sometimes an old policy is not changed because staff do not take the initiative to have it changed. This can create frustration, especially if staff members are trying to implement an unrealistic policy.

Nursing services should also reflect agency priorities, which should coincide with communities' needs. If a community has a high geriatric population, a health department may place priority on delivering service, such as home health care to the elderly. If an agency places a high priority on home health services, the staff nurse will have to schedule other health supervision visits (maternal-child health, school health, mental health) around home health services. If, on the other hand, community statistics reflect high infant and maternal mortality rates, maternal-child health cases at risk may receive top priority for follow-up. Priorities may vary from one census tract to another, depending on the needs evident in each census tract.

Legal Mandates. Communicable disease followup by the official health department is mandated by law and as such must receive priority when caseload needs are analyzed. Communicable disease follow-up is also a high priority because of its potential threat to the community.

Agency Resources

1. *Staffing.* The availability of health personnel influences the type of services that can be provided. Where limited personnel and other resources exist, only clinic and crisis intervention services may be provided. If only limited resources are available, the community health nurse will have to examine carefully what nursing services are essential and how the most people can be reached in the time available. Some agencies have increased clinic services and group work and decreased home visits because of personnel shortages. If changes such as these do not meet the needs of the population being served, careful documentation may help the agency to obtain additional resources. Too often, however, nurses and other health professionals accept their current state and fail to document the need for increased resources.

2. *Funding.* Financing can affect the type and amount of staffing available within a health agency and also the type of services provided by a particular department. When nursing divisions in a health agency contract for special services, such as school health, family planning, and home health services, they often can expand their nursing staff, but there usually are conditions for the type of services that need to be provided, as well as a time frame designating when these services should be delivered. Health departments, for example, are sometimes paid for school health services

by the board of education. Nurses in these instances may be required to visit the schools at least once a week from September through June.

Use Data from Time and Cost Studies

Data from time and cost studies are useful for determining the average time needed to accomplish certain nursing activities and costs related to these activities. Time studies help a new nurse to be more realistic about the quantity of service that can be provided and the cost of the service being delivered. Time studies are not designed to evaluate the performance of an individual staff nurse. They are done to analyze the average time it takes for all staff members to accomplish certain activities. Even though they are time-consuming and taxing, time studies are extremely valuable because they help a staff nurse and the nursing division to gain a better perspective on the cost-effectiveness of nursing service. In addition, time studies can provide the documentation needed to request additional funding for increased personnel and resources. They also provide guidelines that help a nurse to schedule nursing activities more efficiently.

Now as never before nurses must be aware of the relationship between their productivity and the success of a health care organization. Since the income of an agency is based upon the number of visits each nurse makes, the emphasis in this chapter on time management and prioritizing is based on the simple fact that, in community health, time is money. To believe that caring nurses do not concern themselves with money but with giving quality care is to miss the fact that success with clients is dependent on the financial health of an organization. Nurses, rightly so, are demanding to be adequately reimbursed for their work. Concommitantly they need to understand that the overall economic issues facing health care organizations are their responsibility. Though this issue concerns all areas in nursing, it is most obvious in community health/home health nursing, where each nursing visit is billed separately, unlike the situation in the hospital setting. In the increasingly competitive health care environment, only fiscally sound agencies will survive. Sound agencies will provide all employees with orientation to the funding sources for the various services that are provided, as well as the revenue amounts for these services and the costs of providing them.

Factors to Consider When Scheduling Community Health Nursing Activities

The community health nurse has a work schedule that frequently changes. As previously discussed, there are guidelines that help the nurse to give priority to work. Establishing priorities helps the nurse to schedule activities more effectively. Several other factors need to be considered as the nurse schedules work. Ideally, at the beginning of each month the nurse will develop a calendar that identifies her or his scheduled activities for the month and allows the nurse to see how much time is available for other requests such as new referrals. If new demands for service exceed the time available, the nurse will then have an organized calendar to share with the nursing supervisor that documents the excess demand and that helps to rearrange priorities as necessary. Figure 22-4 presents a portion of a monthly calendar to illustrate how a community health nurse uses it to schedule activities. As can be seen, the nurse's workload for this week is heavy. If too many new referrals are received, the nurse should seek assistance from the supervisor. Staff nurses may use the time set aside for office work to handle excess workload. It is not wise to do this consistently, because office time is essential for appropriate planning, adequate follow-up, and high-quality recording.

Nurses in a home health agency typically list all clients to be seen each day on a weekly calendar; they then daily inform the nurse manager of their plans for that day as priorities become apparent, such as referrals for new clients that must be seen immediately and early morning visits to check the effects of new medication orders. The nurse in this situation makes constant, urgent decisions about priorities, with flexibility as a guiding principle.

The community health nurse should consider the following parameters when scheduling community nursing activities for the coming month/week:

1. Schedule every case and activity requiring service during the month/week.
2. Schedule new visits around scheduled commitments.
3. Make daily visits at the same time each day, if possible.
4. Establish priorities for visits according to need and timing of visits, as illustrated by the following examples:
   A. Families with new babies: around feeding or bath time, to assess how these activities are handled by the family
   B. Crisis cases: as soon as possible
   C. IV medications: provide at specified times
   D. Infectious diseases: last in the day, if possible, to decrease potential for exposure to other families
5. Provide for follow-up of families with long-term and chronic diseases.
   A. Handicapped or ill individuals
   B. Chronic problems
6. Set time aside for shared home visits, when care is delegated to:
   A. Home health aides
   B. Licensed practical nurses
7. Plan time for:
   A. Office activities
      1. Planning visits for the week; planning activities for the next week
      2. Assignment of cases
      3. Supervisory conferences
         a. Ancillary personnel
         b. Supervisor
      4. Recording and reporting
      5. Follow-up
         a. Referrals
         b. Phone calls to agencies, physicians, families
      6. Team meetings
      7. Interdisciplinary conferences, i.e., hospice or case conferences
   B. Clinic activities
      1. Setting up
      2. Time in clinic
      3. Follow-up and evaluation
   C. School activities
   D. Agency or community committee activities

Organizational Staffing Patterns for Community Health Nurses

Another area of concern to nurses who are managing the care of families and groups is the staffing pattern used in a health care organization. Some agencies use a system of primary nursing whereas others use a team nursing system or a case management model. The method of staffing selected by an agency will determine how the nurse schedules and implements monthly activities.

Primary Nursing. If this pattern of organization is used, the community health nurse is assigned a geographical area and is responsible for all open cases, new referrals, and schools in that district. The advantages of this

A.M.	Monday	Tuesday		Wednesday	Thursday	Friday
8:30	Prepare for conferences with personnel regarding assigned cases			Office Preparation Conferences with team TCs Recording		Prepare for shared home visits
9:00	TC Lerner, Mayor, and Vinant families re: time for home visit	School		↓	Mary Jones, 16-year-old AP	Shared visit with LPN to Johnson family—diabetic
10:00	Hartsford family, cleft lip and palate, new parents	Gilbert child, recheck vision, TC to parents if indicated		Hartsford family follow-up visit		
11:00		↓		Vinant family, premie in hospital	Spartan, first baby	Shared visit with HHA—White family
12:00 P.M.	Lunch ——					
1:00	Mayor family, threatened abortion	Mayor family, follow-up visit		Well-child conference set up by RN in A.M.	Endicott family, new in area, multiple sclerosis	Bond family, follow-up visit
2:00	Bond family, new TB	Lerner family, new parents		Conference		Make necessary TCs in relation to referrals or family needs
3:00				Follow-up on referrals from the well-child conference	Staff meeting	Complete recording
4:00	Recording and referrals if any; TCs to MDs or sources of referral	Ring family, rheumatic fever child		Hastings family, TB contacts encourage to go to clinic for exam		Plan for next week's work
5:00						

Figure 22-4 A sample weekly calendar of a staff community health nurse in a county health department that provides both home health care and health supervision services.

method of assignment are several. First, the same nurse follows all clients over time, which results in better continuity of care. Second, this method allows for independent planning and decision-making, which is often less time-consuming and, therefore, less expensive than group decisions. Last, one person serves a geographical area, which requires less travel time than if the same person would have to travel in several different geographic areas.

The greatest disadvantage for primary nursing is the lack of flexibility of work assignment. If an indi-

vidual nurse becomes very busy with referrals or if the nurse becomes ill, coverage for the workload is difficult.

The primary nursing organizational pattern does not, or should not, eliminate peer and supervisory guidance with case analysis. Weekly team conferences (refer to Figure 22-5) can be very important to the successful implementation of the primary nursing concept. The nurse can use weekly conferences to increase knowledge in specific areas, such as available community resources, or to analyze the needs of

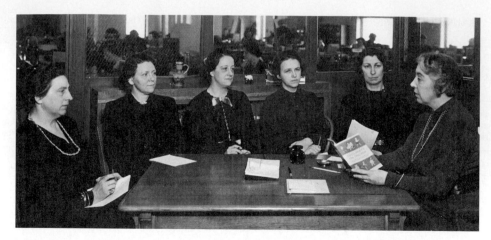

Figure 22-5   The value of team conferences to deal with caseload management concerns, community needs, and agency issues has long been recognized in the field of community nursing. Depicted above is a staff conference being conducted by Alma Haupt (first right in picture), the director of Metropolitan's nursing service. This nursing service was founded in 1909 and significantly influenced the development of management practices in the field of public health nursing. Currently, with the trend toward decreasing the amount of time community health nurses spend in the office, there is a renewed interest in having regular staff meetings in community health agencies. Community health nurses at all levels find it essential to maintain supportive communication with their colleagues. This communication helps them to deal with workload demands, to maintain an objective perspective about practice issues, and to achieve cohesiveness among agency personnel. (Courtesy Metropolitan Life Insurance Company.)

complex families, such as failure-to-thrive families or families with limited resources who are dealing with complicated physical requirements.

Team Nursing. Other agencies use a team nursing method to deliver nursing services to clients in the community. This involves assigning a personnel team consisting of one or more community health nurses, RNs, LPNs, and HHAs to serve a larger geographical area or larger caseload than that in a primary nursing assignment. Each member of the team covers the same geographical area. Team nursing offers the advantage of lending more flexibility to work assignments because there are several team members to share new referrals or care of clients. Perhaps its greatest advantage is that quality of service can improve as a result of the shared planning and problem-solving that occurs in regularly planned team conferences. Disadvantages are that more time is needed for planning because of the number of people involved and travel expenses are often increased.

If cases are divided between nurses who job-share or between part-time nurses, lack of continuity of care may result; this is a major complaint from clients who "see a different nurse every time" and their physicians. When cases are shared, the number of different personnel sharing cases should be minimized and mechanisms to maintain effective and efficient communication should be established.

Case Management. Case management aims, by case type, to achieve quality care at low cost. This is accomplished by standardizing resources with a very clear direction toward specific client interventions for like problems, and with specific expected caregiver and system outcomes. Case managers promote collaboration among all disciplines to provide ongoing care from preadmission to postdischarge while involving the family in the process. Though this sounds like typical community health nursing, emphasis in case management models used by many community agencies is on *case types.* Illustrative of this concept is the case management focus on high-risk children at the Gloucester County Health Department in New Jersey. This health department uses the case management model to promote early identification, evaluation, diagnosis, and treatment of children with special needs and potentially handicapping conditions. The case manager, a nurse who has a caseload of 300 families, is responsible for a team that counsels families, assesses the need for services, promotes and facilitates communication among the team providing services, and monitors the services received (ANA, 1988). With this model, nursing personnel are used efficiently, expected client outcomes are well delineated, timely discharge is facilitated, material resources are used appropriately, and collaborative practice is promoted. (Refer to Chapter 20 for further discussion of case management from a generalized perspective.) The disadvantage is that this model is case-specific rather than general in scope.

Team nursing, primary nursing, and case management can work. Some advantages and disadvantages of each were shared so that nurses will recognize the importance of analyzing strengths and limitations of different organizational patterns. Examining both strengths and limitations helps nurses to identify mechanisms that would minimize limitations when an agency selects a particular organizational pattern. It is possible to mix the patterns within an organization to fit the needs of various clients, nurse teams, and geographical areas.

Determining Priorities in Community Health Nursing Practice

When setting up a calendar for the month, the staff nurse may find that there is not enough time to carry out all the activities that she or he would like to be able to do. Community health nurses cannot meet all the health needs that are evidenced in the community setting. Money, time, and personnel are not limitless, and all three, in fact, are becoming scarcer commodities. As was indicated in Chapters 2, 11, and 12, responsibilities to aggregates in need are based on their vulnerability and their degree of risk. Thus one way of determining whom community health nurses will service is to set priorities for service. Several factors to consider when establishing priorities have already been discussed in the section that addresses how the community health nurse uses the planning function of management in the work setting. In addition to the variables mentioned in that section, such as funding, legal mandates, community needs, and agency priorities, determining priorities based on client needs is useful. In 1953 Ruth Rives wrote a classic

work for public health nurses on the establishment of priorities according to client needs; it was updated in 1958. An update of Rives's article, which provides a basis for determining priorities for nursing services, is provided in Appendix 22-2. Many priorities defined by Rives are still entirely appropriate. Others have been added and some have been deleted.

USING VARIOUS LEVELS OF HEALTH PERSONNEL*

A variety of staffing patterns are used in agencies to deliver community health nursing services. In nearly any community health setting, staff members are involved in offering nursing services who are prepared at various levels. In some agencies RNs (BSN-, AD-, and diploma-prepared), LPNs, and home health aides (HHAs) are hired. In others only RNs and HHAs are available. In yet others, only BSN-prepared RNs are used. Knowledge of the educational preparation of these persons and the agency job descriptions are most helpful tools when nurses need to decide how to use personnel appropriately and determine what type of orientation and staff development is needed. Understanding a state's nurse practice act and the regulations regarding the practice of different levels of personnel is also essential.

Home health aides (HHAs) are often prepared with noncredit courses that last from 8 weeks to 1 year. Coursework usually includes classroom activities and in-hospital clinical preparation. Recent Medicare regulations require that home health aides complete training and competency evaluation programs and have at least 12 hours of in-service per calendar year (HCFA, 1991). In the community setting HHAs can give personal care and assist with housekeeping, marketing, and preparation of meals. Home health aides can give the kinds of personal care that can be taught easily to a family member if there is someone to teach.

The licensed practical nurse (LPN) is prepared to give physical care, to make observations about physical conditions, to carry out special rehabilitative measures after being instructed by the community health nurse, to continue the teaching of clients begun by the registered nurse, and to contribute to the nursing care plan of a client. There is a significant difference in the

*We are indebted to Ruth Carey, former Vice President of Clinical Services, Michigan Home Health Care, Traverse City, Michigan, for the use of this material.

level of care given by LPNs and HHAs. The licensed practical nurse has knowledge and skill that helps in making limited patient assessments and contributing to the development of nursing interventions. Home health aides have knowledge and skill to provide *unskilled* patient care. Both the LPN and HHA, however, are prepared to function under the supervision of a registered nurse. They both make valuable contributions on the health care team.

The registered nurse (RN) prepared at the AD or diploma level has been prepared mostly in acute care institutions where there is a patient-centered approach to care. The RN is usually highly skilled in the care of home health service clients who are ill and who need expert care and observations in the home. Because the RN often has developed expertise in technical procedures, she or he can teach these techniques to other staff and family members. The RN has skill and knowledge to assist in the development of the nursing care plan, especially with clients who have disease conditions. Because the registered nurse's preparation has been primarily patient-centered, she or he should receive orientation in relation to family-centered nursing practice, concepts related to analyzing the needs of populations, and principles relative to the coordination of care and prevention, if she or he is expected to implement all the services provided by community health nurses in a health department. This orientation is a necessity. It is unfair to expect the registered nurse, prepared at the AD or diploma level, to provide comprehensive community health nursing services. She or he has not been prepared to do so. If circumstances exist where only these registered nurses are available, an agency has the responsibility to provide them with orientation and staff development opportunities which adequately prepare them to carry out the demands of the job.

The community health nurse has been prepared at the baccalaureate level in community health, with an emphasis in the educational program on wellness and prevention and experience in the community health setting. She or he is expected to have a family-centered focus and to function in a comprehensive fashion. This entails identifying client strengths and needs and all variables that affect health and illness (physical, social, and emotional), facilitating identification of family health goals, and assisting families to reach their goals. The community health nurse initiates, plans, and evaluates care. In addition, she or he participates in planning for the health needs of the community and works in schools, clinics, and community groups, giving service and functioning as a planning participant to see that needed services are provided.

However, since most graduates begin their work experience in an institutional setting, an orientation that assists them in adapting to the independence of the community is essential. Important elements of this orientation are how to travel safely and efficiently including how to use a map, best routes to use, time management and safety issues, and management of care from a community-based perspective.

The agency job description is a helpful tool for nurses who are in positions where they have to delegate care to various levels of personnel. A job description defines what tasks or functions are appropriate for each level of personnel, based on their educational preparation. Identifying tasks and functions that different levels of staff are capable of handling facilitates the use of all personnel and also the delegation process. The following example illustrates how this is so: in the well-child, immunization, or STD clinic many tasks need to be done, including taking histories, weighing and measuring children, teaching clients, giving immunizations or injections of medication, and drawing blood samples. Some of these tasks are best done by the community health nurse, but others can be done effectively by the LPN or HHA. Knowledge of the educational preparation of personnel and agency job descriptions can help the nurse to decide what may be delegated or assigned. For instance, in one large health department there were five kinds of personnel working in the well-child clinic because activities to be accomplished could be handled by nurses prepared at various levels: the HHA weighed and measured children and set up the equipment needed to run the clinic; the LPNs and RNs gave immunizations; the RNs and community health nurses took immunization histories (determining with parents what their child had had and what was to be given that day); the community health nurse took health and illness histories and counseled and provided education for parents. The pediatric nurse practitioner on the staff carried her own caseload of clients, doing physical examinations and teaching and counseling with parents. Assignments in this situation were based on the complexity of the tasks involved and the preparation each staff member had. Pediatric nurse practitioners, for example, usually have more in-depth preparation to handle complete physicals than does the generalized community health nurse.

Another example of how various levels of personnel can be used to implement nursing services in the community setting is in following up on children with vision and hearing failures from schools. Health departments often have hearing and vision technicians who screen school children, retest those who failed, and then refer the retest failures to the community health nurse for follow-up and referral. It is then the community health nurse's responsibility to see that the follow-up is done. However, lesser-prepared personnel, such as an LPN or clerk, may be taught how to appropriately do the initial contacting of parents by phone to ascertain whether medical care has been obtained and, if so, what the results were. Using lower-level personnel to handle these activities provides more time for the community health nurse to follow up with families who are having difficulty obtaining medical care. In addition to clinic and school activities, home health activities are commonly implemented by differing levels of personnel.

Many home health service clients need to be visited two or three times a week. After the nurse has established a plan of care, visits can often be shared with other personnel, such as the LPN or HHA. Remember, though, that when care is delegated to other personnel, responsibility for care of that client or family remains with the community health nurse. The community health nurse must plan adequate time in her or his schedule to supervise the care delegated to other personnel. Some third-party payors, such as Medicare, require that supervisory visits be made by an RN in a specified time period, such as every two weeks for an HHA when skilled care is being provided (HCFA, 1991).

After orientation, nurses begin to develop familiarity with an organization's policies, procedures, and expectations. For the contemporary professional in the community setting, learning continues. The rapidly changing health care system and resulting complexities of care requirements make it important to have a sound staff development program in an organization.

NURSING STAFF DEVELOPMENT

The American Nurses Association (1990, p. 3) defines nursing staff development as "a process consisting of orientation, in-service education, and continuing education, for the purpose of promoting the development of personnel within any employment setting, consistent with the goals and responsibilities of the employer." The acuity level of client/family care and the rapidity of change in treatment modalities

mandate that nurses in the community setting address their own professional growth. The ANA has developed standards to guide the development of a quality staff development program (refer to the box on p. 862). Nurses can use these standards to judge an employing agency's commitment to the care of clients and the professional growth of its staff.

Using Delegation as a Management Function in Community Health Nursing

In order to carry out the diverse responsibilities of the position, the community health nurse frequently needs to delegate tasks to other health care personnel. When planning responsibilities for others, the community health nurse should:

1. Analyze the nature of the task to be delegated, considering the complexity and the time involved to complete it
2. Determine the capability of the individual staff member to handle the assigned responsibility, especially noting the staff member's educational and experience background and other workload responsibilities
3. Identify the willingness of the staff member to accept responsibility for the assigned activity
4. Determine how much time will be needed to supervise if tasks are delegated to others

Delegation is the process of designating tasks and bestowing on others the authority needed to accomplish these assigned tasks. Delegation does not mean, however, that the community health nurse negates personal responsibility for providing quality care to the families she or he serves. Care given by home health aides or LPNs should never be increased so rapidly that it is impossible for the community health nurse to adequately supervise the care delegated to them. The community health nurse must have sufficient time available to apply the principles of the five management functions when carrying out the following supervisory activities with HHAs and LPNs:

1. Shared home visits with the LPN or HHA on the initial visit to a family (planning, organizing)
2. Development of nursing care plans on each family in the caseload, based on assessment data and input from the LPN or HHA (planning, organizing)
3. Regular conferences with the LPN or HHA to determine guidance and assistance needed in

◄   *ANA Standards for Nursing Staff Development*   ►

Standard I. Organization and Administration

The Nursing Service Department and the nursing staff development unit philosophy, purpose, and goals address the staff development needs of nursing personnel. The organizational structure facilitates the provision of learning experiences for nursing service personnel.

Standard II. Human Resources

Qualified administrative, educational, and support personnel are provided to meet the learning and developmental needs of nursing service personnel.

Standard III. Learner

Nursing staff development educators assist nursing personnel in identifying their learning needs and planning learning activities to meet those needs.

Standard IV. Program Planning

The provider unit systematically plans and evaluates the overall nursing staff development program in response to health care needs, health care trends, nursing personnel's learning needs, and organizational needs and goals.

Standard V. Educational Design

Educational offerings and learning experiences are designed through the use of educational processes and incorporate adult education and learning principles.

Standard VI. Material Resources and Facilities

Material resources and facilities are adequate to achieve the goals and implement the functions of the overall nursing staff development unit.

Standard VII. Records and Reports

The nursing staff development unit establishes and maintains a record keeping and report system.

Standard VIII. Evaluation

Evaluation is an integral, ongoing, and systematic process which includes measuring its impact on the learner, patient, and organization.

Standard IX. Consultation

Nursing staff development educators use the consultation process to facilitate and enhance achievement of individual departmental and organizational goals.

Standard X. Climate

Nursing staff development educators foster a climate which promotes open communication, learning, and professional growth.

Standard XI. Systematic Inquiry

Nursing staff development educators encourage systematic inquiry and applications of the results into nursing practice.

From American Nurses Association: *Standards for nursing staff development,* Washington, D.C., 1990, The Association, pp. 7-13. Reprinted with permission from the American Nurses Association.

specific situations (directing, organizing, coordinating)

4. Periodic shared visits with the LPN or HHA for supervision and reevaluation of the status of the family (directing, coordinating, controlling)
5. Periodic review of family records to evaluate the status of the family and the level of nursing service (controlling)
6. In-service education related to the needs of the staff and the families in the nurse's caseload (directing) when working with home health paraprofessionals; research shows that supervision is a critical component of assuring quality (Moore, 1990; Spiegle, 1987) and per-

sonnel retention (Donovan, 1989; Feldman, 1990).

In community health nursing, management functions are used daily by nurses at every level. The five functions of management—planning, organizing, directing, coordinating, and controlling—are useful tools as nurses work with peers, ancillary personnel, supervisors, and the community in providing nursing care.

Summary

Community health nurses have multiple and diverse responsibilities to handle in the practice setting.

They have found that by applying the principles of management they are more effective in dealing with the multiple and diverse demands in the work environment. Knowledge of the five functions of management is especially helpful. These functions are planning, organizing, directing, coordinating, and controlling. The use of a management information system supports these management functions by using data effectively and efficiently.

The development of management thought has changed over time. Reviewing the historical evolution of management helps nurses to understand why it is useful to implement the five functions of management in the work setting. Analysis of this evolution is also beneficial because it provides a basis for defining a personal philosophy of management.

The use of management concepts in the community health nursing setting is essential. Management principles help the community health nurse to organize and schedule activities, to establish priorities for nursing service, to effectively and efficiently utilize time, and to appropriately delegate responsibilities. All these tasks must be accomplished if the community health nurse is going to deliver quality care to clients in the community.

◀ *An Exercise in Critical Thinking* ▶

Lieutenant General William G. Pagonis led 40,000 men and women who ran the theater logistics during the Persian Gulf War. Following are his remarks about leadership: "To lead successfully, a person must demonstrate two active, essential, and interrelated traits: expertise and empathy. In my experience, both of these traits can be deliberately and systematically cultivated; this personal development is the first important building block of leadership. . . . The good news is that leaders are made, not born. I'm convinced that anyone who wants to work hard enough and develop these traits can lead" (1992, p. 118).

Describe the type of expertise you look for in a leader and share your perceptions of the concept *empathy* as it relates to leadership. Identify your strengths and needs in terms of these two leadership traits and discuss how you would cultivate your leadership abilities.

APPENDIX 22-1
High-Risk Infant and Well Child, Birth to 12 Months

County of San Bernardino

Department of Public Health

163 HRI Program |‾|
164 CHS Program |‾|

1 Name _____

2 Address _____ 3 Census Tract_____

4 Birthdate _____ 5 Gest. Age_____

6 Referring Hospital_____

7 Initial Assessment |‾|

8 Follow Up Assessment |‾|

9 PHN _____

10 Date Planned
   For Next HV_____

11 Flowsheet Closed |‾|

12 Date_____

A = Assessment
√ = WNL
P = Problem
+ = Optimal Problem
    Management

I = Intervention and
Anticipatory Guidance
T = Teach   S = Supervise
D = Demonstrate   C = Contract
L = Literature   P = Physical Care
R = Refer

I = Outcome
1=Goal Met
2=Goal Not Met At This
  Time
3=Lost to Follow Up
4=Refused
5=Client Failed to
  Follow Thru
6=Referred to Another
  Dist. or Co.
7=Continue on Appro-
  priate Flow Sheet

I. PHYSICAL ASSESSMENT A

13 General____
14 Hygiene ____
15 Alert ____
16 Lusty Cry ____

Skin
17 Condition ____
18 Color ____
19 Temp. ____
20 Turgor ____
21 Birth Marks____

Head
22 Shape ____
23 Fontanels ____
24 Scalp ____

Eyes
25 Pupillary
   Response ____
26 Clear ____

Ears
27 Responds to
   Voice ____
28 Nose ____
29 Mouth ____
30 Throat ____
31 Neck Supple____
43 Heart Rate ____

Abdomen
33 Shape ____

34 Cord ____
35 B.Sounds ____

Chest
36 Symmetrical
   Movement ____

Lungs
37 Clear ____

Back
38 Spinal Cord ____

Genitalia
39 Penis/Scrotum ____
   Testes ____
40 Vulva ____

Extremities
41 Symmetrical
   Movements ____
42 Muscle Tone ____
43 ROM ____
44 Gluteal folds ____

Neuro Reflex
45 Palmar Grasp
   (0-4 mos.) ____
46 Rooting
   (0-4 mos.) ____
47 Fencing
   (0-7 mos.) ____
48 Moro
   (1-4 MOs.) ____

Anticipatory Guidance 1
49 Fever Management ____
50 Colic Management ____
51 Thermom. Use ____
52 URI ____
53 Ear Infect____

Goal   0
54 P.A. will be WNL ____
55 Optimal Management
   of Problems ____

Interventions
56 Identify   1
   Abnormalities ____
57 Physical Care
   Required ____
58 PMD Coordination ____

II. GROWTH
   Birth Today % A
59 Ht ____
60 Wt ____
61 HC ____
Goal
62 Growth Components 0
   Within 5-95% ____
63 Demonstrate growth ____
Interventions   1
64 Normal Growth Curve ____
65 PMD Coordination ____
66 Nutrition ____

III. NUTRITION
              Data A
67 Breast-min ____
68   Freq. ____
69 Formula type ____
70   Amt. ____
71   Freq. ____
72 NCAST ____

Anticipatory Guidance
                     I
73 ____
74 ____
75 ____
76 ____
77 ____
78 ____
Goal
79 Age Appropriate   0
   Diet ____
Intervention
80 Nec. Nutrition   1
   Components ____
81 Feeding Tech. ____
82 Equip/BreastCare ____
83 Feeding Sched ____

IV. ELIMINATION A
84 Stool ____
85 Urine ____
Anticipatory Guidance 1
86 Diaper Care ____
87 Constipation
   Management ____
88 Diarrhea Manage. ____
Goal
89 Elimination Pattern 0
   WNL ____
90 Optimal Management
   of problems ____
Interventions
91 Normal Elimination 1
   Patterns ____
92 Diet & Fluids ____
93 PMD Coordination ____

V. DEVELOPMENT A
94 DDST-ADj ____
95 DDST-Chrono ____
96 Phn Assess. ____
Anticipatory Guidance 1
97 Emotional Exp. ____
98 Social Exp. ____
99 Physical Exp. ____
100 Sleeping/Crying ____
101 ____
102 ____
103 ____
104 ____
105 ____
106 ____
107 ____
108 ____
Goal
109 Overall Development 0
    WNL ____
Intervention   1
110 Normal Development ____
111 Stimulation ____
112 PMD Coordination ____

VI. BONDING A
113 Harrison ____
114 Phn Assess ____
115 NCAST ____
Goal
116 Bonding will be   0
    WNL ____
Intervention   1
117 Parenting Skills ____
118 Caregiver Needs ____
VII. CAN POTENTIAL A
119 CAN Scale ____
120 Phn Assess ____
Goal   0
162 CAN Absent ____
121 Low Risk for CAN ____
Intervention   1
122 CAN Flow Sheet ____
123 Agency Coord. ____
124 Mandated Report ____
VIII. SAFETY A
125 Phn Assess ____
Anticipatory Guidance 1
126 ____
127 ____
128 ____
129 ____
Goal
130 Physically Safe   0
    Environment ____
Interventions   1
131 Basic Corrections ____
132 Agency Coord. ____
IX. HEALTH CARE SYS.
                Data A
133 Source ____
134 ER Source ____
135 FIND ____
Goal   0
136 Reg. Health Care ____
Intervention   1
137 Correction of
    Barriers ____
138 PMD/Agency Coord. |‾|

IMMUNIZATIONS (Date Received)
139 DPT _____ 144 HGb ____
140 _____   145 ____
141 _____   146 ____
142 Polio _____ 147 PPD ____
143 _____

REFERRALS

Prob. No.	Ref. Agency	Appt. Date	Appt. Kept	Consult
148				
149				
150				
151				

MEDICAL HISTORY
Severe Illness   152 1_____
                  153 2_____
Hospitalizations 154 _____
165 Preventable |‾| 155 1_____
166 Nonprevent |‾| 156 2_____
Meds-Dose   157 3_____

Prob. No.	Pathology/Deviation	Clinical Notes/Plan	Anticipated Date of Goal Completion
158			
159			
160			
161			

Copyright 1983 County of San Bernardino - Department of Public Health - Division of Community Health Services.
Principal Developer: Janet Buelow, M.S., R.N.   For HRI Program: Original - Chart

High-Risk Infant and Well Child, Birth to 12 Months—cont'd

**SAN BERNARDINO COUNTY DEPARTMENT OF PUBLIC HEALTH
DIVISION OF COMMUNITY HEALTH SERVICES**

Definition of Legend — High Risk Infant and Well Child Flow Sheet

Assessment

Problem = deviation from definition of WNL
+ = deviation from definition of WNL, except problem is being managed
by caregiver following health care provider guidelines and expectations.

Outcome

1 - Goal met: Achievement of WNL and/or optimum problem management of appropriate assessment areas.

2 - Goal not met at this time: Goal not met at this time, caregiver and PHN have initiated interventions to achieve goal.

3 - Lost to follow-up: All resources to locate client have been exhausted.

4 - Refused: Client/caregiver unwilling to plan interventions for goal achievement.

5 - Client failed to follow thru: Client/caregiver appears willing to follow thru with plans but no action is evident.

6 - Referred to another district or county: Client/caregiver has moved and a referral has been initiated.

7 - Continue on appropriate flow sheet: Problem area indicates need for more intensive assessments and interventions than can be documented on this flow sheet.

**SAN BERNARDINO COUNTY DEPARTMENT OF PUBLIC HEALTH
DIVISION OF COMMUNITY HEALTH SERVICES**

Anticipatory Guidance Categories - High Risk Infant and Well Child Flow Sheet

Age	Safety	Nutrition	Development
0-3 months	S-0-1 Bathing S-0-2 Bedding S-0-3 Car and infant seat S-0-4 Prevent falls	N-0-1 Bottle care N-0-2 Bottle carries N-0-3 Bottle propping N-0-4 Breast/formula N-0-5 Burping N-0-6 Vol. Exp.	D-0-1 Bonding D-0-2 Eye tracking D-0-3 Infant swing D-0-4 Mobile D-0-5 Muscle exercise D-0-6 Sibling jealousy D-0-7 Smile response D-0-8 Tactile stimulation
3-6 months	S-3-1 Baby proofing S-3-2 Choking S-3-3 Prevent falls S-3-4 Toy selection	N-3-1 Intro of solids N-3-2 Review formula or Breast feeding N-3-3 Spoon vs bottle N-3-4 Teething	D-3-1 Cradle gym D-3-2 Hand toys D-3-3 Imitates sounds D-3-4 Roll over D-3-5 Sitting Exp. D-3-6 Stranger distrust
6-9 months	S-6-1 Baby proofing S-6-2 Food aspiration S-6-3 Toy selection S-6-4 Walker risks	N-6-1 Cup drinking N-6-2 Finger foods N-6-3 Food selection N-6-4 3 meals/day	D-6-1 Babbling D-6-2 Busy Box D-6-3 Crawling D-6-4 Exploration D-6-5 Object permanence D-6-6 Pincer grasping D-6-7 Separation anxiety
9-12 months	S-9-1 Climbing S-9-2 Poison prevention S-9-3 Streets S-9-4 Wall/floor heater	N-9-1 Dental Hygiene N-9-2 Finger feeding N-9-3 Table foods N-9-4 Weaning N-9-5 16-24 oz. formula	D-9-1 Body parts D-9-2 Consistent limits D-9-3 Discipline D-9-4 Midline activities D-9-5 Nesting toys D-9-6 Nursery rhymes D-9-7 Push and pull

Continued

APPENDIX 22-1

High-Risk Infant and Well Child, Birth to 12 Months—cont'd

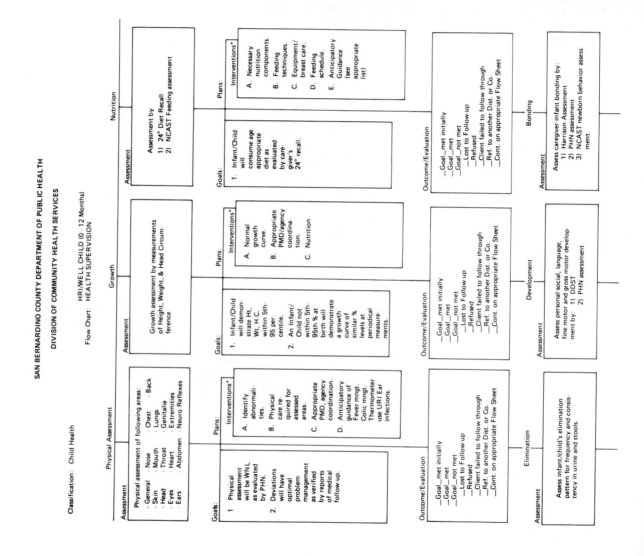

SAN BERNARDINO COUNTY DEPARTMENT OF PUBLIC HEALTH

DIVISION OF COMMUNITY HEALTH SERVICES

Classification: Child Health

HRI/WELL CHILD (0 - 12 Months)
Flow Chart: HEALTH SUPERVISION

Physical Assessment

Assessment

Physical assessment of following areas:

- General - Chest - Back
- Skin - Nose - Lungs
- Head - Mouth - Genitalia
- Eyes - Throat - Extremities
- Ears - Heart - Neuro Reflexes
          - Abdomen

Goals:

1. Physical assessment will be WNL as evaluated by PHN.
2. Deviations will have optimal problem management as verified by reports of medical follow-up.

Plans:

Interventions*

A. Identify abnormalities.
B. Physical care required for assessed areas.
C. Appropriate PMD, agency coordination.
D. Anticipatory guidance of Fever mngt. Colic mngt. Thermometer use URI Ear infections.

Outcome/Evaluation

__Goal met initially
__Goal met
__Goal not met
__Lost to Follow-up
__Refused
__Client failed to follow through
__Ref. to another Dist. or Co.
__Cont. on appropriate Flow Sheet

Growth

Assessment

Growth assessment by measurements of Height, Weight, & Head Circumference

Goals:

1. Infant/Child will demonstrate Ht, Wt, H.C. within 5th-95th percentile.
2. An Infant/Child not within 5th-95th % at birth will demonstrate a growth curve of similar % levels at periodical measurements.

Plans:

Interventions*

A. Normal growth curve.
B. Appropriate PMD/agency coordination.
C. Nutrition

Outcome/Evaluation

__Goal met initially
__Goal met
__Goal not met
__Lost to Follow-up
__Refused
__Client failed to follow through
__Ref. to another Dist. or Co.
__Cont. on appropriate Flow Sheet

Nutrition

Assessment

Assessment by
1) 24° Diet Recall
2) NCAST Feeding assessment

Goals:

1. Infant/Child will consume age appropriate diet as evaluated by caregiver's 24° recall.

Plans:

Interventions*

A. Necessary nutrition components.
B. Feeding techniques.
C. Equipment/breast care.
D. Feeding schedule.
E. Anticipatory Guidance (see appropriate list)

Outcome/Evaluation

__Goal met initially
__Goal met
__Goal not met
__Lost to Follow-up
__Refused
__Client failed to follow through
__Ref. to another Dist. or Co.
__Cont. on appropriate Flow Sheet

Elimination

Assessment

Assess infant/child's elimination pattern for frequency and consistency in urine and stools.

Development

Assessment

Assess personal-social, language, fine motor and gross motor development by: 1) DDST
2) PHN assessment

Bonding

Assessment

Assess caregiver-infant bonding by:
1) Harrison Assessment
2) PHN assessment
3) NCAST newborn behavior assessment.

APPENDIX 22-1
High-Risk Infant and Well Child, Birth to 12 Months—cont'd

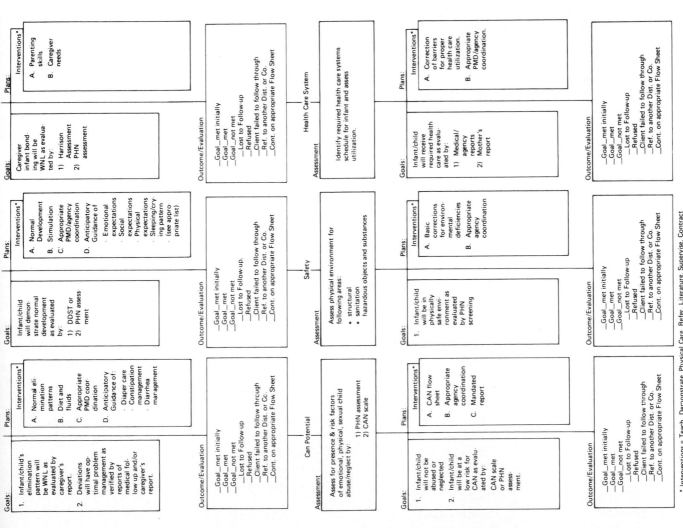

Goals:

1. Infant/child's elimination pattern will be WNL as evaluated by caregiver's report.
2. Deviations will have optimal problem management as verified by reports of medical follow up and/or caregiver's report.

Plans:

Interventions*

A. Normal elimination patterns
B. Diet and fluids
C. Appropriate PMD coordination
D. Anticipatory Guidance of:
 - Diaper care
 - Constipation management
 - Diarrhea management

Goals:

Infant/child will demonstrate normal development as evaluated by:
1) DDST or
2) PHN assessment

Plans:

Interventions*

A. Normal Development
B. Stimulation
C. Appropriate PMD/agency coordination
D. Anticipatory Guidance of
 - Emotional expectations
 - Social expectations
 - Physical expectations
 - Sleeping/crying pattern (see appropriate list)

Goals:

Caregiver infant bonding will be WNL as evaluated by:
1) Harrison Assessment
2) PHN assessment

Plans:

Interventions*

A. Parenting skills
B. Caregiver needs

Outcome/Evaluation

___Goal__met initially
___Goal__met
___Goal__not met
___Lost to Follow-up
___Refused
___Client failed to follow through
___Ref. to another Dist. or Co.
___Cont. on appropriate Flow Sheet

Outcome/Evaluation

___Goal__met initially
___Goal__met
___Goal__not met
___Lost to Follow-up.
___Refused
___Client failed to follow through
___Ref. to another Dist. or Co.
___Cont. on appropriate Flow Sheet

Outcome/Evaluation

___Goal__met initially
___Goal__met
___Goal__not met
___Lost to Follow-up
___Refused
___Client failed to follow through
___Ref. to another Dist. or Co.
___Cont. on appropriate Flow Sheet

Can Potential

Assessment

Assess for presence & risk factors of emotional, physical, sexual child abuse/neglect by:
1) PHN assessment
2) CAN scale

Safety

Assessment

Assess physical environment for following areas:
- structural
- sanitation
- hazardous objects and substances

Health Care System

Assessment

Identify required health care systems schedule for infant and assess utilization.

Goals:

1. Infant/child will not be abused or neglected
2. Infant/child will be at a low risk for CAN as evaluated by: CAN scale or PHN assessment.

Plans:

Interventions*

A. CAN flow sheet
B. Appropriate agency coordination
C. Mandated report

Goals:

1. Infant/child will be in physically safe environment as evaluated by PHN screening

Plans:

Interventions*

A. Basic corrections for environmental deficiencies
B. Appropriate agency coordination

Goals:

Infant/child will receive required health care as evaluated by:
1) Medical/agency reports
2) Mother's report

Plans:

Interventions*

A. Correction of barriers for proper health care utilization.
B. Appropriate PMD/agency coordination.

Outcome/Evaluation

___Goal__met initially
___Goal__met
___Goal__not met
___Lost to Follow-up
___Refused
___Client failed to follow through
___Ref. to another Dist. or Co.
___Cont. on appropriate Flow Sheet

Outcome/Evaluation

___Goal__met initially
___Goal__met
___Goal__not met
___Refused
___Client failed to follow through
___Ref. to another Dist. or Co.
___Cont. on appropriate Flow Sheet

Outcome/Evaluation

___Goal__met initially
___Goal__met
___Goal__not met
___Lost to Follow-up
___Refused
___Client failed to follow through
___Ref. to another Dist. or Co.
___Cont. on appropriate Flow Sheet

* Interventions = Teach, Demonstrate, Physical Care, Refer, Literature, Supervise, Contract

© Copyright 1983 San Bernardino County Public Health Department

APPENDIX 22-2
Priorities in Community Health Nursing

PURPOSES:
1. To identify target population groups requiring community health nursing service
2. To identify realistic spacing of nurse service contacts according to identified target population group
3. To use levels of prevention and health promotion in planning nursing service to a community

CODE
- *Classification I: intensive visiting* is defined as visits spaced daily to 3 times a week
- *Classification II: periodic visiting* is defined as visits spaced every 1 to 2 weeks
- *Classification III: widely spaced visiting* is defined as visits spaced every 2 to 3 months

	I. Intensive visiting	II. Periodic visiting	III. Widely spaced visiting
Communicable Disease			
A. Tuberculosis (by law a priority)	To families who 1. Have young adults and unexamined contacts living in crowded home conditions with a patient who has positive sputum 2. Have a recently diagnosed patient with positive sputum 3. Have a diagnosed patient with positive sputum, who is recalcitrant 4. Have a recently diagnosed patient without positive sputum 5. Have a patient receiving chemotherapy	To families who 1. Have the patient with positive sputum hospitalized; have no young adults in the family; have good living standards but have some unexamined contacts 2. Need preparation for the hospital admission of the patient 3. Need preparation for the discharge of the patient	To families who 1. Have an arrested patient returned to good home conditions 2. Have had all contacts examined and the patient hospitalized, under adequate medical supervision 3. Are under adequate medical supervision, with the source of infection located
B. Acute reportable dangerous communicable diseases	To families who 1. Have been contacts to reportable dangerous communicable disease 2. Have a diagnosed patient needing home care 3. Have food handlers as a case/contact to *Salmonella*	To families who 1. Are unimmunized 2. Have a patient under medical care but complications develop 3. Need follow-up for defects after recovery from acute stage	To families who 1. Are known to have immunization against communicable disease 2. Are receiving adequate medical care 3. Have a typhoid carrier in the home
C. Sexually transmissible diseases	To clients who 1. Need treatments and education on the prevention and spread of disease	To clients who 1. Need follow-up clinical examinations (for example, spinal taps)	

Modified from Rives R: Priorities according to needs, *Nurs Outlook* 6:404-408, 1958. Copyright American Journal of Nursing Company. Updated for the 3rd edition, by F. Armignacco, Director of Patient Services and Community Nursing, Monroe Co. Department of Health, Rochester, NY; updated for this edition by L. Randar, RN, MPH, Director, Division of Nursing, Philadelphia Department of Health, Philadelphia, Penn.

APPENDIX 22-2
Priorities in Community Health Nursing—cont'd

	I. Intensive visiting	II. Periodic visiting	III. Widely spaced visiting
	2. Have known contacts they will name 3. Need examination, advice on treatment, and education on how to arrest and prevent the transfer of infection 4. Need posttreatment observation 5. Need to be convinced of the necessity of the treatment ordered by the doctor 6. Need to be taught how to prevent further manifestations of the disease 7. Have babies born of mothers with active STD 8. To families who need instruction and assistance to care for a person with AIDS		
Home Care of the Sick			
A. Cardiovascular disease	To clients who 1. Have cardiac failure or have had an acute cardiac episode from any cause 2. Have a chronic cardiac disability requiring active treatment: medical, nursing, dietetic 3. Have had a CVA and require active treatment: medical, nursing, occupational, and physical therapy 4. Have cardiac surgery	To clients who 1. Have a congenital heart disease: nonoperable, postoperative 2. Have a murmur of undetermined origin with a history of rheumatic fever 3. Have congenital heart disease (to be followed until a thorough medical evaluation is completed) 4. Have diagnosed, untreated, uncontrolled hypertension	To clients who 1. Have a history of rheumatic fever, but no clinical heart disease 2. Are under medical care, stabilized for cardiovascular diagnoses
B. Diabetes	To clients who 1. Are newly diagnosed, not stabilized by diet or insulin 2. Cannot take own insulin (blind, aged, low mentality, and so forth)	To clients who 1. Are newly diagnosed, administering own insulin but still needing supervision 2. Are suspected of having diabetes	To clients who 1. Are under medical care, stabilized as to diet or insulin, or both

Continued

APPENDIX 22-2
Priorities in Community Health Nursing—cont'd

	I. Intensive visiting	II. Periodic visiting	III. Widely spaced visiting
B. Diabetes (cont'd)	3. Have difficulty understanding diet or administering their own insulin 4. Have uncontrolled diabetes 5. Have diabetes with gangrene 6. Have diabetes complicated by an infection		
C. Kidney disease	To clients who 1. Are on dialysis 2. Need help with medications and diet and understanding disease	To clients who 1. Understand medications and diet but are not stabilized	To clients who 1. Are under medical care and are stabilized
D. Cancer	To clients who 1. Are discharged from a hospital and need active nursing care, instruction for themselves, and interpretation of their physical and emotional needs to the family 2. Have symptoms suspicious of cancer; need medical supervision, completion of all tests and examinations, and, if required, treatment on the earliest possible date 3. Are diagnosed but who, without consulting the physicians, have interrupted their treatment or discontinued having medical checkups 4. Are under observation for malignancy but delinquent from regular medical supervision (the urgency of a patient's problem can be determined only by the attending physician) 5. Have hospice/terminal care needs	To clients who 1. Have precancerous lesions and are delinquent for periodic checkups (cervical erosions, leukoplakias, keratoses, mastitis, and others) 2. Have cancer apparently treated successfully but are not reporting for medical reexamination (cancer of the skin with no apparent recurrence) 3. Have advanced disease and need care (some of these patients may need to be in classification I) 4. Have families that have been taught to carry out medical orders but need support in continuing medical supervision	To clients about whom 1. Information is needed for statistical purposes (cured, deceased, or other)

Priorities in Community Health Nursing—cont'd

	I. Intensive visiting	II. Periodic visiting	III. Widely spaced visiting
	6. Need complex, high technology interventions such as TPN intravenous feedings		
E. Other noncommunicable diseases, acute or chronic	To clients who 1. Are acutely ill and need nursing care 2. Are helpless or bedridden and need nursing service 3. Are senile and do not receive adequate home care 4. Are acutely ill or helpless but have families who can be taught how to give the necessary care 5. Are receiving terminal care	To clients who 1. Are acutely ill or helpless but whose families can provide care under nursing supervision 2. Need encouragement to continue medical care 3. Need emotional support to carry out health instructions	To clients who 1. Are under adequate medical supervision and are given good home care (by the family, a registered nurse, or a practical nurse)
Health Teaching and Supervision			
A. Maternity-antepartum	To women who 1. Are primiparas 2. Are under 17 or over 40 years of age 3. Are single parents 4. Are of low socio-economic status 5. Are hypertensive 6. Have poor nutrition 7. Are not under medical care 8. Have had six or more pregnancies 9. Have had conditions associated with pregnancy resulting in infant deaths 10. Have had complications in past pregnancies or have signs of complications in the present pregnancy, including psychosomatic disturbances	To women who 1. Have adequate medical supervision for apparently normal pregnancies 2. Are in good physical and mental condition 3. Are able to follow advice 4. Have questions and desire help	(No antepartum patients in this category)

Continued

APPENDIX 22-2

Priorities in Community Health Nursing—cont'd

	I. Intensive visiting	II. Periodic visiting	III. Widely spaced visiting
A. Maternity-antepartum (cont'd)	11. Have a chronic disease, such as tuberculosis, diabetes, syphilis, anemia, nephritis, cardiac disease, or rheumatic fever 12. Have previously had premature deliveries 13. Are HIV+ and/or drug abusers		
B. Maternity-postpartum	To women who 1. Have nursing problems or breast complications, such as engorgement or abscess 2. Are not receiving adequate medical supervision or competent nursing care 3. Had complications or accidents of labor: stillbirths, abortions, or other difficulties resulting in a mishap to the mother or baby 4. Delivered prematurely 5. Had multiple births 6. Delivered a baby with a congenital defect 7. Had a baby that died during the first month of life 8. Evidence poor maternal-infant bonding 9. Have no or few support systems 10. Are economically stressed (low socioeconomic status)	To women who 1. Had problems but are making normal progress 7 days after delivery 2. Have adequate medical supervision 3. Are coping but need guidance and support related to care of the baby, the family's adjustment, and socioeconomic variables	To women who 1. Are receiving good care and supervision 2. Stabilizing in parenting skills and family adjustment
C. Infancy (higher priority is given to infants, regardless of whether they are first-born, when they live in low economic districts where the mortality rate is highest)	To infants who 1. Are premature 2. Are newborn, especially if firstborn 3. Have difficulty in breastfeeding 4. Have consistently lost weight	To infants who 1. Are past the first month and are gaining weight slowly 2. Are not being fed properly 3. Have questionable physical and emotional delays	To infants who 1. Are receiving adequate medical supervision 2. Are receiving good home care

APPENDIX 22-2

Priorities in Community Health Nursing—cont'd

	I. Intensive visiting	II. Periodic visiting	III. Widely spaced visiting
	5. Are being weaned		
	6. Have inadequate medical care		
	7. Have a reportable dangerous communicable disease		
	8. Have a physical handicap resulting from a birth injury or a congenital defect—"high tech" babies such as those on respirators and who have been hospitalized at length		
	9. Need immunization		
	10. Are from substandard poorly managed homes, or homes where there are problems of inadequate parenting		
	11. Are considered difficult babies by parents		
	12. Are born to drug abusers		
	13. Are born to mothers who are HIV positive		
	14. Fail to thrive		
	15. Are low birthweight		
D. Preschool period	To children who	To children who	To children who
	1. Have a reportable dangerous communicable disease	1. Are insecure	1. Have adequate medical supervision
	2. Have a physical defect	2. Have lost weight	2. Have good home care
	3. Need immunization	3. Lack medical supervision	
	4. Need dental care	4. Have poor health habits	
	5. Have nutritional deficiencies	5. Deviate from normal physical and emotional behavior	
	6. Are inconsistently disciplined		
	7. Are from homes where there is inadequate parenting		
	8. Are reported for suspected child abuse and neglect		

Continued

APPENDIX 22-2
Priorities in Community Health Nursing—cont'd

	I. Intensive visiting	II. Periodic visiting	III. Widely spaced visiting

E. School health	To children who
	1. Have acute health problems
	  a. Communicable diseases: immunization reactions or complications developing from acute communicable diseases
	  b. Skin conditions: scabies, impetigo, ringworm, pediculosis
	  c. Other: pregnancy, unexpected loss or gain of weight, abuse, neglect, diabetes, epilepsy
	2. Have had an accident in school requiring hospitalization
	3. Need immediate attention for defects discovered on physical examination: vision, hearing, cardiac, kidney, scoliosis, or other serious defects
	4. Need follow-up of incidents indicating intense or serious emotional disturbance
	5. Need follow-up as a contact of a diagnosed dangerous communicable disease
	6. Have growth and other developmental delays
		To children who
		1. Need follow-up of allergies: hives, eczema, asthma
		2. Have inadequate medical care
		3. Have not had diagnosed defects corrected within a reasonable period of time
		4. Are on medication for more than 3 weeks' duration during the school year
		5. Need to be observed in relation to their growth pattern (those with structural scoliosis, those wearing braces, and so forth)
		6. Need follow-up of minor defects: poor eating and health habits, poor dental and personal hygiene, foot and posture problems
			To children who
			1. Have a chronic health condition that is stabilized and under medical care
			2. Have a congenital defect which does not require remedial work at the time

F. Adult health	To clients who 1. Are in situational or maturational crisis 2. Are disorganized as a family and at risk for abuse and neglect of children or spouse	To clients who 1. Are in crisis but have support systems 2. Recognize their disorganization and are working on ordering their lives	To clients who 1. Have needed nursing care, are currently coping well, but are at risk for physical, emotional, and psychosocial problems

Priorities in Community Health Nursing—cont'd

	I. Intensive visiting	**II. Periodic visiting**	**III. Widely spaced visiting**
	3. Are homeless, in need of health and welfare services, but have not yet established contact with community resources 4. Have suspected dangerous communicable or chronic disease symptoms 5. Have no medical supervision for diagnosed physical, emotional, psychosocial problems 6. Are needing help adapting to chronic illness: heart disease, arthritis, multiple sclerosis, depression, etc.	3. Are recently established in a home environment and are working with community resources 4. Have diagnosed disease and are receiving medical treatment; need help with referral to resources 5. Are needing help dealing with developmental tasks of parenting: sexuality and death education tasks of their children	
G. Health of aging people	To clients who 1. Have no medical supervision 2. Have symptoms of a dangerous communicable, nutritional, or chronic disease 3. Have a diagnosed disease and need help following the treatment plan 4. Have no support systems 5. Have evidence of situational or maturational crisis especially in relation to: loss of income, loss of spouse, loss of friends 6. Have evidence of intentional or unintentional alcohol or drug abuse 7. Are unable to maintain an environmentally safe housing situation	To clients who 1. Have a diagnosed medical problem 2. Have a complex treatment regimen and are following it 3. Are able to live independently but need referral sources and support	To clients who 1. Are under medical supervision 2. Have readily available support systems

References

American Nurses Association (ANA): *Nursing case management,* Kansas City, Mo., 1988, The Association.

American Nurses Association: *Standards for nursing staff development,* Washington, D.C., 1990, The Association.

American Nurses Association: *Standards for organized nursing services and responsibilities of nurse administrators across all settings,* Washington, D.C., 1991, The Association.

Buelow J: *A computerized format of the nursing process in community health,* unpublished paper presented to the American Public Health Association, Dallas, Tx., November 1983.

Clark CC and Shea CA: *Management in nursing: a vital link in the health care systems,* New York, 1979, McGraw-Hill.

Davis GD: *Management information systems: conceptual foundations, structure and development,* New York, 1974, McGraw-Hill.

Donovan R: Worker stress and job satisfaction: a study of home care workers in New York City, *Home Health Care Serv Q* 16:97-114, 1989.

Douglass LM: *The effective nurse: leader and manager,* ed 3, St. Louis, 1988, Mosby.

Feldman P: *Who cares for them? Workers in the home care industry,* New York, 1990, Greenwood.

Freedman DH: Is management a science? *Harvard Business Review,* November-December 1992, pp. 26-38.

Freeman RB: *Techniques of supervision in public health nursing,* ed 2, Philadelphia, 1949, Saunders.

Gilbert N: Supervision of home health paraprofessionals: a quality of care issue, *Caring* 11:10-14, 1992.

Gleick J: *Chaos: making a new science,* New York, 1987, Viking.

Harris M: *Home health agency policy manual,* Baltimore, Md., 1990, National Health Publishing.

Health Care Financing Administration (HCFA): Conditions of participation: home health agencies, *Federal Register* 56:32967-32975, 1991, July 18.

Keyes G: Why we need nursing statistics. In *Management information systems for public health/community health agencies,* NLN Pub. No. 21-1506, New York, 1974, National League for Nursing, pp. 56-57.

Koontz H, O'Donnell C, and Weihrich H: *Essentials of management,* ed 4, New York, 1986, McGraw-Hill.

Maslow AH: *Motivation and personality,* New York, 1954, Harper & Row.

McGregor D: *The human side of enterprise,* New York, 1960, McGraw-Hill.

Moore F: What about the quality of care, *Caring* 9:16-26, 1990.

National Association for Home Care (NAHC): NAHC reports results of a computer services survey, *Caring* 2:14-15, 1983.

Ouchi WG: *Theory Z: how American business can meet the Japanese challenge,* Reading, Mass, 1981, Addison-Wesley.

Pagonis, WG: The work of the leader, *Harvard Business Review,* November/December, 1992, pp. 118-126.

Parks SJ: *Introduction to health care facility: food service administration,* University Park, Pa, 1982, Pennsylvania State University.

Rives R: Priorities according to needs. In Stewart DM and Vincent PA, eds: *Public health nursing,* Dubuque, Ia, 1958, Wm C Brown, Copyright 1958. American Journal of Nursing Company, Reproduced with permission from *Nurs Outlook* 6:404-408, July 1958.

Schmele JA, Allen ME, Butler S, and Gresham D: Quality circles in the public health sector: implementation and effect, *Public Health Nursing* 8(3):190-195, 1991.

Senge PM: *The fifth discipline: the art and practice of the learning organization,* New York, 1990, Doubleday.

Simmons DA, Martin KS, Crews CC, and Scheet NJ: *Client management information system for community health nursing agencies,* NTIS accession No. HRP-0907023, Springfield, Va., 1986, National Technical Information Service.

Spiegle A: *Home health care,* ed 2, Owing Mills, Md., 1987, National Health Publishing.

Study Group on Nursing Information Systems: Computerized nursing information systems: an urgent need, *Res Nurs Health* 6:101-106, 1983.

Visiting Nurse Association of Greater Philadelphia: *Software requirements, evaluation and selection for the voluntary home health agency,* Philadelphia, 1990-1992, The Association.

Selected Bibliography

Anglin LT: Caseload management: a model for agencies and staff nurses, *Home Health Care Nurse* 10(3):26-31, 1992.

Bly JL: Measuring productivity for home health nurses, *Home Health Care Serv Q* 2:23-39, 1981.

Bohan GP: Building a high-performance team, *Health Care Superv* 8(4):15-21, 1990.

Churness VH, Kleffel D, Onodera ML, and Jacobson J: Reliability and validity testing of a home health patient classification system. *Public Health Nurs* 5:135-139, 1988.

Corriveau, CL and Rowney RH: What is a day's work? *Nurs Outlook* 31:335-339, 1983.

Crown W, MacAdam M, and Sadowsky E: A national profile of home care workers, *Caring* 11:34-38, 1992.

Epting LA, Glover SH, and Boyd SA: Managing diversity, *Health Care Superv* 12(4):73-83, 1994.

Gleeson S: Helping nurses through the management threshold, *Nurs Administration Q* 7(2):11-16, 1983.

Hays BJ: Nursing care requirements and resource consumption in home health care, *Nurs Research* 41(3):138-143, 1992.

Hedtcke CS, MacQueen L, and Carr A: How do home health nurses spend their time? *JONA* 22:18-22, 1992.

Knollmueller RN: *Community health nursing supervisor: a handbook for community/homecare managers.* New York, 1986, National League for Nursing.

Marriner-Tomey A: *Guide to nursing management,* ed 4, St Louis, 1992, Mosby.

Peters DA: Development of a community health intensity rating scale, *Nurs Research* 37:202-207, 1988.

Saba VK and McCormick KA: *Essentials of computers for nurses,* Philadelphia, 1986, Lippincott.

Stanfill P: Participative management becomes shared management, *Nurs Manage* 18(6):69-70, 1987.

Tappen RM: *Nursing leadership and management: concepts and practice,* ed 2, Philadelphia, 1989, Davis.

23

Quality Processes in Community Health Nursing Practice

OBJECTIVES

Upon completion of this chapter, the reader should be able to:

1. Identify reasons why quality processes are increasingly important in health care systems.
2. Discuss the concept of *total quality management* or *continuous quality improvement.*
3. Explain the concept of client as it is defined under a total quality management model.
4. Describe the components of a total quality management program.
5. Explain how values held by health care professionals influence implementation of quality improvement strategies.
6. Discuss the terms *structure, process,* and *outcome* as they relate to quality processes in community health nursing practice.
7. Identify several types of measurement tools and procedures used to assess quality of care.
8. Identify data display techniques for summarizing quality improvement data.
9. Identify the community health nurse's role in a total quality management program.

One characteristic of a profession is the presence of a professional association that is cohesive, self-governing, and a source of professional self-discipline, standards, and ethics.

JEROME P. LYSAUGHT, 1970, P. 41

Professionals have entered an era of quality improvement in health care delivery. Increasingly they are being challenged by legislative action, third-party payors, and consumers to assume accountability for the services delivered by members of their profession. Legislative emphasis on quality began in the 1970s. The professional standard review organizations (PSROs) established by the 1972 amendments to the Social Security Act were developed to ensure that federal monies spent for Medicaid, Medicare, and other federal health care programs would be used effectively, efficiently, and economically. The PSRO law (Public Law 92-603) mandated review of health care delivered by physicians and nonphysician health practitioners when such care was paid for by federal funds (Public Law 92-603, 1972). This necessitated the development of standards for practice, because the review examined current practice to determine how it compared with established norms for quality care.

The passage of the National Health Planning and Resources Development Act of 1974 (refer to Chapter 13), like the PSRO legislation, also provided an impetus for the development of quality monitoring programs. This law mandated that health care professionals promote activities that improve the quality of health care services to all segments of the population. It set forth as a national priority "equal access to quality health care at a reasonable cost" (Papers on the National Health Guidelines, 1977, p. 1). It called for the development of national health planning goals and standards.

Quality became a major focus among legislators in the 1980s and a resulting avalanche of new requirements to protect the quality of client services emerged. Illustrative of this was the establishment of the peer review organizations (PROs), which were mandated by the 1982 Tax Equity and Fiscal Responsibility Act (TEFRA). These structures were charged by the Health Care Financing Administration (HCFA) to review medical records for appropriateness, quality of care, and compliance with practice standards (Brecker, 1990; Bull, 1985). The competency evaluation stipula-

tions for home health aides and the patient rights requirements mandated by the Omnibus Budget Reconciliation Act of 1987 (refer to Chapters 4, 9, and 20) are other examples of legislative involvement in regulating quality in the health care industry.

Federal involvement in the assessment and monitoring of quality care also increased in the 1980s. In 1986 results of a quality assurance investigation by the House Select Committee on Aging and the American Bar Association's Commission on Legal Problems of the Elderly were presented to the House of Representatives. The document summarizing the findings of this investigation, known as the "Black Box" report on home care quality, raised questions about the quality of care provided to vulnerable groups in our society (Sabatino, 1986). This has resulted in increased governmental involvement in the monitoring of quality in the health care delivery system. For example, the establishment of a home health toll-free hotline and investigative unit, which clients may call if they have complaints about local home health agencies, was mandated in the Omnibus Budget Reconciliation Act of 1986. The Medicare Conditions of Participation require home health agencies to inform their patients how they can reach this hotline (HCFA, 1989).

In addition to federal influences, private nonprofit third-party payors (refer to Chapter 4) have encouraged professionals to monitor both the cost and the quality of health services. They have established criteria for the type of care they will reimburse, and they require as well that health services be audited by professional audit committees.

Consumers are also motivating health care professionals to evaluate the care they provide. Consumers are becoming more sophisticated about the health care they desire and are demanding that current practice keep up with societal changes and needs. In addition, through legislative action, they are becoming more actively involved in reviewing services delivered by health care professionals. Influential organizations, such as the American Association of Retired Persons (AARP), are spearheading this involvement.

Nurses share with all health care professionals the need to examine carefully the delivery of their services in light of changing societal demands. To validate itself as a profession and to maintain the right to govern nursing practice, nursing must take the responsibility to control the activities of its members. There is no question that if nursing does not assume accountability for its actions, others will control nurses' actions for them in this era of quality improvement. The challenge for the 1990s will be to ensure quality while containing health care costs.

EVOLUTION OF QUALITY PROCESSES IN NURSING

Quality in the delivery of nursing services has been stressed since Florence Nightingale's time. As was discussed in Chapter 1, Nightingale insisted that educated nurses were essential to perform the nurse's role. She promoted the use of the nursing process, a scientific method designed to establish appropriate client goals and effective and efficient nursing interventions. Nightingale also advocated for standards in practice that would guide all nurses in the delivery of sound professional nursing services.

Since its origin, the American Nurses Association (ANA) has emphasized the importance of quality assurance in nursing practice. The first objectives for the Nurses' Associated Alumnae of the United States and Canada, established in 1897 and known as the ANA since 1911, focused on lack of standardization in nurses' training, as well as the need for licensure laws to protect the public from inadequately trained nurses. By 1912 there were 33 nurses' associations that had secured nurse practice acts (Christy, 1971, pp. 1778-1779).

Following ANA's focus, early public health nursing leaders pushed for standardization of public health/community health practice. As this specialty-based practice rapidly evolved in the United States around the beginning of the century, its leaders emphasized the importance of developing generally accepted standards for nursing care in the community (Gardner, 1948). The National Organization for Public Health Nursing (NOPHN), founded in 1912, grew out of a concern for the right of clients to receive care from qualified people. One of the major purposes of this organization was to promote standardized quality in practice.

The American Nurses Association has assumed a major leadership role in setting standards for the profession for the past thirty years (Tilbury, 1992, p. 10). Since 1966 the American Nurses Association has diligently pursued the development of a quality assurance program for nurses. At that time the divisions of practice, including community health nursing, geriatric nursing, maternal and child health nursing, medical-surgical nursing, and psychiatric and mental health nursing, were established with a mandate to consider the development of standards for nursing practice as their major priority. After 6 years of concentrated efforts, all divisions on practice presented standards of care for their division, based on their beliefs about nursing practice, at the 1972 biennial ANA convention in Detroit (American Nurses Association, 1975, p. 1). In 1973 the community health nursing standards were made available for distribution to all members of the community health nursing division. The most recent standards for community health nursing practice are delineated in the box on p. 888. They address the responsibility of the nurse for assuring quality of nursing practice.

The ANA's standards of home health nursing practice are listed in Chapter 20. Quality assurance is emphasized in these standards under the concepts of evaluation and the organization of home health services. The ANA believes that managers must assume responsibility for creating an environment that promotes quality assurance and for establishing a quality assurance program that measures both the clinical and administrative aspects of the organization (American Nurses Association, 1986a, pp. 5-6). The ANA standard documents provide a valuable framework for developing a quality assurance program.

The focus of quality efforts in the 1970s and 1980s was on quality assurance. This process was viewed as a dynamic one through which health care professionals assumed accountability for the quality of care they provided. It was a commitment to excellence with an emphasis on ensuring that all health care professionals provided safe clinical care and that all clients received quality care. It involved a series of actions aimed at governing clinical practice so that all clients received clinical services that were *equal to* or *better than* the standard of care designated appropriate for clients who had like characteristics.

Selected definitions of quality assurance used in the past two decades are presented in Table 23-1. Schmadl proposed an additional definition after analyzing what nurses should be assuring, for whom nurses are assuring quality, and what measures identify quality nursing care. His definition is presented below because it is clearly stated, comprehensive, and provides direction for the development of a quality assurance program. It also focuses on several concepts currently considered important when quality in clinical practice is examined.

◀ *Standards of Community Health Nursing Practice* ▶

Standard I. Theory

The nurse applies theoretical concepts as a basis for decisions in practice.

Standard II. Data Collection

The nurse systematically collects data that are comprehensive and accurate.

Standard III. Diagnosis

The nurse analyzes data collected about the community, family, and individual to determine diagnosis.

Standard IV. Planning

At each level of prevention, the nurse develops plans that specify nursing actions unique to client needs.

Standard V. Intervention

The nurse, guided by the plan, intervenes to promote, maintain, or restore health, to prevent illness, and to effect rehabilitation.

Standard VI. Evaluation

The nurse evaluates responses of the community, family, and individual to interventions in order to determine

progress toward goal achievement and to revise the data base, diagnoses, and plan.

Standard VII. Quality Assurance and Professional Development

The nurse participates in peer review and other means of evaluation to assure quality of nursing practice. The nurse assumes responsibility for professional development and contributes to the professional growth of others.

Standard VIII. Interdisciplinary Collaboration

The nurse collaborates with other health care providers, professionals, and community representatives in assessing, planning, implementing, and evaluating programs for community health.

Standard IX. Research

The nurse contributes to theory and practice in community health nursing through research.

From American Nurses Association, Council of Community Health Nurses: *Standards of community health nursing practice,* Kansas City, Mo., 1986b, The Association. Reprinted with permission of the American Nurses Association.

Quality assurance involves assuring the consumer of a specified degree of excellence through continuous measurement and evaluation of structural components, goal-directed nursing process, and/or consumer outcome, using preestablished criteria and standards and available norms, and followed by appropriate alteration with the purpose of improvement. (Schmadl, 1979, p. 465)

During the 1980s the notion of quality *assessment* versus quality assurance emerged. O'Leary (1991) believes that the term *quality assurance* was an "unfortunate semantic selection" because quality cannot be assured but only improved. The terminology preferred by the Joint Commission for Accreditation of Healthcare Organizations (JCAHO) in its 1992 accreditation standards is *quality assessment and improvement.* The 1992 National League for Nursing Accreditation Standards also examine these concepts when the Community Health Accreditation Program, Inc. (CHAP), an independent subsidiary of the NLN, conducts its accreditation visits (NLN, 1992). *Quality assessment* is currently being used synonymously with

quality assurance by many health care professionals.

Beliefs and standards for nursing practice should never be static. As societal changes, expansion of knowledge, and technological advances occur, beliefs and standards should be reevaluated to determine whether they reflect the values of the profession and society. The ANA Standards for Practice of 1973 were presented only as a working document to be continually evaluated and revised. This has been done twice since they were initially developed. ANA's concept of *quality assurance* has also been evaluated and broadened in recent years.

TOTAL QUALITY MANAGEMENT: THE EMPHASIS FOR THE 1990S

As we advance toward the year 2000, the concept of total quality management (TQM) or continuous quality improvement (CQI) has come to the forefront and represents a significant philosophical shift in

23-1 Selected Definitions of Quality Assurance

Author	Definitions
American Nurses Association	Estimation of the degree of excellence in (1) the alteration of the health status of consumers attained through providers' performances of (2) diagnostic, therapeutic, prognostic, and other health care activities,[1,2]
	Quality assurance is a relatively new term conveying the broad idea that superiority or excellence in care is made secure or certain.[3]
	A program executed to make secure or certain the excellence of health care; the term is applied to programs as limited as that of an administrative unit of a health care agency or as broad as that of a community, a region, a state, or a nation. The program must have two major components:
	1. The securing of measurements and ascertaining of the degree to which stated standards are met;
	2. The introduction of changes based on information supplied by the measurements, with the view to improvement of the total effort and product of the unit or agency.[4]
	Quality assurance is an ongoing program in the nursing profession, constructed and executed to secure and implement the excellence of health care.[5]
Brown	Quality assurance, when used in reference to health care, refers to the accountability of health personnel for the quality of care they provide.[6]
Davidson	Quality assurance is a process for attainment of the highest degree of excellence in the delivery of patient or client care.[7]
	A commitment to excellence of care; an estimation of the health status of consumers attained through nursing performance.[8]
Lang	Activities done to determine the extent to which a phenomenon fulfills certain values and activities done to assure changes in practice which will fulfill the highest levels of values.[9]
Mayers	Quality assurance has as its central goal making certain that care practices will produce good patient outcomes.[10]
Nichols	The term quality assurance is used to describe a process in which standards are set and action is taken to ensure achievement of the standards.[11] It involves the description of the level of quality desired and feasible, and a system for ensuring its achievement.[12]
Zimmer	Quality assurance is estimation of the degree of excellence in patient health outcomes and in activity and other resource cost outcomes.[13]

1. American Nurses Association (ANA): *Guidelines for review of nursing care at the local level,* Publ. NP-54, Kansas City, Mo., 1976, The Association, p. A-2.
2. ANA: *Standards of home health nursing practice,* Kansas City, Mo., 1986, The Association.
3. ANA: *A plan for implementation of the standards of nursing practice,* Publ. NP-51, Kansas City, Mo., 1975, The Association, p. 5.
4. Ibid, p. 30.
5. Ibid, p. 6.
6. Brown B: Quality assurance (editorial), *Nurs Admin Q* 1:(5), Spring 1977.
7. Davidson SVS: *PSRO: utilization and audit in patient care,* St Louis, 1976, Mosby, p. 5.
8. Davidson SVS: *Nursing care evaluation: concurrent and retrospective review criteria,* St. Louis, 1977, Mosby, p. 408.
9. Lang N: *A model for quality assurance in nursing,* Milwaukee, 1974, Marquette University, p. 11 (unpublished doctoral dissertation).
10. Mayers MG: *Quality assurance for patient care: nursing perspectives,* New York, 1977, Appleton-Century-Crofts, p. 3.
11. Nichols ME and Wessells VG, eds: *Nursing standards and nursing process,* Wakefield, Mass, 1977, Contemporary Publishers, pp. 1-2.
12. Ibid, p. 37.
13. Zimmer MJ: Quality assurance in the provision of hospital care: a model for evaluation nursing care, *Hospitals* 48:(91)131, 1979.
From Schmadl JC: Quality assurance: examination of the concept, *Nurs Outlook* 27:462-465. Copyright 1979, American Journal of Nursing Company. Reproduced with permission from *Nursing Outlook.*

terms of the concept of quality. TQM moves away from the premise that problems are the result of errors by individual clinical professionals to the notion that the majority of problems arise from defects in the design of systems, products, and processes of production (Donabedian, 1993). Deming (1986) estimates that at least 85% of the problems in organizations are system problems rather than the type of random errors and mistakes introduced by individuals. In keeping with this idea, total quality management is viewed as a strategic mission shared by the entire organization (McLaughlin and Kaluzny, 1990).

"Participative management is a predominant theme under TQM" (Smith, Discenza, and Piland, 1993, p. 35). Leaders at all levels in the organization set the direction for TQM by promoting a shared vision, shared goals, and TQM values throughout the organization, empowering all employees to monitor their own work, evaluating and recognizing TQM progress, and acting as role models for TQM behavior (Melum and Sinioris, 1993, p. 60). TQM puts responsibility for quality control in the province of frontline managers and employees through the use of quality circles and employee education and training in the methods of monitoring (Donabedian, 1993; McLaughlin and Kaluzny, 1990). Quality circles are small, structured problem-solving groups of employees from the same area who work on improving productivity, efficiency, and quality, using a sound data base (McLaughlin and Kaluzny; Mullins and Schmele, 1993). Under TQM staff development, training, and educational activities have a different focus than the traditional models of human resource development. Emphasis is placed on helping employees to deal with innovation and change. Training and educational activities are focused on reinforcing quality improvement processes rather than imparting skills or knowledge to individuals (Smith, Discenza, and Piland).

In addition to creating a style of management that facilitates organization-wide involvement in quality improvement, TQM challenges the prevailing concept of *customer.* It demands that change be based on the needs of the customer, not the values of the providers (McLaughlin and Kaluzny, 1990). "A customer is anyone who receives and benefits from the product of someone else's labor" (Melum and Sinioris, 1993, p. 60), including *internal* consumers of one's labor. Within this context the recipient of clinical services—the client—is not the only focus when implementing job responsibilities. Attention is placed on meeting the needs of all customers, such as personnel from other divisions within an organization, physicians and nurses in private practice, referral agencies, and third-party payors. In line with this philosophy, evaluation of customer satisfaction is seen as a significant component of the quality assessment process.

"Total quality management (TQM) is a management system designed to create customer-focused, high performing organizations by involving all employees in process improvement efforts" (Gaucher and Kratochwill, 1993, p. 10). It is a synergistic approach between all components in an organization that promotes high quality health care. It requires an integrated program (refer to Figure 23-1) that includes but is not limited to the following components (Koch and Fairly, 1993, p. 4):

1. Quality assessment and improvement
2. Infection control
3. Utilization management
4. Risk management/safety

An integrated quality management program is a broad and encompassing endeavor that presents many challenges, as well as opportunities, for an organization.

COMPONENTS OF A QUALITY MANAGEMENT PROGRAM

A well-established, integrated TQM program helps agencies to monitor problems and their trends, review organizational processes and services, protect the consumer from adverse outcomes, and guard the agency from loss. It also assists agencies in maximizing resource management and educating the consumer and agency staff about reasonable and acceptable health care services at affordable prices (Koch and Fairly, 1993, pp. 5-6). An organization that cultivates an environment facilitating the achievement of these goals will maintain a competitive edge in the coming decade.

Quality Assurance/Assessment

It has long been recognized that quality assurance/assessment is a complex process which involves more than the development of standards for practice. Donabedian, a renowned authority on health care quality, stressed that quality assurance efforts should be focused on evaluating the structure, process, and outcome aspects of health care delivery, as well as on the implementation of measures to improve care when

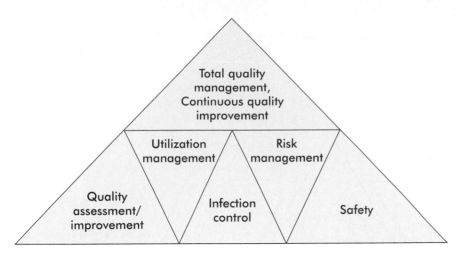

Figure 23-1 Integrated quality management. (From Koch MW and Fairly TM: *Integrated quality management: the key to improving nursing care quality,* St. Louis, 1993, Mosby, p. 5)

warranted (Donabedian, 1966, 1980). Actions to improve care in the community health setting include such elements as securing more nursing staff, hiring better-prepared personnel, strengthening interdisciplinary collaboration, providing additional continuing education, increasing the frequency of home visits to given families, and planning health programs for at-risk aggregates. All aspects of community health nursing practice, including services to individuals, families, aggregates, and the community as a whole, must be evaluated when a total quality management program is implemented.

In 1974 the American Nurses Association adopted a quality assurance model, developed by Dr. Norma Lang, to depict the multiple components of quality assurance. As Figure 23-2 shows, shared responsibility between nurses in all settings and consumers is essential to improve quality in health care delivery. Shared responsibility with other health care providers such as physicians, social workers, and dieticians is also essential. TQM promotes interdisciplinary participation in the quality improvement process (Moran and Johnson, 1992).

When depicted graphically, the assessment of quality appears simple. In reality, it is a complicated process requiring time, effort, a commitment to continuous quality improvement, and involvement of all personnel in an organization.

"Quality assessment and improvement (QA/QI) is the systematic monitoring process that identifies opportunities for improvement in *patient (client)* care delivery, designs ways to improve the service, and continues to evaluate follow-up actions to make certain that improvement occurs" (Koch and Fairly, 1993,

p. 17). Use of a conceptual framework or model for organizing quality assessment and improvement activities facilitates the development and implementation of a meaningful quality assessment plan in the practice setting. Such a model is presented in Figure 23-2. Tilbury (1992, p. 13) believes this generic model can be applied to continuous quality improvement with the addition of activities to maintain the new, higher level of quality after taking action. The Joint Commission on Accreditation of Healthcare Organizations (JCAHO) notes that the concept of continuous quality improvement incorporates the strengths of quality assurance while broadening its scope (JCAHO, 1991). Including these advanced CQI ideas, the basic components of quality assessment/improvement would then involve the following steps (Model shows dynamic concept of quality assurance, 1976; Tilbury):

- Identify values
- Write standards and criteria (structure, process, and outcome)
- Secure measurements
- Make interpretations
- Identify courses of action
- Choose action
- Take action
- Monitor quality improvement actions

Tilbury (1992) contends that the "differences in how the model is applied lie more in how the quality assessment and improvement processes are implemented than in the particular steps undertaken." For example, concurrent and terminal monitoring of performance, involving staff at all levels, is the norm under the continuous quality improvement system.

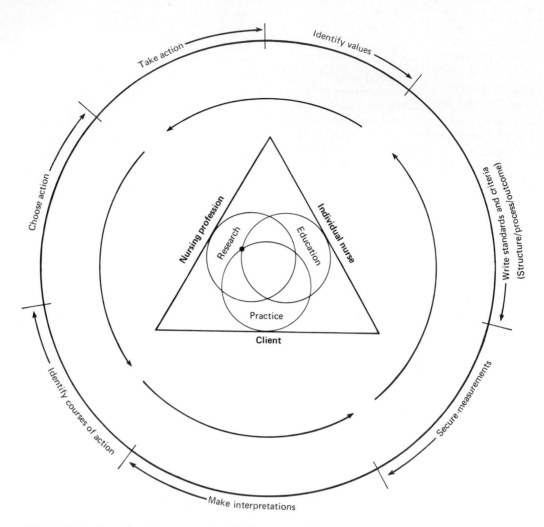

Figure 23-2   A quality assurance model. (From Model shows dynamic concept of quality assurance, *Am Nurse* 9:23, 1976. Adapted from *ANA: Quality assurance model, a plan for implementation of the standards of nursing practice,* Kansas City, Mo., 1975, The Association, p. 15.)

Under the quality assurance (QA) structure, retrospective review of charts by QA personnel is emphasized (Tilbury, 1992).

It is crucial that careful attention be given to how each aspect of a quality assessment program is initiated. Since many of the changes being proposed under a total quality management program are foreign to staff, continuing education for all personnel is the essential first step in developing a quality assessment program. As indicated earlier, staff development activities should focus on helping employees to deal with innovation and change and quality improvement processes (Smith, Discenza, and Piland, 1993). These activities also need to empower the staff to gather data, analyze and solve problems, and develop interdisciplinary team-building skills (McLaughlin and Kaluzny, 1990).

As was previously mentioned, there are several components of quality assessment. Factors to consider when implementing each of these components will be discussed in the following section of this chapter. By using the model presented in Figure 23-2 and the information presented below, the reader should be able to evaluate the progress made in implementing a quality assessment and improvement program in specific practice settings.

Identify Values

Attitudes, beliefs, and values influence how we think, how we act, and how we evaluate events and actions. In terms of quality assessment, they affect commitment to the concept and how quality is defined based on beliefs about health, humanity, and the nature of clinical practice. Identifying values in relation to quality, however, is a difficult task because many factors influence how clinical services are delivered. Available resources, consumer needs and wants, and professional philosophies all determine the scope of practice in a particular community. It is unrealistic, for instance, to assume that an agency can plan clinical services without taking into consideration the restrictions of limited resources. Providing fragmented services for all is not assuring quality.

Establishing a philosophy of nursing practice is fundamental to the identification of quality in health care. A philosophy provides direction for the nature and scope of services provided by both an agency and an individual practitioner. Based on available resources, it identifies clients' needs, the reason activities are being carried out, and the population to be served. A philosophy also describes the type of relationship the practitioner and client will have.

When a philosophy for clinical practice is being defined, discussion related to key general concepts should occur. Often concepts are accepted as truths, but their meaning to each practitioner varies. Concepts such as "clients' right of self-determination," "active client participation," "individualization of client care plans," and a "family-centered preventive approach" to the delivery of health care are difficult to internalize. Practitioners need time to analyze how these concepts can be applied in the practice setting. They need to understand what it means to their practice when they subscribe to a broad concept such as "the right of self-determination." When dealing with this concept, for example, health care providers need time to share feelings about client situations where their value systems differ from their clients' value orientations.

It was said in Chapter 2 that a community health nurse's "dominant responsibility is to the population as a whole" (American Nurses Association, 1986b, Standards of Community Health). This concept, like the concepts just mentioned is difficult to grasp and to apply. An agency that has limited resources and subscribes to this belief must identify ways in which it can implement this concept. It is impossible for any agency to provide direct service to all individuals within a community. However, a community health agency can identify clinical services it can provide and then apply the principles of health planning to see that gaps in services are met by other community agencies.

Agencies must determine realistic goals in view of the resources available or potentially available to them. If this is not done, they will never be able to determine when quality has been achieved. Being "all things to all people" is an impossible goal, but defining what one can do is not impossible. For instance, in the accompanying statement of philosophy (refer to box on p. 886), the Visiting Nurse Association of Hartford, Inc., clearly spelled out that they would provide *skilled* nursing services, including instruction in prevention of disease and preservation of health and other therapeutic services, on a part-time basis. They meet the needs of the population as a whole by referring individuals to other community agencies and by participating in health planning activities when unmet needs are recognized. Although developed in the late 1960s, this agency philosophy statement remains a good model to follow when examining what is realistic for an agency to achieve.

It should not be assumed that all employees have a clear understanding of or an appreciation for their agency's philosophy and beliefs about quality improvement. Even when an agency has a written philosophy statement, staff members should discourse with one another periodically so that a common framework for practice becomes explicit to all. A philosophy document given to new employees may receive little attention. This frequently happens because new employees are naturally more interested in finding out what they have to do to achieve success in their new job situation than in the philosophy behind what they are doing. Thus agency philosophy and beliefs about clinical practice must be reinforced by supervisors as new employees become comfortable with their job responsibilities. These beliefs must also be reexamined by staff who have been employed for a length of time. When the demands of the workload become heavy it is easy to lose sight of the beliefs and goals of the agency.

Write Standards and Criteria: Structure, Process, and Outcome

A philosophy of practice states the values and beliefs of an agency and guides the activities of all agency staff. It does not provide measurable elements

Statement of Philosophy: Visiting Nurse Association of Hartford, Incorporated

In 1969 a committee composed of Board members, supervisors and administrators was formed to develop the following Statement of Philosophy of the Visiting Nurse Association of Hartford, Inc. This was approved by all staff members and the Board of Directors.

The VNA of Hartford exists to provide services to people. It draws its authority from a 1923 Constitution in which the purpose "... to furnish ... skilled services of a Visiting Nurse ... including instruction in prevention of disease and preservation of health" is stated.

More specifically, the nature of the service is:

1. To provide, with a family centered approach, skilled nursing and other therapeutic services on a part-time basis in the home or other appropriate place.
2. To promote health and prevent illness—both mental and physical.
3. To help individuals get other necessary community services appropriate to their needs.
4. To recognize and bring to the attention of appropriate people unmet needs of the community and to participate in planning to meet these needs.

We believe:

1. The agency has a responsibility to honor all requests for services and to do an assessment of the situation involving the patient and the family and other appropriate professions or agencies, e.g., doctors, social workers, etc.
2. All planning and goal setting is done with the individual being served, his family and others involved in implementing care.
3. Planning and goal setting is a continuing process between nurse, patient and family, one of the goals being maximum independence of patient and family in taking care of their health needs.
4. Plans for the termination of VNA services should be made with the individual, family and all others in-

volved when family needs exceed the capabilities of the nursing agency and the family.

5. All planning includes the giving of consideration to the coordination of services, the appropriate use of manpower and the avoidance of duplication of effort.
6. We believe the above can be best achieved through the practice of primary nursing.
   A. The designation of the primary nurse for each patient/family will be based on geography, nurses' skill and nurses' availability.
   B. The primary nurse will interpret her role to the patient/family. The primary nurse is responsible and accountable for the nursing care delivered on a 24 hour basis until the patient is discharged. Her responsibility for directing and evaluating the care of other nurses mandates holding other nurses accountable and responsible for the care they give.
   C. The responsibilities of the primary nurse include:
      (1) Assessment of patient's/family's condition.
      (2) Identification of patient's/family's problems on the problem list.
      (3) Development of the nursing care plan to meet the identified needs.
      (4) Maintenance of the current problem list and plans, based on continuing assessment of the patient's/family's status.
      (5) Implementation of the plan of care to the extent possible.
      (6) Collaboration with nursing staff, physicians and other health workers in the care of the patient/family.
      (7) Evaluation of the effectiveness of nursing intervention.

Reproduced with permission of the Visiting Nurse Association of Hartford, Inc., 80 Coventry Street, Hartford, Connecticut, undated.

by which a practitioner can judge the quality of care given by health care providers. Standards and criteria must be developed so that the measurement of quality is possible.

Standards are norms "that express an agreed-upon level of performance that has been developed to characterize, measure, and provide guidance for achieving excellence in practice" (ANA, 1986b, p. 18). They are rules that help the practitioner to establish a consistent data base in an organized manner so that

consistencies and deficiencies of care are easily identified. They are specific statements that reflect the outcomes or goals toward which an agency is working. For example, in the ANA community health nursing standards, one identified goal is "to promote, maintain, or restore health, to prevent illness, and to effect rehabilitation" (standard V).

Criteria are predetermined measurable elements which reflect the intent of a standard (ANA, 1975, p. 16). They identify expected levels of performance by practitioners (process criteria) or clients (outcome criteria) or organizations (structure criteria). One process criterion for measuring ANA community health nursing standard V might be "community health nurse provides instruction in the prevention of disease and the preservation of health when client situation warrants such activities."

The term *indicator* is used synonymously with criteria by the Joint Commission on the Accreditation of Healthcare Organizations and many other health care organizations. "An indicator is an objective, measurable, well-defined variable relating to the structure, process, or outcome of care" (JCAHO, 1990, p. 29). Indicators/criteria facilitate data collection during the quality assessment process and help health care providers to make informed decisions regarding the quality or appropriateness of care or service (JCAHO).

The development of standards and criteria for evaluation of nursing care should occur from three perspectives: structure, process, and outcome. Donabedian (1966, pp. 169-170), in his classic article on health care quality, saw *structure* standards as those which appraise the environment in which health care is provided. Such things as the organizational framework, the availability of resources, the qualifications of staff, and the adherence to legal mandates are examined with structural standards. The American Nurses Association, the National League for Nursing, and the Joint Commission on Accreditation of Healthcare Organizations have been actively engaged in the development of structural standards. Licensure, certification, and accreditation standards provide guidelines for agencies by which to evaluate their structural characteristics. One such standard requires that agencies have adequate resources to achieve their stated goals. Criteria in relation to such things as numbers of staff and amount of funding are used to measure this standard.

Process standards and criteria/indicators describe how care should be delivered (Donabedian, 1969, p. 1833). They focus on reviewing the activities carried out by health care providers in order to help clients meet their specific health care needs. They are designed *to evaluate the use of the clinical process* to determine if it was appropriately applied with individual clients. Process standards and criteria help health care providers to examine their behavior and skills in relation to client-nurse interactions, the formulation of clinical diagnoses and client goals, the implementation of various intervention strategies, the process of evaluation, and the coordination of care with other health professionals. Process standards and criteria determine if clinical services were appropriate to the needs of the family or a specified at-risk group. They also identify where clinical intervention was needed but not implemented. The ANA community health standards listed earlier are process standards. "Community health nurse documents a biopsychosocial health history on the client service record" could be one process criterion used to determine whether the ANA standard II, in relation to data collection, has been achieved.

Outcome standards and criteria/indicators focus attention on the end results of care (Donabedian, 1969, p. 1833). They measure the behavioral changes within the client rather than the process health care providers used to effect client change. They evaluate what a client has learned, not what or how the professional has taught. For example, an outcome standard might read, "Caregiver demonstrates knowledge of parenting skills." Some outcome criteria to measure achievement of this standard could be (1) caregiver appropriately discusses three safety needs of infants; (2) caregiver verbalizes four basic physical care needs of infants; (3) caregiver appropriately discusses the recommended preventive health care schedule for infants. "Reduce infant mortality by the year 2000" is an aggregate-focused outcome standard. An outcome criteria/indicator to measure this standard might read "reduce the infant mortality rate to no more than 7 per 1,000 live births—baseline: 10.1 per 1,000 live births in 1987" (USDHHS, 1991, p. 368).

There are limitations in all three approaches—structure, process, and outcome—to the evaluation of nursing care. Structural standards and criteria define essential system characteristics necessary for successful implementation of clinical care in a particular setting. They do not ensure that system resources are used effectively or efficiently in the delivery of care. Having sufficient staff, for instance, does not guarantee that quality care will be provided. Process standards and criteria appraise only how health care providers carry out their functions to effect change. They do not evaluate if change has occurred as a result of clinical activities. Outcome standards and criteria are difficult to articulate because client health outcomes are influenced by multiple interrelated factors. The biopsychosocial characteristics of a client, the environmental conditions of the client's setting, and the contributions of various disciplines all affect the health outcome status of a client. Outcome criteria do not specify which contributing factor was most relevant (Donabedian, 1966, pp. 167-169). It takes considerable skill to isolate elements to measure client outcomes that have occurred as a result of clinical actions alone. "The outcome of care can be compared to the picture on a puzzle box: it is what the consumer and provider see as a result of the structure (the pieces) and process (fitting the pieces together)" (Peters and Eigsti, 1991, p. 45).

Outcome standards and criteria/indicators are being used to monitor the process of care (success, failure, or complication of an intervention), the client's health status (short-term or long-term functional level of the client), and organizational outcomes including the cost of quality care (Finnigan, Abel, Dobler, Hudon and Terry, 1993; JCAHO, 1990; Peters and Eigsti, 1991). A futuristic challenge is to develop health care industry outcomes that can be used by organizations to compare themselves to each other and by consumers to identify agencies which provide quality service. The NLN Community Health Accreditation Program's "In Search For Excellence in Home Care" project, funded by the W.K. Kellogg Foundation, is designed to address this challenge (Peters and Eigsti, 1991; Peters, 1992).

When outcome, process, and structure criteria/indicators are developed, thresholds for evaluation and a time frame for goal achievement are also established. A "threshold for evaluation is a level or point at which the results of data collection in monitoring and evaluation trigger intensive evaluation of a particular important aspect of care to determine whether an actual problem or opportunity for improvement exists" (JCAHO, 1990, p. 141). In other words, a threshold is the percentage of time the criteria/indicator should be met within a given time period (Anderson and Singleton, 1992). Thresholds for evaluation can range from 100% of the time to 0% of the time. However, JCAHO (1990) believes that since thresholds of evaluation are designed to take into account the multiple factors that affect health care delivery—such as socioeconomic and educational status of clients and caregivers, severity of a client's illness, and professional experience of staff—it is not effective or productive to set all thresholds for evaluation at 100%. For example, taking into consideration the varying characteristics of family caregivers, it is not realistic to expect that instruction to caregivers on appropriate pain management strategies be completed by the third home visit 100% of the time.

It is apparent that all three approaches to the evaluation of care are essential if quality is to be ensured. When using any of these approaches, it is important to be realistic about what can be accomplished. The realities of an agency's situation should be analyzed carefully to determine what is possible to operationalize. *Standards and criteria/indicators that are all-inclusive can seldom be reached and tend to cause frustration and anxiety among staff.* In the community health setting it is often stated, for instance, that comprehensive health care services will be provided to clients in the home, school, and clinic settings. Resources, however, are frequently not sufficient to achieve this goal. When this is the case, services to all clients are diluted because the available work force is not adequate to meet all the health care needs in each of these settings. It would be more realistic to identify selected services, such as consultation to teachers and follow-up on children with chronic health problems, that will be provided in any one setting.

Developing standards and criteria/indicators presents special challenges to the nurse in the community health setting. A goal of community health nursing practice is to help groups (families, aggregates, and communities) to obtain their maximal level of functioning. Groups in all stages of the life span are the recipients of community health nursing services. Health supervision activities versus curative treatment are the major orientation when community health nurses are working with many of these groups. However, measurement of health supervision activities with groups is not a well-defined art.

Quantitative counts such as numbers of home, school, and clinic visits, changes in mortality and morbidity statistics, and figures obtained from cost-benefit studies have traditionally been used to determine the effectiveness of nursing services in community health. *None of these measurements evaluates quality.* These measurements do not take into consideration the types of services required based on client needs, how well services are provided, and the results of nursing interventions.

Measuring health supervision activities is not an easy task, because often psychosocial variables have a greater impact on health outcomes than do biological variables. There are few absolutes when it comes to defining healthy psychosocial functioning. This is increasingly true as societal values change, allowing for and accepting various lifestyles. Although it is not easy to develop health supervision standards, it is not impossible. The ANA community health standards are designed to evaluate *process* with all types of nursing activities, including health promotion ones. The Ervin Quality Assessment Measurement Instrument (Ervin, Chen, and Upshaw, 1989) is another example of a process-oriented quality assessment tool appropriate for evaluating community health nursing service delivery.

Outcome standards for health supervision visits are also being developed by some agencies. These have been written in a variety of ways: according to developmental age categories such as infant, preschool, school, adolescent, adult, and aging; according to like conditions or health-related phenomena such as pregnancy, parenthood, mental retardation, or child abuse; or according to disease categories such as cancer, arthritis, or heart problems (Buck, 1988; Lalonde, 1988; Minnesota Department of Health, 1979; More and Masterson, 1987; Rinke and Wilson, 1988a and 1988b).

If community health nurses choose to organize standards of care according to disease categories, it is extremely important to guard against focusing attention on the disease process. How the client is *coping* with the disease condition, as well as the client's current health status, should be the major emphasis in these types of standards. The role of the community health nurse is to provide information, to help the client solve problems, and to improve the client's self-care capabilities in a way that will facilitate adaptation to stresses being experienced.

Developmental and family health supervision standards are needed in the community health setting, even when condition or disease standards are available. This is necessary since a major role of the community health nurse is to encourage health-promotion activities, even if disease is not present, among individuals, families, and aggregates across the life span. In order to implement this role, community health nurses need a framework for assessing family structure, functions, and processes and for analyzing strengths and needs of family functioning. They also need a framework that will help them to identify strengths and needs of individuals across the life spectrum and to modify intervention strategies according to the individual needs of a developmental age group.

Health supervision standards must be sufficiently broad so that cultural differences are not discounted. They must be flexible enough to allow for professional judgment and client participation in the formulation of specific outcomes. They should be individualized by providers in each health care setting, based on the needs of the community and the resources of the particular organization. Use of a conceptual framework is more likely to ensure that these provisions will be included in standard forumulation. Maslow's hierarchy of needs, for instance, postulates that people must meet their physical needs before they will achieve self-esteem or self-actualization. Based on this belief, a family health supervision standard that states "the family provides for the basic needs of its members" could be developed and used with families from all cultures. Such a standard does not provide specific directives for how a family should accomplish this goal. This is important because cultures vary as to how food, shelter, and clothing are provided, as well as how health care is obtained. One criterion for evaluation of this standard could be "family members have an adequate intake of iron, which is demonstrated by all family members having a normal hemoglobin value." This criterion does not specify that a particular type of food must be eaten, and thus takes into consideration cultural variations in relation to eating patterns. There are several other criteria that could be used to measure whether this standard has been achieved. For any standard there will likely be many criteria measurements used to evaluate how well the standard has been met.

A strong knowledge base about specific cultural values and religious beliefs is essential in order for the community health nurse to use standards of care appropriately. Factors such as dietary patterns, traditional ways of dealing with child rearing, allocation of family roles, methods for obtaining health care and treating illness, and rituals during periods of joy or sadness must be known. Only when a community health nurse has this information can she or he make accurate professional judgments about a family's pattern of functioning. Judaism, for example, has a complex set of rituals during mourning that allows for various levels of grief and that encourages the release of emotional tension. A memorial prayer, the *kaddish,* is recited by many Jewish families at daily services for 11 months after the death of a loved one (Kensky, 1977, p. 199). This is *normal, traditional* behavior. A community health nurse who is not aware of these rituals may erroneously label this behavior "a prolonged grief reaction."

The importance of having an appreciation for the

inherent worth of different cultural values and religious beliefs cannot be overemphasized. A community health nurse's ability to work effectively with families from different cultural groups is dependent upon the ability to understand them in terms of their background as they view it. Cultural values and religious beliefs dictate behavior and must be respected.

Secure Measurements

Total quality management is a *factual* problem-solving process. After standards and criteria/indicators are specified, tools and methods for evaluating and measuring quality must be selected. Record audits, utilization review procedures, interviews, observation of clients, peer review procedures, client satisfaction surveys, and staff self-reviews are some of the methods used for collecting factual data about quality clinical care.

Four evaluation tools—the Quality Patient Care Scale (Qualpacs), the Slater Nursing Competencies Rating Scale, the Phaneuf Audit, and the Medicus tool—were developed in the 1970s to assist practitioners in evaluating client care or staff performance. The Qualpacs instrument (Wandelt and Ager, 1974) is designed to evaluate care as it is being given. The Slater Scale (Wandelt and Stewart, 1974) was developed to evaluate individual nurse performance. The Phaneuf Audit (Phaneuf, 1976) is constructed to appraise quality of care retrospectively, as it is reflected in the patient care records of discharged patients. The Medicus tool relates processes of care to outcomes of care (Wilbert, 1985). The Medicus tool is widely used in inpatient settings and has been refined over time. It depends on computer support for utilization (Wilbert, 1985) (refer to Figure 23-3). Phaneuf's record audit concept is used in the community health nursing setting but is modified to address both the unique processes involved in the specialty field and changing philosophies about quality monitoring. Quality management uses the skills or methods of quality assurance but focuses on quality measurement to improve it through support, innovation, and creativity, not to ensure it through threats (Peters, 1992, p. 24).

Record Audit

Both concurrent and retrospective record auditing are carried out in community health agencies. Organizations subscribing to total quality management or continuous quality improvement emphasize concurrent review to learn about the process of care and services rather than the performance of individuals (Anderson and Singleton, 1992, p. 69; Peters, 1992). In other words, emphasis is placed on learning how the system is currently functioning with a focus on identifying how it can be improved. The concept underlying this emphasis is that there is always room for improvement (Peters, p. 22).

A record audit encompasses a systematic review of a specified number of service records in a given period of time and the development and implementation of interventions to improve the quality of care provided when system changes are needed. For example, an agency may find that there is a need to develop new criteria/indicators as new services are added. This may be identified through a record review audit or a service review process.

Record audits are used to examine the process of care, as well as outcomes of care. They are structured to ensure consistency of interpretation by all reviewers; this structure is obtained through the use of an audit tool that has a set of care standards, criteria/indicator measurements for each care standard, and a quality rating scale. Criteria/indicators are predetermined, measurable characteristics of a variable (care standard) that are used to make judgments about the quality of care provided. One process criteria/indicator used to determine how well nurses complete assessments might read, "community health nurses collect and record data in relation to a client's family history." An outcome criteria/indicator used to assess continuity of care could be "all clients will be visited within 24 hours of referral to agency."

Each agency should have its own set of criteria/indicators for its quality improvement program. JCAHO requires that client satisfaction be used as an indicator of the quality and appropriateness of care (JCAHO, 1990). An agency functioning under a total quality management philosophy empowers staff to select appropriate quality criteria/indicators, based on a review of the professional literature.

As previously mentioned, record audits are not used to evaluate individual staff performance but rather system problems that inhibit the delivery of effective and efficient clinical services. With this philosophy, staff are encouraged to identify opportunities for improvement in clinical practice and to actively participate in matters affecting delivery of client care (Mills, 1992). This is not meant to imply that staff do not appraise their own performance; all staff are responsible for continuous quality improvement, including examining ways to improve their own performance.

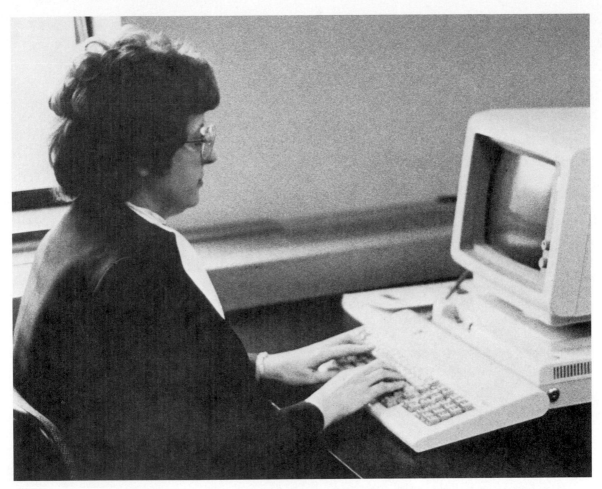

Figure 23-3 Community health nurses across the country use computers to facilitate recording, quality assessment and improvement efforts, and other documentation processes. Computerized information systems help health care providers to effectively and efficiently document client data and clinical services and to obtain easy access to planning data. This, in turn, provides administrators with information needed to support current or projected staffing patterns and relevant clinical programs. (Courtesy Henry Parks, photographer.)

Staff Performance Appraisals

All health care providers have the responsibility to evaluate the quality of care they are providing. Indirectly, the audit approach aids individual providers in examining their practice in relation to standards established for care. Direct mechanisms are also used to evaluate if clients served by the agency receive care equal to or better than established standards. Ongoing evaluation of one's professional performance is important, because it can provide a safeguard for quality client care, promote professional development, and facilitate the identification of professional strengths and opportunities for professional improvement.

Staff evaluation processes also aid employers in identifying system barriers that impede effective and efficient delivery of clinical services. Under a total quality management system, a performance planning and reward system recognizes teamwork in addition to individual accountability, and examines how to change to make the team more effective (Diederich and Eisenberg, 1993).

All nursing personnel must be evaluated on the basis of specified criteria; these criteria should reflect all aspects of nursing performance expected in a given setting, including teamwork. Careful attention must be given to the development of criteria that identify

TABLE 23-2   Milwaukee Visiting Nurse Association's Job and Personnel Specifications for a Public Health Nurse II

Section A—job description and specifications

Job Summary: Under supervision, has responsibility for case management of patients and families with a wide variety of complex health and social problems, including multiproblem families. Is expected to be able to function independently in most situations. Identifies need for consultation or supervisory help. May be assigned additional responsibilities which require leadership ability.

Duties and responsibilities	Basic requirements
1. Functions independently in case management of complex situations, using supervision appropriately.	Interviewing skills. Physical assessment skills.
2. Admits patients and family members and gives service utilizing the nursing process.	Knowledge of health problems and illnesses.
a. Assessment—collects physiological, psychosocial, and financial data. Can identify the need for further data and pursues sources of data independently.	Knowledge of normal growth and development. Ability to make nursing judgments based on scientific nursing principles.
b. Assesses family members' health status and coping ability. Able to evaluate the family as a unit.	Knowledge of data sources within the community.
c. Identifies covert and overt nursing health and social problems of patients and families based on data collection.	Knowledge of family dynamics. Ability to see and interpret relationships in data and to arrive at a nursing care plan.
d. Implements nursing care plan as outlined. Adapts nursing procedures to the home setting.	Ability to identify objective parameters for evaluation of nursing care plan.
e. Evaluates results of care plan in terms of expected outcomes and takes appropriate action.	
3. Recognizes and interprets behavior patterns as influenced by basic physical and emotional needs, cultural and socioeconomic differences. Sensitive and accepting of these needs and differences and adapts plan of care accordingly.	Knowledge of cultural and socioeconomic factors. Knowledge of behavioral principles. Knowledge of self. Sensitivity and ability to listen. Knowledge of dependent and independent nursing functions.
4. Contacts physician to report alterations in patient's health status, to secure and share information, or to obtain medical orders.	Ability to collaborate with other disciplines regarding health care.
5. Independently identifies need for consultation and initiates referral.	Knowledge of consultants available and their role in the agency.
6. Independently refers patients and families to other VNA or community services.	
7. Communicates with other disciplines and services inter-agency and intra-agency to promote continuity and coordination of services.	Knowledge of community resources. Knowledge of agency procedures. Ability to write clear, concise, informative reports.
8. Teaches patients and families nursing procedures and good health practices. Interprets to patient and family the implications of the diagnosis—includes the patient and family in goal setting and plan of care according to their ability.	Knows teaching/learning principles. Ability to adapt to patient and family level of understanding and ability.

Reproduced by permission of the Milwaukee Visiting Nurse Association, Milwaukee, Wis, undated.

23-2 Milwaukee Visiting Nurse Association's Job and Personnel Specifications for a Public Health Nurse II—cont'd

Duties and responsibilities	Basic requirements
9. Plans for the use of ancillary agency personnel and supervises their performance.	Knowledge of the legal functions of the RN, LPN, H-HHA. Knowledge of the legal functions of the RN, LPN, H-HHA in the agency.
10. Organizes and manages caseload efficiently. a. Plans travel routes for optimum economy and efficiency. b. Establishes priorities within own caseload. c. Plans frequency of visits. d. Completes necessary records and reports as required within set time limits.	Good organizational skills. Knowledge of area and travel routes. Ability to use maps.
11. May be assigned additional responsibilities. (Committees, research, etc.)	

Professional Conduct:

1. Accepts agency philosophy, purpose, and objectives.	Knowledge of philosophy, purpose, and objectives.
2. Follows agency policies and procedures.	Knowledge of policies and procedures.
3. Demonstrates good inter-personal relationships.	Recognizes how behavior affects others.
4. Uses proper resources to deal with stress.	

Professional Growth:

1. Participates in performance evaluation.	Motivated towards self-improvement.
2. Takes responsibility for own professional growth.	

Section B—personnel specifications

1. Wisconsin professional nurse registration.
2. Graduate of baccalaureate program accredited by the National League of Nursing and American Public Health Association.
3. Two years current experience in community health nursing.

how well a nurse uses the nursing process. Often greater emphasis is placed on personal appearance, quantitative counts of visits, and adherence to time policies than to nursing care given. These factors should not be ignored when reviewing staff performance, but they should not be the only focus of the staff evaluation process.

Developing job and personnel specifications that focus on the critical components of nursing practice is the first step in developing appropriate evaluation criteria that reflect all aspects of nursing performance. An example of such specifications developed by one Visiting Nurse Association for a Public Health Nurse II

position is presented in Table 23-2. Note particularly in these specifications that the nurse's duties and responsibilities emphasize nursing functions and specifically identify what the community health nurse needs to accomplish in relation to client care. This type of delineation aids in the identification of relevant evaluation categories when nurses are developing evaluation tools.

Community health nurses at all levels, from administrators to staff, have a responsibility to become involved in the evaluation process. Nurses who actively participate in the development of tools for measurement of care and the evaluation process will be more satisfied with the results. Take the initiative to become involved. It will be a learning experience that will have long-lasting effects on the delivery of your nursing care.

Implementation of Evaluation Measurements

Developing measurement tools and procedures to facilitate use of those tools takes time and a commitment to the concept of continuous quality improvement. Administrative support during the development and implementation phases of a quality improvement program is essential. Without administrative support, it is highly unlikely that staff will be allowed sufficient time to prepare adequate measurement tools and evaluation procedures. Administrators can also help to reduce the resistance to change and to obtain funds for staff development activities. Many agencies have found that nurses feel threatened when new evaluation measurements are instituted; staff development programs can reduce this threat.

When implementing a quality improvement program, staff members should be oriented to the use of the tools in addition to the *process* procedures. They should be allowed to verbalize their anxieties and lack of understanding in a supportive atmosphere. At times, committee members who have had the chief responsibility for developing the measurement tools become frustrated when all staff members do not seem to accept the tools as readily as they have. This occurs particularly when committee members forget how long it took them to accomplish their task and to understand the process involved. Members of evaluation committees must recognize that all personnel need time to air their concerns, just as committee members had time during the development phase. It should not be expected that staff will grasp the concepts of quality improvement without thought, debate, and resistance. This type of discourse helps staff to develop ownership of a continuous quality improvement program.

As was discussed in Chapter 13, when any program is planned, implementation occurs more smoothly if a master plan is developed that identifies what is to be done, how it will be done, who will assume primary leadership and accountability, when it will be done, and how the results will be documented. This type of plan assists staff in implementing quality assessment activities in a systematic and timely manner. While certification and accrediting agencies generally require documentation of quality assessment activities, in most states these activities are protected and considered confidential (Koch and Fairly, 1993). Measures need to be established to protect the confidentiality of data collected during the clinical assessment review process.

Make Interpretations

Data from all clinical assessment procedures should be examined to make interpretations about the quality of nursing care being provided in a particular setting. One tool alone, such as the record audit, cannot provide a sufficient data base to determine if quality is high or needs improving. In addition, data from multiple sources are often needed to identify the real reasons for inadequate care.

The purpose of quality assessment activities is to identify discrepancies between established standards and criteria and actual clinical practice. Evaluation assessments should be specific enough to identify both strengths and areas needing improvement in the current level of clinical care. In general, most agencies have found that both strengths and opportunities for improvement do exist. If either is found lacking when analyzing evaluation data, the measurement tools and the process for using these tools should be reevaluated. The tools may be too general and broad to discriminate between safe and unsafe care. On the other hand, the tools may be appropriate, but staff may need additional orientation to use them effectively. When they are using the record audit for the first time, it is not uncommon to find nurses assuming that certain care was given, even if it was not documented in the family service record. This may be an inappropriate assumption that covers up deficiencies in nursing care.

In order to make interpretations about discrepancies between standards and actual practice, measurement data must be organized and grouped so that a composite picture is clearly presented. Summary reports should be developed so that the combined results of multiple efforts can be examined and patterns of care identified. Interpretations about overall agency quality must be based on *patterns* occurring over time, rather than on selected record reviews at a given time. Figure 23-4 is a sample of a summary report that displays the results of multiple records audits. This summary report helps agency staff to quickly identify strengths and areas needing improvement. It also allows for comparisons from one audit review to another, because change is depicted numerically.

Monthly summary report

Nursing audit report _____
(Month) (Day) (Year)

_____
/s/ Chairman, Nursing Audit Committee

Number of family folders reviewed ☐

Overall evaluation by
number of family folders

Outstanding	Satisfactory	Incomplete	Unsatisfactory
☐	☐	☐	☐

Category name	Outstanding	Satisfactory	Incomplete	Unsatisfactory	Total
I. Observation of situation					
II. Evaluate total situation and draw up plans for nursing plans					
III. Implementation of nursing plans					
IV. Coordination of other services—intra- and interagency					
V. Recording format					

Function	Outstanding	Satisfactory	Incomplete	Unsatisfactory
I	49–64	33–48	17–32	0–16
II	49–64	33–48	17–32	0–16
III	28–36	19–27	10–18	0–9
IV	15–20	10–14	5–9	0–4
V	12–14	8–11	4–7	0–3

Record score range

149–198 = Outstanding
100–148 = Satisfactory
51– 99 = Incomplete
0– 50 = Unsatisfactory

Summary of comments:

Figure 23-4 Oakland County Division of Health, Public Health Nurse Family Record Audit: Monthly Summary Report. (Reproduced by permission of the Nursing Division, Oakland County Division of Health, Pontiac, Mich.)

There are several ways to display and summarize data such as the use of tables, histograms, graphs, and charts (refer to Chapter 12). Presented in the box on p. 896 is a brief discussion of some common tools used to help understand the underlying causes of assessments results. A case study analysis using the "fishbone" cause-and-effect diagram is presented later in this chapter.

Identify Course of Action

Once strengths and needed improvements in the delivery of clinical practice have been delineated, alternative interventions should be identified to improve care. In addition, health care providers should receive positive feedback about their strengths. Staff members who receive only negative feedback can become discouraged and may be

◀ *Data Display Tools* ▶

Flow Charts

A flow chart graphically represents the sequence of events or steps that are required in a particular process or to produce a specific output.

Cause-and-effect Diagram

The cause-and-effect diagram looks like a fishbone with the effect being the desired outcome and the causes represented by the "spines." The causes are usually divided into four categories: materials, methods, manpower, and machines. This tool is referred to as a fishbone diagram or Ishikawa, named after a leading QI authority in Japan.

Run Chart

The run chart displays events or observations over time.

Pareto Chart

The pareto chart displays data in a ranking order comparing factors used to determine priorities, a way to sort out the "vital few" from the "trivial many."

Histogram

The histogram displays a graphic summary of how frequently something occurs.

Control Chart

The control chart distinguishes common cause and special cause variation. It appears as a run chart with statistically determined upper and lower limits above and below the average.

Scatter Diagram

The scatter diagram demonstrates the relationship between two variables.

From Koch MW and Fairly TM: *Integrated quality management: the key to improving nursing care quality,* St. Louis, 1993, Mosby, p. 65.

less motivated to make necessary changes.

To identify alternative courses of action for improving care, health care providers must first analyze why certain problems are occurring. For example, perhaps the recording of the nursing staff demonstrates very little follow-up and evaluation of nursing interventions. There are several reasons why this may be happening, including lack of knowledge, insufficient time allocated for recording, inadequate caseload management skills, unshared values, limited resources, and poor staff morale. Discourse among nurses to find the reasons for the problems should occur before change actions are identified. If the problem is due to inadequate resources to meet client needs rather than lack of knowledge, planning for continuing education programs would be inappropriate. Time allocated for continuing education in this situation would probably only increase the probability that all client needs were not being met. Administrative action to secure further resources or to reevaluate job expectations would be more appropriate.

Input from all staff is essential for determining the best course of action to improve the delivery of clinical services. An administrative mandate specifying that changes must occur immediately will frustrate staff members if they have not been allowed to voice their

opinions about the help they need to alter their actions. Most health care providers are interested in providing quality care. They will resist change, however, if they are not actively involved in selecting the appropriate course for change.

Choose Action

Two major activities should occur when choosing change actions: (1) discussion about the advantages and disadvantages of suggested remedial actions and (2) development of a plan for implementing the selected change strategy. Refer again to the situation in which record audits reflect inadequate follow-up and evaluation of nursing interventions. If the major problem identified in this situation is poor documentation due to lack of skill, remedial actions might include conducting a total staff continuing education program that focuses on recording skills, weekly individual supervisory and staff conferences to discuss strengths and areas needing improvement relative to recording, or self-study by individual staff members. If the majority of the nurses are having difficulty with recording, it probably would be most advantageous to initiate a staff development program. If, on the other hand, only a few nurses are having problems, a staff development program might be very costly to the agency in time and money. If it is determined that a staff continuing education activity is needed, a plan should be developed to ensure that this selected action is implemented.

When discussing the pros and cons of alternate change strategies, agency and community resources should be examined. Often existing resources are not used because it is felt that an "outside expert" or a consultant could produce more positive results. Frequently this is not the case. Nurses are more motivated to make necessary changes when their talents and skills are recognized and supported. They also become committed to helping others during the change process when they are actively involved, because they believe they have something to contribute. The outside expert frequently does not become actively involved in the change process. This person often shares knowledge and then agency personnel are left to decide how to make changes based on newly gained information. There are times when outside resources should be used; however, such help should be used with discretion because it can be costly and may not help an agency to accomplish what it hopes to achieve.

Planning for change increases the probability that change will occur. It also increases the likelihood that activities will be orderly and predictable and less stressful to staff. Although the entire staff should be involved in developing action plans, it is important to identify who or what is expected to change, who is responsible for implementing the action plan, and when the change is expected to occur (Koch and Fairly, 1993, p. 65). Without such a plan it is difficult to coordinate change activities and to monitor their progress.

Take Action

Improvement of clinical care is the primary objective of any quality assessment program. Action must be taken if this is to occur; merely defining areas needing improvement is not enough. Decisions about various alternative approaches must be made and improvement measures implemented, because merely having a discussion about change produces few results.

Taking action to alter practice is one of the most significant components of a quality assurance program. It demonstrates that health care providers really do assume accountability for the care provided by members of their profession. It supports the belief that qual-

ity assessment should be the responsibility of a profession rather than the responsibility of legal authorities.

Improvement action must be carefully documented and evaluated to determine whether or not it has altered practice. Other actions may be needed if the selected one does not result in desired change. If, for instance, a staff development program does not improve the documentation on client service records, supervisors may have to increase their conference time with individual staff members or examine the documentation system being used. The quality assessment cycle should continue even if change does occur. Ongoing monitoring is essential in order to maintain quality standards for practice over time.

Monitor Quality Improvement Actions

Ongoing monitoring is essential to maintain quality practice over time. Emphasis should be placed on continuous improvement rather than on simply solving identified problems (Anderson and Singleton, 1992). A sound quality assessment program sets in place strategies to identify if improvement is sustained or if new or additional improvement actions are needed. Such a program also maintains a focus on the future and continuously examines the need for new quality measurements, or for actions and educational programs that will help staff members to gain the skills needed to handle job requirements and quality assessment activities.

"Continuous improvement is like a chain reaction. Improvement in one area contributes to improvement in another area" (Smith, Discenza, and Piland, 1993, p. 44). For example, poor quality is costly to an organization from both a direct and indirect perspective. Poor quality control can directly increase financial outlays for malpractice insurance, and can cause costly insurance billing errors, excessive overtime and the ordering of unnecessary clinical procedures. Indirectly poor quality can lead to such things as dissatisfied or lost clients, a bad reputation in the community, lack of client care follow-up, and upset or frustrated staff (Milakovich, 1991). Improving quality can help to reduce both visible (direct) and hidden (indirect) costs for an organization.

Continuous quality monitoring helps an organization to prevent problems and to maintain the gains achieved through improvement actions. The continuous quality improvement process encourages staff to actively participate in identifying potential and actual problems and to examine how environmental factors make an impact on service delivery. Environmental factors such as the evolutionary nature of the treatment of disease and changing technology, demographic characteristics of the population, and socioeconomic conditions in society continuously influence the health care delivery process (Cesta, 1993). This in turn requires a continuous focus on how the system can improve to address these changes.

Integrated Quality Management Processes

Escalating health care costs and complex changes in health care delivery have resulted in increased concern over cost containment and legal issues affecting community-based health care agencies. This has led to an emphasis on utilization review, risk and safety management, and infection control activities.

Utilization review is a process designed to evaluate "the appropriateness of client admissions and discharges; the appropriate and adequate use of personnel; and over- and under-utilization of services" (NLN, 1985, p. 48). This process focuses on the delivery of services in a cost-effective and efficient manner and uses a client record review to identify if the amount and type of services provided were appropriate to the needs of the clients and appropriate for the agency to provide. Patient classification systems assist agencies in predicting the kind and amount of service needed by client groups with specific characteristics. Although patient classification systems have been more widely used in acute care settings, there are several available community-oriented classification systems designed to predict service needs (Ballard and McNamara, 1983; Churness, Kleffel, Onodera, and Jacobson, 1988; Daubert, 1979; Hardy, 1984; Harris, Santoferraro, and Silva, 1985; Sienkiewicz, 1984).

Risk and safety management is a process designed to identify, evaluate, address, and prevent potential and actual risks that increase the chances of legal liability (Tehan and Colegrove, 1987). Tehan and Colegrove (p. 71) believe that home care agencies face significant risk in relation to the delivery of patient care services, assessment of caregiver competency, and employee health and safety. Nonprofit and public community agencies face similar risks (Knapp, 1989). Community-based agencies are currently placed in a position of improving quality care with limited resources while delivering increasingly complex client services and containing costs. This position has exposed agencies to increased risks and safety issues and has provided a stimulus for agencies to expand their risk and safety management programs. A risk and safety management program focuses on such matters as the monitoring of staff selection, orientation, and on-going educational processes; the development of policies to ensure client and employee safety; the evaluation of unsafe client and employee incidents; and the development of educational materials to enhance caregiver/client competency.

Infection control is a process focused on disease prevention, intervention, and recognition (Koch and Fairly, 1993). The concepts and principles of epidemiology discussed in Chapter 11 form a foundation for an effective infection control program. Control actions are generally directed toward breaking the chain of transmission for infection (refer to Figure 11-10). Examples of infection control activities are reporting and monitoring infection rates; maintaining an infection control surveillance system; orienting or providing inservice for staff about infection control issues; establishing infection control policies and procedures, including policies regarding the disposal of infectious wastes and universal precautions; and instructing clients on infection control techniques (Koch and Fairly, 1993). Community health nurses have numerous opportunities for exposure to infectious diseases. It is imperative that infection control policies and procedures be followed in all community-based settings.

While utilization review, risk and safety management, infection control, and quality assessment programs have distinctive and separate foci, they are interrelated and have a significant impact on each other. For example, selected aspects of utilization review focus on the provision of optimal or quality care. Underutilization of clinical services such as limited referral to other community agencies and too few home visits can seriously affect the quality of care provided to clients. Underutilization of resources can impede client progress.

An ultimate goal of each of these continuous quality improvement (CQI) programs is improved or positive outcomes (refer to Figure 23-5). In order to accomplish this goal, all CQI should be integrated and coordinated to achieve a balance among the goals of the four programs. If this coordination is lacking, an agency may neglect aspects of each of these programs (Harris, 1988, p. 400). Integrated quality management is the key to improving nursing care quality (Koch and Fairly, 1993).

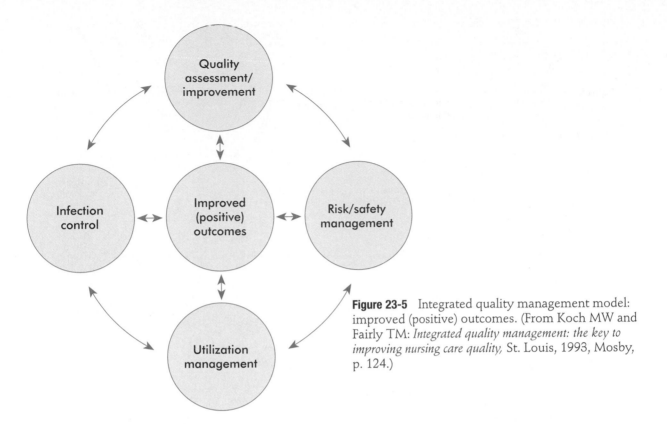

Figure 23-5   Integrated quality management model: improved (positive) outcomes. (From Koch MW and Fairly TM: *Integrated quality management: the key to improving nursing care quality,* St. Louis, 1993, Mosby, p. 124.)

The following case study represents a typical home care client (Koch and Fairly, 1993, pp. 235-236).

▶ **Mr. N. is a 55-year-old white male who retired early from a lucrative law practice because of a debilitating stroke (Fig. 23-6). He has a history of hypertension and workaholic behavior. He has been in a rehabilitation center and has now returned home for continued support.**

He is overweight and has been unable to care for himself since the cardiovascular accident. He has several children in town, including a son who is a nurse at a local hospital. His wife employs an attendant from 10 PM to 6 AM each day to care for Mr. N. She also has a housekeeper who is available for light assistance to Mr. N. during the day. There is good family support. Mr. N.'s private insurance covers intermittent visits by a home care nurse each week.

Figure 23-6 demonstrates the proactive CQI planning process for this case, utilizing the fishbone cause-and-effect diagram described earlier in this chapter. According to Koch and Fairly (1993), this process

"analyzes the possible root causes to produce a positive patient care outcome in each case" (p. 234). The possible root causes of positive outcomes for Mr. N. were defined in terms of issues related to infection control, risk/safety management, utilization management, and quality assessment and improvement (QA/QI). Under the QA/QI component, the authors identified a need to examine the important aspects of Mr. N's care using three priority indicators: high volume (HV), high risk (HR), and problem-prone (PP). According to JCAHO (1990, p. 29), *high volume* means that the client was receiving aspects of care which occur frequently or affect large numbers of clients; *high risk* indicators mean that Mr. N was at risk of serious consequences or would be deprived of substantial benefit if his care is not provided correctly; and *problem-prone* means that aspects of care for Mr. N have tended to produce problems for staff or clients in the past. Though Mr. N had excellent supports and was doing well, the fishbone diagram demonstrated potential risk factors. Koch and Fairly's book is an excellent resource for expanding knowledge of these concepts, as well as the concept of total quality management.

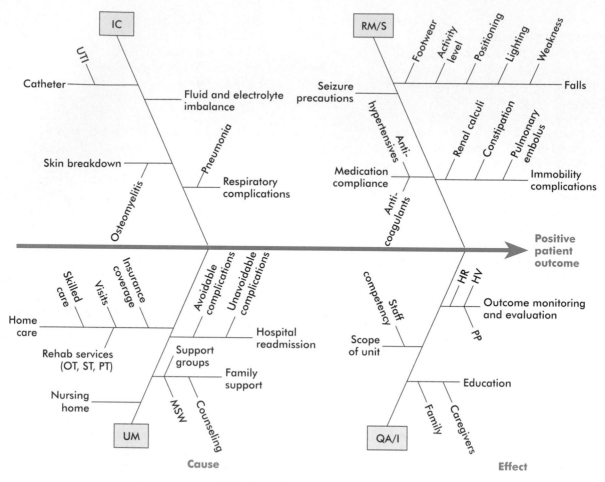

Mr. N.: Home care case study

Figure 23-6   Integrated quality management fishbone diagram: home care case study. *IC,* infection control; *UM,* utilization management; *RM/S,* risk management/safety; *QA/I,* quality assessment/improvement; *HV,* high volume; *HR,* high risk; *PP,* problem-prone. (Redrawn from Koch MW and Fairly TM: *Integrated quality management: the key to improving nursing care quality,* St. Louis, 1993, Mosby, p. 238.)

PARTNERS IN QUALITY IMPROVEMENT

The quality assurance/assessment model (Figure 23-1) presented at the beginning of this chapter illustrates that individual health care providers, professional organizations, and clients all share responsibility for maintaining and improving quality standards for clinical practice. Input from the client is essential for determining values important to recipients of care. Client feedback is also crucial for the identification of improvements needed in practice on an ongoing basis. It is important that clients affect all components of a continuous quality improvement program, because client needs form a foundation from which client services emerge. Organizations that remain viable in the marketplace are ones that are customer-focused in all aspects of health care delivery.

Organizations are using a variety of methods to obtain client input about quality care. Telephone or face-to-face interviews, client satisfaction tools, and client representation on advisory boards are a few examples of ways in which community agencies involve clients in quality assessment. Again, it is important to mention that the term *client* is not limited to the actual recipient of care: community health agencies have multiple clients such as physicians, hospital discharge planners, community groups, third-party payors, and consumers of care. They also have internal clients/customers who benefit from their efforts. Methods should be established to obtain input and feedback from all client groups.

Implementing a total quality management program is an exciting, challenging endeavor that promotes a client-focused system, team-building, and interdisciplinary functioning. All members of the health care team work with the client to improve health care quality. Through collaborative efforts all members of the health care team, including the client, can help an organization to maintain a competitive edge in the health care market. Such a challenge is worth working towards.

Summary

As we advance toward the year 2000, emphasis on quality in health care delivery is increasing. Nurses share with all health care professionals the need to examine carefully the delivery of their services in light of changing societal demands. An exciting approach to quality appraisal and monitoring, *total quality management* or *continuous quality improvement,* has emerged. This concept is client-oriented with a focus on identifying system problems versus individual staff problems. It promotes team-building and interdisciplinary functioning.

Total quality management is a dynamic process that examines both administrative and clinical service aspects of quality care. Quality assessment, utilization review, risk and safety management, and infection control activities are systematically implemented with a focus on improving client and system outcomes. An integrated and coordinated approach is essential to achieve a balance among all quality management components. Quality management is a factual problem-solving process that uses a variety of methods for assessing and improving quality. Crucial to the successful implementation of a total quality management program is an organizational philosophy that promotes a commitment to quality improvement, a participative management leadership style, and a shared vision that places the client in the forefront.

◀ *An Exercise in Critical Thinking* ▶

Using data from a client situation in which you have been involved, identify issues related to infection control, risk/safety management, utilization management, and quality assessment and improvement that needed to be addressed (refer to Figure 23-6). Taking into consideration the environmental conditions existing when you were caring for the identified client, discuss strategies that would improve quality service delivery.

References

American Nurses Association (ANA): *Quality assurance model: a plan for implementation of the standards of nursing practice,* Kansas City, Mo., 1975, The Association.

American Nurses Association: *Standards of home health nursing practice,* Kansas City, Mo., 1986a, The Association.

American Nurses Association, Council of Community Health Nurses: *Standards of community health nursing practice,* Kansas City, Mo., 1986b, The Association.

Anderson P and Singleton EK: From QA to QI in a home health agency. In Dieneman J: *CQI: continuous quality improvement in nursing,* Washington, D.C., 1992, American Nurses Publishing, pp. 63-73.

Ballard S and McNamara R: Quantifying nursing needs in home health care. *Nurs Res* 32(4):236-241, 1983.

Brecker C: The government's role in health care. In Kouner A, ed: *Health care delivery in the United States,* New York, 1990, Springer, pp. 297-328.

Buck JN: Measuring the success of home health care, *Home Health Nurse* 6(3):17-23, 1988.

Bull M: Quality assurance: its origins, transformation, and prospects. In Meisenheimer C, ed: *Quality assurance: a complete guide to effective programs,* Rockville, Md., 1985, Aspens, pp. 8-12.

Cesta TG: The link between continuous quality improvement and case management, *JONA* 23:55-61, 1993.

Christy TE: The first 50 years, *Am J Nurs* 71:1778-1784, 1971.

Churness UH, Kleffel D, Onodera ML, and Jacobson J: Reliability and validity testing of a home health patient classification system, *Public Health Nurs* 5:135-139, 1988.

Daubert EA: Patient classification system and outcome criteria, *Nurs Outlook* 27:450-454, 1979.

Deming WE: *Out of crisis,* Cambridge, Mass., 1986, MIT Press.

Diederich JJ and Eisenberg M: Providing leadership to a decentralized total quality process, *Quality Manage Health Care* 1:19-30, 1993.

Donabedian A: Evaluating the quality of medical care, *Milbank Q* 44:166-206, 1966.

Donabedian A: Some issues in evaluating the quality of nursing care, *Am J Public Health* 59:1833-1836, 1969.

Donabedian A: *The definition of quality and approaches to its assessment,* Ann Arbor, Mich, 1980, Health Administration Press.

Donabedian A: *Models of quality assurance,* materials prepared for the Eighth National Nursing Symposium on Home Health Care, The University of Michigan School of Nursing, Ann Arbor, Mich, June 1993.

Ervin NE, Chen SPC, and Upshaw H: Development of a public health nursing quality assessment measure, *Quality Rev Bull* 15(5):138-143, 1989.

Finnigan SA, Abel M, Dobler T, Hudon L, and Terry B: Automated patient acuity: linking nursing systems and quality measurement with patient outcomes, *JONA* 23:62-71, 1993.

Gardner MS: Typewritten remiscences, Feb. 5, 1948, NOPHN Archive Microfilm #25. In Fitzpatrick ML, ed: *The national organization for public health nursing 1912-1952: development of a practice field,* New York, 1975, National League for Nursing, p. 17.

Gaucher E and Kratochwill EW: The leader's role in implementing total quality management, *Quality Manage Health Care* 1:10-18, 1993.

Hardy JA: A patient classification system for home health patients, *Caring* 3(9):26-27, 1984.

Harris MD: *Home health administration,* Owings Mills, Md., 1988, National Health.

Harris MD, Santoferraro C, and Silva S: A patient classification system in home health care, *Nurs Economics* 3:276-282, 1985.

Health Care Financing Administration (HCFA): *Conditions of participation: home health agencies,* 42CFR, Part 484, Sections 484.1-484.52, Washington, D.C., 1989, U.S. Department of Health and Human Services.

Joint Commission on Accreditation of Healthcare Organizations (JCAHO): *Quality assurance in home care and hospice organizations,* Oakbrook Terrace, Ill., 1990, The Commission.

JCAHO: *Transitions: from QA to CQI—using CQI approaches to monitor, evaluate, and improve quality,* Oakbrook Terrace, Ill., 1991, The Commission.

JCAHO: *Hospice self-assessment and survey guide,* Chicago, 1983, The Commission.

Kensky AD: Cultural influences on the Jewish patient. In Clemen S and Will M, eds: *Family and community health nursing: a workbook,* Ann Arbor, Mich., 1977, University of Michigan.

Knapp MB: Legal concerns affecting nonprofit community agencies that serve the elderly, *Quality Rev Bull* 15(3):86-91, 1989.

Koch MW and Fairly TM: *Integrated quality management: the key to improving nursing care quality,* St. Louis, 1993, Mosby.

Lalonde B: Assuring the quality of home care via the assessment of client outcomes, *Caring* 7(1):20-24, 1988.

Lysaught JP: *An abstract for action,* New York, 1970, McGraw-Hill.

McCann BA and Rooney AL: Striving for excellence in home care: a quality assurance approach, *Caring* 7(10):15-19, 1988.

McLaughlin CP and Kaluzny AD: Total quality management in health: making it work, *Health Care Manage Rev* 15:7-14, 1990.

Melum MM and Sinioris ME: Total quality management in health care: taking stock, *Quality Manage Health Care* 1(4):59-63, 1993.

Milakovich ME: Creating a total quality health care environment, *Health Care Manage Rev* 16:9-20, 1991.

Mills MEC: Some implications of CQI for nursing administration. In Dienemann J: *CQI: continuous quality improvement in nursing,* Washington, DC, 1992, American Nurses Publishing, pp. 31-43.

Minnesota Department of Health, Office of Community Health Services, Section of Community Nursing: *Outcome criteria: public health nursing services and home health care services,* Minneapolis, 1979, The Department.

Model shows dynamic concept of quality assurance, *Am Nurse* 9:23, 1976.

Moran MJ and Johnson JE: Quality improvement: the nurse's role. In Dienemann J, ed: *CQI: continuous quality improvement in nursing,* Washington, D.C., 1992, American Nurses Publishing, pp. 45-61.

More V and Masterson AS: *Hospice care systems, structures, process, costs, and outcomes,* New York, 1987, Springer.

Mullins D and Schmele JA: Reconsideration of the quality circle process as a contemporary management strategy, *Health Care Superv* 12:14-22, 1993.

National League for Nursing (NLN), Council of Home Health Agencies and Community Health Services: *Administrator's handbook for the structure, operation and expansion of home health agencies,* New York, 1985, The League.

NLN: *CHAP, quality through accreditation,* New York, 1992, The League.

O'Leary DS: CQI—a step beyond QA, *Quality Review Bull* 17(1):4-5, 1991.

Papers on the National Health Guidelines: *Baselines for setting health goals and standards,* DHEW Pub No HRA 77-640, Washington, D.C., 1977, Health Resources Administration.

Peters DA and Eigsti D: Utilizing outcomes in home care, *Caring* 10:44-51, 1991.

Peters DA: A new look for quality in home care, *JONA* 22:11-26, 1992.

Phaneuf MC: *The nursing audit: self-regulation in nursing practice,* New York, 1976, Appleton-Century-Crofts.

Public Law 92-603, Section 246E, Title XI, General Provisions and (B) Professional Standards Review, Social Security Amendments of 1972, Ninety-Second Congress HRI, October 30, 1972.

Rinke LT and Wilson AA: *Outcome measures in home care; vol II Service,* New York, 1988a, National League for Nursing.

Rinke LT and Wilson AA: Client-oriented project objectives, *Caring* 7(1):25-29, 1988b.

Sabatino CP: *The "Black Box" of home care quality: a report of the American Bar Association,* presented by Chairman Select Committee, U.S. House of Representatives, Pub No 99-537, Washington, D.C., August 1986, U.S. Government Printing Office.

Schmadl JC: Quality assurance: examination of the concept, *Nurs Outlook* 27:462-465, 1979.

Sienkiewicz JI: Patient classification in community health nursing, *Nurs Outlook* 32:319-321, 1984.

Smith HL, Discenza R, and Piland NF: Reflections on total quality management and health care supervisors, *Health Care Superv* 12:32-45, 1993.

Tehan J and Colegrove SL: Risk management and home health care: the time is now. In Fisher K and Gardner K, eds: *Quality and home health care. redefining the tradition,* Chicago, 1987, Joint Commission on Accreditation of Healthcare Organizations.

Tilbury MS: From QA to CQI: a retrospective review. In Dienemann J, ed: *CQI: continuous quality improvement in nursing,* Washington, D.C., 1992, American Nurses Publishing, pp. 3-14.

USDHHS: *Healthy people 2000: national health promotion and disease prevention objectives, full report, with commentary,* Washington, D.C., 1991, U.S. Government Printing Office.

Visiting Nurse Association of Hartford, Inc.: *Statement of philosophy,* Hartford, Conn., undated.

Wandelt MA and Ager JW: *Quality patient care scale,* New York, 1974, Appleton-Century-Crofts.

Wandelt MA and Stewart DS: *Slater nursing competencies rating scale,* New York, 1974, Appleton-Century-Crofts.

Wilbert C: Computers: quality assurance applications. In Meisenheimer C, ed: *Quality assurance: a complete guide to effective programs,* Rockville, Md., 1985, Aspen, pp. 212-228.

Selected Bibliography

Agency for Health Care Policy and Research: *Report to Congress: progress of research on outcomes of health care services and procedures,* Rockville, Md., 1991, The Agency.

Bernal H: Levels of practice in a community health agency, *Nurs Outlook* 23:364-369, 1978.

Berwick DM, Godfrey AB, and Roessner J: *Caring health care: new strategies for quality improvement,* San Francisco, 1990, Jossey-Bass.

Ceglarek JE and Rife JK: Developing a public health nursing audit, *J Nurs Adm* 10:37-43, 1977.

Daniels K: Planning for quality in the home care system. In Fisher K and Gardner K, eds: *Quality and home health care: redefining the tradition,* Chicago, Ill., 1987, Joint Commission on Accreditation of Healthcare Organizations, pp 38-42.

Deming WE: *Quality, productivity and competitive position,* Cambridge, Mass., 1982, Massachusetts Institute of Technology.

Flynn BC and Ray DW: Current perspectives in quality assurance and community health nursing, *J Community Health Nurs* 4:187-197, 1987.

Gottlieb HJ: Quality assurance: a blueprint for improved patient care and service, *Home Health Nurse* 6(3):11-12, 1988.

Gould EJ and DiPasquale Ruane N: Quality assurance in home health. In Harris MD, ed: *Home health administration,* Ownings Mills, Md., 1988, National Health, pp. 393-439.

Harrington C: Quality, access, and costs: public policy and home health care, *Nurs Outlook* 36:164-166, 1988.

Juran J: *Juran on leadership for quality,* New York, 1989, The Free Press.

Lang NM and Clinton JF: Assessment of quality of nursing care. In Werley HH and Fitzpatrick JJ, eds: *Annual review of nursing research, vol 2,* New York, 1984, Springer.

Masters F and Schmele: Total quality management: an idea whose time has come, *J N Qual Assur* 5:7-16, 1991.

McManis G: Challenges of new decade demand break with tradition, *Modern Healthcare* 20:60, 1990.

New JCAHO Standards emphasize continuous quality improvement, *Hospitals* 5:41-44, 1991, August.

Rice R and Jordan J: Implementing an infection control program for the community-based healthcare facility, *JONA* 22:18-22, 1992.

Sahhey UK and Warden GL: The role of CQI in the strategic planning process, *Quality Manage Health Care* 1:1-11, 1993.

Twardon C, Gartner M, and Cherry C: A competency achievement orientation program: professional development of the home health nurse, *JONA* 23:20-25, 1993.

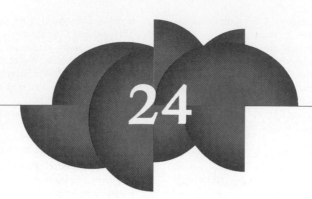

Challenges for the Future

OBJECTIVES

Upon completion of this chapter, the reader should be able to:

1. Describe how technology will change the health care delivery system.
2. Relate changes in the acute care delivery system to service provision in the home setting.
3. Discuss significant nursing challenges in the next decade.
4. List the priority research areas of the National Institute for Nursing Research.

5. Identify ethical issues encountered by community health nurses and the role of an ethics committee in addressing these issues.
6. Explain how political involvement can shape the health care system.
7. Discuss the concept of *health care for all.*

*If you do not think about the future, you cannot
have one.*

JOHN GALSWORTHY
SWAN SONG, 1928

What is the future for community health nursing? The one certainty is that profound change for the health care system lies ahead; where it will lead for providers and consumers alike is not clear. As this chapter is being written, Hillary Rodham Clinton's task force, appointed at the beginning of President Bill Clinton's term in 1993 to address issues in health care reform, had just disbanded and the group's report has been prepared for Congressional hearings. The reform centers on two major issues: health care for all Americans and controlling the growth of health care costs in the future. The White House asked a group of 47 health professionals to critically review the work of this task force: 12 of the 47 members are nurses (Twelve Nurses, 1993, p. 2).

As Chapter 1 demonstrated, nursing developed in response to the needs of society. Florence Nightingale, the pioneer health nurse from England, and Lillian Wald, the first public health nurse, practiced what we know today as primary nursing. They realized that all persons have the right to care, that the community both creates and solves its citizens' health problems, that many disciplines and professions need to work together to solve health problems, and that the focus of care needs to be on prevention. In the years following Wald's work, as increasing technology developed, nursing began to focus on education, research, and practice that was illness-, individual-, and cure-centered. Specialization of nursing roles became important and the legacy of those first public health nursing pioneers was forgotten (Shoulz, Hatcher, and Hurrell, 1992, p. 58). However, health care reform is already moving much illness care to the community and prevention, as well as care, is emphasized for vulnerable populations. The skills and knowledge that are used by past and present community health/public health nurses will again be models for the health care system.

The care of communities conceptualized by contemporary nurses includes the globe: both old and new public health problems make an impact on populations on an international scale. Some concerns such as hurricanes and floods are sudden and affect small areas. Others, including the cholera and AIDS epidem-

ics, as well as the use of guns and drugs, are long-term and have violent implications for all of humankind. Part of our responsibility as public health/community health professionals is to search for innovative approaches to address these problems in our country and to respond to them around the world (Roper, 1992).

The "nurse of the future" requires "consideration of the many issues facing nurses today as health care reform looms. We have many issues to consider—jobs and professional growth, quality of patient care, education—as we face the likelihood of the first major restructuring of the U.S. health care system and the enormous implications for nursing" (Scott, 1993, p. 1). Already there are growing reports of RN layoffs in hospitals around the country in anticipation of changes in health care. The American Nurses Association is calling for a transition plan to help the health care industry deal with the concerns that result from changes in delivering and financing health care (Scott, p. 3).

It remains to be seen how community health nursing will meet growing challenges, such as health care financing, delivery, and accessibility issues, consumer accountability, nursing reimbursement and role changes, changing demands in nursing education, expanding need for nursing research, ethical issues, and politics and nursing. There is a certain amount of risk-taking in predicting and planning the future, because "in an era of change we now face in health care, a forecast based on the past ten to fifteen years experience is the one most likely to be wrong" (Bezold, 1987, p. 94). However, community health nursing will be viable and relevant only as we are willing to take these risks. These challenges and risks will be introduced in this chapter.

HEALTH CARE FINANCING, DELIVERY, ACCESSIBILITY, AND TECHNOLOGY

Throughout this text both the high cost and the lack of availability of health care for many persons has been discussed. More than 60 million Americans are either underinsured or uninsured. Health care costs are nearly 12% of the gross national product. Clinton's Task Force on Health Care Reform addressed both of these problems and, even without legislation, proposed plans to deal with them have already changed the face of nursing. Nursing's Agenda for Health Care Reform promotes the concept of managed care in both public and private plans. Large insurance companies like Cigna are "betting the farm on managed care" (Kerr, 1993, p. 1). Such companies have the power to say who gets what kind of care, how much the providers are paid, and whether health care costs can be controlled. Often nurses are case managers for these companies, functioning as the liaison between the provider, the payor, and the client and taking the leadership role in designing and managing the complete care plan. Experienced community health nurses recognize the description of case manager as their role description. A further method that is already underway to reduce health care costs is the tremendous growth of HMOs and PPOs (discussed in Chapters 4 and 5).

Another trend underway is the changing diversity of primary health care providers. The number of nurse-midwives, nurse practitioners, acupuncturists, and chiropractors is expanding. Dissatisfaction with traditional health care services and the sophistication of consumers who want to have a part in receiving quality care, accompanied by educated practitioners who desire independence from medical institutions, are combining to bring about amazing changes that will benefit clients and the nursing profession. Bezold (1987, p. 93) writes that nurses have a great potential for developing their role in settings that focus on cost containment, high touch (as opposed to high-tech) care delivery, an examination of the outcomes of their care, and quality. Nurses also have a significant potential for helping to build health care systems that are accessible to clients.

The accessibility of health care for all segments of society has also been addressed throughout this text. Lack of accessibility to health care service often results from the service not existing in the first place, lack of knowledge about the service, inability to pay for the service, or inability/difficulty in accessing the services (e.g., transportation problems). The cost of health care is a critical obstacle to accessibility, and we have reached a point in the United States at which the average person cannot afford to be sick. Accessibility of health care for many at-risk and underserved populations, such as inner city and rural residents, the aged, people who are handicapped, and the medically indigent, is an urgent need that must be addressed.

Of all the technologies making an impact on the health care system in the future, the greatest impact will come from telematics (Bezold, 1987, p. 78). The field of telematics includes diagnostic software, record-keeping, the communication of knowledge about health care and individual client observations to almost anywhere in the world, and the capability of developing a client profile that includes biochemical definitions of illness, health, and wellness for that person. Artificial intelligence will, in the coming years, be able to duplicate the reasoning capacity of the brain and software will be produced that can diagnose specific health problems. Medical record-keeping will continue to become more sophisticated and systems will be able to monitor the outcomes of different modalities of care. Likely one of the more astonding scenarios for the future will be the "shaping of health care to the biochemical uniqueness of individuals . . . Current definitions of illness are standardized. . . . Yet the uniqueness of the chemical factories in each of our bodies is as great as the uniqueness of our fingerprints" (Bezold, p. 79). Telematics will allow consumers to be involved both in their own health care and in monitoring the outcomes produced by various providers. Therapies, including drugs, that are deemed to be successful or unsuccessful will be quickly apparent to the public. Questions of privacy, accuracy, and liability will become paramount for ethics committees in health care organizations, as well as for consumers who are currently demanding to become more involved in their own care.

CONSUMER INVOLVEMENT

Consumers of health care, as well as health care professionals, are recognizing the importance of finding ways to meet the needs of underserved populations in our society. Sophisticated consumers are having more to say about the type of care they receive and are increasingly being seen as key members of the health care team. Consumer groups such as the American Association of Retired Persons (AARP) are advocating needed services for their members. This has prompted providers of care to be more responsive to consumer demands and needs.

Maraldo (1990) writes that the "era of the consumer will prevail in the 90s. Consumers will increasingly make their own choices about health services and decisions that affect their health." Nursing also has taken a strong position that the consumer will be the central focus in the new delivery system that develops with the coming health care reform (Betts, 1993). Consumers' needs should determine how health care professionals are educated. This stance says that no longer do doctors and nurses "know what is best for their patients." Rather, professionals and clients will together decide a plan of care. Clients will not be viewed as noncompliant if they do not choose a method of treatment deemed appropriate by the health care professional. Experienced community health nurses have long practiced under this principle, which we call the client's right to self-determination.

Effectiveness and efficiency in the delivery of quality health care services are prime foci for improvement in all health care settings. In this era of limited resources, these foci are essential. Evidence of unmet health care need is prevalent among many segments of the American population and will continue to exist until more appropriate health care delivery patterns are developed. This challenge for the future cannot be ignored. Involving consumers in addressing this challenge can strengthen the position of health care professionals who are advocating needed changes.

NURSING REIMBURSEMENT AND EXPANDED ROLES

Nurses have recognized that changes must occur in traditional nursing roles in order to address the current challenges in the health care delivery system. The role of the nurse is expanding and greater opportunities for nurses are available. Nurses are providing many preventive health services for the "healthy" population, and cost-effective fee-for-service activities. "The American Nurses Association believes that approximately 60 to 80 percent of the primary and preventive care traditionally performed by doctors can be performed by nurses for less money" (Casserta, 1993). Barriers to this kind of practice include limited malpractice insurance, lack of direct reimbursement, and admitting privileges; however, more states are enacting legislation that allows reimbursement for nursing services. The nursing profession can expect resistance from organized medicine in relation to this "competition" and nursing's expanded role, especially as the medical profession faces a personpower surplus with the potential of lost revenue (Ten trends, 1986, p. 18).

An interesting nursing role predicted for the 1990s and beyond is that of the *traveling nurse*. The idea originated with TravCorps, Inc. of Massachusetts in 1978. In 1981 Humana Corporation established its Mobile Nurse Corps to enable its numerous hospitals in 20 states to have adequate nursing staff during periods of high admission and emergencies; there are now more than 70 mobile nurse agencies in the United States (Baumann, 1990a). Traveling nurses go from one assignment to another around the country and are being used in community-based and institutional settings. *Working Woman* listed the traveling nurse as one of the 25 "hottest" careers of the 1990s (Baumann, 1990b). Nursing roles and job opportunities in occupational health, gerontology, preventive health, health education, and long-term care are expanding, many nurses are needed in these areas, and many academic programs are increasingly addressing the need to prepare nurses for such roles.

It will be a challenge to nursing to adapt to the roles necessary to meet increasingly complex and diverse health care needs. As interesting and exciting new roles emerge and traditional roles change, continuing education will be an integral part of role fulfillment.

NURSING EDUCATION

Educators will need to rise to the challenges and prepare nurses to function in the new health care delivery system. All nurses will also have to stand firm as training programs for physician assistants and technicians are suggested as a solution to resolving the personpower shortage. These types of personnel are not prepared to provide nursing care and thus cannot alleviate nursing shortages.

Changes in nursing roles will increase the opportunities for nurses in advanced practice. As roles change, so do the skills needed to effectively facilitate change. The Pew Health Commission's study examined the future needs of health professionals and their educational basis. The Commission identified 17 competencies needed by health professionals in the year 2005; they are presented in the box on p. 908. Throughout this text these concepts have been emphasized as integral to the practice of community health nursing; nurses can use the wonderful history of this specialty area to again regain our preeminence.

There is also a need for continuing education to help nursing faculty and other nurses keep up to date on advances and technology. Issues such as level of entry into practice, funding of nursing education, and continuing education must be addressed in the 21st century. Nursing research will also be a key element in nursing education and practice.

NURSING RESEARCH

As was discussed in Chapter 1, nursing research reached new heights with the establishment of the National Center for Nursing Research (NCNR) within

◀ *Competencies Needed By* ▶
Practitioners For 2005

Practitioners for 2005 should:
- Care for the Community's Health
- Expand Access to Effective Care
- Provide Contemporary Clinical Care
- Emphasize Primary Care
- Participate in Coordinated Care
- Ensure Cost-Effective and Appropriate Care
- Practice Prevention
- Involve Patients and Families in the Decision-Making Process
- Promote Healthy Lifestyles
- Assess and Use Technology Appropriately
- Improve the Health Care System
- Manage Information
- Understand the Role of the Physical Environment
- Provide Counseling on Ethical Issues
- Accommodate Expanded Accountability
- Participate in a Racially and Culturally Diverse Society
- Continue to Learn

From Shugars DA, O'Neil EH, and Bader JD, eds: *Healthy America: practitioners for 2005, an agenda for action for U.S. health professional schools,* Durham, N.C., 1991, The Pew Health Professions Commission, p. x.

the National Institutes of Health in 1986. Its potential for advancing nursing practice and the health of communities is even greater since the establishment of the National Institute of Nursing Research (NINR) on June 10, 1993. The emphasis on nursing research has been impressively supported by the major nursing organizations, has broadened the theoretical basis of nursing, and has added to the prestige of the profession.

In 1989 the National Center for Nursing Research reaffirmed the need to focus research activities on health promotion across the life span, nursing care needs of vulnerable groups, and the development of health care delivery systems to meet the nursing needs of at-risk aggregates. The priority research areas for the NCNR (now the National Institute of Nursing Research) address these areas. Research is an exciting area of nursing that should make great strides during the next decade. The box on p. 909 lists the current priority areas of the NCNR.

Community health nursing, by definition, deals with populations across all age groups and focuses on

prevention and health planning for vulnerable groups. Thus nurses in this practice area are in a unique position to identify significant, researchable questions relative to the ANA's and NINR's priorities. Participating in research activities is one way for the practitioner to begin to address the challenges of the future. Becoming involved in political activities and ethical decision-making are other ways to ensure that cost-effective, quality health care is available to people in need.

ETHICS IN COMMUNITY HEALTH NURSING PRACTICE

Rapid changes in the health care delivery system have made life more complex and have provoked dilemmas never before faced by consumers or health care providers. It is becoming increasingly difficult for professionals in many situations to discern what should or should not be done. Appendix 10-1 (p. 365) is a scenario demonstrating some of the questions raised by the participants in sophisticated health care of a child: should a child have to live her or his life in a hospital? Is such a life of enough quality to make it meaningful? Is the terrible expense for the care of one such child possible, and what will happen when increasing numbers of children need the same care? How justly are the rest of the children in the family being treated when one family member consumes so much time?

The ability to preserve lives that once could not be saved and governmental cutbacks in health care spending have forced community health care nurses to examine the concept of human rights and choices. Cost containment has produced many ethical questions in health care and is forcing this country into a two-tiered system of health care—one for those who can pay and one for those who cannot (ANA, 1991; Ten trends, 1986; The Medicaid Access Study Group, 1994).

Community health nurses must make decisions about whose rights prevail and which client they should serve when resources are not sufficient for meeting the needs of *all* client groups. They must also examine how their choices about the delivery of health care services have affected various consumers and consumer groups. Gaining an understanding of ethics can assist nurses to better deal with these complex and often confusing practice issues.

◀ *Priorities Resulting from Second Conference on Research Priorities* ▶
in Nursing Practice

National Center for Nursing Research

1—Community-based Nursing Models (1995)

Develop and test community-based nursing models designed to promote access to, utilization of, and quality of health services by rural and other underserved populations.

2—Health-promoting Behavior and HIV/AIDS (1996)

Assess the effectiveness of bio-behavioral nursing interventions to foster health-promoting behaviors of individuals of different cultural backgrounds—especially women—who are at high risk for HIV/AIDS, incorporating bio-behavioral markers.

3—Cognitive Impairment (1997)

Develop and test bio-behavioral and environmental approaches to remediating cognitive impairment.

4—Living with Chronic Illness (1998)

Test interventions to strengthen individuals' personal resources in dealing with their chronic illness.

5—Bio-behavioral Factors Related to Immunocompetence (1999)

Identify bio-behavioral factors and test interventions to promote immunocompetence.

From National Center for Nursing Research: *Priorities resulting from second conference on research priorities in nursing practice*, Bethesda, Md., February 1993, The Center.

Ethics is the study of choices made by individuals and groups in their relationships with one another. The development of a code of ethics is basic to a profession because it provides a means for that profession to regulate its practice. It also helps its members to make choices relative to clinical practice concerns.

A code indicates a profession's acceptance of the responsibility and trust with which it has been invested by society. Upon entering the profession of nursing, each person inherits a measure of the responsibility and trust that has accrued to nursing over the years and the corresponding obligation to adhere to the profession's code of conduct and relationships for ethical practice (ANA, 1985).

The American Nurses Association adopted its code in 1950; it is revised periodically. The most recent revision was published in 1985.

Professional codes of ethics are statements encompassing rules that apply to persons in professional roles and that are *voluntarily* adopted by the group themselves (Beauchamp, 1982). Many national organizations involved in promoting quality health and health-related services are increasingly developing a code of ethics for their membership. These codes are designed to preserve the basic rights of clients in an honest and ethical manner. For example, the National

Association for Home Care (NAHC) adopted its Code of Ethics in 1982 to demonstrate to the general public that NAHC and its individual members stand for integrity and the highest ethical standards. NAHC's Code of Ethics elaborates on patient rights and responsibilities: relationships to other provider agencies; member's responsibility to NAHC; fiscal responsibilities; marketing and public relations; responsibilities to employees; and processes for handling code violations (NAHC, 1982).

In a perfect world, everyone's rights and choices are respected. However, in the real world, some people are more respected than others (lawyers receive more respect than sanitation workers), and some people are often not respected at all (the poor and the disabled). Human choices are affected by one's attitude and environment. For example, some nurses believe that selective abortion should be the right of all women. Others believe, due to cultural influences or to personal or religious beliefs, that abortion is categorically wrong. Changes in our society are making choices such as these much more difficult. Naisbitt (1984) describes one of the megatrends in the United States as a move from an either/or option to a multiple-options situation: there is no longer any objectively "right" answer to many questions, which presents ethical dilemmas for professionals in all health care settings.

These dilemmas include multiple-option situations such as how to deal with conflicting needs of patients and caregivers; when to hospitalize a terminally ill client; resolving conflicts between what is ordered and what is needed; allowing "death with dignity"; maintaining agency standards of productivity while competently meeting increasingly complex care needs of clients; giving pain medication even if early death might be an unavoidable consequence of pain control; and provision of service based on payor regulations (Lund, 1989; Michigan Home Health Association, 1990; Pignatello, Moulton, and Eng, 1988).

Ethics attempts to identify, examine, and justify human acts by applying certain principles to determine the right thing to do in specific situations (Wellman, 1975, p. 317). Curtain and Flaherty (1982) write that there are two ethical approaches that influence decision-making: normative and nonnormative. Individuals using normative approaches work within definite interpretations of right and wrong. In contrast, individuals who support nonnormative approaches deny that universal rules for making decisions exist. They use basically subjective internal processes such as emotivism, skepticism, and relativism. Rightness and wrongness are determined within situations and not by them. Using the nonnormative approach, a decision to abort a fetus might be considered unethical for a woman at one point and completely ethical for the *same woman* at another point. Those who use the normative approach state that there are universal principles of right and wrong that should not be broken and would not consider abortion wrong at one time and right at another. However, this view also holds that general principles are interpreted differently by different people. Each approach has its strengths and weaknesses and neither one is completely adequate for all ethical decision-making.

To discuss complex ethical issues, some writers are advocating the development of ethics committees that can deal with complex questions of client care in addition to policy-making and budget and personnel decisions (Aroskar, 1984). Roles and functions of such a committee could include the following (Lynn, 1983):

1. Identifying the types of cases that should be reviewed
2. Assuring correct determination of decision-making competence
3. Providing a responsive mechanism that assures that the interests of all parties, especially those of the patient, have been adequately repre-

sented in decision-making (thus protecting the competent patient)
4. Reviewing surrogate applicants for patients who cannot make their own decisions
5. Protecting the incompetent patient's interests
6. Reviewing and revising institutional decision-making policies related to ethical concerns
7. Educating the committee and others in the institution
8. Determining which cases need attention from outside the institution, such as from the courts
9. Considering how economic costs will be considered in making patient care decisions and in the development of related policies

Ethics committees are most often found in inpatient settings. This, however, should not be the norm. Community health nurses regularly encounter ethical dilemmas that are difficult to resolve, such as when to allow adolescents the right to make choices about health care that differ from their parents' choices and when to ask for legal intervention when parents are neglecting their children. Assistance from an ethics committee can help nurses in the community to more effectively handle these and other complex issues. At times, nurses leave a practice field, because they have not been successful in resolving the ethical dilemmas which they encounter in that field. Support from colleagues might prevent this.

Ethics committees have assisted community health nursing agencies in the development of policies for advance directives and living wills. A *living will* is a written statement in which clients inform caregivers and family members about the type of care they wish to receive should they become terminally ill or permanently unconscious and unable to make or communicate decisions about their care. An *advance directive* is the written document which specifies the care desired in the future. In December 1991 a federal law was passed requiring that health care organizations receiving federal funds must inform their clients about their rights to consent to treatment or to refuse treatment. By 1991 41 states had passed laws making living wills legally binding. A *durable power of attorney,* or *health care proxy,* is a document that gives another person power to make care decisions for a person who is unable to participate in decision-making. The Council of Community Health Nurses of the American Nurses Association (ANA, 1986) has written that "communities, families, and individuals have the right to a clear explanation of proposed health care, due consideration of their wishes, and an opportunity to ask questions prior to making decisions about care. The rights of the individual client include the right to be autonomous, the right to make an informed decision, and the right to one's domain, including one's body; life, property, and privacy. Competent clients have the right to deny access to their home and the right not to seek or follow health care recommendations." Policies designed to use advance directives and living wills help to insure the autonomy of clients. They can, however, produce ethical dilemmas because nurses are taught to offer and provide treatment, not to facilitate death. Dubler (1993) writes compellingly on the need to bring patients' preferences and *rights,* family concerns, legal rules, and ethical principles into harmony in the coming decade. Health care professionals need to understand the concepts of ethics so that their own prejudices do not affect the care that they give to clients when the wishes of clients differs from their own perspective.

An in-depth discussion about ethics and ethical issues in community health nursing practice is beyond the scope of this text. A pamphlet issued by the American Nurses Association in 1982, *Ethics References for Nurses,* provides a valuable guide for identifying resources available in the field of ethics. Use of these resources and others (Haddad and Kapp, 1991) is encouraged; ethical dilemmas cannot be avoided in the community health setting.

POLITICAL INVOLVEMENT

The most powerful approach that nurses can take to shape the future is the political approach. It is vital that nurses understand, actively participate in, and provide leadership in politics and the political process. Nurses make up the largest group of health care providers in the country, and numbers alone give them a powerful majority. Today's nurses are becoming more politically active, visible, and powerful and are providing leadership in health care delivery. They must continue to grow in their sophistication and use of politics and expand their involvement in political activities.

Politics can be defined as the art of influencing the actions of others for the purposes of promoting specified goals and protecting one's interests (Kalisch and Kalisch, 1981). Political action usually involves activities directed toward influencing the behavior of gov-

ernmental officials and other individuals in powerful positions. Politics and nursing are inseparable and, in fact, politics *is* an integral part of nursing. The relationship between federal legislation and health care (costs, programs, education and services) cannot be denied. The federal government is heavily involved in health care and has a great influence on it through legislation and funding.

The political arena is where health care decisions are made, decisions that will bear on health care for all of us. More than 2500 health-related bills and resolutions are introduced into every 2-year federal congressional session (Davis, Oakley, and Sochalski, 1982). Not all of these are major pieces of legislation, and only a few will be enacted into law, but it is evident that the federal government is involved in health care. Nurses need to have an impact on this legislation! Thus they need to keep abreast of what is happening and disseminate this information to others, and they must be persistent in their efforts to influence decisions about health care policy.

Politics involve people. Nurses have highly developed people-oriented skills that present a real political advantage. Use these skills when working with legislators and officials. Getting to know people in politically influential positions can help one to achieve community health goals.

Politicians are open to the opinions of their constituents, even if they do not agree with them. They know they may not be reelected if their constituency is ignored or does not like what they are doing. Many members of Congress are more impressed with a constituent's story than they are with the sophisticated analyses or extensive reports that pass before them (Donley, 1979, p. 1948).

There are many levels of political involvement for nurses. Kalisch and Kalisch (1981) have described levels ranging from spectator to gladiator. The spectators have gone one level above political apathy and are in the process of exposing themselves to political stimuli and collecting political information. From spectator, one moves into transitional activities such as writing letters, sending telegrams, making phone calls, arranging meetings with officials and legislators, making political contributions, and attending political meetings. This is usually done on an individual basis. Once the nurse moves into group or collective activities, he or she is moving into the gladiator role. Gladiator activities can include political campaign work such as helping a candidate to be elected or

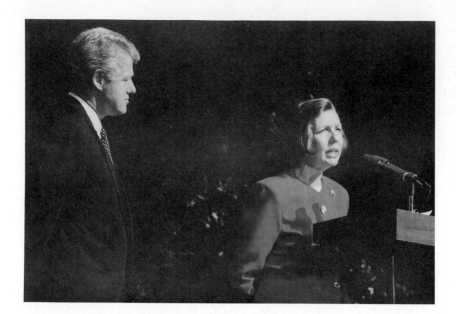

Figure 24-1 Kristine M. Gebbie accepted her appointment as AIDS Policy Coordinator while President Clinton looked on in 1993. While she is no longer in this position, it was significant to have a nurse appointed to a prominent federal-level health policy position.

working against the election of an unresponsive candidate, running for political office, taking an active role in the political aspects of professional organizations, lobbying, and seeking to get legislation passed or changed.

Nurses need to support the organized political activities that already exist through their professional organizations. The American Nurses Association and the National League for Nursing are very active politically. The ANA has established congressional district coordinators in each of the nation's 435 congressional districts to ensure that all nurses in each district are registered to vote, that they have all the necessary information about candidates and issues, and mainly that they *vote*.

In 1992 the American Nurses Association launched a Federal Appointments Project to place more registered nurses in high-level government positions (Meehan, 1993, p. 1). One year later President Clinton appointed two nurses to high-level positions in the Department of Veterans' Affairs. A further illustration of the widening political power of nurses is that in June 1993 Kristine M. Gebbie was appointed as the White House AIDS Coordinator (refer to Figure 24-1). *The New York Times* (Hilts, 1993, p. 10) wrote that "Ms. Gebbie has been given the authority she will need. Her appointment comes with the advantage of a budget proposal by the President that would raise AIDS spending by almost $500 million, the biggest increase ever proposed by a President, to more than $2 billion."

Nurses also sit on local and state boards of health, in policy positions for local, state, national, and international governments and organizations, and in the executive offices of many corporations. Meyer (1992) has developed three case studies that demonstrate how nurses use the skills of the profession and the political process to produce change for themselves, nursing, and their patients. They are worth reviewing because they show how the political process is real and usable for all nurses.

HEALTH CARE FOR ALL: A MAJOR CHALLENGE FOR THE 1990s

The American Public Health Association (APHA) has openly and aggressively championed the right to health care for all in the United States. This is a noble goal, and one that will take much time and effort to achieve. In 1963 President Lyndon Johnson shared with the American public that "Yesterday is not ours to recover but tomorrow is ours to win or lose." This statement is wholly applicable to the state of health care. We must move ahead to a better health care delivery system. We must focus on the future rather than lament about the past, and we must learn from our mistakes. Although data suggest that there are significant difficulties in our health care system that presently prevent the nation from providing comprehensive health care, these obstacles can be overcome. The United States has had a long list of accomplishments in health care delivery and has a strong potential for achieving major public health accomplishments.

The 1990s will bring many challenges as well as opportunities. "Health for all" will be a major battle to win in the next decade. This will involve *taking action* to address emerging threats to the health of the public while containing continuing long-existing threats. These threats include *immediate crises,* such as the AIDS epidemic and inadequate health care for disadvantaged aggregates; *enduring problems,* such as injuries, chronic illness, and infant mortality; and *impending crises* such as long-term care needs of populations across the life span and control of toxic wastes (Institute of Medicine, 1988, p. 1).

The "health for all" challenge emphasizes access to health care that will enable all people to lead productive and satisfying lives. It involves addressing the inequities in society and within the health care system that prevent people from achieving health, and it focuses on the shared responsibility of people for their own health. This battle requires implementing strategies that promote broad-based planning for health and development rather than for health services only. It demands a strong emphasis on political action, policy formulation, multidisciplinary practice, sound managerial functioning, and constituency building (Maglacas, 1988; Institute of Medicine, 1988). Constituency building is a "must." Current and future threats to our nation's public health will require collective action if they are to be resolved.

In 1993, 100 years of public health/community health nursing was celebrated. This is a splendid opportunity to reflect on the rich heritage which Florence Nightingale, Lillian Wald, and many others provided for us. The health problems of today are much like the ones these women faced: communicable diseases, high infant mortality, and poverty. Wald and Nightingale viewed these problems as po-

litical ones, and emphasized that the public's health had to improve to change these problems. That fact is as true today as it was 100 years ago. Let us take on the mantle of developing a scientific basis for the nursing care of aggregates. Let us also use the stories of our sisters of the past to guide us in our future!

Summary

Community health professionals face many challenges. They are being asked to assume responsibility for care of unprecedented complexity and to plan services for multiple, diverse population groups. They must make some difficult decisions about the best means of allocating scarce resources, which often presents ethical dilemmas not easily solved. Competition has increased the number of selected types of community-based services, especially reimbursable home health care, but has not necessarily strengthened services for those most in need. There is, for example, a limited supply of appropriate long-term care resources, even though the demand for these resources is dramatically increasing.

Sophisticated technology, spiraling health care costs, demographic changes, and political decisions are dramatically influencing future directions in the health care delivery system. Community-based care is emphasized, preventive health services are promoted, self-care is stressed, and competition among health care providers is fostered. These trends present both challenges and opportunities for health care providers and consumers alike. To shape the future, health professionals must be risk takers. They must handle ethical dilemmas and engage in research activities to document the need for and the effectiveness of preventive health services, and they must be politically *active.*

Let us as community health nurses think about the future so that we have the very best one possible! Let us follow Lillian Wald and lead the way.

◀ *An Exercise in Critical Thinking* ▶

Appendix 24-1 is a news release about a nurse who was "the first nurse ever appointed director of a county health district in Texas . . ." (Mikulencak, 1993). The title of the article is "Public health stands as a proven model for future delivery systems." Do you believe this is feasible? Can community health nurses make a significant impact on the health care systems of this country? Justify your answers.

APPENDIX 24-1
Public Health Stands as a Proven Model for Future Delivery Systems*

When Karen Wilson became the first nurse ever appointed director of a county health district in Texas, a headline in an area newspaper read "Nursing the Public Health."

The headline captures the essence of what many nurses feel is part of the solution to America's health care crisis— the utilization of public health nurses in existing public health structures.

"Public health nurses are experts at immunization, prenatal care, well child care, screening programs, outreach into the community, education—all that is critical in a health care reform package," said Wilson, MPH, MN, RN, who now directs a staff of 43 at the Williamson County and Cities Health District in Georgetown, Texas. "The emphasis must be reshifted to preventive care and early identification of problems, and that's been the business of public health for decades."

Mike Nilsson, RN, a public health nurse from Clearwater, Fla., firmly believes that the Administration's task force on health care reform must take into account a proven model of delivery.

"We don't need a new model. We know what works. We may fine tune it. We may upgrade it. We may computerize it. But the basis is there," he said. "I want Hillary's task force to come out and say that prevention is needed from the very beginning, and in order to make that work we're going to put 'x' amount of dollars, whether it's millions or billions or whatever, into rebuilding the public health system in this country."

Wilson believes that public health nurses should have a greater voice in health care reform discussions because of their expertise. She says that not only does the public health structure emphasize wellness and prevention, but it addresses issues of access and how to provide care to underserved populations. Ensuring access is a key tenet of *Nursing's Agenda for Health Care Reform* and continues to be one of the greatest challenges facing the President's Task Force on National Health Care Reform.

"Public health nurses just laugh when they hear that the new buzzwords are case management and care coordination because that's what public health nurses have done

since day one. It's helping clients get into the health programs they need," Wilson said.

In Wilson's district, a case management team of nurses, social workers, nutrition staff and clerical staff meet often to solve problems jointly. Wilson notes that the "the more people who can form that safety net, the less likely that someone will fall through the cracks in the system."

Yet, often the groups who need health care the most will not seek it out in the present medical model of delivery, said Nilsson. "Before it was vogue, we were out in the minority communities, the communities with inadequate transportation, in the schools. We went into the homes to speak to teenagers and young women about prenatal and postnatal care or well-baby services. We discussed the whole spectrum of care."

Nilsson said, however, he has witnessed a "deterioration" of the public health system in his state and elsewhere due to a number of factors such as inadequate funding. "If the legislators and decision-makers don't value or understand prevention—if they don't see the value of public health nurses—they eliminate them." He said that legislators may not understand the "whole theory behind upfront prevention dollars—that it may take five years and cost in the short-term, but it will save you from spending thousands of dollars on the other end to take care of crack babies or a child who develops a chronic problem because of a measles outbreak."

Wilson said that current systems make it difficult for some populations to receive all the services they need— where clients must apply for Medicare and Medicaid in one office, health screenings in another office, and housing subsidies in still another location. She advocates a system where clients can "come in and tell their story one time to determine eligibility for a multiplicity of programs at once." A strength of public health nurses, she adds, is that they recognize the "needs of the whole person" and that some health care needs must wait until a family deals with more urgent social or survival needs.

Nilsson said that he hopes the administration recognizes the untapped resources of public health because "the potential is so great and we've got so much to offer."

"Our country has a lot of strong programs and a lot of experts" already available to address issues related to reform, Wilson added. "This doesn't have to be reinvented."

*From Mikulencak M: Public health stands as a proven model for future delivery systems, *Am Nurse* 25(6):18, 1993.

References

American Nurses Association (ANA): *Code for nurses with interpretive statements,* ANA Pub Code No G-58, Kansas City, Mo., 1985, The Association.

ANA: *Ethics references for nurses,* ANA Pub Code No G-159, 3M, Kansas City, Mo., 1982, The Association.

ANA: *Nursing's agenda for health care reform,* Washington, D.C., 1991, The Association.

ANA: *Standards of community health nursing practice,* Washington, D.C., 1986, The Association.

Aroskar M: Institutional ethics committees and nursing administration, *Nurs Economics* 2:132-136, 1984.

Baumann JR: Nursing opportunities in America—Traveling nurses: trend of the 90s, *USA Today,* p. 8D, January 25, 1990a.

Baumann LA: Nursing opportunities in America: international nurses, *USA Today,* p 8D, January 25, 1990b.

Beauchamp TL: *Philosophical ethics,* New York, 1982, McGraw-Hill.

Betts VT: Nursing education for tomorrow's nurse, *American Nurse* 25(5):5, 1993.

Bezold C: Health trends and scenarios: implications for the health care professions. In Meyers JA and Lewin ME, eds: *Charting the future of health care: policy, politics, and public health,* Washington, D.C., 1987, American Enterprise Institute for Public Policy Research.

Casserta RA: Opening doors for advanced practice, *American Nurse* 25(6):18, 1993.

Curtain L and Flaherty J: *Nursing ethics: theories and pragmatics,* Bowie, Md., 1982, Brady.

Davis CK, Oakley D, and Sochalski JA: Leadership for expanding nursing influence on health policy, *J Nurs Adm* 12:15-21, 1982.

Donley R: An inside view of the Washington health scene, *Am J Nurs* 79:1946-1952, 1979.

Donley R: *Health policy and nursing practice—a vision of the 21st century,* Paper presented at conference. New Directions for Nursing: The Future is Now, University of Tennessee (Knoxville) College of Nursing, June 16, 1984.

Dubler NN: Commentary: balancing life and death—proceed with caution, *Amer J Public Health* 83(1):23-25, 1993.

Haddad AM and Kapp MB: *Ethical and legal issues in home health care,* Norwalk, Conn., 1991, Appleton & Lange.

Hilts PJ: Into the maelstrom: new chief of AIDS policy considers the political pitfalls that await her, *The New York Times, National section,* p. 10, June 27, 1993.

Institute of Medicine: *The future of public health,* Washington, D.C., 1988, National Academy Press.

Kalisch BJ and Kalisch PA: *Politics of nursing,* Philadelphia, 1981, Lippincott.

Kerr P: Betting the farm on managed care, *New York Times, Business section,* June 27, 1993, pp. 1,6.

Lund M: Nursing home dilemmas, *Geriat Nurs* 10:298-300, 1989

Lynn J: *The role and functions of institutional ethics committees: the President's commission view,* paper presented at the Conference on Institutional Ethics Committees: Their Role in Medical Decision Making, Washington, D.C., April 21, 1983.

Maglacas AM: Health for all: nursing's role, *Nurs Outlook* 36:66-71, 1988.

Maraldo PJ: The nineties: a decade in search of meaning, *Nurs Health Care* 11(1):11-14, January 1990.

Meehan J: Clinton appoints nurses to high-level posts at DVA, *Am Nurse* 25(5):1, 8, 1993.

Meyer C: Nursing on the political front, *Am J Nurs* 92(10):56-64, 1992.

Michigan Home Health Association, Ethics Committee: *Ethical dilemmas experienced by professionals in home health care,* unpublished research project, East Lansing, Mich., 1990, The Association.

Mikulencak M: Public health stands as a proven model for future delivery systems, *Am Nurse* 25(6):18, 1993.

Naisbitt J: *Megatrends: ten new directions transforming our lives,* New York, 1984, Warner.

National Association for Home Care (NAHC): *Code of ethics,* Washington, D.C., 1982, The Association.

National Center for Nursing Research: *Priorities resulting from second conference on research priorities in nursing practice,* Bethesda, Md., February 1993, The Center.

Office of Information and Legislative Affairs: *National Center for Nursing Research: facts about funding,* Bethesda, Md, 1989, National Center for Nursing Research.

Pignatello CH, Moulton P, and Eng MA: Ethical concerns of home health administration: the day-to-day issues. In Harris MD, ed: *Home health administration,* Owings Mills, Md., 1988, National Health.

Roper WL: Public health surveillance and international health, *MMWR* 41(No. SS-1):ix, March 1992.

Scott K: ANA: making health care reform work for all nurses, *American Nurse,* 25:1, 3, June 1993.

Shoulz J, Hatcher PA, and Hurrell M: Growing edges of a new paradigm: the future of nursing in the health of the nation, *Nursing Outlook* 40(2):57-61, 1992.

Shugars DA, O'Neil EH, and Bader JD, eds: *Healthy America: practitioners for 2005, an agenda for action for U.S. health professional schools,* Durham, N.C., 1991, The Pew Health Professions Commission.

Ten trends to watch, *Nurs Health Care* 7(1):17-19, 1986.

The Medicaid Access Study Group: Access of Medicaid recipients to outpatient care, *N Engl J Med* 330(20):1426-1430, 1994.

Twelve nurses on panel to review Clinton reform proposal, *Am Nurse* 25:2, 6, June 1993.

Wellman C: *Morals and ethics,* Glenview, Ill., 1975, Scott, Foresman.

Selected Bibliography

Davis AJ: Clinical nurses' ethical decision making in situation of informed consent, *Adv Nurs Sci* 11(3):63-69, 1989.

Duffy ME: The research process in baccalaureate nursing education: a ten-year review, *Image* 19(2):87-91, 1987.

Fry ST: Toward a theory of nursing ethics, *Adv Nurs Sci* 11(4):9-22, 1989.

Fry S: Dilemma in community health ethics, *Nurs Outlook* 31:176-179, 1983.

Fry S: Rationing health care, *Nurs Econ* 1:165-169, 1983.

Gortner SR and Nahm H: An overview of nursing research in the United States, *Nurs Res* 26(1):10-33, 1977.

Jecker NS: Futility and rationing, *Am J Med* 92:189-196, 1992.

McManus RL: Nursing research—its evolution, *Am J Nurs* 61(4):76-79, 1961.

McManus RL: Today and tomorrow in nursing research, *Am J Nurs* 61(5):68-71, 1961.

Maraldo PJ: *Nursing as a political force—making our own destiny,* paper presented at conference New Directions for Nursing, The Future Is Now, University of Tennessee (Knoxville) College of Nursing, June 16, 1984.

Milio N: The realities of policymaking: can nurses have an impact? *J Nurs Adm* 14:18-23, 1984.

Rosner D: Health care for the "truly needy": nineteenth-century origins of the concept, *Milbank Q* 60:355-385, 1982.

See EM: The ANA and research in nursing, *Nurs Res* 26(3):165-174, 1977.

Sharp JW and Roncagli T: Home parenteral nutrition in advanced cancer: ethical and psychosocial aspects, *Cancer Practice* 1(2):119-123, 1993.

Silva M: Ethics, scarce resources, and the nurse executive, *Nurs Economics* 2:11-18, 1984.

Stewart MJ: From provider to partner: a conceptual framework for nursing education based on primary health care premises, *Adv Nurs Sci* 12:9-23, 1990.

Stoddard JJ, St. Peter RF, and Newacheck PW: Health insurance status and ambulatory care for children, *N Engl J Med* 330(20):1421-1425, 1994.

Taylor SD: Bibliography on nursing research 1950-1974, *Nurs Res* 24(3):207-225, 1975.

Viens DC: A history of nursing's code of ethics, *Nurs Outlook* 37(1):45-49, 1989.

Ward P: Public health nursing and the future of public health, *Public Health Nurs* 6:163-168, 1989.

Wayne J: Healthcare education 2000: visions for the future, *Healthcare Trends and Transition* 5:10-32, 1994.

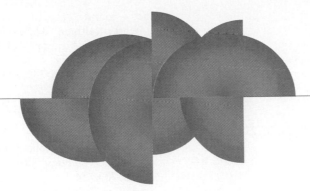

Index

Socialization
  community and, 81
  in group approach, 820
Sociocultural environment, 79, 271, 388
Socioeconomic status
  epidemiology and, 383
  life expectancy and, 621
  minority deaths and, 616
Soil
  contamination of, 177
  lead poisoning and, 188
Soil and Water Resources Conservation Act, 201
Soilborne disease, 185-186
Solid waste
  disposal of, 195
  environmental health programs and, 183
  Healthy People 2000 and, 177
Solid Waste Disposal Act, 200
Solid Waste Disposal Act Amendments, 201
Son, role of, 610-611
Soot, 685
Sorrow, chronic, 711
South America, United States population born in, 213
Spectinomycin, 421
Speech therapist
  in long-term health care team, 808
  school health team role of, 598
Sporadic frequency, in epidemiology, 386
Sports injury, 562
Spouse
  death of, 270
  role of, 610
SSA; *see* Social Security Administration
Staff personnel
  development of, 861, 862
  evaluation of, 891-894
  in organizational structure, 841, 842
Standards, in quality assurance, 886, 887
Standards of Community Health Nursing Practice, 54
Standards of nursing practice
  administration and, 843, 844
  community health, 880
  gerontological, 757, 758
  occupational, 675
  staff development, 862
Standards of School Nursing Practice, 582, 583
State health authority, 153-159
  administration in, 154-158
  in communicable disease control, 157
  in community data collection, 443
  environmental health and, 180, 182
  health education and training and, 159
  laboratory services and, 158-159
  number of nurses working in, 64

State health authority—cont'd
  in occupational health, 158
  organizational chart of, 155
  personal health services and, 157-158
  research and, 159
  special medical services and, 159
  staff of, 159
  vital statistics and, 158
State Workers' Compensation Acts, 109
Statistics
  in community assessment, 436-438
  in epidemiology, 391-392
  mortality, 389
  vital, 389, 393
Status Report: State Progress on 1990 Health Objectives for the Nation, 141, 142
STD Action Coalition, 570
STDs; *see* Sexually transmitted diseases
Stepping-stone neighborhood, 87
Stewart, AM, 48, 672
Stewart, IM, 48
Stewart B. McKinney Homeless Assistance Act, 108, 643
Stimulants, 570
Stress
  career changes and, 613
  families and, 262-267
    culture in, 264-267
    handicapped member of, 708-710
    nursing intervention in, 277-283
  marital, 648
  normative, 634
  physiological and psychological signs of, 262, 263, 264
  unemployment and, 641
Stressors
  community, 82
  families in crisis and, 269-270
  in workplace, 682
Stroke, 618, 619, 624-625
Structural-functional approach in family-centered nursing, 216, 217, 222
Struthers, LR, 49
Student health service, 64
Subclinical symptoms, in epidemiology, 387, 388
Sudden infant death syndrome, 495, 503
Sudden Infant Death Syndrome Act, 133
Suicide
  child, 558-560
  death rates and, 618, 619
  depression and, 636
  in elderly, 739-740
Sulfur dioxide, 193
Sunlight, cancer and, 626
Superfund Amendments and Reauthorization Act of 1986, 202